D1674518

The Chinese Herb Selection Guide:
A Traditional and Modern Clinical Repertory
with
A Summary Materia Medica
for the Health Care Practitioner

The Chinese Herb Selection Guide

A Traditional and Modern Clinical Repertory
with
A Summary Materia Medica
for the Health Care Practitioner

Charles A. Belanger, L.Ac., M.S.

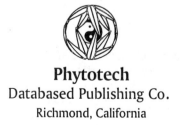

Phytotech
Databased Publishing Co.
Richmond, California

The Chinese Herb Selection Guide

A Traditional and Modern Clinical Repertory with
A Summary Materia Medica
for the Health Care Practitioner
by Charles A. Belanger

DISCLAIMER

This book is a reference work not intended to treat, diagnose or prescribe. The information contained herein is in no way to be considered as a substitute for consultation with a duly licensed health-care professional.

Published by: Phytotech
                 1620 Olive Ave.
                 Richmond, CA 94805-1626 USA

Library of Congress Catalog Card Number: 97-91745
International Standard Book Number: 0-965731-3-0
Printed in the United States of America

Acknowledgements

First and foremost, a compiled reference such as this could not come about without the hard work of the source authors listed in the **Introduction**. To those pioneers who culled and translated the Chinese Medicine texts and journals to create their English text books, I humbly offer my thanks and the thanks of the health care practitioners who may use this book. I encourage all who use this book to have copies of these source books on hand.

Dr. Cheung, one of the source authors, was my Chinese herb instructor at the American College of Traditional Chinese Medicine (ACTCM). He is the one who initially suggested that I might try such a computer project which later became this book. It is Dr. Cheung's unstoppable giving spirit which inspired me to commit to this project in the hope that this book will help other health care practitioners.

Having said that, I can also add that this book has been tremendously difficult to create and I could not have done it without the help and support of many people. First on that list has been my family and especially my wife, Joyce, who not only put up with my late nights and vacation work for the past eight years but also helped in editing and developing the overall look-and-feel of the book. Second in importance has been the members of the acupuncture community, most notably my former classmates at ACTCM. In general many students have continued to give moral support and encouraged me to continue for years even though I was ready to abandon the project several times.

The most notable help, editing and comments have come from Douglas Ball, L.Ac., acupuncturist in Terryville, CT, Jeffery Lee, L.Ac., acupuncturist in Berkeley, CA, and Andrew Ellis, instructor at ACTCM, proprietor of *Spring Wind Herb Company* in Berkely, CA, and extensive author of several import works in Traditional Chinese Medicine (*Fundamentals of Chinese Medicine*, *Grasping the Wind*, and others). Without Doug's regular email companionship on this project I doubt that I would have finished. Jefferey Lee, L.Ac. and Nian-Peng (Mike) Shi, L.Ac. took the time and trouble to look over my Chinese characters to make sure they are correct.

Lastly, I would like to thank the various members and sysops of Compuserve's Ventura Forum (desk top publishing software) for helping me with the particularly troublesome, technical issues with creating the book. This book definitely tested the upper limits of Corel Ventura (version 5.0)!

Thanks, Brother Dharmananda, for letting me know I'd **better** get this book done!

Contents at a Glance

PART I
INDICATIONS &
APPLICATIONS INDEX
(Main Topics)

PART II
HERB SYNOPSIS
(Herb Groups)

Table of Contents

PART I
Indications &
Applications
Index

The table of contents for the **Indication & Application Index** include those entries with more than five occurances in the index. They are listed as the more general starting points for a search. Note that there are many thousands of entries with fewer than five herbal references, so please check the Index itself for a specific entry. Besides these, there are many minor and detailed variations of the main entries in the index.

ABDOMEN/ GASTROINTESTINAL TOPICS

Pertains to organs associated with area
See: **Individual organs in area** for related topics
See: **BOWEL** for related topics
See: **STOMACH/DIGESTION** for related topics

BLOOD RELATED DISORDERS/ TOPICS

TCM as well as biomedically defined conditions/topics
See: **CIRCULATION** for related topics
See: **HEART** for related topics
See: **LIVER** for TCM related topics
See: **SPLEEN** for TCM related topics

BOWEL RELATED DISORDERS

Bowel, rectal and anal related disorders and topics
See: ABDOMEN/GASTROINTESTINAL for related topics

CANCER/ TUMORS/ SWELLINGS/ LUMPS

All referenced Cancers, Tumors, etc. Some are redundantly listed under the associated organ, too.

CHEST

Mostly biomedical conditions of the chest and mediastinum
See: ABDOMEN/GASTROINTESTINAL for related topics
See: HEART for related topics
See: LUNGS for related topics
See: QI for TCM related topics

CHILDHOOD DISORDERS

Many topics, all having a specific reference to infants or children.
See: Any related topic, for adult-viewed treatment

CIRCULATION DISORDERS

Biomedically defined conditions
See: BLOOD for related topics
See: HEART for related topics

COLD

TCM term implying either external cold or
more likely the body acting like it is cold
because of an internal disorder.

EARS/ HEARING DISORDERS

See: GALL BLADDER for TCM related topics
See: HEAD/NECK for related topics
See: INFECTIOUS DISEASES for related
topics
See: KIDNEYS for TCM related topics
See: LIVER for TCM related topics

ENDOCRINE RELATED DISORDERS

DIABETES, references to HORMONES, etc.

ENERGETIC STATE

Mostly disorders of the overall sense of
strength, energy
See: BLOOD for TCM related topics
See: QI for TCM related topics
See: SPLEEN for TCM related topics

EXTERIOR CONDITIONS

TCM conditions which have not affected
the inner organs yet; could be
environmental effects on the body or early
disease states.
See: INFECTIOUS DISEASES for related
topics
See: LUNGS for TCM related topics
See: SKIN for related topics
See: WIND for TCM related topics

EXTREMITIES

Topic includes: Legs, Arms, Hands, Feet
disorders and topics.
See: MUSCULOSKELETAL topic;
See: SKIN topic;
See: PAIN topic;
See: TRAUMA topic;
for related topics and disorders.

EYES

All eye related problems and diseases
See: LIVER topic for other TCM related
syndromes which may be eye related.

FEVERS

All fevers. TCM breaks down fevers into
several main types; some are below; all are
in the index.
See: HEAT for TCM related topics
See: INFECTIOUS DISEASES for related
topics

FLUID DISORDERS

Edema, thirst and TCM Wetness or
Dampness
See: KIDNEYS for related topics
See: LUNGS for related topics
See: STOMACH for related topics
See: TRIPLE WARMER for TCM related
topics
See: URINARY BLADDER for related topics

GALL BLADDER

Mostly Biomedically defined GALL
BLADDER disorders
See: LIVER for related topics;
See: ABDOMEN/GASTROINTESTINAL for
related topics

GERIATRIC TOPICS

This topic includes disorders or topics
with specific mention of effect on the

INFECTIOUS DISEASES

Most acute diseases caused by microscopic organisms, such as Cold, Flu, Pneumonia, Malaria, etc. Many, if associated with a major organ, will be doubly listed under that organ, too.
See: **All major organs** for related topics
See: **ABDOMEN/GASTROINTESTINAL** for related topics
See: **BLOOD** for related topics
See: **BOWEL** for related topics
See: **CANCER/TUMORS/SWELLINGS** for related topics
See: **EXTERIOR CONDITIONS** for TCM related topics
See: **FEVERS** for related topics
See: **HEAT** for TCM related topics
See: **HEAD/NECK** for related topics
See: **IMMUNE SYSTEM** for related topics
See: **LUNGS** for TCM related topics
See: **NOSE** for related topics
See: **PARASITES** for related topics
See: **PHLEGM** for related topics
See: **SIX STAGES** for TCM related topics
See: **SKIN** for related topics
See: **WIND** for TCM related topics

KIDNEYS

All Kidney related disorders or syndromes
See: **URINARY BLADDER** for related topics;
See: **FLUID DISORDERS** for related topics;
See: **INFECTIOUS DISEASES** for related topics;
See: **MUSCULOSKELETAL** for related topics;
See: **SEXUALITY** topics, too
for biomedical or TCM related disorders of the Kidney

LIVER

All Liver related disorders, both TCM syndromes and biomedical conditions
See: **MENTAL STATE** for TCM related topics;
See: **WIND** for TCM related topics;
See: **KIDNEYS** for TCM related topics, too

LUNGS

All Lung related disorders, complexes or topics
See: SKIN for this aspect of TCM Lung organ
See: INFECTIOUS DISEASES topic

MENTAL STATE/ NEUROLOGICAL DISORDERS

All psychological states such as Anger, Irritability, Lassitude, etc. plus conventional psychosis, such as Psychosis, Schizophrenia, Manic states, etc. and Insomnia, dreams, etc.
See: HEART for TCM related topics
See: LIVER for TCM related topics
See: WIND for TCM related topics
See: PHLEGM for TCM related topics

MUSCULOSKELETAL/ CONNECTIVE TISSUE

Joint, Muscular and Bone related disorders
See: EXTREMITIES topic for some Hand,
Arm, Feet, Leg related symptoms or
See: PAIN topic for more generalized pain
syndromes

NOSE

See: HEAD/NECK for related topics
See: IMMUNE SYSTEM for related topics
See: INFECTIOUS DISEASES for related
topics
See: LUNGS for TCM related topics
See: ORAL for related topics

NUTRITIONAL/ METABOLIC DISORDERS/ TOPICS

See: SPLEEN for TCM related topics
See: STOMACH/DIGESTIVE for related
topics

ORAL CAVITY

This includes the Lips, Mouth, Teeth,
Gums, Tongue, Throat
See: STOMACH/DIGESTIVE for related
topics
See: HEAD/NECK for related topics
See: NOSE for related topics

PAIN/ NUMBNESS/ GENERAL DISCOMFORT

This is the general topic for Pain where source was not clear on specific site of pain or numbness. This topic includes "Bi" disorders.
See: **Various specific organs or locations** for related topics
See: **BLOOD** for TCM related topics
See: **EXTREMITIES** for related topics
See: **MUSCULOSKELETAL** for related topics
See: **QI** for TCM related topics
See: **TRAUMA** for related topics

PARASITES

All parasitic diseases or conditions of any part of the body
See: **INFECTIOUS DISEASES**
See: **Specific Organ (e.g. LIVER)**
See: **BOWEL RELATED DISORDERS**

PHLEGM

Primarily TCM disorders
See: **LUNGS** for related topics
See: **MENTAL STATE** for TCM related topics
See: **SPLEEN** for TCM related topics
See: **WIND** for TCM related topics

QI RELATED DISORDERS/ TOPICS

TCM energetic state; functional state of body and organs
See: **ENERGETIC STATE** for related topics
See: **SPLEEN** for related topics
See: **STOMACH/DIGESTION** for related topics

SEXUALITY, EITHER SEX

See: **KIDNEYS** for TCM related topics
See: **SEXUALITY, FEMALE or MALE** for related topics

SEXUALITY, FEMALE: GYNECOLOGICAL

All Female sexual disorders and topics, including those of the Breasts, Uterus, Menstruation, Menopause, Ovaries, Organ related cancers, Pregnancy, Postpartum.
See: SEXUALITY, EITHER SEX, too.
See: KIDNEYS for TCM related topics

SEXUALITY, MALE: UROLOGICAL TOPICS

See: KIDNEYS for TCM related topics
See: URINARY BLADDER for related topics

SIX STAGES/ CHANNELS

Channel pairs used in one particular TCM diagnostic terminology from the **Shan Han Lun.**

SKIN

All Skin related disorders
See: HEAD topic;
See: LUNG topic for TCM related disorders

SPLEEN

TCM disorders usually involving digestion and proper assimilation; may involve immune system, fluid retention, blood.

See: ABDOMEN/GASTROINTESTINAL for related topics
See: BLOOD for TCM related topics
See: ENERGETIC STATE for TCM related topics
See: FLUID DISORDERS for TCM related topics
See: IMMUNE SYSTEM for related topics
See: KIDNEYS for TCM related topics
See: QI for TCM related topics
See: STOMACH/DIGESTIVE for related topics

STOMACH/ DIGESTIVE DISORDERS

See: ABDOMEN/GASTROINTESTINAL for related topics
See: BOWEL for related topics
See: GALL BLADDER for related topics
See: SPLEEN for related topics

TRAUMA, BITES, POISONINGS

Anything, which as an external agent, affects the body
See: **MUSCULOSKELETAL** for related topics
See: **Specific Organs** if they have been affected

TRIPLE WARMER (SAN JIAO)

A TCM "organ" which regulates Qi and Fluids in the body. Recently, one author suggested that it may even be the fascia connective tissue which spreads over the entire body.

URINARY BLADDER

Primarily, biomedical disorders of the Urinary Bladder and tract
See: **KIDNEY** for related topics
See: **SEXUALITY, MALE: UROLOGICAL TOPICS** for related topics
See: **TRIPLE WARMER** for TCM related topics
See: **FLUID DISORDERS** for related topics

WIND DISORDERS

TCM environmental pathogen, the
symptoms of which mimic wind; see
entries for examples
See: EXTERIOR CONDITIONS for TCM
related topics
See: HEAT for TCM related topics
See: INFECTIOUS DISEASES for related
topics
See: MENTAL STATE for related topics
See: PHLEGM for TCM related topics

YANG RELATED DISORDERS/ TOPICS

TCM defined disorders
See: KIDNEYS for TCM related topics

YIN RELATED DISORDERS/ TOPICS

TCM defined disorders
See: HEART for TCM related topics
See: KIDNEYS for TCM related topics
See: LIVER for TCM related topics
See: LUNGS for TCM related topics

PART II
Herb
Synopsis

The herbs are listed by alphabetical order
for their *Pin Yin*, or Romanized Chinese
name, followed by their pharmaceutical
name. The order for the herb groups is
consistent with most of the source texts.

RELEASE EXTERIOR CONDITIONS: SPICY, WARM

RELEASE EXTERIOR CONDITIONS: SPICY, COOL

PURGATIVES

PURGATIVES: MOIST LAXATIVES

PURGATIVES: CATHARTICS TO TRANSFORM WATER

EXPEL WIND DAMPNESS

FRAGRANT HERBS THAT TRANSFORM DAMPNESS

DRAINS DAMPNESS

WARM THE INTERIOR AND EXPEL COLD

NOURISH THE HEART AND CALMS THE SPIRIT

STRONGLY PACIFY AND STABILIZE THE SPIRIT

PACIFIES LIVER, EXTINGUISHES WIND

FRAGRANT HERBS FOR OPENING THE ORIFICES

TONIFY THE QI

TONIFY THE YANG

TONIFY THE BLOOD

TONIFY THE YIN

ASTRINGENT HERBS

Introduction

What you are holding in your hand is essentially a computer generated book. Most Chinese herb books present the herbs one at a time, detailing their application in the context of Traditional Chinese Medicine (TCM). This organization is fine for students of herbology, but as an acupuncturist I found it particularly cumbersome when I began treating patients. As health practitioners, it's much easier to be presented with a list of possible herbs and herbal formulas and then select from them based on the differentiating symptom pattern than to recall all the possible herb combinations which may be useful. The *Chinese Herb Selection Guide* attempts to achieve this by setting out to give the reader a Chinese herb book in reverse—an application and indication index with over 28,000 entries in front and an individual herb synopsis for over 540 herbs in the back.

Purpose of Book

This book's primary purpose is to be "user friendly" to the practitioner who wants to discriminate between the various herbs that he/she may use for a biomedical or a traditionally defined condition. As an acupuncturist and Chinese herbalist, I wrote this book primarily for other herbalists familiar with the Chinese paradigm. Such readers will get the most out of this book, but lack of such training will not make the book any less valuable to herbalists not learned in Chinese diagnosis or herbology. There are ample Western biomedical entries to satisfy the herbalist treating such pathologies. In addition, I have included a few references at the end of this introduction that may be helpful to anyone wishing more information about TCM and Chinese herbology.

It took over seven years of compiling information from multiple sources into a database to create this book. By using a computer to generate the book's files, it allowed me to concentrate on the integrity of the information instead of the drudgery of creating the thousands of tables that comprise this book. It will also allow easier revision of the book at a later date should I decide to continue adding still more information to the Chinese herb database.

Source Material for Book–*Bibliography*

There is a limited number of sources available about Chinese herbs in English, since I do not read Chinese. Below are the ones I selected early in the preparation of this book. Please note that apparent inconsistencies of terms throughout the book came from the use of multiple sources. At no time have I tried to change the English translations offered by the authors. Likewise, if the use of an herb and its context seem to be incomplete or even confusing, it is because that is how the original source presented the information. In such instances, see the herb's entry in the **Herb Synopsis**. There, one can more easily deduce the herb's use and application context because of the multiple entries.

1. Class Notes from various instructors at ACTCM (1988-1990)

2. Bensky, Dan and Andrew Gamble. *Chinese Herbal Medicine, Materia Medica*. Seattle: Eastland Press, 1986.

3. Chang, Hson-Mou and Paul Pui-Hay But, editors. *Pharmacology and Applications of Chinese Materia Medica, Vol I & II*. Translated from the Chinese by Sih-Cheng Yao, Lai-Ling Wang and Shem Chang-Shing Yeung. Singapore: World Scientific Publishing Co. Pte Ltd., 1986, 1987.

4. Cheung, C. S. (Translator and compiler) *Clinical Manual: Selection of Herbs According to Symptom-Sign Complexes*. San Francisco: Harmonious Sunshine Cultural Center, 1987.

5. Cheung, C. S. and U Aik Kaw. Traditional Chinese Medicine *Self-Study Series I: Synopsis of The Pharmacopoeia*. San Francisco: American College of Traditional Chinese Medicine, 1984.

6. Hsu, Hong-Yen, and others. *Oriental Materia Medica: A Concise Guide*. Long Beach: Oriental Healing Arts Institute, 1986

7. Junying, Geng and others. *Practical Traditional Chinese Medicine & Pharmacology: Medicinal Herbs*. Beijing: New World Press, 1991.

8. Yeung, Him-che. *Handbook of Chinese Herbs and Formulas, Vol. I*. Los Angeles: Institute of Chinese Medicine, 1985.

Book's Features

First and foremost is the **Herb Application Index** in Part I. True, other books have an index with a particular indication then page number to the various herbs. However, the *Chinese Herb Selection Guide* offers the application with the herb name in its TCM context, when that information is available in the source material, directly in the index itself. By giving the herb name instead of merely a page number, this feature of the book reduces the tedious process of looking up each page number listed to see which herb is being referenced. In the herb application index the page number is given but is meant to be used to obtain a more complete picture of the herb. By looking up the herb in the herb synopsis, one will find its precautions, contraindications, dosage, broad functional application, traditional properties, and detailed indication and clinical research information.

The **Herb Application Index** has each entry organized either by a biomedically defined application, pharmacological action or TCM diagnosis or condition. The application index is divided into 50 major topics, all in alphabetical order, and then within each topic the applications are listed alphabetically. Yet, each frequently listed indication is also kept in the main sort at the same level as the major topics with a reference to the proper topic under which it falls, thus allowing easier access when one casually uses the book and is not familiar with the topics used to organize the index. I have attempted to cross-reference items as often as possible in as many ways as I could think of. Hopefully, these redundant cross-reference entries will reduce the need for each user to become familiar with any one specific terminology set.

Included in the **Index** are about 2000 herb group entries. These herb groups are principally from Chinese classical medicine. They represent either complete or, as in most cases, partial herb formulas.

The **Herb Synopsis** information in Part II is in a dense, but organized table structure. These tables allow quick scanning for any necessary information such as all the traditional, as well as modern, clinical applications information, dosages, precautions, contraindications and possible side effects. I chose the herbs based on whether they are available in the United States. Some herbs are available by their Western herb name and a few are included, in spite of their lack of general availability, because they are commonly discussed in TCM schools (e.g. Rhinoceros horn (Xi Jiao), bear gall bladder (Xiong Dan))

Included in both the **Index** and the **Synopsis** are the results and clinical directives based on many Chinese clinical studies. When available, the information is concise, though detailed, allowing the practitioner to see how modern Chinese hospitals use these herbs. Often these modern clinical uses of Chinese herbs are not included in any traditional indication listing, leading one to possible new, alternative uses of the herbs.

Since some herbs grow in different soils, climates and are even slightly different variations of the same plant, their functions and properties can vary somewhat. In spite of this fact, as a compilation, I have included all the properties and functions of the several variations of the same herb as it appears in the sources' texts. My combined, consensual approach to resolving slight differences among herb descriptions probably works for most herbs but there are exceptions. One good example is the difference between Chai Hu (Radix Burpleurum) obtained from Southern China and that of Northern China. One tends to "raise the Qi" much more strongly than the other, thus causing headaches in those so prone. Herbalists familiar with this variety tend to use only small amounts, whereas the second variety "circulates the Qi" better and they can use higher doses without problems.

THIS IS NOT A MEDICAL GUIDE

I repeat, this is not a medical guide, rather it is a guide to the selection of the proper herb, ideally, by someone already familiar with Chinese herbs. This book is a compilation of information from multiple sources with the goal of presenting as much information to achieve this selection of an herb as simply and efficiently as possible. The book's purpose is not necessarily to indicate the suitability of any treatment mentioned for a particular condition.

There will be readers, I'm sure, who will use the information in here for self-treatment or treatment of their friends or family. Be forewarned: many of the Chinese clinical studies included have questionable clinical reliability based on the methodology used. In other words, clinical information may show anecdotal evidence of a trend in an herb's application but may not be considered conclusive or reliable enough for consistent success with one's clients. Dosage information is sometimes lacking in these studies, too.

Also of note is the references to "effectiveness." Often authors of a study deemed the results "effective" if any symptom of a particular condition was helped to any degree without necessarily alleviating the overall condition.

The other important point to remember is that, generally, Chinese herbs are not used singly but in tandem with multiple herbs in a formula. An herb said to be used for, let's say, tuberculosis (TB) may in fact be utilized to reduce only one of many presenting symptoms of TB, not necessarily as a cure for TB. Also, it is possible that the herb is generally found in formulas which are used to treat TB, when in fact, the herb itself may have no bio-activity against TB or any of its symptoms. Rather, the herb synergises the other herbs which do have activity against the TB condition.

Chinese traditional hospitals have managed to integrate Western biomedical treatment and procedures more completely with TCM treatment than our country's medical establishment has or probably will. There are many conditions and procedures where the Chinese use herbs in conjunction with conventional biomedical support. Examples include the injection of sterile herb extracts, the treatment of cancer, abortion, gall bladder stones and many others. Whenever the source text is clear, I have included the mode of herb administration of the clinical entries.

Please be advised: if you are an unlicensed health practitioner or anyone without a MD license, do not try without proper medical oversight to substitute Chinese herbs for any treatment which in our culture is normally a surgical procedure. One specific example of a treatment that some readers may try is the use of herbs to induce abortion. Under some unfortunate circumstances it is possible for a woman to bleed to death using such an herb treatment. Abortion is properly a hospital procedure because of the possibility of such complications as heavy bleeding and infection.

Help with Traditional Chinese Medicine Terms, Diagnosis and Herbology

The following are a few of the books that should help those without any TCM training or familiarity to understand traditional Chinese diagnosis and herbology. Also, included is an excellent book (#2) that explains TCM herbal formulas. This book, plus one of the source books by Bensky, has much to offer the neophyte Chinese herbalist.

1. Beinfield, Harriet and Efrem Korngold. *Between Heaven and Earth: A Guide to Chinese Medicine*. Ballantine Books: New York, 1991.

2. Bensky, Dan and Randall Barolet. *Chinese Herbal Medicine: Formulas & Strategies*. Seattle: Eastland Press, 1990.

3. Kaptchuk, Ted. *The Web That Has No Weaver: Understanding Chinese Medicine*. New York: Congdon & Weed, 1983.

4. Maciocia, Giovanni. *The Foundations of Chinese Medicine*. Churchill Livingstone, 1990.

5. Dharmanda, Subhuti. *Foundations of Chinese Herb Prescribing*. Portland: Institute for Traditional Medicine, 1989.

How This Book Came About

I started working on the *Chinese Herb Selection Guide* in its vestigial form as a computer database soon after starting my herbal studies at the American College of Traditional Chinese Medicine in the Spring of 1988. As a student I became quickly overwhelmed by the amount of information that we needed to memorize about each herb. The database thus began as a learning tool. I created flash cards and distributed them to my follow students. By the time I graduated I had enough information from my class notes and the text book we used to create a modest sized book. I distributed that book, published with a limited printing of about 100, to my classmates at the American College. It was the first edition of what was later to become this much more comprehensive rewritten edition.

After graduation in 1990, I began in earnest to select and then slowly add more information from as many sources as I could. Using multiple translated sources compounded the complexity of the task, but the end result, I believe, is a comprehensive and yet usable handbook for the clinic.

It is my sincerest desire that this book help you in your herbal treatments. I would like to hear any suggestions or comments you may have about the *Chinese Herb Selection Guide*. I will carefully consider all such comments when preparing any future revision.

Chuck Belanger, 1997
email: 72050.2415@compuserve.com

Phytotech
1620 Olive Ave.
Richmond, CA 94805
(510) 215-9525

About the Author

Chuck Belanger began studying herbs in 1975 after a friend helped him get over a flu with some goldenseal and echinacea. Soon after he started making simple herb formulae from common Western herbs. 1976 marked the year he entered into a monastic order, although he left sometime later, marrying in 1978. His interest in herbs continued and he built a small laboratory on his property to study herb extraction techniques.

In 1987, Chuck began Chinese herbal and acupuncture post graduate studies at the American College of Traditional Chinese Medicine in San Francisco, graduating in 1990. After passing the National Commission for the Certification of Acupuncturists and the California State licensing exams, he started his Oriental medical practice. Having spent the last five years developing herb extraction techniques for Chinese herbs, he has recently launched **Phytotech Herb Extracts** as a custom herb extract manufacturer for health care practitioners.*

Besides his medical practice he also is a technical support person at Bryant Laboratory, Inc in Berkeley, California, a small distributor of laboratory supplies and chemicals. In this capacity he won the grand prize in the 1994 Corel World Design contest, Ventura category, for the catalog he prepared for Bryant Laboratory using databased publishing techniques which he developed. Much of what he learned producing that catalog has been used to create this book. Lastly, he also runs a part time FoxPro™(Microsoft) application development business.

* If interested please email, write or call **Phytotech**.

Publication Information

For those who are interested, this book was created using a PC Clone with a 90 mhz Pentium CPU with 32 mbs of RAM, 17 inch Nanao F550iW Monitor, Matrox Impression Plus video card with 2 mbs of video ram. I used Windows 3.1 with FoxPro 2.6a™ to develop the data files and programs that created the pre-tagged files for Corel Ventura 5.0 Desk Top Publishing software. To create the Chinese characters, I used TwinBridge, version 3.3. The screen captures for the "How to Use This Book" chapter were produced by SnagIt 2.2.

How to Use This Book

This book is designed to help you find clinically significant information about your patients' or your own conditions as quickly as possible. To accomplish this, the book has many similar entries allowing easy lookup and more than one way to access the information. With the book's densely printed page, I believe I have approached the limits of an acceptable sized "handbook" and readable small typeface–any other typography would have made the book too unwieldy.

I wrote the book to help other practitioners, as well as myself, quickly modify or assemble their own herbal formulas and to show, when the information is available, the modern clinical use of the herbs. I hope the following few pages help you more quickly and efficiently find the best herb for use by laying out the book's overall design and organization

Tips for Selecting Chinese Herbs

For those not trained in Traditional Chinese herbology, please keep the following in mind:

1. Single herbs are not usually used in Traditional practice, but rather a group of herbs, called a "formula," are selected to balance each other and achieve the necessary effect against the pathogen, disease state of the patient, or energetic imbalance. (See the herb group listings in the *Indication/Application Index*. These herb groups are taken from the more commonly used formulae.)

2. Herbs can be used to:
 a) treat a particular complex of symptoms and signs, either individual symptoms or the entire complex,
 b) help clear the underlying disorder, or
 c) act as synergistic or balancing agents within the context of the formula without specifically contributing to the therapeutic effect.

3. As taught in most US. Traditional Chinese Medical (TCM) schools, often diagnosis is a description of the symptom/sign patterns of a disease, not usually a specific disease name as in Western medicine. Thus, there can be several possible bio-medical diseases which will match a particular TCM diagnosis. Likewise, it is possible that a Western disease term may have several diagnoses in TCM, depending on the phase of the disease or its specific manifestation in one's patient.

4. Although the *Indication/Application Index* has many entries of bio-medical conditions referencing the appropriate Chinese herb, keep in mind that the

condition indicated by its bio-medical term must have the proper TCM context for the herb to have the greatest effect. Whenever possible, I've included that context of use. If not present, because the source texts did not include the context, review the herb's main entry in the *Herb Synopsis* section to get a better picture of how the herb is used.

5. Traditional use of herbs treats the TCM pattern of imbalance, not necessarily the bio-medical defined condition. The emphasis is on helping the body to heal itself, although the herbs may in fact have active ingredients which can directly affect a physiological change or attack the particular bio-medical defined infecting agent. Usually this effect is milder than bio-medical pharmaceutical agents. Likewise there are less side effects, but it is also true that some uses of herbs have large enough doses to introduce a pharmacological effect similar to a modern drug.

It will be tempting for those educated in biomedical science to select an herb based on pharmacological research which shows a particular active ingredient, but keep in mind that often the concentration of the ingredient may not be pharmacologically significant in the normal traditional dosage range. Instead, either the accumulative effect over days or weeks may be effective or there may be other synergistic ingredients which support the referenced ingredient's bio-medical role. In either case, the side effects are usually less than modern drugs and the onset of action is generally slower.

For me herbs fall on a continuum of action, depending on the specifics of which herbs are selected, between homeopathic remedies (almost purely energetic) to nutritional supplements and then on to modern drugs (almost exclusively biochemical action). Consequently, by adjusting the dose and the herbs used, one can create an energetic balancing formula, a nutritively supporting formula, or a formula with strong drug-like effects.

6. It is possible for one to over-generalize in selecting herbs for what should be a specific herb for a definite application within the context of an herb formula. My TCM herb teacher, Dr. C.S. Cheung, addresses this issue with the following quote:

Based on an herb's overall functional classification, one may choose among several possible herbs for treatment, but in fact, there is still one herb that is best. The ability to select this single, most efficacious herb comes from the experience of the practitioner and the accumulated clinical experience of others.

So, here in this book is a compilation of a portion of that collected "experience." Use it for your patient's health.

Using this Book to Create an Herb Formula

In the above section I have outlined the criteria for selecting individual herbs for a condition. Without question, it is beyond the scope of this book to train the reader in selecting and creating proper Chinese herb formulas. Since diagnosis and proper formula selection go hand-in-hand in Traditional Chinese Medicine (TCM), it would be necessary for the reader to be at least familiar with the various TCM diagnostic systems (e.g. Zang Fu, Wei, Qi, Yin, Xue, Triple Burner, Five Element, etc.). I believe the key to herb formula creation is to properly identify the most important complaints of the patient and to have a general understanding of the TCM description of the overall symptom-sign complex. If you feel up to the challenge, below is an outline of how to use this book to create an acceptable formula.

Five-Step "Building Block" method to create Chinese herb formulas.

1. **Select for wholistic treatment.** Find the herb group/partial formula in the *Index* which treats the overall condition and symptom-sign complex. There are about 2000 of these entries throughout the *Index*. You may need to search for a more generalized topic describing your patient's condition to find a topic which has one or more herb groups listed. Finding an herb group is important for building a good formula since it will address the underlying as well as the general bio-medical condition. Remember a "formula" is not simply a collection of many single herbs. Ideally, each herb should contribute to the overall treatment plan and support or ameliorate the unpleasant side effects of the other herbs selected. Classical Chinese herb formulas have been successfully used for centuries for various conditions. Try to start making your formula with one or at least part of one of these formulas.

2. **Select traditional single herbs.** Continue building the formula with commonly used herbs for the key biomedical or TCM diagnosis and complaint of the patient. Avoid trying to treat too many separate complaints in one formula, unless they have an underlying common diagnosis. Doing so will make the resultant formula too large and consequently unfocused and less effective. Also, large herbal forumulas tend to be much harder to stomach.

3. **Select modern clinical herbs.** Add to or substitute for the previously selected herbs with any herbs listed in the *Index* which have clinical studies supporting their effectiveness.

4. **Eliminate redundant herbs.** Exclude herbs with duplicate traditional or modern functions, unless these similarly functioning herbs act synergistically. Find herbs which can affect multiple symptoms, while having the least side effects. Use the *Herb Synopsis* section information to help determine this. When finished, the herb formula should have no more than 10-12 herbs, and even this number is probably too many unless the practitioner is very experienced with the effects of the various herbs involved. My experience is that you would be better off to have fewer herbs but larger doses.

5. **Adjust dose.** When deciding the dose of the individual herbs in a formula, consider the clinical information available in the book's *Index* section, the possibility of side effects in your particular patient, and the dose given in the *"Herb Synopsis"* section. If you wish to emphasize a particular herb's function in the formula, then choose an amount near the larger amount given in the dose range. On the other hand, if you wish to merely support the overall effect of the formula or offset some side effect, use the smaller figure given in the dose range.

Dose will vary depending on the mode of ingestion, too. Most doses are for *"Tang"* (which means "soup"or decoction) but can be for ground herbs taken with liquid (a *"San"*). Many herbs require less if taken ground or as an extract. Recently, a Chinese doctor told me that he uses only one-tenth the decoction amount when giving powdered herbs to his patients and he reported that his patients showed definite progress with this amount. Other commercial preparations such as extracts, powders, etc. require adjustments based on the supplier's concentration or raw herb equivalent guidelines.

The book's overall organization

Table of Contents
This is preceded by a two page abbreviated contents.

Part I: Indication/Application Index
Here you find a lengthy listing of all the various applications of the Chinese herbs in this book, organized both alphabetically and topically with fifty such topics.

Part II: Herb Synopsis
This section describes individual herb properties, uses, dose and precautions presented in table format, organized by traditional herb functional groupings.

Appendices
Contained here is an herb cross reference, listed alphabetically by either Pin Yin or pharmaceutical name with the page number of the herb location in the *Herb Synopsis*

How to find a specific <u>Application</u> or <u>Indication</u>

For the quickest access to a specific application or indication take a few moments and review both the *Contents at a Glance* (see Figure 1) abbreviated table of contents to get a feeling for the overall organization of the book and then the actual *Table of Contents* itself for a more detailed view of the structure and contents of the *Indication index* and *Herb synopsis*.

The primary *Table of Contents* has two main sections which correspond to the two main parts of the book, *Part I: Indication and Application Index* and *Part II: Herb Synopsis.* The *Indication and Application Index* section of the *Table of Contents* covers almost eleven pages by itself.

Figure 2: Detailed Table of Contents: Showing Part I, Indication and Application Index

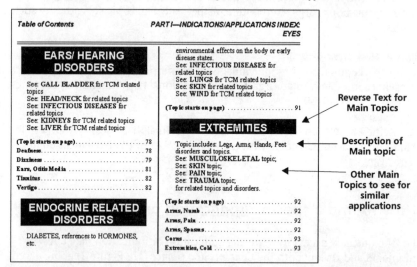

If you can become familiar with the various topic sections and their order in the first part of the *Table of Contents,* you will more quickly find the specific indication/application for which you seek without the tedium of following the path from several cross references. Otherwise, this section of the *Table of*

Contents gives a good overview of the main indications to be found in the ·*Index*. I include in the *Table of Contents* any herb use which has four or more citings in the main *Index*. (see Figure 2)

The second part of the *Table of Contents* (see Figure 3) has a complete alphabetical listing of all the herbs, organized by their functional group. This listing can help one locate an herb of similar application. I find such a listing particularly helpful as a memory aid, reminding me of what other herbs might be useful in a formula I am assembling.

Figure 3: Table of Contents: Listing of herbs by functional group

The *Table of Contents* helps to consolidate the detailed and sometimes numerous listings of the *Indication and Application Index* into a more accessible, easier-to-scan listing of the major topics. In fact, one can choose to look up the application, indication or pharmaceutical function directly in the Index, too, skipping the *Table of Contents* . I have retained all the main entries in the *Index* in alphabetical order without any topical organization. When found, a cross reference will direct you to the proper topic and page number on which the more specific indication, etc. is located.

Note that the order of the herbs beneath a topic and application is alphabetical by Pin Yin Romanization of the Chinese herb names. I learned the herb names by their Pin Yin names, so I am biased in this way. In any case, if I had used the Latin pharmaceutical names instead, it would have made the book even longer, since most Latin herb names are much longer than their Pin Yin counterparts.

Please note also, that if there are herb groups commonly used for the particular application, they will appear first in the list in bold, followed by single herbs. If you are assembling an herb formula, the herb groups make a

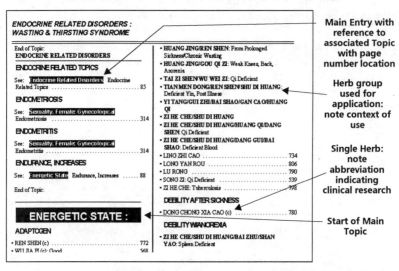

Figure 4: Application/Indication Index: Alphabetical by Main Entry or Topic

good starting point. However, be prepared to distinguish the patient's condition according to TCM differential diagnosis to properly select the best matching herb group. To help with this end, I have included the classical formula name in parentheses after the group and the TCM clinical differentiation for the herb groups whenever the source texts offered this information. The single herbs listed have the page number on which their synopsis begins in *Part II: Herb Synopsis* so that you can quickly look up each herb for more detailed information and review its context of use. (see Figure 4)

How to find a specific <u>Herb</u>

The second section, the *Herb Synopsis*, is organized by the general function of the herb and then alphabetically by its Pin Yin name within that group. The order of the general functions is common to other Chinese herb texts, and anyone familiar with these books will have no problem finding the proper section, then the herb. On the other hand, if you are new to Chinese herbs you may find the organization difficult to comprehend. In which case, you may be better off using one of the *Appendices* (see Figure 5 or 6) to locate a specific herb by using either its Pin Yin or pharmaceutical name or by scanning for the herb in the second part of the *Table of Contents* where the herbs are listed according to their common functional group (see Figure 3). Both lists in the *Appendices* cross over to either the Latin or the Pin Yin name. Furthermore, both lists include the page number for each herb's location in the *Herb Synopsis* and include the herb's alternate names as well.

The *Herb Synopsis* (see Figures 7 and 8) is primarily a series of tables. The *Herb Synopsis* includes the Pin Yin and Latin names as well as the Chinese characters

Figure 5: Finding a specific herb using the Chinese to Pharmaceutical Name cross reference.

Chinese to Pharmaceutical Name					Bei Xing Ren
Pin Yin (Chinese) Herb Name	Pharmaceutical Herb Name	Page No.	Pin Yin (Chinese) Herb Name	Pharmaceutical Herb Name	Page No.
A Jiao.........	Gelatinum Asini	803	Bai Ju........	Scolopendra Subspinipes	755
A Wei.........	Asafoetida	633			
A Xian Yao.....	Acacia Seu Uncaria/Gambir	847	Bai Lian........	Radix Ampelopsis	505
Ai Ye	Folium Artemisiae Vulgaris/Argyi	648	Bai Mao Gen....	Rhizoma Imperatae Cylindricae	650
An Xi Xiang....	Benzoinum	757	Bai Mao Gen Hua	Flos Imperatae Cylindriae	651
Ba Dou.........	Semen Crotonis	543	Bai Mao Teng...	Herba Solani Lyrati	527
Ba Ji..........	Radix Morindae Officinalis	778			
Ba Ji Tian	Radix Morindae Officinalis	778	Bai Mu Er	Fructificatio Tremellae Fuciformis	810
Ba Jiao Gen.....	Musae Caudex	501			
Ba Jiao Hui Xiang	Fructus Illicius	603	Bai Qian........	Rhizoma Cynanchii Stautoni	710
Ba Jiao Lian	Rhizoma Podophylli	501	Bai Shao........	Radix Paeoniae Lactiflorae/Alba	800
Ba Jiao Wu Tong	Folium Clerondendri, Ramulus Et	553	Bai Shao Yao....	Radix Paeoniae Lactiflorae/Alba	800
Bai Bian Dou....	Semen Dolichoris Lablab	496	Bai Shi Zhi......	Halloysitum Rubrum/Album	825
			Bai Tou Weng	Radix Pulsatillae	505

for the herb. If the herb's Chinese name has a simplified character, then I show both the simplified as well as the complex characters. This should help one recognize herb names if one is looking at herb books from mainland China or Taiwan where each uses the simplified or the complex characters respectively. Also included are the properties and entering channels, both of which use abbreviations listed in the table on the last page of this chapter (*How to Use*, p 9).

Figure 6: Finding a specific herb using the Pharmaceutical to Chinese name cross reference.

Pharmaceutical to Chinese Name					Argyi, Folium
Pharmaceutical Herb Name	Pin Yin (Chinese) Herb Name	Page No.	Pharmaceutical Herb Name	Pin Yin (Chinese) Herb Name	Page No.
Abri, Herba	Ji Gu Cao	557	Allii Fistulosi, Herba	Cong Bai	430
Abutiloni, Semen	Dong Kui Zi	588			
Acacia	Er Cha/Hai Er Cha/A Xian Yao	847	Allii, Bulbus	Xie Bai/Jiu Bai/Hai Bai	629
Acanthopanacis Radicis, Cortex	Wu Jia Pi	568	Allii Tuberosi, Semen	Jiu Cai Zi/Jiu Zi	788
Acanthopanax Senticosus, Radix	Wu Jia Shen/Ci Wu Jia	775	Aloes, Herba	Lu Hui	537
			Alpiniae Katsumadai, Semen	Cao Dou Kou/Dou Kou	573
Achyranthis, Radix	Tu Niu Xi	529	Alpiniae Officinari, Rhizoma	Gao Liang Jiang	610
Achyranthis Bidentatae, Radix	Niu Xi/Huai Niu Xi	683	Alpiniae Oxyphyllae, Fructus	Yi Zhi Ren	796
Aconiti Carmichaeli Praeparata, Radix	Fu Zi	608	Alum	Bai Fan/Ming Fan	844
			Amomi Cardamomi, Fructus	Bai Dou Kou/Dou Kou	571
Aconiti Coreani, Rhizoma	Bai Fu Zi/Guan Bai Fu	709	Amomi, Fructus/Semen	Sha Ren/Suo Sha	578
Aconiti Kusnezoffii, Radix	Cao Wu/Tsao Wu	604	Amomi Tsao-ko, Fructus	Cao Guo	574

In order to give the appearance of a free-flowing, multi-columned text describing the uses, clinical applications and clinical notes or precautions, I

Figure 7: Herb Synopsis: Detail herb information in table format.

			Page Header showing Main Functional Group and Herb name on that page.

Clear Heat   **Dan Zhu Ye**

Clear Heat, Subdues Fire ←   — Functional Group

— Chinese name for herb: Complex and Simplified (in parentheses)

DAN ZHU YE   淡竹葉   **HERBA**
(淡竹叶)   **LOPHATHERI GRACILIS**

Traditional Functions:

1. Clears Heat and reduces restlessness
2. Clears Stomach or Heart fire
3. Promotes urination and clears wet Heat
4. Disperses Wind Heat
5. Clears blazing Stomach or Heart fire

Traditional Properties:

Enters: ST, HT, SI

Properties: SW, BL, C

Abbreviations can be found in the table on page 19.

Indications:

ABDOMEN/	NEUROLOGICAL DISORDERS	DISORDERS
GASTROINTESTINAL TOPICS	• IRRITABILITY	• STOMACH HEART HEAT
• HEAT IN SMALL INTESTINE	ORAL CAVITY	URINARY BLADDER

had to use the particular desktop publishing software's "table format." This works well in most cases, except where a table "breaks" at the end of a page and carries over to the next page. Notice (see example in Figure 8) that unlike normal multi-column text which snakes from the bottom of one column to the top of another and finally the last text in the last column on the right continues to the top of the next page on the left, **this book's "text columns" do not snake from column to column when there is a break across a page. Rather, the left column ends at the bottom of the page and then continues on the next page in the left column.** This is important to know about this book's layout. Without this tidbit of information, you may think you're missing something or not know to turn the page. To help matters, I've included a footer which lets you know that the table continues on the next page.

Please see next page for **Figure 8**, showing page and column continuation from an herb table

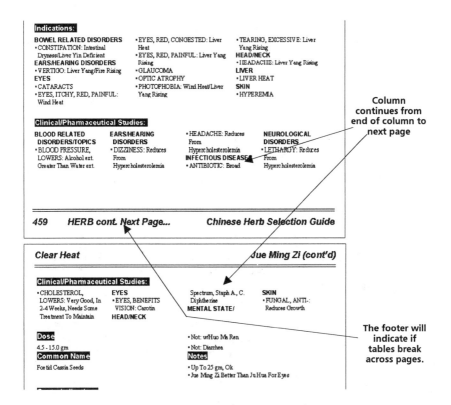

Figure 8: PLEASE NOTE: Table columns continue each column to the next page, not across columns.

Indications:

BOWEL RELATED DISORDERS
• CONSTIPATION: Intestinal Dryness/Liver Yin Deficient
EARS/HEARING DISORDERS
• VERTIGO: Liver Yang/Fire Rising
EYES
• CATARACTS
• EYES, ITCHY, RED, PAINFUL: Wind Heat

• EYES, RED, CONGESTED: Liver Heat
• EYES, RED, PAINFUL: Liver Yang Rising
• GLAUCOMA
• OPTIC ATROPHY
• PHOTOPHOBIA: Wind Heat/Liver Yang Rising

• TEARING, EXCESSIVE: Liver Yang Rising
HEAD/NECK
• HEADACHE: Liver Yang Rising
LIVER
• LIVER HEAT
SKIN
• HYPEREMIA

Clinical/Pharmaceutical Studies:

BLOOD RELATED DISORDERS/TOPICS
• BLOOD PRESSURE, LOWERS: Alcohol ext. Greater Than Water ext.

EARS/HEARING DISORDERS
• DIZZINESS: Reduces From Hypercholesterolemia

• HEADACHE: Reduces From Hypercholesterolemia
INFECTIOUS DISEASE
• ANTIBIOTIC: Broad

NEUROLOGICAL DISORDERS
• LETHARGY: Reduces From Hypercholesterolemia

Column continues from end of column to next page

459   **HERB cont. Next Page...**   *Chinese Herb Selection Guide*

Clear Heat   *Jue Ming Zi (cont'd)*

Clinical/Pharmaceutical Studies:

• CHOLESTEROL, LOWERS: Very Good, In 2-4 Weeks, Needs Some Treatment To Maintain

EYES
• EYES, BENEFITS VISION: Carotin
HEAD/NECK

Spectrum, Staph A., C. Diphtheriae
MENTAL STATE/

SKIN
• FUNGAL, ANTI-: Reduces Growth

The footer will indicate if tables break across pages.

Dose
4.5 - 15.0 gm

Common Name
Foetid Cassia Seeds

• Not: w/Huo Ma Ren
• Not: Diarrhea
Notes
• Up To 25 gm, Ok
• Jue Ming Zi Better Than Ju Hua For Eyes

The next page has a **"Table of Commonly Used Abbreviations."**

Table of Commonly Used Abbreviations

Abbre-viation	Text
Organ or Entering Channels	
GB	Gall Bladder
HT	Heart
KI	Kidney
LI	Large Intestine
LU	Lung
LV	Liver
PC	Pericardium (Circulation sex)
SI	Small Intestine
SJ	San Jiao (Triple Warmer)
SP	Spleen (Pancreas)
ST	Stomach
UB	Urinary Bladder
DU	Du (Governing)
REN	Ren (Conception)
Herbal Properties	
<	Slightly
>	Very
A	Astringent
ARO	Aromatic
BIT	Bitter
BL	Bland
C	Cold
CL	Cool
H	Hot
W	Warm
N	Neutral
SA	Salty
SO	Sour
SP	Spicy
SW	Sweet
TX	Toxic
Text Abbreviations	
*	used as a divider in clinical application information for instances where there is more than one clinical entry for the same application/function.

/	"Or" or "And/or" or as herb group separator in Index
,	(comma) "And" or "with" or as in "library card file style" of Index listings
:	anything following is an explanation, context or function.
(c)	Application determined by clinical or pharmaceutical research.
AKA	"Also known as"
Alc	alcohol (generally ETOH)
AM	Morning
ATP	Adenosine TriPhosphate
BM	Bowel Movement
BP	Blood Pressure
CNS	Central Nervous System
DDT	(Powerful pesticide)
DEF	Deficient/Deficiency
DMSO	Solvent: Dimethyl Sulfoxide
DU	Du (Governing) Acupuncture Channel
e.g.	(such as)
et al	(and others)
etc.	(and so on)
ETOH	Ethyl Alcohol
ext	Extract
g	gram
GB	Gall Bladder
GI	GastroIntestinal
gm	gram
HT	Heart
IM	Intramuscular(ly)
IP	Intraperitoneal
IV	Intravenous(aly)
kg	kilogram
KI	Kidney
lb	pound
LI	Large Intestine
LU	Lung
LV	Liver

MEOH	Methanol/Methyl alcohol/Wood Alcohol
mg	milligram
ml	milliliter
mm	millimeter
oz	ounce
PAF	Platelet Activation Factor
PC	Pericardium (Circulation Sex) acupuncture channel
PM	Afternoon/Evening
PO	Per Os (by mouth)
pwdr	powder
RBC	Red Blood Cells
REN	Ren (Conception) acupuncture channel
S/S	Symptoms & signs
SGOT	Liver enzyme: serum glutamic-oxalacetic transaminase
SGPT	Liver enzyme: serum glutamic pyruvic transaminase
SI	Small Intestine
SJ	San Jiao (Triple Warmer)
SP	Spleen
ST	Stomach
TB	Tuberculosis
UB	Urinary Bladder
vs	versus
w/	with
w/o	with out
WBC	White Blood Cells

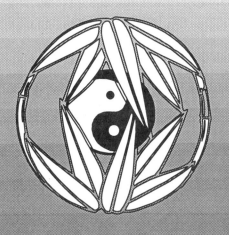

PART I
Indications &
Applications
Index

ABDOMEN MASS, CANCER

See: Cancer/Tumors/Swellings/Lumps Abdomen
Mass, Cancer 66

ABDOMEN, DISTENTION OF, IN CHILDREN

See: Childhood Disorders Abdomen, Distention
Of, Childhood 80

ABDOMEN, PAIN OF IN CHILDHOOD NUTRITIONAL IMPAIRMENT

See: Childhood Disorders Abdomen, Pain Of In
Childhood Nutritional Impairment 80

ABDOMEN/ABDOMINAL AREA RELATED TOPICS

See: Abdomen/Gastrointestinal Topics
Abdomen/Abdominal Area Related Topics 21

End of Topic:
ABDOMEN/ABDOMINAL AREA RELATED TOPICS

ABDOMEN/ GASTROINTESTINAL TOPICS :

See: Bowel Related Disorders 51

ABDOMEN AREA, SUDDEN, SEVERE PAIN

• SHE XIANG/MU XIANG/TAO REN/(VITALIZE BLOOD HERBS)

ABDOMEN REGION, DISTENTION, PAIN

• SHI CHANG PU/HOU PO/CHEN PI: Turbid Damp In Middle Jiao

ABDOMEN, ACCUMULATION, MASS

• WEI LING XIAN 572

ABDOMEN, BLOATING

• CHAI HU: Liver Stomach Disharmony 457

ABDOMEN, COLD

• LU JIAO JIAO 783
• XIAN MAO 788
• YI TANG 772

ABDOMEN, COLD, PAIN

• AI YE/DANG GUI/XIANG FU/CHUAN XIONG/WU YAO: Cold, Deficiency In Lower Jiao
• FU ZI/BAI ZHU: Yang Deficient w/Excess Cold Damp
• YI ZHI REN/DANG SHEN/BAN XIA/FU LING : Spleen Stomach Cold Deficiency
• GAN JIANG: Cold, Deficiency 614

ABDOMEN, COLD/PAIN

• LU JIAO SHUANG 784

ABDOMEN, DISCOMFORT

• SHI HU/MAI MEN DONG/TIAN HUA FEN: Stomach Yin Deficiency/Diabetes

ABDOMEN, DISCOMFORT, VAGUE

• GAN JIANG/HUANG LIAN

ABDOMEN, DISTENTION OF

• BAI ZHU/REN SHEN/FU LING /(SI JUN ZI TANG): Spleen Weakness In Water Metabolism
• BAN XIA/CHEN PI: Stomach Qi Disharmony
• BAN XIA/HOU PO: Phlegm
• CAO DOU KOU/HOU PO/CANG ZHU/BAN XIA: Spleen Stomach, Cold Very Damp Blockage
• CAO DOU KOU/ROU GUI/GAN JIANG: Spleen Stomach, Very Cold Damp Blockage
• CAO GUO/CANG ZHU/HOU PO/BAN XIA: Cold Spleen Stomach Blockage
• CHEN PI/QING PI: Liver Qi Stagnation
• DA FU PI/HOU PO: Qi Stagnation, Dampness
• FO SHOU/MU XIANG/ZHI KE: Spleen Stomach Qi Stagnation
• HOU PO/ZHI KE: Food Stagnation
• HOU PO/BAN XIA: Excess
• HOU PO/DA HUANG/ZHI SHI/(DA CHENG QI TANG): Spleen Stomach Dampness, w/Constipation
• HUO XIANG/BAN XIA: Dampness Blocking Middle Jiao
• HUO XIANG/CANG ZHU/HOU PO/BAN XIA/(BU HUAN JIN ZHEN QI SAN): Spleen Stomach Dampness
• JI NEI JIN/MAI YA/SHAN ZHA
• JI NEI JIN/BIE JIA
• JING DA JI/GAN JIANG
• LAI FU ZI/SHAN ZHA: Stagnant Stomach/Intestines
• LAI FU ZI/BAN XIA: Food Stagnation
• MU XIANG/BING LANG: Stomach/Intestines Stagnation
• MU XIANG/FU LING /ZHI KE/CHEN PI: Spleen Stomach Qi Stagnation
• PEI LAN/HUO XIANG/CANG ZHU/HOU PO/BAI DOU KOU: Spleen Stomach, Dampness Blocking
• QIAN NIU ZI/CHEN XIANG/ROU GUI: Deficient Spleen Kidney Yang
• ROU DOU KOU/BAN XIA/GAN JIANG: Spleen Stomach Cold Deficient
• SHA REN/CANG ZHU/BAI DOU KOU/HOU PO: Spleen Stomach, Dampness Blocking
• SHAN ZHA/MAI YA/SHEN QU: Food Stagnation
• SHAN ZHA/ZHI KE
• SHI CHANG PU/MU XIANG/WU ZHU YU/XIANG FU: Dampness, Qi Obstruction
• SHUI ZHI/MANG XIAO/DA HUANG: Blood Stasis/Ecchymosis From Heat Invasion
• XIANG FU/ZI SU YE: Exterior Pathogen
• ZE XIE/SHA REN
• ZHU LING/DA FU PI
• ZHU LING/MU TONG/HUA SHI: Heat
• BAI DOU KOU: Damp Heat 577
• BAI ZHU 760
• BAN XIA: Damp Heat 710
• BING LANG: Damp Heat 643
• CANG ZHU: Damp Heat 578
• CAO DOU KOU: Damp Heat 579

- CHEN PI: Damp Heat 621
- CHEN PI (c) 621
- DA FU PI: Food Stagnation 624
- DA HUANG: Yang Ming Stage/Excess Heat In Intestine
  542
- E ZHU (c): Stimulates GI Tract 673
- FU LING 594
- FU LING PI 595
- GAN SUI 551
- GE HUA 521
- HAN FANG JI 596
- HOU PO HUA: Food Stagnation/Stagnant Qi/Turbid
  Dampness 580
- HOU PO: Damp Heat/Dampness 581
- HOU PO (c): With Qing Pi, 9 g Each, Da Huang, 6 g, Oral
  Decoction 581
- HU HUANG LIAN: Chronic Childhood
  Malnutrition/Damp Heat 484
- HUA SHI: Damp Heat 597
- HUANG BAI: Damp Heat 485
- HUANG LIAN: Damp Heat 486
- HUANG QIN: Damp Heat 489
- HUO XIANG: Dampness From Spleen Transportation
  Function Loss/Damp Heat 582
- JI NEI JIN 638
- JI NEI JIN (c): Used With Mai Ya, Shan Zha, Bai Zhu,
  Chen Pi 638
- JING DA JI 552
- JU HONG 626
- LAI FU ZI (c): Stir Fried Herb With Shan Zha, Mai Ya,
  Shen Qu 639
- LU LU TONG 681
- LUO BU MA 748
- MA BIAN CAO 682
- MEI GUI HUA 627
- PEI LAN: Damp Heat 583
- QIAN NIU ZI: Excess Heat In Stomach/Intestines 553
- REN SHEN 767
- SANG BAI PI 703
- SHA REN: Damp Heat 584
- SHAN ZHI ZI: Damp Heat 476
- SHANG LU 554
- SHI CHANG PU: Damp Heat 757
- WU JIU GEN PI 555
- XU SUI ZI 556
- YI YI REN: Damp Heat 602
- YUAN HUA 556
- ZE XIE 605

ABDOMEN, DISTENTION OF W/CONSTIPATION, FULLNESS

- ZHI SHI/HOU PO/DA HUANG

ABDOMEN, DISTENTION OF W/EDEMA

- DA FU PI 624

ABDOMEN, DISTENTION OF W/GAS

- MAI YA/(with tonifying herbs)

ABDOMEN, DISTENTION OF, ASCITES

- GAN SUI/GAN CAO: Topical To Navel

ABDOMEN, DISTENTION OF, CHILDHOOD

- ROU DOU KOU/BAN XIA/GAN JIANG/SHEN QU/SHA REN: Spleen Stomach Cold Deficient

ABDOMEN, DISTENTION OF, FOCAL

- LAI FU ZI/ZHI KE: Food Stagnation
- SHEN QU/BING LANG: Food Stagnation

ABDOMEN, DISTENTION OF, FULLNESS

- XIANG FU/SU GENG

ABDOMEN, DISTENTION OF, FULLNESS AFTER MEALS

- ZHI SHI/BAI ZHU/(ZHI ZHU WAN): Spleen Stomach Weakness

ABDOMEN, DISTENTION OF, GAS DURING PANHYSTERECTOMY

- HOU PO (c): 5-7.5 g Powdered If Less Than 50 kg/7.5-10, If Greater Than 50 kg 581

ABDOMEN, DISTENTION OF, LOWER

- CHE QIAN ZI/MU TONG/SHAN ZHI ZI/HUA SHI/(BA ZHENG SAN)
- YI MU CAO/CHI SHAO YAO/DANG GUI/MU XIANG: Blood Stasis

ABDOMEN, DISTENTION OF, PAIN

- E ZHU/SAN LENG/SHAN ZHA/MU XIANG/ZHI SHI
- SAN LENG/E ZHU/QING PI/MAI YA
- SHAN ZHA/MU XIANG/ROU DOU KOU/BAI BIAN DOU/(all toasted)
- XIANG FU/MU XIANG/(XIANG YUAN-CITRON)/FO SHOU: Liver Attacking Stomach
- BAN XIA 710
- CANG ZHU 578
- MAI YA 640

ABDOMEN, DISTENTION OF, POSTOPERATIVE

- QING PI (c): Zhi PO Er Qing Tang (Qing Pi, Hou PO, Zhi Shi, Qing Mu Xiang, 1-2 Doses, Helped Patients To Pass Gas In 24 Hrs 629

ABDOMEN, DISTENTION OF, PRESSURE

- ZHI KE: Food Stagnation 635

ABDOMEN, DISTENTION OF, RESTLESS

- DONG GUA REN 593

ABDOMEN, DISTENTION OF, SEVERE

- CHEN PI (c): With Cang Zhu, Hou PO As In Ping Wei San 621
- DA HUANG (c): External Plaster With Vinegar On K1, Every 2 Hours 542

ABDOMEN, DISTENTION OF, UPPER

- CANG ZHU (c): Ping Wei San (Cang Zhu, Hou PO, Chen Pi, Gan Cao), With Ginger Soup Or Boiled Water 578

ABDOMEN, MASS, IMMOBILE W/PAIN

• HU PO/SAN LENG/E ZHU/BIE JIA: Blood Stasis

ABDOMEN, MASS, IMMOBILE, PALPABLE

• CHUAN SHAN JIA/SAN LENG/E ZHU
• SHUI ZHI/SAN LENG/E ZHU/DANG GUI

ABDOMEN, MASS, IMMOBILE/MOBILE

ABDOMEN, MASS, IN WOMEN

ABDOMEN, MASS, PAIN OF

ABDOMEN, MASS/TUMOR

ABDOMEN, PAIN FROM DYSENTERY

• BAI SHAO/HUANG LIAN/MU XIANG/ZHI KE

ABDOMEN, PAIN OF

• AI YE/XIANG FU: Cold, Deficient/Stagnant Qi
• AI YE/GAN JIANG: Cold
• BAI SHAO/GAN CAO: Liver Stomach Disharmony
• BI BA/GAO LIANG JIANG: Stomach Cold
• CAN SHA/WU ZHU YU/MU GUA: Dampness
• CANG ZHU/XIANG FU: Blocked Qi, Dampness
• CAO DOU KOU/WU ZHU YU: Stomach Cold
• CHAI HU/ZHI KE: Cold Damp
• CHAN SU/XIONG HUANG/CANG ZHU/DING XIANG: Summer Heatstroke
• CHI SHAO YAO/XIANG FU: Qi/Blood Blocked
• CHUAN JIAO/GAN JIANG/DANG SHEN/YI TANG/(DA JIAN ZHONG TANG): Spleen Stomach Cold, Deficient
• DAN SHEN/TAN XIANG/SHA REN/(DAN SHEN YIN): Qi/Blood Stagnation
• DAN SHEN/YI MU CAO/TAO REN/HONG HUA/DANG GUI: Blood Stagnation
• DING XIANG/WU ZHU YU: Cold Stomach
• DOU CHI JIANG/XIANG FU/YI MU CAO/DAN SHEN: Deficient Cold
• DU ZHONG/XU DUAN/SHAN YAO: Threatened Miscarriage/Restless Fetus
• E ZHU/MU XIANG: Food Stagnation
• E ZHU/MU XIANG/HUANG QI/DANG SHEN: Food Stagnation/Deficiency
• E ZHU/QING PI: Qi Stagnation
• GAN CAO/BAI SHAO
• GAN JIANG/GAO LIANG JIANG: Cold Stomach
• GAO BEN/WU ZHU YU: Cold Damp
• GAO BEN/WU ZHU YU/XIAO HUI XIANG: Cold Damp
• GAO LIANG JIANG/XIANG FU/(LIANG FU WAN): Cold, Qi Stagnation
• GUI ZHI/WU ZHU YU: Chong Ren Cold, Deficient
• HONG HUA/CHUAN XIONG: Blood, Qi Stagnation
• HONG HUA/YI MU CAO: Blood Stasis
• HU JIAO/GAO LIANG JIANG: Stomach Cold

• HU LU BA/XIAO HUI XIANG: Cold, Deficient Hernia-Like
• JIANG XIANG/HUO XIANG/MU XIANG: Internal Dampness
• MO YAO/YAN HU SUO/WU LING ZHI/XIANG FU: Qi, Blood Stagnation
• MO YAO/HONG HUA: Blood Stasis
• MU DAN PI/TAO REN: Blood Stasis
• MU DAN PI/GUI ZHI: Blood Stasis Blocking Channels
• MU XIANG/SHA REN: Qi Blockage/Food Stagnation
• PU HUANG/WU LING ZHI/(SHI XIAO SAN): Blood Stagnation
• REN SHEN/BAI ZHU: Spleen Stomach Deficient Qi
• ROU DOU KOU/MU XIANG/SHENG JIANG/BAN XIA: Spleen Stomach Qi Stagnation w/Cold, Deficient
• ROU GUI/GAN JIANG/BAI ZHU/FU ZI/(GUI FU LI ZHONG WAN): Spleen Kidney Yang Deficiency
• ROU GUI/GAN JIANG/WU ZHU YU/DANG GUI/CHUAN XIONG: Cold Stagnation
• SHA REN/BAI ZHU: Spleen Stomach Damp Obstructing
• SHEN QU/MU XIANG/SHA REN: Food Stagnation
• SHUI ZHI/DA HUANG/QIAN NIU ZI/(DUO MING DAN): Blood Stagnation Trauma
• TAN XIANG/SHA REN/DING XIANG/HUO XIANG: Stagnant Qi
• TAN XIANG/SHA REN/WU YAO: Cold, Qi Stagnation
• WU LING ZHI/(quick fried ginger): Deficient Cold, Blood Stasis
• WU MEI/BING LANG: Roundworms In Intestines/Bile Duct
• WU MEI/XI XIN/HUANG LIAN/(WU MEI WAN): Roundworms In Biliary Tract
• WU YAO/WU ZHU YU: Spleen Kidney Deficient, Cold
• WU YAO/MU XIANG: Cold Stagnation, Qi Blockage
• WU ZHU YU/GAN JIANG: Cold Stomach
• WU ZHU YU/GAN JIANG/MU XIANG: Cold Attacking Spleen, Stomach
• XIANG FU/MU XIANG: Liver Spleen Qi Blockage
• XIAO HUI XIANG/ROU GUI: Cold
• XIAO HUI XIANG/LI ZHI HE: Cold
• XIONG HUANG/BING LANG/QIAN NIU ZI: Accumulation Of Worms
• YAN HU SUO/WU LING ZHI: Congealed Blood
• YAN HU SUO/XIAO HUI XIANG: Cold, Qi/Blood Stasis
• YANG JIN HUA/CHUAN XIONG/HAN FANG JI
• YI TANG/GUI ZHI/BAI SHAO/GAN CAO: Cold Deficient In Middle Jiao
• YI ZHI REN/DANG SHEN/BAI ZHU/GAN JIANG: Cold Invading Spleen And Kidneys
• YU JIN/DAN SHEN/XIANG FU/CHAI HU/ZHI KE: Qi/Blood Stagnation Pain
• ZHI SHI/DA HUANG: Damp Heat Obstruction
• ZHI SHI/BAI SHAO: Qi And Blood Stasis

ABDOMEN, PAIN OF W/AMENORRHEA

ABDOMEN, PAIN OF, ACUTE

ABDOMEN, PAIN OF, ASCARIASIS

ABDOMEN, PAIN OF, BELCHING

ABDOMEN, PAIN OF, BELOW UMBILICUS.

ABDOMEN, PAIN OF, CHILDHOOD NUTRITIONAL IMPAIRMENT

ABDOMEN, PAIN OF, CHRONIC COLITIS

- PU HUANG (c): With Wu Ling Zhi, Baked Ge Gen, Baked
  Rou Dou Dou 660

ABDOMEN, PAIN OF, CHRONIC W/EXCESS SALIVA

- YI TANG: Middle Jiao Deficient Cold 772

ABDOMEN, PAIN OF, COLD

- BAI ZHU/GAN JIANG/REN SHEN/(LI ZHONG WAN):
  Spleen Stomach Deficiency Cold
- ROU DOU KOU/MU XIANG: Spleen Stomach Deficiency
  Cold
- ROU GUI/FU ZI: Spleen Kidney Yang Deficiency
- CI WEI PI 819
- SAN QI: Throbbing, Blood Stasis 663

ABDOMEN, PAIN OF, COLD, AT UMBILICUS

- BI CHENG QIE: Spleen Deficient 609

ABDOMEN, PAIN OF, COLD, PAIN IN LOWER, ESPECIALLY

- WU YAO/ROU GUI

ABDOMEN, PAIN OF, CONSTIPATION

- BA DOU/DA HUANG/GAN JIANG/(SAN WU BEI JI WAN):
  Cold/Food Retention

ABDOMEN, PAIN OF, DIARRHEA

- MU GUA/WU ZHU YU/XIAO HUI XIANG/SHENG JIANG:
  Cold Damp
- GAO BEN 444

ABDOMEN, PAIN OF, DISTENTION

- BAI ZHU/GAN JIANG: Cold Deficient Middle Jiao
- CAO DOU KOU/GAO LIANG JIANG: Spleen Deficient
  w/Qi/Dampness Obstruction
- MU XIANG/QING PI
- SHA REN/HOU PO: Spleen Stomach Qi Obstructing
- XIANG FU/CANG ZHU
- BA DOU 550
- E ZHU: Food Stagnation 673
- FO SHOU 624
- MAI YA (c): 9-12 g In Decoction For Mild Cases,
  *Serious Cases—Mai Ya, Stir Fried, Gu Ya, Stir Fried,
  Shan Zha, Browned, 9 g Each, Lai Fu Zi, Stir Fried, 6g,
  *Herb Extract, 10 ml, 3x/Day 640
- ROU DOU KOU: Cold 826
- SU GENG 451
- XIAO HUI XIANG: Stomach Cold 619
- YUE JI HUA 696

ABDOMEN, PAIN OF, DISTENTION W/IRREGULAR BOWEL MOVEMENT

- LU LU TONG/WU YAO/MU XIANG/ZHI KE

ABDOMEN, PAIN OF, DISTENTION, SEVERE

- SAN LENG: Food Stagnation, Qi Stagnation 686

ABDOMEN, PAIN OF, DULL

- BAI SHAO: Liver Qi Stagnation/Liver Spleen
  Disharmony 794

ABDOMEN, PAIN OF, DYSENTERY DISORDERS

- HUANG LIAN/WU ZHU YU/BAI SHAO

ABDOMEN, PAIN OF, FEVER

- BAI JIANG CAO/CHI SHAO YAO: Postpartum Blood Stasis

ABDOMEN, PAIN OF, FULLNESS

- LING LING XIANG 850

ABDOMEN, PAIN OF, HERNIA-LIKE

- BI BA: Cold 608
- BING LANG: Cold 643
- CAO WU: Cold 609
- CHEN XIANG: Cold 622
- CHUAN LIAN ZI: Cold 623
- CHUAN WU: Cold 611
- DING XIANG: Cold 612
- FO SHOU: Cold 624
- FU ZI: Cold 613
- GAN JIANG: Cold 614
- HU LU BA: Cold 781
- JIANG HUANG: Cold 678
- JU HE: Cold 626
- LI ZHI HE: Cold 626
- QING PI: Cold 629
- ROU GUI: Cold 616
- SHAN ZHA: Cold 641
- WU YAO: Cold 632
- WU ZHU YU: Cold 618
- XIAO HUI XIANG: Cold 619
- YAN HU SUO: Cold 693

ABDOMEN, PAIN OF, IN MENSTRUATION

- YU JIN/XIANG FU/DANG GUI/BAI SHAO

ABDOMEN, PAIN OF, LOWER

- XIANG FU/WU YAO: Liver Kidney Qi Blockage, Cold
- AI YE: Cold 651
- BA JI TIAN: Cold 773
- WU YAO: Cold/Qi Stagnation 632
- XIAO HUI XIANG: Cold 619

ABDOMEN, PAIN OF, LOWER, COLD

- HU LU BA/FU ZI/BU GU ZHI

ABDOMEN, PAIN OF, LOWER, ESPECIALLY W/COLD, TENSION

- CHEN XIANG/WU YAO

ABDOMEN, PAIN OF, MILD

- GOU QI ZI: Yin/Blood Deficient 798

ABDOMEN, PAIN OF, OBSTRUCTION

- BAI JIANG CAO: Heat Induced Stagnant Blood 512
- HU PO 737

ABSCESS, LARGE INTESTINE/LUNG

ACCUMULATION

ACCUMULATION, OVERNIGHT

ANALGESIC, IN LARGE INTESTINE

APPENDICEAL ABSCESS

APPENDICITIS

APPENDICITIS W/DIFFUSE PERITONITIS

APPENDICITIS W/FEVER, PAIN

APPENDICITIS W/PAIN

APPENDICITIS W/PERFORATION

APPENDICITIS, ACUTE

APPENDICITIS, ACUTE, PAIN

APPENDICITIS, ACUTE, SIMPLE

- BAI HUA SHE SHE CAO (c): 60 g, 2-3 Doses/Day, Cure 6-8 Days, Severe Cases Add Ye Ju Hua, Hai Jin Sha Or Da Huang, Chi Shao/Liver Heat Purgative Decoction Of Long Dan Cao, Life-Saving Immortal Decotion 511

APPENDICITIS, ACUTE/CHRONIC

- HONG TENG 497
- MU DAN PI (c): Da Huang Mu Dan Pi Tang, 2x/Day, 10 Days 499

APPENDICITIS, BLEEDING

- JIN YIN HUA/DI YU/HUANG QIN

APPENDICITIS, SUPPURATIVE

- BAI JIANG CAO/YI YI REN/FU ZI: Without Heat

APPENDICITIS, UNSUPPURATED

- MU DAN PI/DA HUANG

APPENDICITIS, UNSUPPURATED W/IMMOBILE MASS

- BAI JIANG CAO/CHI SHAO YAO

BLOATING

- CHEN PI: Spleen Stomach Qi Stagnation 621
- HOU PO HUA: Food Stagnation 580
- HOU PO 581

BLOATING, CHILD MALNUTRITION

- WU LING ZHI 691

BORBORYGMUS

- FU LING /MU XIANG: Dampness
- LAI FU ZI/SHAN ZHA: Stagnant Stomach/Intestines
- MU XIANG/FU LING /ZHI KE/CHEN PI: Spleen Stomach Qi Stagnation
- BI BA 608
- BI CHENG QIE: Stomach Cold 609
- BU GU ZHI 773
- CAN SHA: Severe Dampness 558
- CANG ZHU (c): Ping Wei San (Cang Zhu, Hou PO, Chen Pi, Gan Cao) , With Ginger Soup Or Boiled Water 578
- CHEN XIANG 622
- HAN FANG JI 596
- MU XIANG 628

CONGESTION/FULLNESS IN ABDOMEN, CHEST

- ZI SU YE/SHA REN

CRAMPS

- See: Abdomen/Gastrointestinal Topics Abdominal Pain 27

CRAMPS, ABDOMINAL

- CAN SHA/HUANG QIN/MU GUA/WU ZHU YU/(CAN SHI TANG): Spleen Stomach, Turbid Dampness Blocking

CROHN'S DISEASE

- See: Abdomen/Gastrointestinal Topics Enteritis 29
- See: Abdomen/Gastrointestinal Topics Inflammatory Bowel Disease 33
- See: Bowel Related Disorders Irritable Bowel Syndrome 63
- SAN QI (c): Powdered, 10 Days For Acute Condition To Pass 663

ENTERITIS

- See: Abdomen/Gastrointestinal Topics Crohn's Disease 29
- See: Abdomen/Gastrointestinal Topics Inflammatory Bowel Syndrome 33
- BAI HUA SHE SHE CAO (c): Yan Ning Infusion (Bai Hua She She Cao, Herba Monochasmae Savatieri, Ya Zhi Cao) 511
- BAI TOU WENG (c) 514
- BAN BIAN LIAN 586
- CHUAN XIN LIAN (c) 518
- GUI ZHEN CAO 462
- HE ZI (c): Protects Ulceration From 822
- HUANG QIN 489
- JIN YIN HUA 524
- LAO GUAN CAO 565
- MU XIANG 628
- SHAN DOU GEN (c) 532
- WEI LING XIAN (c) 572
- XIAN HE CAO (c) 665
- YE JU HUA (c): (Intestinal Inflammation, Especially The Mucous Lining) With Pu Gong Ying, Wei Ling Xian, Hai Jin Sha, Bai Mao Gen, Jin Yin Hua 468

ENTERITIS, ACUTE

- CHUAN XIN LIAN 518
- HOU PO (c) 581
- HUANG BAI (c): Bai Tou Weng Tang 485
- HUANG LIAN 486
- QIAN LI GUANG (c): Very Good, 4.5 g Of Crude Herb 4x/Day 474

ENTERITIS, CHRONIC

- GAO LIANG JIANG 615
- WU MEI (c): Seeded Fruit 830

FLANK ACCUMULATIONS, PAIN

- BIE JIA 805

FLANK DISTENTION

- QING PI/CHAI HU/YU JIN: Liver Stomach Disharmony

FLANK DISTENTION/PAIN

- HU LU BA 781

FLANK PAIN

- CHEN PI/QING PI: Liver Qi Stagnation
- CHI SHAO YAO/XIANG FU: Qi/Blood Blocked
- GOU QI ZI/DANG GUI/SHU DI HUANG/BEI SHA SHEN/CHUAN LIAN ZI: Yin Deficiency And Liver Qi Stagnation

PERISTALSIS, INCREASES LARGE INTESTINES

PERISTALSIS, INCREASES SMALL INTESTINES

PERISTALSIS, INHIBITS

PERITONITIS

PERITONITIS, MILD LOCAL

POSTPARTUM ABDOMINAL PAIN

SMALL INTESTINE

SMALL INTESTINE, BLEEDING

SMALL INTESTINE, CONTRACTS SMOOTH MUSCLES OF

SMALL INTESTINE, DAMP HEAT

SMALL INTESTINE, HEAT

SMALL INTESTINE, ILEUM, INDUCES CONTRACTIONS

SMALL INTESTINE, JEJUNUM, INCREASES ELASTICITY

SMALL INTESTINES, SPASMS, RELIEVES

SPLANCHNOPTOSIS

SUBCOSTAL

SUBCOSTAL AREA, MASS BELOW

SUBCOSTAL DISTENDED PAIN

SUBCOSTAL DISTENTION

SUBCOSTAL FULLNESS, DISTENTION

SUBCOSTAL LUMPS

SUBCOSTAL PAIN

SUBCOSTAL PAIN, DISTENTION

SUBCOSTAL PAIN/SWELLING

SUBCOSTAL REGION, SOFT PHLEGM MASS

SUBCOSTAL, FOCAL DISTENTION

SWELLINGS, NODULAR OF GI TRACT

TRYPSIN INHIBITION

ULCERS, DUODENAL

ULCERS, INTESTINAL

WAIST, PAIN

WAIST, PAIN, SORE

WAIST, WEAK

- CHEN XIANG: Cold 622
- NU ZHEN ZI 812

End of Topic:
ABDOMEN/GASTROINTESTINAL TOPICS

ABDOMINAL QI STAGNATION

See: Qi Related Disorders/Topics Abdominal Qi
Stagnation 314

ABORTIFACIENT

See: Sexuality, Female: Gynecological
Abortifacient 319

ABORTION RELATED TOPICS

See: Sexuality, Female: Gynecological Abortion
Related Topics 320

ABSCESS IN ORAL CAVITY

See: Oral Cavity Abscess, Tongue, Mouth 283

ABSCESS RELATED TOPICS

See: Skin Abscess Related Topics 349

ABSCESS, INTESTINAL RELATED TOPICS

See: Abdomen/Gastrointestinal Topics Abscess,
Intestinal Related Topics 27

ABSCESS, LIVER

See: Liver Liver, Abscess 211

ABSCESS, LUNG

See: Lungs Abscess, Lung 213

ACCUMULATION OF BLOOD

See: Blood Related Disorders/Topics
Accumulation Of Blood 42

ACCUMULATION TOPICS

See: Abdomen/Gastrointestinal Topics
Accumulation Topics 28

ACETYLCHOLINE

See: Mental State/Neurological Disorders
Acetylcholine 240

ACHES, PAINS, GENERAL

See: Pain/Numbness/General Discomfort Aches,
Pains, General 296

ACID REGURGITATION

See: Stomach/Digestive Disorders Acid
Regurgitation 385

ACNE

See: Skin Acne 350

ACTH, STIMULATES

See: Endocrine Related Disorders Acth,
Stimulates 100

ADAPTOGEN

See: Energetic State Adaptogen 103

ADDICTIVE

See: Mental State/Neurological Disorders
Addictive 240

ADDISON'S DISEASE

See: Endocrine Related Disorders Addison's
Disease 100

ADENITIS

See: Immune System Related Disorders/Topics
Adenitis 175

ADIAPHORESIS

See: Skin Adiaphoresis 350

ADNEXITIS

See: Sexuality, Female: Gynecological
Adnexitis 320

ADRENAL RELATED TOPICS

See: Endocrine Related Disorders Adrenal
Related Topics 100

ADRENALIN RELATED TOPICS

See: Endocrine Related Disorders Adrenalin
Related Topics 100

AFTERNOON SWEATS

See: Skin Afternoon Sweats 350

AGALACTIA

See: Sexuality, Female: Gynecological
Agalactia 320

AGGREGATION EFFECT ON RBC

See: Blood Related Disorders/Topics
Aggregation Effect On RBC 42

AGING RELATED TOPICS

See: Geriatric Topics Aging Related Topics 143

AGITATION

See: Mental State/Neurological Disorders
Agitation 240

ALBINISM

See: Skin Albinism 350

ALBUMINURIA

See: Urinary Bladder Albuminuria 419

ALCOHOLIC INTOXICATION

See: Trauma, Bites, Poisonings Alcoholic
Intoxication 407

ALDOSTERONE RELATED TOPICS

See: Endocrine Related Disorders Aldosterone
Related Topics 100

ALLERGIC DERMATITIS

See: Immune System Related Disorders/Topics
Allergic Dermatitis 175

ALLERGIC RHINITIS

See: Nose Allergic Rhinitis 278

ALLERGIES AND RELATED TOPICS

See: Immune System Related Disorders/Topics
Allergies And Related Topics 175

ALLERGIES, SKIN

See: Skin Allergic/Allergies 350

ALOPECIA

See: Head/Neck Alopecia 144

ALTITUDE SICKNESS

See: Trauma, Bites, Poisonings Altitude Sickness
.... 407

ALZHEIMER'S DISEASE

See: Mental State/Neurological Disorders
Alzheimer's Disease 240

AMENORRHEA RELATED TOPICS

See: Sexuality, Female: Gynecological
Amenorrhea Related Topics 320

AMNESIA

See: Mental State/Neurological Disorders
Amnesia 240

AMOEBA AND RELATED TOPICS

See: Parasites Amoeba And Related Topics 303

AMOEBIC DYSENTERY

See: Parasites Amoebic Dysentery 303

AMYLASE INHIBITION

See: Stomach/Digestive Disorders Amylase
Inhibition 385

ANAL FISSURES

See: Bowel Related Disorders Anal Fissures 51

ANAL PAIN

See: Bowel Related Disorders Anal Pain 51

ANAL PROLAPSE

See: Bowel Related Disorders Anal Prolapse ... 51

ANALGESIC RELATED TOPICS

See: Pain/Numbness/General Discomfort
Analgesic Related Topics 296

ANALGESIC, DENTAL

See: Oral Cavity Analgesic, Dental 283

ANALGESIC, IN LARGE INTESTINE

See: Abdomen/Gastrointestinal Topics
Analgesic, In Large Intestine 28

ANAPHYLACTIC PURPURA

See: Skin Anaphylactic Purpura 351
See: Immune System Related Disorders/Topics
Anaphylactic Purpura 176

ANAPHYLACTIC SHOCK

See: Trauma, Bites, Poisonings Anaphylactic
Shock 407
See: Immune System Related Disorders/Topics
Anaphylactic Shock 176

ANCYLOSTOMIASIS

See: Parasites Ancylostomiasis 303

ANDROGEN-LIKE EFFECT

See: Endocrine Related Disorders Androgen-Like
Effect 100

ANDRONERGIC

See: Endocrine Related Disorders Andronergic
.... 100

ANEMIA RELATED TOPICS

See: Blood Related Disorders/Topics Anemia
Related Topics 43

ANESTHETIC RELATED TOPICS

See: Pain/Numbness/General Discomfort
Anesthetic Related Topics 297

ANGER

See: Mental State/Neurological Disorders
Anger 241

ANGINA PECTORIS

See: Heart Angina Pectoris 151

ANGIOMA, CONGENITAL

See: Heart Angioma, Congenital 152

ANKLE JOINT SWELLINGS

See: Musculoskeletal/Connective Tissue Ankle
Joint Swellings 261

ANKYLOSING SPONDYLITIS

See: Musculoskeletal/Connective Tissue
Ankylosing Spondylitis 261

ANOREXIA RELATED TOPICS

See: Stomach/Digestive Disorders Anorexia
Related Topics 385

ANOREXIA, IN CHILDREN

See: Childhood Disorders Anorexia, Childhood . 80

ANTIACID

See: Stomach/Digestive Disorders Antiacid ... 386

BLOOD RELATED DISORDERS/ TOPICS :

ACCUMULATION OF BLOOD

AGGREGATION EFFECT ON RBC

ANEMIA

ANEMIA, APLASTIC

ANEMIA, APLASTIC, CHRONIC

ANEMIA, PERNICIOUS

ANEMIA, POST HEMORRHAGE

ANTICOAGULANT

BLOOD

BLOOD ACCUMULATION

BLOOD BI

BLOOD CELLS, WHITE

BLOOD CELLS, WHITE, INCREASES

BLOOD CLOTS, REDUCES

BLOOD CLOTTING TIME, LENGHTHENS

BLOOD CLOTTING TIME, SHORTENS

BLOOD CLOTTING, ENHANCES

BLOOD COAGULATION

BLOOD DEFICIENCY SYNDROME

BLOOD, COAGULATON REDUCES

BLOOD, CONGEALED

See: Blood Related Disorders/Topics Blood
Stasis 47
• DAN SHEN/RU XIANG: Pain Swelling
• SHAN ZHA/CHUAN XIONG/DANG GUI: Postpartum Pain
• YAN HU SUO/WU LING ZHI: Chest/Abdomen Pain
• YAN HU SUO/CHUAN XIONG: Headache, Body Aches

BLOOD, CONGEALED MASSES

BLOOD, CONGEALED W/STAGNANT QI

BLOOD, ESSENSE, SEVERE DEFICIENCY

• LU RONG/DANG GUI/SHENG DI HUANG

BLOOD, FLUIDS DEFICIENCY

• SANG SHEN ZI/MAI MEN DONG: Dry Throat/Mouth,
Irritability

BLOOD, HARMONIZE IN LIVER QI STAGNATION

• CHAI HU/BAI SHAO/DANG GUI/CHUAN XIONG

BLOOD, HELPS TO GENERATE

BLOOD, INCREASES PRODUCTION OF

BLOOD, INCREASES RBC

BLOOD, INCREASES RBC, HEMOGLOBIN, DECREASES WBC

BLOOD, INCREASES RBC/WBC

BLOOD, INCREASES WBC

BLOOD, LEUKOCYTES

BLOOD, PLASMA SUBSTITUTE

BLOOD, PLATELETS, PROTECTANT

BLOOD, QI DEFICIENCY

BLOOD, QI DEFICIENCY, CHRONIC

BLOOD, QI, SLUGGISH FLOW OF

BLOOD, QI, VERY DEFICIENCY

• HUANG JING/DANG GUI: Jaundice, Muscular Atrophy

BLOOD, RBC

BLOOD, RECKLESS HOT

BLOOD, RED, REDUCES HEMOLYSIS OF

BLOOD, SEVERE LOSS OF

• REN SHEN/FU ZI/(SHEN FU TANG): Collapsing Syndrome

BLOOD, SPLEEN DEFICIENCY

• SHU DI HUANG/SHA REN

BLOOD, TRIGLYCERIDES

BLOOD, TRIGLYCERIDES, LOWERS

BLOOD, VITALIZES IN VENA PORTAE

BLOOD, WBC

BLOOD, WITHERING OF

THROMBOCYTOPENIC PURPURA HEMORRHAGICA

• E JIAO (c): Xin Jia Fu Mai Tang (E Jiao, Mai Dong, Sheng Di, Bai Shao, Dang Gui, Huang Qi, Zhi Gan Cao, *Jiao Ai Si Wu Tang (Ai Ye, E Jiao, SI Wu Tang, Zhi Gan Cao) .. 797

THROMBOCYTOPENIC PURPURA, BLEEDING OF

• LING YANG JIAO (c): Ling Yang San Huang Decoction (Ling Yang Jiao, Sheng Di, Jin Yin Hua, Mu Dan Pi, Chen Pi, Huang Bai, Huang Lian, Shan Zhi Zi, Bai Shao, Bai Mao Gen, Gan Cao, E Jiao) , Bleeding Stopped 3-7 Days
.... 747

End of Topic:
BLOOD RELATED DISORDERS/TOPICS

BLOOD RELATED TOPICS

See: Blood Related Disorders/Topics   Blood Related Topics 43

BLOOD VESSELS AND RELATED TOPICS

See: Circulation Disorders   Blood Vessels And Related Topics 85

BM

See: Bowel Related Disorders   Bowel Movement
.... 52

BODY ACHES/PAIN RELATED TOPICS

See: Pain/Numbness/General Discomfort   Body Aches/Pain Related Topics 300

BODY ODOR, UNDERARM

See: Skin   Body Odor, Underarm 351

BODY TEMPERATURE, LOWERS

See: Nutritional/Metabolic Disorders/Topics
Body Temperature, Lowers 281

BODY TEMPERATURE, RAISES

See: Nutritional/Metabolic Disorders/Topics
Body Temperature, Raises 281

BODY WEIGHT, DECREASES

See: Nutritional/Metabolic Disorders/Topics
Body Weight, Decreases 281

BODY WEIGHT, INCREASES

See: Nutritional/Metabolic Disorders/Topics
Body Weight, Increases 281

BODY, COLD

See: Nutritional/Metabolic Disorders/Topics
Body, Cold 281

BODY, WEAKNESS RELATED TOPICS

See: Energetic State   Body, Weakness Related Topics 104

BOILS AND RELATED TOPICS

See: Skin   Boils And Related Topics 351

BOILS, INTERNAL

See: Infectious Diseases   Boils, Internal 182

BOILS, PIMPLE INFECTIONS/SUSCEPTIBILITY OF W/WEAK CONSTITUTIONS, IN CHILDREN

See: Childhood Disorders   Boils, Pimple Infections/Susceptibility Of w/Weak Constitutions, In Children 81

BONE STEAMING FEVER

See: Fevers   Bone Steaming Fever 126

BONE/TENDONS TOPICS

See: Musculoskeletal/Connective Tissue   Bone/Tendons Topics 267

BONES, SMALL FISH LODGED IN THROAT

See: Trauma, Bites, Poisonings   Bones, Small Fish Lodged In Throat 408

BORBORYGMUS

See: Abdomen/Gastrointestinal Topics   Borborygmus 29

BOWEL DISEASE, INFLAMMATORY

See: Bowel Related Disorders   Bowel Disease, Inflammatory 52

BOWEL MOVEMENT RELATED TOPICS

See: Bowel Related Disorders   Bowel Movement Related Topics 52

End of Topic:
BOWEL MOVEMENT RELATED TOPICS

BOWEL RELATED DISORDERS :

See: Abdomen/Gastrointestinal Topics   21

AMOEBIC DYSENTERY

See: Bowel Related Disorders   Dysentery 59

ANAL FISSURES

• HUANG BAI (c): 10% Solution, Apply Repeatedly With Cotton With Pressure 485
• HUANG LIAN (c): 10% Solution, Apply Repeatedly With Cotton With Pressure 486

ANAL PAIN

• MU BIE ZI 844

ANAL PROLAPSE

See: Bowel Related Disorders   Rectal Prolapse .. 64
• HE ZI/YING SU KE/GAN JIANG/CHEN PI: Deficiency Cold
• HE ZI/HUANG LIAN/MU XIANG/(HE ZI SAN): Heat
• HUANG QI/REN SHEN/BAI ZHU/SHENG MA/(BU ZHONG YI QI TANG): Spleen Stomach Weak w/Qi Sinking

- CHAI HU 457
- CI WEI PI 819
- DANG SHEN: Spleen Qi Collapsed 762
- HE ZI 822
- HUANG QI 765
- SHENG MA 467

APERIENT

- BAI ZI REN (c) 730
- FENG MI (c) 548

BOWEL DISEASE, INFLAMMATORY

- HUANG LIAN (c) 486

BOWEL MOVEMENT, BLOODY

See: **Hemorrhagic Disorders** Hemafecia 167
- HAN LIAN CAO: Yin Deficient With Blood Heat 806
- WU MEI 830

BOWEL MOVEMENT, DECREASED

- QING FEN 845

BOWEL MOVEMENT, DISCOMFORT

- DA FU PI/HOU PO: Qi Stagnation, Dampness

BOWEL MOVEMENT, IRREGULAR

- CHAI HU/ZHI KE
- LU LU TONG 681

BOWEL MOVEMENT, IRREGULAR W/ABDOMINAL PAIN

- LU LU TONG/WU YAO/MU XIANG/ZHI KE

BOWEL MOVEMENT, LOOSE

- FU LING : Dampness/Fluid Stagnation 594
- GAN JIANG 614

BOWEL MOVEMENT, MUSHY

- JI NEI JIN (c): Used With Mai Ya, Shan Zha, Bai Zhu, Chen Pi 638

COLIC

- ROU GUI (c): Oral, 1.0-4.5 g, Topical, Too 616

COLITIS

- JIU BI YING 625
- YU XING CAO 539

COLITIS, ALLERGIC

- LAI FU ZI (c): Retention Enema Of 639

COLITIS, CHRONIC W/ABDOMINAL PAIN

- PU HUANG (c): With Wu Ling Zhi, Baked Ge Gen, Baked Rou Dou Dou 660

COLITIS, CHRONIC, NONSPECIFIC

- BAI JIANG CAO (c): Retention Enema Of Yi Yi Ren, Fu Zi, Herb 512

COLITIS, ULCERATIVE

- HUANG LIAN (c) 486

COLON CONTRACTIONS, STRONG

- LU HUI (c): Oral/Enema Form 544

COLON, BALANTIDIASIS OF

- HUANG LIAN (c): Protozoan Infection Of GI Tract, With Vomiting Abdominal Pain, Weight Loss 486

CONSTIPATION

See: **Bowel Related Disorders** Laxative 63
See: **Bowel Related Disorders** Purgative 64
- BAI ZI REN/HUO MA REN/HU TAO REN: Postpartum: Deficient Blood
- BAI ZI REN/XING REN/YU LI REN/TAO REN/(WU REN WAN): Intestinal Dryness
- BEI SHA SHEN/SHI HU: Stomach Yin Deficient/Post Febrile Disease
- CHEN XIANG/ROU CONG RONG: Deficient Qi, Dry Intestines
- DA HUANG/MANG XIAO/(DA CHENG QI TANG): Excess Heat In Stomach, Intestines
- DA HUANG/FU ZI/GAN JIANG/(WEN PI TANG): Excess Cold Accumulation
- DANG GUI/ROU CONG RONG/HUO MA REN: Intestinal Dryness
- DONG KUI ZI/HUO MA REN: Fluid Lack Intestines
- DONG KUI ZI/DANG GUI/TAO REN/BAI ZI REN/(USE SOME OR ALL)
- FAN XIE YE/HUO XIANG/MU XIANG: Large Intestine Heat Accumulation
- FAN XIE YE/ZHI SHI/HOU PO
- GUA LOU/HUO MA REN/YU LI REN/ZHI KE
- GUA LOU/DAN NAN XING/HUANG QIN/(QING PI HUA TAN WAN): Phlegm Heat
- GUA LOU REN/HUO MA REN/TAO REN/BAI ZI REN: Hot Phlegm Obstruction w/Dry Mouth, Thirst
- HE SHOU WU/DANG GUI/HUO MA REN: Intestinal Dryness
- HEI ZHI MA/SANG YE/(SANG MA WAN): Deficient Blood/Yin
- HEI ZHI MA/DANG GUI/ROU CONG RONG/BAI ZI REN: Intestinal Dryness
- HEI ZHI MA/(chicken egg): Blood Deficiency
- HOU PO/BAN XIA: Abdominal Distension, Excessive
- HU TAO REN/HUO MA REN/ROU CONG RONG: Intestinal Dryness
- HUANG JING/BEI SHA SHEN/MAI MEN DONG/GU YA: Spleen Stomach Yin Deficiency
- HUO MA REN/DANG GUI: Deficient Blood, Fluids
- HUO MA REN/DANG GUI/SHU DI HUANG/XING REN/(YI XUE RUN CHANG WAN): Dryness
- JUE MING ZI/DANG GUI: Intestinal Dryness
- LU HUI/ZHU SHA: Heat Accumulation
- LU HUI/LONG DAN CAO/SHAN ZHI ZI/QING DAI/DANG GUI/(DANG GUI LU HUI WAN): Excess Liver Fire w/Headache, Dizzyness
- MAI MEN DONG/SHENG DI HUANG/XUAN SHEN/(ZENG YE TANG): Intestinal Dryness/Severely Injured Fluids, Post Febrile Disease
- MU XIANG/BING LANG: Stomach/Intestines Stagnation
- QIAN NIU ZI/BING LANG: Intestinal Parasites
- QIN JIAO/HUO MA REN/YU LI REN: Dry Intestines

CONSTIPATION W/ABDOMINAL SWELLING

CONSTIPATION W/BLOOD HEAT

CONSTIPATION W/CARBUNCLES

CONSTIPATION W/DEFICIENT BLOOD

CONSTIPATION W/EDEMA, DYSURIA

CONSTIPATION W/FOOD STAGNATION

CONSTIPATION W/FULLNESS, DISTENTION

• ZHI SHI/HOU PO/DA HUANG

CONSTIPATION W/GI PAIN, DISTENTION

CONSTIPATION W/HEADACHE & RED EYES

CONSTIPATION W/HEAT ACCUMULATION, YIN DAMAGE

• DA HUANG/SHENG DI HUANG/XUAN SHEN/MAI MEN DONG/(ZENG YE CHENG QI TANG)

CONSTIPATION W/HEMORRHOIDS

• HUO MA REN/DA HUANG/HOU PO/(MA ZI REN WAN): Dryness And Heat In Large Instestine

CONSTIPATION W/SEVERE BAD BREATH, RED EYES, SCANTY URINE

• JUE MING ZI/DAN ZHU YE/GUA LOU REN

CONSTIPATION, ACUTE

CONSTIPATION, CAUSES

CONSTIPATION, CHILDHOOD

CONSTIPATION, CHRONIC

• DA HUANG/ROU GUI
• DANG GUI/ROU CONG RONG/HUO MA REN: Deficient Qi/Blood
• LU HUI/ZHU SHA
• TAO REN/XING REN/HUO MA REN: Deficient Or Stagnation
• YU LI REN/HUO MA REN/XING REN: Deficient Qi/Dry Intestines

CONSTIPATION, CHRONIC DEFICIENCY

• SHU DI HUANG/(lean meat)

CONSTIPATION, DRY STOOL

CONSTIPATION, ELDERLY

• BAI ZI REN/HUO MA REN/HU TAO REN: Deficient Blood
• LIU HUANG/BAN XIA: Cold Deficient
• ROU CONG RONG/HUO MA REN/(RUN CHANG WAN): Deficient Qi And Blood

• SANG SHEN ZI/HE SHOU WU

CONSTIPATION, FROM DRYNESS

CONSTIPATION, FROM FEVER W/THIRST

• SHENG DI HUANG/XUAN SHEN/MAI MEN DONG

CONSTIPATION, FROM INTESTINAL DRYNESS

• TAO REN/DANG GUI/BAI ZI REN/HUO MA REN/XING REN

CONSTIPATION, INTRACTABLE

CONSTIPATION, MILD

CONSTIPATION, MOIST

CONSTIPATION, PAIN W/ABDOMINAL DISTENTION

• HOU PO/DA HUANG/ZHI SHI/(DA CHENG QI TANG): Spleen Stomach Dampness

CONSTIPATION, POST FEBRILE DISEASE

CONSTIPATION, POST GYNECOLOGICAL OPERATION

CONSTIPATION, POSTPARTUM

• SANG SHEN ZI/HE SHOU WU

CONSTIPATION, SEVERE

CONSTIPATION, SEVERE W/EDEMA

CONSTIPATION, SEVERE W/EXCESS EDEMA

• SHANG LU/BING LANG

CONSTIPATION, SWELLING OF

CONSTIPATION, W/DRY MOUTH

DEFECATION

DIARRHEA

- BAI BIAN DOU/BAI ZHU/SHAN YAO: Deficient Spleen/Stomach Qi
- BAI BIAN DOU/REN SHEN/BAI ZHU/FU LING /(SHEN LING BAI ZHU SAN): Spleen Deficient, Not Metabolizing Water
- BAI DOU KOU/SHA REN: Qi Obstruction, With Dampness
- BAI DOU KOU/XING REN/YI YI REN/HUA SHI: Early Damp Warm Febrile Diseases
- BAI ZHU/GAN JIANG: Cold Deficient Middle Jiao
- BAI ZHU/GAN JIANG/REN SHEN/(LI ZHONG WAN): Spleen Stomach Deficiency Cold
- BI BA/GAO LIANG JIANG: Stomach Cold
- CAN SHA/WU ZHU YU/MU GUA: Dampness
- CAN SHA/HUANG QIN/MU GUA/WU ZHU YU/(CAN SHI TANG): Spleen Stomach, Turbid Dampness Blocking
- CANG ZHU/HOU PO: Dampness Blocking Middle Jiao
- CANG ZHU/JIN YIN HUA: Summer Heat w/Dampness
- CAO GUO/CANG ZHU/HOU PO/BAN XIA: Spleen Stomach Cold Blockage
- CHAN SU/XIONG HUANG/CANG ZHU/DING XIANG: Summer Heatstroke
- CHE QIAN ZI/FU LING /BAI ZHU/ZE XIE: Damp Heat
- CHEN PI/BAI ZHU/DANG SHEN
- CHUAN JIAO/CANG ZHU/CHEN PI/MU XIANG: Cold Damp
- CHUN PI/HUANG LIAN/HUANG QIN/MU XIANG: Damp Heat
- DA DOU HUANG JUAN/HUA SHI/TONG CAO: Damp Heat, Damp Summer Heat, Damp Bi
- DANG SHEN/HUANG QI: Lung Spleen Qi Deficient
- DING XIANG/SHA REN/BAI ZHU: Spleen Stomach Cold And Weak
- FU LING /MU XIANG: Dampness
- FU LING /DANG SHEN/BAI ZHU/(SI JUN ZI TANG): Spleen Deficient w/Dampness
- FU LONG GAN/BAI ZHU/HUANG QI/ZHI GAN CAO: Cold, Deficient Spleen/Stomach
- FU ZI/BAI ZHU: Yang Deficient w/Excess Cold Damp
- FU ZI/REN SHEN/BAI ZHU/GAN JIANG/(FU ZI LI ZHONG WAN): Spleen Yang Weakness
- GAN JIANG/BAI ZHU: Spleen Deficient
- GAN JIANG/BAI ZHU/FU LING /(LI ZHONG WAN): Spleen Stomach Weakness, Cold
- GAO LIANG JIANG/BI CHENG QIE/ROU GUI: Cold
- GE GEN/SHAN YAO: Deficient Spleen/Stomach Qi
- GE GEN/HUANG LIAN: Hot
- GE GEN/HUANG LIAN/HUANG QIN: Hot
- GE GEN/BAI ZHU/FU LING : Spleen Deficient
- GE GEN/DANG SHEN/BAI ZHU/MU XIANG: Spleen Deficient

- HU JIAO/GAO LIANG JIANG: Stomach Cold
- HUA QI SHEN/SHI GAO/ZHI MU: Febrile Diseases w/Both Qi/Fluids Injured
- HUA SHI/FU LING /YI YI REN: Damp Heat
- HUANG BAI/BAI TOU WENG/HUANG LIAN/HUANG QIN: Damp Heat In Intestines
- HUANG LIAN/GE GEN/HUANG QIN: Damp Heat
- HUANG QIN/HUANG LIAN
- HUO XIANG/BAN XIA: Dampness Blocking Middle Jiao
- HUO XIANG/BAI ZHU: Deficient Spleen Stomach
- HUO XIANG/ZI SU YE/BAN XIA/HOU PO/CHEN PI/(HUO XIAN ZHENG QI SAN): Digestion, Disturbance From Cold, Raw Food
- JIN YIN HUA/HUANG LIAN/BAI TOU WENG: Toxic Heat
- LAI FU ZI/SHAN ZHA: Stagnant Stomach/Intestines
- LONG GU/GUI ZHI/BAI SHAO: Yang Deficient
- MU GUA/WU ZHU YU/XIAO HUI XIANG/SHENG JIANG: Cold Damp
- MU XIANG/SHA REN: Tenesmus, Pain, Anorexia: Food Stagnation
- MU XIANG/FU LING /ZHI KE/CHEN PI: Spleen Stomach Qi Stagnation
- REN SHEN/BAI ZHU: Spleen Stomach Deficient Qi
- ROU DOU KOU/MU XIANG: Spleen Stomach Deficiency Cold
- ROU DOU KOU/BAN XIA/GAN JIANG: Spleen Stomach Cold Deficient
- ROU GUI/FU ZI: Spleen Kidney Yang Deficiency
- ROU GUI/GAN JIANG/BAI ZHU/FU ZI/(GUI FU LI ZHONG WAN): Spleen Kidney Yang Deficiency
- SHA REN/BAI ZHU: Spleen Stomach Damp Obstructing
- SHA REN/CANG ZHU: Cold Damp
- SHAN YAO/FU LING : Deficient Spleen
- SHAN YAO/QIAN SHI: Kidney Deficient
- SHAN YAO/REN SHEN/BAI ZHU/FU LING /(SHEN LING BAI ZHU SAN): Spleen Stomach Weakness
- SHAN ZHA/MU XIANG/ROU DOU KOU/BAI BIAN DOU/(all toasted)
- TU SI ZI/SHAN YAO/FU LING /DANG SHEN: Kidney Spleen Deficient
- TU SI ZI/DANG SHEN/BAI ZHU/SHAN YAO: Spleen Deficiency
- WU MEI/MU GUA: Summer Heat Disease
- WU YAO/WU ZHU YU: Spleen Kidney Deficient, Cold
- XIANG FU/MU XIANG: Liver Spleen Qi Blockage
- YI YI REN/FU LING /BAI ZHU: Spleen Deficient
- YI YI REN/ZE XIE/BAI ZHU: Spleen Deficiency
- YI ZHI REN/DANG SHEN/BAN XIA/FU LING : Spleen Stomach Cold Deficiency
- YI ZHI REN/FU LING /SHAN YAO/DANG SHEN/BAN XIA: Spleen Deficiency
- ZE XIE/FU LING /ZHU LING/BAI ZHU/(WU LING SAN)
- ZHI SHI/DA HUANG
- ZHU LING/FU LING
- ZHU LING/FU LING /ZE XIE/(SI LING SAN)

DIARRHEA FROM INDIGESTION

DIARRHEA FROM PARASITES

DIARRHEA FROM SUMMER HEAT

DIARRHEA W/BLOOD, MUCOUS

- XIE BAI/HUANG BAI

DIARRHEA W/CALF MUSCLE SPASMS

- MU GUA/HUO XIANG/SHA REN: Summer Heat

DIARRHEA W/EXTERNAL PATHOGEN

- SHEN QU/(spicy warm or cool herbs)

DIARRHEA W/FOOD STAGNATION

- SHEN QU/BAI ZHU: Spleen Deficient

DIARRHEA W/INDIGESTION

DIARRHEA W/LESS URINE

- CHE QIAN ZI/BAI ZHU/YI YI REN: Deficient Spleen Or Summer Heat, Damp

DIARRHEA W/STOMACH PAIN

- GAN JIANG/WU ZHU YU/BAN XIA: Cold Attacking Spleen: Stomach

DIARRHEA W/TENESMUS

DIARRHEA W/TENESMUS, DISTENTION, ESPECIALLY

- MU XIANG/HUANG LIAN

DIARRHEA W/UNDIGESTED FOOD PARTICLES

DIARRHEA W/UPPER BODY HEAT

DIARRHEA, ACUTE

DIARRHEA, ACUTE W/PAIN

- HUANG BAI/MU XIANG

DIARRHEA, BLOODY

DIARRHEA, CHILDHOOD

DIARRHEA, CHRONIC

- BI BA/HE ZI/DANG SHEN/GAN JIANG/ROU GUI: Deficient Cold
- CAO DOU KOU/MU XIANG/HE ZI/(both toasted): Deficient Cold
- CHAI HU/REN SHEN/HUANG QI/BAI ZHU/SHENG MA: Spleen/Stomach Qi Sinking
- GU SUI BU/SHAN YAO
- HE ZI/BAI ZHU/QIAN SHI
- HE ZI/YING SU KE/GAN JIANG/CHEN PI: Deficiency Cold
- HE ZI/ROU DOU KOU
- HE ZI/HUANG LIAN/MU XIANG/(HE ZI SAN): Heat
- HU HUANG LIAN/GAN JIANG
- JIN YING ZI/DANG SHEN/BAI ZHU/SHAN YAO: Spleen Deficient
- LIAN ZI/SHAN YAO: Spleen Deficient
- LIAN ZI/BAI ZHU/SHAN YAO/FU LING : Spleen Deficiency

- QIAN SHI/DANG SHEN/FU LING /BAI ZHU: Spleen Deficient
- QIAN SHI/BAI ZHU/SHAN YAO: Spleen Deficiency
- ROU DOU KOU/DANG SHEN/BAI ZHU/GAN JIANG: Spleen Stomach Cold Deficient
- ROU DOU KOU/HE ZI/BAI ZHU/DANG SHEN
- SHI LIU PI/HE ZI/ROU DOU KOU
- WU BEI ZI/ROU DOU KOU/DANG SHEN
- WU MEI/HE ZI/WU WEI ZI
- WU MEI/ROU DOU KOU/HE ZI/YING SU KE
- WU WEI ZI/ROU DOU KOU/WU ZHU YU/(SI SHEN WAN): Spleen Kidney Deficiency
- WU YI/HE ZI/ROU DOU KOU: Childhood Nutritional Impairment
- WU ZHU YU/WU WEI ZI/ROU DOU KOU/(SI SHEN WAN): Spleen Kidney Deficiency, Cold
- YING SU KE/MU XIANG/HUANG LIAN

DIARRHEA, CHRONIC INFANTILE

DIARRHEA, CHRONIC W/ANOREXIA

DIARRHEA, CHRONIC W/BLOODY STOOL, PAIN

- WU BEI ZI/HE ZI

DIARRHEA, CHRONIC W/INCONTINENCE

DIARRHEA, CHRONIC W/NAVEL PAIN

DIARRHEA, CHRONIC W/STOMACH GROWLING

DIARRHEA, CHRONIC, GERIATIRIC

DIARRHEA, CHRONIC, INTERMITTENT W/HARD/SOFT STOOL

DIARRHEA, CHRONIC, INTRACTABLE

DIARRHEA, CHRONIC, NON-INFECTIOUS

DIARRHEA, DAMAGED FLUIDS FROM HEAT

- GE GEN/SHAN YAO

DIARRHEA, EARLY MORNING

- BU GU ZHI/ROU DOU KOU/WU WEI ZI/WU ZHU YU/(SI SHEN WAN): Kidney Spleen Yang Deficient
- GE JIE/REN SHEN/(korean)/HU TAO REN/WU WEI ZI: Kidney Yang Deficient
- ROU DOU KOU/BU GU ZHI: Spleen Kidney Cold Deficient
- WU WEI ZI/BU GU ZHI: Kidney Deficient
- WU ZHU YU/WU WEI ZI: Spleen Kidney Yang Deficient

DIARRHEA, EARLY STAGE

DIARRHEA, INFANTILE

DIARRHEA, LINGERING

- CHI SHI ZHI 818

DIARRHEA, LOOSE STOOL

- BAI ZHU/REN SHEN/FU LING /(SI JUN ZI TANG): Spleen Weakness In Water Metabolism
- REN SHEN/BAI ZHU/FU LING /GAN CAO/(SI JUN ZI TANG): Spleen Stomach Weakness

DIARRHEA, PAINFUL W/BRIGHT BLOOD IN BM

- FANG FENG 444

DIARRHEA, POST COLON OPERATION

- LAI FU ZI (c): Retention Enema Of 639

DIARRHEA, POSTPARTUM

- DENG XIN CAO 592

DIARRHEA, SEVERE

- HE ZI/YING SU KE/GAN JIANG/CHEN PI: Deficient Cold
- SHI CHANG PU 757

DIARRHEA, SEVERE CAUSING COLLAPSING SYNDROME

- REN SHEN/FU ZI/(SHEN FU TANG)

DIARRHEA, SUMMER

- SHI GAO (c) 477

DIARRHEA, UNCONTROLLABLE

- CHI SHI ZHI 818

DIARRHEA, VIOLENT

- FU ZI: Yang Collapse 613

DIARRHEA, VIOLENT W/SPASMS

- MU GUA 567

DIARRHEA, VOMITING

- BAI BIAN DOU/XIANG RU/HOU PO/(XIANG RU SAN): Summer Damp Heat
- XIANG RU/BAI ZHU: Spleen Dampness w/External Cold From Cold, Raw Food

DIARRHEA, WIND COLD W/DAMP SPLEEN

- FANG FENG/CANG ZHU

DRY INTESTINES

- YU LI REN/HUO MA REN/XING REN: Constipation

DUODENUM, ANTISPASMODIC

- FO SHOU (c) 624

DYSENTERY

- CHUAN XIN LIAN/MA CHI XIAN: Damp Heat

- CHUN PI/HUANG LIAN/HUANG QIN/MU XIANG: Damp Heat
- GE GEN/HUANG LIAN: Damp Heat
- GE GEN/HUANG LIAN/HUANG QIN: Damp Heat
- HUANG BAI/BAI TOU WENG/HUANG LIAN/HUANG QIN: Damp Heat In Intestines
- HUANG LIAN/GE GEN/HUANG QIN: Damp Heat
- HUANG QIN/HUANG LIAN
- JIN YIN HUA/HUANG LIAN/BAI TOU WENG: Toxic Heat
- KU SHEN/MU XIANG/GAN CAO: Damp Heat
- SHI CHANG PU/HUANG LIAN: Damp Heat Blocking Middle Jiao
- YA DAN ZI/BAI TOU WENG/HUANG BAI/HUANG LIAN
- ZHI SHI/DA HUANG/HUANG LIAN/HUANG QIN/(ZHI SHI DAO ZHI WAN): Damp Heat Stagnation In Intestines
- A WEI 637
- BAI FAN 836
- BAI HUA SHE SHE CAO (c) 511
- BAI SHAO: Blood Heat 794
- BAI TOU WENG: Blood Heat 514
- BAN BIAN LIAN 586
- CE BAI YE (c): Dry Powder, 7-10 Days 654
- CHA CHI HUANG 517
- CHI FU LING 483
- CHI XIAO DOU: Damp Heat 591
- CHOU WU TONG 560
- DA SUAN: Good 644
- DI YU: Blood Heat 656
- E BU SHI CAO 711
- ER CHA 839
- FENG LA 840
- FENG WEI CAO 496
- GAN LAN: Bacterial 484
- GE GEN 460
- GUI ZHEN CAO 462
- HE ZI (c): Retention Enemas With Oral Administration Of Capsules, 3 Days/Protects Ulceration From 822
- HONG TENG 497
- HOU PO 581
- HU HUANG LIAN: Blood Heat/Damp Heat 484
- HU JIAO 615
- HU ZHANG 497
- HUA SHI: Heat 597
- HUANG BAI: Blood Heat/Damp Heat 485
- HUANG LIAN: Blood Heat 486
- HUANG QIN 489
- JI NEI JIN 638
- JI ZI HUANG 809
- JIN DI LUO 523
- JIN YIN HUA: Toxic Blood Heat 524
- KU DING CHA 809
- KU SHEN: Blood Heat 491
- KU SHEN (c): Intestinal Trichomoniasis 491
- LAO GUAN CAO 565
- LIAN XU 823
- LONG GU 738
- MA BIAN CAO 682
- MA CHI XIAN: Blood Heat 528
- MA CHI XIAN (c): Decoction, Fresh 90% Acute, 60% Chronic, Sulfa-Like Effectiveness 528

DYSENTERY W/ OR W/O BLOOD

DYSENTERY W/ABDOMINAL PAIN

DYSENTERY W/ANOREXIA

DYSENTERY W/DIFFICULTY INGESTION OF FOOD

DYSENTERY, ABDOMINAL PAIN FROM

DYSENTERY, ABDOMINAL PAIN/TENESMUS OF

DYSENTERY, ACUTE

DYSENTERY, ACUTE W/ABDOMINAL PAIN, TENESMUS

DYSENTERY, ACUTE/CHRONIC W/BLEEDING

DYSENTERY, AMOEBIC

DYSENTERY, BACILLARY

DYSENTERY, BACILLARY, ACUTE

LAXATIVE, MILD

- BAN BIAN LIAN (c) 586
- NIU HUANG (c) 755
- PU GONG YING (c) 529

LAXATIVE, STRONG

- FAN XIE YE (c): Contracts Colon, Similar To Da Huang
  544
- QIAN NIU ZI (c) 553

PILES

See: Bowel Related Disorders Hemorrhoids ... 62

PROLAPSE, ANAL

- HE ZI 822

PROLAPSE, RECTAL

- SHI LIU GEN PI 649
- SHI LIU PI 828
- WU BEI ZI 829

PURGATIVE

See: Bowel Related Disorders Constipation ... 52
- BA DOU (c): Very Drastic, Can Last 10-15hrs 550
- BI MA ZI (c): Cathartic, Irritates Small Intestine, 1-2
  Bowel Movements, 2-6 Hrs After, No Colic, Greater
  Dose Does Not Increase Effect 547
- DA HUANG (c): Bacteria In Intestine Increases Effect,
  6-8 Hrs After Oral Intake, May Produce Secondary
  Constipation—Tannin 542
- DONG KUI ZI: Mild 594
- GAN SUI (c): Intense Diarrhea 551
- HE SHOU WU (c): Increases Peristalsis 799
- HONG DA JI (c) 551
- HU ZHANG (c) 497
- JING DA JI (c) 552
- MANG XIAO (c): Increases Water Thru Osmosis-Drink
  Large Amts Water 545
- NIU BANG ZI (c) 465
- NU ZHEN ZI (c) 812
- QING FEN (c) 845
- SANG BAI PI (c): At 3g/kg Causes Watery Stool 703
- SHANG LU (c): Large Dose Of Extract, Intense 554
- XU SUI ZI (c): Intense Diarrhea, Toxic 556
- YUAN HUA (c): Increase Peristalsis—Diarrhea,
  Abdominal Pain 556
- ZHI SHI (c): Flavonoids In Aqueous Extract 635

PURGATIVE, MILD

- LIU HUANG (c): In Intestines Forms Hydrogen Sulfide
  Which Stimulate Peristalsis 840

PURGATIVE, STRONG

- LU HUI (c) 544

RECTAL BLEEDING

- SAN QI 663

RECTAL POLYPS

- WU MEI (c): See Polyps, Various For Rx 830

RECTAL PROLAPSE

See: Bowel Related Disorders Anal Prolapse ... 51
- CHAI HU/REN SHEN/HUANG QI/BAI ZHU/SHENG MA:
  Spleen/Stomach Qi Sinking
- CHI SHI ZHI/GAN JIANG/DANG SHEN/BAI ZHU: Cold And
  Qi Deficient
- HUANG QI/SHENG MA/CHAI HU: Spleen Qi Weak,
  Sunken
- SHENG MA/CHAI HU: Yang Deficient
- SHI LIU PI/HE ZI/ROU DOU KOU
- WU BEI ZI/HE ZI: External/Steam Bath
- WU BEI ZI/HUANG QI/SHENG MA
- WU BEI ZI/BAI FAN: External
- ZHI SHI/BAI ZHU/HUANG QI
- CAO MIAN HUA ZI: From Uterine Bleeding 850
- CHAI HU 457
- CHI SHI ZHI 818
- HE ZI 822
- HU SUI : External Application Of Decoction With A
  Sponge 446
- JUAN BO 679
- LONG GU: Topical 738
- MU ZEI: Topical 464
- REN SHEN 767
- SHENG MA: From Chronic Diarrhea 467
- SHENG MA (c): Bu Zhong Yi Qi Tang 467
- SHI LIU GEN PI 649
- SHI LIU PI 828
- TIAN XIAN ZI 705
- WO NIU 537
- YING SU KE 832
- YU XING CAO 539
- ZHI KE 635
- ZHI SHI 635
- ZHI SHI (c): Chronic Diarrhea, Decoction, 3x/Day, 5-10
  Days 635

RECTAL PROLAPSE W/BLOODY STOOL

- CHI SHI ZHI: Cold Deficient Lower Jiao 818
- WU BEI ZI: Chronic Diarrhea 829
- YU YU LIANG 833

RECTAL PROLAPSE, COLD DEFICIENCY

- CHI SHI ZHI/GAN JIANG

RECTUM, SORES

- WU BEI ZI/HE ZI: External/Steam Bath

SPASTIC COLON

- WU ZHU YU (c): w/Vinegar, Plaster On Navel 618

STOOLS, BLOODY

- CHEN ZONG TAN/BAI MAO GEN/DA JI/XIAO JI/SHAN ZHI
  ZI/(SHI HUI SAN): Heat
- CHEN ZONG TAN/HUANG QI/REN SHEN/BAI ZHU:
  Spleen Deficiency, Not Holding Blood
- E JIAO/AI YE/SHENG DI HUANG/PU HUANG/OU JIE
- HAN LIAN CAO/SHENG DI HUANG/E JIAO/BAI MAO
  GEN/PU HUANG: Yin Deficiency w/Internal Heat

- HUANG QI/REN SHEN/DANG GUI/(GUI PI TANG): Spleen Qi Deficient, Not Controlling Blood
- HUANG QIN/HUANG LIAN/FANG FENG: Intestinal Wind
- HUANG QIN/DI YU
- WU BEI ZI/DI YU/HUAI HUA MI
- CHUN PI 483
- JIN YIN HUA 524

STOOLS, DRY

- DONG KUI ZI 594
- SHENG DI HUANG 500

STOOLS, LOOSE

See: Bowel Related Disorders Diarrhea 55
- BAI BIAN DOU/REN SHEN/BAI ZHU/FU LING /(SHEN LING BAI ZHU SAN): Spleen Deficient, Not Metabolizing Water
- DA ZAO/REN SHEN/BAI ZHU: Spleen Stomach Weakness
- DANG SHEN/BAI ZHU: Spleen Qi Deficient
- GAN CAO/DANG SHEN: Spleen Deficient
- HUANG QI/REN SHEN/BAI ZHU: Spleen Lung Qi Deficient
- CANG ZHU: Spleen Dampness 578
- FU LING : Dampness/Fluid Stagnation 594
- FU ZI: Spleen Kidney Yang Deficient 613

STOOLS, LOOSE, WATERY

- TU SI ZI/SHAN YAO/FU LING /DANG SHEN: Kidney Spleen Deficient

STOOLS, MUSHY

- JI NEI JIN (c): Used With Mai Ya, Shan Zha, Bai Zhu, Chen Pi 638

STOOLS, UNDIGESTED FOOD IN

- JI NEI JIN: Spleen Stomach Cold, Deficient 638

STOOLS, WATERY

- SHAN YAO/DANG SHEN: Kidney Spleen Deficient

TENESMUS

- MU XIANG/SHA REN: Qi Blockage/Food Stagnation
- ZHI SHI/DA HUANG/HUANG LIAN/HUANG QIN/(ZHI SHI DAO ZHI WAN): Damp Heat Stagnation In Intestines
- BING LANG 643
- DA HUANG 542
- HUANG LIAN 486
- MU XIANG 628
- XIE BAI 634
- ZHI MU 480

TENESMUS, DYSENTERY

- BAI SHAO/HUANG LIAN/MU XIANG/ZHI KE
- XIE BAI/ZHI SHI/MU XIANG/BAI SHAO

TENESMUS, FOOD STAGNATION W/DIARRHEA, DISTENTION, ACID REGURGITATION

- LAI FU ZI/SHAN ZHA/SHEN QU/CHEN PI/(BAO HE WAN)

TENESMUS, RECTAL

- LAI FU ZI 639

ULCERATIVE COLITIS

- HUANG LIAN (c): Local Application 486

End of Topic:
BOWEL RELATED DISORDERS

BRADYCARDIA

See: Heart Bradycardia 152

BRAIN CONCUSSION

See: Trauma, Bites, Poisonings Brain Concussion 408

BRAIN RELATED TOPICS

See: Head/Neck Brain Related Topics 145

BRAIN, BLOOD FLOW TO

See: Circulation Disorders Brain, Blood Flow To 85

BRAIN, CYSTICERCOSIS

See: Parasites Brain, Cysticercosis 304

BRAIN, TAPEWORM LARVAE

See: Parasites Brain, Tapeworm Larvae 304

BREAST CANCER

See: Cancer/Tumors/Swellings/Lumps Breast Cancer 66

BREASTS AND RELATED TOPICS

See: Sexuality, Female: Gynecological Breasts And Related Topics 322

BREATH, FOUL

See: Oral Cavity Breath, Foul 283

BREATH, SHORTNESS OF

See: Lungs Breath, Shortness Of 216

BREATHING RELATED TOPICS

See: Lungs Breathing Related Topics 216

BRONCHI RELATED TOPICS

See: Lungs Bronchi Related Topics 216

BRONCHIECTASIS

See: Lungs Bronchiectasis 217

BRONCHITIS

See: Lungs Bronchitis 217

BRONCHODILATORY

See: Lungs Bronchodilatory 219

BROODING, EXCESS

See: Mental State/Neurological Disorders Brooding, Excess 241

BRUCELLOSIS

See: **Infectious Diseases** Brucellosis 182

BRUISES

See: **Trauma, Bites, Poisonings** Bruises 408

BUERGER'S DISEASE

See: **Circulation Disorders** Buerger's Disease ... 85

BUG BITES

See: **Trauma, Bites, Poisonings** Bug Bites 408

BURNS AND RELATED TOPICS

See: **Skin** Burns And Related Topics 353

BURPING

See: **Stomach/Digestive Disorders** Belching ... 387

CAFFEINE-LIKE

See: **Mental State/Neurological Disorders**
Caffeine-Like 241

CALCIUM METABOLISM TOPICS

See: **Nutritional/Metabolic Disorders/Topics**
Calcium Metabolism Topics 281

CALF MUSCLE SPASMS

See: **Extremities** Calf Muscle Spasms 108

CALLOUSES

See: **Skin** Callouses 354

CALMING

See: **Mental State/Neurological Disorders**
Calming 241

CANCER AND RELATED TOPICS

See: **Cancer/Tumors/Swellings/Lumps** Cancer
And Related Topics 67

End of Topic:
CANCER AND RELATED TOPICS

CANCER/ TUMORS/ SWELLINGS/ LUMPS :

ABDOMEN MASS, CANCER

• TU BIE CHONG: Cancers, 9-15 gm 690

ABDOMEN, MASS/TUMORS

• BIE JIA 805
• SAN LENG 686

ABDOMEN, TUMORS

• GUEI YU JIAN 675
• MA BIAN CAO 682
• TAO REN 689

ABDOMINAL MASSES

See: **Cancer/Tumors/Swellings/Lumps** Masses,
Abdominal 69

ANTICARCINOGENIC

• TIAN NAN XING (c): Many Cell Types 712
• XU SUI ZI (c): Acute Monocytic Leukemia 556

ANTINEOPLASTIC

• BAI HUA SHE SHE CAO (c): High Dose-Leukemia 511
• BAN MAO (c): Liver Cancer 837
• BAN XIA (c): Diluted Alcohol/Aqueous Extract 710
• BI MA ZI (c): Cancer Cells Are Very Sensitive To Ricin
.... 547
• BU GU ZHI (c): Volatile Oil 773
• CHAN SU (c): Synergistic With Cyclophosphamide, etc
.... 837
• DA HUANG (c): Melanoma, Breast Tumors, Liver
Cancer 542
• DA SUAN (c): Water Extracts—Liver Cancer With
Ascites, MTK Sarcoma III Cells, Diet Of Fresh Garlic
Prevented Breast Cancer In Mice 644
• E ZHU (c): Granuloma, Injection, Volatile Oil 673
• FU LING (c): High Inhibition Against Sarcoma 594
• GAN CAO (c): Granuloma, Hepatic Cancer 763
• GUA LOU (c): Granuloma, Hepatic Cancer 718
• GUA LOU PI (c): Granuloma, Hepatic Cancer, Husk Most
Potent, ETOH Extract Strongest 719
• GUA LOU REN (c): Granuloma, Hepatic Cancer 720
• HAI FENG TENG (c): Some Effect 562
• HAN FANG JI (c): Marked 596
• HUANG LIAN (c): Slight 486
• JIN YIN HUA (c): Sarcoma 180, Ehrlich Carcinoma ... 524
• KU SHEN (c) 491
• LU HUI (c): Tumors, Liver Cancer, ETOH Extract 544
• QING DAI (c): Indirubin, Moderate Activity, Injections
Stronger, Lung, Breast Cancer 531
• QING MU XIANG (c) 628
• SHAN CI GU (c): Leukemia, Lymphocytic, Granulocytic,
Breast, Cervix, Esophagus, Lung,
Stomach—Colchincine/Cholchicinamide, See Source
Text For More Details (Chang, But) 846
• SHAN DOU GEN (c): Cervical Cancer, et al 532
• SHAN ZHI ZI (c): Inhibits Ascitic Carcinoma, Orally ... 476
• TIAN MEN DONG (c): Leukemia 814
• XING REN (c): Cervical Cancer 705
• XU SUI ZI (c): Acute Monocytic Leukemia 556
• YI YI REN (c): Granuloma, Hepatic Cancer, Believed To
Be Coixenolide 602
• YU XING CAO (c) 539
• ZHU LING (c): Probably From Immune Enhancement
.... 606
• ZI CAO (c): Chorionepithelioma, Chorioadenoma, Acute
Lymphocytic Leukemia, Breast Cancer 504

BREAST CANCER

• BAI HUA SHE SHE CAO (c): Chief Herb 511
• MAN JING ZI 464
• ZI CAO (c): Reduces Rate Of 504

BREASTS, NIPPLE TUMORS

BREASTS, TUMORS

CANCER

CANCER PATIENTS

CANCER, ANTI-

CANCER, EARLY STAGE

CANCER, MALIGNANT-INHIBITS

CANCER, PAIN OF

CANCER, RADIOTHERAPY, LEUCOPENIA FROM

CANCER, RADIOTHERAPY/CHEMOTHERAPY

CANCER, REDUCES OCCURRANCE OF

- WU JIA PI (c) 574

CANCER, SWELLINGS

- BAN ZHI LIAN 516

CARCINOGENIC

- BA DOU (c): (Cofactor) Effect To Mucosa 550

CARCINOMA

See: Cancer/Tumors/Swellings/Lumps Cancer . 67

CARDIAC CANCER

- BAN MAO (c): See Hepatic Cancer For More Details .. 837

CERVICAL CANCER

- BAI HUA SHE SHE CAO (c): Chief Herb 511
- BAN XIA (c): Ban Xia Water Extract Tablet, Plus Pessary In Cervix And Canal, 2 Months 710
- BO HE (c): Infusion Inhibited 456
- CHUAN BEI MU (c) 717
- E ZHU 673
- E ZHU (c): Early Stage (II Or Less) Most Effectively Treated By Local Injection Of 1% Oil/1% Injection With 0.5%Curcumol/Curzerenone Injected Into Mass With Topical Application, Too, Few Toxic Side Effects 673
- KU SHEN (c): Matrine Ingredient 491
- LIAN FANG 659
- LU FENG FANG 841
- SHAN DOU GEN (c) 532
- SHENG MA (c): 90% Inhibition Against, Hot Aqueous Extract, Also Bu Zhong Yi Qi Tang 467
- TIAN NAN XING (c): Oral (15 g, Then Increase To 45 g, Decoction) + Intracervix Application (50 g Pessary Insert Into Cervical Canal, 2ml (10 g Of Herb) 4 ml Injected Into Cervical Area, 1x/1-2 Days, 3-4 Months Course, 78% Effective, With 20% Short Term Cures ... 712
- WU MEI (c): Inhibits Growth 830
- YA DAN ZI (c): Squamous, Oil Injection With IM Dose 538
- YI YI REN (c): Markedly Inhibited 602
- ZAO XIU (c) 540

CHEMOTHERAPY

- DANG SHEN (c): Increases WBC 762
- NU ZHEN ZI (c): Increases WBC 812

CHORIOADENOMA

- ZI CAO (c) 504

CHORIOCARCINOMA

- TIAN HUA FEN (c): (Rare Uterine Cancer) 726

CHORIONEPITHELIOMA

- ZI CAO (c) 504

CRANIOCERVICAL AREA CANCER

- BI MA ZI (c): Ricin As Cream/Ointment, 3-5% And 3% DMSO, Topical Application, 1x/Day, 5-6x/Week For 1-2 Months 547

CYSTS

- CHUAN BEI MU 717

ESOPHAGEAL CANCER

- SHUI ZHI/HAI ZAO
- BAN MAO (c): See Hepatic Cancer For More Details .. 837
- CANG ZHU (c): Volitile Oil Inhibited In Vitro At High Doses 578
- HUANG YAO ZI 723
- JI XING ZI (c): Symptomatic Improvement, Dysphagia, Some Lessening Vomiting, Pain 677
- QU MAI (c): Decoction Fresh Root, 30-40 g (24-30 g Dried) Alone Or With Ren Shen, Fu Ling, Bai Zhu, Gan Cao 600
- SANG BAI PI (c): Sang Pi Ku Jiu/Cu Tang (Sang Bai Pi Bitter Wine/Vinegar Preparation) 703
- SHAN CI GU 846
- SHI SHANG BAI 534
- WEI LING XIAN (c): With Ban Lan Gen, Aerial Part Of Euphorbia Lunulata, Tian Nan Xing, Niu Huang (Artificial) , Sal Ammoniac, 11% Remission, Another 80% Had Some Effect 572
- YA DAN ZI (c) 538
- ZE QI (c): Softens Tumor, Injections Of 20% Extract Of Neutral Saponins 727
- ZHU LING (c): Synergistic With Chemotherapy, Protects Bone Marrow, Immune System Enhanced 606

ESOPHAGEAL POLYPS

- WU MEI (c): See Polyps, Various For Rx 830

ESOPHAGEAL TUMORS

- HUANG YAO ZI (c): Tincture 723

FIBROSARCOMA

- BAI HUA SHE SHE CAO (c): Chief Herb 511

GASTRIC CANCER

- BAN MAO (c): See Hepatic Cancer For More Details .. 837
- LU FENG FANG 841
- SANG BAI PI (c): Sang Pi Ku Jiu/Cu Tang (Sang Bai Pi Bitter Wine/Vinegar Preparation) 703

GASTRIC TUMORS

- HUANG YAO ZI (c): Tincture 723

GASTROINTESTINAL CANCER

- BAI HUA SHE SHE CAO 511

GRANULOMA

- GAN CAO (c): Inhibits 763
- HUANG LIAN (c): Shrinks 486
- SAN LENG (c) 686

HEPATIC CANCER

- BAN MAO (c): Cook With Eggs, 5-6 With Head, Wings, Legs Removed, Add To Egg, Bake To Dry On Low Heat, Grind, Divide Into 2 Packs, Oral 1 Pack, 1-3x/Day, Up To 14 Months, Help Remission, Life Prolonged, *Tablet Of Substance (As Cantharidin, 0.25 mg) , Ba Ji Powder, Aluminum Hydroxide, Magnesium Trisilicate, 2-6 Tabs/Day In 3 Doses, 45-60% Effective 837

TUMOR, ANTI-, NIPPLES ESPECIALLY

TUMORS

TUMORS, ABDOMINAL

TUMORS, BENIGN

TUMORS, CANCER

TUMORS, EARLY

TUMORS, EHRLICH ASCITES CELLS

TUMORS, FIRM

TUMORS, FISTULOUS

TUMORS, GOOD FOR SMALLER

TUMORS, GYNECOLOGICAL

CEREBRAL EMBOLISM

CEREBRAL ISCHEMIA

CEREBRAL PALSY

CEREBRAL THROMBOSIS

CEREBROVASCULAR RELATED TOPICS

CERUMEN

CERVICAL CANCER

CERVICITIS

CERVIX RELATED TOPICS

CESTODIASIS

CHANCERS, SYPHILITIC

CHAPPED SKIN

CHEEK PAIN THAT RADIATES FROM VERTEX

CHEMOTHERAPY

End of Topic:
CHEMOTHERAPY

CHEST :

CHEST BI

• GUA LOU/XIE BAI/BAN XIA

• XIE BAI/GUA LOU/BAN XIA: Pain, Shortness Of Breath, Productive Cough
• XIE BAI/WU LING ZHI: Pain, Shortness Of Breath, Productive Cough
• GUA LOU   718
• HONG HUA: Blood Stasis   675

CHEST PAIN

CHEST, ABDOMEN FLUID ACCUMULATION

• TING LI ZI/HAN FANG JI/DA HUANG/(JI JIAO LI HUANG WAN)

CHEST, ABDOMEN FULLNESS

• ZI SU YE/SHA REN

CHEST, ACCUMULATION OF FLUIDS

• GAN SUI/DA HUANG/MANG XIAO/(DA XIAN XION TANG OR TOPICAL)
• YUAN HUA   556

CHEST, ACCUMULATIONS, PAIN

• BIE JIA   805

CHEST, ASCITES

• YUAN HUA/GAN SUI/JING DA JI/DA ZAO/(SHI ZAO TANG)

CHEST, CHILLS, PAIN

• CAO DOU KOU   579

CHEST, COLD, HEAT IN

• ZI WAN   706

CHEST, COLD, PAINFUL

• GAN JIANG: Cold, Deficiency   614

CHEST, CONGESTED FLUIDS IN

• CHANG SHAN/GAN CAO: Causes Vomiting

CHEST, CONGESTION/ENTANGLEMENT

• CHUAN BEI MU   717

CHEST, CONGESTION/FULLNESS

• HONG DA JI   551

CHEST, CONSTRICTION

• BAI DOU KOU/XING REN/YI YI REN/HUA SHI: Early Damp Warm Febrile Diseases
• BAN XIA/CHEN PI: Damp Phlegm Or Deficient Spleen Qi
• CHAI HU/ZHI KE
• CHEN PI/BAN XIA/FU LING /HOU PO: Damp Phlegm Obstruction
• HUO XIANG/PEI LAN: Summer Heat Dampness
• HUO XIANG/ZI SU YE: Wind Cold w/Dampness In Middle Jiao
• TONG CAO/HUA SHI/YI YI REN: Summer Heat Dampness
• ZHU LI/BAN XIA: Wind Heat Phlegm
• BAI DOU KOU: Damp Warm Febrile Diseases   577
• CHAI HU: Liver Stomach Disharmony/Shao Yang Disorder   457

CHEST, STIFLING

- **BAI DOU KOU/HUA SHI/YI YI REN/SHA REN/(SAN REN TANG):** Damp Heat Febrile Disease, Early Stage

CHEST, STIFLING SENSATION

- **BAI ZHU/GUI ZHI/FU LING /(LING GUI ZHU GAN TANG):** Phlegm Damp Syndrome
- **CHEN PI/HOU PO/CANG ZHU/(PING WEI SAN)**
- **FO SHOU/XIANG FU/(XIANG YUAN-CITRON)/YU JIN:** Liver Qi Stagnation
- **GUA LOU/DAN NAN XING/HUANG QIN/(QING PI HUA TAN WAN):** Phlegm Heat
- **JIANG XIANG/YU JIN/DANG SHEN/TAO REN/SI GUA LUO:** Qi/Blood Stagnation
- **TIAN NAN XING/BAN XIA/CHEN PI/ZHI SHI/(DAO TAN TANG):** Phlegm Damp
- **XIANG FU/CHAI HU/YU JIN/BAI SHAO:** Liver Qi Stagnation
- **ZHU RU/ZHI SHI/CHEN PI/FU LING /(WEN DAN TANG):** Phlegm Heat
- **BAI GUO YE** 817

CHEST, STIFLING SENSATION W/COSTAL PAIN

- **WU YAO/GUA LOU PI/YU JIN/ZHI KE:** Cold And Qi Stagnation

CHEST, STIFLING SENSATION, PAIN

- **SU HE XIANG/BING PIAN/TAN XIANG/DING XIANG/(GUAN XIN SU HE XIANG WAN OR SU BING DI WAN)**

CHEST, STIFLING SENSATION, PAIN, DISTENTION

- **SHI CHANG PU/HOU PO/CHEN PI:** Turbid Damp In Middle Jiao

CHEST, STUFFINESS

- **BAN XIA** 710
- **HUAI JIAO** 676
- **LAI FU ZI** 639
- **XIE BAI** 634
- **ZHU LI** 728
- **ZI SU ZI** 706

CHEST, STUFFINESS W/YELLOW, THICK SPUTUM

- **ZHI KE** 635
- **ZHI SHI** 635

CHEST, STUFFINESS, FULLNESS

- **SHAN ZHA** 641

CHEST, STUFFINESS/FULLNESS

- **CAO GUO** 580
- **DA HUANG** 542
- **DAN DOU CHI** 459

CHEST, TIGHTNESS

- **CHEN PI (c)** 621

CHEST, TIGHTNESS/CONSTRICTION

- **TIAN NAN XING:** Phlegm 712

CHEST, UNCOMFORTABLE FEELING

- **BAI JI LI/CHAI HU/(JU YE-TANGERINE LEAF)/QING PI/XIANG FU:** Liver Qi Stagnation

CHEST, YANG QI DAMAGE

- **GUI ZHI/ZHI GAN CAO**

CHEST/ABDOMEN, SEVERE PAIN

- **SHE XIANG** 756

CHEST/FLANK PAIN

- **CHAI HU:** Liver Qi Stagnation 457

CHEST/RIB DISTENSTION, FULLNESS

- **CHANG SHAN** 518

CONGESTION/FULLNESS IN CHEST AND ABDOMEN

- **ZI SU YE/SHA REN**

COSTAL

See: Chest Ribs 80
See: Chest Intercostal 80

COSTAL REGION, CHONDRITIS

- **GUA LOU (c):** Tricosanthes-Allium Decoction 718

COSTAL REGION, DISTENTION

- **BAN XIA** 710
- **CHANG SHAN** 518
- **HU LU BA** 781
- **XUAN FU HUA** 713

COSTAL REGION, PAIN

See: Abdomen/Gastrointestinal Topics
Hypochondriac Region, Pain 32
- **BAI JIANG CAO/JIN YIN HUA/PU GONG YING**
- **CHAI HU/BAI SHAO:** Liver Qi Stagnation
- **FO SHOU/XIANG FU/(XIANG YUAN-CITRON)/YU JIN:** Liver Qi Stanation
- **LONG DAN CAO/HUANG QIN/SHAN ZHI ZI/CHAI HU/MU TONG:** Liver Fire Rising
- **MEI GUI HUA/FO SHOU/XIANG FU/YU JIN:** Liver, Stomach Qi Stagnation
- **XIANG FU/CHAI HU/YU JIN/BAI SHAO:** Liver Qi Stagnation
- **SAN LENG** 686
- **YU JIN** 695

COSTAL REGION, PAIN, DISTENTION

- **SU GENG** 451

EDEMA

See: Fluid Disorders Edema 133

FLANK

See: Chest Ribs 80
See: Chest Intercostal 80

FOCAL DISTENTION

See: Pain/Numbness/General Discomfort Focal
Distention 301

FOCAL DISTENTION, CHEST, ABDOMEN

• CAO GUO/CANG ZHU/HOU PO/BAN XIA

HYDROTHORAX

• GAN SUI 551

INTERCOSTAL

See: Chest Costal 79
See: Chest Flank 80
See: Chest Costal 79

INTERCOSTAL CHEST PAIN

• JIANG XIANG/YU JIN/TAO REN: Stasis Qi/Blood

INTERCOSTAL DISTENTION

• MAI YA: Liver Qi Stagnation 640

INTERCOSTAL NEURALGIA

• CHAI HU (c) 457
• GUA LOU (c): Tricosanthes-Allium Decoction 718

INTERCOSTAL PAIN

See: Chest Rib Pain 80
See: Abdomen/Gastrointestinal Topics
Hypochondriac Region, Pain 32
• BAI SHAO/CHAI HU: Liver Qi Stagnation
• CHAI HU/QING PI: Liver Qi Stagnation
• BAI SHAO: Liver Qi Stagnation/Liver Spleen
Disharmony 794
• TAO REN 689
• XIANG FU: Liver Qi Stagnation 633

INTERCOSTAL SPRAIN, PAIN

• RU XIANG/NIU XI

INTERCOSTAL/CHEST PAIN

• XIANG FU/CHAI HU

MASS SENSATION IN MEDIASTINUM W/VOMITING

• QIAN HU 725

PAIN, FLANK/INTERCOSTAL

• BAI SHAO/CHAI HU: Liver Qi Stagnation

PAIN, INTERCOSTAL

• CHAI HU/QING PI: Liver Qi Stagnation
• BAI SHAO: Liver Qi Stagnation/Liver Spleen
Disharmony 794

PHLEGM, CHEST OBSTRUCTION

• REN SHEN LU 835

RIB CAGE SPRAIN, PAIN OF

• RU XIANG/NIU XI

RIB DISTENTION

• CHANG SHAN 518

RIB PAIN

See: Chest Intercostal Pain 80
• FO SHOU: Liver Qi Stagnation 624
• YU JIN 695

RIB PAIN, SWELLING

• BAI JIE ZI 708

RIB SORENESS

• DAN SHEN: Liver Qi Stagnation With Blood Stasis ... 672

RIBS

See: Chest Costal 79
See: Chest Flank 80

THORACIC RELATED TOPICS

See: Chest Costal 79

End of Topic:
CHEST

CHEST BI

See: Chest Chest Bi 75

CHEST RELATED TOPICS

See: Chest Chest Related Topics 75

CHICKEN POX

See: Infectious Diseases Chicken Pox 182

CHILBLAIN

See: Trauma, Bites, Poisonings Chilblain 408

CHILDBIRTH RELATED TOPICS

See: Sexuality, Female: Gynecological
Childbirth Related Topics 324

End of Topic:
CHILDBIRTH RELATED TOPICS

CHILDHOOD DISORDERS :

ABDOMEN, DISTENTION OF, CHILDHOOD

• ROU DOU KOU/BAN XIA/GAN JIANG/SHEN QU/SHA
REN: Spleen Stomach Cold Deficient

ABDOMEN, PAIN OF IN CHILDHOOD NUTRITIONAL IMPAIRMENT

• YE MING SHA/BAI ZHU/HU HUANG LIAN/CHEN PI

ANOREXIA, CHILDHOOD

• ROU DOU KOU/BAN XIA/GAN JIANG/SHEN QU/SHA
REN: Spleen Stomach Cold Deficient

ASCARIASIS, CHILDHOOD

• BIAN XU 588

BALANITIS, CHILDHOOD, YOUNG
- WEI LING XIAN (c) 572

BED WETTING
- JI NEI JIN 638

BLOATING, CHILD MALNUTRITION
- WU LING ZHI 691

BOILS, PIMPLE INFECTIONS/SUSCEPTIBILITY OF W/WEAK CONSTITUTIONS, IN CHILDREN
- HAI MA/(lean pork)

CHILDREN
- SHI GAO/DAN ZHU YE: Cough And Fevers In
- GUI BAN: Late Fontanel Closure 806
- TAI ZI SHEN: Summer Heat 770

CONVULSIONS, CHILDHOOD
See: Mental State/Neurological Disorders Convulsions, Childhood 244
- BIE JIA 805
- DAI MAO 743
- HOU ZAO: Heat 722
- HU PO 737
- JIANG CAN 746
- QING DAI 531
- QUAN XIE: Liver Wind Phlegm 749
- SHE TUI 571
- TIAN MA: Liver Wind 750
- TIAN ZHU HUANG 726
- WU GONG 751
- YE MING SHA 480
- ZHEN ZHU 740
- ZHU RU 729
- ZHU SHA: From High Fever 741
- ZHU YE 482

CONVULSIONS, MUSCLE SPASMS, CHILDHOOD
- NIU HUANG 755

CONVULSIONS, SPASMS FROM FEVERS, CHILDHOOD
- ZAO XIU 540

COUGH, CHILDHOOD
See: Lungs Cough In Children 221

CRYING, MORBID, CHILDHOOD
- DENG XIN CAO 592

DEVELOPMENT, MUSCLES, RETARDED, CHILDHOOD
- WU JIA PI/SANG JI SHENG/NIU XI/XU DUAN

DEVELOPMENT, POOR MENTAL/PHYSICAL, CHILDHOOD
- LU RONG 784

DEVELOPMENT, RETARDED SKELETAL, CHILDHOOD
- GUI BAN 806

DEVELOPMENT, RETARDED, CHILDHOOD
- GUI BAN/NIU XI/SUO YANG/HU GU: Liver Kidney Deficient

DIAPER RASH
- QIAN LI GUANG (c) 474

DIARRHEA, INFANTILE/CHILDHOOD
See: Bowel Related Disorders Diarrhea, Childhood 57
See: Bowel Related Disorders Diarrhea, Infantile 58

ENURESIS, CHILDHOOD
See: Urinary Bladder Enuresis, Childhood 421
- FU XIAO MAI 820
- SANG PIAO XIAO 827

EPILEPSY, CHILDHOOD
See: Mental State/Neurological Disorders Epilepsy, Childhood 247
See: Childhood Disorders Epileptic Convulsions, Childhood 81
- HU HUANG LIAN 484

EPILEPTIC CONVULSIONS, CHILDHOOD
- LU HUI 544

FEAR SPASMS, CHILDHOOD
- CHAN TUI 458

FEAR, CHILDHOOD
- DAN NAN XING 718

FEVER OF MALNUTRITION, CHILDHOOD
- YIN CHAI HU 504

FEVER, CONVULSIONS, CHILDHOOD
- GOU TENG 745
- LING YANG JIAO 747

FEVERS, HIGH, CHILDHOOD
- QING DAI 531

FONTANEL, LATE CLOSURE
- GUI BAN 806

FRIGHT CONVULSIONS, CHILDHOOD
- BAI HUA SHE 558
- CI SHI: Best Liver Yin With Yang Rising 735
- DI LONG 744

GROWTH, INSUFFICIENT, CHILDHOOD
- LU RONG: Essence/Blood Deficiency 784

INDIGESTION IMPROPER FEEDING, CHILDHOOD

INDIGESTION IN INFANTS FROM IMPROPER NURSING

INDIGESTION, CHILDHOOD

INDIGESTION, CHILDHOOD MILK STAGNATION

INDIGESTION, DIARRHEA, CHILDHOOD

INDIGESTION, MILK, INFANTILE

INFANTILE CONVULSIONS

INFANTILE DERMATITIS

INFANTILE DIARRHEA

INFANTILE DYSPEPSIA

INFANTILE MALDEVELOPMENT

INFANTILE MALNUTRITION

INFANTILE PARALYSIS

INFANTILE SPASMS/CONVULSIONS

INFANTS, INDIGESTED MILK IN

INFANTS, INDIGESTION IN FROM IMPROPER NURSING

INFANTS, PROFUSE SPUTUM

INFANTS, REGURGITATION OF MILK

INFANTS, RETENTION OF MILK

INFANTS, VOMITING

INSOMNIA, CHILDHOOD

LEARNING DISABILITIES, CHILDHOOD

MALNUTRITION BLOATING, CHILDHOOD

MALNUTRITION FEVER, CHILDHOOD

MALNUTRITION SYNDROME, CHRONIC, CHILDHOOD

MALNUTRITION W/SWOLLEN ABDOMEN AND EMACIATION, CHILDHOOD

MALNUTRITION, CHILDHOOD

MALNUTRITION-ACCUMULATION, CHILDHOOD

MYCOTIC STOMATIS

- SHU FU: (Thrush) 687

NUTRITIONAL IMPAIRMENT W/ABDOMINAL DISTENTION, ANOREXIA, CHILDHOOD

- SHI JUN ZI/HU HUANG LIAN

NUTRITIONAL IMPAIRMENT W/ABDOMINAL PAIN, CHILDHOOD

- WU YI/BING LANG/SHI JUN ZI
- YE MING SHA/BAI ZHU/HU HUANG LIAN/CHEN PI

NUTRITIONAL IMPAIRMENT, CHILDHOOD

- JI NEI JIN/MAI YA/SHAN ZHA
- JI NEI JIN/BIE JIA
- JI NEI JIN/BAI ZHU/SHAN YAO/FU LING : Spleen Weakness
- SHAN ZHA/MAI YA/SHEN QU: From Poor Breast Feeding
- SHEN QU/BING LANG
- WU LING ZHI/SHI JUN ZI/HU HUANG LIAN: Chronic
- WU YI/HE ZI/ROU DOU KOU: Chronic Diarrhea
- E ZHU 673
- JI NEI JIN 638
- LU HUI 544
- SHI JUN ZI 648
- YE MING SHA 480

NUTRITIONAL IMPAIRMENT, CHRONIC W/FEVER, CHILDHOOD

- YIN CHAI HU/SHAN ZHI ZI

NUTRITIONAL IMPAIRMENT, SEVERE W/EMACIATION, JAUNDICE, CHILDHOOD

- SHI JUN ZI/HU HUANG LIAN/DANG SHEN/BAI ZHU

PARALYSIS, INFANTILE

- SANG JI SHENG/YIN YANG HUO

PEDIATRIC MEDICINE

- HU HUANG LIAN 484

PEDIATRICS, FOR FEAR

- DAN NAN XING 718

PNEUMONIAS, VARIOUS, CHILDHOOD

- TU NIU XI (c) 537

PURPURA, CHILDHOOD

- DI YU (c) 656

RETARDED AMBULATION DEVELOPMENT, CHILDHOOD

- WU JIA PI 574

RETARDED PHYSICAL DEVELOPMENT, CHILDHOOD

- LU RONG/SHU DI HUANG

SKELETAL DEFORMITIES, CHILDHOOD

- LU RONG: Essence/Blood Deficiency 784

SLEEP DISORDERS WITH SCANTY URINE, IRRITABILITY, CHILDHOOD

- DENG XIN CAO 592

SUMMER FEVERS, CHILDHOOD

- BAI WEI 495

TOXICOSIS, CHILDHOOD

- GAN CAO 763

TYPHOID FEVER, CHILDHOOD

- BAI HUA SHE SHE CAO (c): With Di Yu 511

URINARY INCONTINENCE, CHILDHOOD

- FU XIAO MAI/SANG PIAO XIAO/YI ZHI REN
- JI NEI JIN/SANG PIAO XIAO/LONG GU/MU LI
- YI ZHI REN/WU YAO/SHAN YAO/(SUO QUAN WAN): Spleen Kidney Cold, Deficient
- SANG PIAO XIAO 827

URINATION, PAINFUL, CHILDHOOD

- DONG KUI ZI/MU TONG

VOMITING, CHILDHOOD

- ROU DOU KOU/BAN XIA/GAN JIANG/SHEN QU/SHA REN: Spleen Stomach Cold Deficient

VOMITING, CHILDHOOD, YOUNG

- BAI DOU KOU/SHA REN/GAN CAO: Cold Stomach

End of Topic:
CHILDHOOD DISORDERS

CHILDREN RELATED TOPICS

See: Childhood Disorders Children Related
Topics 81

CHILLS

See: Cold Chills 90

CHILLS, FEVER

See: Fevers Chills, Fever 126

CHLOROSIS

See: Blood Related Disorders/Topics Chlorosis
.... 49

CHOKING

See: Trauma, Bites, Poisonings Choking 408

CHOLAGOGUE

See: Gall Bladder Cholagogue 140

CHOLANGITIS

See: Gall Bladder Cholangitis 141

CHOLECYSTALGIA

See: Gall Bladder Cholecystalgia 141

CHOLECYSTITIS RELATED TOPICS

See: Gall Bladder Cholecystitis Related Topics ... 141

CHOLELITHIASIS

See: Gall Bladder Cholelithiasis 141

CHOLERA

See: Infectious Diseases Cholera 182

CHOLERETIC

See: Liver Choleretic 203

CHOLESTEROL RELATED TOPICS

See: Blood Related Disorders/Topics Cholesterol
Related Topics 49

CHOLESTEROLEMIA

See: Blood Related Disorders/Topics
Cholesterolemia 49

CHOLINERGIC, CNS

See: Mental State/Neurological Disorders
Cholinergic, CNS 241

CHORIOADENOMA

See: Cancer/Tumors/Swellings/Lumps
Chorioadenoma 68

CHORIOCARCINOMA

See: Cancer/Tumors/Swellings/Lumps
Choriocarcinoma 68

CHORIONEPITHELIOMA

See: Sexuality, Female: Gynecological
Chorionepithelioma 324
See: Cancer/Tumors/Swellings/Lumps
Chorionepithelioma 68

CHRONIC DISEASES, NOURISHMENT

See: Energetic State Chronic Diseases,
Nourishment 104

CHYLURIA

See: Urinary Bladder Chyluria 419

CIRCULATION DISEASES, PERIPHERAL

See: Circulation Disorders Circulation Diseases,
Peripheral 85

End of Topic:
CIRCULATION DISEASES,PERIPHERAL

CIRCULATION DISORDERS :

See: Heart 151

APOPLEXY

See: Circulation Disorders Stroke 87
• QUAN XIE/WU GONG/(ZI JING SAN)

• AN XI XIANG 753
• BAN XIA 710
• BING PIAN 753
• GUA DI 834
• JIANG CAN 746
• LI LU 834
• SHE XIANG 756
• TIAN MA 750
• TIAN NAN XING: Phlegm 712
• WU YAO 632

APOPLEXY W/LOSS OF CONSCIOUSNESS

• ZAO JIAO 715

ARTERIOSCLEROSIS

• DA SUAN 644
• HE SHOU WU (c): Reduces Lipid Deposition 799
• JIANG CAN (c): Heart Disease 746
• JIN YIN HUA (c): w/Ju Hua 524
• YU JIN (c): Decreased Plaque Formation In Arteries ... 695

ARTERITIS, CONSTRICTIVE

• DANG GUI (c) 795

ATHEROSCLEROSIS

• BAI GUO YE (c): "Shu Xue Ning Tablet", 2 Tabs, 3x/Day,
  3 Months 817
• CHUAN SHAN LONG (c) 442
• DA SUAN (c): Oil Of, Not Decoction 644
• DANG GUI (c): Reduces Plaque Formation 795
• DU ZHONG (c): Lowers Blood Pressure Long Term By
  Tincture 775
• GAN CAO (c): Stopped Progression Of Lesions, Reduced
  Cholesterol 763
• GOU QI ZI (c): Slightly Inhibits 798
• HAI ZAO (c) 721
• HUANG JING (c): Helps To Prevent, Mild 764
• JIANG HUANG (c): Curcumin Inhibits Platelet
  Aggregation 678
• JIN YING ZI (c): 2-3 Weeks, Reduces Cholesterol,
  Lesions 823
• KUN BU (c): Can Reduce Lipids In Blood 724
• MAO DONG QING (c) 682
• MO YAO (c): Prevent Plaque Formation 683
• SHAN ZHA (c) 641
• YIN CHAI HU (c) 504
• YIN CHEN (c): Helps Prevent Fatty Accumulation 603
• YU ZHU (c): 100% Decoction, 3x/Day For 1 Month 815

ATHEROSCLEROSIS, INCREASES BLOOD FLOW TO BRAIN

• GE GEN (c) 460

ATHEROSCLEROSIS, LOWERS BLOOD PRESSURE

• JU HUA (c): With Jin Yin Hua, Huai Hua, Shan Zha, With
  Shan Zha For Best Effect 463

ATHEROSCLEROSIS, PREVENTS

• HUANG LIAN (c) 486

CNS, INCREASES ABILITY OF ANALYSIS

CNS, INHIBITOR

CNS, POSSIBLE HALLUCINATIONS

CNS, PROLONGS SLEEPING

CNS, RELAXANT

CNS, SEDATIVE

CNS, STIMULANT

CNS, TRANQUILIZER

End of Topic:
CNS, TRANQUILIZER

COLD :

CHILLS

- FANG FENG: Wind Cold 444
- FU ZI: Devastated Yang, From Severe Vomit 613
- MA HUANG: Wind Cold Exterior Excess Patterns 448
- ZI SU YE: Wind Cold 454

COLD

- FU ZI: Chronic Diseases With 613

COLD ACCUMULATION, PURGES

- BA DOU 550

COLD CONGESTED FLUIDS

- GAN JIANG/BAN XIA: Vomiting

COLD DAMP

- BAI DOU KOU/HUO XIANG: Anorexia
- GAO BEN/WU ZHU YU: Abdominal Pain
- GAO BEN/WU ZHU YU/XIAO HUI XIANG: Abdominal Pain

COLD DAMP ABDOMINAL PAIN, DIARRHEA

- MU GUA/WU ZHU YU/XIAO HUI XIANG/SHENG JIANG

COLD DAMP BI

- HAN FANG JI/GUI ZHI/FU ZI

COLD DAMP LEG QI

- HU LU BA/MU GUA/JI XUE TENG/BU GU ZHI

COLD DAMP PAIN

- XIAN MAO/XI XIN: Legs, Back

COLD DEFICIENCY

- CAO DOU KOU/MU XIANG/HE ZI/(both toasted): Diarrhea
- GAN JIANG/BAN XIA/REN SHEN: Vomiting

COLD DEFICIENCY IN CHONG AND REN CHANNELS

- GUI ZHI/WU ZHU YU: Dysmenorrhea, Menstrual Irregularity

COLD ESSENCE

- XIAN MAO 788

COLD PHLEGM

- XI XIN/WU WEI ZI: Cough, Wheezing

COLD STAGNANT QI

- XI XIN/GUI ZHI/DAN SHEN: Chest Pain

COLD STAGNATION

- SHEN QU/ZHI KE: Stomach/Abdomen Fullness, No Appetite

COLD WIND W/QI EXERTION

- YIN YANG HUO 791

COLD, AVERSION TO

- LU RONG/REN SHEN/SHU DI HUANG/TU SI ZI: Kidney Yang Deficiency
- QIANG HUO 449
- XIANG RU 453

COLD, EXTERNAL

- SHENG JIANG 450

COLD, EXTERNAL W/INTERIOR DAMP

- XIANG RU/BAI BIAN DOU/HOU PO: Fever, No Sweat, Headache, Thirst, Vomiting, Diarrhea

COLD, EXTERNAL W/YANG DEFICIENCY

- XI XIN 452

COLD, INTOLERANCE TO

- LU JIAO 783
- LU RONG 784

EXTERNAL COLD W/YANG DEFICIENCY

- XI XIN 452

EXTERNAL HOT/COLD

- DAN DOU CHI 459

End of Topic:
EARS AND RELATED TOPICS

EARS/ HEARING DISORDERS :

CERUMEN

• KU DING CHA: Ear Wax 809

DEAFNESS

See: Ears/Hearing Disorders Hearing Loss 97
• CHUAN SHAN JIA/SUAN ZAO REN/SHENG DI HUANG
• GU SUI BU/SHU DI HUANG/SHAN ZHU YU: Kidney
  Deficiency
• LONG DAN CAO/CHAI HU: Liver Fire/Damp Heat
• LONG DAN CAO/HUANG QIN/SHAN ZHI ZI/CHAI HU/MU
  TONG: Liver Fire Rising
• MAN JING ZI/REN SHEN/HUANG QI: Deficient
  Conditions
• SANG SHEN ZI/HE SHOU WU/NU ZHEN ZI/HAN LIAN
  CAO/(SHOU WU YAN SHOU DAN): Yin And Blood
  Deficiency
• SHI CHANG PU/YUAN ZHI/FU LING /(AN SHEN DING ZHI
  WAN)
• CHAI HU 457
• CI SHI 735
• JU HUA: Liver Yang Rising 463
• NU ZHEN ZI 812
• SHAN ZHU YU 827
• SHI CHANG PU: Phlegm Blocking Rising Of Clear Yang
  757
• TIAN MA (c): Ear/Neurological Diseases 750

DEAFNESS, COCHLEAR

• BAI GUO YE (c): From Lowered Blood Circulation 817

DEAFNESS, SUDDEN

• GE GEN (c): w/Vit B's 460
• LONG DAN CAO: Damp Heat In Gall Bladder 492

DIZZINESS

See Also: Dizziness (Topics: Gynecology, Phlegm, Blood, Eyes, Mental State, Liver)

- **BAI JI LI/GOU TENG/NIU XI:** Liver Yang Rising
- **BAI JI LI/GOU TENG/JU HUA/BAI SHAO:** Liver Yang Rising
- **BAI SHAO/DANG GUI/SHU DI HUANG:** Deficient/Stagnant Blood
- **BAI SHAO/DANG GUI/SHU DI HUANG/MAI MEN DONG:** Liver Yin Deficient
- **BAI SHAO/GOU TENG/JU HUA:** Liver Yang Rising
- **BAI SHAO/NIU XI/GOU TENG/JU HUA:** Liver Yang Rising
- **CHAI HU/BAI SHAO:** Liver Qi Stagnation
- **CI SHI/NIU XI/DU ZHONG/SHI JUE MING:** Yin Deficient w/Yang Rising
- **CI SHI/LONG GU/MU LI:** Yin Deficient w/Yang Rising
- **CI SHI/SHU DI HUANG/SHAN ZHU YU**
- **DAI ZHE SHI/LONG GU/MU LI/NIU XI:** Liver Yang Rising
- **DAI ZHE SHI/LONG GU/MU LI/BAI SHAO/GUI BAN/NIU XI/(ZHEN GAN XI FENG TANG):** Liver Kidney Yin Deficient w/Yang Rising
- **DANG SHEN/DANG GUI:** Qi And Blood Deficient
- **DI LONG/DAN SHEN/CI SHI:** Liver Yang Rising
- **DONG CHONG XIA CAO/(with meat):** Wei Qi Weakened
- **E JIAO/REN SHEN/DANG GUI/SHU DI HUANG:** Blood Deficiency
- **FU LING /BAI ZHU/GUI ZHI/(LING GUI ZHU GAN TANG):** Phlegm-Fluid Retention
- **GOU QI ZI/SHU DI HUANG/TU SI ZI/DU ZHONG:** Liver Kidney Deficient (Yin/Blood Deficiency)
- **GOU QI ZI/JU HUA/SHU DI HUANG/(QI JU DI HUANG WAN):** Liver Kidney Yin Deficiency
- **GOU TENG/JU HUA/SHI JUE MING/SANG YE:** Liver Wind
- **GOU TENG/JU HUA/SHI JUE MING/SANG YE/SHI GAO/FU SHEN:** Liver Wind, Yang Rising
- **GOU TENG/XIA KU CAO/HUANG QIN/SHI JUE MING/JU HUA:** Liver Yang Rising
- **GUI BAN/BAI SHAO/NIU XI/SHI JUE MING/GOU TENG:** Liver Yang Rising From Liver Kidney Yin Deficiency
- **HAN LIAN CAO/NU ZHEN ZI/(ER ZHI WAN):** Liver Kidney Yin Deficient, Severe, w/Yang Rising
- **HE SHOU WU/GOU QI ZI/BU GU ZHI/TU SI ZI:** Liver Kidney Deficiency
- **HE SHOU WU/SANG JI SHENG/NU ZHEN ZI/NIU XI:** Liver Blood Deficient
- **HE SHOU WU/SHU DI HUANG/NU ZHEN ZI/GOU QI ZI/TU SI ZI/SANG JI SHENG:** Blood Deficiency
- **HEI ZHI MA/SANG YE/(SANG MA WAN):** Liver Kidney Yin Deficient w/Yang Rising
- **HUAI HUA MI/XI XIAN CAO:** Liver Fire Rising
- **HUANG JING/GOU QI ZI/NU ZHEN ZI:** Kidney Essence Deficiency
- **HUANG QIN/XIA KU CAO:** Liver Fire Rising
- **JU HUA/TIAN MA:** Liver Yang Rising
- **JU HUA/JUE MING ZI/GOU TENG/BAI SHAO:** Liver Yang Rising
- **JUE MING ZI/XIA KU CAO:** Liver Kidney Deficient
- **JUE MING ZI/GOU TENG/MU LI:** Liver Yang Rising
- **LING YANG JIAO/SHI JUE MING/XIA KU CAO/JU HUA:** Liver Yang Rising
- **LONG GU/MU LI/NIU XI/DAI ZHE SHI:** Yin Deficiency w/Yang Rising
- **LONG GU/MU LI/DAI ZHE SHI/BAI SHAO/(ZHEN GAN XI FENG TANG):** Liver Kidney Deficiency w/Liver Yang Rising
- **LONG YAN ROU/SHI CHANG PU:** Heart Qi, Blood Deficient
- **LU HUI/LONG DAN CAO/HUANG QIN:** Liver Channel Excess Heat
- **LU RONG/REN SHEN/SHU DI HUANG/TU SI ZI:** Kidney Yang Deficiency
- **LUO BU MA/XIA KU CAO/GOU TENG/JU HUA:** Liver Yang Rising
- **MAN JING ZI/JU HUA:** Wind Heat
- **MAN JING ZI/REN SHEN/HUANG QI:** Deficient Conditions
- **MAN JING ZI/JU HUA/CHAN TUI/BAI JI LI:** Liver Yang Rising
- **MU DAN PI/JU HUA:** Liver Fire Rising
- **MU LI/LONG GU:** Yin Deficient w/Yang Rising
- **MU LI/LONG GU/GUI BAN/BAI SHAO:** Liver Kidney Yin Deficient w/Yang Rising
- **NIU XI/GOU TENG/SANG JI SHENG:** Liver Yang Rising
- **NIU XI/DAI ZHE SHI/MU LI/LONG GU/(ZHEN GAN XI FENG TANG):** Liver Wind Rising
- **NU ZHEN ZI/SHA YUAN ZI:** Liver Kidney Yin Deficient
- **NU ZHEN ZI/BU GU ZHI/TU SI ZI:** Kidney Yin Deficiency
- **QING HAO/BAI BIAN DOU/HUA SHI:** Summer Heat
- **SANG JI SHENG/SHENG DI HUANG/CHI SHAO YAO/JI XUE TENG:** Liver Kidney Yin Deficient w/Yang Rising
- **SANG SHEN ZI/JI XUE TENG:** Yin Deficient
- **SANG SHEN ZI/SHENG DI HUANG/SHU DI HUANG:** Yin And Blood Deficient
- **SANG SHEN ZI/HE SHOU WU/NU ZHEN ZI/HAN LIAN CAO/(SHOU WU YAN SHOU DAN):** Yin And Blood Deficiency
- **SANG YE/JU HUA/SHI JUE MING/MU LI:** Liver Yang Rising
- **SANG YE/NU ZHEN ZI/GOU QI ZI/HEI ZHI MA:** Liver Yin Deficient
- **SHAN ZHU YU/SHU DI HUANG/SHAN YAO:** Kidney Deficient
- **SHAN ZHU YU/SHU DI HUANG/TU SI ZI/GOU QI ZI/DU ZHONG:** Liver Kidney Deficiency
- **SHI CHANG PU/YU JIN:** Damp Heat w/Turbidity Blocks The Orifices
- **SHI JUE MING/MU LI:** Yin Deficient w/Yang Rising
- **SHI JUE MING/XIA KU CAO:** Liver Yang Excess
- **SHI JUE MING/MU LI/BAI SHAO/GUI BAN:** Liver Kidney Yin Deficient w/Liver Yang Rising
- **SHU DI HUANG/SHAN ZHU YU/SHAN YAO/(LIU WEI DIHUNG WAN):** Kidney Deficiency Syndrome
- **SHU DI HUANG/GUI BAN:** Yin Deficient w/Yang Rising
- **SHU DI HUANG/DANG GUI/BAI SHAO/(SI WU TANG):** Blood Deficiency
- **SHU DI HUANG/DANG GUI/BAI SHAO/CHUAN XIONG/(SI WU TANG):** Blood And Yin Deficiency
- **TIAN MA/CHUAN XIONG/(TIAN MA WAN):** Liver Wind From Liver Deficiency
- **TIAN MA/BAN XIA/BAI ZHU:** Phlegm Dampness
- **TIAN MA/GOU TENG:** Liver Yang Rising
- **TIAN MA/GOU TENG/HUANG QIN/NIU XI/(TIAN MA GOU TENG YIN):** Liver Yang Rising
- **TIAN MA/BAN XIA/BAI ZHU/FU LING /(BAN XIA BAI ZHU TIAN MA TANG):** Wind Phlegm Attacking Upper In Spleen Deficient w/Liver Qi Stagnation

- TIAN NAN XING/TIAN MA: Wind Phlegm
- TIAN NAN XING/BAN XIA/TIAN MA/BAI FU ZI: Wind Phlegm
- XI XIAN CAO/XIA KU CAO: Liver Fire Rising
- XIA KU CAO/JU HUA: Liver Fire Rising
- XIA KU CAO/SHI JUE MING/JU HUA: Liver Fire Flaring
- ZE XIE/MU DAN PI
- ZHEN ZHU MU/BAI SHAO/SHENG DI HUANG/SHI JUE MING/LONG GU: Liver Kidney Yin Deficiency w/Liver Yang Rising
- ZHI MU/HUANG BAI: Yin Deficiency Steaming Bone Syndrome
- ZHU SHA/HAI GE KE: Wind Phlegm
- ZI HE CHE/GUI BAN: Liver Kidney Deficient

DIZZINESS, BLURRED VISION

- JU HUA/GOU QI ZI: Liver Kidney Deficiency

DIZZINESS, VERTIGO

- SANG YE/HEI ZHI MA: Liver Kidney Yin Deficient, Fire Rising
- TU SI ZI/SHA YUAN ZI/(tonify yin-blood herbs): Yin And Blood Weak

EAR INFECTION, PURULENT OTITIS MEDIA

EARACHES

EARACHES, CHRONIC

EARS, BLEEDING

EARS, CHRONIC SUPPURATIVE OTITIS MEDIA

EARS, DEAFNESS, SUDDEN, EARLY STAGE

EARS, ECZEMA, VERY EFFECTIVE

EARS, HEARING LOSS FROM STREPTOMYCIN

• GU SUI BU (c): Helped Control With Regular Doses ... 778

EARS, HEARING, POOR

• CHAI HU 457

EARS, HEAT, PAIN, SWELLING, SUPPURATION

• BING PIAN/ZHU SHA/PENG SHA

EARS, INFLAMMATORY DISEASES

• QING MU XIANG (c): Acute Otitis Media, 5% Ear Drops From Equal Amounts Herb, Cheng Xing Shu Powder With Small Amount Borneol, Extracted With Alcohol
.... 628

EARS, MIDDLE, OUTER

• BAI FAN/BING PIAN: Pain, Swelling, Red

EARS, OTITIS EXTERNA

• DAN SHEN (c) 672

EARS, OTITIS EXTERNA, DIFFUSE

• HUANG LIAN (c): 10% Extract Plus 3% Boric Acid 486

EARS, OTITIS MEDIA

• HUANG LIAN 486
• LONG DAN CAO (c): Liver Gall Bladder Damp Heat, Use Modified Long Dan Xie Gan Tang 492
• MU DAN PI (c): 10% Decoction, 50 ml Before Bed For 10 Days 499
• PU GONG YING (c): Milky Juice Of Fresh Plant Into Ear
.... 529
• PU HUANG: Topical 660

EARS, OTITIS MEDIA, CHRONIC/SUPPURATIVE

• HUANG LIAN (c): 10% Extract Plus 3% Boric Acid As Ear Drops 486

EARS, OTITIS MEDIA, SUPPURATIVE

• CHUAN XIN LIAN (c) 518

EARS, OTITIS MEDIA/EXTERNA, ECZEMA W/PUS DISCHARGE

• BING PIAN (c): w/Alum & Boric Acid 753

EARS, PAINFUL, SWOLLEN

• LONG DAN CAO: Damp Heat In Gall Bladder 492

EARS, PROTECTS AGAINST STREPTOMYCIN TOXICITY

• GAN CAO (c) 763

EARS, SUPPURATIVE OTITIS MEDIA

• DA HUANG (c) 542

EARS, SWOLLEN, PAINFUL

• ZI HUA DI DING: Toxic Heat 541

EARS, WAX IN

• KU DING CHA 809

HEARING DIFFICULTY

• SHI CHANG PU/YU JIN: Damp Heat w/Turbidity Blocks The Orifices

HEARING DYSFUNCTION

• SHI CHANG PU/YU JIN: Damp Heat w/Turbidity Blocks The Orifices

HEARING LOSS

See: Ears/Hearing Disorders Deafness 94
• CI SHI/SHU DI HUANG/SHAN ZHU YU
• TU SI ZI 787

HEARING LOSS, GRADUAL

• LU RONG/REN SHEN/SHU DI HUANG/TU SI ZI: Kidney Yang Deficiency

HEARING LOSS, SUDDEN AT EARLY STAGE

• GE GEN (c): ETOH Extract Tablet, Each = 1.5 g Of Herb, 1-2 Tabs, 3x/Day, Some Injected, Too, With Vit B Complex, 1-2 Months, Hearing Improved In 80% Cases
.... 460

HEARING, IMPAIRED/REDUCED ACUITY

• SHAN ZHU YU: Liver Kidney Deficient 827

HEARING, POOR

• CI SHI 735
• LU RONG 784

HEARING, POWER

• WU JIA SHEN (c): Improves In Stressful Conditions ... 771

MENIERES SYNDROME

• WU WEI ZI (c): 4-5 Doses With Da Zao, Dang Gui, Long Yan Rou 831

OTITIS MEDIA

• BAN XIA (c): Tincture 710

OTITIS MEDIA W/PUS

• HAI PIAO XIAO: Topical 821

OTITIS MEDIA, CHRONIC

• BAI FAN (c): 10% Solution, Topical As Drops 836

OTITIS MEDIA, PURULENT

• CHUAN XIN LIAN 518
• JIN DI LUO 523

OTITIS, MEDIA SUPPURATIVE

• HUANG LIAN (c): External Application 486

TINNITUS

• BAI SHAO/DANG GUI/SHU DI HUANG/MAI MEN DONG: Liver Yin Deficient
• CI SHI/SHU DI HUANG/SHAN ZHU YU

- DAI ZHE SHI/LONG GU/MU LI/NIU XI: Liver Yang Rising
- GOU QI ZI/SHU DI HUANG/TU SI ZI/DU ZHONG: Liver Kidney Deficient (Yin/Blood Deficiency)
- GOU QI ZI/JU HUA: Liver Kidney Deficiency
- GU SUI BU/SHAN YAO
- GU SUI BU/SHU DI HUANG/SHAN ZHU YU: Kidney Deficiency
- HEI ZHI MA/SANG YE/(SANG MA WAN): Liver Kidney Yin Deficient w/Yang Rising
- LU RONG/REN SHEN/SHU DI HUANG/TU SI ZI: Kidney Yang Deficiency
- MAN JING ZI/REN SHEN/HUANG QI: Deficient Conditions
- MU LI/LONG GU: Yin Deficient w/Yang Rising
- MU LI/LONG GU/GUI BAN/BAI SHAO: Liver Kidney Yin Deficient w/Yang Rising
- NU ZHEN ZI/SHA YUAN ZI: Liver Kidney Yin Deficient
- NU ZHEN ZI/SANG SHEN ZI/HAN LIAN CAO/GOU QI ZI: Yin Deficiency And Blood Heat
- SANG JI SHENG/SHENG DI HUANG/CHI SHAO YAO/JI XUE TENG: Liver Kidney Yin Deficient w/Yang Rising
- SANG SHEN ZI/JI XUE TENG: Yin Deficient
- SANG SHEN ZI/HE SHOU WU/NU ZHEN ZI/HAN LIAN CAO/(SHOU WU YAN SHOU DAN): Yin And Blood Deficiency
- SHAN ZHU YU/SHU DI HUANG/SHAN YAO: Kidney Deficient
- SHI CHANG PU/YUAN ZHI/FU LING /(AN SHEN DING ZHI WAN)
- SHU DI HUANG/SHAN ZHU YU/SHAN YAO/(LIU WEI DIHUNG WAN): Liver Kidney Deficiency
- SHU DI HUANG/GUI BAN: Yin Deficient w/Yang Rising
- TU SI ZI/SHA YUAN ZI/(tonify yin-blood herbs): Yin And Blood Weak
- ZHEN ZHU MU/BAI SHAO/SHENG DI HUANG/SHI JUE MING/LONG GU: Liver Kidney Yin Deficiency w/Liver Yang Rising
- ZI HE CHE/GUI BAN: Liver Kidney Deficient

TINNITUS, FROM STREPTOMYCIN

VERTIGO

- BAI JI LI/GOU TENG/NIU XI: Liver Yang Rising
- BAI JI LI/GOU TENG/JU HUA/BAI SHAO: Liver Yang Rising
- CHAI HU/BAI SHAO: Liver Qi Stagnation
- CI SHI/LONG GU/MU LI: Yin Deficient w/Yang Rising
- CI SHI/SHU DI HUANG/SHAN ZHU YU
- DAI ZHE SHI/LONG GU/MU LI/NIU XI: Liver Yang Rising
- DAI ZHE SHI/LONG GU/MU LI/BAI SHAO/GUI BAN/NIU XI/(ZHEN GAN XI FENG TANG): Liver Kidney Yin Deficient w/Yang Rising
- GOU TENG/JU HUA/SHI JUE MING/SANG YE: Liver Wind
- GOU TENG/JU HUA/SHI JUE MING/SANG YE/SHI GAO/FU SHEN: Liver Wind
- GOU TENG/XIA KU CAO/HUANG QIN/SHI JUE MING/JU HUA: Liver Yang Rising
- HE SHOU WU/SHU DI HUANG/NU ZHEN ZI/GOU QI ZI/TU SI ZI/SANG JI SHENG: Blood Deficiency
- JI XUE TENG/DAN SHEN/DU ZHONG: Windstroke
- JU HUA/TIAN MA: Liver Yang Rising
- JU HUA/JUE MING ZI/GOU TENG/BAI SHAO: Liver Yang Rising
- JUE MING ZI/GOU TENG/MU LI: Liver Yang Rising
- LING YANG JIAO/SHI JUE MING/JU HUA/HUANG QIN: Liver Fire Uprising
- LONG GU/MU LI/DAI ZHE SHI/BAI SHAO/(ZHEN GAN XI FENG TANG): Liver Kidney Deficiency w/Liver Yang Rising
- LUO BU MA/XIA KU CAO/GOU TENG/JU HUA: Liver Yang Rising
- MU LI/LONG GU/GUI BAN/BAI SHAO: Liver Kidney Yin Deficient w/Yang Rising
- NIU XI/DAI ZHE SHI/MU LI/LONG GU/(ZHEN GAN XI FENG TANG): Liver Wind Rising
- SANG SHEN ZI/HE SHOU WU/NU ZHEN ZI/HAN LIAN CAO/(SHOU WU YAN SHOU DAN): Yin And Blood Deficiency
- SANG YE/JU HUA/SHI JUE MING/MU LI: Liver Yang Rising
- SANG YE/HEI ZHI MA: Liver Kidney Yin Deficient, Fire Rising
- SHI JUE MING/MU LI/BAI SHAO/GUI BAN: Liver Kidney Yin Deficient w/Liver Yang Rising
- SHU DI HUANG/DANG GUI/BAI SHAO/(SI WU TANG): Blood Deficiency
- TIAN MA/CHUAN XIONG/(TIAN MA WAN): Liver Wind From Liver Deficiency
- TIAN MA/BAN XIA/BAI ZHU: Phlegm Dampness
- TIAN MA/GOU TENG: Liver Yang Rising
- TIAN MA/BAN XIA/BAI ZHU/FU LING /(BAN XIA BAI ZHU TIAN MA TANG): Wind Phlegm Attacking Upper In Spleen Deficient w/Liver Qi Stagnation
- TIAN NAN XING/TIAN MA: Wind Phlegm
- TIAN NAN XING/BAN XIA/TIAN MA/BAI FU ZI: Wind Phlegm
- XIA KU CAO/JU HUA: Liver Fire Rising
- ZE XIE/MU DAN PI
- ZHEN ZHU MU/BAI SHAO/SHENG DI HUANG/SHI JUE MING/LONG GU: Liver Kidney Yin Deficiency w/Liver Yang Rising

End of Topic:
ENCEPHALITIS B

ENDOCRINE RELATED DISORDERS :

ACTH, STIMULATES

ADDISON'S DISEASE

ADDISON'S DISEASE, EARLY STAGE

ADRENAL CORTEX

ADRENAL INSUFFICIENCY

ADRENALIN ANTAGONIZING ACTION

ALDOSTERONE EFFECT

ANDROGEN-LIKE EFFECT

ANDRONERGIC

ANTIADRENALINE

CORTISONE, SYNERGIZES

CORTISONE-LIKE

DIABETES

GOITER

- BAN XIA/KUN BU/HAI ZAO/CHUAN BEI MU
- HAI FU SHI/LIAN QIAO/KUN BU/XUAN SHEN
- HAI FU SHI/MU LI/CHUAN BEI MU/XUAN SHEN/KUN BU: Phlegm, Qi Accumulation
- HAI GE KE/KUN BU/HAI ZAO/WA LENG ZI/(HAN HUA WAN)
- HAI LONG/DA ZAO/(winter fungus)
- HAI ZAO/JIANG CAN/XIA KU CAO/XUAN SHEN
- HAI ZAO/GAN CAO
- HAI ZAO/KUN BU/(HAI ZAO YU HU TANG)
- HUANG YAO ZI/XIA KU CAO
- KUN BU/HAI ZAO
- WA LENG ZI/HAI ZAO/KUN BU
- XIA KU CAO/MU LI/XUAN SHEN/KUN BU: Phlegm Fire
- XUAN SHEN/MU LI/ZHE BEI MU: Phlegm
- XUAN SHEN/MU LI/ZHE BEI MU/XIA KU CAO/ZI CAO: Phlegm
- XUAN SHEN/CHUAN BEI MU/MU LI

GOITER, ENDEMIC

GOITER, HYPOTHYROID

GOITER, INHIBITS

GOITER, STIFLING SENSATION IN THROAT

- KUN BU/HAI ZAO/HAI GE KE/(KUN BU WAN)

HORMONE EFFECTS

HORMONE-LIKE

HORMONES

HYPERTHYROID

HYPERTHYROIDISM

HYPOTHYROID

HYPOTHYROID GOITER

INSULIN

ENERGETIC STATE :

ADAPTOGEN

- **BAI DOU KOU/XING REN/YI YI REN/HUA SHI:** Early Damp Warm Febrile Diseases
- **DANG GUI/HUANG QI:** Blood Loss
- **DANG SHEN/HUANG QI:** Lung Spleen Qi Deficient
- **GAN CAO/DANG SHEN:** Spleen Deficient
- **HUANG JING/REN SHEN:** From Prolonged Sickness/Chronic Wasting
- **HUANG JING/DANG GUI:** Very Deficient Qi Blood
- **HUANG QI/REN SHEN:** Qi Deficient
- **HUO XIANG/PEI LAN:** Summer Heat Dampness
- **LONG YAN ROU/SHI CHANG PU:** Heart Qi, Blood Deficient
- **REN SHEN/BAI ZHU:** Spleen Stomach Deficient Qi
- **SHAN YAO/DANG SHEN:** Lung Spleen/Kidney Spleen Deficient
- **WU WEI ZI/DANG SHEN/MAI MEN DONG:** Febrile Disease, Post: Qi And Yin Deficient, Fluid Loss

FATIGUE FROM CHONIC DISEASE

FATIGUE W/LOWER BACK/EXTREMITIES PAIN W/TENDERNESS AND THROBBING BELOW NAVEL

- **LONG GU/GUI ZHI/BAI SHAO:** Cold Deficiency

FATIGUE, DEFICIENCY

FATIGUE, EXTREME W/FEVER, BONE STEAMING

FATIGUE, MENTAL

FATIGUE, REDUCES

HERBS, TONIFYING

ILLNESS, POST

ILLNESS, RECOVERY FROM

ILLNESS, RECOVERY FROM, SEVERE

INDURANCE, INCREASES

OVEREXERTION

PHYSICAL DEBILITY

- **HE SHOU WU/REN SHEN/DANG GUI/BIE JIA/ZHI MU**

POST ILLNESS WEAKNESS

POST ILLNESS, RECOVERY

PROSTRATION

QI, BLOOD, YIN, YANG

See Also: Qi, Blood, Yin, Yang, Geriatric Topics

RECOVERY FROM ILLNESS

RECOVERY, LONG ILLNESS

STRENGTH, INCREASES

STRENGTHENING, GENERAL

THIRST, EXHAUSTION

TIREDNESS, IN LIMBS

- **DANG SHEN/BAI ZHU/FU LING :** Qi Deficiency Of Spleen Stomach

TONIFIES

- LING ZHI CAO (c): Enhanced Protein Synthesis In Liver
.... 731
- LU RONG (c) 784
- NUO DAO GEN (c) 825
- ROU CONG RONG (c) 786

TONIFIES, NUTRITIVE

- SHU DI HUANG (c) 802

WEAK CONSTITUTION

- SHI JUN ZI 648

WEAKNESS

See: Energetic State Debility 104
- DANG SHEN/DANG GUI: Qi And Blood Deficient
- DONG CHONG XIA CAO/(with meat): Wei Qi Weakened
- GUI BAN/LU RONG: Kidney Deficient
- HUANG JING/REN SHEN: From Prolonged
  Sickness/Chronic Wasting
- HUANG JING/GOU QI ZI: General Debility
- HUANG JING/DANG GUI: Very Deficient Qi Blood
- HUANG QI/BAI ZHU: Spleen Qi Deficient
- MA QIAN ZI/CHUAN WU/WEI LING XIAN: Wind Damp Bi
- SHAN YAO/DANG SHEN: Kidney Spleen Deficient
- SUO YANG/HU GU/NIU XI/SHU DI HUANG: Liver Kidney
  Severely Deficient
- BAI BIAN DOU: Qi Deficiency 506
- BAI ZHU: Qi Deficiency 760
- CE BAI YE (c) 654
- DA ZAO: Spleen Stomach Deficient 761
- DANG SHEN: Qi Deficiency 762
- FU LING : Qi Deficiency 594
- GAN CAO: Qi Deficient 763
- HUA QI SHEN: Qi Deficiency 808
- HUANG JING: Long Illness Recovery, Qi Deficiency ... 764
- HUANG QI: Qi Deficiency 765
- LIAN ZI: Qi Deficiency 824
- LU RONG 784
- REN SHEN: Qi Deficiency 767
- SHAN YAO: Qi Deficiency 769
- SHAN ZHU YU: Qi Deficiency 827
- TAI ZI SHEN: Qi Deficiency 770
- WU WEI ZI: Qi Deficiency 831
- ZHI GAN CAO: Qi Deficiency 772
- ZI HE CHE: Qi Deficiency 792

WEAKNESS, CHRONIC

- ZI HE CHE/SHU DI HUANG
- ZI HE CHE/SHU DI HUANG/HUANG QI/DANG SHEN: Qi
  Deficient
- ZI HE CHE/SHU DI HUANG/DANG GUI/BAI SHAO:
  Deficient Blood

WEAKNESS, CHRONIC/BODY

- HE SHOU WU/REN SHEN/DANG GUI/BIE JIA/ZHI MU

WEAKNESS, DEBILITY

- HAI SHEN 781
- LU JIAO 783

WEAKNESS, EXTREME

- REN SHEN 767

WEAKNESS, GENERAL

- E GUAN SHI 777
- YE JIAO TENG: Deficient Blood 733

End of Topic:
ENERGETIC STATE

ENERGY, LACK OF IN LIMBS

See: Energetic State Energy, Lack Of In Limbs ... 104

ENTERITIS

See: Abdomen/Gastrointestinal Topics
Enteritis 29

ENTEROBIASIS

See: Parasites Enterobiasis 304

ENURESIS

See: Urinary Bladder Enuresis 421

ENURESIS, IN CHILDREN

See: Childhood Disorders Enuresis, Childhood . 81

EOSINOPHILIA, TROPICAL

See: Blood Related Disorders/Topics
Eosinophilia, Tropical 49

EPIDEMIC DISEASES

See: Infectious Diseases Epidemic Diseases 185

EPIDIDYMAL STASIS

See: Sexuality, Male: Urological Topics
Epididymal Stasis 343

EPIGASTRIC RELATED TOPICS

See: Stomach/Digestive Disorders Epigastric
Related Topics 390

EPIGLOTTIS SPASMS

See: Oral Cavity Epiglottis Spasms 284

EPILEPSY RELATED TOPICS

See: Mental State/Neurological Disorders
Epilepsy Related Topics 247

EPILEPSY, IN CHILDREN

See: Childhood Disorders Epilepsy, Childhood .. 81

EPISTAXIS

See: Hemorrhagic Disorders Epistaxis 166

ERUCTATION

See: Stomach/Digestive Disorders Belching ... 387

ERYSIPELAS

See: Skin Erysipelas 358

EXTERNAL CONDITIONS :

EXTERIOR COLD W/YANG DEFICIENCY

• XI XIN 452

EXTERIOR CONDITIONS

• DAN DOU CHI/CONG BAI: Initial Stage

EXTERIOR CONDITIONS, EXCESS

• GUI ZHI/MA HUANG: Wind Cold
• JING JIE/FANG FENG

EXTERIOR DEFICIENCY

• HUANG QI 765

EXTERIOR HOT/COLD

• DAN DOU CHI 459

EXTERIOR INVASION

• CANG ZHU/FANG FENG/XI XIN: Wind Cold Damp

EXTERIOR PATHOGEN

• FU PING: Heat w/Head & Body Aches 460
• SHENG JIANG: Relieves Very Little 450

EXTERIOR PATHOGEN W/SPLEEN DISORDERS

• HUO XIANG 582

EXTERIOR PATHOGEN W/SPLEEN WEAKNESS

• PEI LAN 583

EXTERIOR PATHOGENS

• CONG BAI 442

EXTERIOR, RELEASES

• MA HUANG: Very Good 448

End of Topic:
EXTERIOR CONDITIONS

EXTERIOR PATHOGENS/CONDITIONS AND RELATED TOPICS

EXTERNAL COLD W/YANG DEFICIENCY

EXTERNAL HOT/COLD

EXTERNAL INJURIES

EXTERNAL PATHOGEN W/SPLEEN DISORDERS

EXTERNAL WIND

End of Topic:
EXTERNAL WIND

EXTREMITIES :

ARM SPASMS

See: Musculoskeletal/Connective Tissue
Spasms 275

ARMS

See: Extremities Limbs 114
• CHOU WU TONG/XI XIAN CAO/GOU TENG/SANG JI
SHENG: Wind Damp Bi
• CANG ZHU: Wind Damp Bi 578

ARMS, ACHING

• YE JIAO TENG 733

ARMS, CONTORTION OF

• MU GUA 567

ARMS, CONTRACTURE OR NUMBNESS

• SANG ZHI 570

ARMS, CONVULSIONS, PAIN

• HAN FANG JI 596

ARMS, EDEMA

• ZE QI 727

ARMS, MUSCLE ACHES

• HE HUAN PI 731

ARMS, NUMB

• CHUAN XIONG/CHI SHAO YAO/DI LONG/JI XUE TENG:
Blood, Qi Stagnation
• MU GUA/HAN FANG JI/WEI LING XIAN/DANG GUI
• LU LU TONG 681
• TIAN NAN XING: Wind Phlegm 712
• XI XIAN CAO: Bi 575
• YIN YANG HUO 791

ARMS, NUMB, SPASMS

• QIAN NIAN JIAN/JI XUE TENG/GOU QI ZI: Especially In
Elderly

ARMS, NUMB, WEAK

• YIN YANG HUO 791

ARMS, NUMB, WEAK, CHRONIC

• BAI HUA SHE 558

ARMS, PAIN

• CAN SHA/DU HUO/NIU XI: Wind Damp
• YAN HU SUO/ROU GUI
• DU HUO 561
• GU SUI BU: Arthritic Pain 778
• WEI LING XIAN 572

ARMS, PAIN, SORE

• CHAI HU/QIANG HUO/FANG FENG: Spleen Deficient
w/Dampness
• GUI ZHI 445

ARMS, PAIN, SPASMS

• XIAN MAO 788

ARMS, SPASMS

• HAI TONG PI/HAN FANG JI/WEI LING XIAN/HAI FENG
TENG: Bi
• WU JIA PI/WEI LING XIAN/DU HUO/SANG ZHI/MU GUA:
Bi
• HAI FENG TENG 562
• QIN JIAO 569
• SONG JIE: Sudden 572

ARMS, SWELLING

• SANG BAI PI 703

ARMS, TRAUMA, SWELLING, PAIN

• XU DUAN: Topical, Too 789

ATROPHY OF LIMBS

• HUANG BAI 485

CALF MUSCLE SPASMS

• GAN CAO/BAI SHAO
• BAI SHAO 794
• CAN SHA: Severe Dampness 558

CALF, PAIN

• BAI GUO YE (c): Helps Reduce Pain From Intermittent
Claudication 817

CLAUDICATION, INTERMITTENT

• BAI GUO YE (c): Reduces Pain Of, Long Term 817

CORNS

See: Skin Clavus 355
See: Skin Warts 379
• BAN XIA (c): Remove Keratinized Tissue With Knife,
Powder With Untreated Then Cover With Adhesive
Plaster, Sloughed Off In 5-7 Days 710
• BU GU ZHI (c): Alcohol Extract, Topical Application Or
Inject In Center 773
• GU SUI BU 778
• GU SUI BU (c): Repeated Tincture Application, Every 2
Hrs, 15 Days 778
• WU MEI: Soften In Hot Water, Then Topical 830
• WU MEI (c): External, With Vinegar, Salt To Make
Paste, First Soak In Warm Water, Remove Thick Skin
. . . . 830
• YA DAN ZI: Topical 538
• YA DAN ZI (c) 538

CRAMPING

See: Musculoskeletal/Connective Tissue
Cramps 268

CRAMPS, ARMS/LEGS

• TIAN MA 750

CRAMPS, ESPECIALLY EXTREMITIES

• QIN JIAO 569

CRAMPS, LIMBS

- MAN JING ZI/FANG FENG/QIN JIAO/MU GUA: Wind Damp Bi
- CANG ER ZI 559

CRAMPS, SEVERE IN CALVES

- MU GUA 567

EDEMA

EXTREMITIES, COLD

- FU ZI/ROU GUI: Kidney Yang Deficiency
- FU ZI/GAN JIANG/GAN CAO/(SI NI TANG): Yang Collapse
- GAN JIANG/FU ZI/(SI NI TANG): Collapsing Yang
- LU RONG/REN SHEN/SHU DI HUANG/TU SI ZI: Kidney Yang Deficiency
- FU ZI: Devastated Yang, From Severe Adominal Pain: Spleen Kidney Yang Deficient 613
- GAN JIANG 614
- LU RONG 784

EXTREMITIES, CONTRACTURE OF

- SANG ZHI 570

EXTREMITIES, CRAMPS/SPASMS

- TIAN MA: Liver Wind 750

EXTREMITIES, HOT BI

- LUO SHI TENG/REN DONG TENG

EXTREMITIES, ICY COLD

- REN SHEN/FU ZI/(SHEN FU TANG): Collapsed Qi/Devasted Yang Syndrome

EXTREMITIES, LOWER COLD

- FU PEN ZI/DU ZHONG: Kidney Deficient

EXTREMITIES, LOWER, SORE, PAIN, NUMB

- DU HUO/XI XIN/QIN JIAO: Wind Damp Bi

EXTREMITIES, LOWER, SWELLING, POST LONG-TERM DISEASE

- GOU JI/DANG GUI

EXTREMITIES, LOWER, WEAK

- XU DUAN/DU ZHONG: Kidney Deficient/Cold, Damp Bi

EXTREMITIES, LOWER, WEAK, WASTING W/POOR LOCOMOTION

- GUI BAN/NIU XI/SUO YANG/HU GU: Liver Kidney Deficient

EXTREMITIES, NUMB

- BAI SHAO/DANG GUI/SHU DI HUANG/MAI MEN DONG: Liver Yin Deficient
- HE SHOU WU/SANG JI SHENG/NU ZHEN ZI/NIU XI: Liver Blood Deficient
- XI XIAN CAO/WEI LING XIAN: Wind Damp

- YIN YANG HUO/WEI LING XIAN/DU ZHONG/GUI ZHI: Bi, Wind Cold Damp
- CHUAN SHAN LONG 442
- JI XUE TENG 677
- SANG ZHI 570
- TIAN MA: Wind Stroke 750
- TIAN NAN XING: Wind Phlegm 712
- XI XIAN CAO 575

EXTREMITIES, NUMB, PAIN, SPASM

- HAI FENG TENG/WEI LING XIAN: Wind Damp Bi

EXTREMITIES, NUMB, PAIN, SWELLING

- HUANG QI/HAN FANG JI: Wind Edema

EXTREMITIES, PAIN

- CAN SHA/DU HUO/NIU XI: Wind Damp
- GAO BEN/FANG FENG/QIANG HUO/WEI LING XIAN/CANG ZHU: Wind Cold Damp Bi
- GUANG FANG JI/YI YI REN: Damp Heat
- YAN HU SUO/ROU GUI

EXTREMITIES, PAIN W/TENDERNESS, THROBBING BELOW NAVEL

- LONG GU/GUI ZHI/BAI SHAO: Cold Deficiency

EXTREMITIES, PAIN, NUMB, WEAK

- BEI XIE/NIU XI

EXTREMITIES, PAIN, SORE

- XI XIAN CAO/WEI LING XIAN: Wind Damp

EXTREMITIES, PAIN, SPASMS

- LUO SHI TENG/REN DONG TENG: Hot Bi

EXTREMITIES, PAIN/NUMB

- TIAN MA: Wind Damp Bi 750

EXTREMITIES, PARALYSIS OF

- BAI HUA SHE: Wind Damp 558
- DA DOU HUANG JUAN 506
- HU GU 563
- ZHU LI: Phlegm Blocking Orifices 728

EXTREMITIES, SORE

- HE SHOU WU: Yin/Blood Deficient 799

EXTREMITIES, SPASMS

- FANG FENG/QIANG HUO/DANG GUI: Wind Cold Damp Bi
- TIAN NAN XING: Wind Phlegm 712

EXTREMITIES, SPASMS/NUMB

- YIN YANG HUO 791

EXTREMITIES, STIFF

- DI LONG 744

EXTREMITIES, SWELLING

- HUANG QI/HAN FANG JI/FU LING /GUI ZHI: Superficial Floating Edema
- SANG BAI PI 703

EXTREMITIES, TIREDNESS IN

• DANG SHEN/BAI ZHU/FU LING : Qi Deficiency Of Spleen Stomach

EXTREMITIES, WEAK, NUMB

• TIAN MA/NIU XI/SANG JI SHENG

EXTREMITIES, WEAK, SORE

• NU ZHEN ZI/BU GU ZHI/TU SI ZI: Kidney Yin Deficient

EXTREMITIES, WEAKNESS OF IN ELDERLY

• JI XUE TENG 677

EXTREMITIES, WIND DAMP BI

• HAI TONG PI 562

FEET SPASMS

See: Musculoskeletal/Connective Tissue
Spasms 275

FEET, CHRONIC CONVULSIONS

• QUAN XIE/DANG SHEN/BAI ZHU/TIAN MA: Spleen Deficiency Chronic Diarrhea

FEET, CONVULSIONS

• CAO HE CHE 517
• ZAO XIU 540

FEET, CONVULSIONS PAIN OF

• DU HUO 561

FEET, CRACKED

• BAI JI: With Sesame Oil 652

FEET, CRACKED, BLEEDING SKIN

• BAI JI/SHI GAO/(topical)

FEET, DEBILITY OF

• GOU JI 778
• XU DUAN 789

FEET, EDEMA OF

• HAI ZAO/FU LING /ZE XIE
• KUN BU/FU LING /ZE XIE

FEET, HEAT IN

• HUANG JING/GOU QI ZI/NU ZHEN ZI: Kidney Essence Deficiency

FEET, INFECTIONS OF

• DAN SHEN (c) 672

FEET, MUSCLE SPASMS, PAIN

• BAI SHAO/GAN CAO

FEET, NAILS, PARONYCHIA

• HUANG LIAN (c): Topical 20% Vaseline Dressing, 3% Solution With Oral Powder 486

FEET, NUMB

• LU LU TONG 681
• LU XIAN CAO 566

FEET, PAIN

• YAN HU SUO/ROU GUI

FEET, PARALYSIS OF

• ZHU LI: Phlegm Blocking Orifices 728

FEET, POSTPARTUM SWELLING

• NAN GUA ZI 648

FEET, RED, SWOLLEN, PAINFUL

• HUANG BAI: Hot Leg Qi 485

FEET, SEVERE PAIN, WORSE AT NIGHT

• DAN SHEN (c): (Thromboangiitis Obliterans) Tinctures, With Local Applications Concurrently, Herbal Decoction, Ok, Too 672

FEET, SPASMS

• GUI BAN/E JIAO/SHENG DI HUANG/MU LI: Yin Consumed By Fever Causing Malnutrition Of Tendons, Muscles
• TIAN NAN XING: Wind Phlegm 712

FEET, SPASMS, CRAMPS

• BAI SHAO 794

FEET, SPASMS, PAIN

• HAN FANG JI 596

FEET, SPASMS/CRAMPS

• YIN YANG HUO: Wind Cold Damp 791

FEET, SPASMS/TREMBLING OF

• E JIAO/HUANG LIAN/BAI SHAO/GOU TENG/MU LI: Yin Consumed By Febrile Diseases

FEET, TINEA INFECTION

• CHOU WU TONG 560
• YI YI REN 602

FEET, TOES, BLISTERS BETWEEN

• PENG SHA 844

FEET, TREMORS

• FANG FENG 444
• GUI BAN: Liver Kidney Yin Deficient With Wind 806

FEET, WEAKNESS OF

• LU XIAN CAO 566

FINGERS, BOILS ON

• WU GONG/(fish liver oil, topical)

FINGERS, BOILS ON TIP

• ZI HUA DI DING/YE JU HUA
• ZI HUA DI DING/YE JU HUA/JIN YIN HUA/LIAN QIAO

FINGERS, DIGITAL ARTERIAL SPASM

FINGERS, TREMORS

• BIE JIA/MU LI/SHENG DI HUANG/E JIAO/BAI SHAO/(ER JIA FU MAI TANG): Wind Following Febrile Disease, Yin/Fluids Consumed

FINGERTIPS, BOILS ON

• WU GONG/(fish liver oil, topical)
• ZI HUA DI DING/YE JU HUA
• ZI HUA DI DING/YE JU HUA/JIN YIN HUA/LIAN QIAO

GANGRENE IN TOES, FINGERS

GANGRENE, TOES

• WU GONG/(tea, topical)

GOOSE-FOOT TINEA

HAND SPASMS

HANDS, CONVULSIONS

HANDS, CONVULSIONS, CHRONIC

• QUAN XIE/DANG SHEN/BAI ZHU/TIAN MA: Spleen Deficiency Chronic Diarrhea

HANDS, CONVULSIONS, PAIN OF

HANDS, CRACKED BLEEDING SKIN

• BAI JI/SHI GAO/(topical)

HANDS, FUNGAL INFECTIONS OF

HANDS, INFECTIONS OF

HANDS, MUSCLE SPASMS, PAIN

• BAI SHAO/GAN CAO

HANDS, NAILS, PARONYCHIA

HANDS, NUMB

HANDS, PAIN

• YAN HU SUO/ROU GUI

HANDS, PAIN, SORENESS

• CHAI HU/QIANG HUO/FANG FENG: Spleen Deficient w/Dampness

HANDS, PARALYSIS OF

HANDS, POSTPARTUM SWELLING

HANDS, SEVERED FINGER

HANDS, SKIN FUNGI

HANDS, SPASMS

• GUI BAN/E JIAO/SHENG DI HUANG/MU LI: Yin Consumed By Fever Causing Malnutrition Of Tendons, Muscles

HANDS, SPASMS, CRAMPS

HANDS, SPASMS, PAIN

HANDS, SPASMS/CRAMPS

HANDS, SPASMS/TREMORS

• E JIAO/HUANG LIAN/BAI SHAO/GOU TENG/MU LI: Yin Consumed By Febrile Diseases

HANDS, TINEA ON

• DA FENG ZI/(oil)/HU TAO REN/(oil)/(pork lard)

HANDS, TREMORS

LEG QI

LEG QI, COLD, DAMP

• HU LU BA/MU GUA/JI XUE TENG/BU GU ZHI: Pain, Swelling, Heaviness, Cold, Slow Pulse, White, Greasy Fur

LEG QI, DAMP

• BING LANG 643
• HAN FANG JI 596

LEG QI, EDEMA

• CHI XIAO DOU 591
• MU GUA 567

LEG QI, HOT

• HUANG BAI 485

LEG QI, PAIN

• BA JI TIAN 773

LEG QI, SWELLING

• BING LANG/CHEN PI/MU GUA
• HAN FANG JI/FU LING /GUI ZHI

LEG SPASMS

See: Musculoskeletal/Connective Tissue
Spasms 275

LEGS

See: Extremities Limbs 114
• XIAN MAO/XI XIN: Cold, Damp Pain

LEGS & FEET, SWELLING, POST LONG-TERM DISEASE

• GOU JI/DANG GUI

LEGS, ACHING

• SANG JI SHENG: Arthritis 813
• YE JIAO TENG 733

LEGS, ACHING, PAINS

• DU HUO 561

LEGS, ATROPHY OF BONES

• HU GU (c) 563

LEGS, CALVES, CRAMPING

• MU GUA 567

LEGS, COLD

• FU PEN ZI/DU ZHONG: Kidney Deficient
• ROU GUI PI 617
• YANG QI SHI 789

LEGS, COLD PAIN OF

• CAN SHA 558

LEGS, COLD W/UPPER BODY HEAT

• ROU GUI 616

LEGS, COLD, NUMB BI

• XIAN MAO 788

LEGS, COLD, WEAK

• ROU GUI: Kidney Yang Deficient 616

LEGS, CONTRACTURES, WEAK

• XU DUAN/DU ZHONG: Kidney Deficient/Cold, Damp Bi

LEGS, CONTRACTURES/NUMB

• SANG ZHI 570

LEGS, CONVULSIONS, PAIN

• HAN FANG JI 596

LEGS, EDEMA

• DA FU PI: Damp Leg Qi (Vit B1 Deficiency) .. 624
• HU LU BA: Cold Damp 781
• MU BIE ZI (c) 844
• QIAN NIU ZI 553
• SANG ZHI 570
• WU ZHU YU 618
• ZE QI 727
• ZE XIE 605

LEGS, FRACTURE

• BAO YU 804

LEGS, LOWER, WEAK, SORE

• WU JIA PI 574

LEGS, MUSCLE ACHES

• HE HUAN PI 731

LEGS, NUMB

• CHOU WU TONG/XI XIAN CAO/GOU TENG/SANG JI SHENG: Wind Damp Bi
• CHUAN XIONG/CHI SHAO YAO/DI LONG/JI XUE TENG: Blood, Qi Stagnation
• DU HUO/FANG FENG
• MU GUA/HAN FANG JI/WEI LING XIAN/DANG GUI
• JI XUE TENG 677
• LU LU TONG 681
• TIAN NAN XING: Wind Phlegm 712
• WU JIA PI 574
• YIN YANG HUO 791

LEGS, NUMB, SPASMS

• QIAN NIAN JIAN/JI XUE TENG/GOU QI ZI: Especially In Elderly

LEGS, NUMB, WEAK

• XI XIAN CAO 575
• YIN YANG HUO 791

LEGS, NUMB, WEAKNESS, CHRONIC

• BAI HUA SHE 558

LEGS, PAIN

• CAN SHA/DU HUO/NIU XI: Wind Damp
• KUAN JIN TENG/JI XUE TENG: Wind Damp Bi
• YAN HU SUO/ROU GUI
• CANG ZHU: Wind Damp Bi 578

• DANG SHEN: Spleen Qi Deficient 762

LOINS, COLD

• BU GU ZHI 773

LOINS, COLD OBSTRUCTION OF

• ROU CONG RONG 786

LOINS, COLD PAIN OF

• CAN SHA 558

LOINS, DEBILITY OF

• YANG QI SHI 789

LOINS, PAIN

• BA JI TIAN 773
• DONG CHONG XIA CAO 775
• DU ZHONG 775
• GU SUI BU 778
• SHA YUAN ZI 786
• SHAN ZHU YU 827
• TU SI ZI 787
• WEI LING XIAN 572
• XIAN MAO: Cold 788

LOINS, SORE

• HE SHOU WU 799

LOINS, WEAK

• GUI BAN 806
• JIU CAI ZI 782
• SUO YANG 787
• YIN YANG HUO 791

MUSCLE SPASMS OF LIMBS

See: `Pain/Numbness/General Discomfort` Bi
Disorders 297
See: `Musculoskeletal/Connective Tissue` Muscle
Spasms, Bi 272
• WU JIA PI/WEI LING XIAN/DU HUO/SANG ZHI/MU GUA

MUSCLE SPASMS, CALF

• BAI SHAO/GAN CAO: Blood Deficient

NAILS, FUNGAL INFECTION OF

• BU GU ZHI (c): Tinea Unguium (Onychomycosis) ,
Injection Of Equal Amounts Tu SI Zi, Herb 773

PAIN, LEGS/ARMS

• CAN SHA/DU HUO/NIU XI: Wind Damp

PLANTAR WARTS

See: `Skin` Warts 379
• YA DAN ZI: Topical 538
• YI YI REN 602

PUSTULES, FINGERTIPS

• WU GONG/(fish liver oil, topical)

SCIATICA

See: `Musculoskeletal/Connective Tissue`
Sciatica 275

SPASMS

See: `Extremities` Limbs, Legs, Feet, Arms, Hands
Spasm 114

SWELLING, LEG, FEET

• YI YI REN 602

SWELLING, LEGS

• DONG GUA REN 593

THIGHS, INNER, NUMB

• WU JIA PI 574

THIGHS, INNER, PAIN

• BA JI TIAN 773

TOES, BLISTERS BETWEEN

• PENG SHA: Damp Toxin 844

TOES, ULCERS/GANGRENE

• WU GONG/(tea, topical)

TREMORS HAND/FEET

• GUI BAN 806

TREMORS, HANDS, FEET

See: `Mental State/Neurological Disorders`
Tremors 259

ULCERS, LEGS

• QIAN LI GUANG (c): Topical 474

ULCERS, TOES

• WU GONG/(tea, topical)

End of Topic:
EXTREMITIES
_____

EXTREMITIES, WEAKNESS OF, IN ELDERLY

See: `Geriatric Topics` Extremities, Weakness Of, In
Elderly 143

EXTREMITY RELATED TOPICS

See: `Extremities` Extremity Related Topics 109

EYE RELATED TOPICS

See: `Eyes` Eye Related Topics 117

EYEBALL PAIN

See: `Eyes` Eyeball Pain 117

EYELIDS, INFLAMMATION OF

See: `Eyes` Eyelids, Inflammation Of 117

End of Topic:
EYELIDS,INFLAMMATION OF
_____

EYES :

ANTIMYDRIATIC

- BING LANG (c): Constricts Pupils 643

BLEPHARITIS

- LU GAN SHI: (Eyelids Inflammation) Wind 842

BLEPHARITIS ULCEROSA

- ZAO FAN 848

CATARACTS

- CANG ZHU/HEI ZHI MA
- CHE QIAN ZI/SHU DI HUANG/GOU QI ZI/TU SI ZI: Liver Kidney Deficient
- CHE QIAN ZI/SHENG DI HUANG/MAI MEN DONG/GOU QI ZI: Liver Kidney Deficient
- JUE MING ZI/SHA YUAN ZI/BAI JI LI/NU ZHEN ZI/GOU QI ZI: Liver Kidney Yin Deficient
- CHAN TUI (c): 9 g PO/Day Effective Treatment 458
- CHE QIAN ZI: Liver Kidney Deficient 590
- JUE MING ZI 471
- MAN JING ZI 464
- MI MENG HUA 474
- MU ZEI 464
- QIN PI 493
- QING XIANG ZI: Wind Heat/Deficient Yin 475
- SHI JUE MING 750
- YE MING SHA 480
- ZHEN ZHU MU 741

CATARACTS W/IRRITABILITY

- CI SHI/ZHU SHA/SHEN QU: Liver Kidney Deficient

CATARACTS, EARLY

- NU ZHEN ZI (c) 812

CATARACTS, GERIATRIC

- SHA YUAN ZI/SHU DI HUANG/SHI CHANG PU/YE MING SHA

CENTRAL RETINITIS

- DAN SHEN (c) 672
- JU HUA (c): Gou Qi Zi, Ju Hua Shu Di Tang/Wan, Modified 463
- MAO DONG QING (c): IM Injections, Favorable Results 682
- NU ZHEN ZI (c) 812

CENTRAL RETINITIS/EARLY CATARACT

- NU ZHEN ZI (c): Wang Mo Yan Fang (Retinitis Prescription) /Ming Mu Zi Shen Pian (Vision Improving And Kidney Tonic Tablet) 812

CONJUNCTIVITIS

- XIONG DAN/BING PIAN
- BAI JI LI 743
- BI QI 717
- BING PIAN: Topical 753
- BO HE 456
- CHONG WEI ZI 669
- CHONG WEI ZI (c) 669

- E BU SHI CAO 711
- HUANG BAI (c): Best Results From Best Grade 485
- HUANG LIAN 486
- JU HUA (c): With Xia Ku Cao, Jue Ming Zi, Bai Ji LI, Chan Tui Or With Bai Ji LI, Mu Zei, etc For Steam Therapy Of Eyes 463
- LONG DAN CAO 492
- LONG DAN CAO (c): Liver Gall Bladder Damp Heat, Use Modified Long Dan Xie Gan Tang 492
- LU GAN SHI 842
- MANG XIAO 545
- MU ZEI 464
- PU GONG YING (c): Herb, Ju Hua/Ye Ju Hua Decoction Oral, Second Cooking, Luke Warm Use As An Eye Wash 529
- QIN PI (c): Eye Wash From Decoction 5-15 g, Mu Zei, Jue Ming Zi Or Oral Decoction Of Qin Pi, Huang Lian, Dan Zhu Ye 493
- RONG SHU XU 570
- SU XIN HUA 631
- XIAN HE CAO (c): Alcohol/Aqueous Extract, Antiinflammatory, Decoction Reduces Inflammation Of Chemical Or Bacterial Induced 665

CONJUNCTIVITIS, ACUTE

- BAI JIANG CAO 512
- DA HUANG (c) 542
- HUANG BAI (c) 485
- HUANG LIAN (c): Eye Drops With Extract, Borax Or As Ointment, *Washing Eyes With 5% Decoction Several Times, 95% Cured 486
- JIN YIN HUA (c): 6-15 g (15-100 g Of Vine, Ren Dong Teng) As Oral Dose/Day Or As Wash 524
- QIAN LI GUANG 474
- SANG YE 466
- SHI GAO (c) 477
- SHUI ZHI (c): Eye Drops, 1-5 Days 687
- XIA KU CAO 478
- XIONG DAN 479

CONJUNCTIVITIS, ACUTE/SUBACUTE

- QIAN LI GUANG (c): Similar To Chloramphenicol, As Eye Drops, 50% Solution 474

CONJUNCTIVITIS, CHRONIC

- DI LONG (c): External With Paste And Sugar/Eye Drops Of Saline Extract (Trachoma) 744
- JIN YIN HUA (c) 524

CONJUNCTIVITIS, EPIDEMIC

- YE JU HUA (c): With Pu Gong Ying, Wei Ling Xian, Hai Jin Sha, Bai Mao Gen, Jin Yin Hua 468

CONJUNCTIVITIS, FULMINANT

- BAN LAN GEN (c): 10% Eye Drops, Better Than 0.5% Chloramphenicol, 4 Days For Cure 515

CORNEA, INFLAMMATION

- SHAN ZHI ZI 476

CORNEAL

CORNEAL BURNS

CORNEAL DISORDERS

CORNEAL HAZINESS

CORNEAL OPACITY

CORNEAL ULCERS

CORNEAL ULCERS, SERPIGINOUS

DIABETIC RETINITIS

DIZZINESS

See Also: Dizziness (Topics: Gynecology, Phlegm, Blood, Ears, Mental State, Liver)

DIZZINESS, BLURRED VISION

EYEBALL PAIN

EYEBALLS, PAINFULL, PRESSURE

EYELIDS, INFLAMMATION OF

EYES, BENEFITS

EYES, BENEFITS VISION

EYES, BLEEDING IN

EYES, BLEEDING RETINA

EYES, BLEPHARITIS

EYES, BLEPHARITIS MARGINALIS

EYES, BLOOD SHOT

EYES, BLURRED

EYES, BLURRED VISION

EYES, BLURRED, DRY, CORNEAL OPACITY

EYES, BRIGHTENS

EYES, CHRONIC PROGRESSIVE LOSS OF VISION

EYES, CLOUDY

EYES, CONGESTED

EYES, CONGESTED, BLOOD SHOT

EYES, DECREASED VISION

EYES, DEVIATION OF

EYES, DISEASES OF

EYES, DISORDERS

EYES, DISTENDING SENSATION

EYES, DRY

EYES, DRY, SCRATCHY

EYES, EDEMA

EYES, HEAT, PAIN, SWELLING, SUPPURATION

EYES, HOT, SWOLLEN, PAINFUL

EYES, IMPROVES VISION

EYES, INCREASES VISUAL ACUITY

EYES, INFECTIONS

EYES, INFLAMMATION

EYES, INFLAMMATION, CHRONIC

EYES, INFLAMMATORY DISEASES

EYES, IRRITATION

EYES, IRRITATION, REDNESS

EYES, ITCHY, RED, PAINFUL

EYES, LACERATIONS, ETC

EYES, OBSTRUCTIONS W/IRRITABILITY

EYES, PAIN

EYES, PAIN ABOVE

EYES, PAIN W/EXCESS TEARING

EYES, PAIN W/O REDNESS/SWOLLEN

EYES, PAIN WORSE AT NIGHT

• XIA KU CAO/XIANG FU/DANG GUI/BAI SHAO: Liver Deficient

EYES, PAIN, DISTENTION

• DAI ZHE SHI/LONG GU/MU LI/BAI SHAO/GUI BAN/NIU XI/(ZHEN GAN XI FENG TANG): Liver Kidney Yin Deficient w/Yang Rising

EYES, PAIN, INTERNALLY

• MAN JING ZI 464

EYES, PAIN, RED

• JUE MING ZI/JU HUA: Liver Fire/Wind Heat
• LING YANG JIAO/SHI JUE MING/JU HUA/HUANG QIN: Liver Fire Rising
• MI MENG HUA/MU ZEI/GU JING CAO: Wind Heat/Liver Fire
• XIA KU CAO/JU HUA: Liver Fire Rising

EYES, PAIN, RED, DRY

• JU HUA: Wind Heat 463

EYES, PAIN, RED, SWELLING

• BAI JIANG CAO/JIN YIN HUA/PU GONG YING
• CHI SHAO YAO/JU HUA/HUANG QIN
• HONG HUA/SHENG DI HUANG/CHI SHAO YAO/LIAN QIAO
• MU ZEI/JU HUA
• SANG YE/JU HUA/XIA KU CAO/MU ZEI: Liver Fire
• SHI JUE MING/JU HUA: Liver Fire Blazing

EYES, PAIN, RED, SWELLING W/TEARING

• BAI JI LI/JUE MING ZI/JU HUA: Liver Wind

EYES, PAIN, RED, SWOLLEN

• CHE QIAN ZI/HUANG QIN/LONG DAN CAO/JU HUA: Liver Heat
• ZHEN ZHU MU/JU HUA/CHE QIAN ZI: Wind Heat In Liver Channel
• CHI SHAO YAO: Liver Fire 668
• MAN JING ZI: Wind Heat In Liver Channel 464
• MANG XIAO 545
• MI MENG HUA 474
• QING XIANG ZI 475

EYES, PAIN, REDNESS

• QIN PI: Liver Fire 493

EYES, PAIN, SUPRAORBITAL

• TIAN MA (c): 20% Solution Injection, IM, 1-3x/Day, Marked Effects After 1-4 Injections 750

EYES, PAIN, SWELLING

• QING XIANG ZI/HU HUANG LIAN/LONG DAN CAO: Liver Fire

EYES, PAIN, SWOLLEN, RED

• CHE QIAN ZI: Liver Heat 590
• ZI HUA DI DING 541

EYES, PHOTOPHOBIA

• GU JING CAO/JING JIE/LONG DAN CAO/CHI SHAO YAO: Liver Wind Heat
• MI MENG HUA 474

EYES, PRESSURE IN

• BAN XIA (c): Oral Decoction Reduces 710

EYES, PRESSURE SENSATION

• DAI ZHE SHI: Liver Yang Rising 735

EYES, PROBLEMS

• CHE QIAN ZI: Liver Heat/Liver Kidney Deficient 590
• SANG YE: Wind Heat Or Deficient Yin: Red, Sore, Dry, Painful Eyes 466

EYES, PROBLEMS, WIND HEAT SYNDROME

• MU ZEI/CHAN TUI/GU JING CAO/XIA KU CAO/BAI JI LI

EYES, RED

• GU JING CAO/LONG DAN CAO: Liver Fire
• MANG XIAO/PENG SHA/BING PIAN/(TOPICAL)
• MU DAN PI/JU HUA: Liver Fire Rising
• SHI CHANG PU/YU JIN: Damp Heat w/Turbidity Blocks The Orifices
• ZHEN ZHU/NIU HUANG/BING PIAN
• BO HE: Wind Heat 456
• DAI MAO 743
• DI LONG: Wind Heat 744
• GOU TENG: Liver Fire With Liver Yang Rising 745
• HU HUANG LIAN 484
• HUAI HUA MI: Liver Wind Heat 658
• HUAI JIAO: Liver Fire 676
• HUANG BAI: With Wine 485
• LING YANG JIAO: Heat/Liver Yang Rising Creates Wind 747
• LONG DAN CAO: Liver Fire 492
• LU HUI: Heat Accumulation 544
• SHAN ZHI ZI 476
• SHI JUE MING: Liver Fire/Yang Rising 750
• XUAN SHEN 503

EYES, RED & HEADACHE

• HUANG QIN: Liver Yang Rising 489

EYES, RED EXCESSIVE TEARING

• MU ZEI/CHAN TUI/GU JING CAO/XIA KU CAO/BAI JI LI: Wind Heat

EYES, RED, CONGESTED

• BAI JI LI: Liver Heat 743
• BO HE: Liver Heat 456
• CHAN TUI: Liver Heat 458
• CHE QIAN ZI: Liver Heat 590
• GU JING CAO: Liver Heat 461
• HUAI HUA MI: Liver Heat 658
• HUANG LIAN: Liver Heat 486
• JU HUA: Liver Heat 463
• JUE MING ZI: Liver Heat 471

EYES, SWOLLEN, RED

- DA HUANG/HUANG LIAN/HUANG QIN/(XIE XIN TANG): Fire Rising
- MI MENG HUA/JU HUA/SHI JUE MING/BAI JI LI: Liver Heat

EYES, SWOLLEN, RED, PAINFUL

- JUE MING ZI/JU HUA/SANG YE/SHAN ZHI ZI/XIA KU CAO: Liver Fire/Wind Heat
- SHI JUE MING/JU HUA/JUE MING ZI: Liver Fire Flaring

EYES, SWOLLEN, RED, TEARING

- MAN JING ZI/JU HUA/CHAN TUI/BAI JI LI: Liver Yang Rising

EYES, WATERY, PAINFUL

- SANG YE/JU HUA/JUE MING ZI/CHE QIAN ZI: Liver Fire Rising

EYES, WATERY, RED, SWOLLEN

- XIA KU CAO/SHI JUE MING/JU HUA: Liver Fire Flaring

EYES, WIND HEAT IRRITATION

EYES, WIND LACRIMATION

EYESIGHT, DECREASED

- GOU QI ZI/JU HUA/SHU DI HUANG/(QI JU DI HUANG WAN): Liver Kidney Yin Deficiency
- NU ZHEN ZI/SANG SHEN ZI/HAN LIAN CAO/GOU QI ZI: Yin Deficiency And Blood Heat

EYESIGHT, IMPROVES

EYESIGHT, IMPROVES FROM INTERNAL PROBLEMS

FUNDAL HEMORRHAGE

GLAUCOMA

- CANG ZHU/HEI ZHI MA

GLAUCOMA, ACUTE

GLAUCOMA, PAIN OF

HORDEOLUM

HYPEREMIA

INTRAOCULAR HEMORRHAGE

IRIS INFLAMMATION

KERATITIS

KERATITIS, DEEP

KERATITIS, HERPES SIMPLEX

KERATITIS, SUPERFICIAL

LACRIMATION

LENS OPACITY

MACULAR DEGENERATION

MYDRIATIC

NEBULA

NEURALGIA, SUPRAORBITAL

NIGHT BLINDNESS

NYCTALOPIA

OPTHALMOPATHY

OPTIC ATROPHY

OPTIC NERVE DISORDERS

OPTIC NEURITIS

PHOTOPHOBIA

PHOTOSENSITIZING

PTERYGIUM

PUPILS, CONSTRICTS

PUPILS, DILATES

RETINAL HEMORRHAGE

RETINAL PIGMENTARY DEGENERATION OF

RETINITIS, CENTRAL

SEBACEOUS GLAND INFLAMMATION

- SHE TUI (c): Pieces Soaked In Vinegar, 3 Days 571

STYES

See: **Eyes** Hordeolum 121
- QIN PI/HUANG LIAN/DAN ZHU YE

SUPRAORBITAL PAIN

- BAI ZHI 441

TEARING

See: **Eyes** Lacrimation 121

TEARING, EXCESSIVE

- MI MENG HUA/MU ZEI/GU JING CAO: Wind Heat/Liver Fire
- MU ZEI/BAI JI LI
- MU ZEI/CANG ZHU
- BING PIAN: Topical 753
- DAI MAO 743
- GOU QI ZI 798
- JU HUA: Wind Heat 463
- JUE MING ZI: Liver Yang Rising 471
- MAN JING ZI: Wind Heat In Liver Channel 464
- MU ZEI: Wind Heat 464
- QIN PI 493
- XIA KU CAO 478

TEARING, EXCESSIVE, EXCRETION

- MI MENG HUA 474

TEARING, EXCESSIVE, PHOTOPHOBIA

- MI MENG HUA/JU HUA/SHI JUE MING/BAI JI LI: Liver Heat

TEARING, FROM WIND EXPOSURE

- JIANG CAN/JING JIE/SANG YE/MU ZEI/(BAI JIANG CAN SAN)

TRACHOMA

- DI LONG (c): (Chronic Conjunctivitis) External With Paste And Sugar 744
- HUANG LIAN (c): Bathing Eyes With 10% In 3% Boric Acid Solution, Markedly Improved 486
- QIAN LI GUANG (c): Similar To Chloramphenicol, As Eye Drops, 50% Solution 474

ULCERS

- HUANG LIAN (c): Bathing Eyes With 10% In 3% Boric Acid Solution, Markedly Improved 486

ULCERS, CORNEAL

- SHI CHANG PU/GOU QI ZI/JU HUA
- JIN YIN HUA (c) 524

UVEITIS

- MAO DONG QING: (Inflammation Of Iris) 682

VISION

- WU JIA SHEN (c): Improves In Stressful Conditions ... 771

VISION FAILING

- CHE QIAN ZI/SHU DI HUANG/GOU QI ZI/TU SI ZI: Liver Kidney Deficient

VISION IMPROVEMENT

- WU WEI ZI (c): For Night Vision, Too 831

VISION OBSCURED

- SANG SHEN ZI 801

VISION, BLURRED

- BAI SHAO/DANG GUI/SHU DI HUANG: Blood Deficient
- BAI SHAO/DANG GUI/SHU DI HUANG/MAI MEN DONG: Liver Yin Deficient
- CHE QIAN ZI/SHENG DI HUANG/MAI MEN DONG/GOU QI ZI: Liver Kidney Deficient
- CI SHI/SHU DI HUANG/SHAN ZHU YU
- E JIAO/REN SHEN/DANG GUI/SHU DI HUANG: Blood Deficiency
- GOU QI ZI/JU HUA/SHU DI HUANG/(QI JU DI HUANG WAN): Liver Kidney Yin Deficiency
- GOU TENG/XIA KU CAO/HUANG QIN/SHI JUE MING/JU HUA: Liver Yang Rising
- GU JING CAO/FANG FENG: Wind Heat, Liver
- GUI BAN/BAI SHAO/NIU XI/SHI JUE MING/GOU TENG: Liver Yang Rising From Liver Kidney Yin Deficiency
- HAN LIAN CAO/NU ZHEN ZI/(ER ZHI WAN): Liver Kidney Yin Deficient, Severe, w/Yang Rising
- HE SHOU WU/GOU QI ZI/BU GU ZHI/TU SI ZI: Liver Kidney Deficiency
- HE SHOU WU/SANG JI SHENG/NU ZHEN ZI/NIU XI: Liver Blood Deficient
- HEI ZHI MA/SANG YE/(SANG MA WAN): Liver Kidney Yin Deficient w/Yang Rising
- JU HUA/JUE MING ZI/GOU TENG/BAI SHAO: Liver Yang Rising
- JUE MING ZI/XIA KU CAO: Liver Kidney Deficient
- JUE MING ZI/GOU TENG/MU LI: Liver Yang Rising
- JUE MING ZI/SHA YUAN ZI/BAI JI LI/NU ZHEN ZI/GOU QI ZI: Liver Kidney Yin Deficient
- LING YANG JIAO/SHI JUE MING/JU HUA/HUANG QIN: Liver Fire Uprising
- LING YANG JIAO/SHI JUE MING/XIA KU CAO/JU HUA: Liver Yang Rising
- LONG GU/MU LI/NIU XI/DAI ZHE SHI: Yin Deficiency w/Yang Rising
- LONG GU/MU LI/DAI ZHE SHI/BAI SHAO/(ZHEN GAN XI FENG TANG): Liver Kidney Deficiency w/Liver Yang Rising
- MAN JING ZI/JU HUA/CHAN TUI/BAI JI LI: Liver Yang Rising
- MU LI/LONG GU/GUI BAN/BAI SHAO: Liver Kidney Yin Deficient w/Yang Rising
- MU ZEI/CANG ZHU
- MU ZEI/CHAN TUI/GU JING CAO/XIA KU CAO/BAI JI LI: Wind Heat
- NIU XI/GOU TENG/SANG JI SHENG: Liver Yang Rising
- NU ZHEN ZI/SHA YUAN ZI: Liver Kidney Yin Deficient
- SANG SHEN ZI/SHENG DI HUANG/SHU DI HUANG: Yin And Blood Deficient

- SANG SHEN ZI/HE SHOU WU/NU ZHEN ZI/HAN LIAN CAO/(SHOU WU YAN SHOU DAN): Yin And Blood Deficiency
- SANG YE/NU ZHEN ZI/GOU QI ZI/HEI ZHI MA: Liver Yin Deficient
- SHA YUAN ZI/GOU QI ZI/SHU DI HUANG: Liver Kidney Deficiency
- SHA YUAN ZI/NU ZHEN ZI/SHENG DI HUANG: Yin Deficient
- SHA YUAN ZI/JUE MING ZI/JU HUA/GOU QI ZI: Liver Kidney Yin Deficient
- SHA YUAN ZI/TU SI ZI/JU HUA/GOU QI ZI/NU ZHEN ZI: Liver Blood Deficiency
- SHAN ZHU YU/SHU DI HUANG/TU SI ZI/GOU QI ZI/DU ZHONG: Liver Kidney Deficiency
- SHI HU/SHENG DI HUANG/XUAN SHEN/BEI SHA SHEN: Fluid Damage In Late Heat
- SHI JUE MING/MU LI/BAI SHAO/GUI BAN: Liver Kidney Yin Deficient w/Liver Yang Rising
- SHI JUE MING/JU HUA/JUE MING ZI: Liver Fire Flaring
- SHU DI HUANG/SHAN ZHU YU/SHAN YAO/(LIU WEI DIHUNG WAN): Kidney Deficiency Syndrome
- TU SI ZI/CHE QIAN ZI/GOU QI ZI/NU ZHEN ZI: Liver Kidney Deficient
- TU SI ZI/SHA YUAN ZI/(tonify yin-blood herbs): Yin And Blood Weak
- XI XIAN CAO/XIA KU CAO: Liver Fire Rising
- YE MING SHA/SHI JUE MING
- ZHEN ZHU MU/CANG ZHU/(PIG LIVER OR CHICKEN LIVER OR RABBIT LIVER): Liver Blood Deficiency

VISION, BLURRED, CHRONIC

- SHI JUE MING/SHU DI HUANG/(SHI JUE MING WAN): Liver Blood Deficiency

VISION, BLURRED, CHRONIC UTERINE BLEEDING

- DAI ZHE SHI/YU YU LIANG/CHI SHI ZHI/RU XIANG/MO YAO/(ZHEN LING DAN): Blood Deficient

VISION, BLURRED, DIZZINESS

- JU HUA/GOU QI ZI/NU ZHEN ZI: Liver Kidney Yin Deficient
- JU HUA/GOU QI ZI: Liver Kidney Deficient

VISION, BLURRED, DIZZINESS, PREMATURE GREYING OF HAIR

- HAN LIAN CAO/NU ZHEN ZI/(ER ZHI WAN)

VISION, BLURRED, IMPAIRED

- QING XIANG ZI/JUE MING ZI/MI MENG HUA

VISION, CHRONIC, PROGRESSIVE LOSS OF

- SHI JUE MING/CHAN TUI

VISION, DECREASED ACUITY

VISION, IMPAIRED

- GOU QI ZI/JU HUA: Liver Kidney Deficiency
- SHI JUE MING/SHU DI HUANG/SHAN ZHU YU: Liver Kidney Yin Deficient

VISION, IMPAIRED, BLURRED

- MI MENG HUA/GOU QI ZI/TU SI ZI: Liver Kidney Deficient

VISION, OBSTRUCTIONS

VISION, POOR

VISION, PROBLEMS, DIZZINESS

- JUE MING ZI/XIA KU CAO: Liver Kidney Deficiency

VISION, REDUCED ACUITY

VISION, SPOTS BEFORE EYES

- TU SI ZI/CHE QIAN ZI/GOU QI ZI/NU ZHEN ZI: Liver Kidney Deficient

VISION, SUPERFICIAL OBSTRUCTIONS

- HU PO/JU HUA/GOU QI ZI
- MI MENG HUA/MU ZEI/GU JING CAO: Wind Heat/Liver Fire
- QIN PI/HUANG LIAN/DAN ZHU YE
- SHE TUI/CHAN TUI/BAI JI LI
- XIONG DAN/BING PIAN
- YE MING SHA/SHI JUE MING
- ZHEN ZHU/NIU HUANG/BING PIAN

FEVERS :

ANTIPYRETIC

ANTIPYROGENIC

BONE STEAMING

BONE STEAMING FEVER

CHILLS, FEVER

CHILLS, FEVER, ALTERNATING

CHILLS, FEVER, INTERMITTENT

CHILLS, FEVER, MALARIA-LIKE

CHILLS/FEVER

COMA, FROM FEVERS

FEVER

FEVER FROM HOT DISEASES

FEVER W/FLUID DAMAGE

FEVER W/LOSS OF YIN/FLUIDS, THIRST

FEVER, AFTERMATH TO SPIRIT DISTURBANCES

FEVER, AFTERNOON

FEVER, AFTERNOON W/BLOOD HEAT AND YIN DEFICIENCY

FEVER, AFTERNOON, RECURRENT

FEVER, AFTERNOON/LOW GRADE

FEVER, BLOOD HEAT

FEVER, CHILDHOOD CONVULSIONS

FEVER, CHILDHOOD MALNUTRITION

FEVER, CHILLS

FEVER, CHILLS INTERMITTENT

FEVER, CHILLS, CHRONIC INTERMITTENT

• HE SHOU WU/REN SHEN/DANG GUI/BIE JIA/ZHI MU

FEVER, CHRONIC

• BAI WEI/ZHU RU: Blood Deficient

FEVER, CHRONIC, UNABATING

• HUA QI SHEN 808

FEVER, COMMON COLD

• BAI HUA LIAN 511

FEVER, CONTINUAL W/MACULOPAPULE

• SHI GAO/XUAN SHEN/XI JIAO: Qi/Xue Level Heat

FEVER, DAMPNESS

• CAO GUO 580

FEVER, DAMPNESS, JOINT PAIN

• DA DOU HUANG JUAN 506

FEVER, EFFECTS OF AFTERWARDS

• HUA QI SHEN/SHENG DI HUANG/SHI HU/MAI MEN
DONG: Qi/Yin Exhaustion

FEVER, EPIDEMIC HEMORRHAGIC

• DAN SHEN (c) 672
• ZHI MU (c): Bai Hu Tang, Marked Reduction Of Fever
.... 480

FEVER, FROM ACUTE INFECTIONS

• DAN ZHU YE (c): 3-9 g Decoction, Best As Formula, e.g.
Zhu Ye Liu Bang Tang/Zhu Ye Shi Gao Tang 470

FEVER, FROM EXHAUSTION

• GAN CAO 763

FEVER, HECTIC/DEFICIENCY

• XUAN SHEN (c): Yin Def—Yang Ying Qing Fei Tang
(Xuan Shen, Sheng Di, Mai Dong, Bai Shao, Mu Dan Pi,
Gan Cao, Bo He) 503

FEVER, HIGH

• CHAN TUI/QUAN XIE/JIANG CAN/GOU TENG/JU HUA:
Spasms, Convulsions Of
• HAN SHUI SHI/SHI GAO/HUA SHI: Summer Heat
• HOU ZAO/LING YANG JIAO: Phlegm Heat Obstruction
• HUA QI SHEN/SHI GAO/ZHI MU: Febrile Diseases
w/Both Qi/Fluids Injured
• HUANG QIN/HUANG LIAN: Febrile Diseases
• LING YANG JIAO/SHI GAO/XI JIAO/(ZI XUE DAN)
• SHI GAO/XI JIAO: Damp Heat Toxin
• XI JIAO/LING YANG JIAO: Febrile Disease
• XI JIAO/HUANG LIAN: Febrile Disease
• XUAN SHEN/ZHI MU/SHI GAO/XI JIAO:
Unconsciousness, Maculopapule
• ZHU SHA/XI JIAO/NIU HUANG: Internal Wind
• BAI HUA SHE SHE CAO (c) 511
• CHAN TUI (c): From Flu, Chan Tui, Jiang Can 458
• DA HUANG: Yang Ming Stage/Excess Heat In Intestine
.... 542

• DA QING YE 519
• FAN HONG HUA 674
• GE HUA 521
• HAN SHUI SHI: Summer Heat 471
• HUANG LIAN 486
• HUANG QIN 489
• LING YANG JIAO 747
• LING YANG JIAO (c): From Flu, Measles, Pneumonia, et
al, Use Injection 747
• MU DAN PI 499
• QING DAI: Children 531
• SHI GAO 477
• ZHI MU: Lung Stomach Excess Heat 480

FEVER, HIGH FROM INFECTION

• NIU HUANG (c): Use An Gong Niu Huang Wan 755

FEVER, HIGH W/BLEEDING, RESTLESSNESS

• DAN SHEN/MU DAN PI/SHENG DI HUANG

FEVER, HIGH W/CONVULSIONS

See: `Mental State/Neurological Disorders`
Convulsions 243
• DI LONG (c): From Flu, Lung Infection, Pneumonia,
Bronchitis—Injection, 2 ml Amp Of 1: 5, IM, Fast Onset
.... 744
• XIONG DAN 479

FEVER, HIGH W/FLUIDS DAMAGED

• REN SHEN 767

FEVER, HIGH W/LOSS OF CONSCIOUSNESS

• SHAN ZHI ZI/DAN DOU CHI/LIAN QIAO/HUANG QIN
• SHE XIANG 756

FEVER, HIGH W/LOSS OF CONSCIOUSNESS, CONVULSIONS

• NIU HUANG/HUANG LIAN/XI JIAO/SHE XIANG/(AN
GONG NIU HUANG WAN)

FEVER, HIGH W/MACULOPAPULES

• DA QING YE/MU DAN PI

FEVER, HIGH W/MACULOPAPULES, DULL, W/RED TONGUE

• DAN SHEN/SHENG DI HUANG/XUAN SHEN/ZHU YE

FEVER, HIGH W/PROLONG SWEATING, THIRST

• ZHI MU (c): Bai Hu Tang (Zhi Mu 15 g, Shi Gao, 30 g,
Gan Cao 6g) 480

FEVER, HIGH W/RESTLESSNESS, INSOMNIA

• SHAN ZHI ZI 476

FEVER, HIGH W/SPASMS

• GOU TENG/LING YANG JIAO/JU HUA/SHI GAO: Liver
Wind

FEVER, HIGH W/SPASMS, CONVULSIONS

• LING YANG JIAO/GOU TENG/JU HUA/SHENG DI HUANG/(LING JIAO GOU TENG TANG): Endogenous Wind

FEVER, HIGH W/THIRST

• JIN YIN HUA/SHI GAO/ZHI MU
• XI JIAO: Endangered Species! 502

FEVER, HIGH W/THIRST, DELIRIUM

• LIAN QIAO 525

FEVER, HIGH W/THIRST, IRRITABILITY

• SHI GAO/ZHI MU

FEVER, HIGH W/THIRST, RESTLESSNESS

• LU GEN 472
• ZHI MU: Acute Infectious Disease 480

FEVER, HIGH, UNRELENTING

• JIN YIN HUA/LIAN QIAO/HUANG QIN/HUANG LIAN

FEVER, INITIAL STAGE OF

• LIAN QIAO/YE JU HUA

FEVER, INJURED YIN

• YU ZHU 815

FEVER, INTERMITTENT

• BAI WEI/DI GU PI: Deficient Blood Steaming Bone Syndrome

FEVER, INTERMITTENT W/CHILLS

• QING PI 629

FEVER, IRRITABILITY

• MU LI 739
• TIAN ZHU HUANG 726
• ZHU RU 729

FEVER, IRRITABILITY, RESTLESSNESS

• ZHI MU 480

FEVER, IRRITABLE W/THIRST

• ZHEN ZHU 740

FEVER, LINGERING POST FEBRILE DISEASES

• SHI GAO/DAN ZHU YE

FEVER, LOSS OF CONSCIOUSNESS FROM

• BING PIAN 753
• NIU HUANG 755

FEVER, LOW GRADE

• BEI SHA SHEN/SHI HU: Stomach Yin Deficient/Post Febrile Disease
• DANG GUI/HUANG QI: Blood Loss
• MAI MEN DONG/SHENG DI HUANG/XUAN SHEN/(ZENG YE TANG): Severely Injured Fluids, Post Febrile Disease

• NUO DAO GEN /DAN SHEN/NU ZHEN ZI: Deficient Heat
• QIN JIAO/DI GU PI: Def Yin After Prolonged Illness
• SHI HU/SHENG DI HUANG/XUAN SHEN/BEI SHA SHEN: Fluid Damage In Late Heat
• TIAN MEN DONG/REN SHEN/SHU DI HUANG: Deficient Yin, Post Illness
• BAI HE: Post Febrile Diseases 803
• BIE JIA: Deficient Fire 805
• GUI BAN: Deficient Fire 806
• QING HAO: Summer Heat 508
• YIN CHAI HU 504

FEVER, LOW GRADE, AFTERNOON

• HUA QI SHEN 808
• TIAN MEN DONG 814

FEVER, LOW GRADE, CHRONIC

• DI GU PI 495
• HU HUANG LIAN 484

FEVER, LOW GRADE, CHRONIC DISEASES

• QIN JIAO 569

FEVER, LOW GRADE, CONTINUOUS

• SHENG DI HUANG 500

FEVER, LOWERS

• DI GU PI (c): Slightly Less Than Aspirin 495
• HUANG BAI (c) 485
• ZI SU YE (c): Mild 454

FEVER, MALNUTRITION

• LU HUI 544

FEVER, NAUSEA/VOMITING OF

• BAI MAO GEN/GE GEN

FEVER, NIGHT

• MU DAN PI/BIE JIA/ZHI MU/SHENG DI HUANG: Ying Level Heat After Febrile Disease

FEVER, NIGHT, NO SWEAT, NOT IN AM

• SHENG DI HUANG/ZHI MU/QING HAO/BIE JIA

FEVER, POSTPARTUM

See: **Sexuality, Female: Gynecological**
Postpartum, Fever 336
• BAI WEI/ZHU RU: Blood Deficient
• BAI WEI/REN SHEN/DANG GUI: Yin Deficient
• BAI WEI 495
• HUANG QI 765

FEVER, RECURRENT

• SHI HU: Yin Deficient 813

FEVER, RECURRING AFTERNOON

• HU HUANG LIAN/DI GU PI: Steaming Bone

FEVER, REDUCES

• CHANG SHAN (c): Greater Than Aspirin 518

FILARIASIS

See: Parasites Filariasis 304

FINGER RELATED TOPICS

See: Extremities Finger Related Topics 110

FIRE POISON

See: Heat Fire Poison 161

FIRE POISON RASHES

See: Heat Fire Poison Rashes 161

FIRE RISING

See: Heat Fire Rising 161

FIRE, EXCESS, DAMAGED FLUIDS

See: Heat Fire, Excess, Damaged Fluids 161
See: Fluid Disorders Fire, Excess, Damaged Fluids
.... 137

FISH BONES

See: Trauma, Bites, Poisonings Fish Bones 409

FISH TOXINS

See: Trauma, Bites, Poisonings Fish Toxins 409

FISTULA RELATED TOPICS

See: Bowel Related Disorders Fistula Related
Topics 62

FIVE CENTER HEAT

See: Heat Five Center Heat 161

FLANK DISTENTION

See: Abdomen/Gastrointestinal Topics Flank
Distention 29

FLANK PAIN

See: Abdomen/Gastrointestinal Topics Flank
Pain 29

FLANK PAIN FROM ACUTE SPRAIN

See: Trauma, Bites, Poisonings Flank Pain From
Acute Sprain 409

FLAT WORMS

See: Parasites Flat Worms 304

FLATULENCE

See: Bowel Related Disorders Flatulence 62

FLEAS

See: Parasites Fleas 304

FLIES

See: Trauma, Bites, Poisonings Flies 409

FLUID ACCUMULATION TOPICS

See: Fluid Disorders Fluid Accumulation Topics
.... 137

FLUID DAMAGE

See: Fluid Disorders Fluid Damage 137

End of Topic:
FLUID DAMAGE

FLUID DISORDERS :

ANTIDIURETIC

- CHEN PI (c) 621
- HUANG LIAN (c) 486
- REN SHEN (c) 767
- SANG PIAO XIAO (c) 827
- SHA YUAN ZI (c) 786
- WEI LING XIAN (c) 572
- WU JIA SHEN (c) 771
- YI ZHI REN (c) 790

ASCITES

- BA DOU/XING REN
- BAI ZHU/DA FU PI/FU LING : Spleen Stomach
  Dysfunction w/Internal Dampness
- BAN BIAN LIAN/HU LU BA
- GAN SUI/DA HUANG/MANG XIAO/(DA XIAN XION TANG
  OR TOPICAL): Fluid Accumulation In Chest
- JING DA JI/QIAN NIU ZI
- JING DA JI/GAN JIANG
- JING DA JI/DA ZAO/GAN SUI/YUAN HUA/(SHI ZAO TANG)
- QIAN NIU ZI/GAN SUI
- QING FEN/DA HUANG/QIAN NIU ZI: Kidney Yang
  Deficient
- ZE QI/DA ZAO/(pills)
- BAN BIAN LIAN 586
- DONG GUA REN 593
- FU ZI 613
- HAN FANG JI: Dampness In Lower Jiao 596
- HONG DA JI 551
- JING DA JI 552
- MA BIAN CAO (c): Helps To Eliminate In Patients With
  Schistosomiasis 682
- SANG BAI PI 703
- SHANG LU 554
- SHANG LU (c): Good Diuretic Effect 554
- SHENG JIANG PI 600
- SHU YANG QUAN 535
- WU JIU GEN PI 555
- XUAN FU HUA 713
- YI YI REN 602
- YU LI REN 549
- YUAN HUA: From Schistosoma 556
- YUAN HUA (c): Powder, 1.5 -2.5 g/Day For 4-5 Days .. 556
- ZHU LING 606

ASCITES, ABDOMINAL DISTENTION

- GAN SUI/GAN CAO: Topical To Navel

ASCITES, DIFFICULT URINATION

- TING LI ZI: Excess Lung/Bladder Qi Obstruction 555

- BAI MAO GEN/HUANG QI: Deficient Qi
- BAI MAO GEN/CHE QIAN ZI/JIN QIAN CAO
- BAI QIAN/CANG ZHU: Dampness
- BAI QIAN/ZI WAN/DA JI/(BAI QIAN TANG)
- BAI ZHU/FU LING : Spleen Deficient
- BAI ZHU/DA FU PI/FU LING : Spleen Stomach Dysfunction w/Internal Dampness
- BAN BIAN LIAN/HU LU BA
- BING LANG/SHANG LU/MU TONG/ZE XIE: Excess Caused
- BING LANG/FU LING PI/ZE XIE
- CHE QIAN ZI/ZE XIE
- CHE QIAN ZI/NIU XI: Deficient Kidney
- CHI XIAO DOU/(with carp in soup): Deficient Spleen/Kidneys
- CHI XIAO DOU/BAI MAO GEN/SANG BAI PI
- DA DOU HUANG JUAN/HUA SHI/TONG CAO: Damp Heat, Damp Summer Heat, Damp Bi
- DI LONG/NIU XI/DONG KUI ZI/JIN QIAN CAO
- DONG GUA PI/CHI XIAO DOU/BAI MAO GEN/FU LING /(DONG GUA WAN)
- DONG KUI ZI/FU LING /BAI ZHU
- FU LING /ZHU LING/ZE XIE/BAI ZHU/(WU LING SAN)
- FU ZI/BAI ZHU: Yang Deficient w/Excess Cold Damp
- GUANG FANG JI/HUANG QI
- GUANG FANG JI/DANG SHEN/GUI ZHI
- GUI ZHI/FU LING : Deficient Yang w/Congested Dampness From Blocked Yang
- GUI ZHI/FU LING /BAI ZHU: Spleen Heart Yang Deficient
- HUANG QI/HAN FANG JI/BAI ZHU/(FANG JI HUANG QI TANG): Spleen Deficient w/Poor Water Metabolism
- KU SHEN/FU LING : Damp Heat Urinary Tract Dysfunction
- LU LU TONG/FU LING PI/SANG BAI PI
- MA HUANG/FU ZI. Yang Deficient w/Common Cold
- MU TONG/CHE QIAN ZI: Heart Small Intestine Channel Heat
- MU TONG/FU LING /ZHU LING
- QING FEN/DA HUANG/QIAN NIU ZI: Kidney Yang Deficient
- TING LI ZI/HAN FANG JI/DA HUANG/(JI JIAO LI HUANG WAN)
- WU JIA PI/FU LING PI/DA FU PI/(WU PI YIN)
- XIANG RU/BAI ZHU: Damp Cold
- XIANG RU/BAI MAO GEN/YI MU CAO: Fever, No Sweat, Dark Urine
- YI YI REN/ZE XIE/BAI ZHU: Spleen Deficiency
- YU LI REN/SANG BAI PI/CHI XIAO DOU/BAI MAO GEN/(YU LI REN TANG)
- ZE QI/DA ZAO/(pills)
- ZE XIE/FU LING /ZHU LING/BAI ZHU/(WU LING SAN)
- ZHU LING/FU LING
- ZHU LING/DA FU PI
- ZHU LING/FU LING /ZE XIE/(SI LING SAN)

EDEMA, FULLNESS, DISTENTION

EDEMA, GENERALIZED

EDEMA, GENERALIZED W/YELLOWISH SKIN

EDEMA, HEAD & FACE, CHRONIC

EDEMA, HEAT

EDEMA, HEAT SIGNS

EDEMA, HEMATURIA

EDEMA, HOT SUPERFICIAL

EDEMA, IN WEAK PATIENTS

EDEMA, INHIBITS IN LOWER TRUNK

EDEMA, JAUNDICE

EDEMA, LEG QI

EDEMA, LEGS

EDEMA, LEGS/LOWER BODY

EDEMA, LIMBS

EDEMA, LIVER CIRROSIS, CARDIAC, RENAL

EDEMA, MILD

EDEMA, NEPHRITIC

EDEMA, NEPHRITIC, ACUTE/CHRONIC

EDEMA, NEPHRITIC/CARDIAC

EDEMA, PAIN OF

EDEMA, POSTPARTUM

EDEMA, PREGNANCY

EDEMA, PULMONARY

EDEMA, REDUCES

EDEMA, RENAL

EDEMA, SCANTY URINE

EDEMA, SEVERE

EDEMA, SEVERE OF HYPOTHORAX

- **REN SHEN/SHU DI HUANG/TIAN MEN DONG:** Qi & Yin Deficiency
- **SHAN YAO/TIAN HUA FEN:** Diabetes
- **SHI GAO/SHENG DI HUANG:** Excess Fire Damaged Fluids
- **SHI HU/SHENG DI HUANG/XUAN SHEN/BEI SHA SHEN:** Fluid Damage In Late Heat
- **TAI ZI SHEN/SHI HU/TIAN HUA FEN:** Stomach Yin Deficient
- **TIAN HUA FEN/LU GEN:** Injured Fluids From Heat
- **TIAN HUA FEN/BEI SHA SHEN/MAI MEN DONG/LU GEN:** Febrile Diseases
- **TIAN MEN DONG/MAI MEN DONG/(ER DONG GAO):** Deficient Yin
- **TIAN MEN DONG/SHENG DI HUANG/REN SHEN/(SAN CAI TANG):** Yin/Qi Consumption By Febrile Disease
- **WU MEI/HUANG LIAN/HUANG QIN:** Internal Heat From Injured Fluids From Chronic Dysentery
- **WU MEI/TIAN HUA FEN:** Diabetes/Febrile Disease
- **WU WEI ZI/DANG SHEN/MAI MEN DONG:** Febrile Disease, Post: Qi And Yin Deficient, Fluid Loss
- **XUAN SHEN/SHENG DI HUANG/MAI MEN DONG:** Ying Xue Level Heat
- **YU ZHU/BEI SHA SHEN/MAI MEN DONG/TIAN MEN DONG:** Stomach Yin Deficient
- **ZHI MU/TIAN HUA FEN/MAI MEN DONG:** Lung Stomach Dryness/Diabetes
- **ZHU RU/LU GEN:** Fluids Damaged By Heat
- **ZHU YE/SHI GAO/MAI MEN DONG:** Febrile Diseases

THIRST, CONSTIPATION

- **MAI MEN DONG/SHENG DI HUANG/XUAN SHEN/(ZENG YE TANG):** Late Stage Heat

THIRST, CONSUMPTIVE

THIRST, DEFICIENT YIN

THIRST, DIABETES

- **GE GEN/TIAN HUA FEN/MAI MEN DONG/SHENG DI HUANG**

THIRST, DRY MOUTH

- **SANG SHEN ZI/MAI MEN DONG/NU ZHEN ZI/TIAN HUA FEN:** Deficient Body Fluids

THIRST, DRY TONGUE

- **MAI MEN DONG/YU ZHU/BEI SHA SHEN/SHENG DI HUANG:** Stomach Yin Deficiency

THIRST, DRYNESS

- **BEI SHA SHEN/MAI MEN DONG:** Stomach Yin Deficient

THIRST, ESPECIALLY IN SUMMER

THIRST, EXCESSIVE

- **SHENG DI HUANG/XUAN SHEN:** Ying Stage Heat

GALL BLADDER :

GALL BLADDER, BILIARY TRACT INFECTION

GALL BLADDER, CHOLAGOGUE

GALL BLADDER, CHOLECYSTITIS

GALL BLADDER, SPASMS

GALL BLADDER, STIMULATES CONTRACTION

GALL BLADDER, STONES

GALL BLADDER, STONES/INFECTION

End of Topic:
GALL BLADDER

GALL BLADDER RELATED TOPICS

GANGRENE IN TOES, FINGERS

GANGRENE, SPONTANEOUS PRESENILE

GAS, DIGESTIVE, ELIMINATES

GAS, GASTROINTESTINAL

GASTRALGIA

GASTRIC CANCER

GASTRIC TOPICS

GASTRITIS

GASTROENTERIC DISEASES, ACUTE/CHRONIC

GASTROENTERITIS

GASTROINTESTINAL BLEEDING

GASTROINTESTINAL CANCER

GASTROINTESTINAL DISORDERS

GASTROINTESTINAL RELATED TOPICS

See: Abdomen/Gastrointestinal Topics
Gastrointestinal Related Topics 30

GASTROPTOSIS

See: Stomach/Digestive Disorders Gastroptosis
. . . . 392

GASTROSIS

See: Stomach/Digestive Disorders Gastrosis . . . 393

GENITALS, EITHER SEX AND RELATED TOPICS

See: Sexuality, Either Sex Genitals, Either Sex And
Related Topics 318

GENITALS, FEMALE RELATED TOPICS

See: Sexuality, Female: Gynecological Genitals,
Female Related Topics 326

GENITALS, SWOLLEN, SORE SCROTUM

See: Sexuality, Male: Urological Topics Genitals,
Swollen, Sore Scrotum 343

GERIATRIC TONIC

See: Geriatric Topics Geriatric Tonic 143

End of Topic:
GERIATRIC TONIC

GERIATRIC TOPICS :

AGING PROCESS

• HUANG QI (c): Reduced At Cell Level 765

AGING, PREMATURE

• HE SHOU WU/GOU QI ZI/BU GU ZHI/TU SI ZI

CONSTIPATION, IN ELDERLY-IMPROVES YIN

• HUO MA REN 548

DEBILITY, IN ELDERLY

• HAI LONG 779
• HAI MA 780

DEFICIENCY, IN ELDERLY

• HAI MA 780

EMOLLIENT FOR ELDERLY

• BAI GUO YE (c): Ginkgetin Extract Increases Sebaceous
Secretion, Helping Senile Skin 817

EXTREMITIES, WEAKNESS OF, IN ELDERLY

• JI XUE TENG 677

GERIATRIC TONIC

• LU RONG (c) 784

IMPOTENCE, IN ELDERLY

• HAI LONG 779

JOINT PAIN, ELDERLY

• QIAN NIAN JIAN/JI XUE TENG/GOU QI ZI

JOINT PAIN, IN ELDERLY

• QIAN NIAN JIAN/JI XUE TENG/GOU QI ZI: Joint, Low
Back, Spasms, Numbness
• QIAN NIAN JIAN/HU GU/NIU XI/WU JIA PI/(in wine):
Joint, Low Back, Spasms

STANDING, PROLONGED, IN ELDERLY

• WU JIA PI: Prolonged Standing 574

WIND COLD BI, IN ELDERLY

• QIAN NIAN JIAN: Wind Cold Damp Bi, Topical, Too . . 568

WIND DAMP BI, IN ELDERLY

• QIAN NIAN JIAN: Wind Cold Damp Bi, Topical, Too . . 568

WIND DAMP COLD BI, IN ELDERLY

• WU JIA PI: Wind Damp Cold Bi 574

End of Topic:
GERIATRIC TOPICS

GIARDIA

See: Parasites Giardia 304

GINGIVITIS

See: Oral Cavity Gingivitis 284

GLANDS, SWOLLEN

See: Immune System Related Disorders/Topics
Glands, Swollen 176

GLAUCOMA

See: Eyes Glaucoma 121

GLOBUS HYSTERICUS

See: Oral Cavity Globus Hystericus 284

GLOMERULONEPHRITIS

See: Kidneys Glomerulonephritis 199

GLOTTIS, EDEMA

See: Oral Cavity Glottis, Edema 284

GLUCOCORTICOID EFFECT

See: Endocrine Related Disorders Glucocorticoid
Effect 101

GLUCOSURIA

See: Urinary Bladder Glucosuria 421

GLYCOGEN, LIVER REDUCES DEPLETION

See: Liver Glycogen, Liver Reduces Depletion 203

GOITER RELATED TOPICS

See: Endocrine Related Disorders Goiter Related Topics 102

GONORRHEA

See: Infectious Diseases Gonorrhea 188

GOOSE-FOOT TINEA

See: Extremities Goose-Foot Tinea 111
See: Infectious Diseases Goose-Foot Tinea 188

GOUT

See: Musculoskeletal/Connective Tissue Gout 268

GRANULOMA

See: Cancer/Tumors/Swellings/Lumps Granuloma 68

GRIEF

See: Mental State/Neurological Disorders Grief 248

GROIN AREA PAIN

See: Abdomen/Gastrointestinal Topics Groin Area Pain 31

GROWTH, DELAYED

See: Nutritional/Metabolic Disorders/Topics Growth, Delayed 281

GROWTH, INCREASES

See: Nutritional/Metabolic Disorders/Topics Growth, Increases 281

GROWTH, INSUFFICIENT, IN CHILDREN

See: Childhood Disorders Growth, Insufficient, Childhood 81

GUIDING HERB

See: Herbal Functions Guiding Herb 173

GUMS AND RELATED TOPICS

See: Oral Cavity Gums And Related Topics 284

GYNECOLOGICAL RELATED TOPICS

See: Sexuality, Female: Gynecological Gynecological Related Topics 326

HAIR

See: Head/Neck Hair 146

HAIR, PREMATURE GREYING

See: Head/Neck Hair, Premature Greying 146

HALF-EXTERNAL, HALF-INTERNAL PATHOGEN

See: Six Stages/Channels Half-External, Half-Internal Pathogen 348

HALITOSIS

See: Oral Cavity Halitosis 285

HALLUCINATIONS

See: Mental State/Neurological Disorders Hallucinations 248

HALLUCINOGENIC

See: Mental State/Neurological Disorders Hallucinogenic 248

HAND RELATED TOPICS

See: Extremities Hand Related Topics 111

HANGOVER

See: Trauma, Bites, Poisonings Hangover 410

HEAD RELATED TOPICS

See: Head/Neck Head Related Topics 146

HEAD, TRAUMA

See: Trauma, Bites, Poisonings Head, Trauma 410

HEAD/BODY ACHES

See: Pain/Numbness/General Discomfort Head/Body Aches 301

End of Topic:
HEAD/BODY ACHES

HEAD/ NECK :

ALOPECIA

See: Head/Neck Hair 146
See: Head/Neck Baldness 145
• BAI SHAO: Deficiency Complex 794
• BAN MAO: Topical Application 837
• BU GU ZHI: Topical Application 773
• BU GU ZHI (c): Inject w/Uv Exposure—Six Months For Significant Re-Growth 773
• CE BAI YE: Blood Heat Complex 654
• CE BAI YE (c): Tincture (ETOH) Of Fresh Material, Hair Growth Proportional To Frequency Of Application, Rub Onto Bald Areas 654
• CHI SHAO YAO: Blood Heat Complex 668
• DANG GUI: Deficiency Complex 795
• DANG SHEN: Deficiency Complex 762
• GU SUI BU: Topical Application 778
• HAN LIAN CAO: Blood Heat Complex/Deficiency Complex 806
• HE SHOU WU: Deficiency Complex 799
• HE SHOU WU (c) 799
• HEI ZHI MA: Deficiency Complex 808
• HUANG JING: Deficiency Complex 764
• HUANG QI: Deficiency Complex 765
• LU JIAO JIAO: Deficiency Complex 783
• MU DAN PI: Blood Heat Complex 499
• NU ZHEN ZI: Deficiency Complex 812
• SANG SHEN ZI: Deficiency Complex 801

- TIAN NAN XING/BAN XIA/TIAN MA/BAI FU ZI: Wind Phlegm
- WU GONG/QUAN XIE/JIANG CAN/GOU TENG: Wind
- BAI FU ZI: Wind Phlegm 708
- BAI HUA SHE: Windstroke 558
- BI MA ZI 547
- CAO WU (c): San Wu Syrup (He Shou Wu, Fu Zi, Cao Wu) , 90% Cure Rate 609
- JIANG CAN 746
- MA QIAN ZI (c): Topical Paste, Cut Seeds Into Thin Slices, 18-24 Slices/3.5 g Of Seeds, Set On Zinc Oxide Plaster, Apply To Paralyzed Parts Of Face, Change Every 7-10 Days Until Better, Usually 2 Applications Enough 842
- QUAN XIE 749
- TIAN MA 750
- TIAN NAN XING: Wind Phlegm 712
- TIAN NAN XING (c): Fresh Herb With Vinegar, Ground, Juice Rubbed On Affected Side Of Neck, Nightly, Covered With Gauze 712
- WU SHAO SHE 574
- XI XIAN CAO 575

FACE, PARALYSIS OF

- BA DOU (c) 550

FACE, PARALYSIS W/SUDDEN LOSS OF CONSCIOUSNESS

- ZAO JIAO 715

FACE, RED

- SHI JUE MING/GOU TENG/JU HUA/XIA KU CAO: Liver Kidney Yin Deficient w/Liver Yang Rising

FACE, SALLOW COMPLEXION

- HE SHOU WU/SHU DI HUANG/NU ZHEN ZI/GOU QI ZI/TU SI ZI/SANG JI SHENG: Blood Deficiency
- E JIAO: Blood Deficient 797

FACE, SCARRING

- SHAN CI GU/QING FEN/PENG SHA

FACE, SORES

- SHAN ZHI ZI: Damp Heat Of Gall Bladder/San Jiao Channels 476

FACE, SPASMS OF

- GUI BAN: Liver Kidney Yin Deficient With Wind 806

FACE, WEAKNESS

- BAI FU ZI: Wind Damp/Cold Damp 708

FLUSHING

- MU DAN PI: Liver Fire 499

FOLLICULITIS

- DA HUANG (c): Especially Staph A. Caused 542

HAIR

See: Head/Neck Baldness 145
See: Head/Neck Alopecia 144

- LIU HUANG (c): Can Cause To Fall Out When Applied Topically 840

HAIR GROWTH

- MAN JING ZI (c): Promotes Beard Growth 464
- SANG ZHI (c): Increases In Rabbits, Sheep, Extract, (Yang Mao Sang Zhi Jin Chu Ye) 570

HAIR LOSS

- CE BAI YE (c): Tincture (ETOH) Of Fresh Material, Hair Growth Proportional To Frequency Of Application, Rub Onto Bald Areas 654

HAIR LOSS FROM RADIATION

- CHAN SU (c): Protected 837

HAIR, PREMATURE GREYING

- HAN LIAN CAO/NU ZHEN ZI/(ER ZHI WAN): Liver Kidney Yin Deficient, Severe, w/Yang Rising
- HE SHOU WU/GOU QI ZI/BU GU ZHI/TU SI ZI: Liver Kidney Deficiency
- HE SHOU WU/SHU DI HUANG/NU ZHEN ZI/GOU QI ZI/TU SI ZI/SANG JI SHENG: Blood Deficiency
- HEI ZHI MA/SANG YE/(SANG MA WAN): Blood And Essence Deficiency
- NU ZHEN ZI/SANG SHEN ZI/HAN LIAN CAO/GOU QI ZI: Liver Kidney Yin Deficiency
- SANG SHEN ZI/HE SHOU WU: Liver Kidney Deficiency
- SANG SHEN ZI/HE SHOU WU/NU ZHEN ZI/HAN LIAN CAO/(SHOU WU YAN SHOU DAN): Yin And Blood Deficiency
- FU PEN ZI 820
- HAN LIAN CAO: Liver Kidney Yin Deficient/Blood Heat 806
- HE SHOU WU: Yin/Blood Deficient 799
- NU ZHEN ZI: Liver Kidney Yin Deficient 812
- SANG SHEN ZI: Blood Deficient 801
- SANG SHEN ZI (c): Sang Shen With Honey 801

HAIR, PREMATURE WHITENING

- CE BAI YE: Blood Heat 654
- CHI SHAO YAO: Blood Heat 668
- DANG GUI 795
- GOU QI ZI 798
- HE SHOU WU 799
- MU DAN PI: Blood Heat 499
- SHENG DI HUANG: Blood Heat 500
- SHU DI HUANG 802

HEAD

- BAI ZHI: Any Problem From Wind In Yang Ming 441

HEAD, DISTENDING SENSATION

- LING YANG JIAO/SHI JUE MING/XIA KU CAO/JU HUA: Liver Yang Rising
- SHI JUE MING/GOU TENG/JU HUA/XIA KU CAO: Liver Kidney Yin Deficient w/Liver Yang Rising

HEAD, FUNGAL INFECTIONS

- KU LIAN GEN PI 646

HEAD, HEAVY

- CI SHI/NIU XI/DU ZHONG/SHI JUE MING: Yin Deficient w/Yang Rising
- MAN JING ZI 464

HEAD, INJURY, SEQUELAE OF

- HE SHOU WU (c) 799

HEAD, PAIN, ANY

- BAI FU ZI: Wind Damp/Cold Damp 708

HEAD, PAIN, DISTENTION

- BAI JI LI/GOU TENG/JU HUA/BAI SHAO: Liver Yang Rising
- DAI ZHE SHI/LONG GU/MU LI/BAI SHAO/GUI BAN/NIU XI/(ZHEN GAN XI FENG TANG): Liver Kidney Yin Deficient w/Yang Rising
- GUI BAN/BAI SHAO/NIU XI/SHI JUE MING/GOU TENG: Liver Yang Rising From Liver Kidney Yin Deficiency

HEAD, PRESSURE

- LONG DAN CAO/HUANG QIN/SHAN ZHI ZI/CHAI HU/MU TONG: Liver Fire Rising

HEAD, SCALDED

- LIU HUANG 840
- WU GONG 751

HEAD, SORES

- GUAN ZHONG 521
- WU GONG: Topical 751

HEAD, SORES/ABSCESSES

- ZI HUA DI DING 541

HEAD, TRAUMA

- SAN QI (c): Good For Mild To Moderate Cases 663

HEAD, ULCERS

- SHAN DOU GEN: Topical 532

HEAD, WIND

- WEI LING XIAN 572

HEAD, WIND IN, RELEASES

- JING JIE/BO HE

HEAD/BODY ACHES

- XI XIN: Very Good 452

HEADACHE

- BAI DOU KOU/XING REN/YI YI REN/HUA SHI: Early Damp Warm Febrile Diseases
- BAI FU ZI/BAI ZHI/TIAN MA/TIAN NAN XING: Wind Phlegm Rising
- BAI JI LI/GOU TENG/NIU XI: Liver Yang Rising
- BAI SHAO/GOU TENG/JU HUA: Liver Yang Rising
- BAI SHAO/NIU XI/GOU TENG/JU HUA: Liver Yang Rising
- BAI ZHI/GAO BEN: Wind Cold At Vertex
- BAI ZHI/XI XIN: Wind Cold
- BAI ZHI/CHUAN XIONG/JING JIE/ZI SU YE: Wind Cold
- BAI ZHI/CHUAN XIONG/JU HUA/(tea leaves): Wind Heat

- BAI ZHI/HUANG QIN: Wind Heat
- BO HE/JU HUA: Wind Heat
- CANG ER ZI/XIN YI HUA
- CANG ER ZI/XIN YI HUA/SHI GAO/HUANG QIN: Wind Heat, Acute
- CANG ER ZI/XIN YI HUA/QIAN CAO GEN/JIN YIN HUA: Wind Heat, Chronic
- CHUAN XIONG/FANG FENG/JING JIE: Wind Cold
- CHUAN XIONG/CHAI HU/CHI SHAO YAO: Liver Qi Stag And Blood Stasis
- CHUAN XIONG/JU HUA/SHI GAO/JIANG CAN/(CHUAN XIONG SAN): Wind Heat
- CHUAN XIONG/QIANG HUO/GAO BEN/FANG FENG/(QIANG HUO SHENG SHI TANG): Wind Damp
- CHUAN XIONG/CHI SHAO YAO/DAN SHEN/HONG HUA: Blood Stagnation
- CHUAN XIONG/DANG GUI/BAI SHAO: Deficient Blood
- DAI ZHE SHI/LONG GU/MU LI/NIU XI: Liver Yang Rising
- DI LONG/DAN SHEN/CI SHI: Liver Yang Rising
- DU HUO/QIANG HUO/GAO BEN/MAN JING ZI: Wind Cold, Dampness
- FU PING/BAI JI LI/NIU BANG ZI/BO HE: Common Cold
- GOU QI ZI/JU HUA: Liver Kidney Deficiency
- GOU TENG/XIA KU CAO/HUANG QIN/SHI JUE MING/JU HUA: Liver Yang Rising
- GU JING CAO/LONG DAN CAO: Liver Fire
- HEI ZHI MA/SANG YE/(SANG MA WAN): Liver Kidney Yin Deficient w/Yang Rising
- HUANG QIN/XIA KU CAO: Liver Fire Rising
- HUO XIANG/ZI SU YE/BAN XIA/HOU PO/CHEN PI/(HUO XIAN ZHENG QI SAN): Digestion, Disturbance From Cold, Raw Food
- JU HUA/CHUAN XIONG: Liver Yang Rising
- JU HUA/TIAN MA: Liver Yang Rising
- LING YANG JIAO/SHI JUE MING/JU HUA/HUANG QIN: Liver Fire Uprising
- LING YANG JIAO/SHAN ZHI ZI/LONG DAN CAO/JUE MING ZI/(LING YAN JIAO SAN): Liver Fire Flaring
- LONG DAN CAO/HUANG QIN/SHAN ZHI ZI/CHAI HU/MU TONG: Liver Fire Rising
- LU HUI/LONG DAN CAO/HUANG QIN: Liver Channel Excess Heat
- LUO BU MA/XIA KU CAO/GOU TENG/JU HUA: Liver Yang Rising
- MAN JING ZI/CHUAN XIONG/FANG FENG: External Wind Damp
- MAN JING ZI/FANG FENG/JU HUA/CHUAN XIONG: Wind Heat
- MU LI/LONG GU: Yin Deficient w/Yang Rising
- NIU XI/GOU TENG/SANG JI SHENG: Liver Yang Rising
- NIU XI/DAI ZHE SHI/MU LI/LONG GU/(ZHEN GAN XI FENG TANG): Liver Wind Rising
- QIAN HU/JIE GENG: External Wind Heat
- QUAN XIE/DANG GUI/CHUAN XIONG/BAI ZHI: Bi Type
- SANG JI SHENG/SHENG DI HUANG/CHI SHAO YAO/JI XUE TENG: Liver Kidney Yin Deficient w/Yang Rising
- SHAN ZHI ZI/MU DAN PI: Heat From Deficient Liver Blood
- SHENG MA/BAI ZHI: Yang Ming Channel
- SHENG MA/HUANG LIAN/SHENG DI HUANG/SHI GAO/MU DAN PI: Stomach Heat
- SHI GAO/SHU DI HUANG: Yin Deficient, Fire Rising

- SHI GAO/ZHI MU/SHENG DI HUANG: Stomach Fire Rising
- SHI JUE MING/MU LI: Yin Deficient w/Yang Rising
- SHI JUE MING/XIA KU CAO: Liver Yang Excess
- SHI JUE MING/GOU TENG/JU HUA/XIA KU CAO: Liver Kidney Yin Deficient w/Liver Yang Rising
- TIAN MA/GOU TENG/HUANG QIN/NIU XI/(TIAN MA GOU TENG YIN): Liver Yang Rising
- TIAN NAN XING/BAI FU ZI: Wind Phlegm Obstructing Channels
- TONG CAO/HUA SHI/YI YI REN: Summer Heat Dampness
- WU ZHU YU/SHENG JIANG: Jue Yin/Shao Yin
- XI XIAN CAO/XIA KU CAO: Liver Fire Rising
- XI XIN/CHUAN XIONG/(CHUAN XIONG CHA TIAO SAN): Wind Cold
- XI XIN/CHAI HU: Wind Cold Blocks Channels
- XIA KU CAO/JU HUA: Liver Fire Rising
- XIA KU CAO/SHI JUE MING/JU HUA: Liver Fire Flaring
- YAN HU SUO/CHUAN XIONG: Congealed Blood

- BA JIAO GEN 510
- BAI FU ZI: Cold Phlegm 708
- BAI HUA LIAN 511
- BAI JI LI: Hypertensive/Liver Wind/Heat 743
- BAI SHAO: Hypertension/Liver Yang Rising 794
- BAI ZHI: Wind Cold 441
- BAI ZHI (c): w/Bing Pian And Inhaled Through Nostrils
.... 441
- BAN XIA 710
- BI BA 608
- BO HE: Wind Heat 456
- BO HE (c): Topically As Menthol 456
- CANG ER ZI: Wind Cold/Damp 559
- CANG ZHU: Wind Cold Damp Evil 578
- CHA YE 589
- CHUAN WU 611
- CHUAN XIONG: Wind, Heat, Cold, Deficient Blood/Brain Concussion 671
- CHUAN XIONG (c): 3-9 g Daily Of Oral Decoction, Extract, Tincture 671
- DAN DOU CHI: Wind Heat 459
- DANG GUI: Blood Deficient 795
- DU HUO: Common Cold/Wind Cold Damp 561
- FANG FENG: Wind Cold 444
- FU LING : Spleen Deficient, Congested Fluids With Phlegm Rising 594
- FU PING: Exterior Heat 460
- GAO BEN: Vertex Pain/Wind Cold 444
- GE GEN: External Heat/Hypertension 460
- GE GEN (c): Hypertension, Reduces 460
- GE HUA: Stomach Heat 521
- GOU TENG: Liver Fire With Liver Rising/Nervous/Hypertensive/Wind Heat 745
- GUI ZHI (c): From Blood Vessel Spasms 445
- HEI ZHI MA: Blood Def/Yin Deficient 808
- HU ZHANG 497
- HUAI JIAO: Liver Fire 676
- HUO TAN MU CAO: From General Debility 498
- HUO XIANG 582
- JIANG CAN 746
- JIN YIN HUA: Wind Heat 524
- JING JIE 447
- JU HUA: Liver Yang Rising/Wind Heat 463
- JUE MING ZI: Liver Yang Rising 471
- JUE MING ZI (c): Reduces From Hypercholesterolemia
.... 471
- KU DING CHA 809
- LIAN QIAO: Wind Heat 525
- LING YANG JIAO: Heat/Liver Yang Rising Creates Wind
.... 747
- LONG DAN CAO: Liver Fire 492
- LONG GU: Hypertension Caused 738
- LU HUI: Excess Liver Channel Heat 544
- MA HUANG: Wind Cold Exterior Excess Patterns 448
- MAN JING ZI: Good For Yang Rising Pattern 464
- MU DAN PI: Liver Fire 499
- MU LI: Yin Deficient With Yang Rising 739
- MU ZEI 464
- NAO YANG HUA 740
- NIU XI: Liver Yang Rising 684
- PEI LAN 583
- SANG YE: Wind Heat 466
- SHENG MA: From Common Cold 467
- SHENG MA (c): Analgesic 467
- SHI GAO: Stomach Fire 477
- SHI JUE MING: Liver Fire/Yang Rising 750
- TIAN MA: Liver Wind/Wind Phlegm 750
- WU JIA SHEN (c) 771
- WU ZHU YU: Liver Stomach Phlegm Disorder, Jue Yin Stage 618
- XI XIAN CAO: Liver Yang Rising 575
- XI XIN: Wind Cold 452
- XI XIN (c): 1-3 g In Decoction 452
- XIA KU CAO: Liver Fire 478
- XIANG RU: Summer Heat/Damp 453
- YAN HU SUO (c): 60-120 mg 1-4x/Day Of L-Tetrahydropalmatine, Active Ingredient 693
- YE JU HUA 468
- ZI SU YE: Wind Cold 454

HEADACHE, ANTE, POSTPARTUM

HEADACHE, BODY ACHES

- BAI ZHI/CHUAN XIONG: Bi/Common Cold
- QIANG HUO/CHUAN XIONG: Bi/Common Cold

HEADACHE, BODY ACHES, NUMBNESS

- FANG FENG/TIAN NAN XING/(Zhen Yu San): Wind, Phlegm Obstructing Channel

HEADACHE, CHILL, FEVER

HEADACHE, DISTENTION

- GUI BAN/BAI SHAO/NIU XI/SHI JUE MING/GOU TENG: Liver Yang Rising From Liver Kidney Yin Deficiency

HEADACHE, DIZZY

- MAN JING ZI/JU HUA: Wind Heat

HEADACHE, DYSMENORRHEA

- DANG GUI/BAI SHAO/SHU DI HUANG/CHUAN XIONG/(SI WU TANG)

HEADACHE, FROM BRAIN CONCUSSION

- YAN HU SUO (c): 60-120 mg 1-4x/Day Of L-Tetrahydropalmatine, Active Ingredient 693

HEADACHE, FRONTAL

- TIAN MA/CHUAN XIONG/(TIAN MA WAN)
- BAI ZHI 441

HEADACHE, HYPERTENSIVE

- DAI ZHE SHI 735
- LUO BU MA 748
- ZHEN ZHU MU: Liver Yang Rising 741

HEADACHE, LATERAL

- CHUAN XIONG/QIANG HUO/JIANG CAN: Wind Damp

HEADACHE, MIGRAINE

See: Head/Neck Migraine 150
- GAO BEN/CHUAN XIONG
- CHUAN WU 611
- FANG FENG 444
- GAO BEN 444
- WEI LING XIAN 572

HEADACHE, MIGRAINE W/COMMON COLD

- MAN JING ZI 464

HEADACHE, NEURASTHENIA

- WU WEI ZI (c): Alcohol Extractions 831

HEADACHE, NEUROGENIC

- QI YE LIAN (c): (See "Pain/Numbness/General Discomfort Topic, Analgesic" Entry For Details) 568

HEADACHE, NEUROTIC

- WU WEI ZI (c): 40-100% Tincture, 2.5 ml/2-3x/Day For 2-4 Weeks 831

HEADACHE, OCCIPITAL PAIN

- QIANG HUO: In Wind Cold Damp 449

HEADACHE, OCCIPTIAL NEURALGIA

- QI YE LIAN (c): (See "Pain/Numbness/General Discomfort Topic, Analgesic" Entry For Details) 568

HEADACHE, ORBITAL

- BAI ZHI/XI XIN

HEADACHE, PAIN AT VERTEX

- GAO BEN/CHUAN XIONG: Wind Cold

HEADACHE, PERSISTENT

- WU GONG 751

HEADACHE, POSSIBLE VOMITING

- WU ZHU YU/REN SHEN/SHENG JIANG/(WU ZHU YU TANG): Weak Spleen Stomach w/Liver Qi Rising

HEADACHE, RADIATING FROM VERTEX TO TEETH

- GAO BEN 444

HEADACHE, RED EYES

- JIANG CAN/SANG ZHI/JU HUA/JING JIE

HEADACHE, RED EYES, IRRITABILITY

- HUANG QIN: Liver Yang Rising 489

HEADACHE, SEVERE

- QUAN XIE 749

HEADACHE, SEVERE INTERMITTENT

- CHOU WU TONG 560
- FU ZI 613
- GU JING CAO: Wind 461

HEADACHE, SEVERE LATERAL

- BAI FU ZI: Wind Damp/Cold Damp 708

HEADACHE, SINUSITIS

- BAI ZHI/XI XIN
- XIN YI HUA/CANG ER ZI
- XIN YI HUA/CANG ER ZI/BAI ZHI/XI XIN: Cold Type
- XIN YI HUA/CANG ER ZI/SHI GAO/BO HE/HUANG QIN: Heat
- CANG ER ZI 559
- XIN YI HUA 453

HEADACHE, SORE THROAT

- BO HE 456

HEADACHE, SPLITTING RADIATING TO BACK OF NECK

- CANG ER ZI: Exterior 559

HEADACHE, STUBBORN

- QUAN XIE/WU GONG/JIANG CAN
- WU GONG/QUAN XIE/TIAN MA/JIANG CAN/CHUAN XIONG

HEADACHE, TEMPORAL

- JUE MING ZI/CHUAN XIONG/MAN JING ZI: Wind Heat

HEADACHE, TOOTHACHE

- XI XIN/SHENG DI HUANG: Wind Heat

HEADACHE, TRAUMA INDUCED

- XI XIN/CHAI HU

HEADACHE, UNILATERAL

- BAI FU ZI/CHUAN XIONG/BAI ZHI
- MAN JING ZI/FANG FENG/JU HUA/CHUAN XIONG: Wind Heat
- TIAN MA/CHUAN XIONG/(TIAN MA WAN): Liver Wind From Liver Deficient

• CHOU WU TONG 560

HEADACHE, VASCULAR

• SHE XIANG (c): Sublingual Tabs, 1.5 mg (Muscone) /Tab, 2-3x/Day, Take At First Indication Of Attack, Then 1+ Tabs During Attack, 80% Improved 756

HEADACHE, VERTEX, W/STIFF NECK

• GAO BEN/XI XIN: Wind Cold Damp

HEADACHE, WIND HEAT

• JIANG CAN/JING JIE/SANG YE/MU ZEI/(BAI JIANG CAN SAN)

LOCKJAW

• TIAN NAN XING/BAI FU ZI: Wind Phlegm Obstruction
• FANG FENG 444
• NIU HUANG 755
• SHI CHANG PU 757
• TIAN NAN XING: Wind Phlegm 712
• WU GONG 751

LOCKJAW, SUDDEN SYNCOPE

• ZAO JIAO /XI XIN/(nasal inhalant)

MALAR FLUSH

• SHENG DI HUANG 500

MIGRAINE

See: **Head/Neck** Headache, Migraine 149
• BAI FU ZI/CHUAN XIONG/BAI ZHI
• GAO BEN/CHUAN XIONG
• BAI FU ZI 708
• CHOU WU TONG 560
• CHUAN WU 611
• FANG FENG 444
• GAO BEN 444
• GE GEN (c) 460
• QI YE LIAN (c): (See "Pain/Numbness/General Discomfort Topic, Analgesic" Entry For Details) 568
• QUAN XIE 749
• SHE XIANG (c) 756
• TIAN MA: Wind Phlegm 750
• WEI LING XIAN 572
• WU ZHU YU (c): Wu Zhu Yu Tang (Herb, Ren Shen, Da Zao, Sheng Jiang) , Eye Pain, Headache Disappeared, No Recurrence After 4 Months 618

NECK, ACUTE SUBMANDIBULAR LYMPHADENITIS

• WU GONG (c): Decoctions, Good 751

NECK, CELLULITIS OF

• PU GONG YING (c): Topical Paste Of Fresh Herb/Ointment Of Herb Root 529

NECK, LUMPS

• HE SHOU WU 799
• LIAN QIAO 525
• WU GONG: Topical 751

NECK, LYMPH GLANDS SWOLLEN

• JIANG CAN (c) 746
• XIA KU CAO: Phlegm Fire 478
• XUAN SHEN: Phlegm Fire 503

NECK, NODULES

• XIA KU CAO/CHAI HU: Liver Qi Stagnation
• BAN XIA: Phlegm 710
• LUO HAN GUO: Phlegm 810

NECK, PAIN

• QIANG HUO 449

NECK, PAIN, SWELLING

• MA BO/SHAN DOU GEN/XUAN SHEN

NECK, RIGID

• JIANG HUANG/QIANG HUO/FANG FENG/DANG GUI/(SHU JING TANG): Wind Damp Bi

NECK, SORE, PAINFUL, NUMBNESS

• DU HUO/XI XIN/QIN JIAO: Wind Damp Bi

NECK, SPASMS, STIFF

• GE GEN 460

NECK, STIFFNESS

• GE GEN/MA HUANG/GUI ZHI/BAI SHAO: Wind Cold

NECK, STIFFNESS/PAIN

• GE GEN (c): From Common Cold/Hypertension 460

NECK, SWELLINGS

• YUE JI HUA: Auxillary Herb 696
• ZHE BEI MU: Phlegm Fire 728

OCCIPITAL NEURALGIA

• DANG GUI (c) 795

PALLOR

• DANG GUI/HUANG QI: Blood Loss
• GAN JIANG 614

PLUM SEED QI

See: **Oral Cavity** Globus Hystericus 284
• BAN XIA 710
• LA MEI HUA 680

TEMPOROMANDIBULAR JOINT DISORDER

• DANG GUI (c): Injection 795

TENDO-MANDIBULAR JOINT DISLOCATION

• CHE QIAN ZI (c) 590

TICS

• DI LONG: With High Fever 744
• QUAN XIE: Liver Wind Phlegm 749
• WU GONG 751

ANGIOMA, CONGENITAL

AORTITIS, CONSTRICTIVE

ARRHYTHMIAS

BRADYCARDIA W/SLIGHT LOWERING BLOOD PRESSURE

CARDIAC BLOOD FLOW, INCREASES

CARDIAC CANCER

CARDIAC DISEASE

CARDIAC FUNCTION DEFICIENCY

CARDIAC INHIBITOR

CARDIAC OUTPUT INCREASES

CARDIAC PAIN

CARDIAC PAIN IN WOMEN

CARDIAC PAIN, ACUTE

CARDIAC STIMULANT

CARDIOGLYCOSIDE-LIKE

CARDIOTONIC

HEART ATTACK

- GE GEN (c): Increases Blood Flow, Helps Metabolism Of Myocardium, Reduces Platelet Aggregation 460
- LU XIAN CAO (c): Improved Symptoms After Treatment 566
- MAO DONG QING (c): Injection + Oral 682

HEART BI

- GUA LOU REN/BAN XIA/XIE BAI/(GUA LOU XIE BAI TANG)
- BAI GUO YE 817

HEART BI, W/DEFICIENT YIN, QI

- YU ZHU/DANG SHEN

HEART BLOOD DEFICIENCY

- BAI ZI REN/YUAN ZHI/SUAN ZAO REN: Palpitations, Insomnia
- DAN SHEN/SUAN ZAO REN/BAI ZI REN: Palpitations, Insomnia
- YE JIAO TENG/SUAN ZAO REN/BAI ZI REN: Insomnia w/Frightening Dreams
- YUAN ZHI/FU SHEN/SUAN ZAO REN: Palpitations w/Anxiety, Mental Disorientation, Insomnia, Irritability
- ZHU SHA/(pig's heart): Restless, Palpitations, Anxiety
- ZI SHI YING/FU SHEN/SUAN ZAO REN/HUANG QI/DANG GUI: Restless, Palpitations, Anxiety, Insomnia
- BAI ZI REN 730

HEART BLOOD DEFICIENCY W/SPLEEN QI DEFICIENCY

- LONG YAN ROU/SUAN ZAO REN: Palpitations, Insomnia

HEART BLOOD, SPLEEN QI DEFICIENCY

- SUAN ZAO REN/DANG SHEN/FU LING /LONG YAN ROU: Insomnia, Palpitations, Irritability

HEART BLOOD, YIN DEFICIENCY

- SUAN ZAO REN/SHU DI HUANG/DANG GUI/BAI ZI REN: Insomnia, Palpitations, With Anxiety, Irritability

HEART CHANNEL FIRE W/PAINFUL URINATION, INSOMNIA, IRRITABILITY

- DENG XIN CAO/DAN ZHU YE

HEART CHANNEL HEAT

- DAN ZHU YE/MU TONG/SHENG DI HUANG: Mouth, Tongue Sores w/Dysuria

HEART DEFICIENCY

- WU WEI ZI/SUAN ZAO REN: Insomnia, Irritablility, Forgetfulness
- FU SHEN: Poor Memory, Anger, Fright Palpitation, Insomnia 736
- HAN FANG JI 596
- HUA QI SHEN 808

HEART DISEASE

- CHEN PI (c): Hespiridin Reduces Capillary Fragility, Unreliable Though 621

- CHUAN SHAN LONG (c): Tabs, 160 mg Each, 2 Tabs 3x/Day, 92% Remission From Angina, *With Huai Hua Mi, Rz Hemsleya Macrosperma 442
- DAN SHEN (c): 1-9 Months, Extract Tablet 672
- DANG GUI: Coronary 795
- HONG HUA 675
- HUANG JING (c): With Bai Shao 764
- JIN QIAN CAO (c): Can Help Reduce Cholesterol Plague In Arteriosclerosis 598
- LING ZHI CAO (c): Satisfactory Results 731
- MAO DONG QING (c): Decoction, Tablet, Granule Infusion, 60-150 g/Day, 6-8 Weeks Or 1-3 Months 682
- REN SHEN (c): Helps To Utilize Nutrients And Improves Function 767
- SHE XIANG (c) 756
- SU HE XIANG 758
- TING LI ZI (c): Chronic Cor Pulmonale With Cardiac Failure 555
- WU JIA SHEN (c): Injection, 66% Effective Rate For Symptom Improvement, *Tablet, 1.5 g, 3x/Day, In 14 Days Improvement Of Angina, Mental State, Sleep, Appetite, 77% Improvement 771
- YI MU CAO (c): Injection IM Or IV In Glucose, Marked Symptom Improvement 694

HEART DISEASE, KESHAN DISEASE (ENLARGED HEART)

- LING ZHI CAO (c): Ling Zhi Syrup, 45 g Crude Herb, 1.5-3 Months 731

HEART DISEASE, RHEUMATIC W/HEART FAILURE

- LUO BU MA (c) 748

HEART DISORDERS, KESHAN DISEASES(ENLARGED HEART)

- SHAN ZHA (c): Shan Zha, Wu Wei Zi, Eliminated Most Symptoms With Treatment 641

HEART FAILURE

- CHAN SU (c): 4-8 mg, 2-3x/Day, Improvement In 2-48 Hrs, *Cardiotonic Powder (Chan Su, Fu Ling, 1: 9) , 87% Effective 837
- CHUAN SHAN LONG (c) 442
- FU ZI (c): Injection/SI Ni San/Ren Shen Fu Zi Tang 613
- YU ZHU (c): From Rheumatic, Coronary, Pulmonary Heart Disease—5-10 Days Control, 25 g, 1x/Day As Decoction, Able To Discontinue Digitalis 815
- ZHANG NAO (c) 849
- ZHI SHI (c): Injection 635

HEART FAILURE, CHRONIC CONGESTIVE

- LUO BU MA (c): 8% Decoction, 100 ml, 2x/Day Or 5 ml Of Fluid Extract (8 g Crude Herb) , 2x/Day, When Heart Slowed Reduce To 50 ml/3 ml Respectively 748

HEART FIRE FLARING

- ZHU YE/MU TONG/SHENG DI HUANG: Mouth, Tongue Ulcers
- ZHU YE: Mouth, Tongue Ulcers 482

HEART FIRE W/KIDNEY YIN DEFICIENCY

- DENG XIN CAO 592

HEART FIRE, EXCESS

- MU TONG/DAN ZHU YE/SHENG DI HUANG/GAN CAO/(DAO CHI SAN): Restless, Insomnia, Mouth Sores, Throat Pain, Hematuria
- ZHU SHA/SHENG DI HUANG/DANG GUI/SUAN ZAO REN: Palpitations, Insomnia, Irritability

HEART FIRE, EXCESS, MILD

- LIAN ZI/BAI HE/YI YI REN/BEI SHA SHEN: Insominia, Palpitations, Irritability, Nocturnal Emissions w/Thirst, Oliguria

HEART KIDNEY DEFICIENCY

- ROU GUI/REN SHEN/SHU DI HUANG: Palpitations, Shortness Of Breath

HEART KIDNEY DEFICIENCY, SEVERE

- LU RONG/REN SHEN

HEART KIDNEY DISCOMMUNICATION

- LIAN ZI/HUANG LIAN/DANG SHEN: Insomnia, Palpitations, Noctrnl Emissions, Thirst, Irritability

HEART KIDNEY DISHARMONY

- DENG XIN CAO 592

HEART KIDNEY YIN DEFICIENCY PATTERNS

- DAN SHEN 672

HEART LIVER BLOOD DEFICIENCY

- SUAN ZAO REN/DANG GUI/YUAN ZHI/BAI SHAO/HE SHOU WU/LONG YAN ROU: Irritability, Insomnia, Palpitations, Forgetfulnes

HEART LUNG DEFICIENCY, SEVERE

- MAI MEN DONG/REN SHEN/WU WEI ZI: Profuse Sweating, Wheezing, Exhaustion, Increased Heart Rate

HEART MUSCLE, INHIBITS

- SHI HU (c) 813

HEART MUSCLE, REDUCED OXYGEN NEEDS

- LING ZHI CAO (c) 731

HEART ORIFICE BLOCKED BY PHLEGM

- ZHU LI 728

HEART PAIN

- HAI GE KE 721
- SHAN ZHA 641
- TAN XIANG 632
- YING SU KE 832

HEART PAIN, FULLNESS

- LING LING XIANG 850

HEART PAIN, SHARP

- PU HUANG 660

HEART PAIN, VIOLENT

- SHE XIANG 756

HEART QI DEF-KIDNEY YIN DEFICIENCY

- DAN SHEN 672

HEART QI DEFICIENCY

- GAN CAO/DANG SHEN: Palpitations
- GAN CAO/DANG SHEN/GUI ZHI: Palpitations

HEART QI OBSTRUCTED

- TAN XIANG/DAN SHEN: Chest Pain

HEART QI STAGNATION

- LONG GU 738

HEART QI, BLOOD DEFICIENCY

- LONG YAN ROU/SHI CHANG PU: Forgetful, Dizzy, Fatigue

HEART RATE, INCREASES

- MAI MEN DONG/REN SHEN/WU WEI ZI: Severe Heart Lung Deficiency
- HOU PO (c) 581

HEART RATE, REDUCES

- DI GU PI (c) 495
- GOU QI ZI (c): Reduces Output Volume, Too 798
- KU SHEN (c) 491
- LI LU (c) 834
- LUO BU MA (c): Orally, Recovers In 30 Minutes 748
- NAO YANG HUA (c) 740
- XUAN FU HUA (c): Slows Heart Rate 713

HEART RESTLESSNESS

- HUANG LIAN 486

HEART SPIRIT, DISTURBED

- HE HUAN PI 731

HEART SPLEEN DEFICIENCY

- REN SHEN/FU LING /YUAN ZHI: Palpitations, Shortness Of Breath, Insomnia
- DA ZAO 761
- LONG YAN ROU: Insomnia, Dizziness, etc 800

HEART SPLEEN FIRE

- SHENG MA/HUANG LIAN: Gums, Toothache, Mouth/Tongue Ulcers

HEART SPLEEN YANG DEFICIENCY

- GUI ZHI/FU LING /BAI ZHU: Shortness Of Breath, Edema, Palpitations

HEART YANG DEFICIENCY

- FU ZI/REN SHEN/GUI ZHI: Palpitations, Chest Pain, Short Of Breath
- GUI ZHI/FU LING : Palpitations, Dyspnea
- GUI ZHI/MU LI/LONG GU: Floats In Upper, Damaged Yin In Lower: Insomnia, Irritable

HEART YANG DEFICIENCY W/BLOOD STASIS BI IN CHANNELS

ORIFICE, HEART BLOCKED BY PHLEGM

PALPITATIONS

- **BAI HE/SHENG DI HUANG:** Lingering Heat
- **BAI HE/ZHI MU/SHENG DI HUANG/(BAI HE DI HUANG TANG):** Febrile Diseases, Later Stage w/Heat
- **BAI MU ER/TAI ZI SHEN/(rock candy)**
- **BAI ZHU/GUI ZHI/FU LING /(LING GUI ZHU GAN TANG):** Phlegm Damp Syndrome
- **BAI ZI REN/YUAN ZHI/SUAN ZAO REN:** Heart Blood Deficient
- **BAI ZI REN/SUAN ZAO REN/WU WEI ZI:** Heart Blood Deficient
- **CI SHI/NIU XI/DU ZHONG/SHI JUE MING:** Yin Deficient w/Yang Rising
- **DAN SHEN/SUAN ZAO REN/BAI ZI REN:** Deficient Heart Blood
- **E JIAO/REN SHEN/DANG GUI/SHU DI HUANG:** Blood Deficiency
- **FU LING /GAN CAO:** Spleen Heat Deficient
- **FU LING /BAI ZHU/GUI ZHI/(LING GUI ZHU GAN TANG):** Phlegm-Fluid Retention
- **FU ZI/REN SHEN/GUI ZHI:** Heart Yang Deficiency
- **GAN CAO/DANG SHEN:** Heart Qi Deficient
- **GAN CAO/DANG SHEN/GUI ZHI:** Heart Qi Deficient
- **GUI ZHI/FU LING /BAI ZHU:** Spleen Heart Yang Deficient
- **HU PO/SUAN ZAO REN/YE JIAO TENG**
- **HUANG QI/LONG YAN ROU/SUAN ZAO REN/YUAN ZHI/(GUI PI TANG):** Qi And Blood Deficient
- **LIAN ZI/BAI HE/YI YI REN/BEI SHA SHEN:** Excess Heart Fire
- **LIAN ZI/HUANG LIAN/DANG SHEN:** Heart Kidney Discommunication
- **LIAN ZI/SUAN ZAO REN/BAI ZI REN/FU SHEN**
- **LONG GU/YUAN ZHI/GUI BAN**
- **LONG GU/MU LI/YUAN ZHI/SUAN ZAO REN**
- **LONG YAN ROU/SUAN ZAO REN:** Heart Blood Deficient w/Spleen Qi Deficient
- **LONG YAN ROU/REN SHEN/HUANG QI/DANG GUI/SUAN ZAO REN/(GUI PI TANG):** Qi And Blood Deficiency
- **LU RONG/REN SHEN:** Severely Deficient Heart Kidney
- **MU LI/LONG GU**
- **MU LI/LONG GU/GUI BAN/BAI SHAO:** Liver Kidney Yin Deficient w/Yang Rising
- **QIAN DAN/CHAI HU/HUANG QIN/LONG GU/MU LI**
- **REN SHEN/FU LING /YUAN ZHI:** Heart Spleen Deficiency
- **REN SHEN/SUAN ZAO REN/DANG GUI/(GUI PI TANG):** Mental Restlessness
- **ROU GUI/REN SHEN/SHU DI HUANG:** Heart Kidney Deficiency
- **SANG JI SHENG/SHENG DI HUANG/CHI SHAO YAO/JI XUE TENG:** Liver Kidney Yin Deficient w/Yang Rising
- **SHAN ZHU YU/WU WEI ZI:** Liver Kidney Yin And Yang Deficient
- **SHU DI HUANG/DANG GUI/BAI SHAO/(SI WU TANG):** Blood Deficiency
- **SHU DI HUANG/DANG GUI/BAI SHAO/CHUAN XIONG/(SI WU TANG):** Blood And Yin Deficiency

- SUAN ZAO REN/DANG SHEN/FU LING /LONG YAN ROU: Spleen Qi, Heart Blood Deficient
- SUAN ZAO REN/DANG GUI/YUAN ZHI/BAI SHAO/HE SHOU WU/LONG YAN ROU: Heat Liver Blood Deficiency
- TAI ZI SHEN/SUAN ZAO REN/WU WEI ZI: Spleen Qi Deficiency w/Blood Deficient
- WU WEI ZI/REN SHEN/MAI MEN DONG/(SHENG MAI SAN): Qi And Fluid Deficient
- WU WEI ZI/SHENG DI HUANG/MAI MEN DONG/SUAN ZAO REN/(TIAN WANG BU XIN DAN): Heart Kidney Yin/Blood Deficient
- YUAN ZHI/SUAN ZAO REN/LONG GU
- ZHU RU/BAN XIA/ZHI SHI: Hot Phlegm
- ZHU RU/ZHI SHI/CHEN PI/FU LING /(WEN DAN TANG): Phlegm Heat
- ZHU SHA/SHENG DI HUANG/DANG GUI/SUAN ZAO REN: Heart Fire, Excess

PALPITATIONS W/ANXIETY

- HU PO/YUAN ZHI/SHI CHANG PU/SUAN ZAO REN
- SUAN ZAO REN/SHU DI HUANG/DANG GUI/BAI ZI REN: Heart Blood/Yin Deficient
- YUAN ZHI/FU SHEN/SUAN ZAO REN: Heart Blood Deficient/Stagnant Qi
- ZHEN ZHU/LONG GU/MU LI/ZHU SHA
- ZHU SHA/(pig's heart): Heart Blood Deficient
- ZI SHI YING/FU SHEN/SUAN ZAO REN/HUANG QI/DANG GUI: Heart Blood Deficient/Liver Yang Rising

PALPITATIONS W/ANXIETY, RAPID BEATS

PALPITATIONS W/CHEST PAIN

- GUI ZHI/DAN SHEN: Heart Yang Deficiency w/Blood Stasis

PALPITATIONS W/DYSPNEA

- GUI ZHI/FU LING : Heart Yang Deficient

PALPITATIONS W/INSOMNIA

- FU LING /SUAN ZAO REN/YUAN ZHI/WU WEI ZI

PALPITATIONS, FROM FLUID RETENTION

- ZE XIE/FU LING /ZHU LING/BAI ZHU/(WU LING SAN)

PALPITATIONS, NEURASTHENIA

PALPITATIONS, SHORTNESS OF BREATH

- GUI ZIII/ZIII GAN CAO: Yang Qi Damage
- SHU DI HUANG/DANG GUI/BAI SHAO/CHUAN XIONG/BAI ZI REN/SUAN ZAO REN: Blood And Yin Deficiency

PERICARDIUM, HEAT CRUSHING

- NIU HUANG/HUANG LIAN/SHAN ZHI ZI/ZHU SHA: Delirium, Irritability

PERICARDIUM, HEAT IN

PERICARDIUM, HEAT PHLEGM

PULMONARY HEART DISEASE

RESTLESS HEART

SHEN DISTURBANCES

- YUAN ZHI/FU SHEN/SUAN ZAO REN: Heart Blood Deficient

SHOCK, CARDIOGENIC, INFECTIOUS, ANAPHYLACTIC

- ZHI SHI (c): Injection, Increases Blood Pressure, Does Not Work With Oral Dose 635

SHOCK, CARDIOGENIC/SEPTIC

- REN SHEN (c): Sheng Mai Zhu She Ye, Injection Gave Excellent Results 767

SHORTNESS OF BREATH

See: Lungs Shortness Of Breath 236

SYNCOPE W/HEART PAIN

- CHUAN LIAN ZI: Heat 623

TACHYCARDIA, SINUS

- CANG ZHU (c): IM Injection Of Herb Preparation (Not Mentioned) , 3-5 Days Treatment 578

End of Topic:
HEART

HEART ATTACK

See: Heart Heart Attack 154

HEART BI

See: Heart Heart Bi 154

HEART RELATED TOPICS

See: Heart Heart Related Topics 155

End of Topic:
HEART RELATED TOPICS

HEAT :

BLOOD HEAT

See: Blood Related Disorders/Topics Blood Heat
.... 45

BLOOD HEAT BLEEDING

- HUANG QIN/SHENG DI HUANG/BAI MAO GEN/CE BAI YE: Hematemesis, Epistaxis, Hematuria, Uterine Bleeding
- SHAN ZHI ZI/BAI MAO GEN/SHENG DI HUANG/HUANG QIN: Hematemesis, Epistaxis, Hematuria

BLOOD HEAT BLOTCHES/ERUPTIONS IN THROAT, MOUTH, SKIN

- DA QING YE 519

BLOOD HEAT FEBRILE DISEASE

- MU DAN PI/SHENG DI HUANG/XI JIAO/CHI SHAO YAO: Deep Red Tongue

BLOOD HEAT LEVEL

See: Blood Related Disorders/Topics Blood Heat
.... 45
See: Heat Xue Level Heat 164
- SHENG DI HUANG 500

BLOOD HEAT W/BLOOD STASIS

- YU JIN/MU DAN PI: Bleeding

BLOOD HEAT W/EXCESS TOXINS

- SHENG DI HUANG/XI JIAO/MU DAN PI/CHI SHAO YAO

BLOOD HEAT W/HIGH FEVER, MACULOPAPULE

- XUAN SHEN/ZHI MU/SHI GAO/XI JIAO

BLOOD HEAT W/YIN DEFICIENCY

- DI GU PI/ZHI MU/BIE JIA

BLOOD HEAT-YING STAGE

- CHI SHAO YAO 668

DAMP HEAT

See: Bowel Related Disorders Dysentery 59
See: Heat Wet Heat 164
- BAI JIANG CAO/YI YI REN: Suppurations
- BAI SHAO/HUANG QIN/HUANG LIAN: Dysentery: Like
- BEI XIE/HUANG BAI/YI YI REN: Skin Lesions
- DI FU ZI/KU SHEN: Pruritus
- DI FU ZI/SHENG DI HUANG/BAI XIAN PI: Pruritus
- GE GEN/HUANG LIAN: Dysentery
- GE GEN/HUANG LIAN/HUANG QIN: Dysentery
- GUANG FANG JI/YI YI REN: Pain In Extremities
- HUA SHI/FU LING /YI YI REN: Diarrhea
- TU FU LING/BEI XIE: Painful Joints
- BAI XIAN PI 515
- HUANG BAI: Leukorrhea 485
- KU SHEN 491
- QIN PI: Dysentary 493
- ZE XIE 605

DAMP HEAT BI

- HAN FANG JI/YI YI REN/HUA SHI/CAN SHA/MU GUA

DAMP HEAT BLOCKAGE

- LUO SHI TENG/MU DAN PI: Pain, Swelling

DAMP HEAT CONDITIONS W/GREASY TONGUE, DIGESTIVE PROBLEMS

- YI YI REN 602

DAMP HEAT CONGESTED AS JAUNDICE

- HUANG BAI/SHAN ZHI ZI/YIN CHEN

DAMP HEAT CONGESTED IN INTESTINES

- HUANG BAI/BAI TOU WENG/HUANG LIAN/HUANG QIN: Diarrhea, Dysentery

DAMP HEAT DISCHARGING TO INTERIOR

- HAI TONG PI 562

DAMP HEAT DISEASES

- BAI DOU KOU/XING REN/YI YI REN/HUA SHI: Early Stage
- DA DOU HUANG JUAN/HUA SHI/TONG CAO

DAMP HEAT DISORDERS

DAMP HEAT DYSENTERY

• HUANG QIN/BAI SHAO
• JIN YIN HUA/DI YU/HUANG QIN
• WU MEI/HUANG LIAN/HUANG QIN

DAMP HEAT DYSENTERY, W/TENESMUS, PAIN

• MU XIANG/BING LANG/DA HUANG/(MU XIANG BING LANG WAN)

DAMP HEAT FEBRILE DISEASE W/TURBID DAMP BLOCKS ORIFICES

• SHI CHANG PU/YU JIN: Disorientation, Unconsciousness, Irritability, Respiratory Difficulty, Flushed Face, Red Eyes, Dizziness, Auditory Dysfunction

DAMP HEAT FEBRILE DISEASE, EARLY STAGE

• BAI DOU KOU/HUA SHI/YI YI REN/SHA REN/(SAN REN TANG): Chest Stifling, Anorexia, Sticky Tongue

DAMP HEAT FEBRILE DISEASES

• HUANG QIN/HUA SHI/TONG CAO

DAMP HEAT FEVER, EARLY

• PEI LAN/HUO XIANG/QING HAO/HUA SHI/YI YI REN: Low Hunger, Low Fever, Chest Stifling

DAMP HEAT IN BLADDER

• PU HUANG/XIAO JI: Dysuria, Hematuria

DAMP HEAT IN HEART, URINARY BLADDER, LUNG CHANNELS

• DENG XIN CAO/HUA SHI: Painful, Incomplete Urine, Restless

DAMP HEAT IN INTESTINES

• ZHI SHI/DA HUANG/HUANG LIAN/HUANG QIN/(ZHI SHI DAO ZHI WAN): Dysentery, Tenesmus, Pain

DAMP HEAT IN LIVER GALL BLADDER

• BAN LAN GEN/YIN CHEN
• LONG DAN CAO/CHAI HU
• TU FU LING/PU GONG YING: Jaundice

DAMP HEAT IN LOWER BURNER

• DI YU/QIAN CAO GEN: Bleeding
• HUA SHI/DONG KUI ZI
• QU MAI/SHAN ZHI ZI
• SHI WEI/QU MAI/HUA SHI: Dysuria

DAMP HEAT IN LUNG/INTESTINES

DAMP HEAT IN URINARY BLADDER

• SHAN ZHI ZI/HUA SHI: Hot, Painful Urinary Dysfunction

DAMP HEAT INVADING MIDDLE BURNER

• XI GUA/(JUICE OF: FRESH DI HUANG,PEAR,SUGAR CANE)

DAMP HEAT JAUNDICE

• BAI HUA SHE SHE CAO/SHAN ZHI ZI/HUANG BAI/YIN CHEN
• HUANG QIN/BAI SHAO/SHAN ZHI ZI/YIN CHEN/HUANG BAI
• LONG DAN CAO/YIN CHEN

DAMP HEAT OBSTRUCTION

• TONG CAO/DA FU PI: Edema, Distension
• ZHI SHI/DA HUANG: Abdominal Pain

DAMP HEAT PAINFUL URINARY DYSFUNCTION

• HAI JIN SHA CAO/BIAN XU
• YU XING CAO/CHE QIAN ZI/BAI MAO GEN

DAMP HEAT POISONS

• TU FU LING/YI YI REN: Joint Pain

DAMP HEAT SORES

DAMP HEAT SORES, ITCHY

• BAI XIAN PI/KU SHEN

DAMP HEAT TOXIN

• SHI GAO/XI JIAO: High Fever, Rash, Unconsciousness, Epistaxis

DAMP HEAT W/LINGERING HEAT

• CHAI HU/HUANG QIN

DAMP HEAT, ANY

DAMP HEAT, DEFICIENT SPLEEN

• CHE QIAN ZI/CANG ZHU: Leukorrhea

DAMP HEAT, DOWNWARD FLOW TO LEGS

• CANG ZHU/HUANG BAI/NIU XI/(SAN MIAO WAN)

DAMP HEAT, GI

DAMP HEAT, JAUNDICE, MILD

• CHI XIAO DOU/MA HUANG/LIAN QIAO/SANG BAI PI

DAMP HEAT, QI LEVEL

• YI YI REN/HUA SHI/ZHU YE/TONG CAO/(SAN REN TANG)

DEFICIENT FIRE

See: Yin Related Disorders/Topics   Yin Deficiency,

DEFICIENT FIRE RISING

DEFICIENT HEAT/DEFICIENT YIN/QI/FLUID INJURY

DRYNESS, HEAT

EMACIATION W/HEAT IN FIVE CENTERS

EXCESS FIRE, DAMAGED FLUIDS

• SHI GAO/SHENG DI HUANG

EXTERNAL HOT/COLD

FIRE POISON

FIRE POISON RASHES

• SHENG MA/NIU BANG ZI

FIRE RISING

• DA HUANG/HUANG LIAN/HUANG QIN/(XIE XIN TANG): Swollen, Red Eyes, Sore Throat, Painful Gums

FIRE RISING, DEFICIENT

FIRE, EXCESS, DAMAGED FLUIDS

• SHI GAO/SHENG DI HUANG

FIVE CENTER HEAT

• SHU DI HUANG/GUI BAN/HUANG BAI/ZHI MU/(ZHI BAI DI HUANG WAN): Yin Deficiency w/Excess Fire

FLUIDS DAMAGED BY FIRE

• SHI GAO/SHENG DI HUANG

FLUIDS DAMAGED FROM HEAT DISEASE

• ZHU RU/LU GEN: Thirst, Vomit, Restless

FLUIDS DAMAGED IN LATE HEAT DISEASE

• SHI HU/SHENG DI HUANG/XUAN SHEN/BEI SHA SHEN: Low Grade Fever, Thirst, Blurred Vision, Achy Muscles

HEAT

HEAT ABOVE, COLD BELOW

HEAT ACCUMULATION W/DISTENTION

• DA HUANG/HUANG LIAN

HEAT CRUSHING PERICARDIUM

• NIU HUANG/HUANG LIAN/SHAN ZHI ZI/ZHU SHA: Warm Febrile Disease, Delirium, Irritability

HEAT DISEASES

HEAT DISEASES W/ACUTE ONSET

HEAT DISEASES, ANY

HEAT DISEASES, FLUIDS DAMAGED

• ZHU RU/LU GEN

HEAT DISEASES, LATE STAGE

• SHI HU/SHENG DI HUANG/XUAN SHEN/BEI SHA SHEN: Low Grade Fever, Thirst, Blurred Vision, Achy Muscles

HEAT DISEASES, LATE STAGE W/DEFICIENT YIN/LINGERING HEAT

• BAI HE/ZHI MU: Irritability, Mental Disorientation

HEAT IN FIVE CENTERS

HEAT IN HEART CHANNEL

• DAN ZHU YE/MU TONG/SHENG DI HUANG

HEAT IN KIDNEY

HEAT IN LOWER BURNER

• CHE QIAN ZI/HAI JIN SHA CAO: Dysuria

HEAT IN PERICARDIUM

HEAT IN QI/BLOOD STAGE

• XI JIAO/SHI GAO

HEAT IN SMALL INTESTINE CHANNEL

HEAT IN WEI QI LEVEL

• LIAN QIAO/NIU BANG ZI/BO HE

HEAT PHLEGM

HEAT POISON

• DONG BEI GUAN ZHONG/JIN YIN HUA/LIAN QIAO/PU GONG YING: Mumps, Abscess

HEAT SENSATION

HEAT STROKE

HEAT STROKE, SUMMER

HEAT, ACCUMULATED

HEAT, ANALGESIC FOR

HEAT, BLOOD LEVEL

HEAT, DEFICIENT

HEAT, DEFICIENT BLOOD

• SHENG DI HUANG/BAI SHAO

HEAT, DEFICIENT(W/SHAN YAO TO PREVENT AS SIDE EFFECT)

• YI ZHI REN/SHAN YAO

HEAT, EXCESS

HEAT, EXCESS AND TOXIC HEAT FROM YANG MING

• SHENG MA/SHI GAO

HEAT, EXHAUSTION W/SURFACE COMPLEX

HEAT, EXTERIOR W/SORE THROAT, IRRITABILITY

• DA QING YE/JIN YIN HUA/SHI GAO

HEAT, FEVER, HIGH & CONVULSIONS

HEAT, FLUID DAMAGE

HEAT, ILLUSIONARY & TRUE COLD

HEAT, INJURED FLUIDS

• TIAN HUA FEN/LU GEN

HEAT, INTERNAL

HEAT, LINGERING

• BAI HE/SHENG DI HUANG: Irritability, Palpitations, Insomnia, Scanty Urine

HEAT, LINGERING DAMP HEAT

• CHAI HU/HUANG QIN

HEAT, LINGERING W/DEFICIENT RESTLESSNESS

• SHAN ZHI ZI/DAN DOU CHI

HEAT, RESTLESS

HEAT, RESTLESS W/CONSUMPTION THIRST

HEAT, RESTLESS W/VOMITING

HEAT, SEVERE W/NEUROLOGICAL SYMPTOMS

HEAT, SHAO YANG CHANNELS

• CHAI HU/HUANG QIN

HEAT, TOXIC

SUMMER HEAT W/URINARY DYSFUNCTION
• HUA SHI/GAN CAO/(LIU YI SAN)

SUMMER HEAT, EXPELS
• JIN YIN HUA 524

SUMMER HEAT, EXTERIOR
• DA DOU HUANG JUAN/ZI SU YE

SUMMER HEAT, EXTREMELY TURBID
• CHAN SU: Abdominal Pain, Nausea/Vomiting 837

SUMMER HEAT/DAMPNESS W/VOMITING, DIARRHEA
• BAI BIAN DOU/XIANG RU/HOU PO/(XIANG RU SAN)

SUMMER HEATSTROKE
• CHAN SU/XIONG HUANG/CANG ZHU/DING XIANG: Heat/Dampness: Abdominal Pain, Vomit, Diarrhea

SUNSTROKE W/FEVER, THIRST
• BAI BIAN DOU 506

TOXIC HEAT
See: Heat Fire Poison 161
• ZI CAO/DA QING YE: Purpuric Rash
• DA QING YE 519
• JIN YIN HUA 524

TOXIC HEAT CONDITIONS
• DA QING YE/JIN YIN HUA: Sores, etc

TOXIC HEAT, INTERIOR SEVERE
• ZI CAO/GUA LOU REN: Carbuncles, Constipation

TOXIC HEAT, RASHES
• JIN YIN HUA/LIAN QIAO/DA QING YE/ZI CAO

TOXIC HEAT, SWELLING, PAIN OF
• SHENG MA/CHAI HU/(clear heat herbs)

WEI & QI STAGE HEAT
• JIN YIN HUA/LIAN QIAO/NIU BANG ZI
• LIAN QIAO 525

WEI STAGE HEAT
• JIN YIN HUA 524

WET HEAT
See: Heat Damp Heat 159

XUE LEVEL HEAT
See: Heat Blood Heat Level 159
• DA QING YE 519
• SHUI NIU JIAO: High Fever 501
• XI JIAO: High Fever 502

YING & BLOOD STAGE HEAT DISORDERS
• XUAN SHEN 503

YING & XUE STAGE HEAT
• JIN YIN HUA/MU DAN PI/SHENG DI HUANG

YING STAGE HEAT
• BAI WEI/DI GU PI: Steaming Bone Syndrome
• DAN SHEN/MU DAN PI/SHENG DI HUANG: High Fever, Subcutaneous Bleeding, Other Bleeding
• HUANG LIAN/SHENG DI HUANG: Insomnia, Delirium
• MAI MEN DONG/SHENG DI HUANG/ZHU YE/HUANG LIAN/(QING YING TANG): Insomnia, Irritability
• MU DAN PI/BIE JIA/ZHI MU/SHENG DI HUANG: Fevers In Afternoon, Evening
• SHENG DI HUANG/XUAN SHEN: Excess Thirst, Irritability
• DAN SHEN: Insomnia, Palpitations, Restlessness, Irritability 672
• QING HAO 508
• SHENG DI HUANG 500
• SHUI NIU JIAO: High Fever 501
• XI JIAO: High Fever 502

YING STAGE HEAT W/WIND
• DAN SHEN/SHENG DI HUANG/XUAN SHEN/ZHU YE

YING STAGE, BLOOD HEAT
• CHI SHAO YAO 668

YING/XUE HEAT DAMAGE
• MU DAN PI/CHI SHAO YAO: Rashes, Hematemesis

YING/XUE HEAT W/SUSTAINED FEVER
• BAI WEI/DI GU PI/SHENG DI HUANG

YING/XUE STAGE HEAT
• SHENG DI HUANG/XUAN SHEN/XI JIAO/MAI MEN DONG
• XUAN SHEN/SHENG DI HUANG/MAI MEN DONG: Thirst, Deep Red Tongue, Insomnia, Fever

End of Topic:
HEAT

HEAT IN HEART CHANNEL
See: Heart Heat In Heart Channel 157

HEAT IN KIDNEY
See: Kidneys Heat In Kidney 199

HEAT IN PERICARDIUM
See: Heart Heat In Pericardium 157

HEAT IN SMALL INTESTINE CHANNEL
See: Abdomen/Gastrointestinal Topics Heat In Small Intestine Channel 32

HEAT RELATED TOPICS
See: Heat Heat Related Topics 161

HEATSTROKE
See: Heat Heatstroke 163

HEAVINESS SENSATION

See: Pain/Numbness/General Discomfort
Heaviness Sensation 301

HEMAFECIA RELATED TOPICS

See: Hemorrhagic Disorders Hemafecia Related
Topics 167

HEMATEMESIS

See: Hemorrhagic Disorders Hematemesis 168

HEMATINIC

See: Blood Related Disorders/Topics Hematinic
.... 49

HEMATURIA RELATED TOPICS

See: Hemorrhagic Disorders Hematuria Related
Topics 169

HEMIPLEGIA RELATED TOPICS

See: Mental State/Neurological Disorders
Hemiplegia Related Topics 248

HEMOLYTIC

See: Blood Related Disorders/Topics Hemolytic
.... 49

HEMOPHILIA

See: Hemorrhagic Disorders Hemophilia 170

HEMOPTYSIS

See: Hemorrhagic Disorders Hemoptysis 170

HEMORRHAGE TOPICS

See: Hemorrhagic Disorders Hemorrhage Topics
.... 171

End of Topic:
HEMORRHAGE TOPICS

HEMORRHAGIC DISORDERS :

BLEEDING

See: Trauma, Bites, Poisonings Wounds 417
See: Hemorrhagic Disorders Hemorrhage 171
• CE BAI YE/AI YE/GAN JIANG: Cold Deficient
• DA JI/XIAO JI/CE BAI YE: Heat
• HAI PIAO XIAO/QIAN CAO GEN/CHEN ZONG TAN/E JIAO
• QIAN CAO GEN/DA JI/XIAO JI/CE BAI YE: Heat
• SHENG DI HUANG/CE BAI YE/HE YE: Blood Heat
• XIAO JI/BAI MAO GEN/PU HUANG/CE BAI YE: Blood Heat
• CE BAI YE: Hot Blood 654
• CHE QIAN CAO 589
• CHI FU LING: Deficient 483
• CHI SHAO YAO: Blood Heat 668
• DI GU PI: Blood Heat 495
• JIANG XIANG (c): Clotting Time, Mildly Lengthens From
Oral Dose 659
• JING JIE: Mild Hemostat 447

• PU HUANG (c): Hemostatic 660
• QIAN CAO GEN: Blood Heat 662
• SHAN ZHI ZI: Heat 476
• XI JIAO (c): Blood Heat Types, With Sheng Di, Chi Shao
(e.g. Xi Jiao Sheng Di Tang) 502
• XUE JIE: Topical 692

BLEEDING FROM TRAUMA

• SAN QI/LONG GU/WU BEI ZI/(topical)

BLEEDING GUMS

• CE BAI YE 654
• NIU XI: Yin Deficient With Fire Rising 684

BLEEDING, ANY TYPE

• DI YU: Hot, Cold, Deficient, *Use w/Huai Hua Mi For
Lower Jiao Bleedng 656
• E JIAO: (Best Consumptive Types) 797
• XIAN HE CAO: Hot, Cold, Deficient 665

BLEEDING, CHRONIC

• FU LONG GAN/ROU GUI/AI YE/DANG GUI: Cold,
Deficient Spleen
• DANG SHEN 762
• OU JIE 660

BLEEDING, DURING PREGNANCY

• DU ZHONG 775

BLEEDING, EXTERNAL

• PU HUANG/HAI PIAO XIAO/(topical)

BLEEDING, FUNCTIONAL

• CHEN ZONG TAN 655
• LING XIAO HUA 680
• XIAO JI 666

BLEEDING, GENERAL INTERNAL/EXTERNAL

• SAN QI 663

BLEEDING, GENITALS

• XUE YU TAN 666

BLEEDING, IN LOWER JIAO

• HE YE: Heat/Stagnation 507

BLEEDING, INTERNAL/EXTERNAL

• ZI ZHU CAO 667

BLEEDING, LIPS/ORAL CAVITY

• MA BO: Topical 528

BLEEDING, LOCAL

• SHAN ZHI ZI (c): Powder 476

BLEEDING, MANY KINDS

• XUE YU TAN 666

BLEEDING, POSTPARTUM

• SHAN ZHA 641

HEMAFECIA W/DIARRHEA, PAINFUL STOOLS

HEMAFECIA W/HEMORRHOIDS

- HUANG QIN/HUANG LIAN/FANG FENG

HEMAFECIA, CHRONIC

- FU LONG GAN/ROU GUI/AI YE/DANG GUI: Cold, Deficient Spleen
- HAN LIAN CAO/DI YU: Cold Deficient SP/KI
- PU HUANG/(quick fried ginger): Cold Deficient Spleen Kidneys

HEMATEMESIS

See: Stomach/Digestive Disorders Vomiting, Blood In 402
- BAI JI/HAI PIAO XIAO/(WU JI SAN)
- CE BAI YE/DA JI/XIAO JI/BAI MAO GEN: Heat
- CHEN ZONG TAN/BAI MAO GEN/DA JI/XIAO JI/SHAN ZHI ZI/(SHI HUI SAN): Heat
- DA HUANG/HUANG LIAN/HUANG QIN/(XIE XIN TANG): Hot Blood
- DAI ZHE SHI/SHENG DI HUANG/MU DAN PI: Blood Heat In Liver Stomach Disharmony w/Rebellious Qi
- DAI ZHE SHI/SHENG DI HUANG/MU DAN PI/ZI WAN/KUAN DONG HUA/XING REN: Lungs, Hot Blood
- Hemoptysis: Lungs, Hot Blood
- Liver Stomach Disharmony w/Hot Blood: Hematemesis, Hemoptosis: Especially Cough
- DAI ZHE SHI/BAI SHAO/ZHU RU/NIU BANG ZI/(HAN JIANG TANG): Blood Heat

- DI GU PI/MU DAN PI: Steaming Bone Syndrome, From Deficient Blood
- E JIAO/SHENG DI HUANG: Blood Heat
- E JIAO/AI YE/SHENG DI HUANG/PU HUANG/OU JIE
- GUAN ZHONG/CE BAI YE/XIAN HE CAO/CHEN ZONG TAN: Heat
- HAN LIAN CAO/CE BAI YE
- HAN LIAN CAO/SHENG DI HUANG: Blood Heat
- HAN LIAN CAO/SHENG DI HUANG/E JIAO/BAI MAO GEN/PU HUANG: Yin Deficiency w/Internal Heat
- HUANG QIN/BAI SHAO/SHAN ZHI ZI/YIN CHEN/HUANG BAI/MU DAN PI/DA HUANG
- HUANG QIN/SHENG DI HUANG/BAI MAO GEN/CE BAI YE: Blood Heat
- MU DAN PI/CHI SHAO YAO: Ying/Xue Level Heat
- MU DAN PI/BAI MAO GEN: Febrile Diseases
- NIU XI/XIAO JI/CE BAI YE/BAI MAO GEN: Blood Heat
- OU JIE/BAI JI/QIAN CAO GEN
- OU JIE/BAI JI/CE BAI YE/BAI MAO GEN
- PI PA YE/BAI MAO GEN: Heat
- PU HUANG/XIAN HE CAO/CE BAI YE/HAN LIAN CAO
- QING DAI/CE BAI YE/BAI MAO GEN: Blood Heat
- SAN QI/BAI JI
- SAN QI/HUA RUI SHI/XUE YU TAN/(HUA XUE DAN)
- SHAN ZHI ZI/CE BAI YE/SHENG DI HUANG: Heat Induced
- SHAN ZHI ZI/BAI MAO GEN
- SHAN ZHI ZI/BAI MAO GEN/SHENG DI HUANG/HUANG QIN: Blood Heat
- SHENG DI HUANG/E JIAO: Deficient Heat
- SHENG DI HUANG/BAI SHAO/BAI MAO GEN/DI YU: Blood Heat
- XI JIAO/SHENG DI HUANG: Blood Heat
- XI JIAO/SHENG DI HUANG/MU DAN PI/CHI SHAO YAO/DA QING YE/ZI CAO: Blood Heat
- XI JIAO/SHENG DI HUANG/MU DAN PI/CHI SHAO YAO: Blood Heat
- XIAN HE CAO/CE BAI YE
- XIAN HE CAO/SHENG DI HUANG/MU DAN PI/SHAN ZHI ZI/CE BAI YE: Heat
- YIN CHAI HU/HU HUANG LIAN: Blood Heat
- ZI ZHU CAO/XIAN HE CAO/HAN LIAN CAO

HEMATEMESIS, W/BLOOD STAGNATION

HEMATEMESIS, W/CONSTIPATION

HEMATOCHEZIA

HEMATURIA

HEMATURIA W/OLIGURIA

HEMATURIA W/PAIN

HEMATURIA W/STABBING PAIN

HEMATURIA W/URINATION DISTURBANCE

HEMATURIA, CHRONIC

HEMATURIA, DYSURIA

HEMATURIA, URINARY STONES W/LOW BACK PAIN

HEMOPHILIA

HEMOPTYSIS

- BAI MAO GEN/SHENG DI HUANG/OU JIE: Heat
- BAI MU ER/BAI HE/BEI SHA SHEN/(rock candy)
- CE BAI YE/DA JI/XIAO JI/BAI MAO GEN: Heat
- CHEN ZONG TAN/BAI MAO GEN/DA JI/XIAO JI/SHAN ZHI ZI/(SHI HUI SAN): Heat
- DAI ZHE SHI/SHENG DI HUANG/MU DAN PI: Blood Heat In Liver Stomach Disharmony w/Rebellious Qi
- DAN SHEN/MU DAN PI/SHENG DI HUANG: Ying Level Heat
- DONG CHONG XIA CAO/XING REN/CHUAN BEI MU/E JIAO: Lung Yin Deficient
- HAI PIAO XIAO/BAI JI/CHUAN BEI MU
- HAN LIAN CAO/SHENG DI HUANG: Lung Deficiency
- HUA RUI SHI/BAI JI: Consumptive Lung
- HUAI HUA MI/CE BAI YE
- HUAI HUA MI/CE BAI YE/BAI MAO GEN/XIAN HE CAO
- OU JIE/SHENG DI HUANG/E JIAO/CHUAN BEI MU: Lung Heat
- OU JIE/BAI JI/CE BAI YE/BAI MAO GEN
- PU HUANG/XIAN HE CAO/CE BAI YE/HAN LIAN CAO
- QIAN CAO GEN/SHENG DI HUANG/BAI JI: Heat
- QING DAI/CE BAI YE/BAI MAO GEN: Blood Heat
- SAN QI/BAI JI
- SAN QI/HUA RUI SHI/XUE YU TAN/(HUA XUE DAN)
- SHENG DI HUANG/E JIAO: Deficient Heat
- SHI WEI/DI YU: Lung Heat
- XIAN HE CAO/E JIAO: Deficient Lung Yin
- XIAN HE CAO/SHENG DI HUANG/MU DAN PI/SHAN ZHI ZI/CE BAI YE: Heat
- XUE YU TAN/DANG GUI/YI MU CAO: Deficiency
- YU JIN/MU DAN PI: Blood Heat/Blood Stagnation
- ZHU SHA/HAI GE KE: Lung Heat
- ZI WAN/BAI BU: Cough, Chronic/Acute
- ZI ZHU CAO/XIAN HE CAO/HAN LIAN CAO

- ZI ZHU CAO (c): Increased Platelets, Shortens Bleeding Time 667

HEMOSTATIC, MILD

- QIAN CAO GEN (c): Local Application With Gauze For 35 Seconds, Charred Herb Better 662

INTESTINAL BLEEDING

- CI WEI PI 819

INTESTINAL BLEEDING IN WOMEN

- QIN PI 493

INTESTINAL HEMORRHAGE

- CHEN ZONG TAN 655
- GE HUA 521

INTESTINAL WIND W/BLOODY STOOL

- HUAI HUA MI/JING JIE/ZHI KE: Hemafecia
- HUANG QIN/HUANG LIAN/FANG FENG
- HUANG QIN/DI YU

INTESTINAL WIND W/MELENA

- HE ZI 822

MELENA

- XIAN HE CAO 665

PURPURA

See: Skin Purpura 364

SHOCK, HEMORRHAGE

- REN SHEN (c): Du Shen Tang (Ren Shen + Fu Zi) 767

UTERINE BLEEDING

See: Sexuality, Female: Gynecological Uterine Bleeding 338

End of Topic:
HEMORRHAGIC DISORDERS

HEMORRHOIDS

See: Bowel Related Disorders Hemorrhoids . . . 62

HEMOSTATIC

See: Hemorrhagic Disorders Hemostatic 172

HEPATIC CANCER

See: Cancer/Tumors/Swellings/Lumps Hepatic Cancer 68

HEPATIC CANCER RELATED TOPICS

See: Liver Hepatic Cancer Related Topics 203

HEPATITIS RELATED TOPICS

See: Liver Hepatitis Related Topics 203

HEPATOLITHIASIS

See: Liver Hepatolithiasis 205

HEPATOMEGALY

See: Liver Hepatomegaly 205

End of Topic:
HEPATOMEGALY

HERBAL FUNCTIONS :

DU CHANNEL GUIDING HERB

- QIANG HUO 449

GUIDING HERB

- QIANG HUO: Qi To Tai Yang And Du Ch's 449

GUIDING HERB TO HEAD/FACE

- SHENG MA 467

HERBAL PREPARATION

- FENG MI 548

HERBS, DIRECTS UPWARDS

- JIE GENG 711

HERBS, GUIDING TO ALL 12 CH

- GAN CAO 763

HERBS, HARMONIZES OTHER

- SHENG JIANG/DA ZAO

HERBS, HARSH

- DA ZAO: Harmonizes And Moderates 761

HERBS, MODERATING, HARMONIZES

- GAN CAO 763

SWELLING, FROM USE OF THESE HERBS, ADD CHEN PI

- CHEN PI/DANG SHEN/HUANG QI

TAI YANG CHANNEL GUIDING HERB

- QIANG HUO 449

End of Topic:
HERBAL FUNCTIONS

HERBAL PREPARATION

See: Herbal Functions Herbal Preparation 173

HERBS, DIRECTS/GUIDES/HARMONIZES TOPICS

See: Herbal Functions Herbs, Directs/Guides/Harmonizes Topics 173

HERBS, TONIFYING

See: Energetic State Herbs, Tonifying 105

HERNIA RELATED TOPICS

See: Abdomen/Gastrointestinal Topics Hernia Related Topics 32

HERPES RELATED TOPICS

See: Infectious Diseases Herpes Related Topics 188

HYPOGONADISM

See: **Sexuality, Either Sex** Hypogonadism 319

HYPOTENSION

See: **Circulation Disorders** Hypotension 87

HYPOTHERMIA

See: **Nutritional/Metabolic Disorders/Topics**
Hypothermia 281

HYPOTHYROID

See: **Endocrine Related Disorders** Hypothyroid
.... 102

HYPOXIA PROTECTION

See: **Nutritional/Metabolic Disorders/Topics**
Hypoxia Protection 282

HYSTERIA

See: **Mental State/Neurological Disorders**
Hysteria 249

ILLNESS, RECOVERY FROM

See: **Energetic State** Illness, Recovery From 105

IMMUNE EFFECT RELATED TOPICS

See: **Immune System Related Disorders/Topics**
Immune Effect Related Topics 176

End of Topic:
IMMUNE EFFECT RELATED TOPICS

IMMUNE SYSTEM RELATED DISORDERS/ TOPICS :

ADENITIS

• SHI SHANG BAI: (Inflammation Of Lymph Gland) 534

ALLERGIC DERMATITIS

• BO HE (c): Modify Jing Feng Bai Du Tang 456
• JING JIE (c): Jing Fang Bai Du Tang/Wu Wei Xiao Du Yin,
Modified Helped 447

ALLERGIC DISORDERS

• GAN CAO (c): Inhibits Histamine Induced Capillary
Permeability 763
• HUANG QIN (c): Oral, Inhibits Mast Cells' Release Of
Enzymes 489
• LING ZHI CAO (c): Markedly Inhibits Reaction 731
• LU LU TONG (c) 681
• WU MEI (c): Counteracts Histamine Shock, Protein
Sensitization 830

ALLERGIC INFLAMMATION

• QIN JIAO 569

ALLERGIC REACTIONS

• CHAN TUI (c) 458

ALLERGIC RESPONSE, ARTHUS PHENOMENON, DECREASES

• HUAI HUA MI (c) 658

ALLERGIC RHINITIS

• CANG ER ZI (c): Herb Powder Macerate In ETOH, 12
Days, Percolate With ETOH, Evaporate, Make Tablets
Each Equivalent To 1.5 g Of Crude Herb, Dose—2 Tabs,
3x/Day For 2 Weeks, 72% Effective 559
• MAO DONG QING (c): Decoction 682

ALLERGIC TRACHEAL CONSTRICTION

• HUANG QIN (c) 489

ALLERGIC, ANTI-

• AI YE (c): Oral, Oil, Inhibits Histamines 651
• CHEN PI (c) 621
• DA HUANG (c) 542
• DA ZAO (c): Cyclic-Amp In Aqueous Extract 761
• DI GU PI (c): No Side Effects, More For Skin, Mucous
Membranes Than Internal Organs 495
• GAN CAO (c) 763
• GUI ZHI (c): Strong 445
• HAN FANG JI (c): Inhibits Allergic Reactions, Wheezing
.... 596
• HUANG QIN (c): Skin 489
• LONG KUI (c) 526
• MA HUANG (c): Release Of Mediators Suppressed By
ETOH/Aqueous Extract 448
• MU DAN PI (c): ETOH ext 499
• NIU XI (c): Aqueous Extract 684
• WU MEI (c) 830
• XI XIN (c): Aqueous/ETOH Extract 452
• XIONG DAN (c) 479
• ZHEN ZHU (c) 740
• ZHI SHI (c): Inhibits Histamine Release 635

ALLERGIES

See: **Skin** Allergies 351
See: **Nose** Rhinitis, Allergic 279
See: **Immune System Related Disorders/Topics**
Mast Cell Inhibitor 178
• BAI GUO YE (c): Respiratory Effects Of 817
• CHAN SU (c): Antihypersensitivity Effect 837
• DA ZAO 761
• LING ZHI CAO 731
• NIU XI (c): Aqueous Extract Helps 684
• REN SHEN (c): Reduces Anaphylactic Shock, Inhibits
Alllergic Edema, Antihistamine Action 767
• SHAN DOU GEN (c): Markedly Suppressed With
Injection 532
• SHAN ZHU YU (c): Antihistamine Effect 827
• ZI HE CHE (c) 792

ALLERGIES, ANTIANAPHYLACTIC, ANTIHISTAMINE

• LONG DAN CAO (c): Gentianine 492

ALLERGIES, ASTHMA

• ZI HE CHE 792

ALLERGIES, HAYFEVER

• LU LU TONG/CANG ER ZI/XIN YI HUA: Allergic Rhinitis

ALLERGIES, ITCHING

• MU ZEI/BAI JI LI

ALLERGIES, PROTECTS AGAINST

• LONG KUI (c) 526

ALLERGIES, REDUCES REACTION TO

• LING ZHI CAO (c) 731

ALLERGIES, RHINITIS

• CANG ER ZI/XIN YI HUA/WU WEI ZI/JIN YING ZI
• LU LU TONG/CANG ER ZI/XIN YI HUA
• CANG ER ZI 559

ALLERGIES, TO CLAMS

• NIU HUANG (c): 0.1 g Tab, 3 Tabs 3x/Day 755

ALLERGY, TO DRUGS

• AI YE (c): Decoction 651

ANAPHLACTIC, ANTI-

• HUANG QIN (c) 489

ANAPHYLACTIC PURPURA

• DA ZAO 761
• DI GU PI (c): Di Gu Pi, 50 g, Xu Chang Qing
(Radix/Herba Cynanchu Paniculatum) , 25 g) 495
• SHANG LU (c) 554

ANAPHYLACTIC SHOCK

• QIN JIAO (c): IP Injection 569

ANTIBODY FORMATION, INHANCES

• SHU YANG QUAN (c): With 1: 1 Da Zao 535

ANTIGENIC, STRONG

• TIAN HUA FEN (c) 726

COLITIS, ALLERGIC

• LAI FU ZI (c): Retention Enema Of 639

GLANDS, SWOLLEN

• XIA KU CAO/MU LI/XUAN SHEN/KUN BU: Phlegm Fire
• CHUAN BEI MU 717
• HAI ZAO: Phlegm 721
• HUANG YAO ZI 723
• KUN BU: Hot Phlegm 724
• XIA KU CAO: Phlegm Fire 478

HIV+

• LING ZHI CAO 731

HIVES

• BAI XIAN PI/FANG FENG/BAI JI LI
• BAI JI LI 743

HIVES, ITCHING

• MU ZEI/BAI JI LI

IMMUNE EFFECT

• SANG ZHI (c): Increases Lymphocyte Production, 30
g/Day As Decoction With Other Herbs 570
• WU JIA PI (c): Reduces Loss Of Lymphocytes 574

IMMUNE REACTION

• BI MA ZI (c): Strongly Antigenic, Increases Antibody
Production, Allergic Reaction 547

IMMUNE RESPONSE

• DA SUAN (c): Paste With Mang Xiao, On Lower Right
Quad, Increases Peristalsis, Activated Immune
Response 644
• DAN SHEN (c): Increases 672
• LONG KUI (c): Stimulates Antibody Formation 526
• LU RONG (c): Desensitizing On Reexposure Of
Presensitized Animals 784
• MU TONG (c): Increases Ability Of Phagocytosis 599
• REN SHEN (c): Increases WBC Production And Reduces
Their Decrease, *Long Term, Small Dose Helps
Reticuloendothelial System Where Large Doses Hinders
Response, *Inflammatory Response Lowered 767
• SHUI NIU JIAO (c): Raises White Blood Cell Count,
Increase Tissue Activity In Spleen, Lymph Nodes 501
• XI JIAO (c): Raises White Blood Cell Count, Increase
Tissue Activity In Spleen, Lymph Nodes 502

IMMUNE SYSTEM

• BAN MAO (c): Stimulates Bone Marrow To Produce
White Blood Cells 837
• CHUAN SHAN JIA (c): Raises WBC Count 670
• CHUAN XIN LIAN (c): Increase WBC Activity 518
• HUANG LIAN (c): Increases WBC Phagocytosis 486
• LONG DAN CAO (c): Suppressed Antibody Formation
.... 492
• MANG XIAO (c): Increases Phagocytosis 545
• TAN XIANG (c): Increases White Blood Cells 632
• YU XING CAO (c): Very Good, Increases WBC
Phagocytosis, Other Activity 539

IMMUNE SYSTEM ENHANCEMENT

• AI YE (c): Increased Phagocytosis 651
• BAI HUA SHE SHE CAO (c): Increases Phagocytic
Activity Of Leukocytes, Antiinfective 511
• BAI ZHU (c) 760
• CHAN SU (c) 837
• DAN SHEN (c): Increases Macrophage Activity 672
• DANG SHEN (c): Oral, 0.25 g/Day 1-2 Weeks, Increased
Phagocytosis, Similar To Huang Qi, Ling Zhi Cao,
Synergistic With Ling Zhi 762
• DU ZHONG (c): Increased Phagocytosis, Similar To
Huang Qi/Dang Shen, But Different Route 775
• E ZHU (c): Contributes To Antineoplastic Effects 673
• FU LING (c): Oral With Dang Shen, Bai Zhu Significantly
Increased 594
• GOU QI ZI (c): Aqueous Extract Orally/100% ETOH
Extract IM Injection Markedly Increased Phagocytosis,
*Use With Dang Shen, 1: 2, Also 798

- HUANG BAI (c): Markedly Increases Antibody Formation 485
- HUANG QI (c): Increases Phagocytosis, Size Of Spleen, Plasma Cells And Antibodies, 32% Decoction PO For 2 Weeks, Use As Ling Zhi Cao Mixture (Herb, Dang Shen, Ling Zhi Cao) , Resembled Interferon Mediator, Tilorone 765
- JIE GENG (c): Aqueous Extract Enhances Phagocytosis 711
- JIN YIN HUA (c): Increased Phagocytosis 524
- LIAN QIAO (c): Antiinflammatory, Increased Antibody Formation, Qing Dan Injection (Lian Qiao, Jin Yin Hua, Pu Gong Ying, Chai Hu, Huang Qin, Qing Pi, Da Huang, Long Dan Cao, Dan Shen, Ban Xia (Treated) , Dan Zhu Ye) 525
- LING ZHI CAO (c): Enhanced Phagocytic Function, Herb With Dang Shen Particularly Effective 731
- LU RONG (c): Promotes Lymphocyte Transformation 784
- MA DOU LING (c): Increases Phagocytosis 701
- PU GONG YING (c) 529
- QING MU XIANG (c): Increases Nonspecific Antibodies, Phagocytic Activity 628
- REN SHEN (c) 767
- SAN QI (c) 663
- SANG SHEN ZI (c): Modest 801
- SANG YE (c): Increased Phagocytosis, Sang Ju Yin 466
- SHU YANG QUAN (c): With (1: 1) Da Jao, Increase Antibody Formation And Non-Specific Immune Response 535
- WU JIA SHEN (c): Enhanced Phagocytosis, Increased Antibody Formation 771
- WU MEI (c) 830
- YE JU HUA (c): Increased Phagocytic Function Of WBC 468
- YIN YANG HUO (c): Increased Phagocytosis 791
- ZHU LING (c): Extract, ETOH Extract Helps Phagocytosis, T-Cell Transformation 606
- ZI HE CHE (c): Oral Administration, Injected Contains Gamma-Globulin, Interferon 792

IMMUNE SYSTEM ENHANCEMENT, PHAGOCYTOSIS

- DANG GUI (c) 795

IMMUNE SYSTEM, INHIBITS

- DANG GUI (c): Similar To Azathioprine 795

IMMUNE SYSTEM, STRENGTHENS

- CHAI HU (c): Inhibits Effect Of Histamine On Capillary Permeability, Other Antibody Formation 457
- WU JIA SHEN (c) 771

IMMUNE SYSTEM, WEAKENED

- DONG CHONG XIA CAO/(with meat): We Qi Weakened

IMMUNOLOGICAL DISEASE

- SHENG DI HUANG (c) 500

INFLAMMATION

See: Trauma, Bites, Poisonings Inflammation .. 410

JOINTS, PAINFUL, SWOLLEN FROM ALLERGIC RESPONSE

- DANG GUI (c): Yi Shen Tang (Dang Gui, Chi Shao, Chuan Xiong, Hong Hua, Dan Shen, Tao Ren) 795

LUPUS ERYTHEMATOSUS

- QING HAO (c): Active Ingredient, Arteannuin, Given Orally, 0.1 g, 2x/Day, 1ST Month, 0.1 g, 3x/Day, 2nd Month, 0.1 g, 4x/Day, 3rd Month, Achieve Some Remission In All Patients, But First Few Days Worsened With Tingling Sensation, Ok After 2 Weeks, Takes 50 Days To See Improvement, *May Use 36-54 g Honeyed Herb Powder, Took 1 Month For Rash To Subside, 2-3 Months To Disappear 508

LYMPH GLANDS

See: Cancer/Tumors/Swellings/Lumps
Lymphatic Cancer 69

LYMPH GLANDS, ENLARGEMENT, CHRONIC

- CHUAN BEI MU: Phlegm Nodules 717
- CHUAN SHAN JIA: Phlegm Nodules 670
- HAI FU SHI: Phlegm Nodules 720
- HAI GE KE: Phlegm Nodules 721
- HAI ZAO: Phlegm Nodules 721
- HE SHOU WU: Phlegm Nodules 799
- HONG DA JI: Phlegm Nodules 551
- KUN BU: Phlegm Nodules 724
- LIAN QIAO: Phlegm Nodules 525
- MU LI: Phlegm Nodules 739
- SHE XIANG: Phlegm Nodules 756
- WA LENG ZI: Phlegm Nodules 690
- XIA KU CAO: Phlegm Nodules 478
- XUAN SHEN: Phlegm Nodules 503

LYMPH GLANDS, SWOLLEN

- BAN MAO: Topical 837

LYMPH NODES, CHRONIC SWOLLEN INFLAMMATION OF

- KUN BU 724

LYMPH NODES, INFLAMED

- LIAN QIAO 525

LYMPH NODES, PAIN

- DI LONG: Wind 744
- TU FU LING 536

LYMPH NODES, SWELLING

- BAI JIE ZI 708
- BI MA ZI: Topical 547
- BO HE 456
- DAI MAO: Wind Pain 743
- HAI FU SHI: Phlegm Fire 720
- HAI ZAO: Phlegm 721
- HE SHOU WU 799
- HUANG YAO ZI 723
- MU LI 739
- PU GONG YING 529

End of Topic:
INFECTIONS AND RELATED TOPICS

INFECTIOUS DISEASES :

ANTIBIOTIC

- XI HE LIU (c): Inhibits Pneumococcus, Strep, Staph .. 451
- XIANG FU (c) 633
- XIANG RU (c): Broad Spectrum 453
- XING REN (c): B.Typhi, B.Paratyphi, etc 705
- XIONG HUANG (c) 848
- XUAN FU HUA (c): Strongly Inhibits Staph Aureus, Bacillus Anthracis, Shigella, Salmonella, Pseudomonas, Proteus, C.Diphtheriae 713
- XUAN SHEN (c): Pseud.Aeruginosa 503
- YE JU HUA (c): 1 : 5 Decoction Staph Aureus, Shigella, Many Others, Fresh More Potent, Heat Reduced Effect 468
- YI MU CAO (c) 694
- YI YI REN (c): Decoction Of Root, Staph Aureus, Strep, B.Anthracis, Corynebacterium Diphtheriae 602
- YIN CHEN (c): Staph Aureus, Strep., B.Dysenteriae, Pneumococci, C.Diphteriae, B.Typhi, B.Subtilis, Mycobacteria, et al 603
- YU JIN (c) 695
- YUAN HUA (c) 556
- YUAN ZHI (c): ETOH Extract—Staph, Shigella, B.Tuberculosis, Diplococcus Pneumoniae 734
- ZAO XIU (c): B.Dysenteriae, B.Typhi, B.Paratyphi, Streptococci, Meningococci, etc, (May Be Stonger Than Huang Lian) 540
- ZE XIE (c): Staph, Pneumococci, Mycobacteria, etc ... 605
- ZHI XUE CAO (c): Water Extract 697
- ZHU LING (c): Staph, E.Coli 606
- ZHU SHA (c): Topical 741

BACTERIOSTATIC

- XIONG DAN (c) 479

BOILS, INTERNAL

- FENG LA 840

BRUCELLOSIS

- HUANG LIAN (c) 486

BRUCELLOSIS, CHRONIC

- CHUAN SHAN LONG (c): Decoction Helped 442
- SANG ZHI (c): Sang Liu Tang/Wan (Sang Zhi, Dang Gui, Mo Yao, Mu Gua, Hong Hua, Fang Feng, Liu Zhi (Willow) , Herba Geranii Seu Erodii (Geranium) , Wu Jia Pi) Helped Cases Unresponsive To Antibiotics 570

CANDIDA

- DA SUAN (c): Oral With Sugar As Paste, Multivitamins 644

CANDIDA ALBICANS

- BAI FAN (c) 836
- BAI TOU WENG (c): Bai Tou Weng Decoction 514

CANDIDIASIS, ORAL

- CHAI HU (c): Even Not Responsive To Nystatin, Trichomycin, Amphotericin Effectively Treated With Chai Hu Qing Gan Tang 457
- WU ZHU YU (c): Apply Powder Mixed With Wax To Soles Of Feet At Bedtime, Good Results 618

CANDIDIASIS, VAGINAL

- HU ZHANG (c) 497

- PENG SHA: Severe 844

CELLULITIS

- DA HUANG (c) 542
- DAN SHEN (c) 672
- HUANG LIAN (c): Topical 20% Vaseline Dressing, 3% Solution With Oral Powder 486
- QIAN LI GUANG (c): Topical 474

CHANCERS, SYPHILITIC

- QING FEN: Topical Wash 845

CHICKEN POX

- BAN LAN GEN (c): IM Injection Of 50% Solution, 2 ml/Day, Lowered Temperature In 1-3 Days 515
- CHUAN XIN LIAN (c) 518
- ZI CAO 504

CHOLERA

- HU JIAO 615
- HUANG LIAN (c): Controls Diarrhea In Mild Cases, In Early Stage Helped Disease, Too 486

CHOLERA, CALF MUSCLE SPASMS

- CAN SHA 558

COMMON COLD

See: Wind Disorders   Wind Heat 434
See: Wind Disorders   Wind Cold 432
See: Exterior Conditions   Exterior Conditions ... 107
See: Infectious Diseases   Flu 185
- BAI BU/JING JIE/JIE GENG/ZI WAN: Cough Of
- CANG ZHU/FANG FENG/XI XIN: Wind Cold Damp
- CHAN TUI/PANG DA HAI/NIU BANG ZI/JIE GENG: Wind Heat w/Hoarse Voice
- CHUAN XIONG/FANG FENG/JING JIE: Headache
- DAN DOU CHI/CONG BAI: Deficient Yin
- DOU CHI JIANG/JING JIE/ZI SU YE: Wind Cold
- DU HUO/QIANG HUO/(QIANG HUO SHENG SHI TANG): Wind Cold
- FANG FENG/JING JIE/QIANG HUO: Wind Cold w/General Pain
- FU PING/BAI JI LI/NIU BANG ZI/BO HE: Fever, Headache
- FU ZI/MA HUANG/XI XIN/(MA HUANG FU ZI XI XIN TANG): Wind Cold In Person w/Deficient Yang
- GE GEN/CHAI HU/HUANG QIN: Wind Heat w/Dry Throat, Painful Eyes
- GUAN ZHONG/JIN YIN HUA/LIAN QIAO/DA QING YE/BAN LAN GEN: Wind Heat
- JIN YIN HUA/LIAN QIAO/NIU BANG ZI: Wind Heat
- JING JIE/BO HE/FANG FENG/QIANG HUO: Wind Cold
- JING JIE/BO HE/SANG YE/JU HUA: Wind Heat
- LIAN QIAO/BAN LAN GEN/JING JIE/BO HE
- LIAN QIAO/NIU BANG ZI/BO HE: Wind Heat
- MA HUANG/GUI ZHI: Wind Cold Exterior Excess
- QIAN HU/JIE GENG: Wind Heat-Cough, Runny Nose
- SANG YE/JU HUA/BO HE/JING JIE: Wind Heat
- SHENG JIANG/DA ZAO: Wind Cold
- TU NIU XI/JIN YIN HUA/LIAN QIAO: Fever From
- XIANG FU/ZI SU YE: Stomach/Abdominal Distension, Discomfort From
- BAI ZHI: Wind Cold 441

COMMON COLD W/BODY ACHES, NO SWEAT

- DU HUO/MA HUANG

COMMON COLD W/CHRONIC ILLNESS

- YI TANG/GUI ZHI/BAI SHAO/GAN CAO
- YI TANG/GUI ZHI/BAI SHAO/GAN CAO/HUANG QI

COMMON COLD W/COPIOUS SPUTUM

COMMON COLD W/COUGH

- ZI SU YE/JIE GENG/XING REN/QIANG HUO

COMMON COLD W/DAMPNESS

COMMON COLD W/DEFICIENT QI

- REN SHEN/ZI SU YE: Wind Cold

COMMON COLD W/FEVER

COMMON COLD W/FEVER, HEADACHE, HEAVY SENSATION

COMMON COLD W/FEVER, HEADACHE, SORE THROAT

COMMON COLD W/FEVER, HOARSENESS

COMMON COLD W/GENERAL PAIN

- XI XIN/QIANG HUO/FANG FENG/(JIU WEI QIANG HUO TANG): Wind Cold Syndrome

COMMON COLD W/HEADACHE, BODYACHE, STIFF NECK

COMMON COLD W/HEADACHE, SEVERE GENERAL PAIN
• QIANG HUO/FANG FENG/BAI ZHI/CANG ZHU

COMMON COLD W/HEADACHE, SORE THROAT

COMMON COLD W/INDIGESTION

COMMON COLD W/MAINLY HEAD, BODY ACHES

COMMON COLD W/MIGRAINE HEADACHE

COMMON COLD W/NECK, BACK PAIN, STIFF

COMMON COLD W/O SWEAT

COMMON COLD W/PRODUCTIVE COUGH, NASAL CONGESTION
• ZI SU YE/JIE GENG

COMMON COLD W/SORE THROAT, COUGH
• SANG YE/JU HUA/JIE GENG/BO HE/LIAN QIAO

COMMON COLD W/SUPRAORBITAL PAIN, NASAL OBSTRUCTION
• BAI ZHI/CONG BAI/DAN DOU CHI/SHENG JIANG

COMMON COLD W/YANG DEFICIENCY

COMMON COLD, BI
• BAI ZHI/CHUAN XIONG: Headache, Body Aches

COMMON COLD, EARLY STAGE

COMMON COLD, EDEMA FROM DEFICIENCY YANG
• MA HUANG/FU ZI

COMMON COLD, FEVER OF

COMMON COLD, FLU W/VOMITING, ABDOMINAL PAIN
• ZI SU YE/HUO XIANG: Wind Cold Damp

COMMON COLD, FREQUENT

COMMON COLD, HEADACHES, BODY ACHES
• QIANG HUO/CHUAN XIONG

COMMON COLD, IN SUMMER

COMMON COLD, IN SUMMER W/DAMPNESS

COMMON COLD, INITIAL STAGE
• CONG BAI/DAN DOU CHI: w/Nasal Congestion, Fever Chills, No Sweat
• CONG BAI/DAN DOU CHI/SHENG JIANG

COMMON COLD, PATIENTS W/YIN DEFICIENCY

COMMON COLD, REDUCES FREQUENCY OF

COMMON COLD, W/NASAL OBSTRUCTION, HEADACHE, COUGH
• ZI SU YE/SHENG JIANG/CHEN PI/XIANG FU/XING REN: Wind Cold

COMMON COLD, WIND HEAT SYNDROME
• DAN DOU CHI/NIU BANG ZI/LIAN QIAO
• JING JIE/LIAN QIAO/BO HE/JIE GENG

COMMON COLD, WIND HEAT W/HEADACHE, RED EYES
• FANG FENG/JING JIE/HUANG QIN/BO HE/LIAN QIAO

COMMON COLD, WIND HEAT W/RED, SORE EYES
• BO HE/JIE GENG/NIU BANG ZI/JU HUA

FEBRILE DISEASES, FAINTING

• ZHANG NAO 849

FEBRILE DISEASES, FLUID LOSS, IRRITABILITY

• SHAN YAO/TIAN HUA FEN

FEBRILE DISEASES, LATE STAGE

• BAI HE/ZHI MU/SHENG DI HUANG/(BAI HE DI HUANG TANG): w/Irritability, Palpitations, Insomnia, Dreamful Sleep
• DAN ZHU YE/SHI GAO
• MAI MEN DONG/SHENG DI HUANG/XUAN SHEN/(ZENG YE TANG): Thirst, Constipation

FEBRILE DISEASES, LATE STAGE W/YIN LOSS

• SHENG DI HUANG/ZHI MU/QING HAO/BIE JIA

FEBRILE DISEASES, LATE STAGE W/YIN/FLUID DAMAGE

• QING HAO/BIE JIA/MU DAN PI/SHENG DI HUANG/(HING HAO BIE JIA TANG)

FEBRILE DISEASES, LATE STAGE W/YIN/FLUID DEPLETION, NO SWEATING

• MU DAN PI/ZHI MU/SHENG DI HUANG/BIE JIA/QING HAO

FEBRILE DISEASES, MACULOPAPULE IN

• ZI CAO/CHI SHAO YAO/MU DAN PI/JIN YIN HUA/LIAN QIAO

FEBRILE DISEASES, SEASONAL W/DEPLETION OF BODILY FLUIDS

• XUAN SHEN (c): Zeng Ye Tang (Xuan Shen, Sheng Di, Mai Dong) , Has Laxative Effect, Too, 9-15 g, Max 30 g/Dose 503

FEBRILE DISEASES, SEQUELAE

• PI PA YE/LU GEN: Irritable, Vomiting

FEBRILE DISEASES, SEQUELAE OF

• BAI WEI 495
• DAI MAO 743
• E JIAO 797
• XUAN SHEN 503

FEBRILE DISEASES, SPASMS, CONVULSIONS

• GUI BAN/E JIAO/SHENG DI HUANG/MU LI: Yin Consumed Causing Malnutrition Of Tendons, Muscles

FEBRILE DISEASES, SYNCOPE DURING

• JI ZI HUANG 809

FEBRILE DISEASES, THIRST

• GE GEN/TIAN HUA FEN/MAI MEN DONG/SHENG DI HUANG

FEBRILE DISEASES, THIRST, FLUID DAMAGE AFTER

• TAI ZI SHEN 770

FEBRILE DISEASES, THIRST, IRRITABILITY

• WU MEI/TIAN HUA FEN

FEBRILE DISEASES, WARM

• GOU TENG/TIAN MA/QUAN XIE/SHI JUE MING: Liver Wind Convulsions
• HUANG QIN/HUANG LIAN
• NIU HUANG/HUANG LIAN/SHAN ZHI ZI/ZHU SHA: Heat Crushing Pericardium, Delirium, Irritabililty
• XI JIAO/LING YANG JIAO: High Fever, Delirium, Convulsions
• XI JIAO/HUANG LIAN: High Fever, Delirium, With Bleeding
• BAN LAN GEN 515
• DI LONG: Convulsions/Seizures From 744

FEBRILE DISEASES, WARM W/HEMATURIA, HEMTAEMESIS, EPISTAXIS

• MU DAN PI/BAI MAO GEN

FEBRILE DISEASES, WARM, INITIAL STAGE

• CANG ZHU/SHI GAO
• LIAN QIAO/YE JU HUA

FEBRILE DISEASES, YIN CONSUMED

• E JIAO/HUANG LIAN/BAI SHAO/GOU TENG/MU LI: Irritability, Insomnia, Spasms Of Hands/Feet

FEBRILE DISEASES, YIN/FLUIDS CONSUMED W/WIND

• BIE JIA/MU LI/SHENG DI HUANG/E JIAO/BAI SHAO/(ER JIA FU MAI TANG): Spasms, Convulsions, Trembling Fingers, Pulse-Thready, Rapid, Dry Tongue

FLU

See: Infectious Diseases Influenza 188
See: Infectious Diseases Common Cold 182
See: Infectious Diseases Viral, Anti- 195

FOCAL INFECTIONS

See: Skin Boils 351
• CAO HE CHE 517
• LIAN QIAO: Boils, Abscesses 525

FUNGAL

See: Skin Fungal 358

FUNGAL INFECTIONS

• LU HUI: Damp, Use Topical 544

FUNGAL INFECTIONS, HANDS

• DA FENG ZI/(oil)/HU TAO REN/(oil)/(pork lard)
• DI GU PI (c): 30 g Decocted With Gan Cao, 15 g, Use As Wash 495

• YU XING CAO (c) 539

GONORRHEA

• BIAN XU 588
• CHE QIAN CAO 589
• CHE QIAN ZI 590
• CHI FU LING 483
• DA HUANG (c): Used Rhein From Da Huang 542
• DENG XIN CAO 592
• DONG KUI ZI 594
• FENG WEI CAO 496
• HAN FANG JI 596
• LIAN QIAO 525
• SHI WEI 601
• ZHU MA GEN 607

GOOSE-FOOT TINEA

• CHOU WU TONG 560

HERPES

• CE BAI YE (c): Especially Good For 654

HERPES SIMPLEX

• BAN LAN GEN (c): 50% Herb Injection 2 ml IM, 1-2x/Day
.... 515
• HU ZHANG (c): Decoction 497
• YU XING CAO (c): Very Effective, Use Distilled Topical
.... 539

HERPES ZOSTER

See: Skin Shingles 368
• XIONG HUANG/BING PIAN/(tincture,external)
• BAN BIAN LIAN (c): Apply Crushed Herb And She Mei
(Herba Duchesneae) To Skin 586
• BAN LAN GEN (c): 50% Herb Injection 2 ml IM, 1-2x/Day
.... 515
• CHUAN XIN LIAN (c) 518
• DA HUANG (c) 542
• DANG GUI (c): Tablet Of Extract 795
• DI LONG (c): External With Paste And Sugar 744
• HU ZHANG (c) 497
• JIN QIAN CAO (c): Fresh Herb, 250 g Macerated In 100
ml 75% ETOH, 1 Week, Mix Filtrate With Realgar, Apply
Topically, 2-3x/Day, Not If Broken Skin 598
• WANG BU LIU XING (c): Pain/Cleared—Toasted,
Powdered, With Sesame Oil, Local, Not Open Sores,
1-2x/Day For 30 Minutes, Pain Gone In 10-20 Minutes
.... 691

HERPES, ON LIPS

• ER CHA 839

INFECTIONS

See: Skin Skin, Infections 368
• BAN LAN GEN 515
• DA HUANG: Topical, Too 542
• GAN CAO: Topical, Too 763
• PU GONG YING (c): Especially Effective Against Those
Caused By Gram+ Bacteria Or Drug Resistant Strains Of
Staph, Strep 529
• ZI HE CHE (c): A-Globulin-Like Substance 792

INFECTIONS W/HIGH FEVER, COMA, DELIRUIUM

• NIU HUANG (c): Use An Gong Niu Huang Wan 755

INFECTIONS W/PUS

• BAI ZHI 441
• WU BEI ZI 829

INFECTIONS, ACUTE SUPPURATIVE

• CHAN SU (c) 837

INFECTIONS, EPIDEMIC

• SHENG MA 467

INFECTIONS, LOCALIZED

• CHI SHAO YAO 668

INFECTIONS, POSTOPERATIVE

• DAN SHEN (c) 672

INFECTIONS, PYOGENIC

• PU GONG YING: (With Pus) 529

INFECTIONS, SEVERE

• CAO HE CHE 517

INFECTIONS, SUPPURATIVE

• DAN SHEN (c) 672
• HAI PIAO XIAO 821
• HUANG LIAN (c): Topical 20% Vaseline Dressing, 3%
Solution With Oral Powder 486

INFECTIOUS DISEASES

See: Infectious Diseases Infectious Diseases 188
• CHUAN XIN LIAN (c): Many (Listed Individually) , ETOH
Extract 518
• MA DOU LING (c): Use With Antibiotics 701

INFECTIOUS DISEASES, ACUTE

• LIAN QIAO/BAN LAN GEN/HUANG LIAN

INFLUENZA

See: Wind Disorders Wind Heat 434
• LIAN QIAO/BAN LAN GEN/JING JIE/BO HE
• ZI SU YE/HUO XIANG: Wind Cold Damp
• BAI JIANG CAO (c): Antipyretic In Granule Infusion
Form 512
• BAI TOU WENG (c): Weak Inhibitory Effect, Aqueous
Extract 514
• BAN LAN GEN (c): Injection Can Prevent 515
• BING LANG (c): Apply Extract Into Nose, * Also Drink
Water Mixed With 643
• CHUAN XIN LIAN (c): Powder/Aqueous Extract, Powder
More Effective 518
• DA QING YE 519
• GUAN ZHONG 521
• GUAN ZHONG (c): Gui Guan Xiang—Incense Made Of
Gui Zhi/Guan Zhong With Or Without Moxa, Used As
Fumigant When Flu Present 521
• GUI ZHEN CAO 462

MENINGITIS, LYMPHOCYTIC CHORIO

MONONUCLEOSIS, INFECTIOUS

MUMPS

MUMPS W/PAIN, SWELLING

MUMPS, ACUTE

MUMPS, ORCHITIS FROM

MUMPS, SUBCUTANEOUS

MYCOBACTERIAL, ANTI-

NAILS, FUNGAL INFECTION OF

PAROTITIS

PAROTITIS, ACUTE

PAROTITIS, EPIDEMIC

PAROTITIS, HEAT TOXIN

PERTUSSIS

PERTUSSIS, COUGH PAROXYSMS

PESTILENT DISEASES

PNEUMONIA

See: Lungs Pneumonia 234

POLIOMYELITIS

• DANG GUI (c): Volatile Oil, 0.5 g/ml Injection In Acupoints, Shen Shu, Xia Qu, Zu San LI, Da Zui, Jian Jin , Nei Guan, 1 ml/Point, Every 5 Days, Good Results 795

POLIOMYELITIS, ACUTE

• YIN YANG HUO (c): 10% Injection 2 ml IM Injection, 1x/Day For 10 Days, *Antiparalytic Injection (Herb, Sang Ji Sheng) For Sequelae, Acute Stase, 2 ml IM 2x/Day For 20 Days 791

POLIOMYELITIS, INHIBITS

• BAO YU (c) 804

POLIOMYELITIS, SEQUELAE OF

• REN SHEN (c): Acupoint Injection—Helped Affect Limbs Improve 767

PULMONARY TUBERCULOSIS

• LIAN QIAO (c): Lian Qiao, Xia Ku Cao, Xuan Dong, Mu LI, May Be Also Ground With Sesame Seeds, Take 5 g, 3x/Day, May Take Herb Alone 525

PURULENT

See: Skin Pus 365

PURULENT DISEASES

• JIN YIN HUA (c) 524

PYEMIA

See: Blood Related Disorders/Topics Pyemia .. 50

RABIES

• BAN MAO: Topical On Swollen Glands 837

RHEUMATIC FEVER

• CHEN PI (c) 621
• DA QING YE (c) 519

RUBELLA

See: Infectious Diseases Measles 191
• BAI JI LI/JING JIE/CHAN TUI: (German Measles) Wind Heat In Blood
• JIANG CAN/CHAN TUI/BO HE
• BAI XIAN PI 515
• JIANG CAN 746

SCARLET FEVER

• HUANG LIAN (c): 10% Solution, Equal To Penicillin/Sulfa 486
• HUANG QIN (c): Oral Decoction, Markedly Reduced Incidence 489

SCARLET FEVER, PREVENTATIVE

• YE JU HUA (c): Spray Throat With 2 ml, 50% Decoction For 3 Days 468

SCROFULA

• BAN XIA/ZHE BEI MU

• BAN XIA/KUN BU/HAI ZAO/CHUAN BEI MU
• BO HE/XIA KU CAO
• CHUAN BEI MU/ZHE BEI MU
• CHUAN BEI MU/XUAN SHEN/MU LI
• HAI FU SHI/LIAN QIAO/KUN BU/XUAN SHEN
• HAI FU SHI/MU LI/CHUAN BEI MU/XUAN SHEN/KUN BU: Phlegm, Qi Accumulation
• HAI GE KE/KUN BU/HAI ZAO/WA LENG ZI/(HAN HUA WAN)
• HAI LONG/DA ZAO/(winter fungus)
• HAI ZAO/JIANG CAN/XIA KU CAO/XUAN SHEN
• HAI ZAO/GAN CAO
• HAI ZAO/XIA KU CAO/XUAN SHEN/CHUAN BEI MU/(NEI XIAO LEI LI WAN)
• HE SHOU WU/XUAN SHEN/LIAN QIAO
• HE SHOU WU/XIA KU CAO/CHUAN BEI MU
• HUANG QIN/XIA KU CAO/MU LI: Liver Fire Obstruction
• JIANG CAN/XIA KU CAO/(chuan or zhi bei mu)/MU LI
• JING DA JI/SHAN CI GU/(QIAN JIN ZI)/(ZI JIN DING-EXTL OR INTL)
• KUN BU/HAI ZAO
• LIAN QIAO/XIA KU CAO/XUAN SHEN/CHUAN BEI MU
• LUO HAN GUO/ZHE BEI MU/XIA KU CAO
• MU LI/XUAN SHEN/XIA KU CAO/ZHE BEI MU
• MU LI/ZHE BEI MU/XUAN SHEN/(XIAO LEI WAN): Phlegm Fire
• QUAN XIE/SHAN ZHI ZI/(beeswax-topical)
• SHAN CI GU/SHE XIANG/WU BEI ZI
• SHAN CI GU/GAO LIANG JIANG
• WA LENG ZI/HAI ZAO/KUN BU
• WU GONG/GAN CAO/(beeswax, topical)
• XIA KU CAO/MU LI/XUAN SHEN/KUN BU: Phlegm Fire
• XUAN SHEN/MU LI/ZHE BEI MU: Phlegm
• XUAN SHEN/MU LI/ZHE BEI MU/XIA KU CAO/ZI CAO: Phlegm
• XUAN SHEN/CHUAN BEI MU/MU LI
• YUE JI HUA/XIA KU CAO/MU LI
• YUE JI HUA/XIA KU CAO/MU LI/CHUAN BEI MU
• ZHE BEI MU/XUAN SHEN/MU LI/XIA KU CAO: Phlegm Fire w/Pain
• BA JIAO LIAN 510
• BAI FU ZI 708
• BAI LIAN 513
• BAN MAO: Topical 837
• BAN XIA 710
• BAN ZHI LIAN 516
• BI MA ZI 547
• CAO HE CHE 517
• CHUAN BEI MU: Phlegm Fire 717
• CHUAN SHAN JIA 670
• HAI FU SHI: Phlegm Fire 720
• HAI GE KE: Phlegm Fire 721
• HAI LONG 779
• HAI MA 780
• HAI ZAO: Phlegm 721
• HE SHOU WU 799
• HOU ZAO 722
• JIANG CAN: Phlegm Heat 746
• KUN BU: Hot Phlegm 724
• LIAN QIAO 525
• LOU LU 527

SCROFULA, EARLY, NONULCERATED

SCROFULA, ULCERATED

SCROFULA, ULCERATED, SLOW HEALING

SEPTICEMIA

SHIGELOSIS, LEUKOPENIA OF

SHOCK, CARDIOGENIC, INFECTIOUS, ANAPHYLACTIC

SHOCK, CARDIOGENIC/SEPTIC

SPIROCHETTES, ANTI-

SURGICAL INFECTIONS

SWEATING, POST FEBRILE

SWEATING, POST LONG ILLNESS, TUBERCULOSIS

SYPHILIS

SYPHILIS, CONGENITAL

SYPHILITIC CHANCRES

SYPHILITIC NEURALGIA

TETANUS

Poliomyelitis, Coxsackie, Encephalitis B, 20% Solution,
Hepatitis B 497
• HUANG LIAN (c): Flu, Newcastle 486
• HUANG QI (c): In Sense That Could Inhibit
Pathogenicity Of Virus 765
• HUANG QIN (c): Extract, Decoction Inhibited Some Flu
.... 489
• JIANG HUANG (c): Many 678
• JIN YIN HUA (c): Strong: Flu (Pr8) 524
• JIN YING ZI (c): Some Flu 823
• JING JIE (c): None Noted Against Flu 447
• JU HUA (c): Flu 463
• LAO GUAN CAO (c) 565
• LIAN QIAO (c): Flu 525
• LIAN XU (c): Flu, Strong 823
• MA HUANG (c): Essential Oil, Influenza, Therapeutic
Effect 448
• MIAN HUA GEN (c): Inhibits Several, Inhibits Flu Greater
Than Amantadine 851
• MU DAN PI (c): Flu: Decoction Inhibited, Inconsistent,
Though 499
• PANG DA HAI (c): Flu-Strong, Pr3 724
• PEI LAN (c): Hepatitis, Flu 583
• PI PA YE (c): Flu 703
• PU GONG YING (c): Echo 529
• QIAN CAO GEN (c): Some Flu 662
• QIAN HU (c): 1: 1 Herb Decoction Inhibited Asian Flu
.... 725
• SAN QI (c) 663
• SANG JI SHENG (c): Echo, Coxsackie, Polio (More
Pronounced With Yin Yang Huo) , Flu 813
• SHAN CI GU (c): Flu Virus 846
• SHANG LU (c): Tobacco Mosaic 554
• SHE CHUANG ZI (c): Flu, etc 847
• SHE GAN (c): Pharyngitis Causing 533
• SHENG MA (c) 467
• SHI LIU PI (c): Flu, Some Other Common 828
• SHUI XIAN GEN (c): Lymphocytic Choriomeningitis ... 535
• TU YIN CHEN (c): 1: 10 Decoction Inhibits Echo Virus,
Not Any Others 602
• WU BEI ZI (c): Flu, et al 829
• WU ZHU YU (c) 618
• XI HE LIU (c): Flu 451
• XIAN HE CAO (c): Alcohol Extract—Columbia Sk Virus
.... 665
• XIANG RU (c) 453
• YE JU HUA (c): Echo, Herpes, Some Influenza, Not Some
Cold 468
• YIN CHEN (c): ETOH Extract Strongly Inhibits Flu 603
• YIN YANG HUO (c): Inhibits Polio, Echo, Coxsackie ... 791
• YU XING CAO (c): Decoction, Flu, Echo 539
• ZI WAN (c): Markedly Inhibited Flu 706

WHOOPING COUGH
See: Lungs Whooping Cough 238

YEAST
• BAI TOU WENG (c): Bai Tou Weng Decoction 514

End of Topic:
INFECTIOUS DISEASES

INFERTILITY, FEMALE
See: Sexuality, Female: Gynecological
Infertility, Female 327

INFERTILITY, MALE
See: Sexuality, Male: Urological Topics
Infertility, Male 344

INFERTILITY, MEN/WOMEN
See: Sexuality, Either Sex Infertility, Men/Women
.... 319

INFLAMMATION
See: Skin Inflammation 361

INFLAMMATION RELATED TOPICS
See: Trauma, Bites, Poisonings Inflammation
Related Topics 410

INFLAMMATORY BOWEL DISEASE
See: Abdomen/Gastrointestinal Topics
Inflammatory Bowel Disease 33

INFLUENZA RELATED TOPICS
See: Infectious Diseases Influenza Related Topics
.... 188

INGUINAL CANAL NODULES
See: Cancer/Tumors/Swellings/Lumps Inguinal
Canal Nodules 69
See: Abdomen/Gastrointestinal Topics Inguinal
Canal Nodules 33

INJURIES AND RELATED TOPICS
See: Trauma, Bites, Poisonings Injuries And
Related Topics 411

INSANITY
See: Mental State/Neurological Disorders
Insanity 249

INSECT BITES
See: Trauma, Bites, Poisonings Insect Bites ... 411

INSOMNIA RELATED TOPICS
See: Mental State/Neurological Disorders
Insomnia Related Topics 249

INSOMNIA, CHILDHOOD
See: Childhood Disorders Insomnia, Childhood
.... 82

INSULIN
See: Endocrine Related Disorders Insulin 102

INTERCOSTAL RELATED TOPICS
See: Chest Intercostal Related Topics 80

INTESTINAL BLEEDING
See: Hemorrhagic Disorders Intestinal Bleeding
.... 173

INTESTINAL CANCER

See: Cancer/Tumors/Swellings/Lumps Intestinal Cancer 69

INTESTINAL FUNGI AFTER ANTIBIOTIC TREATMENT

See: Infectious Diseases Intestinal Fungi After Antibiotic Treatment 189

INTESTINAL GAS, FROM PANHYSTERECTOMY

See: Sexuality, Female: Gynecological Intestinal Gas, From Panhysterectomy 327

INTESTINAL PARASITES

See: Parasites Intestinal Parasites 305

INTESTINAL WIND

See: Hemorrhagic Disorders Intestinal Wind ... 173
See: Abdomen/Gastrointestinal Topics Intestinal Wind 33

INTESTINE, LARGE, INCREASES PERISTALSIS

See: Abdomen/Gastrointestinal Topics Intestine, Large, Increases Peristalsis 33

INTESTINES AND RELATED TOPICS

See: Abdomen/Gastrointestinal Topics Intestines And Related Topics 33

INTESTINES, TRICHOMONIASIS

See: Parasites Intestines, Trichomoniasis 305

INTOXICATION, ALCOHOLIC

See: Mental State/Neurological Disorders Intoxication, Alcoholic 251

INTRAOCULAR HEMORRHAGE

See: Eyes Intraocular Hemorrhage 121

INVOLUNTARY EMISSION

See: Sexuality, Male: Urological Topics Involuntary Emission 344

IRIS INFLAMMATION

See: Eyes Iris Inflammation 121

IRRITABILITY RELATED TOPICS

See: Mental State/Neurological Disorders Irritability Related Topics 251

IRRITABLE BOWEL SYNDROME

See: Bowel Related Disorders Irritable Bowel Syndrome 63

ISCHEMIC PAIN

See: Circulation Disorders Ischemic Pain 87

ITCHING

See: Skin Itching 361

ITCHING, GENITAL

See: Sexuality, Either Sex Itching, Genital 319

JAUNDICE RELATED TOPICS

See: Liver Jaundice Related Topics 205

JOINT BI

See: Musculoskeletal/Connective Tissue Joint Bi 268

JOINT CAPSULES, TIGHTENS IF LOOSE W/RECURRENT DISLOCATION

See: Musculoskeletal/Connective Tissue Joint Capsules, Tightens If Loose w/Recurrent Dislocation 268

JOINT PAIN, ELDERLY

See: Geriatric Topics Joint Pain, Elderly 143

JOINT RELATED TOPICS

See: Musculoskeletal/Connective Tissue Joint Related Topics 268

JOINT TUBERCULOSIS

See: Infectious Diseases Joint Tuberculosis 189

JOINTS, INFECTIONS OF

See: Infectious Diseases Joints, Infections Of ... 189

JOINTS, PAINFUL, SWOLLEN FROM ALLERGIC RESPONSE

See: Immune System Related Disorders/Topics Joints, Painful, Swollen From Allergic Response 177

JUE YIN STAGE DISEASE

See: Six Stages/Channels Jue Yin Stage Disease 348

KELOIDS

See: Skin Keloids 361

KERATITIS

See: Eyes Keratitis 121

KESHAN DISEASE

See: Heart Keshan Disease 157

KIDNEY RELATED TOPICS

See: Kidneys Kidney Related Topics 199

End of Topic:
KIDNEY RELATED TOPICS

KIDNEYS :

BACK PAIN FROM KIDNEY STONES

• HU TAO REN/DU ZHONG/BU GU ZHI/JIN QIAN CAO/HAI JIN SHA CAO

DIURESIS, INHIBITS

- BAI SHAO (c) 794

DIURETIC

- BAI JI LI (c) 743
- BAI MAO GEN (c): Aqueous Extract, Most Prominent After 5-10 Hrs Of Taking 653
- BAI WEI (c) 495
- BAI ZHU (c): Significant, Prolonged 760
- BAI ZHU: Mild 760
- BAN BIAN LIAN (c): Prolonged, Strong 586
- BIAN XU (c) 588
- CHAI HU (c): Oral Small Doses, Large Doses May Cause Edema 457
- CHAN SU (c) 837
- CHE QIAN CAO (c) 589
- CHE QIAN ZI (c): Unknown Ingredient, Recently No Evidence Seen 590
- CHI SHAO YAO (c) 668
- CHI XIAO DOU (c) 591
- CHONG WEI ZI (c): Significant 669
- CHUAN SHAN LONG (c) 442
- CONG BAI (c) 442
- DA HUANG (c) 542
- DA JI (c) 655
- DANG GUI (c) 795
- DI DAN TOU (c) 520
- DI FU ZI: Mild 592
- DI FU ZI (c) 592
- DONG GUA PI (c) 593
- DU ZHONG (c) 775
- FU LING (c): Slow, Prolonged, But Not Shown In Normal Doses (Slight At 15+g), More ETOH Extract 594
- FU LONG GAN (c) 657
- FU PING (c) 460
- GAN SUI (c): Effect Not Shown For Herb 551
- HAI JIN SHA (c) 522
- HAI JIN SHA CAO (c) 522
- HAN FANG JI (c) 596
- HE HUAN PI (c) 731
- HONG DA JI (c) 551
- HUA SHI: Good 597
- HUANG BAI (c) 485
- HUANG QI (c): Moderate, Prolonged 765
- HUANG QIN (c): Orally Given ETOH Extract 489
- JIN QIAN CAO (c): Calcium/Potassium Salts 598
- JIN YIN HUA (c) 524
- KU SHEN (c) 491
- LIAN QIAO (c) 525
- LONG DAN CAO (c) 492
- LU FENG FANG (c) 841
- LU GEN (c) 472
- LU RONG (c) 784
- LUO BU MA (c): Renal Or Cardiac Edema Or Ascites Of Cirrhosis 748
- MA CHI XIAN (c) 528
- MA HUANG (c): Marked 448
- MAI MEN DONG (c) 810
- MANG XIAO (c): When Injected 545
- MI MENG HUA (c): Slightly 474
- MU GUA (c): Dramatic Increase 567
- MU ZEI (c) 464
- NIU BANG ZI (c) 465
- NIU XI (c) 684
- NU ZHEN ZI (c) 812
- PANG DA HAI (c) 724
- PEI LAN (c) 583
- PU GONG YING (c) 529
- PU HUANG (c) 660
- QIAN CAO GEN (c) 662
- QIAN NIU ZI (c) 553
- QIN PI (c): Short Term 493
- QING FEN (c) 845
- REN DONG TENG (c): Mild 531
- SAN QI (c): Increase Urine Output 5x 663
- SANG BAI PI (c): For 6 Hours 703
- SANG JI SHENG (c): Marked 813
- SHAN ZHU YU (c): Marked 827
- SHAN ZI CAO (c) 664
- SHANG LU (c): Mixed Findings 554
- SHE XIANG (c) 756
- SHENG DI HUANG (c) 500
- SHI CHANG PU (c) 757
- SHU DI HUANG (c) 802
- SI GUA LUO (c) 688
- TAN XIANG (c) 632
- TIAN MEN DONG (c) 814
- TING LI ZI (c) 555
- TONG CAO (c) 601
- TU YIN CHEN (c) 602
- WU JIA PI (c) 574
- XI GUA (c): Increases Urea Formation In Liver 509
- XI XIN (c) 452
- XIA KU CAO (c) 478
- XIANG RU (c): Essential Oil 453
- XUE YU TAN (c) 666
- YI MU CAO (c): Significant 694
- YIN CHEN (c) 603
- YIN YANG HUO (c): Low Doses 791
- YU JIN (c) 695
- YU LI REN (c): For Edema 549
- YU XING CAO (c) 539
- YU ZHU (c) 815
- YUAN HUA (c): Not With Large Doses And With Diarrhea 556
- ZE LAN (c) 696
- ZE XIE (c): Varies With Season Harvested, Can Be Marked, Winter Collection Stronger, Salt Treated Herb Not Diuretic 605
- ZHEN ZHU (c) 740
- ZHI MU (c) 480
- ZHI SHI (c) 635
- ZHU LING (c): Stronger Than Caffeine, Mu Tong, Fu Ling As A Decoction, No Diuresis If As ETOH Extract 606
- ZI WAN (c): Marked 706

DIURETIC, MILD

DIURETIC, NOT SHOWN

DIURETIC, STRONG

DIURETIC, WEAK

EDEMA

ESSENCE DEFICIENCY

ESSENCE, RETENTION

ESSENCE/KI QI DEFICIENCY

GLOMERULO-NEPHRITIS

GLOMERULO-NEPHRITIS, ACUTE

GLOMERULO-NEPHRITIS, ACUTE/CHRONIC

GLOMERULO-NEPHRITIS, PROTEINURIA, REDUCES

HEAT IN KIDNEY

HYPERTENSION, ACUTE RENAL

KIDNEY DEFICIENCY

KIDNEY DEFICIENCY, COLD

KIDNEY DEFICIENCY, ESSENCE LOSS

KIDNEY DEFICIENCY, LOWER BACK

KIDNEY DEFICIENCY, SEVERE

KIDNEY DISEASES

KIDNEY FAILURE, CHRONIC

KIDNEY FIRE

KIDNEY HEART DISCOMMUNICATION

KIDNEY HEART DISHARMONY

- HUANG LIAN/ROU GUI: Insomnia
- DENG XIN CAO 592

KIDNEY HEAT

- ZE XIE 605
- ZHI MU 480

KIDNEY LIVER DEFICIENCY

- SHAN ZHU YU 827

KIDNEY LUNG QI DEFICIENCY

- LIU HUANG/FU ZI/ROU GUI: Unable To Hold Qi, Waning Life Gate Fire

KIDNEY QI DEFICIENCY

- QIAN SHI/JIN YING ZI: Nocturnal Emission, Spermatorrhea, Premature Ejaculation, Frequent Urination
- QIAN SHI 826

KIDNEY QI DEFICIENCY, COLD

- HAI MA 780

KIDNEY SPLEEN DEFICIENCY W/ANOREXIA, DIARRHEA

- TU SI ZI/SHAN YAO/FU LING /DANG SHEN

KIDNEY SPLEEN YANG DEFICIENCY

- FU ZI/GAN JIANG/GAN CAO/(SI NI TANG)

KIDNEY STONES

- HU PO/HAI JIN SHA CAO/JIN QIAN CAO: Urine Retention From
- HU TAO REN/DU ZHONG/BU GU ZHI/JIN QIAN CAO/HAI JIN SHA CAO: Back Pain
- JIN QIAN CAO/HAI JIN SHA CAO/JI NEI JIN/(SAN JIN TANG)
- YI MU CAO/HUANG JING/SHI WEI/DONG KUI ZI
- CHE QIAN CAO (c): 15-30 g 589
- CHE QIAN ZI (c): 3-10 g 590
- HUA SHI 597
- JIN QIAN CAO 598
- QIAN CAO GEN (c): Helps Prevent Formation Of 662
- SHI WEI 601

KIDNEY STONES W/HEMATURIA

- NIU XI/JIN QIAN CAO

KIDNEY UNABLE TO GRASP QI

See: Lungs Asthma 214
- REN SHEN/GE JIE/(REN SHEN GE JIE TANG): Wheezing

KIDNEY YANG DEFICIENCY

- BA JI TIAN/BU GU ZHI/FU PEN ZI: Urinary Problems
- BU GU ZHI/ROU DOU KOU/WU WEI ZI/WU ZHU YU/(SI SHEN WAN): Early AM Diarrhea
- BU GU ZHI/TU SI ZI/YI ZHI REN: Urinary Frequency
- BU GU ZHI/HU TAO REN: Wheezing, Low Back Pain, Premature Ejaculation
- DONG CHONG XIA CAO/DU ZHONG/YIN YANG HUO/ROU CONG RONG: Legs, Sore, Sore Back, Spermatorrhea
- DU ZHONG/BU GU ZHI: Lower Back Pain, Wheezing
- FU ZI/ROU GUI: Failing Life Gate Fire
- ROU CONG RONG/TU SI ZI: Lower Back Cold, Pain, Impotence
- ROU GUI/FU ZI/SHU DI HUANG/SHAN ZHU YU/(GUI FU BA WEI WAN)
- SUO YANG/SANG PIAO XIAO: Urinary Problems
- BU GU ZHI 773
- FU PEN ZI: Urination, Urogenital Symptoms 820
- GE JIE 777
- GU SUI BU 778
- HU LU BA: Cold 781
- LIU HUANG 840
- LU JIAO 783
- LU RONG 784
- ROU GUI 616
- ROU GUI PI 617
- SANG PIAO XIAO 827
- SHA YUAN ZI 786
- TU SI ZI 787
- YIN YANG HUO 791

KIDNEY YANG DEFICIENCY W/EDEMA, ASCITES, CONSTIPATION

- QING FEN/DA HUANG/QIAN NIU ZI

KIDNEY YANG DEFICIENCY W/FIRE REDUCED

- FU ZI/ROU GUI/SHAN ZHU YU/SHU DI HUANG/(GUI FU BA WEI WAN)

KIDNEY YANG DEFICIENCY W/LOW LIFE GATE FIRE

- BA JI TIAN/TU SI ZI/ROU CONG RONG/REN SHEN
- GE JIE/REN SHEN/(korean)/HU TAO REN/WU WEI ZI
- ROU GUI/FU ZI
- YANG QI SHI/BU GU ZHI/TU SI ZI/LU RONG

KIDNEY YANG WEAKNESS W/WIND COLD DAMP BI

- XIAN MAO/YIN YANG HUO

KIDNEY YIN DEFICIENCY

- MA HUANG/SHU DI HUANG: Cough/Wheezing
- NU ZHEN ZI/BU GU ZHI/TU SI ZI: Sore Back, Legs, Dizziness
- GUI BAN 806
- HAN LIAN CAO: Dizziness, Vertigo, Blurred Vision ... 806

KIDNEY YIN DEFICIENCY WITH HEAT

- ZE XIE: Tinnitus, Dizziness 605

KIDNEY YIN, INSUFFICIENT

- GUI BAN 806

KIDNEYS, ACUTE GLOMERULONEPHRITS

- YI MU CAO (c): Decoctions, 5-36 Days For Cure 694

PYELONEPHRITIS, CHRONIC

- HUANG QI (c) 765

RENAL DISEASES

- LUO LE 583
- YU MI XU 605

VASODILATOR IN KIDNEY

- HAN FANG JI (c) 596
- YU XING CAO (c) 539

End of Topic:
KIDNEYS

KNEE RELATED TOPICS

See: Musculoskeletal/Connective Tissue Knee Related Topics 270

LABOR, DIFFICULT

See: Sexuality, Female: Gynecological Labor, Difficult 327

LABOR, INDUCES

See: Sexuality, Female: Gynecological Labor, Induces 327

LACERATIONS

See: Trauma, Bites, Poisonings Lacerations 412

LACRIMATION

See: Eyes Lacrimation 121

LACTATION RELATED TOPICS

See: Sexuality, Female: Gynecological Lactation Related Topics 327

LARGE INTESTINE QI STAGNATION

See: Qi Related Disorders/Topics Large Intestine Qi Stagnation 314

LARGE INTESTINE RELATED TOPICS

See: Abdomen/Gastrointestinal Topics Large Intestine Related Topics 36

LARYNGEAL NODULES

See: Oral Cavity Laryngeal Nodules 285

LARYNGITIS

See: Oral Cavity Laryngitis 285

LASSITUDE

See: Mental State/Neurological Disorders Lassitude 253

LAXATIVE

See: Bowel Related Disorders Laxative 63

LEAD POISONING

See: Trauma, Bites, Poisonings Lead Poisoning 412

LEARNING ABILITY

See: Mental State/Neurological Disorders Learning Ability 253

LEARNING DISABILITIES, IN CHILDREN

See: Childhood Disorders Learning Disabilities, Childhood 82

LEG QI

See: Extremities Leg Qi 111

LEG RELATED TOPICS

See: Extremities Leg Related Topics 111

LENS OPACITY

See: Eyes Lens Opacity 121

LEPROSY

See: Infectious Diseases Leprosy 189

LEPTOSPIROSIS

See: Infectious Diseases Leptospirosis 189

LESIONS

See: Skin Lesions 361

LETHARGY

See: Mental State/Neurological Disorders Lethargy 253

LEUKEMIA

See: Cancer/Tumors/Swellings/Lumps Leukemia 69

LEUKOCYTOSIS

See: Blood Related Disorders/Topics Leukocytosis 50

LEUKODERMA

See: Skin Leukoderma 362

LEUKOPENIA

See: Sexuality, Female: Gynecological Leukopenia 328
See: Blood Related Disorders/Topics Leukopenia 50

LEUKORRHAGIA

See: Sexuality, Female: Gynecological Leukorrhagia 328

LEUKORRHEA RELATED TOPICS

See: Sexuality, Female: Gynecological Leukorrhea Related Topics 328

LI, HOT

See: Urinary Bladder LI, Hot 421

LI, W/STONES

See: Urinary Bladder LI, w/Stones 421

LICE

See: **Parasites** Lice 305

LIFE GATE FIRE

See: **Kidneys** Life Gate Fire 201

LIGAMENTS

See: **Musculoskeletal/Connective Tissue**
Ligaments 272

LIMB RELATED TOPICS

See: **Extremities** Limb Related Topics 114

LIMB, SEVERED (FINGER)

See: **Trauma, Bites, Poisonings** Limb, Severed
(Finger) 412

LIN DISEASE, PAINFUL URINATION SYNDROME

See: **Urinary Bladder** Lin Disease, Painful Urination
Syndrome 421

LIPEMIA

See: **Blood Related Disorders/Topics** Lipemia .. 50

LIPOMA

See: **Cancer/Tumors/Swellings/Lumps** Lipoma
.... 69

LIPS AND RELATED TOPICS

See: **Oral Cavity** Lips And Related Topics 285

LISTLESSNESS

See: **Mental State/Neurological Disorders**
Listlessness 253

End of Topic:
LISTLESSNESS

LIVER :

See: **Gall Bladder** 140

ASCITES

See: **Fluid Disorders** Ascites 132

ASCITES, LIVER CIRRHOSIS

• LUO BU MA (c) 748
• SHI SHANG BAI: Damp Heat 534

BILE SECRETION

See: **Gall Bladder** Bile Secretion 140

CHOLERETIC

• SHAN ZHI ZI (c): (Increases Liver Bile Secretion) 476

CIRRHOSIS

See: **Liver** Liver, Cirrhosis 211

CIRRHOSIS, ASCITIC

See: **Fluid Disorders** Edema 133

DIZZINESS

❚ See Also: Dizziness (Topics: Gynecology, Phlegm,
Blood, Eyes, Mental State, Ears)

EDEMA

See: **Fluid Disorders** Edema 133

GLYCOGEN, LIVER REDUCES DEPLETION

• SHENG DI HUANG (c) 500

HEPATIC CANCER, ASCITIC

• GAN CAO (c): Inhibits 763

HEPATIC CARCINOMA

• BAN MAO (c): Cook With Eggs, 5-6 With Head, Wings,
Legs Removed, Add To Egg, Bake To Dry On Low Heat,
Grind, Divide Into 2 Packs, Oral 1 Pack, 1-3x/Day, Up To
14 Months, Help Remission, Life Prolonged, *Tablet Of
Substance (As Cantharidin, 0.25 mg) , Ba Ji Powder,
Aluminum Hydroxide, Magnesium Trisilicate, 2-6
Tabs/Day In 3 Doses, 45-60% Effective 837

HEPATITIS

• BAI FAN 836
• BAN ZHI LIAN 516
• CHUAN LIAN ZI: Pain 623
• CHUAN XIN LIAN (c) 518
• DA HUANG (c): Yin Chen Tang w/Da Huang 542
• DI DAN TOU 520
• GUI ZHEN CAO 462
• HAI JIN SHA CAO 522
• HONG HUA (c): IM Injection, Lowered SGPT 675
• HU HUANG LIAN (c) 484
• HU ZHANG 497
• HU ZHANG (c): Better For Acute, Icteric Viral, Some
What Effective In Chronic Persistent, Ineffective In
Chronic Hepatitis, Use Herb, Syrup, Or
Compound—With Yin Chen, Tian Ji Huang, et al 497
• JI GU CAO 564
• JI ZI HUANG 809
• JIN QIAN CAO 598
• LING ZHI CAO (c): Best In Cases With High SGPT But
Liver Still Functioning, 15-106 Days, Ling Zhi Syrup
(Alcohol Extract, 10%) 20 ml, 2x/Day For 1-3 Months
.... 731
• LONG DAN CAO (c): Long Dan Xie Gan Tang (Long Dan
Cao, Shan Zhi Zi, Huang Qin, Chai Hu, Dang Gui, Sheng
Di, Ze Xie, Gan Cao, Che Qian Zi, Mu Tong) , 62 Doses
.... 492
• LUO BU MA 748
• MEI GUI HUA 627
• MU TONG (c) 599
• PU GONG YING 529
• QIN JIAO 569
• SHAN ZHA (c): Acute Viral/Chronic, Powder, 3g 3x/Day
Oral, 10 Days/Course, 2-4 Courses Required For
Cure/Marked Improvement, Lowers SGPT 641
• SHUI NIU JIAO (c) 501

- SHAN ZHI ZI (c): 30 Days Of Treatment 476
- TU YIN CHEN (c) ...., ... 602
- YIN CHEN (c): 1-1.5 Liang, 3x/Day, 7 Days/Wih Gan Cao, Da Zao, Sugar 10 Days, For Young Children, *30-45 g, 7 Days PO, Gives Rapid Reduction Of Jaundice, Fever, Size Of Liver, *Yin Chen, Huang Bai, Xhan Zhi Zi, Ban Lan Gen, *Prophylaxis Use Against Viral—Yin Chen, Dan Shen, Ba Qing Ye, Da Zao/With Serissa Serissoides, Tian Ji Huang, Bai Jian Cao, Gan Cao 603
- YU MI XU 605

HEPATITIS, ICTERIC/ANICTERIC

- DA QING YE/DAN SHEN
- DA QING YE/DAN SHEN/YU JIN/LONG DAN CAO

HEPATITIS, IMPROVES APPETITE

- LIU JI NU (c) 681

HEPATITIS, INFECTIOUS

- CHAI HU (c): Injection, 1: 2, 10-20 ml In 50% Glucose, IV, 1-2x/Day/20-30 ml In 250-500 ml 10% Glucose For IV Infusion, 1x/Day, 10 Courses 457
- FO SHOU 624
- GAN CAO (c): 100% Decoction, 15-20 ml, 3x/Day For 10-20 Days, Helped Jaundice, Bile, Hepatomegaly, Pain 763
- HUANG QIN (c): Icteric/Non-Icteric, Improved Symptoms, Restored Liver Functions 489
- NUO DAO GEN 825
- REN DONG TENG 531
- REN DONG TENG (c): 60 g Decoction, 2x/Day, 15 Days, Helps Symptoms, Recovered Liver Functions 531
- SHENG DI HUANG (c): IM Injection, 12 g Of Herb With 6 g Gan Cao, 10 Day Course, SGPT Lowering, Or Decoction Of Same Works 500

HEPATITIS, INFECTIOUS, IN CHILDREN

- FO SHOU (c): Helpful For Symptomatic Treatment, Used With Fruit Of Bai Jiang Cao 624

HEPATITIS, NONICTERIC

- YU MI XU (c): Fluid Extract, 30-40 Drops/Tablet 0.8 g, 3-4x/Day 605

HEPATITIS, PAIN

- CHAI HU/GAN CAO

HEPATITIS, REDUCES SYMPTOMS OF

- LING ZHI CAO (c) 731

HEPATITIS, SEVERE

- XIONG DAN/YIN CHEN

HEPATITIS, STOMACH PAIN IN

- JI NEI JIN/DAN SHEN

HEPATITIS, TOXIC

- HUANG LIAN (c): From Industrial Toxins 486
- HUANG QI (c): Oral 100% Decoction Protects Liver ... 765

HEPATITIS, VIRAL

- BAN MAO (c) 837
- QING DAI (c) 531

- REN SHEN (c): Helps Cure, And Keeps From Becoming Chronic, Reduced Jaundice 767

HEPATITIS, W/HEPATOMEGALY

- DA QING YE/DAN SHEN/YU JIN/LONG DAN CAO/TAO REN/HONG HUA/BIE JIA

HEPATOLITHIASIS

- HU ZHANG (c) 497

HEPATOMEGALY

- DA QING YE/DAN SHEN/YU JIN/LONG DAN CAO/TAO REN/HONG HUA/BIE JIA
- E ZHU/SAN LENG/(E ZHU WAN): Strong Constitution
- QING PI/CHAI HU/YU JIN/BIE JIA/DAN SHEN
- BAI SHAO 794
- BIE JIA 805
- CHI SHAO YAO 668
- DAN SHEN 672
- E ZHU 673
- HAI ZAO 721
- HONG HUA 675
- JI NEI JIN 638
- KUN BU 724
- MU LI 739
- QIAN CAO GEN 662
- SAN LENG 686
- TU BIE CHONG: Hypochondriac Pain 690
- WA LENG ZI 690
- YU JIN 695

HEPATOMEGALY W/HEAT

- E ZHU/SAN LENG/SHAN ZHI ZI/SHENG DI HUANG

HEPATOMEGALY, PAIN OF

- TU BIE CHONG/YU JIN/SAN QI/JI NEI JIN

JAUNDICE

- BAI HUA SHE SHE CAO/SHAN ZHI ZI/HUANG BAI/YIN CHEN: Damp Heat
- BAI MAO GEN/CHE QIAN ZI/JIN QIAN CAO: Damp Heat
- BAN LAN GEN/YIN CHEN: Damp Heat
- CHI XIAO DOU/MA HUANG/LIAN QIAO/SANG BAI PI: Damp Heat, Mild
- CHI XIAO DOU/YIN CHEN/SHAN ZHI ZI: Damp Heat
- HUANG BAI/SHAN ZHI ZI/YIN CHEN: Damp Heat Congested
- HUANG JING/DANG GUI: Very Deficient Qi Blood
- HUANG QIN/BAI SHAO/SHAN ZHI ZI/YIN CHEN/HUANG BAI: Damp Heat
- HUANG QIN/SHAN ZHI ZI/YIN CHEN/ZHU YE: Damp Heat
- JIN QIAN CAO/YIN CHEN/SHAN ZHI ZI: Damp Heat
- KU SHEN/MU XIANG/GAN CAO: Damp Heat
- KU SHEN/LONG DAN CAO/HUANG BAI/SHAN ZHI ZI/YIN CHEN: Damp Heat
- LONG DAN CAO/YIN CHEN: Damp Heat
- LONG DAN CAO/YIN CHEN/SHAN ZHI ZI: Damp Heat
- PU GONG YING/YIN CHEN: Damp Heat
- QIN JIAO/HUANG QIN/CANG ZHU: Damp Heat Especially In Children
- QIN JIAO/YIN CHEN/SHAN ZHI ZI: Damp Heat

- TU FU LING/PU GONG YING: Liver Gall Bladder Damp Heat
- YIN CHEN/SHAN ZHI ZI/DA HUANG/(YIN CHEN HAO TANG): Damp Heat Yang-Fever, Constipation, Urinary Problems
- YIN CHEN/GAN JIANG/FU ZI/FU LING /(YIN CHEN SI NI TANG): Damp Cold, Yin
- YIN CHEN/HOU PO
- YIN CHEN/HUA SHI: Summer Heat/Fever, Hot
- YU JIN/YIN CHEN/SHAN ZHI ZI: Damp Heat
- ZI HUA DI DING/PU GONG YING: Damp Heat

JAUNDICE W/EDEMA

- BAI MAO GEN/CHI XIAO DOU

JAUNDICE W/FEVER, DYSURIA

- SHAN ZHI ZI/YIN CHEN/DA HUANG/HUANG BAI

JAUNDICE W/FLANK PAIN

- YU JIN/YIN CHEN: Damp Heat Diseases

JAUNDICE W/INTERCOSTAL/FLANK PAIN

- DA HUANG/YIN CHEN/SHAN ZHI ZI

JAUNDICE, ACUTE

JAUNDICE, ACUTE/INFANTS

JAUNDICE, ICTERIC

JAUNDICE, NEONATAL

JAUNDICE, POSTPARTUM

JAUNDICE, YIN

LIVER ATTACKING SPLEEN/STOMACH

LIVER ATTACKING STOMACH

LIVER BLOOD DEFICIENCY

- HE SHOU WU/SANG JI SHENG/NU ZHEN ZI/NIU XI: Blurred Vision, Dizziness, Numbness

LIVER BLOOD DEFICIENCY W/HEAT

- SHAN ZHI ZI/MU DAN PI

LIVER BLOOD DEFICIENCY/STAGNATION

- CHAI HU/BO HE: Depression, Chest Constriction, Irregular Menses

LIVER CHANNEL COLD STAGNATION

- WU ZHU YU/XIAO HUI XIANG/WU YAO: Hernia, Pulling Sensation

LIVER CHANNEL HEAT

- CHE QIAN ZI/HUANG QIN/LONG DAN CAO/JU HUA: Painful, Red Eyes

LIVER CHANNEL HEAT W/CONSTIPATION

- LU HUI 544

LIVER CHANNEL HEAT, EXCESS

- LU HUI/LONG DAN CAO/HUANG QIN: Dizzy, Headache, Restless, Stomach Pain

LIVER CHANNEL PAIN

- XIAO HUI XIANG: Hernia-Like Disorders 619

LIVER CHANNEL WIND

- BAI JI LI/JUE MING ZI/JU HUA: Eye Problems w/Tearing

LIVER CHANNEL WIND HEAT

- MU ZEI/CHAN TUI/GU JING CAO/XIA KU CAO/BAI JI LI: Eye Problems—

Eyes, Red Excessive Tearing, Blurred Vision, Corneal Opacity

LIVER CHANNEL, COLD

- WU ZHU YU: Hernia-Like Pain 618

LIVER CHANNEL, COLD STAGNATION

- XIANG FU/XIAO HUI XIANG/WU YAO: Hernia, Testicle Pain

LIVER CHANNEL, WIND HEAT IN EYES

- CHAN TUI/JU HUA/MU ZEI

LIVER COLD STAGNATION

- QING PI/WU YAO/XIAO HUI XIANG/MU XIANG/(TIAN TAI WU YAO SAN): Hernia, Testicular Or Scrotal Pain

LIVER DEFICIENCY EYE PAIN

- XIA KU CAO/XIANG FU/DANG GUI/BAI SHAO: Worse At Night
- XIA KU CAO: No Red, Pain More Afternoon 478

LIVER FIRE

- GU JING CAO/LONG DAN CAO: Red Eyes, Pterygium, Headache, Toothache
- JU HUA/SANG YE/CHAN TUI/XIA KU CAO: Red, Painful Eyes
- JUE MING ZI/JU HUA: Eye Pain
- MI MENG HUA/MU ZEI/GU JING CAO: Tearing

- QING XIANG ZI/HU HUANG LIAN/LONG DAN CAO: Eye Pain, Swelling
- SANG YE/JU HUA/XIA KU CAO/MU ZEI: Eye Pain, Redness
- MU DAN PI: Headache, Eye Pain, Flank Pain, Flushing, Dysmenorrhea 499
- SHI JUE MING 750

LIVER FIRE ATTACKING STOMACH

- HUANG LIAN/WU ZHU YU: Vomiting

LIVER FIRE BLAZING

- SHI JUE MING/JU HUA: Eye Red, Swelling, Pain
- LING YANG JIAO 747
- LONG DAN CAO 492
- SHI JUE MING 750
- XIA KU CAO 478

LIVER FIRE FLARING

- QING XIANG ZI/JUE MING ZI/JU HUA/CHE QIAN ZI: Eye Problems
- SHI JUE MING/JU HUA/JUE MING ZI: Eyes, Red Painful, Vision Blurred
- XIA KU CAO/SHI JUE MING/JU HUA: Red, Painful, Swollen, Watery Eyes, Headache, Dizziness

LIVER FIRE OBSTRUCTION

- HUANG QIN/XIA KU CAO/MU LI: Scrofula
- LONG DAN CAO/CHAI HU: Scrofula

LIVER FIRE RISING

- HUAI HUA MI/XI XIAN CAO: Dizzy, Insomnia
- HUANG QIN/XIA KU CAO: Dizzy, Headache
- LING YANG JIAO/SHI JUE MING/JU HUA/HUANG QIN: Headache, Vertigo, N/V
- LONG DAN CAO/HUANG QIN/SHAN ZHI ZI/CHAI HU/MU TONG: Headache, Head Pressure, Red Eyes
- MU DAN PI/JU HUA: Dizzy, Red Eyes
- SANG YE/JU HUA/JUE MING ZI/CHE QIAN ZI: Watery, Painful Eyes
- XI XIAN CAO/XIA KU CAO: Headache, Dizzy, Blurred Vision
- XIA KU CAO/JU HUA: Red Painful Eyes, Headache, Dizziness, Vertigo
- LING YANG JIAO (c): Glaucoma Pain, With Che Qian Zi, Huang Qin, Xuan Shen, Zhi Mu, Fu Ling, Fang Feng, Xi Xin 747

LIVER FIRE W/YANG RISING

- GOU TENG 745

LIVER FIRE, EXCESS

- BO HE/JU HUA: Eye Congestion, Headache

LIVER FIRE, PHLEGM CONVULSIONS, ESPECIALLY CHILDREN

- LONG DAN CAO/NIU HUANG/GOU TENG

LIVER FLUKES

See: **Parasites** Liver Flukes 305

LIVER GALL BLADDER AREA PAIN

- CHAI HU/GAN CAO

LIVER GALL BLADDER DAMP HEAT

- BAN LAN GEN/YIN CHEN
- LONG DAN CAO/YIN CHEN: Bitter Taste, Chest Fullness, Pain
- TU FU LING/PU GONG YING: Jaundice
- SHAN ZHI ZI 476

LIVER GALL BLADDER DYSFUNCTION

- CHAI HU/HUANG QIN

LIVER GALL BLADDER EXCESS FIRE

- CHUAN LIAN ZI/YAN HU SUO/(JIN LING ZI SAN): Flank Pain

LIVER HEART SPASMS

- SHUI NIU JIAO 501
- XI JIAO 502

LIVER HEAT

- JUE MING ZI 471
- PU GONG YING: Red, Swollen Eyes 529
- YE JU HUA: Hypertension 468

LIVER HEAT IN EYES

- SHI JUE MING 750

LIVER HEAT W/RED, SWOLLEN EYES

- MI MENG HUA/JU HUA/SHI JUE MING/BAI JI LI

LIVER HEAT W/WIND

- GOU TENG 745

LIVER HEAT, EXCESS W/YANG RISING

- GOU TENG/XIA KU CAO/HUANG QIN/SHI JUE MING/JU HUA: Dizziness, Vertigo, Blurred Vision, Headache

LIVER HEAT, MILD CLEARING

- MI MENG HUA 474

LIVER KIDNEY BLOOD DEFICIENCY

- SANG SHEN ZI 801

LIVER KIDNEY DEFICIENCY

- CHE QIAN ZI/SHU DI HUANG/GOU QI ZI/TU SI ZI: Vision Poor, Cataracts
- CI SHI/ZHU SHA/SHEN QU: Visual Obstructions w/Irritability
- GOU JI/DU ZHONG/NIU XI/XU DUAN: Leg Weakness
- GUI BAN/NIU XI/SUO YANG/HU GU: Wasting/Weakness Of Lower Extremities, Retarded Development In Children
- HE SHOU WU/GOU QI ZI/BU GU ZHI/TU SI ZI: Premature Aging
- HUANG JING/XU DUAN: Low Back, Knees
- JU HUA/GOU QI ZI: Dizziness, Blurred Vision
- JUE MING ZI/XIA KU CAO: Dizziness, Vision Problems
- MI MENG HUA/GOU QI ZI/TU SI ZI: Vision Impairment
- NIU XI/SANG JI SHENG/DU ZHONG/GOU JI

- SANG SHEN ZI/HE SHOU WU: Premature Greying Of Hair
- SHA YUAN ZI/GOU QI ZI/SHU DI HUANG: Vision Blurred
- SHAN ZHU YU/SHU DI HUANG/TU SI ZI/GOU QI ZI/DU ZHONG: Dizziness, Blurred Vision, Low Back Pain
- SHU DI HUANG/SHAN ZHU YU/SHAN YAO/(LIU WEI DIHUNG WAN): Low Back, Knees
- TU SI ZI/CHE QIAN ZI/GOU QI ZI/NU ZHEN ZI: Vision Blurred, Spotty
- WU JIA PI/DU ZHONG/NIU XI/SANG JI SHENG/XU DUAN: Low Back, Knee Pain
- ZI HE CHE/GUI BAN: Dizziness, Tinnitus
- DU ZHONG 775
- FU PEN ZI 820

LIVER KIDNEY DEFICIENCY W/LIVER YANG RISING

- LONG GU/MU LI/DAI ZHE SHI/BAI SHAO/(ZHEN GAN XI FENG TANG): Dizziness, Vertigo, Blurred Vision, Irritability

LIVER KIDNEY DEFICIENCY W/WIND DAMP

- SANG JI SHENG/DU HUO/NIU XI

LIVER KIDNEY DEFICIENCY(YIN/BLOOD DEFICIENCY)

- GOU QI ZI/SHU DI HUANG/TU SI ZI/DU ZHONG: Dizziness, Impotence, Spermatorrhea, Tinnitus

LIVER KIDNEY DEFICIENCY, ESSENCE LEAKAGE

- SHA YUAN ZI/FU PEN ZI: Enuresis, Leukorrhea, Spermatorrhea

LIVER KIDNEY DEFICIENCY, SEVERE

- SUO YANG/HU GU/NIU XI/SHU DI HUANG: Muscular Atrophy

LIVER KIDNEY DEFICIENCY, SEVERE W/LOW BACK PAIN

- SHA YUAN ZI/DU ZHONG

LIVER KIDNEY INSUFFICIENCY

- SHA YUAN ZI 786

LIVER KIDNEY QI BLOCKAGE, COLD

- XIANG FU/WU YAO: Lower Abdominal Pain, Prolapse

LIVER KIDNEY YIN DEFICIENCY

- CHE QIAN ZI/SHENG DI HUANG/MAI MEN DONG/GOU QI ZI: Blurred Vision, Cataracts
- JU HUA/GOU QI ZI/NU ZHEN ZI: Blurred Vision, Dizziness
- SHA YUAN ZI/JUE MING ZI/JU HUA/GOU QI ZI: Vision Blurred
- SHI JUE MING/SHU DI HUANG/SHAN ZHU YU: Vision Impairment
- HE SHOU WU 799
- HEI ZHI MA: Blurred Vision, Tinnitus, Dizzines 808
- NU ZHEN ZI 812
- SHU DI HUANG 802

LIVER KIDNEY YIN DEFICIENCY W/LIVER YANG RISING

- GOU TENG/XIA KU CAO/HUANG QIN/SHI JUE MING/JU HUA: Dizziness, Vertigo, Blurred Vision, Headache
- SHI JUE MING/GOU TENG/JU HUA/XIA KU CAO: Eye Pain, Red Face, Headache
- ZHEN ZHU MU/BAI SHAO/SHENG DI HUANG/SHI JUE MING/LONG GU: Dizziness, Vertigo, Tinnitus, Irritability, Insomnia

LIVER KIDNEY YIN DEFICIENCY W/YANG RISING

- HEI ZHI MA/SANG YE/(SANG MA WAN): Dizziness, Blurred Vision, Tinnitus, Headache
- SANG JI SHENG/SHENG DI HUANG/CHI SHAO YAO/JI XUE TENG
- YIN YANG HUO/XIAN MAO/HUANG BAI/ZHI MU: Menopause

LIVER KIDNEY YIN DEFICIENCY W/YANG RISING FOR MEN

- YIN YANG HUO/XIAN MAO/HUANG BAI/ZHI MU

LIVER KIDNEY YIN DEFICIENCY, FIRE RISING

- SANG YE/HEI ZHI MA: Dizziness, Vertigo

LIVER KIDNEY YIN DEFICIENCY, SEVERE, W/YANG RISING

- HAN LIAN CAO/NU ZHEN ZI/(ER ZHI WAN)

LIVER KIDNEY YIN, YANG DEFICIENCY

- SHAN ZHU YU/WU WEI ZI: Abnormal Sweat, Palpitations, Shortness Of Breath, Spermatorrhea

LIVER QI ATTACKING STOMACH

- XIANG FU/MU XIANG/(XIANG YUAN-CITRON)/FO SHOU: Distension, Pain

LIVER QI CONGESTION

- XIA KU CAO/CHAI HU: Neck Nodules

LIVER QI CONGESTION W/SUBCOSTAL PAIN

LIVER QI CONGESTION, BLOOD STASIS

- YU JIN/CHAI HU: Menstruation Problems

LIVER QI CONSTRAINED

LIVER QI OBSTRUCTED

- QING PI/XIANG FU: Flank Pain/Distension

LIVER QI STAGNATION

- BAI JI LI/QING PI/XIANG FU: Chest, Flank Pain, Swelling
- BAI SHAO/CHAI HU: Flank Pain
- BO HE/BAI SHAO/CHAI HU
- CHAI HU/BAI SHAO: Vertigo, Dizzy, Costal Pain, Menstrual Irregularity
- CHAI HU/BAI SHAO/DANG GUI/CHUAN XIONG: Harmonize Blood
- CHAI HU/BAI SHAO/DANG SHEN/BAI ZHU: Qi Deficient
- CHAI HU/QING PI: Intercostal Pain
- CHAi HU/XIANG FU/ZHI KE/QING PI: Irregular Menstruation, Chest Pain
- CHEN PI/QING PI: Intercostal Pain, Abdominal Distension
- CHUAN LIAN ZI/YAN HU SUO/(JIN LING ZI SAN): Flank, Stomach Pain
- MEI GUI HUA/XIANG FU/CHUAN LIAN ZI: Flank Pain, Stomach Pain
- QING PI/CHAI HU/YU JIN/XIANG FU/(QING JU YE): Distension, Pain In Breast, Hypochondrium
- XIANG FU/CHAI HU/YU JIN/XIANG FU/BAI SHAO: Costal Pain, Stifling Sensation In The Chest
- XIANG FU/CHAI HU/DANG GUI/CHUAN XIONG: Irregular Menstration, Dysmenorrhea

LIVER QI STAGNATION LUMPS

LIVER QI STAGNATION W/COSTAL PAIN, STIFLING SENSATION

- FO SHOU/XIANG FU/(XIANG YUAN-CITRON)/YU JIN

LIVER QI STAGNATION W/HEAT

LIVER QI STAGNATION, DEFICIENCY BLOOD

- CHAI HU/DANG GUI/BAI SHAO

LIVER QI STAGNATION, YIN DEFICIENCY

• GOU QI ZI/DANG GUI/SHU DI HUANG/BEI SHA SHEN/CHUAN LIAN ZI: Stomach/Flank Pain w/Dry Throat, Regurgitation, Bitterness

LIVER QI STAGNATION/LIVER SPLEEN DISHARMONY

LIVER QI, BLOOD STAGNATION

• CHUAN XIONG/CHAI HU/CHI SHAO YAO: Headache

LIVER SPLEEN DISHARMONY

LIVER SPLEEN QI BLOCKAGE

• XIANG FU/MU XIANG: Stomach, Abdominal Pain, Indigestion, Diarrhea

LIVER SPLEEN/STOMACH DISHARMONY

LIVER STOMACH DEFICIENCY

LIVER STOMACH DISHARMONY

LIVER STOMACH DISHARMONY, REBELLIOUS QI W/HOT BLOOD

• DAI ZHE SHI/SHENG DI HUANG/MU DAN PI: Hematemesis, Hemoptosis

LIVER STOMACH HEAT DISHARMONY

• WU ZHU YU/HUANG LIAN/(ZUO JIN WAN): Vomit, Stomach Pain, Regurgitation

LIVER STOMACH QI STAGNATION

• CHUAN LIAN ZI/YAN HU SUO/(JIN LING ZI SAN)
• MAI YA/CHAI HU/ZHI SHI/CHUAN LIAN ZI: Epigastric Pain, Distension/Fullness In Chest/Hypochondium

LIVER WIND

• GOU TENG/JU HUA/SHI JUE MING/SANG YE: Dizzy, Vertigo
• GOU TENG/JU HUA/SHI JUE MING/SANG YE/SHI GAO/FU SHEN: Dizzy, Vertigo
• JU HUA/TIAN MA: Childhood Seizures
• SANG YE/JU HUA/LING YANG JIAO/GOU TENG: Cramps And Spasms

LIVER WIND FROM DEFICIENCY

• TIAN MA/CHUAN XIONG/(TIAN MA WAN): Headache, Dizzy, Vertigo

LIVER WIND HEAT

• GU JING CAO/JING JIE/LONG DAN CAO/CHI SHAO YAO: Red, Swollen Eyes, Tearing, etc
• JU HUA/SANG YE/CHAN TUI/XIA KU CAO: Red, Painful Eyes

LIVER WIND PHLEGM

LIVER WIND RISING

• NIU XI/DAI ZHE SHI/MU LI/LONG GU/(ZHEN GAN XI FENG TANG): Yin Deficiency w/Yang Rising

LIVER WIND W/HEAT

• GOU TENG/LING YANG JIAO/JU HUA/SHI GAO

LIVER WIND, YANG RISING

• GOU TENG/JU HUA/SHI JUE MING/SANG YE/SHI GAO/FU SHEN: Dizziness, Veritgo w/Short Temper, Wiry Pulse, Facial Flush

LIVER YANG EXCESS

• SHI JUE MING/XIA KU CAO: Headache, Dizzy

LIVER YANG RISING

• BAI JI LI/GOU TENG/NIU XI: Headache, Vertigo, Dizziness
• BAI SHAO/GOU TENG/JU HUA: Headache, Dizziness
• DAI ZHE SHI/LONG GU/MU LI/NIU XI: Headache, Vertigo, Dizziness, Tinnitus
• DI LONG/DAN SHEN/CI SHI
• JU HUA/TIAN MA: Headache, Vertigo, Dizziness
• JU HUA/JUE MING ZI/GOU TENG/BAI SHAO: Dizziness, Vertigo, Blurred Vision
• MAN JING ZI/JU HUA/CHAN TUI/BAI JI LI: Swollen, Red Eyes, Dizziness, Blurred Vision
• NIU XI/GOU TENG/SANG JI SHENG: Headache, Dizziness, Blurred Vision
• SANG JI SHENG/GOU TENG/JU HUA/GOU QI ZI/CHOU WU TONG: Hypertension
• SANG YE/JU HUA/SHI JUE MING/MU LI: Vertigo, Dizziness
• TIAN MA/GOU TENG: Vertigo, Dizziness
• XI XIAN CAO/GOU TENG/CHOU WU TONG: Hypertension
• ZI SHI YING/FU SHEN/SUAN ZAO REN/HUANG QI/DANG GUI: Restless, Palpitations, Anxiety, Insomnia

ASTHMA

- QING PI (c): Less Than Isoproterenol, Aminophylline 629
- SHAN DOU GEN (c): Pure Alkaloid In 100 mg Caps, 3x/Day For 10 Days, 88-100% Effective, Some Short Term Dizziness, Stomach Discomfort 532
- SHI CHANG PU (c): Volatile Oil Preparations, 120 mg 1x/Day, For Greater Than 20 Days 757
- YIN YANG HUO (c): Yang Huo Gan Chuan Ping Tablet (Yin Yang Huo, Mu Li, Hai Piao Xiao, Yuan Zhi, Qian Cao Gen, Xiao Hui Xiang, Lycorine, Clorprenaline Glycyrrhizinate) 791
- ZHI SHI (c): (Synephrine) 635

ASTHMA, BRONCHIAL W/STICKY SPUTUM

- ZAO JIAO 715

ASTHMA, BRONCHIAL, CHRONIC

- GAN CAO (c): Powdered, 3-11 Days 763

ASTHMA, BRONCHODILATORY

- HUANG QIN (c) 489

ASTHMA, CARDIAC

- YUAN HUA 556

ASTHMA, CHRONIC

- DONG CHONG XIA CAO/BEI SHA SHEN/E JIAO/CHUAN BEI MU: Lung Deficiency
- CI SHI: Kidneys Unable To Grasp Qi 735
- GE JIE: Kidney Qi Type/Weak LU/KI Qi 777
- HE ZI 822
- LIU HUANG: Spleen Kidney Deficient, Cold 840

ASTHMA, CHRONIC WORSENED BY SLIGHT EXERTION

- WU WEI ZI/SHAN ZHU YU/SHU DI HUANG/MAI MEN DONG/(BA XIAN CHANG SHOU WAN)

ASTHMA, COUGH

- QING DAI/GUA LOU/CHUAN BEI MU/HAI FU SHI/(QING DAI HAI SHI WAN): Lung Heat
- TIAN XIAN ZI 705
- XIE BAI 634

ASTHMA, COUGH OF, W/PHLEGM

- BAI GUO YE 817

ASTHMA, COUGH W/COPIOUS SPUTUM

- XUAN FU HUA 713

ASTHMA, COUGH W/PHLEGM RETENTION

- ZE QI 727

ASTHMA, DYSPNEA

- SHU DI HUANG 802

ASTHMA, ELDERLY

- ZI SHI YING 742

ASTHMA, IN CHILDREN

- MA HUANG (c): In Ma Xing Shi Gan Tang 448

ASTHMA, IN WHICH PATIENT CANNOT LIE FLAT

- TING LI ZI/DA ZAO/(TING LI DA ZAO XIE FEI TANG)

ASTHMA, POST ATTACK

- DAI ZHE SHI/BAN XIA/XUAN FU HUA/SHENG JIANG/(XUAN FU BAI ZHE TANG)

ASTHMA, PROFUSE, YELLOW SPUTUM

- MA DOU LING/PI PA YE/QIAN HU/SANG BAI PI/HUANG QIN: Lung Heat

ASTHMA, WITH PROFUSE PHLEGM

- HOU PO 581

ASTHMA/WHEEZING

- CHEN XIANG: Kidney Deficient 622

ASTHMATICUS, STATUS

- DANG GUI (c): Ether Extract, No Other Medication, 2-10 Hrs To Get Benefit 795

BREATH, SHORTNESS OF

- REN SHEN/WU WEI ZI/MAI MEN DONG: Febrile Diseases, Exhaustion Of Qi And Fluids
- DA ZAO: Spleen Stomach Deficient 761
- DANG SHEN: Lung Deficient 762

BREATH, SHORTNESS OF W/LASSITUDE, SPONTANEOUS SWEATING

- REN SHEN/GE JIE/(REN SHEN GE JIE TANG): Lung Qi Deficiency

BREATHING DIFFICULTLY

- GUANG FANG JI/DANG SHEN/GUI ZHI

BREATHING RATE

- ROU CONG RONG (c): Slows Respiration By Paralysis 786

BREATHING, LABORED

- HONG DA JI: Ascites 551

BREATHING, LOWERS RATE

- FU ZI (c) 613

BREATHING, RAPID

- BA DOU: pwdr Blown In Throat To Cause Vomiting .. 550

BRONCHI, CONTRACTS SMOOTH MUSCLES OF

- SHAN ZI CAO (c) 664

BRONCHI, INHIBITS SECRETION

- MO YAO (c) 683

BRONCHITIS, CHRONIC

- YUAN HUA/DA ZAO: Cold Damp
- AI YE (c): Caps Of Oil, 2 Courses Of 10 Days Each/Decoction 651
- BAI BU (c): 50% Syrup, 15-100 ml And Extract Tab, 0.5 g 3-4 Tabs, 3x/Day, For 10 Day Course, Each, 1/2 Improved 699
- BAI GUO (c): With Di Long, Huang Qin Or Di Long, Pu Gong Ying, 90-100% Effective, 1ST Group Better As Tablet, *Antiasthmatic Decoction (Yin Guo, Ma Huang, Ban Xia, Kuan Dong Hua, Sang Bai Pi, Zi Su Zi, Xing Ren, Huang Qin) 818
- BAI HUA SHE SHE CAO (c): Mild/Simple Cases Cured Easier, With Crude Extract, Pig Bile/Deoxycholic Acid 511
- BAI JIE ZI (c): (Injection Into Accu-Pts) 708
- BAN XIA (c): With Jie Geng, Fu Ling, Gan Cao (Ju Fang Er Chen Tang) 710
- BAO MA ZI 700
- BAO MA ZI (c) 700
- CANG ER ZI (c): With Oral Dose Of Stir Fried Seeds, 83% Even A Year After Treatment 559
- CANG ZHU (c): Use Of Incense Of Cang Zhu, Ai Ye, 7-14 Days Improved Cough, Dyspnea, Expectoration 578
- CE BAI YE 654
- CE BAI YE (c): 70-95% Effective Rate, Herb Plus e.g. Shan Yao, Yin Yang Huo, 15 g Ea, SIGA Levels Increased, *60 g/Day In 2 Doses Of Cone, 15 Days=Course, 81% Effective 654
- CHOU WU TONG (c): Fresh Herb, 200 g As Decoction, 3 Doses/Day, 10=1 Course, 3 Courses Markedly Effective, But Slow, Unstable 560
- CHUAN BEI MU 717
- CHUAN SHAN LONG 442
- CHUAN SHAN LONG (c): Decoction/Tablet With Herb, Huang Qin, Jie Geng, Zi Wan, Bai Bu, Wu Wei Zi, *Tablet/Decoction Of Herb, Huang Qin, Chuan Bei Mu 442
- DI LONG (c): Chuan Shu Ning Pian (Di Long, Ammonium Chloride) , 1-2 Tabs/Day/Di Long Powder, 3-4 g, 3-4x/Day, Orally/Compound Ephedra-Pheretima Tablet (Ma Huang, Fried Di Long, Dan Nan Xing, Ye Qiao Mai, Pu Gong Ying, Rough Extract With Alcohol, Then Made Into Tabs) , 10 Day Courses 744
- DU HUO (c): Decoction, 74% Showed Some Response, 7% Marked, Some Cough Suppressing Effects 561
- FO SHOU (c): With Ban Xia, Fu Ling, etc, *30 g With Honey As Tea, 2 Months 624
- GAN JIANG: Thin, White, Foamy Sputum 614
- GUAN ZHONG (c) 521
- HAI ZAO 721
- HE SHOU WU (c) 799
- HU ZHANG (c): Singly Or With Yu Xing Cao, Folium Elaeagnus Pungens 497
- HUANG QI (c) 765
- HUANG QIN (c): Huang Qin, Gan Cao, Lime Water (Calcium Hydroxide Solution) , Good Response In Simple Disease 489
- JIANG CAN (c): Alleviated Cough, Thinned Sputum, Did Not Cure, Though 746
- KU SHEN (c) 491

- KUAN DONG HUA (c): Cough Of, With Zi Wan As Decoction, 5-10 g Each, *Kuan Dong Hua, Di Long Injection Helped After 3-4 Days 700
- LAI FU ZI 639
- LAI FU ZI (c): San Zi Yang Qin Tang (Lai Fu Zi, Bai Jie Zi, Zi Su Zi) , *Often With Phlegm Use Tan Yin Wan With Cang Zhu, Bai Zhu, Gan Jiang, Rou Gui Pi, Gan Cao, Fu Zi, Especially For Kidney Spleen Deficient Patterns ... 639
- LING ZHI CAO 731
- LING ZHI CAO (c): Spleen Deficiency Type, Treated With Preparations For 4 Months, Reduced Excitability Of Parasympathetic Nerves, *Concentrated Solution, 2 ml, 4 Weeks Of Herb Plus Bai Mu Er Spores Helped Regenerate Bronchial Epithelium, *After Months Of Treatment A General Increase Of Iga, *Best For Bronchitis Of "Old Age", Asthmatic Type, Deficiency-Cold Type, 1-2 Weeks To Marked Effects, Ling Zhi Syrup Tablet 731
- LONG KUI 526
- LONG KUI (c): Compound Long Kui Tablet (Long Kui 30 g, Jie Geng 10 g, Gan Cao 3 g Daily Dose) Divide, Take 3x/Day, For 10 Days, Best Results In Simple Type, Fruit May Be Better 526
- LUO BU MA (c): Cigarette From Leaves Useful In Prevention/Treatment, Help Cough And Other Symptoms 748
- MA DOU LING (c): With Gan Cao Pi, Effective 701
- MA QIAN ZI (c): Brucine Tablet, 10-50 mg, 3x/Day For 10 Days With 3 Day Rest Mid-Course, 3 Courses Needed To Cure, Better After 3 Days 842
- MAN SHAN HONG 851
- MIAN HUA GEN (c): Symptomatic Treatment, Good For Cough, Expectoration 851
- MO YAO (c) 683
- NU ZHEN ZI (c): Equivalent 50 g Of Raw Herb Or Nu Zhen Zi, Dong Gua Ren, Promethazine 812
- PI PA YE (c): Short Term Control 703
- QIAN CAO GEN 662
- QIAN CAO GEN (c): Decoction With Qing Pi, More Effective With Asthmatic Than Simple Type, Controlled Rales, Wheezing 662
- QIN PI (c): 1: 1 Aerosol, 2 ml Each Time For 10x, Generally 2 Courses, *Extract Tablet, 0.3 g Or Extract/Tab, 2 Tabs, 3x/Day For 3 Course, 10 Days/Course, Both Treatments Very Effective For Short-Term Control Of Dyspnea 493
- QING HAO (c): Volatile Oil 508
- QING MU XIANG (c): Cleared Up Purulent Sputum ... 628
- SHANG LU (c): Best In Simple Type, ETOH Extract Tablet, Honey Pill, ETOH Extract Best At 87-95% Short-Term Control 554
- SHI WEI (c): Helps Symptoms, Cell Changes 601
- XI HE LIU 451
- XING REN (c): Paste Made With Sugar, 3-4 Days 705
- XUAN FU HUA (c): With Sang Bai Pi, Jie Geng, Pu Yan Pian (Radix Rhois Chinensis) 713
- YANG JIN HUA (c): Injection Was Highly Efficacious, Control 70%, High Rate Of Side Effects, Less With Liquor, Tablet, Herb Cigarette, Suppository (Keep Dose At 0.01 mg/kg) , *Clinical Control Acheived 63% For Tablet, 0.01 mg/kg Taken At Bed For 5 Courses Of 10 Days Each 714
- YE JU HUA (c): Reduces Acute Attacks 468
- YIN YANG HUO 791

COUGH IN CHILDREN

COUGH, ACUTE

COUGH, ACUTE FROM EXTERNAL WIND PATHOGENS

- JING JIE/BO HE/JIE GENG/GAN CAO

COUGH, ACUTE/CHRONIC W/BLOODY SPUTUM

- ZI WAN/BAI BU

COUGH, ALL KINDS

COUGH, ASTHMA

See: Lungs Asthma 214
- HOU PO/XING REN/(GUI ZHI JIA HOU PO XING ZI TANG)
- SHI GAO/MA HUANG/XING REN: Lung Heat

COUGH, ASTHMA W/COPIOUS SPUTUM

COUGH, ASTHMA W/PHLEGM

COUGH, ASTHMATIC

COUGH, BLOOD

- BAI JI/E JIAO/OU JIE/PI PA YE: Lung Deficient Yin
- CE BAI YE/DA JI/XIAO JI/BAI MAO GEN: Heat
- CHEN ZONG TAN/BAI MAO GEN/DA JI/XIAO JI/SHAN ZHI ZI/(SHI HUI SAN): Heat
- DA JI/XIAO JI/CE BAI YE: Blood Heat
- DI GU PI/BAI MAO GEN/CE BAI YE: Yin Deficiency w/Heat
- GUI BAN/SHU DI HUANG/(DA BU YIN WAN): Yin Deficiency w/Excess Fire
- HUAI HUA MI/CE BAI YE/BAI MAO GEN/XIAN HE CAO
- OU JIE/BAI JI/CE BAI YE/BAI MAO GEN
- XIAN HE CAO/SHENG DI HUANG/MU DAN PI/SHAN ZHI ZI/CE BAI YE: Heat

COUGH, BLOOD STREAKED SPUTUM

COUGH, BLOOD, PUS

- JIE GENG/YU XING CAO/DONG GUA REN/GUA LOU: Lung Abscess, Toxic Heat

COUGH, BLOODY SPUTUM

- BAI JI/PI PA YE
- DONG CHONG XIA CAO/BEI SHA SHEN/E JIAO/CHUAN BEI MU: Lung Deficiency
- HUA QI SHEN/MAI MEN DONG/E JIAO/ZHI MU/CHUAN BEI MU: Lung Yin Deficiency w/Excess Fire
- MA DOU LING/E JIAO: Yin Damage From Heat, Lung Deficient
- MAI MEN DONG/BEI SHA SHEN/TIAN MEN DONG/CHUAN BEI MU/SHENG DI HUANG: Lung Yin Deficiency w/Heat, Dryness
- TIAN MEN DONG/MAI MEN DONG/(ER DONG GAO): Lung Kidney Yin Deficiency w/Fire Flaring
- ZI WAN/ZHI MU/CHUAN BEI MU/E JIAO/(ZI WAN TANG): Lung Deficiency

COUGH, BLOODY SPUTUM W/SHORTNESS OF BREATH

- MA DOU LING/BEI SHA SHEN/MAI MEN DONG/ZI WAN/E JIAO: Lung Deficiency

COUGH, BLOODY SPUTUM, DRY MOUTH

- E JIAO/BEI SHA SHEN/MAI MEN DONG/XING REN/CHUAN BEI MU: Yin Deficient

COUGH, BLOODY, DIFFICULT TO EXPECTORATE SPUTUM

COUGH, BRONCHIAL

COUGH, CHEST CONSTRICTION

COUGH, CHEST FULLNESS

COUGH, CHEST PAIN

- BAI BU/CHUAN BEI MU: Phlegm Heat

COUGH, CHEST PAIN, DIFFICULT EXPECTORATION

- BAN XIA/GUA LOU: Phlegm Heat Blocking Interior
- GUA LOU REN/BAN XIA/HUANG LIAN/(XIAO XIAN XIONG TANG)

COUGH, CHEST PAIN, PROFUSE SPUTUM

- FO SHOU/PI PA YE/SI GUA LUO/XING REN

COUGH, CHEST, RIB PAIN

COUGH, CHEST/DIAPHRAGM CONSTRICTION, COPIOUS SPUTUM

COUGH, CHRONIC

- CHUAN BEI MU/PI PA YE/MAI MEN DONG/YU ZHU: w/Fatigue, Irritability, Sputum, Excess/Bloody, Chest Constriction/Distension, Anorexia
- DONG CHONG XIA CAO/BEI SHA SHEN/E JIAO/CHUAN BEI MU: Lung Deficiency
- HE ZI/WU WEI ZI/BEI SHA SHEN/BAI HE: Deficient Lungs
- SHAN YAO/BEI SHA SHEN/MAI MEN DONG/WU WEI ZI: Lung Deficiency
- WU BEI ZI/WU WEI ZI: Deficient Lungs
- WU MEI/XING REN/BAN XIA: Deficient Lungs
- WU MEI/HE ZI/WU WEI ZI
- WU MEI/YING SU KE/E JIAO/XING REN: Lung Deficiency
- ZI WAN/TIAN MEN DONG/HUANG QIN/SANG BAI PI: w/Heat—Bloody Sputum w/Pus

COUGH, DIFFICULT EXPECTORATION, CHEST PAIN

- TIAN ZHU HUANG/BAN XIA: Hot Phlegm

COUGH, DRY

- BEI SHA SHEN/MAI MEN DONG/CHUAN BEI MU: Lung Yin Deficiency w/Heat
- E JIAO/XING REN/NIU BANG ZI: Heat Damage Fluids
- GAN CAO/XING REN/CHUAN BEI MU: Heat
- HUANG JING/BEI SHA SHEN/MAI MEN DONG: Deficient Lung Qi/Yin
- PI PA YE/XING REN: Lung Heat
- TAI ZI SHEN/BEI SHA SHEN/MAI MEN DONG: Lung Yin Deficiency
- TIAN HUA FEN/SANG BAI PI/CHUAN BEI MU/JIE GENG: Lung Heat
- XING REN/ZI SU YE: Wind Cold
- XING REN/MAI MEN DONG: Lung Heat, Dryness
- XING REN/SANG YE: Wind Heat
- ZHI MU/CHUAN BEI MU: Yin Deficient

COUGH, DRY THROAT

- MU HU DIE/PANG DA HAI/CHAN TUI

COUGH, DRY THROAT, YELLOW SPUTUM

- BO HE/NIU BANG ZI

COUGH, DRY W/BLOODY SPUTUM

- E JIAO/MAI MEN DONG/BEI SHA SHEN: Lung Yin Deficient
- KUAN DONG HUA/BAI HE

COUGH, DRY W/SCANTY SPUTUM

- YU ZHU/BEI SHA SHEN/MAI MEN DONG/TIAN MEN DONG: Lung Yin Deficiency

COUGH, DRY W/THICK SPUTUM

- YU ZHU/YI YI REN: Lung Abscess

COUGH, DRY W/THIN/BLOODY SPUTUM

COUGH, DRY W/WEAK VOICE, WHEEZING

- YI TANG/BAI BU/XING REN: Lung Deficient

COUGH, DRY, CHRONIC

- BAI HE/MAI MEN DONG/XUAN SHEN/CHUAN BEI MU: Lung Yin Deficient
- BEI SHA SHEN/MAI MEN DONG: Decreased Fluids, Lung Yin Deficient
- MAI MEN DONG/BAN XIA/DANG SHEN: Deficient Lung Yin
- TIAN MEN DONG/SHENG DI HUANG/CHUAN BEI MU/BAI HE: Heat, Lung Yin Deficient
- TIAN MEN DONG/MAI MEN DONG/(ER DONG GAO): Lung Kidney Yin Deficiency w/Fire Flaring/Injured Fluids

COUGH, DRY, CHRONIC, NON-PRODUCTIVE

- CE BAI YE/DA ZAO: Hot

COUGH, DRY, DIFFICULT EXPECTORATION

- BEI SHA SHEN/CHUAN BEI MU: Lung Yin Deficient

COUGH, DRY, DIFFICULT SPUTUM

COUGH, DRY, NON-PRODUCTIVE

COUGH, DRY, PAROXYSMAL

- BAI QIAN/BAI BU

COUGH, DRY, STICKY SPUTUM

COUGH, DRY, THICK SPUTUM

COUGH, DRY/BLOODY SPUTUM

COUGH, DURING COMMON COLD

- ZI SU YE/JIE GENG/XING REN/QIANG HUO

COUGH, DYSPNEA

COUGH, EXCESS SPUTUM

- BAI ZHU/GUI ZHI/FU LING /(LING GUI ZHU GAN TANG): Phlegm Damp Syndrome
- SANG BAI PI/DI GU PI/GAN CAO/(XIE BAI SAN): Lung Heat

COUGH, EXCESS, THICK PHLEGM

• YUAN ZHI/XING REN/JIE GENG/GAN CAO

COUGH, EXHAUSTION W/STEAMING BONE FEVER

• ZHI MU 480

COUGH, EXTREME HEAT

• GUA LOU REN/BAN XIA/HUANG LIAN/CHAI HU/HUANG QIN: w/Chest Pain, Difficult Expectoration

COUGH, FEVER IN CHILDREN

• SHI GAO/DAN ZHU YE

COUGH, FEVER, CHEST PAIN

• SI GUA LUO: Lung Heat 688

COUGH, FROM EXOGENEOUS FACTORS

• BAI QIAN/JING JIE/JIE GENG/(ZHI SUO SAN)

COUGH, FROM FATIGUE

• ZHI MU 480

COUGH, FROM FLUID RETENTION

• ZE XIE/FU LING /ZHU LING/BAI ZHU/(WU LING SAN)

COUGH, FROM TUBERCULOSIS

• BAI BU/MAI MEN DONG/SHENG DI HUANG

COUGH, GASPING

• JUAN BO 679

COUGH, GENERAL

• XING REN: Hot/Cold, Best Dry 705

COUGH, HEADACHE

• SHENG JIANG/ZHU LI: Hot Phlegm

COUGH, HEMOPTYSIS

See: Hemorrhagic Disorders Hemoptysis 170
• BAI HE/XUAN SHEN/CHUAN BEI MU/SHENG DI HUANG/(BAI HE GU JIN TANG): Lung Yin Deficiency w/Excess Fire
• XUAN SHEN (c): Yang Ying Qing Fei Tang (Xuan Shen, Sheng Di, Mai Dong, Bai Shao, Mu Dan Pi, Gan Cao, Bo He) 503

COUGH, LUNG EXHAUSTION

• BAI BU: Tuberculosis 699
• BAI HE: Tuberculosis 803
• BAI JI: Tuberculosis 652
• BEI SHA SHEN: Tuberculosis 804
• CHUAN BEI MU: Tuberculosis 717
• DONG CHONG XIA CAO: Tuberculosis 775
• E JIAO: Tuberculosis 797
• GUI BAN: Tuberculosis 806
• HUANG JING: Tuberculosis 764
• KUAN DONG HUA: Tuberculosis 700
• MAI MEN DONG: Tuberculosis 810
• SANG YE: Tuberculosis 466
• SHAN YAO: Tuberculosis 769

• SHENG DI HUANG: Tuberculosis 500
• SHI HU: Tuberculosis 813
• SHU DI HUANG: Tuberculosis 802
• TIAN MEN DONG: Tuberculosis 814
• YU ZHU: Tuberculosis 815
• ZHI MU: Tuberculosis 480
• ZI WAN: Tuberculosis 706

COUGH, LUNG EXHAUSTION W/HEMORRHAGE

• SAN QI 663
• XIAN HE CAO 665

COUGH, NASAL FLARING

• SHI GAO/MA HUANG: Lung Heat

COUGH, NASAL FLARING, WHEEZING

• MA HUANG/SHI GAO/HUANG QIN/SANG BAI PI: Lung Heat

COUGH, NAUSEA

• HUO XIANG/ZI SU YE: Wind Cold w/Dampness In Middle Jiao

COUGH, NO SPUTUM

• YANG JIN HUA 714

COUGH, PERTUSSIS

See: Lungs Cough, Whooping 227
See: Lungs Whooping Cough 238

COUGH, PERTUSSIS PAROXYSMS

• XIONG DAN (c) 479

COUGH, PHLEGM

• CHE QIAN CAO 589

COUGH, PHLEGM HEAT

• BAI QIAN/GUA LOU: Phlegm Blocking Lungs

COUGH, PRODUCTIVE

• BAN XIA/CHEN PI: Damp Phlegm Or Deficient Spleen Qi
• SHENG JIANG/BAN XIA: Damp Phlegm
• ZHE BEI MU: Phlegm Heat/Lung Heat 728

COUGH, PRODUCTIVE W/SORE THROAT

• NIU BANG ZI/JIE GENG: Wind Heat
• NIU BANG ZI/JIE GENG/BO HE: Wind Heat

COUGH, PRODUCTIVE, CLEAR BUBBLY SPUTUM

• JIE GENG/ZI SU YE: Wind Cold

COUGH, PROFUSE SPUTUM

• CHEN PI/BAN XIA/FU LING /(ER CHEN TANG): Excess Dampness, Spleen Deficiency, Turbid Phlegm Blocking Lungs
• TING LI ZI/DA ZAO/(TING LI DA ZAO XIE FEI TANG): Phlegm Fluid In Lungs
• XUAN FU HUA/BAN XIA/XI XIN: Phlegm Fluid Blocking The Lungs
• ZI WAN/JING JIE/BAI QIAN: Exogenous Factors

COUGH, PROFUSE, CLEAR SPUTUM

- XI XIN/MA HUANG/GAN JIANG/(QING LONG TANG): Lungs w/Cold Phlegm Fluid

COUGH, PROFUSE, DILUTE, WHITE SPUTUM

- BAN XIA/CHEN PI/FU LING /(ER CHEN TANG): Phlegm Damp Cough

COUGH, PROFUSE, THICK, YELLOW SPUTUM

- DAN NAN XING/HUANG QIN/GUA LOU: Lung Phlegm Heat

COUGH, PROFUSE, YELLOW SPUTUM

- MA DOU LING/PI PA YE/QIAN HU/SANG BAI PI/HUANG QIN: Lung Heat

COUGH, PROLONGED

COUGH, PULMONARY TUBERCULOSIS

COUGH, RED, PAINFUL EYES

- SANG YE/JU HUA: Wind Heat

COUGH, SCANTY SPUTUM

- BEI SHA SHEN/MAI MEN DONG/CHUAN BEI MU: Lung Yin Deficiency w/Heat
- E JIAO/BEI SHA SHEN/MAI MEN DONG/XING REN/CHUAN BEI MU: Yin Deficient
- MA DOU LING/BEI SHA SHEN/MAI MEN DONG/ZI WAN/E JIAO: Lung Deficiency
- TAI ZI SHEN/BEI SHA SHEN/MAI MEN DONG: Lung Yin Deficiency
- ZI WAN/ZHI MU/CHUAN BEI MU/E JIAO/(ZI WAN TANG): Lung Deficiency

COUGH, SCANTY, STICKY SPUTUM

- MAI MEN DONG/BEI SHA SHEN/TIAN MEN DONG/CHUAN BEI MU/SHENG DI HUANG: Lung Yin Deficiency w/Heat, Dryness

COUGH, SCANTY/DIFFICULT SPUTUM

- CHUAN BEI MU/ZHI MU: Deficient Yin Fire In Lungs

COUGH, SPUTUM

COUGH, SPUTUM, DURING COMMON COLD

- ZI SU YE/JIE GENG

COUGH, SPUTUM, SORE THROAT

COUGH, SPUTUM, SPONTANEOUS SWEAT, WHEEZING

- ZI WAN/WU WEI ZI

COUGH, SPUTUM, WHEEZING, HOARSENESS

- MA DOU LING/XING REN: Lung Heat

COUGH, STICKY PHLEGM

COUGH, SUDDEN

- YUAN HUA/DA ZAO

COUGH, THICK SPUTUM

COUGH, THICK SPUTUM W/CHEST PAIN, DRY THROAT

- PI PA YE/XING REN

COUGH, THICK SPUTUM, CHEST CONSTRICTION, IRRITABILITY

- QIAN HU/SANG BAI PI: Lung Heat

COUGH, THICK SPUTUM, FEVER, RESTLESS, THIRST

- SANG BAI PI/DI GU PI: Phlegm Heat Obstructing Lung

COUGH, THICK, YELLOW SPUTUM

- QING DAI/GUA LOU/CHUAN BEI MU/HAI FU SHI/(QING DAI HAI SHI WAN): Lung Heat

COUGH, THICK, YELLOW SPUTUM W/CHEST PAIN

- ZHU LI/PI PA YE/GUA LOU: Phlegm Heat

COUGH, THICK, YELLOW SPUTUM, CHEST PAIN

- HAI GE KE/HAI FU SHI/BAI QIAN/SANG BAI PI/SHAN ZHI ZI/GUA LOU: Phlegm Heat

COUGH, THICK/BLOODY SPUTUM

COUGH, THIN, WATERY SPUTUM

- SHAN YAO/DANG SHEN: Lung Spleen/Kidney Spleen Deficient

COUGH, TUBERCULOSIS

- BAI QIAN/BAI BU: Bloody Sputm
- CHUAN BEI MU (c): With Pi Pa Ye, Sang Ye, Mai Ya, Yu Zhu (Qing Zao Jiu Fei Tang) 717

COUGH, W/LOSS OF VOICE

COUGH, WHEEZING

See: Lungs Asthma 214
• BU GU ZHI/HU TAO REN: Kidney Yang Deficient
• DI LONG/MA HUANG/XING REN/HUANG QIN: Lung Heat
• DI LONG/HAI PIAO XIAO/TIAN ZHU HUANG/(powder): With Other Decoctions
• E GUAN SHI/HU TAO REN/XING REN/LAI FU ZI: Deficient Kidney Yang
• E GUAN SHI/BEI SHA SHEN: Deficient Zhong Qi
• GAN JIANG/WU WEI ZI: Lung Qi Not Descending From Congested Fluids
• HAI GE KE/HAI FU SHI: Phlegm Fire Obstructing Lung
• HOU PO/XING REN/MA HUANG: Congested Fluids w/Copious Sputum
• KUAN DONG HUA/XING REN: Phlegm Obstruction
• KUAN DONG HUA/WU WEI ZI/BAN XIA: Congested Fluids
• LAI FU ZI/BAN XIA: Damp Phlegm
• MA HUANG/SHU DI HUANG: Deficient Kidney Yin
• WU WEI ZI/SHU DI HUANG/SHAN YAO/SHAN ZHU YU: Lung Kidney Deficiency
• WU WEI ZI/GAN JIANG: Lung Deficient/Cold
• XI XIN/MA HUANG: Wind Cold, Phlegm
• XI XIN/WU WEI ZI: Cold Phlegm
• XING REN/MA HUANG: Excess
• XING REN/MA HUANG/SHI GAO/(MA XING SHI GAN TANG): Lung Heat
• YUAN ZHI/CHUAN BEI MU/BAN XIA: Cold Phlegm
• ZE QI/YU XING CAO/QIAN HU: Lung Heat From Congested Fluids
• ZI HE CHE/WU WEI ZI/MAI MEN DONG: Lung Deficient
• ZI SU ZI/BAN XIA: Rebellious Qi, Phlegm
• ZI SU ZI/BAI QIAN: Qi, Phlegm Obstruction
• ZI WAN/KUAN DONG HUA: Copious Sputum, Rebellious Qi

COUGH, WHEEZING CHRONIC

• LAI FU ZI/ZI SU ZI/BAI JIE ZI/(SAN ZI YANG QING TANG): Especially Excess Phlegm

COUGH, WHEEZING FROM CONGESTED FLUIDS W/EDEMA

• ZE QI/BAN XIA/ZI WAN

COUGH, WHEEZING W/COPIOUS SPUTUM

• CHUAN BEI MU/XING REN

COUGH, WHEEZING W/COPIOUS, THICK SPUTUM

• ZI SU ZI/ZHE BEI MU: Phlegm Obstruction

COUGH, WHEEZING W/DIFFICULT TO EXPECTORATE SPUTUM, GURGLING SOUNDS

• BAI QIAN/ZI WAN/BAN XIA: Phlegm, Damp Obstructing Lungs

COUGH, WHEEZING W/EXCESS YELLOW SPUTUM

• BAI GUO/MA HUANG/XING REN/SANG BAI PI: Deficient Lungs And Hot Phlegm

COUGH, WHEEZING W/HOARSENESS, BLOODY SPUTUM

• GE JIE/SHENG DI HUANG: Lung Kidney Deficient

COUGH, WHEEZING W/SPUTUM OBSTRUCTION

COUGH, WHEEZING(INHALATION DIFFICULT)

• GE JIE/REN SHEN/(korean)/HU TAO REN/WU WEI ZI: Lung Kidney Deficient

COUGH, WHEEZING, CHRONIC

• BAI BU/BAI QIAN: Lung Qi Obstruction
• CI SHI/SHU DI HUANG/SHAN ZHU YU/WU WEI ZI: Kidney Lung Deficient—Kidney Unable To Grasp Lung Qi

COUGH, WHEEZING, CHRONIC W/PHLEGM HEAT

• GE JIE/CHUAN BEI MU: Lung Deficiency

COUGH, WHEEZING, CHRONIC W/SPUTUM

COUGH, WHEEZING, CHRONIC/RECURRENT

COUGH, WHEEZING, W/SPUTUM

• ZI SHI YING/SHU DI HUANG/E JIAO/HU TAO REN: Lungs Cold, Deficient

COUGH, WHITE, PROFUSE SPUTUM

• ZI SU ZI/BAI JIE ZI/LAI FU ZI/(SAN ZI YANG QING TANG): Rebellious Lung Qi From Excess Phlegm Fluid

COUGH, WHOOPING

COUGH, YELLOW SPUTUM

• ZHU RU/ZHI SHI/CHEN PI/FU LING /(WEN DAN TANG): Phlegm Heat

COUGH, YELLOW, THICK SPUTUM

- CHUAN BEI MU/ZHI MU/HUANG QIN/GUA LOU: Phlegm Heat
- GUA LOU/DAN NAN XING/HUANG QIN/(QING PI HUA TAN WAN): Phlegm Heat
- ZHU RU/GUA LOU/HUANG QIN: Lung Heat

COUGH, YELLOW, THICK, STICKY SPUTUM

- HAI FU SHI/HAI GE KE/GUA LOU/SHAN ZHI ZI/QING DAI: Phlegm Heat
- PANG DA HAI/JIE GENG/CHAN TUI/BO HE/GAN CAO: Lung Heat Accumulation

COUGH/DYSPNEA

- BAN XIA 710

COUGH/WHEEZING

- LIU HUANG: Lung Deficiency 840
- QIAN HU: Early Lung Heat w/Thick Sputum 725
- SANG BAI PI: Lung Heat 703
- SHI WEI: Lung Heat 601
- WU WEI ZI: Lung Kidney Deficient 831
- XI XIN: Phlegm Fluid 452
- ZI SHI YING: Lung Cold, Deficient 742
- ZI SU ZI: Copious Phlegm/Exhalation Difficult Compared To Inhalation 706

DYSPNEA

- XIE BAI/GUA LOU/(GUA LOU XIE BAI BAI JIU TANG): Cold Phlegm Stagnation
- BAN BIAN LIAN 586
- BAN XIA 710
- CI SHI: Deficiency 735
- GAN JIANG: Cold 614
- GE JIE 777
- HAI GE KE: Phlegm Heat 721
- HOU PO: Surging Phlegm 581
- HOU ZAO 722
- HU TAO REN: Deficiency Cold 782
- HUA QI SHEN 808
- KUAN DONG HUA 700
- LAI FU ZI: Phlegm 639
- LI LU 834
- MA DOU LING 701
- MA HUANG 448
- QIAN HU 725
- QIAN NIU ZI 553
- REN SHEN: Lung Qi Deficient 767
- SANG BAI PI: Lung Heat 703
- SHAN DOU GEN 532
- SHAN YAO 769
- SHENG JIANG 450
- SHI GAO: Lung Heat 477
- TAI ZI SHEN: Lung Deficiency 770
- WU WEI ZI: Lung Deficient 831
- XI XIN: Phlegm Fluid 452
- XIE BAI: Turbid Phlegm Causing Cold, Damp Chest Bi 634
- XUAN FU HUA 713

- YUAN HUA: Soft Phlegm Mass 556
- ZHU LI 728
- ZI HE CHE 792
- ZI SU ZI: Copious Phlegm 706
- ZI WAN: Cold Phlegm/Lung Heat 706

DYSPNEA, CHEST DISTENTION

- XING REN 705

DYSPNEA, PALPITATIONS

- GUI ZHI/FU LING : Heart Yang Deficient

DYSPNEA, QI REFLUX

- CHEN XIANG 622

EMPHYSEMA

- FO SHOU (c): 30 g With Honey As Tea, 2 Months 624

EMPHYSEMA, PULMONARY

- CHEN XIANG 622

EMPHYSEMA, PULMONARY DUE TO HEART

- ZE QI 727

EXPECTORANT

See: Lungs Cough 219
- A WEI (c): Through Irritation Of Lungs 637
- AI YE (c): Oral Can Reduce Cough 651
- AN XI XIANG (c): Tincture, In Water, Boiled, Direct Inhalation, Watch Irritation 753
- BAI BU (c) 699
- BAI GUO (c): Possible 818
- BAI JIE ZI (c): Oil Slightly Irritates GI, Thus Increasing Secretions Of Bronchi 708
- BAN XIA (c) 710
- BAO MA ZI (c): Similar To Jie Geng 700
- BEI XIE (c) 587
- BO HE (c) 456
- CE BAI YE (c): ETOH Extract 654
- CHE QIAN CAO (c) 589
- CHE QIAN ZI (c) 590
- CHEN PI (c): Volatile Oil 621
- CHUAN BEI MU (c): Decreases Secretion 717
- CHUAN SHAN LONG (c): Oral 442
- CONG BAI (c) 442
- DI JIAO (c) 443
- E BU SHI CAO (c): Tincture 711
- FENG MI (c) 548
- FO SHOU (c) 624
- GAN CAO (c) 763
- GUA LOU PI (c): Good 719
- HU ZHANG (c) 497
- KUAN DONG HUA (c): Thru Irritation Of Lung Mucosa, Less Than Jie Geng Or Less Than Che Qian Cao 700
- KUN BU (c) 724
- LAI FU ZI (c) 639
- LING ZHI CAO (c): Thru Irritation Of Lung Mucosa ... 731
- LONG GU (c) 738
- LONG KUI (c) 526

- MA DOU LING (c): Bronchidilatory, Weak, Less Than Zi Wan, Tian Nan Xing, But Greater Than Ammonium Chloride 701
- MAI MEN DONG (c) 810
- MAN SHAN HONG (c): Alcohol Infusion Dramatic 851
- MAO DONG QING (c) 682
- MIAN HUA GEN (c): Dramatic, Especially ETOH Extract, Resin Fraction 851
- MO YAO (c): Tincture Of 683
- NAN SHA SHEN (c) 811
- PENG SHA (c) 844
- PI PA YE (c): Weak 703
- QIAN CAO GEN (c): Marked From Oral Decoction, Not Tinctures 662
- QIAN HU (c): Similar To Jie Geng 725
- QIN PI (c) 493
- QING PI (c): Volatile Oil 629
- SANG BAI PI (c) 703
- SHANG LU (c): Decoction Strong, IP Stronger, Herb Decoction Stronger Than Jie Geng, Tincture/Aqueous Extract Weaker, Enhances Ciliary Movement 554
- SHI WEI (c): Very Strong 601
- SI GUA LUO (c) 688
- SU HE XIANG (c): Thru Irritation Of Lung Mucosa 758
- TIAN MEN DONG 814
- TIAN MEN DONG (c) 814
- TIAN NAN XING (c): Increases Bronchial Secretion By Irritating GI Mucosa 712
- TING LI ZI (c): Oil Of 555
- TU YIN CHEN (c) 602
- WU JIA SHEN (c) 771
- WU WEI ZI (c): Ether Extract 831
- XIAO HUI XIANG (c) 619
- XING REN (c) 705
- XIONG DAN (c) 479
- XUAN FU HUA (c) 713
- YIN YANG HUO (c) 791
- YUAN HUA (c) 556
- YUAN ZHI (c): Thru Irritation Of Lung Mucosa, Need High Concentration 734
- ZAO JIAO (c): Stomach/Lungs, Increases Secretions, Significant, Less Than Jie Geng 715
- ZHI MU (c) 480
- ZI WAN (c): Increases Respiratory Tract Secretions, Significant, Last Greater Than 4 Hrs 706

EXPECTORANT, SLIGHT

- BEI SHA SHEN (c) 804

EXPECTORANT, STRONG

- JIE GENG (c): Oral Intake Stimulates Mild Nausea, Causing Bronchi To Secrete By Reflex, Similar In Strength To Ammonium Chloride, Stronger Than Yuan Zhi 711

HEMOPTYSIS

See: Hemorrhagic Disorders Hemoptysis 170

HYPERPNEA

- SHE GAN 533
- SHU DI HUANG 802
- TAI ZI SHEN 770

LUNG ATROPHY

- GE JIE 777
- KUAN DONG HUA 700
- LU GEN 472
- YI YI REN 602

LUNG BLEEDING

- BAI JI 652

LUNG CANCER

- DONG CHONG XIA CAO (c): Significant Anticancer Effect, 3 Months 775
- HAN FANG JI (c): Short Term Effect On Advanced, Tetrandrine With Radiotherapy 596
- SHAN DOU GEN 532
- SHI SHANG BAI 534
- ZHU LING (c): With Chemotherapy, Improves Symptoms, Reduces Side Effects Of Chemo, Supports Immune System 606

LUNG COLD PHLEGM

- GAN JIANG/MA HUANG/XI XIN/BAN XIA/(XIAO QING LONG TANG): Chills, Asthma, Cough w/Clear, Profuse Sputum, With Cold Feeling In Upper Back

LUNG CONSUMPTION, BLOODY SPUTUM W/DRY PAROXYSMAL COUGH

- BAI QIAN/BAI BU

LUNG DAMP HEAT

- DONG GUA REN 593

LUNG DEFICIENCY

- HE ZI/WU WEI ZI/BEI SHA SHEN/BAI HE: Chronic Hoarseness, Cough
- LUO HAN GUO/(lean pork): Cough
- WU BEI ZI/WU WEI ZI: Chronic Cough
- WU MEI/XING REN/BAN XIA: Chronic Cough
- YI TANG/BAI BU/XING REN: Cough, Dry, Weak, Wheezing
- ZI HE CHE/WU WEI ZI/MAI MEN DONG: Cough, Wheezing
- HUANG QI 765
- WU WEI ZI: Cough, Dyspnea 831
- YI TANG: Dry Cough 772

LUNG DEFICIENCY W/COUGHING BLOOD

- HAN LIAN CAO/SHENG DI HUANG

LUNG DEFICIENCY W/PHLEGM HEAT

- GE JIE/CHUAN BEI MU: Chronic Cough: Wheezing

LUNG DEFICIENCY, COLD

- WU WEI ZI/GAN JIANG: Cough, Wheezing

LUNG DEFICIENCY, YIN DAMAGED BY HEAT

- MA DOU LING/E JIAO: Cough w/Bloody Sputum

LUNG DISEASES

- HUO TAN MU CAO 498

LUNG DRYNESS

LUNG DRYNESS W/COUGH

LUNG FISTULA

LUNG HEART IMBALANCE

LUNG HEAT

LUNG HEAT INJURES FLUIDS, QI

LUNG HEAT SPUTUM W/DIFFICULT SPUTUM

LUNG HEAT W/CONGESTED FLUIDS

LUNG HEAT W/CONGESTED FLUIDS-WHEEZING

LUNG HEAT W/COUGH, SORE THROAT

LUNG HEAT W/SPUTUM IN COUGH

LUNG HEAT W/THICK YELLOW SPUTUM

LUNG HEAT W/YIN DEFICIENCY

LUNG HEAT WITH COUGH, PHLEGM

LUNG HEAT WITH DRY COUGH AND BLOODY SPUTUM

LUNG HEAT, ACUTE

LUNG HEAT, BLOCKING QI

LUNG HEAT, CHRONIC W/BLOODY SPUTM

LUNG HEAT, DRYNESS

- SANG YE/XING REN/CHUAN BEI MU/MAI MEN DONG: Cough, Dry Nose, Mouth

LUNG INFECTION

LUNG INFECTION W/HOT SPUTUM

LUNG INFLAMMATION, UPPER AREA

LUNG KIDNEY DEFICIENCY

- GE JIE/REN SHEN/(korean)/HU TAO REN/WU WEI ZI: Cough, Wheezing
- HU TAO REN/REN SHEN/GE JIE: Wheezing
- WU WEI ZI/SHU DI HUANG/SHAN YAO/SHAN ZHU YU: Cough, Wheezing

LUNG KIDNEY DEFICIENCY, SEVERE

- GE JIE/SHENG DI HUANG: Cough, Wheezing w/Hoarseness, Bloody Sputum

LUNG KIDNEY QI DEFICIENCY

- REN SHEN/WU WEI ZI/MAI MEN DONG/FU ZI/SHENG DI HUANG/GE JIE: Wheezing

LUNG KIDNEY YIN DEFICIENCY

LUNG KIDNEY YIN DEFICIENCY W/HEAT SIGNS

- ZHI MU/HUANG BAI

LUNG PHLEGM HEAT W/COUGH

- QIAN HU/SANG BAI PI/GUA LOU/CHUAN BEI MU/(QIAN HU SAN)

LUNG QI AND YIN DEFICIENCY

- HUANG JING/BEI SHA SHEN/MAI MEN DONG: Cough

LUNG QI BLOCKAGE & STAGNATION

LUNG QI CONGESTION W/SPUTUM

LUNG QI DEFICIENCY

- DANG SHEN/HUANG QI/WU WEI ZI: Shortness Of Breath, Cough, Asthma, Lassitude, Low Voice, Deficient, Forceless Pulse
- REN SHEN/GE JIE/(REN SHEN GE JIE TANG): Spontaneous Sweating, Lassitude, Shortness Of Breath

LUNG QI DEFICIENCY COUGH

LUNG QI DESCENT, DISRUPTION OF

LUNG QI NOT DESCENDING

- TING LI ZI/DA ZAO/(TING LI DA ZAO XIE FEI TANG): Phlegm Blockage

LUNG QI NOT DESCENDING, COLD CONGESTED FLUIDS

- GAN JIANG/WU WEI ZI: Cough, Wheezing

LUNG QI OBSTRUCTION W/CONGESTED FLUIDS

- QIAN NIU ZI/TING LI ZI/XING REN: Wheezing

LUNG QI OBSTRUCTION, EXTERNAL/INTERNAL

- BAI BU/BAI QIAN: Chronic Cough

LUNG QI, CONSTRAINED

LUNG SPLEEN DEFICIENCY

- DANG SHEN/HUANG QI: Shortness Of Breath, Fatigue, Diarrhea
- SHAN YAO/DANG SHEN: Cough w/Thin Sputum, Anorexia, Fatigue, Weight Loss

LUNG SPUTUM, CHRONIC

LUNG STIMULATES RESPIRATORY CENTER

LUNG STOMACH DRY HEAT

LUNG STOMACH DRYNESS

- ZHI MU/TIAN HUA FEN/MAI MEN DONG: Thirst, Restless

LUNG STOMACH EXCESS HEAT

LUNG TUMORS

- SHI SHANG BAI/(STEW WITH LEAN PORK)

LUNG W/COLD PHLEGM FLUID

- XI XIN/MA HUANG/GAN JIANG/(QING LONG TANG)

LUNG YIN DAMAGE

LUNG YIN DEFICIENCY

- **BAI HE/MAI MEN DONG/XUAN SHEN/CHUAN BEI MU:** Chronic Dry Cough
- **BAI JI/BAI BU:** Hemoptosis
- **BEI SHA SHEN/MAI MEN DONG:** Chronic, Dry Cough
- **BEI SHA SHEN/CHUAN BEI MU:** Dry Cough
- **DONG CHONG XIA CAO/XING REN/CHUAN BEI MU/E JIAO:** Dry Cough w/Blood, Chest Pain, Wheezing
- **E JIAO/MAI MEN DONG/BEI SHA SHEN:** Dry Cough w/Blood
- **HE ZI/HAI FU SHI/GUA LOU PI:** Chronic Cough, Bloody Sputum
- **MAI MEN DONG/BAN XIA/DANG SHEN:** Chronic Dry Cough
- **TAI ZI SHEN/BEI SHA SHEN/MAI MEN DONG:** Dry Cough Or w/Scanty Sputum
- **XIAN HE CAO/E JIAO:** Hemoptosis
- **YU ZHU/BEI SHA SHEN/MAI MEN DONG/TIAN MEN DONG:** Cough, Dry w/Scanty Sputum

LUNG YIN DEFICIENCY COUGH

LUNG YIN DEFICIENCY W/EXCESS FIRE

- **HUA QI SHEN/MAI MEN DONG/E JIAO/ZHI MU/CHUAN BEI MU:** Asthma, Cough w/Blood

LUNG YIN DEFICIENCY W/HEAT

- **TIAN MEN DONG/SHENG DI HUANG/CHUAN BEI MU/BAI HE:** Dry Chronic Cough

LUNG YIN DEFICIENCY, CHRONIC

LUNGS

LUNGS, ABSCESS

- **BAI JI/CHUAN BEI MU:** Hemoptosis
- **BAI MU ER/BAI HE/BEI SHA SHEN/(rock candy)**
- **CHUAN BEI MU/YU XING CAO/YI YI REN**
- **DONG GUA REN/JIE GENG/YU XING CAO/JIN YIN HUA:** Hot Phlegm
- **GUA LOU REN/YU XING CAO/JIE GENG:** Hot
- **HE HUAN PI/DONG GUA REN/YU XING CAO/TAO REN**
- **JIE GENG/GUA LOU REN/YI YI REN**
- **JIE GENG/YU XING CAO/DONG GUA REN/GUA LOU:** Toxic Heat, With Bloody, Pus Cough
- **LU GEN/JIN YIN HUA/YU XING CAO/DONG GUA REN**
- **TAO REN/YI YI REN/DONG GUA REN**
- **TIAN MEN DONG/SHAN CI GU**
- **YI YI REN/LU GEN/DONG GUA REN/TAO REN**
- **YU ZHU/YI YI REN:** Dry Cough w/Thick Sputum
- **ZHE BEI MU/YI YI REN/DONG GUA REN/YU XING CAO**

LUNGS, ABSCESS W/COUGH, PHLEGM, PUS

- **YI YI REN/LU JING/DONG GUA REN/TAO REN/(QIAN JIN WI JING TANG)**

LUNGS, ABSCESS W/FEVER, COUGH, SPUTUM

- **YU XING CAO/JIE GENG**

LUNGS, ABSCESS W/HEMOPTYSIS, PUS

LUNGS, ABSCESS W/PURULENT VOMIT

LUNGS, ABSCESS W/PUS/BLOODY SPUTUM

- **LU GEN/YI YI REN/DONG GUA REN**

LUNGS, ABSCESS, W/COUGH, BLOODY SPUTUM

- **YU XING CAO/JIE GENG/YI YI REN**

LUNGS, ABSCESS, W/PUS, BLOOD

LUNGS, ACUTE INFECTION OF

LUNGS, BLEEDING

LUNGS, BLOCKED BY COLD PHLEGM

LUNGS, BREATHING DIFFICULTY

LUNGS, BRONCHIOLES, CONTRACTS

LUNGS, CANDIDIASIS OF

LUNGS, CHRONIC OBSTRUCTIVE DISEASE

LUNGS, CHRONIC OBSTRUCTIVE PULMONARY DISEASE, SEVERE, RECALCITRANT

LUNGS, COLD

LUNGS, CONSUMPTIVE

LUNGS, DAMAGE TO

LUNGS, DAMP PHLEGM OBSTRUCTING

LUNGS, DEFICIENT W/HOT PHLEGM

LUNGS, DEFICIENT YIN FIRE

LUNGS, DILATES BRONCHII

LUNGS, DRY

LUNGS, DRYNESS AND HEAT

LUNGS, DYSPNEA

LUNGS, HEAT

LUNGS, INCREASES SECRETION

LUNGS, INCREASES SECRETIONS

LUNGS, INCREASES SPUTUM IN

LUNGS, INFLAMMATION OF MUCOSA

RESPIRATORY TRACT INFECTION, UPPER, CHILDREN

RESPIRATORY TRACT, INCREASES SPUTUM IN

RESPIRATORY TRACT, RELAXES

RESPIRATORY TRACT, UPPER INFECTION

RESPIRATORY TRACT, UPPER INFECTION, FEVER OF

SHORTNESS OF BREATH

SHORTNESS OF BREATH W/FEVER

SILICOSIS

STIMULANT, RESPIRATION

SUFFOCATION

TRACHEA, CONSTRICTION, ALLERGIC

TRACHEA, EXCESS SPUTUM BLOCKING

TUBERCULOSIS

- CE BAI YE (c): Fresh Leaves, Branches, 30 g Decoct To 100 ml With 20 ml Honey Added, Less Than 2 Yrs, 15-25 ml, 3x/Day, Increase With Age 654
- CHE QIAN CAO (c): Antitussiuve, Expectorant, 30 gm/Day 589
- CHEN PI (c): In Young Children, With Snake Bile As Powder, 4-16 Days 621
- CHUAN BEI MU (c): Snake Bile-Fritillaria Bulb Powder 717
- DA SUAN 644
- DA SUAN (c): 95% Effective, 60 g Cut, Macerated For 10 Hrs In 300 ml Boiled Cold Water, Filter, Sweetened With Sugar, 5+Yrs 15 ml/2 Hrs, Less Than 5yrs, 1/2 Dose 644
- HUANG LIAN (c): 100% Decoction, 33% Cured, Marked Effect 27%, About 2 Days To Marked Effect 486
- HUANG YAO ZI 723
- MA HUANG (c): 3-5 Years Old, Ma Xing Shi Gan Tang With Bai Bu, Ting LI Zi, Da Zao, Maltose, Effective In Catarrhal, Spastic Stages, *Wen Fei Huay Yin Tang (AKA, Xiao Qing Long Tang) 448
- MU HU DIE 702
- NAN GUA ZI (c): Fine Powder Of Browned Seeds With Brown Sugar Solution, 2-3x/Day 648
- NIU HUANG (c): Mix With Sugar, Less Than 2 Yrs, 0.12-.24 g/Day, 2-5 Years, 0.24-.36 g, 5+Yrs, 0.36-.49 g For 1-2 Weeks 755
- RONG SHU XU 570
- SANG YE (c): Sang Xing Tang (Sang Ye, Xing Ren, Chuan Bei Mu, Nan Sha Shen, Dan Dou Chi, Cortex Gardeniae (Shan Zhi Zi?) , Pericarium Pyri) , Helped With 1 Dose, 3 Doses To Stop Cough In Most Cases 466
- SHE XIANG (c) 756
- SUAN JIANG 852

WHOOPING COUGH PAROXYSMS

- XIONG DAN (c) 479

WIND COLD

See: Wind Disorders Wind Cold 432

WIND HEAT

See: Wind Disorders Wind Heat 434

WINDPIPE, RATTLING SOUND

- TIAN NAN XING/BAN XIA/TIAN MA/BAI FU ZI: Wind Phlegm

End of Topic:
LUNGS

LUPUS ERYTHEMATOSUS

See: Skin Lupus Erythematosus 362
See: Immune System Related Disorders/Topics
Lupus Erythematosus 177

LYMPH GLANDS AND RELATED TOPICS

See: Immune System Related Disorders/Topics
Lymph Glands And Related Topics 177

LYMPHADENITIS

See: Immune System Related Disorders/Topics
Lymphadenitis 178

LYMPHATIC CANCER

See: Cancer/Tumors/Swellings/Lumps
Lymphatic Cancer 69

LYMPHATITIS

See: Immune System Related Disorders/Topics
Lymphatitis 178

LYMPHOCYTES, INCREASES

See: Blood Related Disorders/Topics
Lymphocytes, Increases 50

LYMPHOSARCOMA

See: Cancer/Tumors/Swellings/Lumps
Lymphosarcoma 69

MACROPAPULE W/HIGH FEVER

See: Skin Macropapule w/High Fever 362

MACULA

See: Skin Macula 362

MACULAR DEGENERATION

See: Eyes Macular Degeneration 121

MADNESS

See: Mental State/Neurological Disorders
Madness 253

MALAISE

See: Mental State/Neurological Disorders
Malaise 253

MALAR FLUSH

See: Skin Malar Flush 362
See: Head/Neck Malar Flush 150

MALARIA RELATED TOPICS

See: Infectious Diseases Malaria Related Topics 189

MALIGNANCIES, PAIN OF

See: Cancer/Tumors/Swellings/Lumps
Malignancies, Pain Of 69

MALNUTRITION

See: Nutritional/Metabolic Disorders/Topics
Malnutrition 282

MALNUTRITION IN CHILDREN AND RELATED TOPICS

See: Childhood Disorders Malnutrition, Childhood And Related Topics 82

MALPOSITION OF FETUS(8 MO)

See: Sexuality, Female: Gynecological
Malposition Of Fetus (8 Mo) 330

MANIA RELATED TOPICS

See: Mental State/Neurological Disorders
Mania Related Topics 253

MENTAL STATE/ NEUROLOGICAL DISORDERS :

ACETYLCHOLINE

• BAN XIA (c): Antidote To 710

ADDICTIVE

• BING LANG (c): Causes Peridontal Disease,
Discoloration 643

AGITATION

• BIE JIA: Yin Deficient 805
• GUI BAN: Yin Deficiency Wind 806
• LING YANG JIAO 747
• SHI GAO 477
• SHUI NIU JIAO 501
• XI JIAO 502
• YU JIN: Hot Phlegm Obstructing Heart 695

AGITATION/FRUSTRATION

• LU DOU: Summer Heat 508

ALZHEIMER'S DISEASE

• BAI GUO YE (c): Possible Help In 817

AMNESIA

• BAI ZI REN 730
• LONG YAN ROU 800
• SHI CHANG PU 757
• WU WEI ZI 831
• YUAN ZHI 734

CNS, DEPRESSES

- HOU PO (c): Ether Extract IP Injection, Lessened Stimulation Of Methamphetamine 581

CNS, EFFECTS

- CHAN SU (c): Analgesic, Hallucinogenic—Short Duration, Convulsions, Stimulant 837
- JIANG CAN (c): Hypnotic 746

CNS, ENHANCES ADAPTABILITY

- REN SHEN (c) 767

CNS, ENHANCES CONDITIONED REFLEX

- REN SHEN (c) 767

CNS, EXCITATORY

- HUAI JIAO (c): Respiration, Small Doses 676

CNS, HELPS TO REGULATE EXCITATORY/INHIBITORY CONTROL

- WU JIA SHEN (c) 771

CNS, HYPNOTIC

- SU MU (c): In Large Doses 688

CNS, INCREASES ABILITY OF ANALYSIS

- REN SHEN (c) 767

CNS, INHIBITOR

- BAI SHAO (c) 794
- CHI SHAO YAO (c) 668
- CHUAN BEI MU (c) 717
- HUANG BAI (c): Milder Than Curare 485
- HUANG QIN (c) 489
- YA DAN ZI (c) 538
- YI MU CAO (c) 694

CNS, INHIBITOR/SEDATIVE

- LING ZHI CAO (c): Tincture/Reflux Percolate, Water Soluble Portion 731

CNS, INHIBITS CEREBRAL CORTEX

- HUA QI SHEN (c) 808

CNS, POSSIBLE HALLUCINATIONS

- WU ZHU YU (c): 5-Methoxy-N-Dimethyl-Tryptamine, Rutamine, At High Dose 618

CNS, PROLONGS SLEEPING

- HUANG LIAN (c) 486

CNS, RELAXANT

- SHAN ZHI ZI (c) 476

CNS, SEDATIVE

- CE BAI YE (c): Synergistic w/Barbituates 654
- CHONG WEI ZI (c) 669
- CI SHI (c) 735
- DAN SHEN (c) 672
- DU ZHONG (c): Large Doses, Oral 775

- LING YANG JIAO (c): ETOH Extract 747
- YI YI REN (c): Counteracts Caffeine 602
- ZHU SHA (c) 741

CNS, SEDATIVE, INHIBITS NERVE IMPULSES

- SUAN ZAO REN (c) 732

CNS, STIMULANT

- AI YE (c): Stimulates, May Cause Convulsions In Large Doses 651
- AN XI XIANG (c) 753
- BING PIAN (c) 753
- CHA YE (c) 589
- DANG SHEN (c): 6-7 Mcg/kg 762
- DU HUO (c) 561
- HUANG QI (c) 765
- JIN YIN HUA (c): 1/6th Of Caffeine 524
- LIAN QIAO (c) 525
- LONG DAN CAO (c): At Low Doses, High Doses Anesthetic 492
- LONG KUI (c) 526
- LOU LU (c): Like Strychnine 527
- MA HUANG (c) 448
- MAI YA (c): Hordenine, Similar To Epinephrine, Small Amount, Insoluble In Water 640
- NIU BANG ZI (c): Large Doses Could Produce Convulsions, Then Paralysis 465
- QIN JIAO (c): Large Doses 569
- WU BEI ZI (c): Increases Efficiency 829
- WU WEI ZI (c): Quickens Reflexes, Increases Work Efficiency—Less Than Caffeine, Tincture Strongest ... 831
- WU YAO (c): Cerebral Cortex, Respiration 632
- XUAN FU HUA (c): Caffeine-Like 713
- ZHANG NAO (c): Small Doses 849

CNS, STIMULANT, CEREBRAL CORTEX, SMALL DOSES

- HUANG LIAN (c) 486

CNS, STIMULANT, SUBCORTICAL AREAS

- HUA QI SHEN (c) 808

CNS, TRANQUILIZER

- FU LING (c) 594
- ROU GUI (c): Synergistic With Phenobarbital, Countered Methamphetamine 616

COMA

See: Mental State/Neurological Disorders
Unconsciousness 259
- BING PIAN/SHE XIANG/(AN GONG NIU HUANG WAN): Heat/Phlegm Blocked Orifices
- NIU HUANG/SHE XIANG/XI JIAO: Severe Heat, Choked Orifices
- SHE XIANG/XI JIAO/NIU HUANG/(SHI BAO DAN): From Extreme Heat/Windstroke
- SU HE XIANG/SHE XIANG/DING XIANG/BING PIAN: Phlegm, Qi Obstruction
- TIAN ZHU HUANG/SHI CHANG PU: Heat, Windstroke w/Phlegm Obstruction
- XIONG DAN/YIN CHEN: Hepatic

CONVULSIONS, CHILDHOOD

See: Childhood Disorders Convulsions,
Childhood 81
- BO HE/BAI JIANG CAO/CHAN TUI/QUAN XIE
- HOU ZAO/SHE XIANG/SHI CHANG PU: Wind Heat And Hot Phlegm
- HU PO/ZHU SHA
- JU HUA/TIAN MA: Liver Wind
- LONG DAN CAO/NIU HUANG/GOU TENG: Liver Fire And Phlegm
- QUAN XIE/WU GONG/(ZI JING SAN): Wind
- TIAN ZHU HUANG/JIANG CAN: Wind, Heat, Phlegm
- XIONG HUANG/YU JIN: Phlegm Obstruction
- ZHEN ZHU/LONG GU/MU LI/ZHU SHA
- BIE JIA 805
- CHAN TUI: Febrile Disease Wind 458
- HU PO 737
- JIANG CAN 746
- QING DAI 531
- QUAN XIE: Liver Wind Phlegm 749
- SHE TUI 571
- TIAN MA 750
- TIAN ZHU HUANG 726
- WU GONG 751

CONVULSIONS, CHILDHOOD ACUTE/CHRONIC

- WU GONG/QUAN XIE/JIANG CAN/GOU TENG: Spasms, Contracture, Opisthotonos
- ZHU SHA/TIAN ZHU HUANG/TIAN NAN XING

CONVULSIONS, CHILDHOOD CHRONIC

- JIANG CAN/DANG SHEN/BAI ZHU/TIAN MA: Prolonged Spleen Deficient Diarrhea
- REN SHEN 767

CONVULSIONS, CHILDHOOD CLONIC

- NIU HUANG/QUAN XIE/DAN NAN XING: Extreme Heat

CONVULSIONS, CHILDHOOD FRIGHT

- CI SHI: Best Liver Yin With Yang Rising 735
- DAI MAO 743
- DI LONG 744
- ZHEN ZHU 740

CONVULSIONS, CHILDHOOD FROM FEVERS

- ZAO XIU 540

CONVULSIONS, CHILDHOOD, HIGH FEVER

- ZHU SHA 741

CONVULSIONS, CHRONIC

- FANG FENG 444
- HU PO 737
- TIAN MA 750
- ZHU SHA 741

CONVULSIONS, FEBRILE DISEASES

- DAI MAO 743

CONVULSIONS, FEVER, ACUTE

- DAN NAN XING 718
- DI LONG 744
- GOU TENG 745
- HAI ZAO 721
- HU PO 737
- HUANG LIAN 486
- JIANG CAN 746
- LING YANG JIAO 747
- NIU HUANG 755
- QING DAI 531
- SHI JUE MING 750
- TIAN ZHU HUANG 726
- XIONG DAN 479
- YU JIN 695
- ZHU SHA 741

CONVULSIONS, FRIGHT

- LONG DAN CAO: Liver Wind Heat 492
- LONG GU 738

CONVULSIONS, FRIGHT IN YOUNG CHILDREN

- BAI HUA SHE 558

CONVULSIONS, HAND/FEET

- GUI BAN/E JIAO/SHENG DI HUANG/MU LI: Yin Consumed By Fever Causing Malnutrition Of Tendons, Muscles

CONVULSIONS, HANDS, FEET, CHRONIC

- QUAN XIE/DANG SHEN/BAI ZHU/TIAN MA: Spleen Deficiency Chronic Diarrhea

CONVULSIONS, HIGH FEVER

- GOU TENG/LING YANG JIAO/JU HUA/SHI GAO: Liver Wind
- JIANG CAN/TIAN MA/DAN NAN XING/NIU HUANG/(QIAN JIN SAN)
- LING YANG JIAO/GOU TENG/JU HUA/SHENG DI HUANG/(LING JIAO GOU TENG TANG): Endogenous Wind
- QUAN XIE/WU GONG/(ZI JING SAN)
- LING YANG JIAO (c): Ling Yang Gou Teng Tang, (With Gou Teng, Sheng Di, Ju Hua) 747
- NIU HUANG (c): Use An Gong Niu Huang Wan 755
- TIAN NAN XING 712

CONVULSIONS, HIGH FEVER, LOSS OF CONSCIOUSNESS

- NIU HUANG/HUANG LIAN/XI JIAO/SHE XIANG/(AN GONG NIU HUANG WAN)

CONVULSIONS, HIGH FEVER/TETANUS

- CHAN TUI/QUAN XIE/JIANG CAN/GOU TENG/JU HUA

CONVULSIONS, INFANTILE

- HU PO/WU GONG/QUAN XIE

EXCITABILITY, MILD

• LONG YAN ROU/BAI HE

FACIAL PARALYSIS

See: Head/Neck Face, Paralysis 145

FATIGUE

See: Energetic State Fatigue 104

FATIGUE, MENTAL

• TAI ZI SHEN 770

FEAR

• YUAN ZHI (c): Decoction/Syrup, Yuan Zhi, 9g Plus Wu Wei Zi, 6 g, *3 g Powder, 2x/Day 734

FEAR, IN CHILDREN

• DAN NAN XING 718

FEARFULNESS

• HU GU 563
• MAI MEN DONG 810

FIDGETS

• CHA YE 589
• SHI GAO 477
• SUAN ZAO REN: Deficiency 732

FORGETFULNESS

• HU PO/YUAN ZHI/SHI CHANG PU/SUAN ZAO REN
• HUANG QI/LONG YAN ROU/SUAN ZAO REN/YUAN ZHI/(GUI PI TANG): Qi And Blood Deficient
• LONG GU/YUAN ZHI/GUI BAN
• LONG YAN ROU/SHI CHANG PU: Heart Blood, Qi Deficient
• LONG YAN ROU/REN SHEN/HUANG QI/DANG GUI/SUAN ZAO REN/(GUI PI TANG): Qi And Blood Deficiency
• REN SHEN/SUAN ZAO REN/DANG GUI/(GUI PI TANG): Mental Restlessness
• SHI CHANG PU/YUAN ZHI/FU LING /(AN SHEN DING ZHI WAN)
• SHU DI HUANG/GUI BAN: Yin Deficient w/Yang Rising
• SUAN ZAO REN/DANG GUI/YUAN ZHI/BAI SHAO/HE SHOU WU/LONG YAN ROU: Heat Liver Blood Deficiency
• WU WEI ZI/SUAN ZAO REN: Heart Deficiency Patterns
• WU WEI ZI/SHENG DI HUANG/MAI MEN DONG/SUAN ZAO REN/(TIAN WANG BU XIN DAN): Heart Kidney Yin/Blood Deficiency
• BAI ZI REN: Heart Blood Deficient 730
• FU LING 594
• FU SHEN 736
• HE HUAN HUA 730
• HU PO 737
• LING ZHI CAO: From Hypertension, Neurasthenia 731
• LONG YAN ROU: Heart Spleen Deficient 800
• REN SHEN: Blood/Qi Deficient 767
• WU WEI ZI 831
• XI XIAN CAO 575
• YIN YANG HUO 791
• YUAN ZHI 734

FORGETFULNESS W/INSOMNIA

• YUAN ZHI/REN SHEN/SHI CHANG PU/(BU WANG SAN)

FORGETFULNESS W/MENTAL DERANGEMENT

• GUI BAN/LONG GU/SHI CHANG PU/YUAN ZHI/(KONG SHENG ZHEN ZHONG DAN): Yin/Blood Deficiency

FORGETFULNESS, FROM ANGER/DEPRESSION

• HE HUAN PI/BAI ZI REN/YE JIAO TENG

FRIGHT

• LONG CHI 737

FRIGHT W/MENTAL DERANGEMENT

• GUI BAN/LONG GU/SHI CHANG PU/YUAN ZHI/(KONG SHENG ZHEN ZHONG DAN): Yin/Blood Deficiency

FRIGHT, PALPITATIONS

• BAI HE 803
• ZHU SHA 741
• ZI SHI YING 742

FRIGHTENED EASILY

• ZHEN ZHU 740

GRIEF

• DA ZAO/GAN CAO/FU XIAO MAI/(GAN MAI DA ZAO TANG): Hysteria

HALLUCINATIONS

• YANG JIN HUA (c): Causes 714

HALLUCINOGENIC

• CHAN SU (c): Onset, Disappearance Quicker Than Mescaline 837
• ROU DOU KOU (c) 826

HEMIPLEGIA

• BAI FU ZI/JIANG CAN/QUAN XIE: Wind Stroke/Phlegm Obstruction Of Channels
• BAI HUA SHE/QUAN XIE/DANG GUI/(in wine): Stroke
• CHOU WU TONG/XI XIAN CAO/GOU TENG/SANG JI SHENG: Wind Damp Bi
• DI LONG/HUANG QI/DANG GUI/CHI SHAO YAO: Wind Stroke
• HUANG QI/DANG GUI/CHUAN XIONG/DI LONG/(BU YANG HUAN WU TONG): Qi And Blood Deficient w/Poor Blood Circulation
• BAI FU ZI: Wind Phlegm 708
• BAI HUA SHE: Windstroke 558
• CHOU WU TONG 560
• DAI MAO 743
• DI LONG 744
• FU ZI 613
• QUAN XIE 749
• TIAN MA: Wind Stroke 750
• TIAN NAN XING 712
• XI XIAN CAO 575
• YIN YANG HUO 791

INSOMNIA, CHILDHOOD

INSOMNIA, DISTURBING DREAMS

INSOMNIA, DREAM DISTURBED

INSOMNIA, DREAM TROUBLED

INSOMNIA, DREAMS, ESPECIALLY W/FRIGHTENING

INSOMNIA, DREAMS, FREQUENT

INSOMNIA, FORGETFULNESS

- YUAN ZHI/REN SHEN/SHI CHANG PU/(BU WANG SAN)

INSOMNIA, FROM ANGER/DEPRESSION

- HE HUAN PI/BAI ZI REN/YE JIAO TENG

INSOMNIA, FROM FIDGETS

- JI ZI HUANG 809

INSOMNIA, INTERMITTENT FULLNESS, PAIN

- CHUAN LIAN ZI/YAN HU SUO/(JIN LING ZI SAN): Liver GB Fire/Stagnant Qi

INSOMNIA, IRRITABILITY

- DAN DOU CHI/SHAN ZHI ZI: Post Febrile Disease
- GUI ZHI/MU LI/LONG GU: Deficient Heart Yang
- HUANG LIAN/SHENG DI HUANG: Ying Level Heat

INSOMNIA, MENTAL DERANGEMENT

- GUI BAN/LONG GU/SHI CHANG PU/YUAN ZHI/(KONG SHENG ZHEN ZHONG DAN): Yin/Blood Deficiency

INSOMNIA, MILD

- LIAN ZI/BAI HE/YI YI REN/BEI SHA SHEN: Excess Heart Fire
- LONG YAN ROU/BAI HE

INSOMNIA, NEURASTHENIA

- HE SHOU WU (c): 5-7 Tabs, 2-3x/Day Of 1 g Tabs, For 15-20 Days 799
- WU WEI ZI (c): Alcohol Extractions 831

INSOMNIA, PALPITATIONS

- CHUAN SHAN JIA/SUAN ZAO REN/SHENG DI HUANG

- DAN SHEN/SUAN ZAO REN/BAI ZI REN: Deficient Heart Blood
- FU LING /SUAN ZAO REN/YUAN ZHI/WU WEI ZI
- LONG YAN ROU/SUAN ZAO REN: Heart Blood Deficient w/Spleen Qi Deficient
- SHU DI HUANG/DANG GUI/BAI SHAO/CHUAN XIONG/BAI ZI REN/SUAN ZAO REN: Blood And Yin Deficiency

INSOMNIA, PALPITATIONS, IRRITABILITY

- DAN SHEN/SUAN ZAO REN/YE JIAO TENG: Blood Deficiency w/Internal Heat

INSOMNIA, RESTLESS

- E JIAO/HUANG QIN/BAI SHAO/(egg yolk): Post Febrile Disease w/Fluid Damage
- ZHU RU/BAN XIA/ZHI SHI: Hot Phlegm
- E JIAO 797
- XUAN SHEN: From Heat 503

INTOXICATION, ALCOHOLIC

- GE HUA/DANG SHEN/BAI DOU KOU/CHEN PI
- GE HUA: Fidgets, Thirst 521

IRRITABILITY

- BAI HE/SHENG DI HUANG: Lingering Heat
- BAI HE/ZHI MU: Heat Diseases, Late Stage w/Deficient Yin/Lingering Heat
- BAI HE/ZHI MU/SHENG DI HUANG/(BAI HE DI HUANG TANG): Febrile Diseases, Later Stage w/Heat
- BAI MAO GEN/LU GEN: Fevers
- BAI WEI/ZHU RU: Blood Deficient
- BAI ZI REN/SUAN ZAO REN/WU WEI ZI: Heart Blood Deficient
- BAN LAN GEN/XUAN SHEN/ZHI MU/JIN YIN HUA/LIAN QIAO/SHI GAO: Heat
- DAN DOU CHI/SHAN ZHI ZI: Post Febrile Disease
- DAN SHEN/MU DAN PI/SHENG DI HUANG: Ying Level Heat
- DAN ZHU YE/SHI GAO: Febrile Disease, Late Stage
- DENG XIN CAO/DAN ZHU YE: Heart Fire
- E JIAO/HUANG LIAN/BAI SHAO/GOU TENG/MU LI: Yin Consumed By Febrile Diseases
- FU XIAO MAI/GAN CAO/DA ZAO: Spleen Heart Deficiency, Mild
- HAN SHUI SHI/SHI GAO/HUA SHI: Summer Heat
- HE HUAN PI/DAN SHEN/YE JIAO TENG
- HUA QI SHEN/SHENG DI HUANG/SHI HU/MAI MEN DONG: Febrile Disease, Exhaustion Of Qi/Yin
- HUANG QIN/HUANG LIAN: Febrile Diseases
- LIAN ZI/BAI HE/YI YI REN/BEI SHA SHEN: Excess Heart Fire
- LIAN ZI/HUANG LIAN/DANG SHEN: Heart Kidney Discommunication
- LIAN ZI/SUAN ZAO REN/BAI ZI REN/FU SHEN
- LONG GU/MU LI/NIU XI/DAI ZHE SHI: Yin Deficiency w/Yang Rising
- LONG GU/MU LI/DAI ZHE SHI/BAI SHAO/(ZHEN GAN XI FENG TANG): Liver Kidney Deficiency w/Liver Yang Rising
- LU GEN/ZHU RU/SHENG JIANG: Stomach Heat
- LU HUI/LONG DAN CAO/HUANG QIN: Liver Channel Excess Heat

IRRITABILITY WITH MOUTH SORES/TONGUE

IRRITABILITY, FEVER

IRRITABILITY, FEVER, HIGH

IRRITABILITY, FROM ANGER/DEPRESSION

IRRITABILITY, FROM SEVERE SWEATING

IRRITABILITY, HEAT SENSATION IN CHEST
• MU TONG 599

IRRITABILITY, SPUTUM, GURGLING IN THROAT
• BAI FAN/YU JIN

IRRITABILITY, UNREMITTING
• TAI ZI SHEN/WU WEI ZI: Qi Deficient

IRRITABLILITY, EMOTIONAL W/INTERMITTENT FULLNESS, PAIN
• CHUAN LIAN ZI/YAN HU SUO/(JIN LING ZI SAN): Liver GB Fire/Stagnant Qi

LASSITUDE
See: Mental State/Neurological Disorders Lethargy 253
See: Energetic State Fatigue 104
• BAI BIAN DOU/REN SHEN/BAI ZHU/FU LING /(SHEN LING BAI ZHU SAN): Spleen Deficient, Not Metabolizing Water
• BAI ZHU/REN SHEN/FU LING /(SI JUN ZI TANG): Spleen Weakness In Water Metabolism
• DA ZAO/REN SHEN/BAI ZHU: Spleen Stomach Weakness
• DANG SHEN/DANG GUI: Qi And Blood Deficient
• DANG SHEN/HUANG QI/WU WEI ZI: Lung Qi Deficiency
• FU LING /DANG SHEN/BAI ZHU/(SI JUN ZI TANG): Spleen Deficient w/Dampness
• GAN JIANG/BAI ZHU/FU LING /(LI ZHONG WAN): Spleen Stomach Weakness, Cold
• HUANG JING/DANG SHEN/BAI ZHU: Spleen Stomach Qi Deficient
• HUANG QI/BAI ZHU: Spleen Qi Deficient
• HUANG QI/REN SHEN/BAI ZHU: Spleen Lung Qi Deficient
• REN SHEN/BAI ZHU/FU LING /GAN CAO/(SI JUN ZI TANG): Spleen Stomach Weakness
• SHAN YAO/REN SHEN/BAI ZHU/FU LING /(SHEN LING BAI ZHU SAN): Spleen Stomach Weakness
• SHAN YAO/BAI ZHU/FU LING /QIAN SHI: Excess Dampness From Spleen Deficient
• TAI ZI SHEN/SHAN YAO/BAI BIAN DOU/GU YA/MAI YA: Spleen Deficiency
• DA ZAO: Spleen Stomach Deficient 761
• WU JIA SHEN (c) 771

LEARNING ABILITY
• REN SHEN (c): One Fraction (Rg1) Can Increase 767

LETHARGY
See: Mental State/Neurological Disorders Lassitude 253
• JUE MING ZI (c): Reduces From Hypercholesterolemia 471
• MA HUANG (c): Ma Huang Fu Zi Xi Xin Tang 448
• REN SHEN 767
• TAI ZI SHEN: Spleen Deficiency With Fluid Insufficiency 770

LISTLESSNESS
• LU RONG/REN SHEN/SHU DI HUANG/TU SI ZI: Kidney Yang Deficiency

MADNESS
• YU JIN: Hot Phlegm Obstructing Heart 695

MALAISE
• DA ZAO 761
• GAN CAO: Qi Deficient 763
• HUO XIANG 582
• TAI ZI SHEN 770
• YI TANG 772
• YIN YANG HUO 791

MANIA
• LING YANG JIAO/SHI GAO/XI JIAO/(ZI XUE DAN)
• CI SHI 735
• HONG DA JI (c) 551
• JING DA JI (c) 552
• NIU HUANG 755
• SHI GAO 477
• SHUI NIU JIAO 501
• XI JIAO 502
• ZHEN ZHU MU: Liver Yang Rising 741

MANIA W/DELIRIUM, CONVULSIONS
• YU JIN 695

MANIC AGITATION
• DA HUANG 542
• DAI MAO 743
• MU TONG 599

MANIC BEHAVIOR
• HUANG LIAN 486
• LING YANG JIAO: From High Fever 747

MANIC EMOTIONAL DISORDERS
• SHI CHANG PU/YU JIN/BAI FAN: Phlegm/Qi Obstruction

MANIC PSYCHOSIS
• ZHU LI/SHENG JIANG/(large amounts juice): With Phlegm Obstruction Of Heart

MANIC-DEPRESSIVE STATES
• LONG CHI 737
• LONG GU 738
• ZHU SHA 741

MELANCHOLIA
• JIU JIE CHANG PU 754
• SHI CHANG PU 757

MEMORY LOSS
• BING LANG (c): Inhibits Loss Of Due To Chlorpromazine 643
• REN SHEN (c): Geriatric 767

MEMORY, IMPAIRED

MEMORY, IMPROVES

MEMORY, POOR

MENTAL CLOUDINESS

MENTAL CONFUSION

MENTAL DERANGEMENT

MENTAL DISORDERS

MENTAL DISORIENTATION

MENTAL DULLNESS

MENTAL FATIGUE

MENTAL POWER, IMPROVES

MENTAL RESTLESSNESS

MENTAL RETARDATION, ESPECIALLY CHILDREN

MIND, CLOUDY

MONOAMINE OXIDASE INHIBITOR

MOODY

NEURALGIA

NEURASTHENIA

- GOU QI ZI (c): Kidney And Jing/Blood Deficiency—Herb, Ju Hua, Shu Di, Shan Zhu Yu, Shan Yao, Ze Xie Or You Gui Wan (Herb, Shu Di, Shan Yao, Rou Gui Pi, Fu Zi, Du Zhong, Dang Gui, Tuber Of Colocasia Esculenta) 798
- HAI SHEN 781
- HE SHOU WU 799
- LING ZHI CAO 731
- LING ZHI CAO (c) 731
- LU XIAN CAO 566
- LUO BU MA 748
- MU LI 739
- NU ZHEN ZI 812
- REN SHEN (c) 767
- SUAN ZAO REN (c) 732
- TAI ZI SHEN (c): w/Wuweizi, Good 770
- WU JIA SHEN (c): Marked Amelioration In 20 Days With Tablet, Tincture, Some Cured In 6 Months 771
- WU WEI ZI 831
- WU WEI ZI (c): Alcohol Extractions 831
- YE JIAO TENG 733
- YIN YANG HUO (c) 791
- YUAN ZHI 734
- YUAN ZHI (c): Decoction/Syrup, Yuan Zhi, 9g Plus Wu Wei Zi, 6 g, *3 g Powder, 2x/Day 734

NEURASTHENIA, DREAMFULNESS

- LONG CHI 737
- LONG GU 738

NEUROLOGICAL DISORDERS W/SHAKING

See: Wind Disorders Wind Disorders 433

NEUROLOGICAL PAIN

See: Pain/Numbness/General Discomfort Neuralgia 301
- YAN HU SUO (c): 60-120 mg 1-4x/Day Of L-Tetrahydropalmatine, Active Ingredient 693

NEUROLOGICAL PROBLEMS

- BAI HUA SHE 558

NEUROSIS

- DANG SHEN (c): Injection, Contains 1 g Plus 50 mg Vit B/ml, 2ml/Day IM, 2 Weeks, Some Effectiveness 762
- HAN LIAN CAO 806
- WU JIA SHEN (c): Symptoms Of Insomnia, Dizziness, Headache, Blurred Vision, Palpitation, Frequent Dreaming, Wakefulness, Impaired Memory, Irritability, Lassitude 771
- WU WEI ZI (c): 40-100% Tincture, 2.5 ml/2-3x/Day For 2-4 Weeks, Relieved Insomnia, Headache, Dizziness, Blurred Vision, Palpitation, Nocturnal Emission 831

NICOTINE, DECREASES MUSCULAR TREMORS FROM

- CHAN TUI (c) 458

NIGHTMARES

- ZHU SHA 741

NOCTURNAL CRYING

- DENG XIN CAO 592

OPISTHOTONOS

- LING YANG JIAO/GOU TENG: Liver Wind From Warm Febrile Diseases
- QUAN XIE/TIAN NAN XING/CHAN TUI/(WU HU ZHUI FENG SAN): From Tetanus
- QUAN XIE: Liver Wind Phlegm 749
- TIAN MA: Liver Wind 750
- TIAN NAN XING: Wind Phlegm 712
- WU GONG 751

PARALYSIS

- CHUAN XIONG/DANG GUI: Bi, Wind Damp And Stagnant Qi
- HUANG QI/DANG GUI: Qi Blood Deficient
- JI XUE TENG/DANG GUI/CHUAN XIONG/MU GUA/SANG JI SHENG: Deficient Blood/Tendons, Muscles Not Nourished
- SUO YANG/HU GU/NIU XI/SHU DI HUANG: Liver Kidney Severely Deficient
- E JIAO 797
- FU PING: Wind Damp 460
- HEI ZHI MA: Wind Damp 808
- HUANG BAI 485
- SUO YANG: Essence, Blood Deficient 787
- TIAN NAN XING 712

PARALYSIS W/VERTIGO, WINDSTROKE

- JI XUE TENG: Blood Stasis 677

PARALYSIS, APOPLEXY

- CAO WU 609

PARALYSIS, CEREBROVASCULAR HEMORRAGE/OCCULSION

- HUANG QIN (c): Scutellarin Component 489

PARALYSIS, EXTREMITIES

- BAI HUA SHE: Wind Damp 558
- DA DOU HUANG JUAN 506
- HU GU 563
- ZHU LI: Phlegm Blocking Orifices 728

PARALYSIS, GENERAL

- YIN YANG HUO 791

PARALYSIS, INFANTILE

- SANG JI SHENG/YIN YANG HUO

PARALYTIC EFFECT

- TAN XIANG (c): Oil 632

PARANOIA

- BAN XIA (c): Wen Dan Tang With Suan Zao Ren, Yuan Zhi, Zhu Li 710

PARAPLEGIA

- HE SHOU WU (c) 799

SEDATIVE EFFECT FROM ODOR

SEDATIVE, CNS

SEDATIVE, INHIBITS CNS

SEDATIVE, LARGE DOSES

SEIZURES

- GOU TENG/LING YANG JIAO/QUAN XIE: High Fever
- HU PO/GOU TENG/QUAN XIE
- JIANG CAN/NIU HUANG/HUANG LIAN/DAN NAN XING: Phlegm Heat
- SU HE XIANG/SHE XIANG/DING XIANG/BING PIAN: Phlegm, Qi Obstruction
- TIAN MA/GOU TENG/QUAN XIE: Liver Yang Rising

- **TIAN NAN XING/TIAN MA:** Wind Phlegm
- **YU JIN/BAI FAN:** Phlegm Obstruction
- **YUAN ZHI/QUAN XIE/TIAN MA:** Phlegm Covering Orifices
- **ZHEN ZHU/LONG GU/MU LI/ZHU SHA**

SEIZURES, CHILD/ADULT

- **DI LONG/GOU TENG/QUAN XIE/JIANG CAN:** High Fever

SEIZURES, EPILEPTIC

- **JIANG CAN/CHAN TUI/QUAN XIE/WU GONG**

SEIZURES, REDUCES

SENSES, DULLED

SENSORY ACUITY, INCREASES

SHEN DISTURBANCES

- **YUAN ZHI/FU SHEN/SUAN ZAO REN:** Heart Blood Deficient

SHUT-IN COMPLEX

SIGHING

- **DA ZAO/GAN CAO/FU XIAO MAI/(GAN MAI DA ZAO TANG):** Hysteria

SLEEP

SLEEP W/TOO MANY DREAMS

SLEEP WALKING

SLEEP, DREAM DISTURBED

- **LONG GU/YUAN ZHI/GUI BAN**
- **MU LI/LONG GU**
- **REN SHEN/SUAN ZAO REN/DANG GUI/(GUI PI TANG):** Mental Restlessness

SLEEP, DREAMFUL

- **BAI HE/ZHI MU/SHENG DI HUANG/(BAI HE DI HUANG TANG):** Febrile Diseases, Later Stage w/Heat

SLEEP, RESTLESS

SLEEPINESS

SOMNOLENCE

SPIRIT, CALMS

STIMULANT

STIMULANT, CNS

STIMULANT, CNS, SMALL DOSES

STIMULANT, SMALL DOSES

STRESS

STRESS, ANTI-

STRESS, CAUSING INTERNAL IMPAIRMENT

STRESS, HELPS

STRESS, HELPS REDUCE

STROKE

STRYCHNINE-LIKE TO CNS

STUPOR

TEMPER

TEMPER, SHORT

TOUCH, INCREASES DISCRIMINATION

TRANQUILIZING

TREMORS

TREMORS, HAND/FEET

TRIGEMINAL NEURALGIA

UNCONSCIOUSNESS

- SHI GAO/XI JIAO: Damp Heat Toxin
- SU HE XIANG/SHE XIANG/DING XIANG/AN XI XIANG/(SU HE XIANG WAN): Windstroke
- XI JIAO/DA QING YE/SHI GAO/LING YANG JIAO: Blood Heat
- ZHU SHA/XI JIAO/NIU HUANG: Internal Wind
- BING PIAN: (Mental Cloudiness) , Excess Heat (Shut-In) 753
- CHAN SU: Excess, Mental Cloudiness, (Shut-In Complex) 837
- DAI MAO: (Mental Cloudiness) Use w/Heat Shut-In Herbs 743
- HUANG LIAN: (Mental Cloudiness) Use w/Heat Shut-In Herbs 486
- LING YANG JIAO: From High Fever 747
- NIU HUANG: (Mental Cloudiness) , Excess Heat (Shut-In) 755
- SHAN ZHI ZI: (Mental Cloudiness) Use w/Heat Shut-In Herbs 476
- SHE XIANG: Excess (Shut-In Complex) 756
- SHI CHANG PU: Excess (Shut-In Complex) 757
- SU HE XIANG: Closed Syndrome Stroke 758
- XI JIAO: (Mental Cloudiness) , Use w/Heat Shut-In Herbs 502
- XI XIN: (Mental Cloudiness) Excess (Shut-In Complex) 452
- YU JIN: (Mental Cloudiness) , Excess Heat (Shut-In) . . 695
- ZAO JIAO : Excess (Shut-In Complex) 715
- ZAO JIAO CI: Excess (Shut-In Complex) 716
- ZHANG NAO: Excess (Shut-In Complex) 849
- ZHU LI: (Mental Cloudiness) Use w/Heat Shut-In Herbs/Phlegm Blocking Orifices 728

UNCONSCIOUSNESS W/BLEEDING, PURPURA
- XI JIAO/SHENG DI HUANG: Blood Heat
- XI JIAO/SHENG DI HUANG/MU DAN PI/CHI SHAO YAO/DA QING YE/ZI CAO: Blood Heat

UNCONSCIOUSNESS, (MENTAL CLOUDINESS)
- LING YANG JIAO: Use w/Heat Shut-In Herbs 747

UNCONSCIOUSNESS, FROM HIGH FEVER, APOPLEXY
- SHE XIANG 756

UNCONSCIOUSNESS, FROM WINDSTROKE
- SHE XIANG/SU HE XIANG/DING XIANG/(SU HE XIANG WAN)

UNCONSCIOUSNESS, PHLEGM COVERING THE HEART
- YUAN ZHI/YU JIN/SHI CHANG PU

UNCONSCIOUSNESS, SUDDEN
- CHAN SU/XIONG HUANG/CANG ZHU/DING XIANG: Summer Heatstroke
- SU HE XIANG/SHE XIANG/DING XIANG/BING PIAN: Phlegm, Qi Obstruction
- ZHANG NAO/SHE XIANG/(or)/BING PIAN/(pill or powder)

VEXATION
- XUAN SHEN: 18-30gm 503

WEEPING
- DA ZAO/GAN CAO/FU XIAO MAI/(GAN MAI DA ZAO TANG): Hysteria

WITHDRAWAL, EMOTIONAL
- YIN YANG HUO 791

WORRIES, CONGESTED
- HE HUAN PI 731

End of Topic:
MENTAL STATE/NEUROLOGICAL DISORDERS

MERCURY POISONING, NEUTRALIZES
See: Trauma, Bites, Poisonings Mercury Poisoning, Neutralizes 412

METABOLISM OF LIVER, HELPS
See: Liver Liver, Helps Metabolism 211

METABOLISM RELATED TOPICS
See: Nutritional/Metabolic Disorders/Topics Metabolism Related Topics 282

METRORRHAGIA
See: Sexuality, Female: Gynecological Metrorrhagia 334

MIDDLE BURNER RELATED TOPICS
See: Triple Warmer (San Jiao) Middle Burner Related Topics 418

MIGRAINE
See: Head/Neck Migraine 150

MILIARIA
See: Skin Miliaria 362
See: Heat Miliaria 163

MILK DEFICIENCY
See: Sexuality, Female: Gynecological Milk Deficiency 334

MIND, CLOUDY
See: Mental State/Neurological Disorders Mind, Cloudy 254

MISCARRIAGE RELATED TOPICS
See: Sexuality, Female: Gynecological Miscarriage Related Topics 334

MITRAL VALVULAR DEFECT
See: Heart Mitral Valvular Defect 157

MOLE, MALIGNANT HYDATIDIFORM
See: Sexuality, Female: Gynecological Mole, Malignant Hydatidiform 335

MUSCULOSKELETAL/ CONNECTIVE TISSUE :

ARTHRITIS, RHEUMATIC, RHEUMATOID

ARTHRITIS, RHEUMATIC/RHEUMATOID

ARTHRITIS, RHEUMATOID

ARTHRITIS, SHOULDERS

ARTHRITIS, WHOLE BODY

ARTHRITIS, WHOLE BODY PAIN

ARTHRITIS, WITH WALKING DIFFICULTY

ATROPHIC DEBILITIES

ATROPHY SYNDROME

- SUO YANG/HU GU/NIU XI/SHU DI HUANG: Liver Kidney Severely Deficient

BACK ACHE

BACK, DISK PROBLEMS

BACK, JOINT PAIN

- GAO BEN/CANG ZHU: Bi, Initial Stage

BACK, LOWER

BACK, LOWER COLD PAIN IN

- YIN YANG HUO/WEI LING XIAN/DU ZHONG/GUI ZHI: Bi, Wind Cold Damp

BACK, LOWER COLD, PAIN

- QIAN NIAN JIAN/HU GU/NIU XI/GOU QI ZI
- ROU CONG RONG/TU SI ZI

BACK, LOWER COLD, SORE

- ROU CONG RONG/SUO YANG

BACK, LOWER PAIN

- BU GU ZHI/HU TAO REN: Kidney Yang Deficient
- DI LONG/DANG GUI/ROU GUI: Trauma Induced
- DONG CHONG XIA CAO/SHAN ZHU YU/SHAN YAO/TU SI ZI: Kidney Deficiency
- DU ZHONG/BU GU ZHI: Kidney Deficient Yang
- DU ZHONG/TU SI ZI/SANG JI SHENG: Kidney Deficient
- DU ZHONG/BU GU ZHI/HU TAO REN: Kidney Liver Deficiency
- FU PEN ZI/DU ZHONG: Kidney Deficient/Cold, Damp Bi
- GOU JI/TU SI ZI: Kidney Disorders
- GOU JI/GUI ZHI/QIN JIAO/HAI FENG TENG: Wind Damp Bi w/Liver Kidney Deficiency
- HAI FENG TENG/HAI TONG PI/QIN JIAO/SANG ZHI: Bi, Wind Damp
- HAI TONG PI/HAN FANG JI/WEI LING XIAN/HAI FENG TENG: Bi
- HU TAO REN/DU ZHONG/BU GU ZHI/(QING'E WAN): Kidney Deficiency
- HUANG JING/XU DUAN: Kidney Liver Deficient
- KUAN JIN TENG/JI XUE TENG: Wind Damp Bi
- LIU HUANG/FU ZI/ROU GUI: Lowered Life Gate Fire
- LU RONG/REN SHEN: Severely Deficient Heart Kidney
- LU RONG/REN SHEN/SHU DI HUANG/TU SI ZI: Kidney Yang Deficiency
- QIAN NIAN JIAN/HU GU/NIU XI/WU JIA PI/(in wine): In Elderly
- ROU GUI/GAN JIANG/WU ZHU YU/DANG GUI/CHUAN XIONG: Cold Stagnation
- SANG JI SHENG/DU HUO/CHUAN NIU XI/DU ZHONG/GOU JI/(DU HUO JI SHENG TANG): Pain, Soreness: Wind Damp Bi
- SHA YUAN ZI/DU ZHONG: Severe Deficient Liver Kidney
- SHAN ZHU YU/SHU DI HUANG/SHAN YAO: Kidney Deficient
- SHAN ZHU YU/SHU DI HUANG/TU SI ZI/GOU QI ZI/DU ZHONG: Liver Kidney Deficiency
- TU SI ZI/BU GU ZHI/DU ZHONG: Kidney Deficient
- TU SI ZI/BU GU ZHI/DU ZHONG/LU RONG: Kidney Deficient Yang
- TU SI ZI/BU GU ZHI/DU ZHONG/SHU DI HUANG/SHAN ZHU YU: Kidney Deficient Yin
- TU SI ZI/DU ZHONG/SHAN YAO/GOU JI: Kidney Deficiency
- WU JIA PI/DU ZHONG/NIU XI/SANG JI SHENG/XU DUAN: Liver Kidney Deficiency
- XIAN MAO/XI XIN: Cold, Damp

BACK, LOWER PAIN/SORE

• DONG CHONG XIA CAO (c) 775

BACK, LOWER PAIN/STIFF

• LU LU TONG: Wind Damp Bi 681

BACK, LOWER SORE

See: Musculoskeletal/Connective Tissue Back,
Lower Pain 264
• DONG CHONG XIA CAO/DU ZHONG/YIN YANG
HUO/ROU CONG RONG: Kidney Yang Deficient
• GOU QI ZI/SHU DI HUANG/TIAN MEN DONG: Liver
Kidney Yin Deficiency
• HUANG JING/GOU QI ZI/NU ZHEN ZI: Kidney Essence
Deficiency
• GUI BAN: Kidney Yin Deficient 806

BACK, LOWER SORE, PAIN

• XU DUAN/DU ZHONG/NIU XI: Liver Kidney Weakness
• SANG JI SHENG: Liver Kidney Yin Weak 813
• TU SI ZI 787
• XU DUAN 789

BACK, LOWER SORE, WEAK

• BA JI TIAN/DU ZHONG/XU DUAN: Kidney Yang
Deficiency
• GUI BAN/NIU XI/LONG GU/SHU DI HUANG: Liver Kidney
Yin Deficiency
• HE SHOU WU/SHU DI HUANG/NU ZHEN ZI/GOU QI
ZI/TU SI ZI/SANG JI SHENG: Blood Deficiency
• NIU XI/SANG JI SHENG/DU ZHONG/GOU JI: Liver Kidney
Deficiency
• LU RONG 784
• SANG SHEN ZI (c): Sang Shen With Honey 801

BACK, LOWER SORE/WEAK

• BU GU ZHI/TU SI ZI/ROU CONG RONG/DU ZHONG:
Kidney Deficiency
• NU ZHEN ZI/SANG SHEN ZI/HAN LIAN CAO/GOU QI ZI:
Yin Deficiency And Blood Heat
• SHU DI HUANG/SHAN ZHU YU/SHAN YAO/(LIU WEI
DIHUNG WAN): Liver Kidney Deficiency

BACK, LOWER SPRAIN

• HAI JIN SHA CAO 522

BACK, LOWER STIFF

• HU GU 563

BACK, LOWER WEAK

See: Musculoskeletal/Connective Tissue Back,
Sore 267
• ROU CONG RONG/SHAN ZHU YU: Severely Deficient
Kidneys
• ROU GUI/FU ZI/SHU DI HUANG/SHAN ZHU YU/(GUI FU
BA WEI WAN): Kidney Yang Deficiency
• YIN YANG HUO/XIAN MAO/SHU DI HUANG: Kidney
Yang Deficiency
• GU SUI BU 778
• HE SHOU WU: Yin/Blood Deficient 799
• LU RONG (c) 784
• MU GUA 567

• WU JIA SHEN 771

BACK, LUMBAR MYOSITIS

• CANG ER ZI (c): Injection In Pain Points 559

BACK, LUMBAR STRAIN

• GOU JI 778

BACK, NUMB PAIN OF

• QIAN SHI 826

BACK, NUMB, WEAK

• XI XIAN CAO 575

BACK, PAIN

See: Musculoskeletal/Connective Tissue Back,
Sore 267
• GUANG FANG JI/WEI LING XIAN: Wind Damp
• GUI ZHI/FU ZI: Bi w/Yang Deficiency
• HU LU BA/FU PEN ZI/HUANG JING: Kidney Deficient
• MAN JING ZI/CHUAN XIONG/FANG FENG: Wind Damp Bi
• BA JI TIAN 773
• DU ZHONG: Kidney Liver Deficient 775
• GOU QI ZI: Yin/Blood Deficient 798
• HAI TONG PI: Wind Damp Bi 562
• LAI FU ZI (c): Spondylitis,
Hypertrophic—Osteohyperplasia Pill (See Analgesic
Entry) 639
• QIANG HUO 449
• SHA YUAN ZI 786

BACK, PAIN FROM KIDNEY STONES

• HU TAO REN/DU ZHONG/BU GU ZHI/JIN QIAN CAO/HAI
JIN SHA CAO

BACK, PAIN, COLD

• BEI XIE/NIU XI: Wind Damp
• CHEN XIANG: Deficiency Type 622
• ROU CONG RONG 786

BACK, PAIN, COLD, SWOLLEN FEELING

• DU ZHONG/GUI ZHI/DU HUO/QIN JIAO: Cold Damp Bi

BACK, PAIN, HYPERTOPHIC ARTHIRITIS OF LUMBAR SPINES

• MA QIAN ZI (c): 300 g Of Ma Qian Zi, 35 g Each, Niu Xi,
Gan Cao, Cang Zhu, Ma Huang, Bai Jian Can, Ru Xiang,
Mo Yao, Quan Xie Powder, 1 g Each Night With White
Wine, 20 Days/Course, 90% Marked Effect 842

BACK, PAIN/WEAKNESS

• FU ZI/ROU GUI: Kidney Yang Deficiency

BACK, RHEUMATIC PAIN

• GOU JI 778

BACK, SORE

See: Musculoskeletal/Connective Tissue Back,
Pain 266
See: Musculoskeletal/Connective Tissue Back,
Lower Pain 264

JOINTS, PAIN, SPASMS

- CANG ER ZI/WEI LING XIAN/ROU GUI/CANG ZHU/CHUAN XIONG: Wind Damp Bi

JOINTS, PAIN, STIFF

- HU GU/MU GUA/NIU XI/DANG GUI/(in wine): Wind Damp
- CHUAN SHAN JIA: Wind Damp Bi 670

JOINTS, PAIN, STIFF, LACK OF MOBILITY

- YI YI REN 602

JOINTS, PAIN, STIFF, WEAK

- BAI HUA SHE/QIANG HUO/FANG FENG/QIN JIAO: Wind Damp

JOINTS, PAIN, SWELLING

- CHUAN SHAN JIA/DANG GUI/CHUAN XIONG/QIANG HUO/FANG FENG: Wind Damp
- HAI TONG PI/GUI ZHI/(external wash)
- LU FENG FANG/QIAN NIAN JIAN/WU GONG
- SI GUA LUO/WEI LING XIAN: Wind, Damp
- CHAN SU 837
- GUANG FANG JI 595
- JIU BI YING 625
- LU FENG FANG 841

JOINTS, PAIN, SWELLING FROM ALLERGIC RESPONSE

- DANG GUI (c): Yi Shen Tang (Dang Gui, Chi Shao, Chuan Xiong, Hong Hua, Dan Shen, Tao Ren) 795

JOINTS, PAIN, SWELLING, RED

- DI LONG/SANG ZHI/REN DONG TENG/CHI SHAO YAO: Bi, Damp Heat
- BAI XIAN PI: Hot Bi 515
- BEI XIE: Hot Bi 587
- CANG ZHU: Hot Bi 578
- CHI SHAO YAO: Hot Bi, Toxic Heat With Stasis 668
- CHUAN NIU XI: Hot Bi 669
- DA HUANG: Hot Bi, Toxic Heat With Stasis 542
- DAN SHEN: Hot Bi 672
- HAN FANG JI: Hot Bi 596
- HU ZHANG: Hot Bi 497
- HUANG BAI: Hot Bi 485
- JIN YIN HUA: Hot Bi, Toxic Heat With Stasis 524
- LIAN QIAO: Hot Bi, Toxic Heat With Stasis 525
- LUO SHI TENG: Hot Bi 566
- MU DAN PI: Hot Bi, Toxic Heat With Stasis 499
- MU TONG: Hot Bi 599
- PU GONG YING: Hot Bi, Toxic Heat With Stasis 529
- QIN JIAO: Hot Bi 569
- REN DONG TENG: Hot Bi 531
- SANG ZHI: Hot Bi 570
- SI GUA LUO: Hot Bi 688
- XI XIAN CAO: Hot Bi 575

JOINTS, PAIN, SWELLING, RED, HOT W/FEVER

- HAN FANG JI: Wind Damp Heat 596

JOINTS, PAIN, WEAKNESS IN LEGS

- MU GUA/HU GU/DU HUO

JOINTS, PROBLEMS

- SANG JI SHENG: Liver Kidney Yin Weak 813

JOINTS, REDUCES INFLAMMATION OF

- JI GU CAO (c) 564

JOINTS, SMOOTHES MOVEMENT

- SANG ZHI 570

JOINTS, SORE

- JI XUE TENG: Wind Damp Bi, With Blood Stasis/Deficient 677

JOINTS, SORE, PAINFUL

- RU XIANG: Wind Damp Bi 685
- XUN GU FENG 576

JOINTS, SORE, PAINFUL W/MOTOR IMPAIRMENT

- WEI LING XIAN/DU HUO/SANG JI SHENG/DANG GUI: Wind Damp

JOINTS, SORE, SWELLING

- CANG ZHU: Damp Heat 578

JOINTS, STIFF

- HAI FENG TENG: Wind Cold Damp Bi 562
- SI GUA LUO: Wind Damp Heat In Muscles, Channels 688
- XU DUAN 789

JOINTS, STIFF, PAIN

- HAI FENG TENG/HAI TONG PI/QIN JIAO/SANG ZHI: Bi, Wind Damp
- MU TONG 599

JOINTS, TUBERCULOSIS

- WU GONG 751

KNEES, COLD

- BU GU ZHI 773

KNEES, COLD SENSATION, PAIN

- BA JI TIAN/XU DUAN/SANG JI SHENG/BEI XIE
- YIN YANG HUO/WEI LING XIAN/DU ZHONG/GUI ZHI: Bi, Wind Cold Damp

KNEES, COLD, PAIN

- JIU CAI ZI/ROU CONG RONG/BA JI TIAN: Kidney Yang Deficient

KNEES, DEBILITY

- GOU JI 778

KNEES, DEBILITY, COLD, NUMB

- YANG QI SHI 789

KNEES, JOINTS

- CHE QIAN ZI (c): Helps Recovery Of Joint Capsule, Injected, 5% Solution 590

KNEES, LOINS, PAIN, ACHING OF

- DU HUO 561

KNEES, NUMB

- LU XIAN CAO 566

KNEES, PAIN

- DONG CHONG XIA CAO/SHAN ZHU YU/SHAN YAO/TU SI ZI: Kidney Deficiency
- DU ZHONG/BU GU ZHI/HU TAO REN: Kidney Liver Deficiency
- GOU JI/GUI ZHI/QIN JIAO/HAI FENG TENG: Wind Damp Bi w/Liver Kidney Deficiency
- HAI FENG TENG/HAI TONG PI/QIN JIAO/SANG ZHI: Bi, Wind Damp
- HAI TONG PI/HAN FANG JI/WEI LING XIAN/HAI FENG TENG: Bi
- HUANG JING/XU DUAN: Liver Kidney Deficient
- LU RONG/REN SHEN/SHU DI HUANG/TU SI ZI: Kidney Yang Deficiency
- ROU CONG RONG/DU ZHONG/BA JI TIAN/(JIN GANG WAN): Kidney Deficiency
- WU JIA PI/DU ZHONG/NIU XI/SANG JI SHENG/XU DUAN: Liver Kidney Deficiency
- BA JI TIAN 773
- BEI XIE 587
- DONG CHONG XIA CAO 775
- GOU JI 778
- HAI TONG PI: Wind Damp Bi 562
- HU TAO REN: Cold 782
- NIU XI: Deficiency/Damp Heat Descending/Wind Damp, Wine Treated 684
- SHA YUAN ZI 786
- SHAN ZHU YU: Liver Kidney Deficient ... 827
- TU SI ZI 787
- WEI LING XIAN 572
- XIAN MAO: Obstinate Cold Damp Bi 788
- YAN HU SUO 693

KNEES, PAIN, CHRONIC

- HAI TONG PI/NIU XI/QIANG HUO: Wind Cold Damp

KNEES, PAIN, COLD

- QIAN NIAN JIAN/HU GU/NIU XI/GOU QI ZI
- LIU HUANG 840
- ROU CONG RONG 786
- YIN YANG HUO 791

KNEES, PAIN, NUMB

- QIAN SHI 826

KNEES, PAIN, SORE

- GOU JI/DU ZHONG/NIU XI/XU DUAN: Liver Kidney Deficiency
- SANG JI SHENG/DU HUO/CHUAN NIU XI/DU ZHONG/GOU JI/(DU HUO JI SHENG TANG): Wind Damp Bi

- XU DUAN/DU ZHONG/NIU XI: Liver Kidney Weakness
- SANG JI SHENG: Liver Kidney Yin Weak 813
- TIAN MA 750
- XU DUAN 789

KNEES, PAIN, SWELLING

- CANG ZHU/HUANG BAI/NIU XI/(SAN MIAO WAN): Damp Heat Downward Flow
- CANG ZHU/MU GUA/SANG ZHI/DU HUO: Wind Cold Damp Bi

KNEES, PAIN, SWELLING, RED

- HUANG BAI: Hot Leg Qi 485

KNEES, PAIN/NUMB

- JI XUE TENG 677

KNEES, PAIN/WEAK

- FU ZI/ROU GUI: Kidney Yang Deficiency

KNEES, SORE

- GOU QI ZI/SHU DI HUANG/TIAN MEN DONG: Liver Kidney Yin Deficiency
- HUANG JING/GOU QI ZI: General Debility
- BA JI TIAN 773
- DONG CHONG XIA CAO (c) 775
- HAI FENG TENG: Wind Cold Damp Bi 562
- HE SHOU WU 799
- ROU GUI 616
- ROU GUI PI: Cold 617
- WU JIA PI 574

KNEES, SORE W/WEAKNESS

- GUI BAN 806

KNEES, SORE, WEAK

- BA JI TIAN/DU ZHONG/XU DUAN: Kidney Yang Deficiency
- GUI BAN/NIU XI/LONG GU/SHU DI HUANG: Liver Kidney Yin Deficiency
- HE SHOU WU/SHU DI HUANG/NU ZHEN ZI/GOU QI ZI/TU SI ZI/SANG JI SHENG: Blood Deficiency
- LU RONG 784

KNEES, SORE/WEAK

- BU GU ZHI/TU SI ZI/ROU CONG RONG/DU ZHONG: Kidney Deficiency
- NU ZHEN ZI/SANG SHEN ZI/HAN LIAN CAO/GOU QI ZI: Yin Deficiency And Blood Heat

KNEES, STIFF/PAIN

- LU LU TONG: Wind Damp Bi 681

KNEES, WEAK

- YIN YANG HUO/XIAN MAO/SHU DI HUANG: Kidney Yang Deficiency
- CHEN XIANG: Cold 622
- DU ZHONG: Kidney Liver Deficient 775
- GOU QI ZI 798
- GU SUI BU 778
- GUI BAN 806
- HE SHOU WU: Yin/Blood Deficient 799

MUSCLES, PAIN, SPASMS

- YU ZHU: Wind From Insuffient Fluids 815

MUSCLES, RELAXANT

- HOU PO (c): Lasts 3 Hrs, Injection 581
- HUANG LIAN (c): 3x Potent As Meprobamate 486
- SHAN ZHI ZI (c) 476
- YAN HU SUO (c) 693

MUSCLES, RELAXANT, LOCAL

- WU YAO (c) 632

MUSCLES, RELAXANT, STRIATED MUSCLES

- HAN FANG JI (c): High Dose 596

MUSCLES, RETARDED DEVELOPMENT IN CHILDREN

- WU JIA PI/SANG JI SHENG/NIU XI/XU DUAN

MUSCLES, SKELETAL

- LONG DAN CAO (c): Relaxed 492

MUSCLES, SMOOTH

- GUANG FANG JI (c): Stimulates, Large Doses Paralyze 595
- WU LING ZHI (c): Releases Spasms 691

MUSCLES, SMOOTH RELAXES

- FU LING (c) 594
- XI XIN (c) 452

MUSCLES, SMOOTH RELAXES LU/LI

- HUAI HUA MI (c): Decrease Tension 658

MUSCLES, SMOOTH STIMULATES

- GAO LIANG JIANG (c): At Low Doses 615
- NIU HUANG (c) 755
- WU JIA PI (c): Uterus Esp 574
- XIA KU CAO (c) 478
- XUAN FU HUA (c) 713

MUSCLES, SMOOTH, INHIBITS

- BO HE (c) 456
- CE BAI YE (c) 654
- CHEN PI (c) 621
- CHUAN XIONG (c): Large Doses 671
- DANG GUI (c): Small Intestines 795
- DONG CHONG XIA CAO (c) 775
- KUN BU (c) 724

MUSCLES, SMOOTH, INHIBITS, RELAXES

- XIAN HE CAO (c) 665

MUSCLES, SMOOTH, REDUCES SPASMS

- BAI SHAO (c): Synergistic With Gan Cao 794
- GE GEN (c) 460
- XIONG DAN (c): Action Similar To Papaverine 479

MUSCLES, SORE

- SI GUA LUO: Wind Damp Heat In Muscles, Channels 688

MUSCLES, SPASMS

- BAI SHAO/DANG GUI/SHU DI HUANG/MAI MEN DONG: Liver Yin Deficient
- GAN CAO/BAI SHAO
- HAI FENG TENG/HAI TONG PI/QIN JIAO/SANG ZHI: Bi, Wind Damp
- HAI FENG TENG/GUI ZHI: Wind Damp Bi
- MU GUA/DANG GUI/BAI SHAO: Blood Deficient
- TIAN NAN XING/TIAN MA: Wind Phlegm
- WU MEI/MU GUA: Summer Heat Disease
- CHUAN XIONG 671
- HAI FENG TENG: Wind Cold Damp Bi 562
- LUO SHI TENG 566

MUSCLES, SPASMS OF LIMBS

- WU JIA PI/WEI LING XIAN/DU HUO/SANG ZHI/MU GUA

MUSCLES, SPASMS, CALF

- BAI SHAO/GAN CAO: Blood Deficient
- CAN SHA/WU ZHU YU/MU GUA: Dampness

MUSCLES, SPASMS, CONTRACTURES

- E JIAO/GUI BAN/MU LI: Yin Deficient

MUSCLES, SPASMS, NUMB

- QIAN NIAN JIAN/HU GU/NIU XI/WU JIA PI/(in wine): Elderly

MUSCLES, SPASMS, PAIN

- HAI TONG PI/KUAN JIN TENG/GUI ZHI/(external wash for 1 month): Trauma
- WU JIA PI/WEI LING XIAN/QIANG HUO/QIN JIAO: Wind Damp Bi

MUSCLES, SPASMS, PARAMYOTONIA CONGENITA

- GAN CAO (c): 15 Day Course 763

MUSCLES, SPASMS, STRIATED

- YI YI REN (c): Relaxes 602

MUSCLES, STRENGTH, INCREASES

- DA ZAO (c) 761

MUSCLES, STRIATED, CURARE-LIKE ACTION

- XIN YI HUA (c): When Injected, Or Other Parts Of Plant 453

MUSCLES, STRIATED, STIMULANT

- CHAN SU (c): Bufotenidine, Active Ingredient, Greater Than Nicotine, Less Than Acetylcholine 837

MUSCLES, TENDONS, WEAK/SORE

- GUI BAN/NIU XI/LONG GU/SHU DI HUANG: Liver Kidney Yin Deficiency

MUSCLES, TETANY

MUSCLES, TRAUMA TO

- GU SUI BU/XU DUAN
- GU SUI BU/XU DUAN/RU XIANG/MO YAO/ZI RAN TONG: Strong Combination

MUSCLES, WEAK

MUSCLES, WEAK, ATROPHY

MUSCLES, WEAK, CHRONIC

- BA JI TIAN/DU ZHONG/NIU XI/XU DUAN: Bi, Chronic w/Kidney Deficient

MUSCULAR DYSTROPHY, NUTRITIONAL OR PROGRESSIVE

MUSCULAR DYSTROPHY, PROGRESSIVE/ATROPHIC

MYALGIA

OSTALGIA

OSTEALGIA

OSTEOARTHRITIS

OSTEOMALACIA

OSTEOMYELITIS

OSTEOMYELITIS, CHRONIC

PAIN, JOINT/MUSCLES

- BAN MAO/QUAN XIE/WU GONG/ZHU SHA: Chronic, Persistant

PAIN, JOINTS, SWELLING

- LU FENG FANG/QIAN NIAN JIAN/WU GONG

PAIN, LOW BACK

- QIAN NIAN JIAN/JI XUE TENG/GOU QI ZI: Elderly

PAIN, LOW BACK, LEGS

- KUAN JIN TENG/JI XUE TENG: Wind Damp Bi

PARAMYOTONIA CONGENITA

RHEUMATALGIA

RHEUMATALGIA, CHRONIC, ACUTE

RHEUMATIC ARTHRITIS

RHEUMATIC PAIN

- DANG GUI/GUI ZHI/JI XUE TENG/BAI SHAO
- WU GONG/QUAN XIE/TIAN MA/JIANG CAN/CHUAN XIONG

RHEUMATIC PAIN, STUBBORN

- QUAN XIE/WU GONG/JIANG CAN

RHEUMATIC PAIN, WIND DAMP

- WEI LING XIAN/DU HUO/SANG JI SHENG/DANG GUI

RHEUMATISM

RHEUMATISM, CHRONIC

RHEUMATOID ARTHRITIS

- DANG GUI (c) 795
- SHENG DI HUANG (c): (See Arthritis)
Sedative: Large Doses Potentiate Pentobarbital 500

SCIATICA

- MA QIAN ZI (c): Injection 842
- TIAN MA (c): 20% Solution Injection, IM, 1-3x/Day, Marked Effects After 1-4 Injections 750

SCIATICA IN PREGNANCY

- DANG GUI (c): Dang Gui Bai Shao San 795

SCLERODERMA

See: Skin Scleroderma 367

SHOULDER, ARTHRITIS

- JIANG HUANG 678

SHOULDERS, JOINT PAIN

- GUI ZHI 445

SHOULDERS, PAIN

- GUANG FANG JI/WEI LING XIAN: Wind Damp
- GUI ZHI/FU ZI: Bi w/Yang Deficiency
- JIANG HUANG/GUI ZHI/HUANG QI: Wind Damp, Especially Good
- JIANG HUANG/QIANG HUO/FANG FENG/DANG GUI/(SHU JING TANG): Bi
- MAN JING ZI/CHUAN XIONG/FANG FENG: Wind Damp
- QIANG HUO/FANG FENG/JIANG HUANG
- JIANG HUANG: Wind Damp Bi With Blood Stasis 678
- QIANG HUO 449

SHOULDERS, PAIN, SORENESS

- TIAN NAN XING 712

SHOULDERS, PERIARTHRITIS OF JOINT

- DAN SHEN (c): Injection As Local Block, Followed By Vigorous Massaged With Electropuncture Anesthesia 672

SHOULDERS, REDUCES INFLAMMATION OF

- JI GU CAO (c) 564

SMOOTH MUSCLE, ANTISPASMATIC, NOTED ON GB DUCT

- MI MENG HUA (c) 474

SMOOTH MUSCLE, CONTRACTS(EXCEPT VESSELS)

- HUANG LIAN (c) 486

SMOOTH MUSCLE, INHIBITS

- HE ZI (c) 822
- XIE BAI (c): Oral Extract First Stimulates Short Term, Then Inhibits 634

SMOOTH MUSCLE, RELAXES

- LIAN ZI (c): Uterus, Coronary Arteries 824

SPASMS

See: Musculoskeletal/Connective Tissue
Antispasmodic 261
See: Mental State/Neurological Disorders
Convulsions 243
See: Abdomen/Gastrointestinal Topics
Abdominal Spasms 27
See: Extremities Limb Spasms 114
See: Extremities Leg Spasms 111
See: Extremities Feet Spasms 110
See: Extremities Arm Spasms 108
See: Extremities Hand Spasms 111
See: Musculoskeletal/Connective Tissue
Spasms 275
See: Musculoskeletal/Connective Tissue
Antispasmodic 261
- BAI FU ZI/TIAN NAN XING/BAN XIA/TIAN MA/QUAN XIE: Excess Wind Phlegm
- BIE JIA/MU LI/SHENG DI HUANG/E JIAO/BAI SHAO/(ER JIA FU MAI TANG): Wind Following Febrile Disease, Yin/Fluids Consumed
- LONG DAN CAO/GOU TENG/NIU HUANG
- MA QIAN ZI/CHUAN WU/WEI LING XIAN: Wind Damp Bi
- MU GUA/RU XIANG/MO YAO/(MU GUA JIAN)
- MU LI/GUI BAN/E JIAO/BAI SHAO/BIE JIA/(SAN JIA FU MAI TANG): Late Febrile Disease Yin Depletion
- QUAN XIE/WU GONG/(ZI JING SAN): Tetanus
- RU XIANG/DI LONG/CHUAN WU: Cold, Damp Bi/Windstroke
- TIAN MA/GOU TENG/QUAN XIE: Liver Wind
- BAI HUA SHE: Any Kind 558
- CHAN TUI: High Fever 458
- CHAN TUI (c): Decreased From Tetanus/Other Drugs, Add With Other Herbs 458
- DAN NAN XING: Hot Phlegm 718
- FANG FENG 444
- HU GU 563
- HUO TAN MU CAO: Fever 498
- JIANG CAN 746
- LING YANG JIAO: Heat/Liver Yang Rising Creates Wind 747
- LONG DAN CAO: Liver Wind Heat 492
- MA QIAN ZI 842
- MU GUA: Liver Wind 567
- MU LI 739
- NIU HUANG: Liver Wind 755
- NIU HUANG (c): Relieves 755
- QUAN XIE: Liver Wind Phlegm 749
- RU XIANG 685
- TIAN MA 750
- TIAN ZHU HUANG: Phlegm Heat 726
- WO NIU: Fever 537
- WU GONG 751
- WU LING ZHI: Wind 691
- WU SHAO SHE 574
- YU ZHU: Wind From Insufficient Fluids 815
- ZHEN ZHU 740
- ZHU SHA (c) 741

SPASMS, CHILDHOOD

- CHAN TUI: Febrile Disease Wind 458

NASOSINUSITIS

NAUSEA RELATED TOPICS

NEBULA

NECK LUMPS

NECK RELATED TOPICS

NEPHRITIC EDEMA

NEPHRITIS RELATED TOPICS

NEPHROLITHIASIS

NEURALGIA

NEURALGIA, SUPRAORBITAL

NEURASTHENIA

NEURODERMATITIS

NEUROLOGICAL PAIN

NEUROSIS

NICOTINE

NIGHT BLINDNESS

NIGHT FEVER, NO SWEAT W/RED TONGUE

NIGHT SWEATS

NIGHTMARES

NOCTURIA

NOCTURNAL CRYING

NOCTURNAL EMISSIONS

NODULES AND RELATED TOPICS

End of Topic:
NODULES AND RELATED TOPICS

NOSE :

ALLERGIC RHINITIS

- CANG ER ZI/XIN YI HUA/WU WEI ZI/JIN YING ZI
- LU LU TONG/CANG ER ZI/XIN YI HUA
- CANG ER ZI (c): Herb Powder Macerate In ETOH, 12 Days, Percolate With ETOH, Evaporate, Make Tablets Each Equivalent To 1.5 g Of Crude Herb, Dose—2 Tabs, 3x/Day For 2 Weeks, 72% Effective 559
- CANG ER ZI 559
- MAO DONG QING (c): Decoction 682

EPISTAXIS

See: Hemorrhagic Disorders Epistaxis 166

NASAL CONGESTION

- BAI ZHI/XI XIN/XIN YI HUA/CANG ER ZI
- QIAN HU/JIE GENG: External Wind Heat
- XIANG FU/ZI SU YE
- XIN YI HUA/CANG ER ZI: Wind Cold
- XIN YI HUA/CANG ER ZI/BAI ZHI/XI XIN: Wind Cold
- XIN YI HUA/CANG ER ZI/SHI GAO/BO HE/HUANG QIN: Heat
- BAI ZHI 441
- CONG BAI: Yang Qi Blocked By Cold 442
- XIN YI HUA: Cold 453
- ZI SU YE: Wind Cold 454

NASAL CONGESTION, COMMON COLD

- ZI SU YE/JIE GENG

NASAL DISCHARGE, COPIOUS W/HEADACHE

- XI XIN/BAI ZHI/XIN YI HUA/BO HE

NASAL MUCOSA, CLEARS

- MA HUANG (c): As In Asthma 448

NASAL OBSTRUCTION

- CANG ER ZI/XIN YI HUA
- CANG ER ZI/XIN YI HUA/SHI GAO/HUANG QIN: Wind Heat, Acute
- CANG ER ZI/XIN YI HUA/QIAN CAO GEN/JIN YIN HUA: Wind Heat, Chronic

NASAL OBSTRUCTION, COMMON COLD W/SUPRAORBITAL PAIN

- BAI ZHI/CONG BAI/DAN DOU CHI/SHENG JIANG: Wind Cold

NASAL OBSTRUCTIONS, ANY

- XIN YI HUA 453

NASAL POLYPS

- XIONG HUANG/BAI FAN
- WU MEI (c): See Polyps, Various For Rx 830

NASAL SECRETIONS, DECREASES

- XIN YI HUA (c): Topical, Essential Oil 453

NASAL SECRETIONS, RUNNY

- XIN YI HUA 453

NASOPHARYNGEAL CANCER

- DONG CHONG XIA CAO (c): Inhibits In Humans 775
- SHI SHANG BAI 534
- WU MEI (c) 830

NASOSINUSITIS

- BAI ZHI 441

NOSE

- MA HUANG (c): Vasoconstricts Mucosa, Longer, Stronger Than Pseudoephedrine 448

NOSE INFECTION, SWELLING

- LIAN ZI (c): Reduces 824

NOSE TUMORS

- SHI SHANG BAI/(STEW WITH LEAN PORK)
- SHI SHANG BAI (c) 534

NOSE, DISCHARGE FROM

- BAI ZHI/CANG ER ZI/XIN YI HUA

NOSE, HEAT, PAIN, SWELLING, SUPPURATION

- BING PIAN/ZHU SHA/PENG SHA

NOSE, INFLAMMATION OF

- MA DOU LING 701

NOSE, INFLAMMATORY DISEASES

- QING MU XIANG (c) 628

NOSE, RUNNY

- QIAN HU/JIE GENG: External Wind Heat
- CANG ER ZI 559

NOSE, SORES

- SHAN ZHI ZI: Damp Heat Of Gall Bladder/San Jiao Channels 476

NOSE, STUFFY

- E BU SHI CAO 711
- LING LING XIANG 850

NOSEBLEED

See: Hemorrhagic Disorders Epistaxis 166
- DA QING YE/XI JIAO: Xue Level Heat
- DAI ZHE SHI/BAI ZHU/(quick fried ginger): Cold, Deficient
- HUANG LIAN 486
- SHUI NIU JIAO 501
- XI JIAO 502
- ZHU RU 729

RHINITIS

- BAI ZHI/CANG ER ZI/XIN YI HUA
- BAI ZHI 441
- BI BA 608
- BO HE (c): Menthol Dilutes Thick Mucus, Helping Symptoms 456
- CHAN TUI 458
- MA HUANG (c): As Nose Drops, 100% Decoction 448
- XIN YI HUA 453

RHINITIS, ACUTE/CHRONIC

- E BU SHI CAO 711

RHINITIS, ALLERGIC

See: Immune System Related Disorders/Topics
Allergies 175
- CANG ER ZI/XIN YI HUA/WU WEI ZI/JIN YING ZI
- LU LU TONG/CANG ER ZI/XIN YI HUA
- AI YE (c): Decoction 651
- BAN MAO (c): Symptomatic Relief, Topical To Yin Tang Acupoint 837
- CANG ER ZI 559
- LU LU TONG (c): Cures 681
- MU DAN PI (c): Symptom Removal (ETOH ext) , *10% Decoction, 50 ml Before Bed For 10 Days 499

RHINITIS, ALLERGIC/SIMPLE

- XIN YI HUA (c): Nose Drops Of Water Distillate Of Xin Yi Hua, Extract Of Huang Qin, 2-3x/Day In Nose For 2-3 Weeks, 80% Effective 453

RHINITIS, ATROPHIC

- XIN YI HUA (c): Topical Application Of Ointment From Herb, Chan Su, She Xiang, Bing Pian, Glycerin 453
- YU XING CAO (c): Nose Drop Preparation 539

RHINITIS, CHRONIC

- CANG ER ZI 559

- CANG ER ZI (c): Good 30-40 Seeds Crushed With Ounce Of Sesame Oil, Fry Over Low Heat, Cool, Apply To Nasal Cavities With Cotton Swabs 2-3 X/Day For 2 Weeks, Almost 100% Cure With No Relapse 559
- HUANG LIAN (c): Nasal Inserts Of Gauze Soaked With 10% Solution, 1x/Day For 7-10 Days, Recovers Sense Of Smell, Reduces Secretions 486

RHINITIS, CHRONIC W/HEADACHE

- XIN YI HUA (c) 453

RHINITIS, CHRONIC/ACUTE/ALLERGIC

- XIN YI HUA (c): Xin Yi Hua, Cang Er Zi, Yu Xing Cao, Qian Li Guang (Herba Senecionis) , 150 g Each, Plus Few Drops Menthol, Boiled In Water, Filtered Then Concentrated To 500 ml, 80-90% Effective 453

RHINITIS, HYPERTROPHIC/ACUTE

- XIN YI HUA (c): Volatile Oil Emulsion, *Ointment Of Alcohol Extract Apply In Nasal Cavity With Gauze, Retain 2-3 Hrs, 1x/Day Or 2, 10 Applications, 4-5 Applications To Show Improvement 453

RHINORRHEA

- XI XIN/BAI ZHI/XIN YI HUA/BO HE
- BAI ZHI 441

RHINORRHEA, COLD TYPE

- XIN YI HUA/CANG ER ZI/BAI ZHI/XI XIN

SINUS CONGESTION

- BAI ZHI/XI XIN/XIN YI HUA/CANG ER ZI
- BAI ZHI 441

SINUS HEADACHE

See: Head/Neck Headache, Sinusitis 149

SINUSITIS

- BAI ZHI/CANG ER ZI/XIN YI HUA
- BI BA 608
- FENG MI 548
- HUANG QIN: Heat, Needs Sinusitis Herbs Added 489
- JIN YIN HUA: Heat, Needs Sinusitis Herbs Plus 524
- LIAN QIAO: Heat, Needs Sinusitis Herbs Plus 525
- SHI GAO: Heat, Needs Sinusitis Herbs, Too 477
- XI XIN 452
- XIN YI HUA 453
- XIN YI HUA (c): Xin Yi Hua Repeatedly Soaked In Banana Stump Juice Then Sun Dried Added To Musk, Bing Pian 453

SINUSITIS W/HEADACHE

- BAI ZHI 441
- CANG ER ZI 559
- XI XIN 452
- XIN YI HUA 453

SINUSITIS W/RUNNY NOSE

- XI XIN/BAI ZHI/XIN YI HUA/BO HE

SINUSITIS, FRONTAL

- XIN YI HUA/CANG ER ZI/JU HUA/XI XIAN CAO

SINUSITIS, MAXILLARY

- HUANG LIAN (c): Injection Into Sinus With 2 ml 10% Decotion In 3% Boric Acid, Equally Effective As Penicillin 486

SINUSITIS, MAXILLARY, CHRONIC

- HUANG BAI (c) 485
- HUANG LIAN (c): Injection Into Sinus With 2 ml 30% Decotion 486
- YU XING CAO (c): Perfusion With Extract 539

SINUSITIS, PARANASAL

- E BU SHI CAO 711
- XIN YI HUA (c): With Cang Er Zi, Du Huo, Bo He Or Xi Xin (Cang Er Zi San) , *With Jing Jie, Huang Qin (Xin Yi Jing Jie San) , *Paste Made With Xin Yi Hua, Hai Er Cha, Ru Xiang, Bing Pian, Glycerin, 2-8 Days 453

SINUSITIS, PARANASAL, CHRONIC

- CANG ER ZI (c): As Honey Pill, 3 g/Pill, 1-2 Pills, Or Tab, 1.5 g/Tab, 2 Tabs, 3x/Day For 2 Weeks, *Fluidextract Of Herb With Xin Yi Hua, Jin Yin Hua, Ju Hua, Qian Cao Gen, Orally, Greater Than 80% Effective 559

SINUSITIS, W/HEADACHE/RUNNY NOSE

- CANG ER ZI 559

End of Topic:
NOSE

NOSE AND RELATED TOPICS

See: Nose Nose And Related Topics 279

NOSE TUMORS

See: Cancer/Tumors/Swellings/Lumps Nose Tumors 71

NOSEBLEED

See: Nose Nosebleed 279

NUMB PAIN

See: Pain/Numbness/General Discomfort Numb Pain 301

NUMBNESS

See: Pain/Numbness/General Discomfort Numbness 301

NUTRITIONAL IMPAIRMENT, IN CHILDREN

See: Childhood Disorders Nutritional Impairment, Childhood 83

NUTRITIONAL TOPICS

See: Nutritional/Metabolic Disorders/Topics Nutritional Topics 282

End of Topic:
NUTRITIONAL TOPICS

NUTRITIONAL/ METABOLIC DISORDERS/ TOPICS :

BERIBERI

- BING LANG/CHEN PI/MU GUA: Leg Qi Of
- WU ZHU YU/MU GUA/(EXTERNAL)
- BA JI TIAN 773
- BA JIAO HUI XIANG 608
- BAI JIE ZI 708
- BING LANG 643
- CAN SHA: Cold Dampness 558
- CANG ER ZI: Cold Dampness 559
- CANG ZHU: Cold Dampness 578
- CHEN PI (c): Vit B1 621
- CHI XIAO DOU: Leg Qi 591
- CHUAN JIAO: Cold Dampness 610
- DA FU PI 624
- HAI PIAO XIAO: Cold Dampness 821
- HAN FANG JI: Damp Heat 596
- HU LU BA: Cold Dampness 781
- HU TAO REN 782
- LU XIAN CAO 566
- SHE CHUANG ZI: Cold Dampness 847
- SONG JIE 572
- WU ZHU YU 618
- XIANG RU 453
- YU LI REN 549
- ZE QI 727
- ZE XIE 605
- ZHANG NAO 849

BERIBERI, SWELLING OF

- MU GUA 567
- YU MI XU 605

BODY TEMPERATURE, LOWERS

- See: Fevers Antipyretic 125
- BEI SHA SHEN (c): Alcohol Extracts 804
- MA HUANG (c) 448
- SHI CHANG PU (c) 757
- SUAN ZAO REN (c): Oral/Injected 732

BODY TEMPERATURE, RAISES

- WU ZHU YU (c) 618

BODY WEIGHT, DECREASES

- MO YAO (c) 683

BODY WEIGHT, INCREASES

- ROU CONG RONG (c) 786
- WU JIA SHEN (c): Anabolic 771
- ZHU SHA (c) 741

BODY, COLD

- XI XIN: Interior 452
- XIAN MAO 788

CALCIUM REDUCES, IN SOME GLANDS

- SHI GAO (c): (Pitutary, Pancreas, Adrenals) 477

CALCIUM UPTAKE, INCREASES

- E JIAO (c): From Glycine Content Which Promotes
  Calcium Absorption 797

CALCIUM, INCREASES IN SPLEEN

- SHI GAO (c) 477

DIABETES

See: Nutritional/Metabolic Disorders/Topics
Wasting & Thirsting 283

EDEMA, DEFICIENT FROM MALNUTRITION

- CHI XIAO DOU/(peanuts & red dates)

EMACIATION

- HUANG JING/REN SHEN: Prolonged Illness,
  Consumptive Illness
- TIAN HUA FEN/BEI SHA SHEN/MAI MEN DONG/SHENG
  DI HUANG: Stomach Heat Injured Yin
- ZI HE CHE: Tuberculosis 792

EMACIATION W/HEAT IN FIVE CENTERS

- BAI MU ER 803

GOUT

See: Musculoskeletal/Connective Tissue Gout
. . . . 268

GROWTH STIMULANT

- GOU QI ZI (c): 1: 10 Dang Shen/Herb Oral Decoction
  For 4 Days Markedly Increased Body Weight In Animals,
  Betaine Active Ingredient 798

GROWTH, DELAYED

- GUI BAN: Kidney Yin Deficient 806

GROWTH, INCREASES

- LU RONG (c) 784

GROWTH, INCREASES OF IMMATURE

- ROU CONG RONG (c): Alcohol Extract 786

GROWTH, PROMOTES

- LU RONG (c): Stimulates Bodily Functions 784

HEALING, HELPS

- LU RONG (c) 784

HYPOTHERMIA

- HE SHOU WU (c): Enhances Ability To Withstand 799
- MU DAN PI (c) 499
- SHI CHANG PU (c) 757
- SUAN ZAO REN (c) 732
- YAN HU SUO (c): Helps 693
- YI YI REN (c) 602

HYPOXIA

- YIN YANG HUO (c): Reduces Effects Of, 100% Decoction 791

HYPOXIA PROTECTION

- WU JIA SHEN (c) 771

HYPOXIA TOLERANCE, INCREASES

- MAI MEN DONG (c) 810

HYPOXIA, TOLERANCE TO

- CHUAN SHAN LONG (c): Oral Dose Decreased Oxygen Consumption 442

MALNUTRITION

- LU HUI: From Heat 544
- ZAO FAN 848

MALNUTRITION ACCUMULATION

- KU SHEN 491

MALNUTRITION FEVER

- LU HUI 544

MALNUTRITION FEVER, CHILDHOOD

- YIN CHAI HU 504

MALNUTRITION, CHILDHOOD

- HU HUANG LIAN 484

METABOLISM

- HUANG QI (c): Increased Life Of Cells And Induced Vigorous Growth 765
- LING YANG JIAO (c): Increases Resistance To Lower Oxygen 747
- REN SHEN (c): Increases Protein Synthesis 767
- SANG YE (c): Promotes Anabolism 466

METABOLISM OF PHOSPHATE, INCREASES IN KIDNEYS, UTERUS

- JI XUE TENG (c) 677

METABOLISM, HARMONIZES

- WU JIA PI (c) 574

METABOLISM, HYPOXIA TOLERANCE

- CHAI HU (c): Injection IP Of Flavones 457

METABOLISM, INCREASE PROTEIN SYNTHESIS

- CHAI HU (c) 457

METABOLISM, INCREASES

- DAN SHEN (c): Increase Hypoxia Tolerance, Too 672
- DANG GUI (c) 795
- LU RONG (c) 784
- WU WEI ZI (c) 831

METABOLISM, LIPIDS INCREASES

- GOU QI ZI (c) 798

METABOLISM, PROMOTES

- DANG SHEN (c) 762

METABOLISM, STRONG PROTEIN ANABOLISM ACTION

- NIU XI (c) 684

NUTRITIONAL

- FENG MI (c) 548

NUTRITIONAL TOPICS

See: Energetic State Energetic State 104

NUTRITIVE

- FU LING (c) 594
- SHAN YAO (c) 769

OXYGEN METABOLISM, INCREASED RESISTANCE TO LOW OXYGEN

- LING YANG JIAO (c) 747

PROTEIN SYNTHESIS, INCREASES

- CHAI HU (c) 457
- REN SHEN (c) 767

RICKETS

- GUI BAN 806
- LU RONG: Essence/Blood Deficiency 784

RUTIN MAIN INGREDIENT

- HUAI HUA MI (c) 658

TEMPERATURE EXTREMES

- REN SHEN (c): Helps Body To Withstand 767

TEMPERATURE, BODY

- WU ZHU YU (c): Raises Slightly 618

TEMPERATURE, INCREASES TOLERANCE TO HIGH

- DANG SHEN (c) 762

TEMPERATURE, LOWERS

- BI BA (c): Vasodilator, Cutaneous, Develops Tolerance 608
- FU ZI (c): In Both Febrile/Normal 613
- MU DAN PI (c) 499

THINNESS

- ZI HE CHE 792

TISSUES, PROMOTES REGENERATION OF

- DAN SHEN (c): Promotes Repair, Regeneration 672
- XU DUAN (c) 789

VITAMIN C, INCREASES ABSORPTION

- ER CHA (c) 839

ORAL CAVITY :

CANKERS

CARIES

CARIES, TOOTHACHE

COLD SORES

DROOLING

DRY THROAT

EPIGLOTTIS SPASMS

ESOPHAGEAL CANCER

ESOPHAGITIS

GINGIVA, ULCERS OF

GINGIVITIS

GLOBUS HYSTERICUS

GLOBUS HYSTERICUS W/NAUSEA, CHEST, EPIGASTRIC DISTENTION

GLOTTIS, EDEMA

GUMS

GUMS, ABSCESS

GUMS, BLEEDING

GUMS, BLEEDING FROM FROSTBITE

GUMS, PAIN, SWELLING

GUMS, PAIN, SWELLING AROUND TEETH

GUMS, PAIN, SWELLING, RED

GUMS, PAIN, SWELLING, ULCERS

GUMS, PAIN, SWOLLEN

GUMS, SEVERE SORES

GUMS, SWOLLEN

- NIU XI/SHENG DI HUANG/ZHI MU: Yin Deficiency, Excess Fire
- SHENG MA/HUANG LIAN: Heart/Spleen Fire
- RU XIANG 685
- WU MEI (c): Kidney Qi Weak 830

GUMS, SWOLLEN W/TOOTHACHE

- SHI GAO/XI XIN: Stomach Fire Flaring

GUMS, ULCERS

- ER CHA/QING DAI/HUANG BAI/BING PIAN
- SHENG MA 467

HALITOSIS

See: Oral Cavity Bad Breath 283
- HUANG LIAN 486
- JI NEI JIN (c): Used With Mai Ya, Shan Zha, Bai Zhu, Chen Pi 638
- PEI LAN 583
- SHENG MA (c): Water-Alcohol Extract 467
- ZHU RU: Stomach Heat 729

HEADACHE, TOOTHACHE

- XI XIN/SHENG DI HUANG: Wind Heat

HERPES, ON LIPS

- ER CHA 839

HOARSENESS

- CHAN TUI/PANG DA HAI: Lung Heat
- JIANG CAN/JIE GENG/GAN CAO/BO HE: Wind Heat
- MA DOU LING/XING REN: Lung Heat
- MU HU DIE/PANG DA HAI/CHAN TUI
- PANG DA HAI/SHI CHANG PU/BO HE: Wind Heat In Lungs
- BEI SHA SHEN: Chronic Cough 804
- CHAN TUI 458
- HE ZI 822
- HOU ZAO 722
- MA BO 528
- MU HU DIE 702
- NAN SHA SHEN: Chronic Cough 811
- PANG DA HAI 724
- REN SHEN YE: Lung Heat 769
- XUE YU TAN 666

HOARSENESS, CHRONIC

- HE ZI/JIE GENG/GAN CAO
- HE ZI/WU WEI ZI/BEI SHA SHEN/BAI HE: Deficient Lungs

HOARSENESS, VOICE, COMMON COLD

- CHAN TUI/PANG DA HAI/NIU BANG ZI/JIE GENG: Wind Heat

HOARSENESS, W/SORE THROAT

- JIE GENG/GAN CAO: Wind Heat
- PANG DA HAI/XUAN SHEN: Deficient Yin Fire
- SHE GAN/HUANG QIN/JIE GENG: Fire

HOARSENESS, W/SPUTUM IN THROAT

- SHI CHANG PU/JIE GENG/SHI HU

HOARSENESS, W/SWOLLEN, EDEMOUS VOCAL CORDS

- SHI CHANG PU/JIE GENG/SHI HU

HOARSENESS, WATER DISTENTION OF LARYNX

- MAO DONG QING 682

HOARSENESS, WITH THICK PHLEGM

- PENG SHA **844**

HOARSNESS

See: Oral Cavity Voice, Hoarse 295

LARYNGEAL NODULES

- WU MEI (c): See Polyps, Various For Rx 830

LARYNGEAL POLYPS

- WU MEI (c): See Polyps, Various For Rx 830

LARYNGEAL ULCER

- ZHE BEI MU 728

LARYNGITIS

- BAI HUA SHE SHE CAO 511
- BAI HUA SHE SHE CAO (c) 511
- BING PIAN 753
- BO HE (c): Menthol Dilutes Thick Mucus, Helping Symptoms 456
- CHAN SU 837
- CHAN TUI 458
- ER CHA 839
- GU JING CAO 461
- HUO TAN MU CAO 498
- JIANG CAN 746
- JING JIE 447
- MA BO 528
- MU TONG 599
- PANG DA HAI 724
- REN SHEN YE 769
- SHAN DOU GEN (c) 532

LARYNGITIS, ACUTE

- SHE GAN 533

LARYNX, RATTLING SOUND

- TIAN NAN XING/BAN XIA/TIAN MA/BAI FU ZI: Wind Phlegm

LARYNX, WATER DISTENTION

- MAO DONG QING 682

LIPS, BLEEDING

- MA BO: Topical 528

LIPS, DRY

- SHENG DI HUANG 500

LIPS, ULCERS

- DA HUANG (c) 542

PHARYNGITIS, ACUTE/CHRONIC

PHARYNGITIS, CHRONIC

PHARYNGITIS, SEVERE

PHARYNGO-LARYNGITIS

PHARYNGOLARYNGITIS

PULPITIS, DECREASES PAIN

SALIVATION

SALIVATION, EXCESS

- YI ZHI REN/DANG SHEN/BAN XIA/FU LING : Spleen Stomach Cold Deficiency
- YI ZHI REN/FU LING /SHAN YAO/DANG SHEN/BAN XIA: Spleen Deficiency

SALIVATION, EXCESS W/THICK, UNPLEASANT TASTE

SALIVATION, INCREASES

SALIVATION, INHIBITS

SORES, MOUTH

- NIU HUANG/ZHEN ZHU: Heat

SORES, MOUTH/TONGUE

- DAN ZHU YE/MU TONG/SHENG DI HUANG: Heart Channel Heat
- SHENG MA/HUANG LIAN: Heart/Spleen Fire

SORES, MOUTH/TONGUE/THROAT

SORES, ORAL CAVITY

SORES, PAINFUL—ESPECIALLY THROAT

- SHE XIANG/ZHEN ZHU/XIONG HUANG/NIU HUANG: Severe Heat

SPEECH, DIFFICULTY IN

SPEECH, LOSS OF W/NUMBNESS

- SHENG JIANG/ZHU LI: Windstroke, Phlegm Obstruction

STOMATITIS

STOMATITIS, APHTHOUS

STOMATITIS, MYCOTIC

STOMATITIS, NECROTIC

SWALLOWING, DIFFICULT

- DAI ZHE SHI/DANG SHEN/DANG GUI: Blockage In Throat, Chest

TASTE, BITTER

- LONG DAN CAO/CHAI HU: Liver Fire/Damp Heat

TASTE, DECREASING

TEETH

TEETH, DENTAL CARIES

TEETH, DENTAL CARIES, ACUTE PULPITIS

TEETH, DENTAL CARIES, PAIN OF

TEETH, GUMS

TEETH, GUMS, PAIN, SWELLING, RED

TEETH, LOOSE

TEETH, LOOSE, PAIN

TEETH, LOSS/LOOSE

TEETH, PAIN OF

TEETH, PAIN THAT RADIATES FROM VERTEX

TEETH, PULPITIS

TEETH, SORE

THIRST, DRY MOUTH

THIRST, DRY TONGUE

THROAT ABSCESS

THROAT ABSCESS, EXPELS PUS

THROAT BI W/OBSTRUCTION

THROAT CANCER

THROAT INFECTIONS

THROAT INFECTIONS/SWELLINGS, PAINFUL

THROAT OBSTRUCTION

THROAT OBSTRUCTION, PHLEGM, SALIVA

THROAT PAIN

THROAT SORES

THROAT TUMORS

THROAT ULCERS

THROAT WIND/BI

THROAT, ACUTE INFLAMMATION

THROAT, BI

THROAT, BI PAIN

THROAT, BONE OBSTRUCTION

THROAT, DRY

- GE GEN/CHAI HU/HUANG QIN: Common Cold, Wind Heat
- GOU QI ZI/DANG GUI/SHU DI HUANG/BEI SHA SHEN/CHUAN LIAN ZI: Yin Deficiency And Liver Qi Stagnation
- SANG SHEN ZI/MAI MEN DONG: Blood And Fluids Deficiency
- SHENG DI HUANG/XUAN SHEN: Yin Deficiency w/Fire
- BEI SHA SHEN: Yin Deficiency/Febrile Diseases 804
- GUI BAN 806
- LU GEN 472
- MAI MEN DONG 810
- NAN SHA SHEN: Yin Deficiency/Febrile Diseases 811
- SHI GAO 477
- TIAN MEN DONG 814
- YU ZHU: Yin Deficient 815

THROAT, DRY W/COUGH, THICK SPUTUM

- PI PA YE/XING REN

THROAT, DRY W/COUGH, YELLOW SPUTUM

- BO HE/NIU BANG ZI

THROAT, FEELING OF FOREIGN BODY IN

See: Oral Cavity Globus Hystericus 284
- BAN XIA/HOU PO/ZI SU YE/FU LING /(BAN XIA HOU PO TANG)

THROAT, FISH BONES LODGED IN

- WEI LING XIAN/(vinegar,brown sugar)
- WEI LING XIAN/SHA REN
- WEI LING XIAN (c): Good, Best Extracted With Acetic Acid, Relaxes Spasms, But Increases Peristalsis, Thus Allowing Bone To Dislodge, 30 g, May Add Du Huo, Wu Mei, Gan Cao, Make Concentrated Decoction/Use With Vinegar, Give Slowly By Mouth (30-60 Min) , 1-2 Doses/Day, 88% Effective 572
- WEI LING XIAN 572

THROAT, HEAT, PAIN, SWOLLEN, SUPPURATION

- BING PIAN/ZHU SHA/PENG SHA

THROAT, IMMOBILE, PALPABLE MASSES

- SHUI ZHI/HAI ZAO

THROAT, INFECTION, SWOLLEN

- LIAN ZI (c): Reduces 824

THROAT, INFLAMMATION

- MA DOU LING 701
- YE JU HUA 468

THROAT, INTENSIFIES ESOPHAGEAL PERISTALSIS

- WEI LING XIAN (c) 572

THROAT, NUMB

- DAI MAO 743
- DENG XIN CAO: External 592
- DI LONG 744

- ZHEN ZHU 740

THROAT, OBSTRUCTION

- LUO SHI TENG 566
- NUO DAO GEN 825

THROAT, PAIN W/HOARSENESS

- SHE GAN/HUANG QIN/JIE GENG: Fire

THROAT, PAIN, SWELLING

- GAN CAO/JIE GENG: Acute, Mild
- BAN ZHI LIAN 516

THROAT, PAIN, SWOLLEN

- BAN LAN GEN/XUAN SHEN/ZHI MU
- BO HE/JIE GENG
- LUO SHI TENG/SHE GAN/JIE GENG
- MA BO/SHAN DOU GEN/XUAN SHEN
- MU BIE ZI/SHAN DOU GEN/(blowed powder)
- MU HU DIE/PANG DA HAI/CHAN TUI
- NIU BANG ZI/LIAN QIAO
- PANG DA HAI/XUAN SHEN: Deficient Yin Fire
- SHAN DOU GEN/NIU BANG ZI
- SHAN DOU GEN/BAN LAN GEN
- ZHU SHA/XIONG HUANG/(or)/BING PIAN/(topical,pwdr)
- BO HE 456
- CHI SHAO YAO 668
- DA QING YE 519
- GAN CAO 763
- HAI JIN SHA CAO 522
- HUANG YAO ZI 723
- JIE GENG 711
- JIU BI YING 625
- LIAN QIAO 525
- MA BO 528
- MU DAN PI 499
- MU HU DIE 702
- NIU BANG ZI 465
- PANG DA HAI 724
- PENG SHA: Take Internal/External 844
- SHAN DOU GEN 532
- SHE GAN 533
- XUAN SHEN 503

THROAT, PAIN, SWOLLEN W/MUMPS

- BAN LAN GEN/NIU BANG ZI/BAI JIANG CAO

THROAT, PAIN, SWOLLEN, RED

- ER CHA/JIN YIN HUA/LIAN QIAO

THROAT, PHLEGM IN

- TING LI ZI (c): Oil Alleviates 555

THROAT, PLUM PIT SENSATION

- LA MEI HUA 680

THROAT, RATTLING SOUND IN

- BAI QIAN/ZI WAN/DA JI/(BAI QIAN TANG)

THROAT, RED, SWOLLEN

• MANG XIAO/PENG SHA/(topical): Topical

THROAT, SENSATION OF OBSTRUCTION

• JI XING ZI 677

THROAT, SEVERE PAIN, ULCERS

• ZHEN ZHU/NIU HUANG/BING PIAN: Topical

THROAT, SEVERE SORE, SWELLING

• MA QIAN ZI/SHAN DOU GEN/BAN LAN GEN

THROAT, SEVERE SORES

• CHAN SU/ZHEN ZHU/NIU HUANG/SHE XIANG/XIONG HUANG

THROAT, SORE

See: Oral Cavity Pharyngitis 287
• BING PIAN/PENG SHA/GAN CAO/MANG XIAO/(XUAN MING FEN WITH BING PENG SAN)
• CHUAN XIN LIAN/JIN YIN HUA/JIE GENG/NIU BANG ZI: Wind Heat Early Stage
• DA HUANG/HUANG LIAN/HUANG QIN/(XIE XIN TANG): Fire Rising
• DA QING YE/JIN YIN HUA
• DA QING YE/JIN YIN HUA/SHI GAO: Exterior Heat
• DA QING YE/XUAN SHEN/JIN YIN HUA
• GAN CAO/JIE GENG/XUAN SHEN/NIU BANG ZI: Toxic Heat
• JIANG CAN/JIE GENG/FANG FENG/GAN CAO: Wind Heat
• JIE GENG/XUAN SHEN/GAN CAO/NIU BANG ZI
• LUO SHI TENG/ZAO JIAO CI/GUA LOU/RU XIANG/MO YAO/(ZI TONG LIN BAO SAN)
• MANG XIAO/PENG SHA/BING PIAN/(TOPICAL)
• NIU BANG ZI/JIE GENG/BO HE/JING JIE: Wind Heat
• NIU HUANG/QING DAI/JIN YIN HUA: Toxic Heat
• PANG DA HAI/JIE GENG/CHAN TUI/BO HE/GAN CAO: Lung Heat Accumulation
• SHE GAN/XING REN/JIE GENG: Lung Heat
• SHENG MA/XUAN SHEN/JIE GENG/NIU BANG ZI: Wind Heat
• XUAN SHEN/NIU BANG ZI/JIE GENG/BO HE: Wind
• XUAN SHEN/MAI MEN DONG/JIE GENG/GAN CAO: Excess Internal Heat
• YE JU HUA/JIN YIN HUA/PU GONG YING/ZI HUA DI DING
• BA DOU: pwdr Blown In Throat To Cause Vomiting . . 550
• BAI HE: Lung Heat/Dry 803
• BAI HUA SHE SHE CAO (c) 511
• BAI WEI 495
• BI MA ZI 547
• BO HE (c): Cured With "Modified Solidaga Decurrens Decoction" (Herba Solidago, Bo He, She Gan, Herba Rhodeae, Herba Peristrophis, Zou Ma Tai (Radix Ardisiae) , Gan Cao) , 1-3 Doses Effective, Any Of Herbs May Be Used Singly, Too 456
• CAO HE CHE 517
• CHAN SU: w/Swelling/Pain 837
• CHAN SU (c): Topical Application Of Tincture 837
• CONG BAI 442
• DENG XIN CAO 592
• DI LONG 744

• E BU SHI CAO 711
• FENG MI 548
• FENG WEI CAO 496
• GAN CAO: Topical, Too 763
• GUA LOU REN 720
• HUANG LIAN 486
• HUO TAN MU CAO 498
• JIANG CAN: Wind Heat 746
• JIE GENG: Heat/Hot Phlegm/Deficient Yin Heat 711
• JIE GENG (c): Oral Dose 711
• JIN DI LUO 523
• JIN GUO LAN 523
• JIN YIN HUA: Wind Heat 524
• JU HUA (c): Sang Ju Yin, Two Flowers Decoction (Ju Hua, Jin Yin Hua, Gan Cao, Pang Da Hai) 463
• KUAN DONG HUA: Bi Pain 700
• LI LU 834
• LUO SHI TENG 566
• MU HU DIE 702
• MU TONG 599
• MU TONG (c) 599
• NIU HUANG (c): Topical Spray Powder (Chui Hou San—Niu Huang, Alunite Powder, She Xiang, Borax, Hu PO, Zhu Sha, Bing Pian, Huang Lian, Fructus Malus Asiaticae) , 1-2 X/Day 755
• QING DAI: Topical 531
• SAN QI HUA: Acute 663
• SANG YE: Common Cold 466
• SHAN DOU GEN 532
• SHANG LU 554
• SHE TUI 571
• SHENG DI HUANG: Yin Deficient 500
• SHI SHANG BAI: Lung Heat 534
• TIAN HUA FEN 726
• WO NIU 537
• XIONG DAN 479
• XUAN SHEN (c): Yin Def Heat—Yang Ying Qing Fei Tang (Xuan Shen, Sheng Di, Mai Dong, Bai Shao, Mu Dan Pi, Gan Cao, Bo He) 503
• YI TANG 772
• ZAO FAN 848
• ZAO JIAO 715
• ZAO XIU 540
• ZHEN ZHU: Deficient Heat 740
• ZHI XUE CAO 697
• ZHU SHA: Topical 741

THROAT, SORE, ACUTE

• PU GONG YING (c): See Respiratory Tract Infections (Pu Gong Ying) 529
• SHENG MA (c): Qing Wei San—Sheng Ma, Huang Lian, Sheng Di, Dan Shen, Dang Gui 467

THROAT, SORE, BI NUMBNESS

• SHE GAN 533

THROAT, SORE, BURNING

• MU TONG/DAN ZHU YE/SHENG DI HUANG/GAN CAO/(DAO CHI SAN): Excess Heart Fire

THROAT, SORE, COUGH

- SANG YE/JU HUA/JIE GENG/BO HE/LIAN QIAO: Common Cold: Wind Heat
- SHE GAN/HUANG QIN

THROAT, SORE, ESOPHAGITIS

- SANG YE (c) 466

THROAT, SORE, HEADACHE

- BO HE: Wind Heat 456

THROAT, SORE, INFLAMED

- PANG DA HAI 724

THROAT, SORE, LOWER BODY COLD

- ROU GUI 616

THROAT, SORE, PAINFUL

- CHUAN BEI MU (c): With Lian Qiao, Shan Zhi Zi, Jin Yin Hua, etc 717

THROAT, SORE, PRODUCTIVE COUGH

- NIU BANG ZI/JIE GENG: Wind Heat
- NIU BANG ZI/JIE GENG/BO HE: Wind Heat

THROAT, SORE, RED, PAINFUL, SWELLING/ULCERATED

- NIU HUANG 755

THROAT, SORE, SWOLLEN

- JIE GENG/GAN CAO: Wind Heat
- JIN YIN HUA/LIAN QIAO/JIE GENG/NIU BANG ZI
- XUAN SHEN/NIU BANG ZI: Wind Heat
- BAI HUA LIAN 511
- BAN LAN GEN 515
- CHAN TUI: Wind Heat 458
- DA QING YE 519
- GUI ZHEN CAO 462
- JING JIE 447
- MA QIAN ZI 842
- REN SHEN YE 769
- SHENG MA 467
- TU NIU XI 537
- WU HUAN ZI 538
- ZI HUA DI DING: Toxic Heat 541

THROAT, SORE, SWOLLEN, ACUTE

- XUAN SHEN 503

THROAT, SORE, SWOLLEN, PAINFUL

- DA QING YE/SHE GAN
- DA QING YE/SHE GAN/SHAN DOU GEN

THROAT, SORES

- SHE XIANG/ZHEN ZHU/XIONG HUANG/NIU HUANG: Extreme Heat

THROAT, SWALLOWING DIFFICULTY

- DAI ZHE SHI/DANG SHEN/DANG GUI

THROAT, SWOLLEN

- DI JIAO 443

THROAT, SWOLLEN, PAINFUL

- BAI FAN 836

THROAT, SWOLLEN, SORE

- JIANG CAN/JIE GENG/GAN CAO/BO HE: Wind Heat
- GAN LAN 484
- LONG DAN CAO: Damp Heat In Gall Bladder 492

THROAT, SWOLLEN, SORE, RED

- NIU BANG ZI: Wind Heat 465

THROAT, SWOLLEN, ULCERATED

- MANG XIAO 545

THROAT, SWOLLEN, ULCERATED, PAINFUL

- NIU HUANG/ZHEN ZHU: Heat

THROAT, SWOLLEN/INFLAMMATION

- MU HU DIE 702

THROAT, SWOLLEN/PAIN

- BING PIAN: Topical 753
- SHE GAN: Fire/Toxic Heat/Hot Phlegm Obstruction ... 533

THROAT, ULCERS

- NIU HUANG 755

THROAT, W/SPUTUM, GURGLIN DURING IRRITABILITY, DELIRIUM, CONVULSIONS

- BAI FAN/YU JIN

THRUSH

- QING DAI 531
- SHU FU 687

TONGUE

- NIU XI/SHI GAO: Pain, Swelling, Ulcers

TONGUE CANCER

- MU ZEI (c) 464

TONGUE, INFLAMMATION OF

- HUANG LIAN 486

TONGUE, NUMB, SWOLLEN

- TU BIE CHONG: Congealed Blood 690

TONGUE, RED FROM FEVER

- SHENG DI HUANG 500

TONGUE, SORES

- SHAN DOU GEN/BAN LAN GEN
- SHENG MA/HUANG LIAN: Heart/Spleen Fire
- DAN ZHU YE 470
- MU TONG 599
- NIU HUANG 755

- SHENG DI HUANG: Heart Fire Flaring 500
- SHENG MA 467

TONGUE, SORES W/SCANTY URINE

- DAN ZHU YE/MU TONG/SHENG DI HUANG: Heat In Heart

TONGUE, THICK, GREASY

- FU LING 594

TONGUE, ULCERS

- HUANG LIAN/XI XIN
- HUANG LIAN/XI XIN/SHI GAO
- PENG SHA/BING PIAN/BAI FAN
- SHENG MA/HUANG LIAN/SHENG DI HUANG/SHI GAO/MU DAN PI: Stomach Heat
- XIONG HUANG/PENG SHA
- ZHU SHA/XIONG HUANG/(or)/BING PIAN/(topical,pwdr)
- ZHU YE/MU TONG/SHENG DI HUANG: Heart Fire Flaring
- HUANG LIAN: Topical 486
- MU TONG (c): 3-9 gm Decoction 599
- ZHU YE 482

TONGUE, ULCERS/ABSCESSES OF

- NIU BANG ZI/LIAN QIAO

TONSILLITIS

- LIAN QIAO/BAN LAN GEN/NIU BANG ZI
- BAI HUA SHE SHE CAO 511
- BAI HUA SHE SHE CAO (c): Yan Ning Infusion (Bai Hua She She Cao, Herba Monochasmae Savatieri, Ya Zhi Cao) 511
- BAI JIANG CAO (c): Distillate, 2 Gr/ml, 2-4 ml, 2-4x/Day, IM Injection, 2-15 Days 512
- BAN BIAN LIAN 586
- BING PIAN 753
- CHUAN XIN LIAN 518
- DA QING YE (c): Use Decoction To Cure, 75% Rate ... 519
- HU ZHANG (c) 497
- JIANG CAN 746
- JIE GENG 711
- JIU BI YING 625
- JU HUA (c): 80% Effective As IM Injection Of Distillate Of Fresh Plant, As Volatile Oil, 4-8 mg/2 ml 463
- LA MEI HUA 680
- MA DOU LING (c) 701
- MAO DONG QING 682
- NIU HUANG (c) 755
- PANG DA HAI 724
- QIAN LI GUANG (c): Very Good, 4.5 g Of Crude Herb 4x/Day 474
- RONG SHU XU 570
- SHAN DOU GEN (c) 532
- SHAN ZHI ZI 476
- SHENG MA (c) 467
- TIAN JI HUANG 536
- YE JU HUA (c): With Pu Gong Ying, Wei Ling Xian, Hai Jin Sha, Bai Mao Gen, Jin Yin Hua 468
- ZAO JIAO CI 716

TONSILLITIS, ACUTE

- BAN LAN GEN/XUAN SHEN/ZHI MU
- DA QING YE/SHE GAN
- DA QING YE/SHE GAN/SHAN DOU GEN
- BA JIAO LIAN 510
- BAI HUA SHE SHE CAO (c) 511
- CHAN SU 837
- CHUAN XIN LIAN (c): Powder/Aqueous Extract, Powder More Effective, *May Add Sodium Bisulfite As Adduct, 92% Effective 518
- DAN SHEN (c) 672
- HUANG LIAN (c): Prompt Effect With Oral Dose/Aerosol 486
- JIN YIN HUA (c): IM Injection 524
- NIU BANG ZI 465
- PANG DA HAI (c): 4-8 Seeds To Make Tea, 30 Minutes Steep, Every 4 Hrs 724
- PENG SHA 844
- PU GONG YING (c): See: Lung Topic, Respiratory Tract Infections (Pu Gong Ying) , *Ju Hua Tang (Pu Gong Ying, Ju Hua, Ban Lan Gen, Mai Dong, Jie Geng, Gan Cao ... 529
- SHE GAN 533
- WEI LING XIAN (c): Fresh Leaves, As Tea 572

TONSILLITIS, ACUTE, CHILDHOOD

- HUANG QIN (c): 50% Decoction, Less Than 1 Yr 6 ml, Greater Than 1 8-10 ml, Increase If Greater Than 5 Yrs, 3x/Day, Body Temperature Normal In 3 Days 489

TONSILLITIS, ACUTE, FEVER OF

- SHUI NIU JIAO (c) 501

TONSILLITIS, CHRONIC

- HUANG LIAN (c): Injection Into Tonsils 486

TONSILLITIS, FEVER

- HAI JIN SHA CAO/DA QING YE

TONSILLITIS, IN CHILDREN

- QING MU XIANG (c): Markedly Reduced Recurrence, With Antibiotics 628

TOOTH EXTRACTION

- CHAN SU (c): Anesthesia In 3 Minutes When Tincture Applied To Gingiva, Periodontal Sac Of Tooth, Good Alternative To Procaine 837
- HAI PIAO XIAO (c): Hemostatic, Powdered With Starch 821
- XI XIN (c): Local Injection, With Uncured Tian Nan Xing 452
- ZI ZHU CAO (c): Stops Bleeding 667

TOOTH EXTRACTION, BLEEDING OF

- QIAN CAO GEN (c): Local Application Of Powder, Stopped 1-2 Minutes 662

TOOTHACHE

- BAI ZHI/SHI GAO/SHENG MA
- DU HUO/FANG FENG/BAI ZHI: Wind Cold
- GAO BEN/XI XIN: Wind Cold Damp
- GU JING CAO/LONG DAN CAO: Liver Fire

- GU SUI BU/XI XIN/(with yin tonifiers): Kidney Yin Deficient w/Floating Yang
- GU SUI BU/SHU DI HUANG/SHAN ZHU YU: Kidney Deficiency
- HUANG LIAN/XI XIN
- HUANG LIAN/XI XIN/SHI GAO
- HUANG LIAN/SHENG MA/SHENG DI HUANG: Stomach Fire
- LU GEN/SHI GAO: Stomach Fire
- SHENG MA/HUANG LIAN: Heart/Spleen Fire
- SHI GAO/SHU DI HUANG: Yin Deficient, Fire Rising
- SHI GAO/ZHI MU/SHENG DI HUANG: Stomach Fire Rising
- XI XIN/BAI ZHI: Wind Cold
- XI XIN/SHI GAO/HUANG QIN: Excess Stomach Heat
- BA JIAO GEN: Wind 510
- BAI HUA SHE SHE CAO (c): Crushed Fresh Acted As Analgesic 511
- BAI ZHI 441
- BAI ZHI (c): w/Bing Pian And Inhaled Through Nostrils 441
- BAN XIA (c): Untreated, 30 g Crushed, Soak In 90 ml 90% Alcohol For 1 Day, Soak Cotton Ball, 95% Effective 710
- BI BA: Topical 608
- BING PIAN: External 753
- BO HE 456
- CHAN SU 837
- DI JIAO 443
- DING XIANG (c): Oil 612
- DU HUO: Wind, Cold, Damp 561
- GAN SONG XIANG 580
- GU JING CAO 461
- GU SUI BU: Kidney Deficient 778
- HAI JIN SHA CAO 522
- HAN SHUI SHI · 471
- KU DING CHA 809
- NIU XI: Yin Deficient With Fire Rising 684
- PANG DA HAI: Wind Heat, Fire 724
- SHU FU 687
- WU GONG 751
- XI XIN (c): Patent, Yatonshui (Toothache Liquid—Xi Xin, Bing Pian, Bi Ba, Gao Liang Jiang) Apply With Cotton Ball 452
- XIONG DAN: Wind 479
- XIONG DAN (c): From Dental Carries, Mix With Borneol, Pig Bile, Topical Application 479
- ZE QI 727
- ZHANG NAO 849

TOOTHACHE, ACUTE

- LU FENG FANG: Warm Gargle 841
- SHI GAO: Stomach Fire 477

TOOTHACHE, FROM CARIES

- HAI TONG PI: Gargle 562

TOOTHACHE, HEADACHE

- XI XIN/SHENG DI HUANG: Wind Heat

TOOTHACHE, REFRACTORY

- CANG ER ZI (c) 559

TOOTHACHE, SEVERE

- XI XIN 452

TOOTHACHE, SWELLING GUMS

- SHI GAO/XI XIN: Stomach Fire Flaring

TOOTHACHE, WORSE AT NIGHT WITH LOWER BODY COLD

- ROU GUI 616

ULCERS, ESPECIALLY THROAT

- SHE XIANG/ZHEN ZHU/XIONG HUANG/NIU HUANG: Extreme Heat

ULCERS, MOUTH

- BING PIAN/PENG SHA/GAN CAO/MANG XIAO/(XUAN MING FEN WITH BING PENG SAN)
- MU TONG/DAN ZHU YE/SHENG DI HUANG/GAN CAO/(DAO CHI SAN): Excess Heart Fire
- NIU XI/SHENG DI HUANG/ZHI MU: Yin Deficiency, Excess Fire
- ZHI MU/XUAN SHEN/SHENG DI HUANG
- DA HUANG (c): Topical 542

ULCERS, MOUTH, THROAT, TONGUE

- PENG SHA/BING PIAN/BAI FAN
- XIONG HUANG/PENG SHA

ULCERS, MOUTH, TONGUE

- NIU BANG ZI/LIAN QIAO

ULCERS, MOUTH/TONGUE

- HUANG LIAN/XI XIN
- HUANG LIAN/XI XIN/SHI GAO

ULCERS, ORAL

- ER CHA/QING DAI/HUANG BAI/BING PIAN: Mouth, Gums
- ZHU SHA/XIONG HUANG/(or)/BING PIAN/(topical,pwdr): Tongue And Mouth
- DA QING YE 519
- FENG MI 548
- HUANG BAI 485
- HUANG LIAN: Tongue/Mouth (Topically) 486
- PU HUANG: Topical 660
- WU ZHU YU: Topical 618
- ZHEN ZHU 740

ULCERS, ORAL, IN CHILDREN

- WU ZHU YU (c): Bilateral Powder K1, Good Response In 1 Day 618

VOCAL CORDS, SWOLLEN

- SHI CHANG PU/JIE GENG/SHI HU

VOCAL CORDS, WEAK

- DANG GUI (c): Solution Of Alum, Dang Gui 795

VOICE LOSS

VOICE, HOARSE

VOICE, HOARSE, SORE THROAT

VOICE, HOARSENESS/SORE THROAT

VOICE, LOSS OF

VOICE, LOW, WEAK

VOICE, WEAK

VOICE, WEAK W/DRY COUGH

End of Topic:
ORAL CAVITY

ORAL RELATED TOPICS

ORCHITIS RELATED TOPICS

ORIFICE, HEART BLOCKED BY PHLEGM

ORTHOSTATIC HYPOTENSION, CAUSES

OSTALGIA

OSTEALGIA

OSTEOARTHRITIS

OSTEOMALACIA

OSTEOMYELITIS

OTITIS MEDIA

OVARIAN RELATED TOPICS

OVEREXERTION

OXYGEN METABOLISM, INCREASED RESISTANCE TO LOW OXYGEN

OXYURIASIS

PAIN IN LIVER

PAIN RELATED TOPICS (SEE SPECIFIC ORGAN/LOCATION, TOO)

PAIN, ABDOMINAL

PAIN, ACCUMULATION OF WORMS

PAIN, EPIGASTRIC

PAIN, FLANK/INTERCOSTAL

PAIN, INTERCOSTAL

PAIN, JOINT/MUSCLES

See: Musculoskeletal/Connective Tissue Pain, Joint/Muscles 274

PAIN, LEGS/ARMS

See: Extremities Pain, Legs/Arms 115

PAIN, LOW BACK, LEGS

See: Musculoskeletal/Connective Tissue Pain, Low Back, Legs 274

PAIN, SWELLING, BRUISING

See: Trauma, Bites, Poisonings Pain, Swelling, Bruising 412

End of Topic:
PAIN,SWELLING,BRUISING

PAIN/ NUMBNESS/ GENERAL DISCOMFORT :

ACHES, BODY

- BAI JIE ZI 708
- XI XIN: Good 452

ACHES, HEAD/BODY

- FU PING: External Heat 460

ACHES, PAINS, DIFFUSE W/HEAT

- GUANG FANG JI 595

ACHES, PAINS, GENERAL

- GUI ZHI 445

ACHING, GENERALIZED

- CANG ZHU/SHI GAO: Warm Febrile Disorders
- CANG ZHU 578
- DI JIAO 443
- FANG FENG 444
- QIANG HUO 449

ANALGESIC

- BAI FU ZI (c): Less Than Aconite 708
- BAI HUA SHE (c) 558
- BAI HUA SHE SHE CAO (c) 511
- BAI SHAO (c) 794
- BAI TOU WENG (c): Alcohol Extract 514
- BAI ZHI (c): Local 441
- BEI SHA SHEN (c): ETOH Extract, Tooth Extraction ... 804
- BI BA (c): Helps With Deficient Blood Pain By Stimulating Blood Flow 608
- BING PIAN (c): Topical 753
- BO HE (c): Local Application 456
- CANG ER ZI (c) 559
- CAO WU (c): 1/5 Of Morphine, Processed Herb Did Not Lose Effect 609
- CHAI HU (c): Moderate, Oral 457
- CHAN SU (c): Topical, Local, 90x Cocaine 837
- CHAN TUI (c) 458

- CHEN XIANG (c): Essential Oil 622
- CHI SHAO YAO (c): Abdominal Pain From Small Intestine Smooth Muscle Spasms 668
- CHOU WU TONG (c) 560
- CHUAN LIAN ZI (c) 623
- DANG GUI: Stomach, Muscles, Joints 795
- DANG GUI (c): Not For Acute, Sprains, Infections, Tumors, But All Others, About 1.7 X Aspirin 795
- DI JIAO (c): Thymol 443
- DING XIANG (c): Toothache 612
- DU HUO (c): Heat 561
- DU ZHONG (c) 775
- FANG FENG (c): Significant, In Enema/Subcutaneous Injection, Oral ETOH Extract 444
- FU ZI (c): Enhanced By Scopolamine, Stronger But Shorter Than Morphine 613
- GAN CAO (c): Weak 763
- GAN SUI (c) 551
- GAO BEN (c) 444
- GAO LIANG JIANG (c): Greater Than Dried Ginger 615
- GUAN ZHONG (c) 521
- GUANG FANG JI (c): Less Than Morphine 595
- GUI BAN (c) 806
- GUI ZHI (c): Raises Cerebral Pain Threshold 445
- HAI FENG TENG (c): Arthritic Pain 562
- HAN FANG JI (c): Reduced At High Doses Or w/Yan Hu Suo, Less Potent Than Yan Hu Suo 596
- HE HUAN PI (c) 731
- HU GU (c): 1 g/kg 563
- HUANG LIAN (c) 486
- JIANG HUANG (c) 678
- JIE GENG (c): Inhibits CNS 711
- JU HE: Stomach, Muscles, Joints 626
- LAI FU ZI (c): As In Osteohyperplasia Pill (Shu Di, Yin Yang Huo, Gu Sui Bu, Rou Cong Rong, LU Ti Cao, Lai Fu Zi, Caulis Spatholobi) 639
- LIAO DIAO ZHU (c): Joint Pain, Abdominal Pain 565
- LING YANG JIAO (c): No Relaxation, Some Effect 747
- LING ZHI CAO (c) 731
- LONG KUI (c) 526
- MA BIAN CAO (c) 682
- MAN JING ZI (c) 464
- MU DAN PI (c): Oral/IP Injection 499
- MU LI (c) 739
- MU TONG (c) 599
- NAO YANG HUA (c): Decoction Has Pronounced Effects 740
- PANG DA HAI (c) 724
- PI PA YE (c): Amygdalin Ingredient 703
- QI YE LIAN (c): 80-90%, Induced Sleep, Too, Lasted 8-12 Hours, Less If Infection Involved—Decocted 2x, Then ETOH Extracted/Precipitated-3-5 Tabs Of 0.3 gm Postprandial 568
- QIANG HUO: Stomach, Muscles, Joints 449
- QIANG HUO (c) 449
- QIN JIAO (c): Synergistic w/Yan Hu Suo, Tian Xian Zi, Cao Wu 569
- ROU GUI (c) 616
- ROU GUI PI (c) 617
- SANG BAI PI (c): Aqueous Extract, 2g/kg=0.5 g/kg Of Aspirin 703

ANALGESIC, DENTAL

ANALGESIC, IN LARGE INTESTINE

ANALGESIC, MILD

ANALGESIC, SPRAINS

ANALGESIC, SYNERGISTIC

ANESTHETIC

ANESTHETIC, HERBAL

ANESTHETIC, LOCAL

ANESTHETIC, LOCAL WHEN INJECTED/ETHOH EXTRACT

ANESTHETIC, SURFACE

ARTHRITIS, WHOLE BODY PAIN

BI DISORDERS

- MO YAO: Blood Stasis 683
- SHE XIANG: Topical 756
- WU GONG 751
- XU DUAN 789
- YIN YANG HUO 791

BI DISORDERS, DAMP TYPE

- DA DOU HUANG JUAN/HUA SHI/TONG CAO
- TIAN MA/QUAN XIE/RU XIANG

BI FROM DEFICIENCY LV/KI

- WU JIA PI/SANG JI SHENG/NIU XI/XU DUAN: Prolonged Illness

BI OBSTRUCTIONS

- QUAN XIE/DANG GUI/CHUAN XIONG/BAI ZHI: General Application

BI PAIN

- QIN PI: Hot, Primarily 493

BI PAIN, WIND COLD DAMP

- HAI FENG TENG 562

BI PAIN, WIND DAMP

- LUO SHI TENG 566

BI W/YANG DEFICIENCY

- GUI ZHI/FU ZI: Arthritis, Pain: Joints, Limbs, Shoulders, Back: Bi

BI, BLOOD

- WU ZHU YU: Numbness, Pain 618

BI, CHEST

- HONG HUA: Blood Stasis 675

BI, CHEST W/LUNG SYMPTOMS, ANGINA

- XIE BAI 634

BI, CHRONIC W/KIDNEY DEFICIENCY

- BA JI TIAN/DU ZHONG/NIU XI/XU DUAN

BI, COLD

- XI XIN/MA HUANG/FU ZI: Wind Damp w/Kidney Deficient, Deep Pulse
- CAO WU 609

BI, COLD IN ORGANS

- FU ZI 613

BI, COLD, DAMP

- BAI ZHU/CANG ZHU
- BEI XIE/GUI ZHI/FU ZI
- DU ZHONG/GUI ZHI/DU HUO/QIN JIAO: Back Pain w/Coldness, Swollen Feeling
- FU ZI/GUI ZHI
- FU ZI/GUI ZHI/BAI ZHU/(GAN CAO FU ZI TANG)
- HAN FANG JI/GUI ZHI/FU ZI
- RU XIANG/DI LONG/CHUAN WU
- XIAN MAO/XI XIN: Legs, Back

- XIAN MAO 788

BI, COLD, DAMP CHEST

- XIE BAI: Turbid Phlegm 634

BI, COLD, WIND

- SONG ZI: Rheumatoid Arthritis 546

BI, DAMP

- BAI ZHU: Auxillary Herb 760
- MU GUA: Pain 567

BI, DAMP HEAT

- BEI XIE/SANG ZHI/QIN JIAO/YI YI REN
- DI LONG/SANG ZHI/REN DONG TENG/CHI SHAO YAO: Joints, Painful, Red, Swollen
- HAN FANG JI/YI YI REN/HUA SHI/CAN SHA/MU GUA
- BEI XIE: Mild 587

BI, DAMP HEAT, ESPECIALLY IN UPPER BODY

- CAN SHA/HAN FANG JI/YI YI REN/HUA SHI/(XUAN BI TANG)

BI, DAMP NUMBNESS

- YI YI REN 602

BI, HEADACHE, BODY ACHES

- QIANG HUO/CHUAN XIONG

BI, HOT

- LUO SHI TENG/REN DONG TENG: Pain, Spasms In Extremities
- KUAN JIN TENG: Cramping, Stiffness 564

BI, IN MUSCLES

- HUANG QI/GUI ZHI: Deficient Qi, Blood/Wei, Ying Qi Deficient

BI, INITIAL STAGE

- GAO BEN/CANG ZHU: Back, Joint Pain

BI, JOINT PAIN

- BAI XIAN PI: Damp 515

BI, LEGS W/HEAT

- HAN FANG JI 596

BI, LOW BACK/LIMBS

- TIAN MA 750

BI, LOWER EXTREMITIES, PAIN, PARALYSIS

- YIN YANG HUO/SANG JI SHENG

BI, PAIN

- SHU DI HUANG (c) 802

BI, STIFFNESS OF EXTREMITIES

- DI LONG 744

BI, WIND

- CHUAN SHAN JIA: Joint Pain 670
- CHUAN XIONG 671
- DI DAN TOU: Arthralgia 520
- FANG FENG 444
- LU LU TONG: Knees, Low Back 681
- WEI LING XIAN: Entire Body 572

BI, WIND COLD

- JIANG HUANG/GUI ZHI/HUANG QI
- JING JIE/BO HE/FANG FENG/QIANG HUO
- WU SHAO SHE/QIANG HUO/QIN JIAO: Migratory Joint Pain
- HU GU: Joints 563

BI, WIND DAMP

- BAI HUA SHE/QIANG HUO/FANG FENG/QIN JIAO: Joint Pain, Weakness, Stiff
- BEI XIE/WEI LING XIAN
- CAN SHA/DU HUO/NIU XI: Legs, Arms
- CANG ER ZI/WEI LING XIAN/ROU GUI/CANG ZHU/CHUAN XIONG: Joint Pain, Spasms
- CANG ER ZI: Pain, Numbness
- CHOU WU TONG/XI XIAN CAO/GOU TENG/SANG JI SHENG: As Rheumatic Pain, Numbness, Hemiplegia
- CHUAN SHAN JIA/DANG GUI/CHUAN XIONG/QIANG HUO/FANG FENG: Joint Pain
- CHUAN SHAN JIA/CHUAN XIONG/QIANG HUO/DU HUO/FANG FENG
- CHUAN XIONG/DANG GUI: Pain, Numbness, Paralysis
- CHUAN XIONG/QIANG HUO/DU HUO/FANG FENG/SANG ZHI
- DANG GUI/GUI ZHI
- DANG GUI/GUI ZHI/JI XUE TENG/BAI SHAO
- DU HUO/XI XIN/QIN JIAO: Neck, Back, Legs
- FU ZI/BAI ZHU
- GOU JI/GUI ZHI/QIN JIAO/HAI FENG TENG: Lower Back w/Kidney Liver Deficiency
- HAI FENG TENG/GUI ZHI: Pain, Spasms, Joint Stiffness
- HAI FENG TENG/WEI LING XIAN: Pain, Spasm, Numbness
- HAI FENG TENG/HAI TONG PI/QIN JIAO/SANG ZHI: Joint, Painful, Stiff, Trauma, Spasms
- HAI TONG PI/HAN FANG JI/WEI LING XIAN/HAI FENG TENG: Joint Pain, Spasms, Low Back, Knee Pain
- HU GU/MU GUA/NIU XI/DANG GUI/(in wine): Joint Pain, Stiffness
- JIANG HUANG/QIANG HUO/FANG FENG/DANG GUI/(SHU JING TANG): Shoulder
- KUAN JIN TENG/JI XUE TENG: Low Back/Legs/Joint Pain
- LU LU TONG/QIANG HUO/DU HUO/JI XUE TENG: Joints
- LUO SHI TENG/WU JIA PI/CHUAN NIU XI: Rheumatic Pain, Muscle Spasms, Contractions
- MA QIAN ZI/CHUAN WU/WEI LING XIAN: Spasm, Numbness, Weak
- MAN JING ZI/FANG FENG/QIN JIAO/MU GUA
- MU GUA/HAN FANG JI/WEI LING XIAN/DANG GUI: Joint Pain, Numbness Of Limbs
- MU TONG/GUANG FANG JI/CANG ZHU: Joints
- QIAN CAO GEN/JI XUE TENG/HAI FENG TENG

- QIAN NIAN JIAN/HU GU/NIU XI/GOU QI ZI: Cold, Painful Lower Back
- QIANG HUO/DU HUO
- SANG JI SHENG/DU HUO/CHUAN NIU XI/DU ZHONG/GOU JI/(DU HUO JI SHENG TANG): Rheumatic Pain, Soreness In Low Back And Knees
- SANG ZHI/GUANG FANG JI/WEI LING XIAN
- SANG ZHI/HAN FANG JI/MU GUA/LUO SHI TENG: Pain Or Spasms
- SI GUA LUO/WEI LING XIAN: Joints
- SONG JIE/QIANG HUO/DU HUO/SANG ZHI: General Use
- TIAN NAN XING/CANG ZHU
- WEI LING XIAN/QIANG HUO: Upper Extremeties
- WEI LING XIAN/NIU XI: Legs
- WU JIA PI/WEI LING XIAN/DU HUO/SANG ZHI/MU GUA: Rheumatic Pain, Spasms
- XI XIAN CAO/WEI LING XIAN: Sore Bones, Numb In Extremities
- XI XIAN CAO/CHOU WU TONG/(XI TONG WAN): Rheumatic Pain
- YANG JIN HUA/CHUAN XIONG/HAN FANG JI: Arthritis
- CAN SHA 558
- CANG ER ZI 559
- CANG ZHU: w/Fang Feng 578
- CHUAN NIU XI: Low Back 669
- DOU CHI JIANG 612
- GAO BEN: Shoulders, Extremities 444
- GUI ZHEN CAO 462
- HAI TONG PI: Extremities 562
- MA QIAN ZI: Arthritis 842
- MO YAO: Pain 683
- NAO YANG HUA 740
- QIANG HUO: Shoulders, Extremities 449
- REN DONG TENG 531
- RONG SHU XU: Bone Pain 570
- SANG ZHI: Especially Upper Extremities 570
- SONG JIE: Joints Pain, Sore 572
- SONG XIANG 847
- TIAN MA: Pain, Numb Lower Back/Extremities 750
- YANG JIN HUA 714
- YI YI REN: Joint Pain, Chronic Conditions: Aches, Stiff, Spasms 602

BI, WIND DAMP COLD

- CANG ZHU/MU GUA/SANG ZHI/DU HUO: Knees And Weak Legs
- DI LONG/TIAN NAN XING/CHUAN WU/(XIAO HUO LU DAN)
- DOU CHI JIANG/GU SUI BU/JI XUE TENG
- FANG FENG/QIANG HUO/DANG GUI: With Spasms In Limbs
- GAO BEN/FANG FENG/QIANG HUO/WEI LING XIAN/CANG ZHU: Joint And Limb Pain
- HAI TONG PI/KUAN JIN TENG/GUI ZHI/(external wash for 1 month): Muscle Spasm, Joint Pain
- JI XUE TENG/DANG GUI/CHUAN XIONG/MU GUA/SANG JI SHENG: Painful, Sore Joints
- MA HUANG/GUI ZHI
- MA HUANG/FU ZI
- MO YAO/QIANG HUO/HAI FENG TENG/QIN JIAO/DANG GUI/CHUAN XIONG/(JUAN BI TANG): Joints, General

BI, WIND DAMP COLD W/KIDNEY YANG WEAKNESS

BI, WIND DAMP COLD, CHRONIC

BI, WIND DAMP DISEASES

BI, WIND DAMP DISEASES W/LIVER KIDNEY YIN WEAK

BI, WIND DAMP HEAT

BI, WIND DAMP PAIN

BI, WIND DAMP W/BLOOD STASIS

BI, WIND DAMP W/COLD SIGNS

BI, WIND DAMP W/DEFICIENT BLOOD

BI, WIND DAMP W/HEAT SIGNS

BI, WIND DAMP, CHRONIC

BI, WIND DAMP, EXTREMITIES

BI, WIND DAMP, SEVERE

BODY ACHES

BODY ACHES, PAINS, DIFFUSE W/HEAT

BODY PAIN

BODY SORENESS

BODY, GENERAL PAIN

- YI YI REN/MA HUANG/XING REN/GAN CAO: Wind Damp

BODY, HEAVY FEELING

- CHAI HU/QIANG HUO/FANG FENG: Spleen Deficient w/Dampness
- FU LING /ZE XIE/GUI ZHI/BAI ZHU
- GUANG FANG JI/DANG SHEN/GUI ZHI
- TONG CAO/HUA SHI/YI REN: Summer Heat Dampness
- HUA SHI: Qi Level Heat With Dampness 597

BODY, NUMBNESS

- JI XUE TENG 677
- LU LU TONG 681

BODY, NUMBNESS, PAIN

- CANG ER ZI 559

BODY, PAIN ALL OVER

- MU TONG 599

CRAMPS

See: [Location] Pain

FOCAL DISTENTION

See: Abdomen/Gastrointestinal Topics Focal
Distention 30
See: Stomach/Digestive Disorders Focal
Distention 390
See: Chest Focal Distention 80
- GU YA/CHEN PI/SHA REN: Food Stagnation
- MU XIANG/SHA REN: Qi Blockage/Food Stagnation
- BAN MAO: Blood Stasis 837
- BAN XIA 710
- LAI FU ZI 639

HEAD/BODY ACHES

- XI XIN: Very Good 452

HEAVINESS SENSATION

- MAN JING ZI: Wind Damp, Auxillary Herb 464
- QIANG HUO: In Wind Cold Damp 449

NEURALGIA

See: Mental State/Neurological Disorders
Neurological Pain 255
- BING PIAN (c): Topical 753
- BO HE (c): Topically As Menthol 456
- CAO WU (c): Injection 609
- DANG GUI (c): 25% Injection, Into Acu-Points 795

NEURALGIA, OCCIPITAL

- DANG GUI (c) 795

NEURALGIA, SUPRAORBITAL

- BAI ZHI 441

NUMB PAIN

- BAI JIE ZI: External 708

NUMBNESS

- CHUAN XIONG/DANG GUI: Bi, Wind Damp And Stagnant Qi
- FANG FENG/TIAN NAN XING/(Zhen Yu San): Wind, Phlegm Obstructing Channel
- HEI ZHI MA/SANG YE/(SANG MA WAN): Blood/Yin Deficiency
- MA QIAN ZI/CHUAN WU/WEI LING XIAN: Wind Damp Bi
- YE JIAO TENG/DANG GUI/JI XUE TENG/DAN SHEN: Deficient Blood
- HEI ZHI MA: Blood Def/Yin Deficient 808
- HUANG QI: 30-60 gm 765
- MAN JING ZI: Wind Damp, Auxillary Herb 464
- SANG JI SHENG: Liver Kidney Yin Weak 813
- XIAN MAO 788
- YE JIAO TENG: Blood Deficient 733
- YI YI REN: Damp Bi 602

NUMBNESS W/SPASMS, CONTRACTURES

- BAI SHAO: Blood Deficiency Bi 794
- DANG GUI: Blood Deficiency Bi 795
- DU ZHONG: Blood Deficiency Bi 775
- GAN CAO: Blood Deficiency Bi 763
- JI XUE TENG: Blood Deficiency Bi 677
- MU GUA: Blood Deficiency Bi 567
- SANG JI SHENG: Blood Deficiency Bi 813
- WU JIA PI: Blood Deficiency Bi 574
- YE JIAO TENG: Blood Deficiency Bi 733

NUMBNESS, BODY

- LU LU TONG 681

NUMBNESS, EXTREMITIES

- CHOU WU TONG/XI XIAN CAO/GOU TENG/SANG JI SHENG: Wind Damp Bi
- HAI FENG TENG/WEI LING XIAN: Wind Damp Bi
- MU GUA/HAN FANG JI/WEI LING XIAN/DANG GUI
- TIAN MA/DANG GUI/NIU XI: Blood Deficient In Channels
- XI XIAN CAO/WEI LING XIAN: Wind Damp
- YIN YANG HUO/SANG JI SHENG
- BAI FU ZI 708
- BAI HUA SHE 558
- CHUAN WU 611
- DU HUO 561
- TIAN MA: Wind Stroke/Wind Damp Bi, Stroke, Hypertension 750
- XI XIAN CAO 575

NUMBNESS, LEGS

- HUANG QI/DANG GUI: Qi Blood Deficient

NUMBNESS, LEGS, ARMS, BODY

- JI XUE TENG 677

NUMBNESS, LOINS, LEGS

- WU JIA PI 574

NUMBNESS, PAIN

- CHI SHAO YAO: Blood Stasis 668

PAINFUL URINARY DYSFUNCTION

See: `Urinary Bladder` Painful Urinary Dysfunction
.... 422

PALLOR

See: `Head/Neck` Pallor 150

PALPITATIONS

See: `Heart` Palpitations 157

PANCREAS

See: `Abdomen/Gastrointestinal Topics`
Pancreas 36

PANCREATITIS

See: `Abdomen/Gastrointestinal Topics`
Pancreatitis 36

PAPILLOMAS

See: `Skin` Papillomas 363

PAPULES

See: `Skin` Papules 363

PARALYSIS RELATED TOPICS

See: `Mental State/Neurological Disorders`
Paralysis Related Topics 255

PARALYSIS, INFANTILE

See: `Childhood Disorders` Paralysis, Infantile ... 83

PARAMYOTONIA CONGENITA

See: `Musculoskeletal/Connective Tissue`
Paramyotonia Congenita 274

PARANOIA

See: `Mental State/Neurological Disorders`
Paranoia 255

PARAPLEGIA

See: `Mental State/Neurological Disorders`
Paraplegia 255

End of Topic:
PARAPLEGIA

PARASITES :

AMOEBIC DYSENTERY

• BAI TOU WENG 514

AMOEBIC, ANTI-

• CHANG SHAN (c): Stronger Than Emetine 518
• DA SUAN (c): Strong (Purple Skin Garlic Best) 644
• GUANG FANG JI (c) 595
• HAN FANG JI (c): Stronger Than Berberine 596
• YA DAN ZI (c): Aqueous Extract, Killed On Contact, 1/5
To 1/10 Of Emetine 538

ANCYLOSTOMIASIS

• KU LIAN GEN PI 646
• LEI WAN 647
• LEI WAN (c) 647

ANTIHELMINTIC

• BIAN XU (c) 588
• CHUAN LIAN ZI (c): Kills Various Worms—Earthworms,
Leeches, Ascaris 623
• HOU PO (c): Ascaris 581

ANTIPARASITIC

See: `Parasites` Parasites 305
• A WEI (c) 637
• BAI BU (c): Stronger Than DDT For Lice 699
• BAI FAN (c): Candida Albicans, Trichomonas 836
• BAI TOU WENG (c): Endamoiba Histol. (High Doses) ,
Trichomonas Vaginitis (5% Oral) 514
• BEI XIE (c): Intestinal 587
• CHUAN LIAN ZI (c): Pork Tapeworm, Earthworm, Leech
.... 623
• CHUN PI (c): Trichomonas Vaginalis 483
• DA HUANG (c) 542
• DA SUAN (c): Amoeba: Strong (Purple Skin Garlic Best)
.... 644
• DING XIANG (c): Round Worms (Oil Better) 612
• GUAN ZHONG (c): Roundworms, Flukes, Tapeworm
.... 521
• HAI ZAO (c): Schistosoma 721
• HAN FANG JI (c): Weak 596
• JI GUAN HUA (c): Trichomonas-Very Effective, Extract
Completely Eliminates 10-15 Mins 822
• LIAN QIAO (c): Weak 525
• NAN GUA ZI (c): Intestinal Parasites 648
• QIAN NIU ZI (c): Weak 553
• QING FEN (c) 845
• QU MAI (c): Inhibits Schistosomiasis 600
• SHI LIU PI (c): Strong, Hookworm 828
• WU ZHU YU (c): Ascarisis, Liver Flukes, Tapeworms,
Decoction/Alcohol Extract 618
• XIONG HUANG (c): Ascaris, Blood Fluke, Schistosome
.... 848
• YA DAN ZI (c): Inhibits Amoeba, Malaria, Tapeworm,
Pinworm, Round Worms 538
• ZHU SHA (c): Topical 741

ASCARIASIS

• BAI BU 699
• BING LANG 643
• BING LANG (c) 643
• BO HE (c): Oil Is Effective 456
• GUAN ZHONG (c) 521
• LEI WAN 647
• LEI WAN (c): ETOH Extract Active, Not Aqueous
Extract 647
• LU HUI 544
• NAN GUA ZI 648
• QIAN NIU ZI 553
• SHE CHUANG ZI (c) 847

- SHI JUN ZI (c): The Best 8 Herbs Are: This Herb, He Shi, Wu Yi, Bing Lang, Guang Zhong, Chuan Lian Zi, Lei Wan, Wu Zhu Yu, *Best Chewed, Not As Effective As Decoction, 1 Large Dose Better Than Several Smaller Doses, Fresh Herb Better, Dose-1 g/Year Of Age With 16 g As Maximum, Best To Combine With Bing Lang To Increase Effectiveness, Reduce Side Effects 648
- WU ZHU YU (c): ETOH Extract 618
- XIONG HUANG 848
- YI YI REN (c): 1: 1 Fluid Extract, 50 ml In 1 Or 3 Doses Preprandial 602

ASCARIASIS, ABDOMINAL PAIN

- KU LIAN GEN PI 646
- XIONG DAN 479

ASCARIASIS, BILIARY

- HONG TENG (c) 497
- WU MEI (c): Decoction, Pill, etc 830
- YIN CHEN (c): Oral Decoction, Plus Acupuncture Analgesia Of PC6, Neiguan, "Other Measures", Cure In 4 Days, Pain Gone In 1.5 Days, Much Shorter Than Western Drugs 603

ASCARIASIS, IN BILE DUCT

- BA DOU (c): 100 mg Caps/3-4 Hrs Until Purgation, Colic Is Then Reduced, Do Not Exceed 400 mg/24 Hrs 550

ASCARIASIS, SWINE

- LONG DAN CAO (c): Decoction Paralyzing, Lethal To 492

ASCARIASIS, VOMITING

- WU MEI 830

ASCARIASIS, W/CHOLECYSTITIS

- HUANG QIN (c): IV Infusion 489

ASCITES W/WORMS

- QIAN NIU ZI 553

ASCITES, FROM SCHISTOSOMIASIS

- JING DA JI (c) 552

BRAIN, CYSTICERCOSIS

- CHUAN SHAN JIA 670
- LEI WAN 647
- SHE TUI (c): Long Term, Some Symptoms Releaved .. 571
- XIONG HUANG 848

BRAIN, TAPEWORM LARVAE

- SHE TUI (c) 571

CESTODIASIS

- NAN GUA ZI 648

CYSTICERCOSIS OF THE BRAIN

- SHE TUI (c): Long Term, Some Symptoms Releaved .. 571

ENTEROBIASIS

- BAI BU: (Pinworm Infestation) 699
- SHI JUN ZI: (Pinworm Infestation) 648

FASCIOLOPSIASIS

- BING LANG/WU MEI/GAN CAO
- BING LANG 643

FILARIASIS

- NUO DAO GEN 825
- WEI LING XIAN (c) 572
- XIANG FU (c): Fresh Herb 30-60 g In 2 Doses, One In AM, 1 In PM, Symptoms Controlled 633
- YUAN HUA (c) 556

FLAT WORMS

- QIAN NIU ZI (c) 553

FLEAS

- BAI BU: Topical (Tincture/Decoction) 699

FLUKES

- QIAN NIU ZI (c) 553

FLUKES, BLOOD

- BING LANG 643
- QU MAI (c): Kills 600

FLUKES, LIVER

- WU ZHU YU (c) 618

GIARDIA

- CHANG SHAN (c): Decoction, 3-9 g/Day In 2-3 Doses For 7 Days 518

HOOKWORMS

- DA SUAN/BING LANG/HE SHI/KU LIAN GEN PI: Dislodge, Expel
- FEI ZI/BAI BU: Dislodge, Expel
- FEI ZI/GUAN ZHONG/BING LANG/(GROUND WITH HONEY IN BALL,BEST)
- HE SHI/BING LANG/SHI JUN ZI/KU LIAN GEN PI: Dislodge, Expel
- KU LIAN GEN PI/BING LANG
- LEI WAN/BING LANG/MU XIANG/KU LIAN GEN PI
- BAI BU 699
- BAI BU (c) 699
- BIAN XU 588
- BING LANG 643
- BING LANG (c) 643
- DA SUAN 644
- DONG BEI GUAN ZHONG 645
- FEI ZI 645
- FEI ZI (c): 1 Month, 100-150 Gms, Toasted, No Side Effects 645
- GUAN ZHONG 521
- HE SHI (c): 15 Days, Concentrated Decoctions 646
- KU LIAN GEN PI 646
- LEI WAN 647
- LEI WAN (c): Powder In Glucose Solution, 40-60 g In 1-3 Doses, Inconsistent Results, Though 647
- LU LU TONG (c): Tincture Prevents From Penetration Of Skin 681
- MA CHI XIAN (c): Decoction 528

PINWORMS, ABDOMINAL PAIN

PINWORMS, IN CHILDREN

ROUNDWORMS

ROUNDWORMS, ABDOMINAL PAIN

ROUNDWORMS, CHRONIC W/JAUNDICE, EMACIATION IN CHILDREN

ROUNDWORMS, GENERALIZED INFECTION OF BODY

ROUNDWORMS, IN BILE DUCT

ROUNDWORMS, IN BILIARY TRACT

ROUNDWORMS, IN CHILDREN

ROUNDWORMS, IN CHILDREN, CHRONIC

ROUNDWORMS, PAIN

ROUNDWORMS, VOMIT, PAIN

SCHISTOSOMA

SCHISTOSOMA, ANTI-

SCHISTOSOMIASIS

VOMITING, FROM ROUNDWORMS

• CHUAN JIAO/WU MEI/GAN JIANG/HUANG LIAN/(WU MEI WAN)

WHIPWORMS

• YA DAN ZI (c) 538

WORM POISONING

• YU XING CAO 539

WORMS

• A WEI 637
• BAI TOU WENG (c) 514
• BIAN XU: Kills 588
• BIAN XU (c) 588
• HE HUAN PI (c) 731
• NAN GUA ZI (c) 648

WORMS, ABDOMINAL PAIN

• FEI ZI 645
• HE SHI 646

WORMS, ASCARIASIS

• SHI CHANG PU (c): Kills And Paralyzes 70% In Culture 757

WORMS, CHILDHOOD, CHRONIC

• WU YI/BING LANG/SHI JUN ZI

WORMS, CHILDHOOD, CHRONIC W/DIARRHEA

• WU YI/IIE ZI/ROU DOU KOU

WORMS, FASCIOLOPSIASIS

• BING LANG (c): Decoction 40-50 g, 95% Cured After 3 Treatments, May Add Chillis, Bephenium 643
• BING LANG 643

WORMS, FILARIASIS

• LEI WAN (c): 30 g For 7 Days 647
• NAN GUA ZI (c): 60 g Seeds With 30 g Decoction Of Bing Lang, Mixed In Emulsion, Take On Empty Stomach 648
• WEI LING XIAN (c): Fresh Herb, 500 g, Decoct For 30 Min, Then Boil Liquid With White Wine, 60 g, Brown Sugar 500 g For Short Time, Divide To Take 2x/Day, 5 Days, 75-100% Worm Free 572

WORMS, HELPS TO DRAIN DEAD ONES OUT

• BING LANG 643

WORMS, INTESTINAL ACCUMULATION W/PAIN

• CHUAN LIAN ZI/BING LANG/LEI WAN
• DONG BEI GUAN ZHONG/SHI JUN ZI/KU LIAN GEN PI/BING LANG/HE SHI
• SHI LIU PI/SHI JUN ZI/BING LANG
• XIONG HUANG/BING LANG/QIAN NIU ZI

WORMS, INTESTINAL WITH ABDOMINAL PAIN

• DONG BEI GUAN ZHONG 645

WORMS, TRICHURIASIS

• BING LANG (c) 643

WORMS, W/ASCITES, KILLS

• QIAN NIU ZI 553

End of Topic:
PARASITES

PARASITES AND RELATED TOPICS

See: Parasites Parasites And Related Topics 305

PARASYMPATHETIC STIMULANT

See: Mental State/Neurological Disorders Parasympathetic Stimulant 256

PARASYMPATHOMIMETIC, MILD

See: Mental State/Neurological Disorders Parasympathomimetic, Mild 256

PARKINSON'S DISEASE

See: Mental State/Neurological Disorders Parkinson's Disease 256

PAROTITIS

See: Infectious Diseases Parotitis 192

PEDIATRIC MEDICINE

See: Childhood Disorders Pediatric Medicine ... 83

PEDIATRICS, FOR FEAR

See: Childhood Disorders Pediatrics, For Fear .. 83

PELVIC INFECTIONS

See: Sexuality, Female: Gynecological Pelvic Infections 335

PEMPHIGUS

See: Skin Pemphigus 363

PENILE PAIN

See: Sexuality, Male: Urological Topics Penile Pain 345

PENIS RELATED TOPICS

See: Sexuality, Male: Urological Topics Penis Related Topics 345

PEPTIC ULCER, BLEEDING

See: Stomach/Digestive Disorders Peptic Ulcer, Bleeding 395

PERDONTAL DISEASE

See: Oral Cavity Perdontal Disease 287

PERICARDIUM TOPICS

See: Heart Pericardium Topics 158

PHLEGM :

CONGESTED PHLEGM

DAMP PHLEGM

DAMP PHLEGM COUGH, WHEEZING

• LAI FU ZI/BAN XIA

DAMP PHLEGM OBSTRUCTION

• CHEN PI/BAN XIA/FU LING /(ER CHEN TANG): Chest Constriction, Cough
• CHEN PI/BAN XIA/FU LING /HOU PO: Chest Constriction, Cough

DIZZINESS

See Also: Dizziness (Topics: Gynecology, Ears, Blood, Eyes, Mental State, Liver)

DIZZINESS, FROM FLUID/PHLEGM

• ZE XIE/FU LING /ZHU LING/BAI ZHU/(WU LING SAN)

HOT PHLEGM

OBSTRUCTION BY PHLEGM, QI

• KUAN DONG HUA/BAI QIAN: Cough
• ZI SU ZI/BAI QIAN: Cough, Wheezing

PHLEGM

PHLEGM ACCUMULATION

PHLEGM BLOCKAGE

PHLEGM BLOCKING HEART ORIFICE

PHLEGM COLLAPSE

PHLEGM COLLAPSE W/COMA

PHLEGM CONGESTION

PHLEGM COVERING THE HEART ORIFICES

• YUAN ZHI/YU JIN/SHI CHANG PU: Mental Disorientation

PHLEGM COVERING THE ORIFICES

• YUAN ZHI/QUAN XIE/TIAN MA: Siezures

PHLEGM DAMP

• TIAN MA/BAN XIA/BAI ZHU: Dizziness, Vertigo
• TIAN NAN XING/BAN XIA/CHEN PI/ZHI SHI/(DAO TAN TANG): Cough, Stifling Sensation In Chest
• QING PI: Intermittent Fever, Chills/Breast Abscess ... 629

PHLEGM DAMP COUGH FROM SPLEEN DEFICIENCY

• BAN XIA/CHEN PI/FU LING /(ER CHEN TANG)

PHLEGM DAMP SYNDROME

• BAI ZHU/GUI ZHI/FU LING /(LING GUI ZHU GAN TANG): Palpitation, Asthma, Cough w/Excess Sputum, Stifling Sensation In Chest

PHLEGM DISORDERS

PHLEGM FIRE

- XIA KU CAO 478

PHLEGM FIRE ACCUMULATION

- XIA KU CAO/MU LI/XUAN SHEN/KUN BU: Scrofula, Lipoma, Goiter, etc

PHLEGM FIRE IN LUNG

- HAI FU SHI 720

PHLEGM FIRE, SCROFULA W/PAIN

- ZHE BEI MU/XUAN SHEN/MU LI/XIA KU CAO

PHLEGM FLUID

- BAI ZHU 760
- GAN SUI 551
- QIAN NIU ZI 553
- SHAN ZHA 641
- SHENG JIANG 450
- WEI LING XIAN 572
- XI XIN 452
- ZE XIE 605

PHLEGM FLUID ACCUMULATION

- HONG DA JI 551

PHLEGM FLUID RETENTION

- FU LING /BAI ZHU/GUI ZHI/(LING GUI ZHU GAN TANG): w/Cough, Dizziness, Palpitations
- PI PA YE 703
- XU SUI ZI 556

PHLEGM FLUID SYNDROME

- BAI ZHU/DA FU PI/FU LING : Spleen Stomach Dysfunction w/Internal Dampness

PHLEGM FLUID W/MASS SENSATION

- CAO GUO 580

PHLEGM HEAT

See: Heat   Heat Phlegm 162
- BAI BU/CHUAN BEI MU: Cough, Chest Pain
- BAN XIA/XIA KU CAO: Insomnia
- JIANG CAN/NIU HUANG/HUANG LIAN/DAN NAN XING: Seizure, Convlsion
- PENG SHA/GUA LOU/ZHE BEI MU: Cough w/Difficult Expectoration
- HAI GE KE 721
- HOU ZAO 722

PHLEGM HEAT IN PERICARDIUM

- SHI CHANG PU 757

PHLEGM HEAT OBSTRUCT INTERIOR

- BAN XIA/GUA LOU: Cough, Vomit, Chest Distention

PHLEGM HEAT OBSTRUCTION

- HOU ZAO/LING YANG JIAO: Convulsions, Fever, Wheezing

PHLEGM HEAT SPASMS/CONVULSIONS

- TIAN ZHU HUANG 726

PHLEGM MASKING

- BING PIAN 753

PHLEGM NODULES

- JIANG CAN/XIA KU CAO/(chuan or zhi bei mu)/MU LI
- WA LENG ZI/HAI ZAO/KUN BU
- XUAN SHEN/MU LI/ZHE BEI MU
- XUAN SHEN/MU LI/ZHE BEI MU/XIA KU CAO/ZI CAO
- JIANG CAN 746
- TIAN NAN XING 712
- ZAO JIAO 715

PHLEGM NODULES, SUBCUTANEOUS

- PU GONG YING/XIA KU CAO

PHLEGM OBSTRUCTION

- KUAN DONG HUA/XING REN: Cough, Wheezing
- XIONG HUANG/YU JIN: In Childhood Convulsions
- ZI SU ZI/ZHE BEI MU: Cough, Wheezing w/Thick Sputum
- BING PIAN 753
- HOU PO HUA 580
- SHE GAN 533
- SHE XIANG 756
- ZAO JIAO 715

PHLEGM RETENTION

- QIAN NIU ZI 553
- SHENG JIANG 450

PHLEGM STAGNATION

- FO SHOU 624

PHLEGM STAGNATION, ACCUMULATION IN CHEST

- MANG XIAO 545

PHLEGM SURGING

- WU YAO 632

PHLEGM, BLOODY

- ZI WAN 706

PHLEGM, CHEST OBSTRUCTION

- REN SHEN LU 835

PHLEGM, COLD

- YUAN ZHI/CHUAN BEI MU/BAN XIA: Cough, Wheezing
- HU JIAO 615

PHLEGM, COLD OBSTRUCTING CHEST, FLANKS

- BAI JIE ZI/ZI SU ZI/LAI FU ZI/(SAN ZI YANG QING TANG): Cough w/Clear Copious Sputum

PHLEGM, DAMP

- BAN XIA/ZHE BEI MU: Cough

SPUTUM, EXCESSIVE

SPUTUM, PROFUSE

SPUTUM, THICK, BLOOD STAINED

SPUTUM, THICK, DIFFICULT TO EXPECTORATE

SPUTUM, THIN, WATERY WHITE

SPUTUM, VISCOUS

SWELLING, PHLEGM NODULES

VERTIGO

VERTIGO, FROM FLUID/PHLEGM RETENTION

• ZE XIE/FU LING /ZHU LING/BAI ZHU/(WU LING SAN)

End of Topic:
PHLEGM

PHLEGM FIRE IN LUNG

PHLEGM RELATED TOPICS

PHLEGM, CHEST OBSTRUCTION

PHOTOPHOBIA

PHOTOSENSITIZING

PHYSICAL DEBILITY

PIMPLES

PINWORMS

PITUITARY GLAND RELATED TOPICS

PITYRIASIS ROSEA

PLACENTA RELATED TOPICS

PLANTAR WARTS

PLEURISY

PLEURITIS

PLUM SEED QI

PMS

PNEUMONIA

PNEUMONIAS, VARIOUS, IN CHILDREN

PNEUMOSILICOSIS

POISONING RELATED TOPICS

POLIOMYELITIS

POLYPS, VARIOUS

POLYURIA

POST FEBRILE DISEASE

POST ILLNESS, RECOVERY

POST OPERATIVE TOPICS

POSTNATAL QI DEFICIENCY

POSTPARTUM INSUFFICIENT LACTATION

See: Sexuality, Female: Gynecological
Lactation, Insufficient 327

POSTPARTUM RELATED TOPICS

See: Sexuality, Female: Gynecological
Postpartum Related Topics 335

PREGNANCY RELATED TOPICS

See: Sexuality, Female: Gynecological
Pregnancy Related Topics 337

PREMATURE EJACULATION

See: Sexuality, Male: Urological Topics
Premature Ejaculation 345

PREMENSTRUAL TENSION

See: Sexuality, Female: Gynecological
Premenstrual Tension 338

PREMIERE FIRE, PURGES

See: Kidneys Premiere Fire, Purges 201

PROLAPSE

See: Sexuality, Male: Urological Topics
Prolapse 345

PROLAPSE OF UTERUS

See: Sexuality, Female: Gynecological Prolapse
Of Uterus 338

PROLAPSE, ANAL

See: Bowel Related Disorders Prolapse, Anal ... 64

PROLAPSE, RECTAL

See: Bowel Related Disorders Prolapse, Rectal . 64

PROSTATIC HYPERTROPHY

See: Sexuality, Male: Urological Topics
Prostatic Hypertrophy 345

PROSTATITIS

See: Sexuality, Male: Urological Topics
Prostatitis 345

PROSTRATION

See: Energetic State Prostration 105

PROTEIN SYNTHESIS, INCREASES

See: Nutritional/Metabolic Disorders/Topics
Protein Synthesis, Increases 282

PROTEIN, INHIBITS EXCRETION

See: Kidneys Protein, Inhibits Excretion 201

PROTEINURIA, REDUCES

See: Urinary Bladder Proteinuria, Reduces 422

PROTHROMBIN, INCREASES, DECREASES CLOT TIME

See: Blood Related Disorders/Topics
Prothrombin, Increases, Decreases Clot Time 50

PRURITUS RELATED TOPICS

See: Skin Pruritus Related Topics 363

PRURITUS, GENITAL

See: Sexuality, Either Sex Pruritus, Genital 319

PRURITUS, VAGINAL

See: Sexuality, Female: Gynecological Pruritus,
Vaginal 338

PSORIASIS

See: Skin Psoriasis 364

PSYCHOLOGICAL DISORDERS

See: Mental State/Neurological Disorders
Psychological Disorders 256

PSYCHOSIS

See: Mental State/Neurological Disorders
Psychosis 256

PTERYGIUM

See: Eyes Pterygium 122

PULMONARY HEART DISEASE

See: Heart Pulmonary Heart Disease 158
See: Lungs Pulmonary Heart Disease 235

PULMONARY RELATED TOPICS

See: Lungs Pulmonary Related Topics 235

PULMONARY TUBERCULOSIS

See: Infectious Diseases Pulmonary Tuberculosis
.... 193

PULPITIS

See: Oral Cavity Pulpitis 288

PUPILS, CONSTRICTS

See: Eyes Pupils, Constricts 122

PUPILS, DILATES

See: Eyes Pupils, Dilates 122

PURGATIVE

See: Bowel Related Disorders Purgative 64

PURGES COLD ACCUMULATION, STAGNATION

See: Cold Purges Cold Accumulation, Stagnation .. 91

PURPURA RELATED TOPICS

See: Skin Purpura Related Topics 364

PURPURA, ALLERGENIC

See: Immune System Related Disorders/Topics
Purpura, Allergenic 178

PURPURA, CHILDHOOD

See: Childhood Disorders Purpura, Childhood .. 83

PURULENT DISEASES

See: Infectious Diseases Purulent Diseases 193

PUS

See: Skin Pus 365

PUSTULES, FINGERTIPS

See: Extremities Pustules, Fingertips 115

PYELONEPHRITIS RELATED TOPICS

See: Kidneys Pyelonephritis Related Topics 201

PYEMIA

See: Blood Related Disorders/Topics Pyemia .. 50

PYROGENIC

See: Fevers Pyrogenic 131

QI LEVEL HEAT TOPICS

See: Heat Qi Level Heat Topics 163

End of Topic:
QI LEVEL HEAT TOPICS

QI RELATED DISORDERS/ TOPICS :

ABDOMINAL QI STAGNATION

• LONG GU 738

BLADDER QI OBSTRUCTION

• ZHI MU/HUANG BAI/ROU GUI: Damp Heat In Lower Burner

COLLAPSED QI

• REN SHEN 767

LARGE INTESTINE QI STAGNATION

• YU LI REN 549

PLUM SEED QI

See: Oral Cavity Globus Hystericus 284
• BAN XIA 710
• LA MEI HUA 680

POSTNATAL QI DEFICIENCY

• HUANG QI/FANG FENG/BAI ZHU

QI ACCUMULATION

• ZI WAN 706

QI COLLAPSE

• REN SHEN/FU ZI/(SHEN FU TANG)
• REN SHEN 767

QI DEFICIENCY

• DANG SHEN/HUANG QI: Lung Spleen Deficient
• HUANG QI/REN SHEN: Sweating, Spontaneous
• MU TONG/HUANG QI/DANG GUI: Insufficient Lactation
• TAI ZI SHEN/WU WEI ZI: Insomnia, Debility, Irritability
• YU LI REN/HUO MA REN/XING REN: Chronic Constipation
• DANG SHEN: Sinking Of Central Qi 762
• GAN CAO 763
• HUANG QI: Original Qi 765
• YI TANG: Zhong Qi 772

QI DEFICIENCY BLOOD DETACHMENT

• HUANG QI 765

QI DEFICIENCY FROM CHRONIC DISEASE

• TAI ZI SHEN 770

QI DEFICIENCY W/LIVER QI STAGNATION

• CHAI HU/BAI SHAO/DANG SHEN/BAI ZHU

QI DEFICIENCY, POSTNATAL

• HUANG QI/FANG FENG/BAI ZHU

QI DEFICIENCY, SEVERE

• REN SHEN/FU ZI/(SHEN FU TANG): Collapsing Syndrome

QI DISTENTION

• XIAO HUI XIANG 619

QI FLUSHING UP

• WU YAO 632

QI INSUFFICIENCY

• DA ZAO 761

QI OBSTRUCTION

• BAI DOU KOU/HOU PO: Distension
• DA FU PI 624
• SHI CHANG PU 757
• SU MU 688

QI OBSTRUCTION, DAMPNESS

• BAI DOU KOU/SHA REN: Chest Fullness/Constriction, Diarrhea, Vomit
• CANG ZHU/XIANG FU: Pain In Chest, Stomach, Abdmn

QI STAGNATION

• DONG KUI ZI/SHA REN: Mastalgia, Insufficient Lactation
• E ZHU/QING PI: Chest, Abdomen
• HOU PO/ZHI KE: Distension
• FO SHOU 624
• HU LU BA: Cold 781
• JIANG HUANG 678
• LAI FU ZI 639
• MU XIANG 628

QI STAGNATION, BLOOD STASIS

QI STAGNATION, CONGEALED BLOOD

- DAN SHEN/TAN XIANG/SHA REN/(DAN SHEN YIN): Stomach, Chest, Abdminal Pain

QI STAGNATION, DAMPNESS

- DA FU PI/HOU PO: BM Discomfort, Distension

QI, BLOOD DEFICIENCY

- DANG SHEN/DANG GUI: Dizzy, Weak, Lassitude
- ROU CONG RONG/HUO MA REN/(RUN CHANG WAN): Constipation
- ROU GUI/HUANG QI

QI, BLOOD DEFICIENCY, CHRONIC

QI, BLOOD DEFICIENCY, SEVERE

- HUANG JING/DANG GUI: Jaundice, Muscular Atrophy

QI, BLOOD FLUID INSUFFICIENCY

QI, BLOOD STAGE HEAT

- XI JIAO/SHI GAO: Simultaneous

QI, BLOOD STAGNATION

QI, COLD UP SURGING

QI, CONSTRAINED

- YUAN ZHI/FU SHEN/SUAN ZAO REN: Palpitations w/Anxiety, Mental Disorientation, Insomnia, Irritability

QI, FLUID DEFICIENCY

- WU WEI ZI/REN SHEN/MAI MEN DONG/(SHENG MAI SAN): With Spontaneous Sweating, Thirst, Palpitations, Shortness Of Breath, Weak Pulse

QI, PHLEGM OBSTRUCTION

- ZI SU ZI/BAI QIAN: Cough, Wheezing

QI, REBELLIOUS

- DAI ZHE SHI/BAN XIA/XUAN FU HUA/SHENG JIANG/(XUAN FU BAI ZHE TANG): Vomiting, Hiccup, Belching

QI, YIN DEFICIENCY

- REN SHEN/WU WEI ZI/MAI MEN DONG
- TAI ZI SHEN/BEI SHA SHEN/SHAN YAO: Post Febrile Diseases

QI, YIN EXHAUSTION

- WU WEI ZI/DANG SHEN/MAI MEN DONG: Fluid Loss Febrile Diseases w/Fatigue, Wheezing, Thirst

QI, ZHONG DEFICIENCY

QI/BLOOD BLOCKED

- MO YAO/YAN HU SUO/WU LING ZHI/XIANG FU: Stomach, Abdominal Pain

QI/BLOOD CONGESTION

QI/BLOOD DEFICIENCY

QI/BLOOD INSUFFICIENCY

QI/BLOOD STAGNATION

QI/YIN DEFICIENCY

- REN SHEN/SHU DI HUANG/TIAN MEN DONG: Fever, Thirst, Shortness Of Breath, Restless

REBELLIOUS QI

- See Also: See Related Disorders In Lungs/Stomach Topics
- CHEN XIANG/LAI FU ZI: Wheezing: Lung Qi Def/Kidney Unable To Grasp
- HOU PO/CANG ZHU/FU LING : Stomach
- ZI WAN/KUAN DONG HUA: Cough, Wheezing w/Copious Sputum

REBELLIOUS QI FROM PHLEGM AND HEAT

- BAN XIA/HUANG QIN: Cough, Nausea, Vomit

STAGNANT QI

WEI QI

WEI QI DEFICIENCY

- DONG CHONG XIA CAO/(with meat): Aversion To Cold, Weak Body

WEI QI WEAKNESS

- FU ZI/HUANG QI/GUI ZHI: Spontaneous Sweating

WEI QI, STABILIZES

End of Topic:
QI RELATED DISORDERS/TOPICS

QI RELATED TOPICS

SEXUALITY, EITHER SEX :

ANTIFERTILITY

APHRODISIAC

CONTRACEPTIVE

GENITAL AREA DAMPNESS, PAIN, SWELLING

GENITAL BLEEDING

GENITAL BLEEDING, ABNORMAL

GENITALS, DISEASES OF

GENITALS, ECZEMA

GENITALS, ECZEMA W/ITCHING, WEEPING

GENITALS, PAIN, SWELLING

GENITALS, PRURITUS

GENITALS, PRURITUS, DAMP

GENITALS, PRURITUS, EXTERNAL

GENITALS, PRURITUS, SORES

GENITALS, PRURITUS/ULCERS

GENITALS, UNDERSIZED

HYPOGONADISM

INFERTILITY

INFERTILITY, MEN/WOMEN

ITCHING, GENITAL

PRURITUS, EXTERNAL GENITALIA

PRURITUS, GENITAL

SEX GLANDS, INCREASES WEIGHT OF

SEX HORMONE

SEX HORMONE-LIKE

SEXUAL DRIVE DECREASED

SEXUAL DRIVE, DECREASED

SEXUAL DRIVE, INCREASED ABNORMALLY

SEXUAL EFFECTS

SEXUAL FUNCTION, DECREASED

SEXUAL NERVES, STIMULATES

SEXUAL NEURASTHENIA

SEXUAL RESPONSE, LACKING

STERILITY

ULCERS, PERINEAL REGION

ULCERS/PRURITUS OF EXTERNAL GENITALS

End of Topic:
SEXUALITY, EITHER SEX

SEXUALITY, FEMALE: GYNECOLOGICAL :

ABORTIFACIENT

- QU MAI/DAN SHEN: Blood Stasis
- QU MAI/TAO REN/HONG HUA: Blood Stagnation
- ROU GUI/DANG GUI: Cold Deficient Ren/Chong
- SAN LENG/E ZHU/DANG GUI/HONG HUA/TAO REN: Blood Stagnation
- SHE XIANG/CHI SHAO YAO/DAN SHEN/SAN LENG/E ZHU: Blood Stasis
- SHUI ZHI/TAO REN/SAN LENG/DANG GUI: Blood Stagnation
- SU MU/DANG GUI/CHI SHAO YAO/HONG HUA: Blood Stagnation
- TAO REN/HONG HUA/DANG GUI/CHI SHAO YAO/CHUAN XIONG/(TAO HONG SI WU TANG): Blood Stagnation
- TU BIE CHONG/DA HUANG/TAO REN/(XIA YU XUE TANG): Blood Stasis
- WANG BU LIU XING/DANG GUI/CHUAN XIONG/HONG HUA/YI MU CAO: Blood Stagnation
- YI MU CAO/CHI SHAO YAO/DANG GUI/MU XIANG/CHUAN XIONG/XIANG FU: Blood Stagnation
- YUE JI HUA/DANG GUI/DAN SHEN/(in wine)
- YUE JI HUA/DANG GUI/DAN SHEN/XIANG FU: Liver Qi/Blood Stagnation
- ZE LAN/CHUAN XIONG
- ZE LAN/DANG GUI/DAN SHEN/CHI SHAO YAO: Blood Stagnation

AMENORRHEA, CLOTTING, SCANTY FLOW, PAIN

- TAO REN/HONG HUA: Blood Stagnation

AMENORRHEA, FUNCTIONAL

AMENORRHEA, W/ABDOMINAL PAIN

- CHI SHAO YAO/CHUAN XIONG
- DANG GUI/BAI SHAO/SHU DI HUANG/CHUAN XIONG/(SI WU TANG): Deficient Blood
- GUI ZHI/TAO REN/MU DAN PI/FU LING : Cold, Blood Stasis
- JI XUE TENG/SHU DI HUANG/CHUAN XIONG/DANG GUI: Deficient Blood
- JI XUE TENG: Blood Deficient 677

AMENORRHEA, W/ABDOMINAL PAIN, STRESS, CONSTIPATION

- YUE JI HUA/(brown sugar)

AMENORRHEA, W/CHRONIC MALARIA

• BIE JIA/SAN LENG/E ZHU/MU DAN PI/DA HUANG: Hard Masses In Abdomen, Hypochondriac Pain

AMENORRHEA, W/MASS

• TU BIE CHONG/PU HUANG/WU LING ZHI

AMENORRHEA, W/PAINFUL MASS, DEPRESSION

• E ZHU/DANG GUI/CHI SHAO YAO/CHUAN XIONG

BACK, LOWER, PAIN DURING PREGNANCY

BIRTH

BIRTH, DIFFICULT

BIRTH, INDUCES

BIRTH, PROMOTES

BREASTS, ABSCESS OF

• DAN SHEN/GUA LOU/CHUAN SHAN JIA
• GUA LOU/PU GONG YING/RU XIANG/MO YAO: Initial Stage
• GUA LOU REN/CHUAN SHAN JIA/JIN YIN HUA
• LUO SHI TENG/PU GONG YING
• PU GONG YING/GUA LOU/ZHE BEI MU/MO YAO
• QING PI/CHUAN SHAN JIA/WANG BU LIU XING/JIN YIN HUA/PU GONG YING
• SI GUA LUO/PU GONG YING: Initial Stage
• TIAN HUA FEN/CHUAN SHAN JIA/ZAO JIAO /JIN YIN HUA: Yang Type
• WANG BU LIU XING/CHUAN SHAN JIA/TONG CAO
• WANG BU LIU XING/PU GONG YING
• ZI HUA DI DING/PU GONG YING

BREASTS, CANCER

BREASTS, DISTENTION

• BAI JI LI/CHAI HU/(JU YE-TANGERINE LEAF)/QING PI/XIANG FU: Liver Qi Stagnation
• BAI SHAO/CHAI HU/DANG GUI/(XIAO YAO SAN): Liver Qi Stagnation

BREASTS, DISTENTION FROM CESSATION OF BREAST FEEDING—TREATS PAIN, SWELLING

BREASTS, DISTENTION W/O MILK SECRETION

BREASTS, DISTENTION, PAIN

• DONG KUI ZI/SHA REN/TONG CAO
• MEI GUI HUA/DANG GUI/CHUAN XIONG/BAI SHAO/ZE LAN: Pms: Liver Qi Stagnation, Blood Stagnation
• QING PI/CHAI HU/YU JIN/XIANG FU/(QING JU YE): Liver Qi Stagnation
• XIANG FU/CHAI HU/DANG GUI/CHUAN XIONG: Liver Qi Stagnation

BREASTS, IMMOBILE MASSES

• SHAN CI GU/WANG BU LIU XING/JIN YIN HUA/BING PIAN

BREASTS, INFECTIONS

BREASTS, LACTATION, INSUFFICIENT

• LOU LU/TONG CAO/WANG BU LIU XING

BREASTS, LUMPS, PAINFUL

• XI XIN/DANG GUI/HONG HUA

BREASTS, NIPPLE TUMORS

BREASTS, PAIN

BREASTS, PAIN, PREMENSTRUAL

BREASTS, PAIN, SWELLING

• LOU LU/GUA LOU/ZHE BEI MU/PU GONG YING
• QING PI/XIANG FU/WANG BU LIU XING/DAN SHEN

BREASTS, SORES/SWELLINGS

- JIN YIN HUA 524

BREASTS, SWOLLEN

- WANG BU LIU XING 691
- ZHE BEI MU 728

BREASTS, SWOLLEN, PAINFUL

- GUA LOU/PU GONG YING/RU XIANG/MO YAO
- LOU LU/PU GONG YING/GUA LOU/LIAN QIAO
- SI GUA LUO 688

BREASTS, SWOLLEN, PAINFUL, ABSCESS

- BAI JIANG CAO 512
- BAI ZHI 441
- CHEN PI 621
- CHI SHAO YAO 668
- CHUAN BEI MU 717
- CHUAN LIAN ZI 623
- CHUAN SHAN JIA 670
- DAN SHEN 672
- JIN YIN HUA 524
- LIAN QIAO 525
- MO YAO 683
- MU DAN PI 499
- MU TONG 599
- NIU BANG ZI 465
- PU GONG YING 529
- QING PI 629
- RU XIANG 685
- XUAN SHEN 503
- YE JU HUA 468
- ZAO JIAO CI 716

BREASTS, SWOLLEN, TENDERNESS

- MAI YA/SHEN QU/(toasted,large doses): Post Nursing

BREASTS, TUMORS OF

- WANG BU LIU XING 691

BREASTS, TUMORS, INHIBITS

- DA HUANG (c) 542

CANDIDIASIS, VAGINAL

- HU ZHANG (c) 497
- PENG SHA: Severe 844

CERVICITIS

- BAI HUA SHE SHE CAO (c): 1: 1 Decoction With Pu Yin Gen, Apply Locally To Cervix 511
- DA QING YE (c) 519
- DANG GUI (c): Dang Gui Bai Shao San 795
- HUANG BAI (c): Trichomonas Infections 485
- ZI CAO (c) 504

CERVICITIS, CHRONIC

- QIAN LI GUANG (c) 474
- YE JU HUA (c): Topical 468

- YI MU CAO (c): Xiao Yan Zhi Dai Wan (Yi Mu Cao, Xi Xian Cao, Fried, etc) , 10 Days Treatment, Leucorrhea Became Clear, Scanty, Abdominal Pain Less 694
- YU XING CAO (c): Cotton Impregnated With/Injection Form 539

CERVIX

- NIU XI (c): Dilates, Local Application, Directly Insert Piece Into Cervix 684

CERVIX, CANCINOMA

- BAI HUA SHE SHE CAO (c): Chief Herb 511
- BAN XIA (c): Ban Xia Water Extract Tablet, Plus Pessary In Cervix And Canal, 2 Months 710
- BO HE (c): Infusion Inhibited 456
- CHUAN BEI MU (c) 717
- E ZHU 673
- E ZHU (c): Early Stage (II Or Less) Most Effectively Treated By Local Injection Of 1% Oil/1% Injection With 0.5%Curcumol/Curzerenone Injected Into Mass With Topical Application, Too, Few Toxic Side Effects 673
- KU SHEN (c): Matrine Ingredient 491
- LIAN FANG 659
- LU FENG FANG 841
- SHAN DOU GEN (c) 532
- SHENG MA (c): 90% Inhibition Against, Hot Aqueous Extract, Also Bu Zhong Yi Qi Tang 467
- TIAN NAN XING (c): Oral (15 g, Then Increase To 45 g, Decoction) + Intracervix Application (50 g Pessary Insert Into Cervical Canal, 2ml (10 g Of Herb) 4 ml Injected Into Cervical Area, 1x/1-2 Days, 3-4 Months Course, 78% Effective, With 20% Short Term Cures ... 712
- YA DAN ZI (c): Squamous, Oil Injection With IM Dose 538
- YI YI REN (c): Markedly Inhibited 602
- ZAO XIU (c) 540

CERVIX, CARCINOMA

- WU MEI (c): Inhibits Growth 830

CERVIX, EROSION OF

- CHUAN XIN LIAN (c) 518
- DI YU (c): 2 Pills (Di Yu, Huai Hua, Alum, Long Gu) Inserted Deep Into Vagina In Evening, After 0.1% Potassium Permanganate Solution Cleanse, 1x/2 Days, 4 Applications/Course, Stop For 5 Days Between Courses, Omit Treatment 5 Days Before, After Menstrual Period, Usually 1-3 Courses Needed, About 50% Cured 656
- HU ZHANG (c) 497
- HUANG BAI (c) 485
- HUANG LIAN (c) 486
- JIN YIN HUA (c): Fluid Extract Or Powder Or Herb With Gan Cao, Applied Vaginally With Cotton Balls 524
- LONG KUI (c): Decoction Then Concentrated, Applied With Stringed Cotton Ball, Remove After 24 Hrs, Treat 1-2 X/Week For Minimum 8 Applications 526
- MA QIAN ZI (c): Make Ointment, Local Application, Daily/Alternate Days, 5 Applications 842
- PU GONG YING (c): Solution Of Herb, Ya Zhi Cao/Herb Powder, Zi He Che 529
- SHAN DOU GEN (c): Apply Sterilized, 1-3 Days, 10 Applications, 78% Effective, Foam Spray Of Purified Alkaloids Used, Too, 2x/Week 5 Sprays=Course, Good Effect 532

CERVIX, INFLAMMATION

CERVIX, LYMPH NODE TUBERCULOSIS

CHILDBIRTH, DESCENDS LOCHIA

CHILDBIRTH, DIFFICULT DELIVERY

CHORIONEPITHELIOMA

CLIMACTERIC SYNDROME

CONTRACEPTIVE, IN FEMALE RATS

CONTRACEPTIVE, INHIBITS EGG RELEASE

CRAMPS, DELAYED MENSTRUAL

CRAMPS, MENSTRUAL

DIZZINESS

See Also: Dizziness (Topics: Ears, Phlegm, Blood, Eyes, Mental State, Liver)

DIZZINESS, CHRONIC UTERINE BLEEDING

• DAI ZHE SHI/YU YU LIANG/CHI SHI ZHI/RU XIANG/MO YAO/(ZHEN LING DAN): Blood Deficient

DIZZINESS, POSTPARTUM

DYSMENORRHEA

• BAI SHAO/DANG GUI/SHU DI HUANG: Deficient/Stagnant Blood
• BAI SHAO/DANG GUI/SHU DI HUANG/CHUAN XIONG/(SI WU TANG): Blood Deficiency
• CHI SHAO YAO/XIANG FU: Qi/Blood Blocked
• CHI SHAO YAO/CHUAN XIONG/DANG GUI/TAO REN/HONG HUA: Blood Stagnation
• CHUAN XIONG/DANG GUI: Deficient Blood

• CHUAN XIONG/DANG GUI/CHI SHAO YAO/XIANG FU/YI MU CAO: Blood, Qi Stagnation
• DANG GUI/GUI ZHI: Cold
• DANG GUI/XIANG FU/YAN HU SUO/YI MU CAO
• DOU CHI JIANG/XIANG FU/YI MU CAO/DAN SHEN: Deficient Cold
• E ZHU/DANG GUI/CHI SHAO YAO/CHUAN XIONG: Painful Mass, Depression
• GUI ZHI/WU ZHU YU: Cold Deficient In Chong And Ren
• GUI ZHI/TAO REN: Blood Stasis
• HU LU BA/XIAO HUI XIANG
• HU PO/DANG GUI/E ZHU/WU YAO/(HU PO SAN): Blood Stagnation
• JI XUE TENG/DANG GUI/BAI SHAO/CHUAN XIONG: Blood Deficiency/Stagnation
• JIANG HUANG/ROU GUI: Congealed Blood
• LIU JI NU/DANG GUI/CHI SHAO YAO: Blood Stasis
• LIU JI NU/DANG GUI/YAN HU SUO/CHUAN XIONG: Blood Stagnation
• MO YAO/HONG HUA
• MO YAO/DANG GUI/CHUAN XIONG/XIANG FU: Blood Stagnation
• MU DAN PI/TAO REN/GUI ZHI/CHI SHAO YAO/FU LING /(GUI ZHI FU LING WAN): Blood Stagnation
• NIU XI/HONG HUA/DANG GUI/ROU GUI: Blood Stasis
• NIU XI/TAO REN/HONG HUA/DANG GUI/YAN HU SUO: Blood Stagnation
• PU HUANG/WU LING ZHI/(SHI XIAO SAN): Stagnant Blood, Especially Irregular Menstruation
• ROU GUI/DANG GUI: Cold Deficient Ren/Chong
• ROU GUI/GAN JIANG/WU ZHU YU/DANG GUI/CHUAN XIONG: Cold Stagnation
• RU XIANG/DANG GUI/CHUAN XIONG/XIANG FU: Blood Stagnation
• SHAN ZHA/CHUAN XIONG/DANG GUI: Blood Stagnation
• SHAN ZHI ZI/MU DAN PI: Heat From Deficient Liver Blood
• SHE XIANG/CHI SHAO YAO/DAN SHEN/SAN LENG/E ZHU: Blood Stasis
• SU MU/DANG GUI/CHI SHAO YAO/HONG HUA: Blood Stagnation
• TAO REN/HONG HUA: Blood Stagnation
• TAO REN/HONG HUA/DANG GUI/CHI SHAO YAO/CHUAN XIONG/(TAO HONG SI WU TANG): Blood Stagnation
• WANG BU LIU XING/DANG GUI/CHUAN XIONG/HONG HUA/YI MU CAO: Blood Stagnation
• WU LING ZHI/YAN HU SUO/YI MU CAO: Blood Stasis
• WU YAO/MU XIANG/XIANG FU: Stagnant Qi
• WU YAO/XIANG FU/DANG GUI/CHUAN XIONG: Cold, Qi Stagnation
• XIANG FU/DANG GUI: Qi/Blood Stasis
• XIANG FU/CHAI HU/DANG GUI/CHUAN XIONG: Liver Qi Stagnation
• YAN HU SUO/XIANG FU: Stagnant Qi, Congealed Blood
• YAN HU SUO/ROU GUI
• YI MU CAO/CHI SHAO YAO/DANG GUI/MU XIANG/CHUAN XIONG/XIANG FU: Congealed Blood
• YU JIN/CHAI HU: Liver Qi Congestion, Blood Stasis
• YU JIN/CHAI HU/XIANG FU/BAI SHAO/DANG GUI: Qi/Blood Stagnation
• YUE JI HUA/DANG GUI/DAN SHEN/XIANG FU: Liver Qi/Blood Stagnation

FETUS, ABNORMAL MOVEMENTS

FETUS, DEAD

FETUS, DEAD ABORTION OF

FETUS, DEAD RETENTION

FETUS, MALPOSITION

FETUS, RESTLESS

FETUS, RESTLESS, CALMS

FETUS, RESTLESS, W/ABDOMINAL PAIN/UTERINE BLEEDING

FETUS, RESTLESS, W/CHEST/ABDOMINAL DISTENTION, FULLNESS

FETUS, RESTLESS, W/DIZZINESS, VERTIGO, PALPITATIONS

FETUS, RESTLESS, W/INTERNAL HEAT

FETUS, RESTLESS, W/LUMBAR SORENESS

FETUS, RESTLESS, W/VAGINAL BLEEDING

FETUS, RESTLESS, W/VAGINAL BLEEDING, LOW ABDOMEN PAIN

FETUS, STABILIZES

FRIGIDITY

FUNCTIONAL BLEEDING

GALACTOSTASIS

GENITALS, FEMALE, LEUKOPLAKIA VULVAE

GENITALS, PRURITUS IN WOMEN

GYNECOLOGICAL CONDITIONS, GENERAL

GYNECOLOGICAL INFLAMMATORY DISEASES

GYNECOLOGICAL PROBLEMS FROM BLOOD HEAT

GYNECOLOGICAL PROBLEMS W/BLOOD DEFICIENCY

GYNECOLOGICAL TUMORS

HEADACHE, DYSMENORRHEA

HYDATID MOLE, MALIGNANT

HYPERTENSION, CLIMACTERIC

HYPOGALACTIA

INFERTILITY, FEMALE

INTESTINAL GAS, FROM PANHYSTERECTOMY

LABOR, DIFFICULT

LABOR, INDUCES

LABOR, INDUCES, IN PROLONGED LABOR

LABOR, INDUCES, W/INTRAUTERINE FETAL DEATH

LACTATION

LACTATION, INSUFFICIENT

LACTATION, INCREASES

LACTATION, INHIBITS

LACTATION, INSUFFICIENT

LACTATION, INSUFFICIENT, POSTPARTUM

- LOU LU/WANG BU LIU XING/CHUAN SHAN JIA/TONG CAO

LACTATION, INSUFFICIENT/STOPPED

LACTATION, OBSTRUCTED

- BAI JI LI/CHAI HU/(JU YE-TANGERINE LEAF)/QING PI/XIANG FU: Liver Qi Stagnation
- DONG KUI ZI/SHA REN/TONG CAO

LACTATION, PROMOTES

LACTATION, STAGNATION OF

LEUKOPENIA

LEUKORRHAGIA

- AI YE/DANG GUI/XIANG FU/CHUAN XIONG/WU YAO: Cold, Deficiency In Lower Jiao
- JIN YING ZI/QIAN SHI/TU SI ZI: Kidney Deficient
- LIAN ZI/TU SI ZI/SHAN YAO/QIAN SHI: Kidney Deficiency
- MU LI/LONG GU/SHAN YAO/WU WEI ZI: Chong Ren Deficiency
- TU SI ZI/DU ZHONG/SHAN YAO/GOU JI: Kidney Deficiency
- CHI SHI ZHI 818

LEUKORRHAGIA W/LOWER BACK PAIN

- SHAN YAO/SHAN ZHU YU/TU SI ZI: Deficient Kidneys

LEUKORRHAGIA, THIN, WHITISH

- SHAN YAO/BAI ZHU/FU LING /QIAN SHI: Excess Dampness From Spleen Deficient

LEUKORRHEA

- BAI BIAN DOU/BAI ZHU/SHAN YAO: Spleen Deficient
- BAI GUO/HUANG BAI/QIAN SHI: Damp Heat
- BAI ZHI/HAI PIAO XIAO: Cold Damp

- BAI ZHI/BAI ZHU/HAI PIAO XIAO/FU LING : Damp Cold Type
- BAI ZHI/HUANG BAI/CHE QIAN ZI/KU SHEN: Damp Heat Type
- BEI XIE/SHI CHANG PU/CHE QIAN ZI/HUANG BAI: Dampness
- CHE QIAN ZI/CANG ZHU: Damp Heat And Spleen Deficient
- DI YU/WU MEI: Chronic Damp Heat
- DING XIANG/ROU GUI: Kidney Deficient
- DONG GUA REN/HUANG BAI/BEI XIE: Damp Heat
- HAI GE KE/HUANG BAI
- HAI MA/GOU QI ZI/DA ZAO: Kidney Yang Deficient
- HAI PIAO XIAO/SHAN YAO/BAI ZHI
- HAI PIAO XIAO/SHAN ZHU YU/SHAN YAO/TU SI ZI/MU LI: Kidney Deficient
- HE SHOU WU/GOU QI ZI/BU GU ZHI/TU SI ZI: Liver Kidney Deficiency
- HUANG BAI/CHE QIAN ZI/ZHU YE/MU TONG: Damp Heat Downward Flowing
- JIN YING ZI/QIAN SHI: Kidney Deficient
- JIU CAI ZI/LONG GU/SANG PIAO XIAO: Kidney Yang Deficient
- JIU CAI ZI/BU GU ZHI/SHAN YAO/YI ZHI REN: Kidney Deficiency
- KU SHEN/SHE CHUANG ZI/DAN SHEN: Damp
- KU SHEN/SHE CHUANG ZI/HUANG BAI/LONG DAN CAO: Damp Heat
- LONG GU/GUI ZHI/BAI SHAO: Yang Deficient
- LONG GU/MU LI/SHAN YAO/HAI PIAO XIAO: Kidney Deficiency
- MU LI/LONG GU/E JIAO/CHI SHI ZHI
- QIAN SHI/HUANG BAI/CHE QIAN ZI: Damp Heat And Spleen Deficient
- QIAN SHI/SHAN YAO: Spleen Kidney Deficient
- QIAN SHI/SHA YUAN ZI/JIN YING ZI
- SANG PIAO XIAO/TU SI ZI: Kidney Deficient
- SANG PIAO XIAO/LONG GU/MU LI/TU SI ZI/BU GU ZHI: Kidney Yang Deficient
- SHA YUAN ZI/FU PEN ZI: Liver Kidney Deficiency
- SHA YUAN ZI/LONG GU/MU LI/QIAN SHI: Kidney Deficiency
- SHAN YAO/QIAN SHI: Kidney Deficiency

LEUKORRHEA, BLOOD TINGED

LEUKORRHEA, BLOOD TINGED, CHRONIC

LEUKORRHEA, BLOODY

LEUKORRHEA, CHRONIC W/ITCHING

- BAI FAN/SHE CHUANG ZI/(wash)

LEUKORRHEA, CLEAR

LEUKORRHEA, COLD DAMP

- BAI ZHU/CANG ZHU

LEUKORRHEA, EXCESSIVE

- ER CHA/SHE CHUANG ZI/(external wash)

LEUKORRHEA, FROM DOWNWARD FLOW OF TURBID DAMPNESS

- BAI BIAN DOU/REN SHEN/BAI ZHU/FU LING /(SHEN LING BAI ZHU SAN): Spleen Deficient, Not Metabolizing Water

LEUKORRHEA, ITCHY

- BAI TOU WENG/KU SHEN/(external wash)

LEUKORRHEA, MORBID

LEUKORRHEA, PINK

LEUKORRHEA, PINK/WHITE DISCHARGE

LEUKORRHEA, PINKISH W/WHITE MATTER

LEUKORRHEA, PROFUSE

- ZE XIE/FU LING /ZHU LING/BAI ZHU/(WU LING SAN)
- ZHU LING/FU LING /ZE XIE/(SI LING SAN)
- SHE CHUANG ZI (c): Nontrichomonal, Reduces Leukorrhea Discharge, Alleviates Pruritus 847

LEUKORRHEA, PROFUSE YELLOW

- CANG ZHU (c): Er Miao San (Cang Zhu, Huang Bai) ... 578

LEUKORRHEA, THIN

- LU RONG/SHU DI HUANG: Cold Kidney

LEUKORRHEA, THIN, WHITE

- LU RONG/E JIAO/DANG GUI/SHAN ZHU YU/HAI PIAO XIAO: Chong Ren Channels, Cold And Deficient

LEUKORRHEA, W/PAIN, SWELLING IN GENITALS

- LONG DAN CAO/HUANG BAI/KU SHEN/CHE QIAN ZI: Damp Heat

LEUKORRHEA, WHITE

- LONG GU 738

LEUKORRHEA, WHITE, BLOOD STREAKED

- QIAN CAO GEN/LONG GU

LEUKORRHEA, WHITE, ORDORLESS

- BAI GUO/ROU GUI/HUANG QI/SHAN ZHU YU: Kidney Yang Deficiency

LEUKORRHEA, YELLOW

- CHUN PI/HUANG BAI: Damp Heat
- HUANG BAI/CHE QIAN ZI/SHAN YAO/QIAN SHI/BAI GUO: Damp Heat
- SHAN YAO/HUANG BAI/CHE QIAN ZI/(YI HUANG TANG): Excess Dampness Into Heat

LEUKORRHEA, YELLOW, ODOROUS

- BAI GUO/HUANG BAI/CHE QIAN ZI/(YI HUANG TANG): Downward Flowing Damp Heat

LOCHIA

- SHAN ZHA/DANG GUI/CHUAN XIONG/YI MU CAO: Blood Stagnation
- ROU GUI PI 617
- WU MEI (c): Oral Concentrated Decoction, 3-5 ml, 3x/Day, Not With Blood Stasis 830

LOCHIA, DESCENDS

- QIAN CAO GEN 662

LOCHIA, PROLONGED

- DANG GUI (c): SI Wu Tang 795

LOCHIA, RETENTION

- LIAN FANG 659
- SHAN ZHA 641

- SHE XIANG 756

LOCHIA, RETENTION, PAIN OF

- PU HUANG/(quick fried ginger)
- PU HUANG/WU LING ZHI/(SHI XIAO SAN)

LOCHIOSCHESIS

- DAN SHEN/DANG GUI
- YI MU CAO/PU HUANG
- CHUAN XIONG 671
- DAN SHEN 672
- HONG HUA 675
- NIU XI: Blood Stasis 684
- WU LING ZHI 691

LOCHIOSCHESIS, POSTPARTUM

- HONG HUA/YI MU CAO: Blood Stasis
- WU LING ZHI/PU HUANG: Blood Stasis

MALPOSITION OF FETUS(8 MO)

- CHE QIAN ZI (c) 590

MASTALGIA

See: Sexuality, Female: Gynecological Breasts, Pain 322
See: Sexuality, Female: Gynecological Mastitis 330
- DONG KUI ZI/SHA REN: Qi Stagnation
- DONG KUI ZI/WANG BU LIU XING: Blood Stasis
- QING PI/XIANG FU/WANG BU LIU XING/DAN SHEN
- XI XIN/DANG GUI/HONG HUA
- DONG KUI ZI 594
- LU LU TONG 681

MASTALGIA, W/LACTATION OBSTRUCTED

- DONG KUI ZI/SHA REN/TONG CAO

MASTITIS

See: Sexuality, Female: Gynecological Breasts, Pain 322
See: Sexuality, Female: Gynecological, Mastalgia 330
- CHUAN BEI MU/PU GONG YING/LIAN QIAO
- LOU LU/GUA LOU/ZHE BEI MU/PU GONG YING
- QING PI/GUA LOU/PU GONG YING/JIN YIN HUA/LIAN QIAO
- BAI JI LI 743
- CHUAN BEI MU 717
- CI WEI PI 819
- CONG BAI (c): w/Ban Xia, Ginger Juice Via Enema, 97% Effective 442
- DAN SHEN (c) 672
- DANG GUI (c): Xiao Yao San 795
- DONG KUI ZI 594
- GUA LOU (c): As Adjuvant In Treating, With Pu Gong Ying, Chi Shao, Chuan Shan Jia, Jin Yin Hua, etc 718
- GUA LOU REN 720
- HU ZHANG 497
- HUANG LIAN (c): Topical 20% Vaseline Dressing, 3% Solution With Oral Powder 486
- JU HE 626

MENORRHAGIA W/DEFICIENT BLOOD THIRST, DRYNESS

MENORRHAGIA, INFLAMMATION DURING

MENORRHALGIA

MENSTRUATION, ABNORMAL

MENSTRUATION, CLOTS DURING

MENSTRUATION, CRAMPS OF

MENSTRUATION, DELAYED

MENSTRUATION, DISORDERS OF

MENSTRUATION, EXCESS BLEEDING

MENSTRUATION, EXCESSIVE

MENSTRUATION, FLANK PAIN

MENSTRUATION, FLANK, ABDOMINAL PAIN OF

MENSTRUATION, INHIBITS

MENSTRUATION, IRREGULAR

MOLE, MALIGNANT HYDATIDIFORM

MORNING SICKNESS

OVARIAN INFECTIONS

OVARIAN SURGICAL REMOVAL, POST SYNDROME

OVARIES, OVIDUCT, INFLAMMATION OF

OVULATION, INHIBITS

OVULATION, REDUCES

PELVIC INFECTIONS

PELVIC INFECTIONS, ACUTE

PELVIC INFLAMMATION

PELVIC INFLAMMATORY DISEASE, CHRONIC

PELVIC INFLAMMATORY INFECTION

PERIODS

PLACENTA, FAILING TO EXPELL

PLACENTA, LEAKAGE

PLACENTA, RETENTION

PMS

POSTPARTUM

POSTPARTUM EDEMA

POSTPARTUM, ABDOMINAL CRAMPS

POSTPARTUM, ABDOMINAL PAIN

UTERUS, FIBROSIS

UTERUS, INCOMPLETE INVOLUTION

UTERUS, INCREASES MUSCLE TENSION, RHYTHMIC CONTRACTIONS

UTERUS, INCREASES TONICITY

UTERUS, INCREASES TONICITY, CONTRACTION OF

UTERUS, INHIBITS

UTERUS, INHIBITS CONTRACTION

UTERUS, INHIBITS CONTRACTION, SPASMS

UTERUS, INHIBITS FUNCTION

UTERUS, INHIBITS SECRETION

UTERUS, MUSCLE, STIMULATES

UTERUS, MYOMA

UTERUS, MYOMETRITIS

UTERUS, PAIN

UTERUS, POLYPS

UTERUS, PROLAPSE

UTERUS, RELAXES

UTERUS, SPASMS

UTERUS, STIMULATES

WOMEN'S DISEASES

WOMEN'S DISEASES, BLEEDING

End of Topic:
SEXUALITY, FEMALE: GYNECOLOGICAL

SEXUALITY, MALE: UROLOGICAL TOPICS :

BALANITIS, IN YOUNG CHILDREN

BIRTH CONTROL

CONTRACEPTION, MALE

EJACULATION, PREMATURE

• REN SHEN/LU RONG/ZI HE CHE

EPIDIDYMAL STASIS

GENITALS, SWOLLEN, SORE SCROTUM

HYDROCELE OF TUNICA VAGINALIS

IMPOTENCE

• BA JI TIAN/TU SI ZI/ROU CONG RONG/REN SHEN:
Kidney Yang Deficient
• BU GU ZHI/TU SI ZI/ROU CONG RONG/DU ZHONG:
Kidney Deficiency
• DING XIANG/FU ZI/ROU GUI/BA JI TIAN/YIN YANG HUO:
Kidney Yang Deficiency
• DING XIANG/ROU GUI: Deficient Kidneys
• DONG CHONG XIA CAO/SHAN ZHU YU/SHAN YAO/TU SI
ZI: Kidney Deficiency
• DONG CHONG XIA CAO/DU ZHONG/YIN YANG
HUO/ROU CONG RONG: Deficient Kidney Yang
• DU ZHONG/SHAN ZHU YU/TU SI ZI/WU WEI ZI: Kidney
Deficiency
• FU PEN ZI/TU SI ZI/GOU QI ZI/WU WEI ZI: Kidney
Deficient
• FU ZI/ROU GUI: Kidney Yang Deficiency

• FU ZI/ROU GUI/SHAN ZHU YU/SHU DI HUANG/(GUI FU
BA WEI WAN): Kidney Yang Deficiency
• GE JIE/REN SHEN/(korean)/HU TAO REN/WU WEI ZI:
Kidney Yang Deficient
• GE JIE/REN SHEN/LU RONG/YIN YANG HUO: Kidney
Deficiency
• GOU QI ZI/SHU DI HUANG/TU SI ZI/DU ZHONG: Liver
Kidney Deficient (Yin/Blood Deficiency)
• JIU CAI ZI/ROU CONG RONG/BA JI TIAN: Kidney Yang
Deficient
• LIU HUANG/FU ZI/ROU GUI: Lowered Life Gate Fire
• LU RONG/SHU DI HUANG: Cold Kidney
• LU RONG/REN SHEN/SHU DI HUANG/TU SI ZI: Kidney
Yang Deficiency
• REN SHEN/LU RONG/ZI HE CHE
• ROU CONG RONG/SUO YANG
• ROU CONG RONG/SHAN ZHU YU: Severely Deficient
Kidneys
• ROU CONG RONG/SHU DI HUANG/TU SI ZI/WU WEI
ZI/(ROU CONG RONG WAN): Kidney Deficiency
• ROU CONG RONG/TU SI ZI: Deficient Kidney Yang
• ROU GUI/FU ZI/SHU DI HUANG/SHAN ZHU YU/(GUI FU
BA WEI WAN): Kidney Yang Deficiency
• SHA YUAN ZI/LONG GU/MU LI/QIAN SHI: Kidney
Deficiency
• SHAN ZHU YU/SHU DI HUANG/SHAN YAO/LU RONG/BU
GU ZHI: Deficient Kidney Yang
• SHAN ZHU YU/SHU DI HUANG/TU SI ZI/GOU QI ZI/DU
ZHONG: Liver Kidney Deficiency
• SHE CHUANG ZI/TU SI ZI/WU WEI ZI: Kidney Deficient
• SHU DI HUANG/SHAN ZHU YU/SHAN YAO/(LIU WEI
DIHUNG WAN): Liver Kidney Deficiency
• TU SI ZI/DU ZHONG/SHAN YAO/GOU JI: Kidney
Deficiency
• TU SI ZI/WU WEI ZI/SHE CHUANG ZI/SHA YUAN ZI/NU
ZHEN ZI: Kidney Deficiency
• XIAN MAO/DU ZHONG
• YANG QI SHI/BU GU ZHI/TU SI ZI/LU RONG: Kidney
Yang Deficiency
• YIN YANG HUO/XIAN MAO/SHU DI HUANG: Kidney
Yang Deficiency
• YIN YANG HUO/WU WEI ZI/GOU QI ZI/SHA YUAN ZI:
Deficient Kidneys

ORCHITIS, ACUTE

- SHENG JIANG (c): External Application Of 6-10 Slices Over Testes, Change Daily (Not If Sores!) 450

PENILE PAIN

- BEI XIE 587

PENIS, EDEMA IN PREPUCE, CHILDHOOD

- HUANG BAI (c) 485

PENIS, FIBROTIC CAVERNITIS

- DANG GUI (c): Injection Of 10% Solution 795

PENIS, INFLAMMATION OF PREPUS IN YOUNG CHILDREN

- WEI LING XIAN (c) 572

PENIS, PAIN

- HU PO 737

PREMATURE EJACULATION

- BA JI TIAN/TU SI ZI/ROU CONG RONG/REN SHEN: Kidney Yang Deficient
- BU GU ZHI/HU TAO REN: Kidney Yang Deficient
- JIN YING ZI/LONG GU/MU LI: Deficient Yin
- QIAN SHI/JIN YING ZI: Kidney Qi Deficient
- REN SHEN/LU RONG/ZI HE CHE
- SHA YUAN ZI/FU PEN ZI: Liver Kidney Deficiency
- SHA YUAN ZI/LONG GU/MU LI/QIAN SHI: Kidney Deficiency
- SHAN ZHU YU/SHU DI HUANG/SHAN YAO/LU RONG/BU GU ZHI: Kidney Deficient Yang
- SUO YANG/SANG PIAO XIAO: Kidney Yang Deficient
- TU SI ZI/BU GU ZHI/DU ZHONG: Kidney Deficient
- TU SI ZI/BU GU ZHI/DU ZHONG/LU RONG: Kidney Deficient Yang
- TU SI ZI/BU GU ZHI/DU ZHONG/SHU DI HUANG/SHAN ZHU YU: Kidney Deficient Yin
- TU SI ZI/DU ZHONG/SHAN YAO/GOU JI: Kidney Deficiency
- YANG QI SHI/BU GU ZHI/TU SI ZI/LU RONG: Kidney Yang Deficiency
- BA JI TIAN 773
- BU GU ZHI 773
- FU PEN ZI: Kidney Yang Deficient 820
- HAI PIAO XIAO: Kidney Deficient 821
- QIAN SHI: Kidney Qi Deficient 826
- ROU CONG RONG 786
- SHA YUAN ZI: Kidney Yang Deficient 786
- SUO YANG 787
- TU SI ZI 787

PREMATURE EJACULATION W/SORE/WEAK LOWER BACK/KNEES

- YANG QI SHI 789

PROLAPSE

- SHAN ZHA/XIAO HUI XIANG: Testicular Pain, Swelling

PROSTATIC HYPERTROPHY

- WU MEI (c) 830

PROSTATITIS

- QING MU XIANG (c): Use With Chemotherapy For Better Results 628
- YANG QI SHI 789

SCROTUM, ECZEMA

- WU JIA PI 574

SCROTUM, PAIN

See: **Sexuality, Male: Urological Topics**
Testicles, Pain 347
- QING PI/WU YAO/XIAO HUI XIANG/MU XIANG/(TIAN TAI WU YAO SAN): Cold Liver Stagnation
- XIANG FU/XIAO HUI XIANG/WU YAO: Cold Stagnation In Liver

SCROTUM, PAIN FROM HERNIA

- CHUAN LIAN ZI/XIAO HUI XIANG/WU ZHU YU/MU XIANG/(DAO QI TANG)

SCROTUM, PAIN, SWELLING

- WU YAO/XIAO HUI XIANG/QING PI/(TIAN TAI WU YAO SAN): Cold, Qi Stagnation

SCROTUM, PAIN/SWELLING

- HU PO 737

SCROTUM, PRURITUS

- SHE CHUANG ZI 847

SCROTUM, PRURITUS, DAMP

- LONG GU: Topical 738

SCROTUM, SWELLING, SORE

- LONG DAN CAO 492

SEMEN, INCREASES SECRETION OF

- YIN YANG HUO (c) 791

SEMINAL EMISSIONS

See: **Sexuality, Male: Urological Topics**
Spermatorrhea 346
See: **Sexuality, Male: Urological Topics**
Nocturnal Emissions 344
- DONG CHONG XIA CAO/SHAN ZHU YU/SHAN YAO/TU SI ZI: Kidney Deficiency
- GUI BAN/SHU DI HUANG/(DA BU YIN WAN): Yin Deficiency w/Excess Fire
- HAI PIAO XIAO/SHAN ZHU YU/SHAN YAO/TU SI ZI/MU LI: Kidney Deficient
- JIN YING ZI/QIAN SHI/TU SI ZI: Kidney Deficient
- LIAN ZI/TU SI ZI/SHAN YAO/QIAN SHI: Kidney Deficiency
- LONG GU/MU LI/SHA YUAN ZI/QIAN SHI: Kidney Deficiency
- QIAN SHI/SHA YUAN ZI/JIN YING ZI
- SANG PIAO XIAO/LONG GU/MU LI/TU SI ZI/BU GU ZHI: Kidney Yang Deficient
- SHA YUAN ZI/LONG GU/MU LI/QIAN SHI: Kidney Deficiency

SEMINAL EMISSIONS, IN LUNG TUBERCULOSIS PATIENTS

SEMINAL EMISSIONS, INVOLUTARY

SEMINAL EMISSIONS, NOCTURNAL

SEMINAL EMISSIONS, SPONTANEOUS

SEMINAL FLUID

SEMINAL FLUID INCONTINENCE

SEMINAL FLUID, INCONTINENCE

SEMINAL INCONTINENCE

SEXUAL ACTIVITY, INCREASED

SPERM PRODUCTION INCREASED

SPERM, LACK OF

SPERM, LOSS/INSUFFICIENCY

SPERMATIC VARICOSITY

SPERMATOGENIC, ANTI-

SPERMATORRHEA

- BA JI TIAN/TU SI ZI/ROU CONG RONG/REN SHEN: Kidney Yang Deficient
- DONG CHONG XIA CAO/DU ZHONG/YIN YANG HUO/ROU CONG RONG: Kidney Yang Deficient
- FU PEN ZI/TU SI ZI/GOU QI ZI/WU WEI ZI: Kidney Deficient
- GOU QI ZI/SHU DI HUANG/TU SI ZI/DU ZHONG: Liver Kidney Deficient (Yin/Blood Deficiency)
- HAI PIAO XIAO/SHAN YAO/BAI ZHI
- HE SHOU WU/GOU QI ZI/BU GU ZHI/TU SI ZI: Liver Kidney Deficiency
- HU LU BA/FU PEN ZI/HUANG JING: Kidney Deficient
- JIN YING ZI/QIAN SHI: Kidney Deficient
- JIN YING ZI/LONG GU/MU LI: Deficient Yin
- JIU CAI ZI/LONG GU/SANG PIAO XIAO: Kidney Yang Deficient
- LONG GU/GUI ZHI/BAI SHAO: Yang Deficient
- LU RONG/SHU DI HUANG: Cold Kidney
- MU LI/LONG GU/QIAN SHI/LIAN XU
- QIAN SHI/JIN YING ZI: Kidney Qi Deficient
- ROU CONG RONG/SHAN ZHU YU: Severely Deficient Kidneys
- SANG PIAO XIAO/QIAN SHI/SUO YANG: Kidney Deficient
- SANG PIAO XIAO/TU SI ZI: Kidney Deficient
- SHA YUAN ZI/FU PEN ZI: Liver Kidney Deficiency
- SHA YUAN ZI/QIAN SHI
- SHAN YAO/QIAN SHI: Kidney Deficient
- SHAN ZHU YU/WU WEI ZI: Liver Kidney Yin And Yang Deficient
- SHAN ZHU YU/SHU DI HUANG/TU SI ZI/GOU QI ZI/DU ZHONG: Liver Kidney Deficiency
- SHU DI HUANG/SHAN ZHU YU/SHAN YAO/(LIU WEI DIHUNG WAN): Liver Kidney Deficiency
- TU SI ZI/BU GU ZHI/DU ZHONG: Kidney Deficient
- TU SI ZI/BU GU ZHI/DU ZHONG/LU RONG: Kidney Yang Deficient
- TU SI ZI/BU GU ZHI/DU ZHONG/SHU DI HUANG/SHAN ZHU YU: Kidney Yin Deficient
- XIAN MAO/DU ZHONG

SPERMATORRHEA FROM EXHAUSTION

- GUI ZHI/MU LI/LONG GU/BAI ZHU/SHENG JIANG/DA ZAO/GAN CAO

SPERMATORRHEA FROM EXHAUSTION/KIDNEY DEFICIENCY

- SHAN YAO/SHU DI HUANG/SHAN ZHU YU/(LIU WEI DIHUANG WAN)

SPERMATORRHEA W/SORE/WEAK LOWER BACK/KNEES

SPERMICIDAL ACTION

SWELLING, BREASTS/TESTICLES

TESTICLES

TESTICLES, COLD PAIN IN

TESTICLES, EPIDIDYMIC STASIS

TESTICLES, EPIDIDYMIS, SWOLLEN

TESTICLES, HYDROCELE

TESTICLES, INFLAMED

TESTICLES, INFLAMED, PAIN, SWELLING

TESTICLES, PAIN

See: Sexuality, Male: Urological Topics
- HU LU BA/XIAO HUI XIANG: Cold, Deficient
- QING PI/WU YAO/XIAO HUI XIANG/MU XIANG/(TIAN TAI WU YAO SAN): Cold Liver Stagnation
- XIAO HUI XIANG/LI ZHI HE: Cold

TESTICLES, PAIN, SWELLING

- LI ZHI HE/XIAO HUI XIANG
- LONG DAN CAO/CHAI HU: Liver Fire/Damp Heat
- QING PI/JU HE/XIAO HUI XIANG/CHUAN LIAN ZI
- SHAN ZHA/XIAO HUI XIANG: Prolapse
- WU YAO/XIAO HUI XIANG/QING PI/(TIAN TAI WU YAO. SAN): Cold, Qi Stagnation
- XIANG FU/XIAO HUI XIANG/WU YAO: Cold Stagnation In Liver

TESTICLES, PROLAPSE

TESTICLES, SCROTAL CONTRACTION W/ICY COLD SENSATION

- HU LU BA/XIAO HUI XIANG

TESTICLES, SWELLING

TESTICLES, UNDERDEVELOPMENT, SHEEHAN'S SYNDROME

WET DREAMS

End of Topic:
SEXUALITY, MALE: UROLOGICAL TOPICS

SHAO YANG STAGE DISEASE

SHAO YIN STAGE DISEASE

SHEN DISTURBANCES

SHIGELOSIS, LEUKOPENIA OF

SHINGLES

SHOCK, ANTI-

SHOCK, CARDIOGENIC

SHOCK, CARDIOGENIC, INFECTIOUS, ANAPHYLACTIC

SHOCK, HEMORRHAGE

SHOCK, INSULIN

SHORTNESS OF BREATH

SHOULDERS

SHUT-IN COMPLEX

SIGHING

SILICOSIS

SINUSITIS RELATED TOPICS

End of Topic:
SINUSITIS RELATED TOPICS

SIX STAGES/ CHANNELS :

HALF-EXTERNAL, HALF-INTERNAL

HALF-EXTERNAL, HALF-INTERNAL PATHOGEN

JUE YIN STAGE DISEASE

SHAO YANG STAGE DISEASE

SHAO YIN STAGE DISEASE

TAI YANG STAGE DISEASE

TAI YANG STAGE W/STOMACH ACHE, NAUSEA, ABDOMINAL DISTENTION

YANG MING ORGAN SYNDROME

YANG MING STAGE DISEASE

YANG MING STAGE DISEASE W/IRRITABILITY, EXTREME THIRST

• SHI GAO/ZHI MU

YANG MING STAGE W/QI DEFICIENCY

• HUA QI SHEN/SHI GAO/ZHI MU

End of Topic:
SIX STAGES/CHANNELS

SKELETAL DEFORMITIES, IN CHILDREN

See: Childhood Disorders Skeletal Deformities,
Childhood 83

End of Topic:
SKELETAL DEFORMITIES,IN CHILDREN

SKIN :

ABSCESS

See: Skin Boils 351
• CHAN SU/ZHEN ZHU/NIU HUANG/SHE XIANG/XIONG HUANG: Mouth, Gums, Throat, Severe
• CHI SHAO YAO/CHUAN XIONG
• CHI XIAO DOU/DANG GUI: Topical As Plaster
• CHUAN BEI MU/ZHE BEI MU
• DONG BEI GUAN ZHONG/JIN YIN HUA/LIAN QIAO/PU GONG YING: Heat Toxin
• GAN CAO/PU GONG YING/(ext or intl)
• HE HUAN PI/PU GONG YING/ZAO JIAO CI/CHUAN SHAN JIA
• HE SHOU WU/XUAN SHEN/LIAN QIAO
• LUO SHI TENG/ZAO JIAO CI/GUA LOU/RU XIANG/MO YAO/(ZI TONG LIN BAO SAN)
• MA QIAN ZI/XIONG HUANG/RU XIANG/CHUAN SHAN JIA
• SHAN CI GU/SHE XIANG/WU BEI ZI
• SHI GAO/QING DAI/HUANG BAI
• YU XING CAO/JU HUA/JIN YIN HUA/PU GONG YING: Heat
• BAI JIANG CAO 512
• BAI LIAN 513
• BAI WEI 495
• CAO HE CHE 517
• CHUAN BEI MU 717
• CHUAN SHAN JIA: Helps To Drain 670
• CHUAN XIONG 671
• DA JI: Topical 655
• DAI MAO 743
• DONG BEI GUAN ZHONG 645
• HE SHOU WU 799
• HUANG BAI 485
• HUANG LIAN 486
• HUANG LIAN (c): Topical 20% Vaseline Dressing, 3% Solution With Oral Powder 486
• HUANG QI 765
• HUANG YAO ZI 723
• JIN QIAN CAO 598
• JIN YIN HUA 524
• JING JIE 447
• JING JIE (c): Incrase Healing Process 447
• LIAN QIAO 525

• LONG KUI 526
• MO YAO 683
• NIU BANG ZI: Topical 465
• PU GONG YING 529
• PU HUANG 660
• QIAN LI GUANG (c): Topical 474
• QUAN XIE 749
• RU XIANG: Early Stage 685
• SHAN YAO: Topical Poultice 769
• SHANG LU 554
• SHE XIANG 756
• SHI GAO 477
• TIAN NAN XING: Topical 712
• TU FU LING 536
• TU NIU XI 537
• WANG BU LIU XING: Topical 691
• WU BEI ZI 829
• XIONG HUANG 848
• YE JU HUA (c): Herb/Wu Wei Xiao Du Tang (Ye Ju Hua, Jin Yin Hua, Pu Gong Ying, Zi Hua Di Ding, Tian Kui Zi (Semen Semiaquilegiae) , *Herb, Fu Ling, Shan Zhi Zi, Browned, Sang Ye, Che Qian Cao 468
• ZE LAN: Topical, Too 696

ABSCESS, ACUTE

• LOU LU/LIAN QIAO/DA HUANG: With Redness, Pain, Heat, Swelling

ABSCESS, BREAST

• LUO SHI TENG/PU GONG YING
• DONG KUI ZI 594

ABSCESS, CHRONIC

• MA DOU LING (c) 701
• QING MU XIANG (c) 628

ABSCESS, CHRONIC, RED, HOT, PAINFUL

• MU BIE ZI/HUANG QIN/HUANG BAI/DA HUANG/TIAN HUA FEN

ABSCESS, CONCAVE, CLEAR FLUID

• ROU GUI: Yin 616

ABSCESS, EARLY STAGE

• ZAO JIAO /JIN YIN HUA
• ZHE BEI MU/JIN YIN HUA/PU GONG YING/JU HUA: Firm Swelling, Redness, Pain
• CHI SHAO YAO 668
• QIAN CAO GEN 662

ABSCESS, EXTERNAL

• DI YU 656

ABSCESS, GLUTEAL

• DAN SHEN (c) 672

ABSCESS, HEAD, BACK

• ZI HUA DI DING: Hot, Topical, Too 541

ABSCESS, HELPS TO DRAIN

• BAI ZHI 441

ABSCESS, HOT, PAINFUL, RED

ABSCESS, INFLAMMATION

ABSCESS, INHIBITS PUS FORMATION

ABSCESS, LUNG, BREAST

ABSCESS, LUNG/BREAST

ABSCESS, MULTIPLE

ABSCESS, MULTIPLE, SEPTICEMIA

ABSCESS, PAIN

ABSCESS, PAIN, SWELLING

- CHI SHAO YAO/RU XIANG/MO YAO/JIN YIN HUA/LIAN QIAO
- ZE LAN/DANG GUI/JIN YIN HUA/GAN CAO

ABSCESS, PERINEAL

ABSCESS, SUPERFICIAL

- LUO SHI TENG/RU XIANG/MO YAO

ABSCESS, SUPPURATIVE

- BAI JIANG CAO/JIN YIN HUA

ABSCESS, SWELLING

ABSCESS, SWOLLEN

ABSCESS, ULCERATED W/INSUFFICIENT SUPERATION/CLEAR FLUID

- DANG GUI/HUANG QI

ABSCESS, ULCERATED, SLOWLY SUPPURATIVE

- JIE GENG/BAI ZHI

ABSCESS, UNPERFORATED

- RU XIANG/MO YAO/XIONG HUANG/SHE XIANG

ABSCESS, W/ OR W/O ULCERS TO FORCE SUPPURATION

- XIONG HUANG/SHE XIANG/RU XIANG/MO YAO
- ZAO JIAO /BAI ZHI

ABSCESS, W/MENTAL DULLNESS, HIGH FEVER, SPASMS

ABSCESS, WANDERING

ABSCESS, YANG

- TIAN HUA FEN/CHUAN SHAN JIA/ZAO JIAO /JIN YIN HUA: Type Breast/Intestinal

ABSCESS, YIN, INTERNAL SINKING OF

ABSORBED THROUGH

ABSORBED THROUGH ANY BODY SURFACE

ACNE

- GAN CAO/JIN YIN HUA
- MU BIE ZI/LIU HUANG/QING FEN

ACNE VULGARIS

ADIAPHORESIS

AFTERNOON SWEATS

- YIN CHAI HU/QING HAO/BIE JIA/DI GU PI/(QING GU SAN): Yin Deficiency Heat

ALBINISM

ALLERGIC DERMATITIS

BOILS, CARBUNCLES

- NIU BANG ZI/BAI ZHI/JIE GENG/JIN YIN HUA: Pain, Swelling Of (Unulcerated)
- ZI HUA DI DING/YE JU HUA
- ZI HUA DI DING/YE JU HUA/JIN YIN HUA/LIAN QIAO

BOILS, CHRONIC

- ROU GUI/DANG GUI/HUANG QI/(TUO LI HUANG QI TANG): Yin Type

BOILS, DEEP ROOTED

- LUO SHI TENG/PU GONG YING
- SHAN CI GU/SHE XIANG/WU BEI ZI

BOILS, DEEP ROOTED, HARD

- PU GONG YING/JIN YIN HUA: Hot
- PU GONG YING/JIN YIN HUA/LIAN QIAO/YE JU HUA: Hot

BOILS, HELPS TO DRAIN PUS

BOILS, INITIAL STAGE

- JING JIE/FANG FENG
- ZAO JIAO /JIN YIN HUA
- ZI CAO/HUANG BAI: Heat

BOILS, INTERNAL

BOILS, MALIGNANT

BOILS, MULTIPLE

BOILS, NON-SUPPURATIVE

- JIN YIN HUA/HUANG QIN

BOILS, ON BACK

BOILS, ON FINGERTIPS

- WU GONG/(fish liver oil, topical)

- ZI HUA DI DING/YE JU HUA
- ZI HUA DI DING/YE JU HUA/JIN YIN HUA/LIAN QIAO

BOILS, PAIN, SWELLING

- CHI SHAO YAO/RU XIANG/MO YAO/JIN YIN HUA/LIAN QIAO
- RU XIANG/MO YAO/CHI SHAO YAO/JIN YIN HUA/(XIAN FANG HUO MING YIN)

BOILS, PIMPLE INFECTIONS/SUSCEPTIBILITY

- HAI MA/(lean pork): Children With Weak Constitutions

BOILS, RED, HOT, PAINFUL, SWOLLEN

- BAI JI/JIN YIN HUA/CHUAN BEI MU/TIAN HUA FEN/ZAO JIAO CI/(NEI XIAO SAN)

BOILS, SNAKE HEAD

- WU GONG/(fish liver oil, topical)

BOILS, SUPPURATIVE BUT NO ULCERS

- JIN YIN HUA/HUANG QIN

BOILS, SWELLINGS

- YU XING CAO/PU GONG YING/LIAN QIAO: Toxic Heat

BOILS, TOXIC

BOILS, ULCERATED BUT PUS NOT DISCHARGED

- BAI ZHI/JIE GENG

BOILS, W/PUS BUT NOT HEALED WELL

- HUANG QI/ROU GUI/DANG GUI/REN SHEN: Qi And Blood Deficient

BOILS, YIN TYPE

- BAI JIE ZI/ROU GUI: Deep: Damp Phlegm Obstruct Channels
- ROU GUI/HUANG QI

- ROU GUI 616

BOILS/CARBUNCLES/SKIN, ULCERS

- BAI ZHI/GUA LOU/CHUAN BEI MU/PU GONG YING

BURNS

- DA HUANG/SHI GAO/(topical plaster)
- DI YU/HUANG BAI/(topical)
- DI YU/HUANG LIAN/(TOPICAL)
- HAN SHUI SHI/LU GAN SHI/SHI GAO/(external pwdr)
- QIAN DAN/SHI GAO/(duan)
- SHI GAO/(duan)/HUANG BAI/(external)
- SHI GAO/QING DAI/HUANG BAI
- ZI CAO/HUANG BAI: Heat
- ZI CAO/DANG GUI/BAI ZHI/XUE JIE/(EXTERNAL-SHENG JI YU HONG GAO)

BURNS, ANALGESIC FOR

BURNS, DELIRIUM FROM EXTENSIVE

BURNS, EARLY STAGE

BURNS, EXTENSIVE

BURNS, MILD

BURNS, ON HEAD

BURNS, SCALDS

BURNS, SEPTICEMIA

BURNS, SMALL AREA

BURNS, TOPICAL

BURNS, W/INFECTION

BURNS/SCALDS

CALLOUSES

CARBUNCLES

CARBUNCLES, DAMP, FESTERING

CARBUNCLES, INITIAL STAGE

CARBUNCLES, INITIAL STAGE W/RED, HOT, SWOLLEN SKIN

CARBUNCLES, PAIN

CARBUNCLES, PREMATURE

CARBUNCLES, RED, HOT, PAINFUL, SWOLLEN

CARBUNCLES, SOFT PUS-FILLED

CARBUNCLES, TOXIC

CARBUNCLES, TOXIC HEAT

CARBUNCLES, W/CONSTIPATION

CARBUNCLES, YIN

CHAPPED

CLAVUS

CRACKED, BLEEDING OF HANDS, FEET

DERMATITIS

ECZEMA, CHILDHOOD

ECZEMA, CHILDHOOD/INFANTS

ECZEMA, CHRONIC

ECZEMA, CHRONIC W/ITCHING, WEEPING

ECZEMA, EARLY/SUBACUTE

ECZEMA, GENITALS

ECZEMA, GENITALS W/WEEPY, ITCHY

ECZEMA, INFANTILE

ECZEMA, INFANTILE ACUTE/SUBACUTE, SEBORRHEIC

May Use Cooled 10% Decoction Of Uncured Herb As
Wet Compress 656

ECZEMA, PERINEUM

• KU SHEN (c): Injection Or Tablet, 0.3 g, 5 Tabs/Day ... 491

ECZEMA, PRURITUS OF

• CHUAN JIAO/KU SHEN/DI FU ZI/(external wash)

ECZEMA, SUBACUTE

• BAN BIAN LIAN (c): Wet Compress Or Topical
Application Of Decoction, Prompt 586

EMOLLIENT FOR ELDERLY

• BAI GUO YE (c): Ginkgetin Extract Increases Sebaceous
Secretion, Helping Senile Skin 817

ERUPTIONS OF

• DA QING YE: Blood Heat 519
• MU DAN PI 499
• SHI GAO 477
• XI JIAO 502

ERYSIPELAS

• DA QING YE/JIN YIN HUA
• DA QING YE/XUAN SHEN/JIN YIN HUA
• LIAN QIAO/BAN LAN GEN/DA QING YE
• BAI JIANG CAO 512
• BAN LAN GEN 515
• CE BAI YE 654
• DA QING YE 519
• DAN SHEN 672
• DAN SHEN (c) 672
• DI GU PI (c) 495
• DI LONG: Topical 744
• FU PING: Topical 460
• HAN SHUI SHI 471
• JIANG CAN 746
• JIN QIAN CAO (c): Fresh Herb, 250 g Macerated In 100
ml 75% ETOH, 1 Week, Mix Filtrate With Realgar, Apply
Topically, 2-3x/Day, Not If Broken Skin 598
• JIN YIN HUA (c): 6-15 g (15-100 g Of Vine, Ren Dong
Teng) As Oral Dose/Day Or As Wash 524
• LIAN QIAO 525
• LONG KUI 526
• MA CHI XIAN 528
• MAO DONG QING 682
• QIAN LI GUANG (c): Very Good, 4.5 g Of Crude Herb
4x/Day 474
• QING DAI 531
• SHU YANG QUAN 535
• SHUI NIU JIAO 501
• XI JIAO 502
• ZHU MA GEN 607
• ZI HUA DI DING 541

ERYSIPELAS, HEAD/FACE

• SHENG MA/CHAI HU/(clear heat herbs)
• XUAN SHEN/MU DAN PI: Blood Heat

ERYTHEMA

• DA QING YE 519
• LIAN QIAO 525
• SHUI NIU JIAO 501
• XI JIAO 502

ERYTHEMA MULTIFORME, EXUDATIVE

• HUANG LIAN (c): (Usually On Extremities) Local, Oral
.... 486

ERYTHEMA NODOSUM

• DAN SHEN (c): Injection Alone Or With Spatholobus
Suberectus Stem 672

ERYTHEMA, PURPLE

• HONG HUA 675

ERYTHEMA, UNERUPTED

• NIU BANG ZI 465

EXANTHEMA

• SHENG DI HUANG 500

EXANTHEMA DESQUAMATIVUM

• JING JIE (c): Jing Fang Bai Du Tang/Wu Wei Xiao Du Yin,
Modified Helped 447

EXANTHEMA, EXPRESSION OF

• FU PING 460

FUNGAL INFECTIONS

• AI YE: Topical 651
• BA DOU: Topical 550
• BAI BU: Topical 699
• BAI FU ZI: Topical 708
• BAI HUA SHE 558
• BAI TOU WENG (c): Bai Tou Weng Decoction 514
• BAI XIAN PI 515
• BAN BIAN LIAN (c): Tinea Mannum, Capitis: Wet
Compress Or Topical Application Of Decoction,
Prompt 586
• BIAN XU: Tinea 588
• BING PIAN 753
• CHEN ZONG TAN: External 655
• CHUAN LIAN ZI: Scalp, External 623
• FU PING: Topical 460
• GUAN ZHONG: Tinea 521
• GUAN ZHONG (c): Some 521
• HOU PO (c) 581
• JIN YIN HUA 524
• KU LIAN GEN PI 646
• NAO YANG HUA: Persistent Tinea 740
• QIAN LI GUANG: Moist 474
• SHE TUI 571
• WU SHAO SHE 574
• XU SUI ZI: Topical 556
• YIN CHEN (c): Tinea Corporis, Pedis Treated With 5%
Volatile Oil In ETOH (High Boiling Point Fraction) ,
2x/Day, 4 Weeks, 71% Cured, *Fluid Extract Of 25 g/Day
Helped Various Tinea 603

FURUNCLES

FURUNCLES, DEEP ROOTED

FURUNCLES, DEEP ROOTED, NAIL-LIKE

FURUNCLES, MALIGNANT

- BAN MAO 837
- KU LIAN GEN PI 646
- LU FENG FANG 841
- LU XIAN CAO 566
- MA QIAN ZI 842
- QIAN DAN 845
- XIONG DAN 479

FURUNCLES, ON SHOULDER

- ZHU MA GEN 607

FURUNCLES, PAIN OF

- DANG GUI/MU DAN PI/CHI SHAO YAO/JIN YIN HUA/LIAN QIAO

FURUNCLES, RED THREAD

- ZI HUA DI DING/YE JU HUA
- ZI HUA DI DING/YE JU HUA/JIN YIN HUA/LIAN QIAO

FURUNCLES, SNAKE HEAD

- ZI HUA DI DING/YE JU HUA
- ZI HUA DI DING/YE JU HUA/JIN YIN HUA/LIAN QIAO

FURUNCLES, SWELLING

- RU XIANG/MO YAO/CHI SHAO YAO/JIN YIN HUA/(XIAN FANG HUO MING YIN)
- YUE JI HUA: Topical 696

FURUNCLES, TOXIC

- BEI XIE 587
- DA QING YE 519
- MING DANG SHEN 702
- NIU HUANG 755
- WANG BU LIU XING 691
- XIAN HE CAO 665

FURUNCLES, YIN

- LIU HUANG: Topical 840

FURUNCLES, YIN W/DAMP, COLD BLOCKAGE

- MA HUANG/SHU DI HUANG

HIVES

See: Skin Urticaria 379
- BAI XIAN PI/FANG FENG/BAI JI LI
- BAI JI LI 743

HIVES, ITCHING

- MU ZEI/BAI JI LI

HYPEREMIA

- BAI JIANG CAO 512
- BO HE 456
- DI LONG 744
- HU HUANG LIAN 484
- JIN GUO LAN 523
- JUE MING ZI 471
- MI MENG HUA 474

- MU ZEI 464
- QIN PI 493
- QING XIANG ZI 475
- SANG YE 466
- SHAN ZHI ZI 476
- XIONG DAN 479

HYPEREMIA W/SWELLING

- CHI SHAO YAO 668

HYPERHIDROSIS

- DA DOU HUANG JUAN 506
- DONG CHONG XIA CAO 775

IMPETIGO

- KU SHEN/DANG GUI/BAI XIAN PI/DI FU ZI/CHI SHAO YAO/(INTERNAL OR EXTERNAL)
- HUANG BAI (c) 485

IMPETIGO CONTAGIOSA

- DA HUANG (c) 542

INFLAMMATION

See: Trauma, Bites, Poisonings Inflammation .. 410

INFLAMMATION, ACUTE PURULENT

- CHUAN SHAN JIA 670

ITCHING

See: Skin Pruritus 363
- BEI SHA SHEN/YU ZHU/MAI MEN DONG: Especially From Dry, Cold
- JING JIE/BO HE

ITCHING, ALLERGIC

- MU ZEI/BAI JI LI

ITCHING, CHRONIC

- KU SHEN: Skin Lesions 491

ITCHING, GENERAL

- JING JIE 447
- KU SHEN 491
- LU FENG FANG: Topical 841

ITCHING, SKIN

- GU JING CAO/FANG FENG: Wind Heat, Damp

ITCHING, WIND

- CHAN TUI/BAI JI LI/JING JIE

KELOIDS

- YA DAN ZI (c) 538

LESIONS

See: Skin Sores 373
- BAN ZHI LIAN 516
- BEI XIE: Damp Heat 587

LESIONS, SUPPURATIVE

- XIONG HUANG/SHE XIANG/RU XIANG/MO YAO

LESIONS, SWOLLEN

LESIONS, TOXIC

LEUKODERMA

LUPUS ERYTHEMATOSUS

MACROPAPULE W/HIGH FEVER

- DA QING YE/MU DAN PI

MACULA

MACULA, FROM ACUTE INFECTIOUS DISEASES

MACULATION

MACULOPAPULES

- JIN YIN HUA/MU DAN PI/SHENG DI HUANG: Ying/Xue Heat
- SHENG DI HUANG/XI JIAO/MU DAN PI/CHI SHAO YAO: Blood Heat Toxins

MACULOPAPULES IN FEBRILE DISEASES

- ZI CAO/CHI SHAO YAO/MU DAN PI/JIN YIN HUA/LIAN QIAO

MACULOPAPULES, WARM

- GUAN ZHONG/JIN YIN HUA/LIAN QIAO/DA QING YE/BAN LAN GEN: Heat

MACUPAPULES W/CONTINUAL FEVER

- SHI GAO/XUAN SHEN/XI JIAO: Qi, Xue Level Heat

MALAR FLUSH

MILIARIA

- HUA SHI/SHI GAO/LU GAN SHI/(EXTERNAL): (Sweat Glands, Inflammed, Obstructed-Prickly Heat)

NEURODERMATITIS

NEURODERMATITIS, DISCOID

NIGHT SWEATS

- BAI SHAO/LONG GU/MU LI/FU XIAO MAI: Yin And Blood Deficiency w/Yang Floating
- BAI ZI REN/WU WEI ZI/MU LI/REN SHEN: Yin Deficient
- BIE JIA/DI GU PI/QING HAO: Steaming Bone Syndrome
- BIE JIA/YIN CHAI HU/DI GU PI/(QING GU SAN): Yin Deficient w/Internal Heat
- FU XIAO MAI/MU LI/HUANG QI/MA HUANG GEN/(MU LI SAN): Body Weakness
- GUI BAN/ZHI MU/HUANG BAI/SHENG DI HUANG: Deficient Yin
- GUI BAN/BIE JIA: Yin Deficient w/Yang Rising
- GUI BAN/SHU DI HUANG/(DA BU YIN WAN): Yin Deficiency w/Excess Fire
- HUANG BAI/ZHI MU/SHENG DI HUANG: Yin Deficient
- HUANG QI/SHENG DI HUANG/HUANG BAI/(DANG GUI LIU HUANG TANG): Yin Deficient w/Excess Fire
- HUANG QI/MU LI: Deficient Yang/Yin And Qi
- LONG GU/SHAN ZHU YU/MU LI: Yin Deficient
- LONG GU/MU LI/WU WEI ZI
- MA HUANG/WU WEI ZI/BAI ZI REN
- MA HUANG GEN/SHENG DI HUANG/MU LI
- MU LI/HUANG QI/MA HUANG GEN/FU XIAO MAI/(MU LI SAN): Body Weakness
- MU LI/HUANG QI/FU XIAO MAI
- QING HAO/DI GU PI/BAI WEI
- SHAN YAO/SHU DI HUANG/SHAN ZHU YU/(LIU WEI DIHUANG WAN): Deficient Kidneys
- SHAN ZHU YU/LONG GU/MU LI/FU ZI/REN SHEN/DANG GUI/SHU DI HUANG: Yin Deficient

- SHU DI HUANG/SHAN ZHU YU/SHAN YAO/(LIU WEI DIHUNG WAN): Kidney Deficiency Syndrome
- SHU DI HUANG/GUI BAN/HUANG BAI/ZHI MU/(ZHI BAI DI HUANG WAN): Yin Deficiency w/Excess Fire
- SHU DI HUANG/GUI BAN: Yin Deficient w/Yang Rising
- SUAN ZAO REN/WU WEI ZI/REN SHEN: Bodily Weakness
- SUAN ZAO REN/WU WEI ZI/HUANG QI/MU LI
- WU WEI ZI/REN SHEN/MAI MEN DONG/(SHENG MAI SAN): Qi And Fluid Deficient
- WU WEI ZI/LONG GU: Yin Deficient
- YIN CHAI HU/QING HAO/BIE JIA/DI GU PI/(QING GU SAN): Yin Deficiency Heat
- ZHI MU/HUANG BAI: Yin Deficiency Steaming Bone Syndrome
- BAI ZI REN: Yin Deficients 730
- BIE JIA: Yin Deficient With Heat 805
- DI GU PI 495
- DONG CHONG XIA CAO 775
- GUI BAN: Yin Deficient With Yang Rising 806
- HE ZI 822
- HEI DOU 807
- HUA QI SHEN 808
- HUANG BAI: Yin Deficient 485
- LONG GU: From Fear, Calcined 738
- MU LI 739
- SUAN ZAO REN 732
- TIAN MEN DONG 814
- WU WEI ZI: Yin Deficient 831
- YIN CHAI HU 504
- ZHI MU: Yin Deficiency With Heat 480
- ZI HE CHE: Tuberculosis 792

ODOR, SEVERE UNDERARM

- MI TUO SENG/XIONG HUANG/LIU HUANG

PAPILLOMAS

See: Skin Warts 379
- YA DAN ZI (c): Throat, Ear, Causes Necrosis Of Cells, Topical Application Of Oil 538

PAPULES

- QING DAI 531

PEMPHIGUS

- MI TUO SENG/XIONG HUANG/LIU HUANG: (Disease Of Skin Blisters)
- LIAN FANG: Autoimmune Disease 659

PERSPIRATION

- BAI ZHU (c): Huang Qi, Bai Zhu, Wheat Grain, Or Singly As Powder 760
- MU LI: All Types 739

PERSPIRATION W/THIRST

- DI GU PI 495

PERSPIRATION, DECREASED

- DA DOU HUANG JUAN 506

PERSPIRATION, EXCESS

- BAI FAN (c): Astringent 836
- DONG CHONG XIA CAO 775

PERSPIRATION, FURTIVE

- BAI ZI REN 730
- HE ZI 822
- MA HUANG GEN 825

PERSPIRATION, INHIBITS

- SANG PIAO XIAO (c) 827
- TIAN XIAN ZI (c) 705

PERSPIRATION, NIGHT TIME

- YIN CHAI HU 504

PERSPIRATION, PROFUSE

- YE JIAO TENG 733

PERSPIRATION, RESTING

- REN SHEN 767
- WU WEI ZI 831

PERSPIRATION, RESTING & THIEF

- BAI SHAO 794
- BAI ZHU 760
- BAI ZI REN 730
- FU XIAO MAI 820
- HUANG QI 765
- LONG GU 738
- MA HUANG GEN 825
- MU LI 739
- NUO DAO GEN 825
- SHAN ZHU YU 827
- SUAN ZAO REN 732

PERSPIRATION, SELF

- MA HUANG GEN 825

PERSPIRATION, SPONTANEOUS

- BAI ZHU: Deficient Qi 760
- LONG GU 738

PERSPIRATION, THIEF

- WU WEI ZI 831

PIMPLES

- QIAN LI GUANG 474

PIMPLES ON BACK/SHOULDER

- ZHU MA GEN 607

PITYRIASIS ROSEA

- ZI CAO (c) 504

PRURITIC SORES

- BAI XIAN PI/KU SHEN: Damp Heat

PRURITIC, ANTI-

- XI XIAN CAO (c) 575

PRURITUS

See: Skin Itching 361
See: Infectious Diseases Measles 191

- AI YE/DI FU ZI: Cold, Damp
- BAI JI LI/CHAN TUI/FANG FENG: Wind Heat
- BAI JI LI/JING JIE/CHAN TUI: Wind Heat In Blood
- BAI XIAN PI/KU SHEN/HUANG BAI/CANG ZHU
- BAI XIAN PI/KU SHEN/SHE CHUANG ZI: Wind Cold Damp/Parasites
- BEI SHA SHEN/YU ZHU/MAI MEN DONG: Especially From Dry, Cold
- CHAN TUI/BAI JI LI/JING JIE: Wind Attack
- DI FU ZI/KU SHEN: Damp Heat
- DI FU ZI/SHE CHUANG ZI/(external wash)
- DI FU ZI/SHENG DI HUANG/BAI XIAN PI: Damp Heat/Wind Heat
- FANG FENG/KU SHEN/CHAN TUI
- FU PING/BO HE/NIU BANG ZI: Wind Heat
- JIANG CAN/CHAN TUI/BO HE
- JING JIE/BO HE
- JING JIE/BO HE/MU ZEI/GU JING CAO
- JING JIE/FANG FENG
- KU SHEN/DANG GUI/BAI XIAN PI/DI FU ZI/CHI SHAO YAO/(INTERNAL OR EXTERNAL)
- MU ZEI/BAI JI LI
- ZHANG NAO/LIU HUANG/BAI FAN/(ku fan-calcined)

PRURITUS, ALLEVIATES

- JING JIE/BO HE/NIU BANG ZI/CHAN TUI

PRURITUS, DAMP SORES

PRURITUS, DRY

PRURITUS, ECZEMIC

- CHUAN JIAO/KU SHEN/DI FU ZI/(external wash)

PRURITUS, GENERAL

- LING XIAO HUA/MU DAN PI/SHENG DI HUANG/BAI JI LI/CHAN TUI: Endogenous Wind From Blood Heat

PRURITUS, W/OILY SKIN

PRURITUS, W/RASH

- BO HE/BAI JIANG CAO/CHAN TUI/QUAN XIE
- BO HE/NIU BANG ZI

PSORIASIS

PURPURA

- XI JIAO/SHENG DI HUANG: Blood Heat
- XI JIAO/SHENG DI HUANG/MU DAN PI/CHI SHAO YAO/DA QING YE/ZI CAO: Blood Heat
- XI JIAO/HUANG LIAN: Febrile Disease

PURPURA THROBOPENIC HEMORRHAGICA

PURPURA, ALLERGENIC

PURPURA, ANAPHYLACTIC

PURPURA, ANAPHYLACTOID

PURPURA, CHILDHOOD

PUS

PUS, DRAINAGE FROM OPEN SORES

PUS, HELPS TO DISCHARGE

PUS, HELPS TO EXPEL

RASHES

RASHES, ACUTE FEBRILE MACULOPAPULAR

RASHES, ALLERGIC

RASHES, ALLEVIATES ITCHING

RASHES, CHRONIC

RASHES, DAMP

RASHES, DIAPER

RASHES, DRUG INDUCED

RASHES, ENCOURAGES EXPRESSION OF

RASHES, INCOMPLETE

RASHES, INCOMPLETE ERUPTION

RASHES, INCOMPLETE EXPRESSION OF

RASHES, INCOMPLETE EXPRESSION OF, W/COUGH, DYSPNEA

RASHES, INCOMPLETE FROM FEBRILE DISEASE

- ZI CAO/LIAN QIAO

RASHES, INCOMPLETE, MEASLES

- ZI CAO/CHAN TUI/NIU BANG ZI: Blood Heat

RASHES, INITIAL STAGE

RASHES, LATENT

RASHES, POX

RASHES, PRURITIC

- BO HE/BAI JIANG CAO/CHAN TUI/QUAN XIE
- BO HE/NIU BANG ZI
- JING JIE/BO HE/MU ZEI/GU JING CAO
- JING JIE/FANG FENG

RASHES, PURPURIC

- DI GU PI/MU DAN PI: Deficient Blood Steaming Bone Syndrome
- QING HAO/BIE JIA: Blood Heat
- XUAN SHEN/MU DAN PI: Blood Heat
- XUAN SHEN/NIU BANG ZI: Wind Heat

RASHES, PURPURIC FROM TOXIC HEAT DISEASES

- JIN YIN HUA/LIAN QIAO/DA QING YE/ZI CAO

RASHES, PURPURIC, DENSE

- ZI CAO/DA QING YE: Severe Toxic Heat

RASHES, TOXIC HEAT

- SHENG MA/NIU BANG ZI

RASHES, VERY DARK PURPLE

RASHES, W/PRURITUS

RASHES, WIND

- CHAN TUI/BO HE: Encourages To Surface
- CHAN TUI/BO HE/JU HUA/SANG YE: Encourages To Surface
- FU PING/BO HE/CHAN TUI/SHENG MA: Encourages To Surface
- LU LU TONG/CHAN TUI/BAI XIAN PI

RASHES, WIND ENCOURAGES TO SURFACE

- JING JIE/BO HE

RASHES, WIND W/ITCH

- JIANG CAN/CHAN TUI/FANG FENG/MU DAN PI
- LU FENG FANG/CHAN TUI/(tincture)

RINGWORM

RINGWORM, SCALP

RINGWORM, WHITE/STUBBORN

- YUAN HUA/XIONG HUANG/(PIG FAT OIL-TOPICAL)

ROSACEA

- MI TUO SENG/XUAN SHEN/LIU HUANG/QING FEN

- MU BIE ZI/LIU HUANG/QING FEN
- FANG FENG (c): Fang Feng, Shan Zhi Zi, Chen Pi, Chuan Xiong, Huang Qin, Lian Qiao, Du Huo, Jie Geng, All 9 g, Jing Jie, Huang Lian, Gan Cao, Each 6 g, Decoct Take As 2 Doses In One Day, 3 Treatments/2 Days, Plus Topical Ointment Of Da Feng Zi, Mercury, Xing Ren 1x/Day, 100% Cure Rate 444

SCABIES

- BAI XIAN PI/KU SHEN/SHE CHUANG ZI
- DA FENG ZI/DI FU ZI/LIU HUANG/ZHANG NAO/(topical)
- DI FU ZI/HUANG BAI/KU SHEN/BAI XIAN PI
- HAI TONG PI/SHE CHUANG ZI/(external oil)
- KU SHEN/DANG GUI/BAI XIAN PI/DI FU ZI/CHI SHAO YAO/(INTERNAL OR EXTERNAL)
- LIU HUANG/QING FEN/BAN MAO/BING PIAN
- LU FENG FANG/CHAN TUI/(tincture)
- MI TUO SENG/XIONG HUANG/LIU HUANG
- QING FEN/XIONG HUANG/DA FENG ZI/(topical)
- SHE CHUANG ZI/QING FEN: Itchy, Weepy
- XIONG HUANG/HUANG BAI/BING PIAN
- YUAN HUA/XIONG HUANG/(PIG FAT OIL-TOPICAL)
- ZHANG NAO/LIU HUANG/BAI FAN/(ku fan-calcined)
- AI YE: Topical 651
- BA DOU: Topical 550
- BAI BU: Topical 699
- BAI BU (c): 50% Decoction/Extract 699
- BAI FAN: Damp Rashes 836
- BAI FU ZI: Topical 708
- BAI HUA SHE 558
- BAI XIAN PI 515
- BAN MAO 837
- BIAN XU 588
- BING PIAN: Topical 753
- BO HE 456
- CANG ER ZI: With Pruritus 559
- CANG ER ZI (c) 559
- CHEN ZONG TAN: External 655
- DA FENG ZI 839
- DI FU ZI: Topical, Too 592
- GAO BEN: Topical 444
- HAI TONG PI 562
- HUANG LIAN 486
- JIN YIN HUA 524
- JING JIE 447
- KU LIAN GEN PI 646
- KU LIAN GEN PI (c): Powdered With Vinegar, Apply Topically 646
- KU SHEN 491
- LI LU: Topical 834
- LIU HUANG: Topical 840
- LU FENG FANG: Topical 841
- MI TUO SENG 843
- QING FEN: Topical Wash 845
- QING HAO 508
- QING XIANG ZI 475
- SHAN DOU GEN: Topical 532
- SHE CHUANG ZI 847
- SHE TUI 571
- SHI GAO (c): Fu Ping Shi Gao Decoction 477
- SONG XIANG 847

- SU HE XIANG (c): With Olive Oil 758
- WU HUAN ZI 538
- WU JIU GEN PI 555
- WU SHAO SHE 574
- XIONG HUANG: Topical 848
- XU SUI ZI: Topical 556
- YE JIAO TENG: Topical 733
- YUAN HUA 556
- ZAO FAN 848
- ZE QI 727
- ZHANG NAO: Topical 849
- ZHI XUE CAO 697

SCALDS

See: Skin Burns 353
- BAI LIAN 513
- CE BAI YE 654
- CHUAN LIAN ZI (c) 623
- DA HUANG 542
- DI YU: Topical 656
- DI YU (c): Petroleum Jelly, 3% 656
- FENG LA 840
- FENG MI 548
- HU ZHANG (c) 497
- JI ZI HUANG 809
- MAO DONG QING 682
- PU GONG YING (c): Fresh Root Juice 529
- ZI RAN TONG 698

SCALDS, TOPICAL FOR

- HAN SHUI SHI 471

SCALP, FUNGUS

- HE SHOU WU: Topical 799

SCALP, RINGWORM

- DA SUAN 644

SCALP, SCABBY

- LIU HUANG 840

SCALP, TINEA

- CHUAN LIAN ZI: Topical Powder 623

SCARRING, FACE

- SHAN CI GU/QING FEN/PENG SHA

SCARS

- WU BEI ZI/WU GONG/(black vinegar-external)
- WU BEI ZI: Topical 829

SCARS, FACIAL

- SHAN CI GU/QING FEN/PENG SHA

SCARS, KELOIDS

- YA DAN ZI (c) 538

SCLERODERMA

- DAN SHEN (c): Injection Alone Or With Spatholobus Suberectus Stem 672

- LU RONG 784

SKIN, INFECTIONS, DECUBITUS ULCER

- LIAN QIAO (c): Pu Gong Ying, Jin Yin Hua, Chai Hu, Da Huang, Quan Shen, Tao Ren, Chi Shao, Mu Dan Pi, Externally 1-2x/Day, 8-46 Days 525

SKIN, INFECTIONS, EARLY STAGE TO CAUSE SUPPURATION

- ZAO JIAO CI 716

SKIN, INFECTIONS, LOCAL

- JU HUA 463

SKIN, INFECTIONS, PYROGENIC

- WU BEI ZI 829

SKIN, INFECTIONS, PYROGENIC, ACUTE

- ZI HUA DI DING 541

SKIN, INFECTIONS, SWOLLEN

- XIA KU CAO (c): Inhibits Transplanted Skin Infections
  478

SKIN, INFLAMMATION RESPONSE, REDUCES

- HUAI HUA MI (c) 658

SKIN, INFLAMMATIONS

- CHE QIAN ZI (c): Reduced, Powdered Seed Ointment
  590
- DA HUANG (c): Topical 542
- HUANG QIN 489
- QIN PI (c): Reduced 493
- QUAN XIE 749
- TIAN HUA FEN 726
- YUE JI HUA 696

SKIN, INFLAMMATIONS, SLOW HEALING, SUPPURATIVE

- MU DAN PI/JIN YIN HUA/LIAN QIAO

SKIN, IRRITATES

- BO HE (c) 456
- SHI CHANG PU (c): Topical 757

SKIN, ITCHING

- BAI JI LI/CHAN TUI/FANG FENG: Wind Heat
- BAI XIAN PI/KU SHEN/HUANG BAI/CANG ZHU
- DI FU ZI/SHE CHUANG ZI/(external wash)
- DI FU ZI/SHENG DI HUANG/BAI XIAN PI: Wind Heat/Damp Heat
- FANG FENG/KU SHEN/CHAN TUI
- FU PING/BO HE/NIU BANG ZI: Wind Heat
- GU JING CAO/FANG FENG: Wind Heat, Damp
- JIANG CAN/CHAN TUI/FANG FENG/MU DAN PI: Wind Rash
- ZHANG NAO/LIU HUANG/BAI FAN/(ku fan-calcined)
- CANG ER ZI 559
- MU DAN PI (c) 499
- XIONG HUANG: Soak 848

- YE JU HUA 468
- ZHANG NAO (c) 849

SKIN, ITCHING, IRRITATION

- WU WEI ZI/(in rice wine,160 proof): Wind Rash

SKIN, LACERATIONS

- BAI JI 652
- LU HUI (c): 10% Solution, Topical 544

SKIN, LESIONS

- BEI XIE/HUANG BAI/YI YI REN: Damp Heat
- CANG ZHU/HUANG BAI/NIU XI/(SAN MIAO WAN): Wind Damp
- DI YU/HUANG BAI/(topical): Damp Heat
- ER CHA/LONG GU/QING FEN: Damp
- HUA SHI/HUANG BAI/BAI FAN: Damp
- TU FU LING/BAI XIAN PI: Damp Heat
- DA HUANG: Topical, Too 542
- HUA SHI: Damp—Topical 597
- HUANG BAI: Damp/Toxic Heat 485
- JIANG CAN: Wind Rash 746
- MU BIE ZI (c): Paste Of 844
- QIAN LI GUANG 474
- SHE TUI: Wind 571
- TU FU LING: Damp Heat 536
- XIONG DAN: Hot: Topical 479
- ZAO JIAO CI: Acute Purulent 716
- ZI CAO 504

SKIN, LESIONS PAIN/SWELLING

- SHE GAN 533

SKIN, LESIONS W/CHRONIC ITCHING/SEEPAGE/BLEEDING

- KU SHEN 491

SKIN, LESIONS, EARLY STAGE, SWOLLEN, NODULAR, PAINFUL

- GAN SUI: Topical—Damp Heat 551

SKIN, LESIONS, INFLAMMED, SUPPURATIVE

- CHUAN SHAN JIA/ZAO JIAO CI

SKIN, LESIONS, ITCHY

- AI YE/DI FU ZI: Cold, Damp
- HAI TONG PI/SHE CHUANG ZI/(external oil)
- BAI JI LI 743
- BIAN XU: Damp 588
- HAI TONG PI 562

SKIN, LESIONS, ITCHY, WEEPING

- SHE CHUANG ZI/KU SHEN/BAI BU
- SHE CHUANG ZI 847

SKIN, LESIONS, NO INFLAMMATION

- TIAN JI HUANG 536

SKIN, LESIONS, RED

- MANG XIAO 545

SKIN, SEBORRHEIC DERMATITIS

- KU SHEN (c): Injection Or Tablet, 0.3 g, 5 Tabs/Day ... 491
- QING HAO (c): 10 Catties Of Fresh Herb Decocted To 6-7, Add 30-35 g Borneol Predissolved In Alcohol, Apply With Cotton Swabs, 3-4x/Day 508

SKIN, SOFTENS

- LIU HUANG (c) 840

SKIN, SORE W/MENTAL DULLNESS, HIGH FEVER, SPASMS

- DAI MAO: Blood Heat 743
- LING YANG JIAO: Blood Heat 747
- ZI CAO: Blood Heat 504

SKIN, SORE/CARBUNCLES

- CHUAN XIN LIAN 518

SKIN, SORES

- KU SHEN/SHE CHUANG ZI/DAN SHEN: Damp
- BAI JIANG CAO: Toxic Heat, Topical, Too 512
- BAI XIAN PI: Damp Heat 515
- BEI XIE: Damp Heat 587
- BING LANG: Cold Damp 643
- CAN SHA: Cold Damp 558
- CANG ER ZI: Cold Damp 559
- CANG ZHU: Cold Damp/Damp Heat 578
- CHE QIAN ZI: Damp Heat 590
- CHI SHAO YAO: Damp Heat 668
- CHUAN JIAO: Cold Damp 610
- DA FU PI: Cold Damp 624
- DAN SHEN: Damp Heat 672
- DI FU ZI: Damp Heat 592
- HAI PIAO XIAO: Cold Damp 821
- HAN FANG JI: Damp Heat 596
- HU HUANG LIAN: Damp Heat 484
- HUA SHI: Damp Heat 597
- HUANG LIAN: Damp Heat 486
- HUANG QIN: Damp Heat 489
- KU SHEN: Damp Heat 491
- LONG DAN CAO: Damp Heat 492
- MA CHI XIAN: Damp Heat 528
- MU DAN PI: Damp Heat 499
- MU GUA: Cold Damp 567
- MU TONG: Damp Heat 599
- QIN PI: Damp Heat 493
- SHAN ZHI ZI: Damp Heat 476
- SHE CHUANG ZI: Cold Damp 847
- SU MU: Damp Heat 688
- TU FU LING: Damp Heat 536
- TU NIU XI 537
- WU ZHU YU: Cold Damp 618
- YI MU CAO: Damp Heat 694
- YI YI REN: Damp Heat 602

SKIN, SORES, DAMP

- MI TUO SENG 843

SKIN, SORES, INTRACTABLE

- DA FENG ZI 839
- HE SHOU WU 799
- KU SHEN 491
- WU SHAO SHE 574
- ZAO JIAO 715
- ZAO JIAO CI 716

SKIN, SORES, SUPPURATIVE

- HOU ZAO 722
- MU MIAN HUA 529

SKIN, SORES, SWOLLEN

- BAI JIANG CAO: Heat, Toxins, Swelling 512
- BAI LIAN: Heat, Toxins, Swelling 513
- CHUAN XIN LIAN: Heat, Toxins, Swelling 518
- DA HUANG: Heat, Toxins, Swelling 542
- ER CHA: Heat, Toxins, Swelling 839
- HE SHOU WU: Heat, Toxins, Swelling 799
- HUANG BAI: Heat, Toxins, Swelling/Damp Heat 485
- HUANG LIAN: Heat, Toxins, Swelling 486
- HUANG QIN: Heat, Toxins, Swelling, Topical/Internal 489
- PU GONG YING: Heat, Toxins, Swelling 529
- SHAN ZHI ZI: Heat, Toxins, Swelling, Topical 476
- SHENG MA: Heat, Toxins, Swelling, Relieves Surface Complex 467
- TIAN HUA FEN: Heat, Toxins, Swelling 726
- ZHU SHA: Heat, Toxins, Swelling 741
- ZI HUA DI DING: Heat, Toxins, Swelling 541

SKIN, SORES, SWOLLEN, TOXIC

- BAI ZHI: Relieves Surface Complex 441
- BING PIAN: Topical 753
- CHI SHAO YAO: Blood Stasis, Swelling 668
- CHUAN SHAN JIA: Blood Stasis, Swelling 670
- CHUAN XIONG: Blood Stasis, Swelling 671
- DA HUANG: Topical 542
- DAN SHEN: Blood Stasis, Swelling 672
- DANG GUI: Blood Stasis, Swelling 795
- DANG SHEN: Helps Healing, Deficiency 762
- FANG FENG: Relieves Surface Complex 444
- HONG HUA: Blood Stasis, Swelling 675
- HUANG QI: Helps Healing, Deficiency 765
- JIN YIN HUA: Relieves Surface Complex/Heat, Toxins, Swelling 524
- JING JIE: Relieves Surface Complex 447
- JU HUA: Relieves Surface Complex 463
- LIAN QIAO: Relieves Surface Complex/Heat, Toxins, Swelling 525
- LU GAN SHI: Topical 842
- LU JIAO: Blood Stasis, Swelling 783
- LU JIAO JIAO: Helps Healing, Deficiency 783
- MA CHI XIAN: Topical 528
- MANG XIAO: Topical 545
- MO YAO: Blood Stasis, Swelling 683
- MU DAN PI: Blood Stasis, Swelling 499
- NIU BANG ZI: Relieves Surface Complex 465
- PENG SHA: Topical 844

- NIU HUANG (c): Niu Huang San—Niu Huang, She Xiang, Pearl, Bing Pian, Mercurous Chloride, Xiong Dan, Long Gu, Mu LI, Ru Xiang, Mo Yao, Shi Jui Ming, Huang Lian 755
- ZHEN ZHU: Topical 740

SKIN, ULCERS, CHRONIC, LEGS

- HAI PIAO XIAO 821

SKIN, ULCERS, DAMP

- WU BEI ZI: Topical As Wash/Powder 829

SKIN, ULCERS, DEEP ROOTED SORES

- TIAN NAN XING: Topical 712

SKIN, ULCERS, INHIBITS

- LU HUI (c): Inhibits Histamine Synthesis 544

SKIN, ULCERS, RED BAYBERRY, TOXIC

- TU FU LING 536

SKIN, ULCERS, SWOLLEN

- NIU BANG ZI: Topical 465

SKIN, ULCERS, TOXIC

- ZHU SHA: Topical 741

SKIN, ULCERS, TOXIC EROSIVE

- QU MAI 600

SKIN, URTICARIA

- BA JIAO GEN 510

SKIN, VARICELLA

- MA HUANG (c): Ma Huang Chan Tui Tang, Modified (Ma Huang, Chan Tui, Huai Hua, Huang Lian, Fu Ping, Gan Cao) Or Ma Huang Lian Qiao Chi Xiao Dou Tang (Ma Huang, Lian Qiao, Chi Xiao Dou, Xing Ren, Gan Cao, Sheng Jiang, Da Zao, Zi Bai Pi (Cortex Catalpae Radicis)) 448

SKIN, YELLOW, DULL, DUSKY, SEVERE

- SHUI ZHI/MANG XIAO/DA HUANG

SKIN/SCALP FUNGUS

- HE SHOU WU: Topical 799

SORES

See: Skin Ulcers 377
See: Skin Lesions 361
- BO HE/NIU BANG ZI: Wind Heat
- DA QING YE/JIN YIN HUA
- MA QIAN ZI/XIONG HUANG/RU XIANG/CHUAN SHAN JIA
- QIAN DAN/SHI GAO/(duan)
- QUAN XIE/SHAN ZHI ZI/(beeswax-topical)
- WU GONG/GAN CAO/(beeswax, topical)
- BAI JI: Topical 652
- BAI JIANG CAO: Topical, Too 512
- BAI XIAN PI: Wind Heat/Damp Heat 515
- BAN MAO: Topical 837
- BING PIAN: Topical 753
- CHUAN XIN LIAN 518
- DA HUANG: Toxic Heat In Blood Level 542
- DA JI: Topical 655
- DANG GUI 795
- DI YU: Topical 656
- FU PING: Topical 460
- GAN CAO: Topical, Too 763
- GUAN ZHONG: Damp Heat 521
- HE SHOU WU 799
- HU HUANG LIAN: Damp Heat 484
- HU PO 737
- HUANG BAI: Damp/Toxic Heat 485
- HUANG QIN: Heat (Topical/Internal) 489
- HUANG YAO ZI: Topical 723
- JING JIE 447
- KU LIAN GEN PI 646
- LONG GU: Topical 738
- LU FENG FANG: Topical 841
- LU HUI (c): 10% Solution Shortens Healing Time 544
- MA CHI XIAN: Damp Heat 528
- MO YAO 683
- PANG DA HAI: San Jiao Fire 724
- RU XIANG: Early Stage, Promotes Healing, Reduces Pain 685
- SHAN CI GU: Excess Heat 846
- SHANG LU: Hot—Topical 554
- SHI GAO: Topical/Internal 477
- SHI SHANG BAI: Lung Heat 534
- WU BEI ZI: Topical As Wash/Powder 829
- XI XIAN CAO: Damp Heat 575
- XIONG DAN: Hot: Topical 479
- YE JU HUA 468

SORES, AUXILLARY HERB FOR

- HUO MA REN: Topical, Too 548

SORES, CHRONIC

- YU JIN: Heals 695

SORES, CHRONIC NON-HEALING

- BAI JI 652
- GUI BAN 806
- HUANG QI 765

SORES, CHRONIC, NON-HEALING

- BIE JIA/HUANG QI/LONG GU
- GUI BAN/ZAO JIAO CI/BAI TOU WENG
- HUANG QI/DANG GUI
- LONG GU/(calcined)/BAI FAN/(topical)
- LONG GU: Topical 738
- MO YAO: Topical 683

SORES, DAMP

- HUA SHI: Topical 597

SORES, DAMP, FESTERING

- LIU HUANG: Topical 840

SORES, DAMP, ITCHY

- CANG ER ZI/BAI JI LI

SORES, DEEP ROOTED

SORES, DRAINS PUS LONG TERM

SORES, FIRM, HARD

SORES, HEAD

SORES, HEAD, BACK

SORES, HOT, PAINFUL

- SHANG LU/KU SHEN: Warm Poultice

SORES, INFECTED

SORES, INITIAL STAGE

- YUAN ZHI/(rice wine-topical)

SORES, INTRACTABLE

SORES, ITCHY

- BAI XIAN PI/KU SHEN: Damp Heat

SORES, ITCHY, WEEPING

- SHE CHUANG ZI/KU SHEN/BAI BU

SORES, NON-DRAINING

SORES, NON-HEALING

SORES, OOZING YIN SORES

SORES, PAIN/SWELLING OF

- PU HUANG/(with honey,external)

SORES, POORLY HEALED

- HUANG QI/ROU GUI/DANG GUI/REN SHEN: Qi And
  Blood Deficient

SORES, PUSTULAR

SORES, SLOW HEALING, SUPPURATIVE, INFLAMMED, FLAT

- JU HUA/JIN YIN HUA

SORES, SUPPURATIVE

- SHE XIANG/RU XIANG/MO YAO
- XIONG HUANG/SHE XIANG/RU XIANG/MO YAO

SORES, SUPPURATIVE, BUT UNABLE TO PERFORATE OR THIN DISCHARGE

- HUANG QI/CHUAN SHAN JIA: Yin Type

SORES, SWELLING OF SKIN

- DAN SHEN/GUA LOU/CHUAN SHAN JIA

SORES, SWOLLEN

SORES, SWOLLEN, INITIAL STAGE

SORES, SWOLLEN, TOXIC

SORES, SWOLLEN, TOXIC, PAINFUL

SORES, TOXIC

SORES, TOXIC HEAT

SORES, TOXIC, RED, SWOLLEN, PAINFUL

SORES, ULCERATED, SUPPURATIVE

SORES, W/MENTAL DULLNESS, HIGH FEVER, SPASMS

SORES, W/O SUPPURATION

SWEATING, FURTIVE

- BAI SHAO 794
- HUANG QI 765
- MU LI 739
- WU BEI ZI 829
- ZI HE CHE 792

SWEATING, INCREASES

- BING LANG 643

SWEATING, INHIBITS

- BAI SHAO 794
- CHAN SU 837
- NUO DAO GEN 825
- YANG JIN HUA 714

SWEATING, LACK OF

- QIANG HUO 449
- XIANG RU: Summer Heat/Damp 453

SWEATING, NIGHT

See: **Skin** Night Sweats 362
- LONG GU/SHAN ZHU YU/MU LI: Deficient Yin
- LONG GU/MU LI/WU WEI ZI
- MU LI/HUANG QI/FU XIAO MAI
- BAI SHAO: Floating Yang 794
- DONG CHONG XIA CAO 775
- FU XIAO MAI: Yin Deficient 820
- HE ZI 822
- LONG GU 738
- MA HUANG GEN: Yin Deficient 825
- MU LI: Tuberculosis 739
- NUO DAO GEN 825
- SHU DI HUANG 802
- SUAN ZAO REN 732
- WU BEI ZI: From TB Or TB With Silicosis, Powdered Into Paste On Navel Before Bedtime 829
- WU WEI ZI: Yin Deficient 831

SWEATING, POST FEBRILE

- MU LI 739

SWEATING, POST LONG ILLNESS, TB

- NUO DAO GEN /MU LI/FU XIAO MAI

SWEATING, POSTPARTUM

- MA HUANG GEN 825

SWEATING, PROFUSE

- CANG ZHU/SHI GAO: Warm Febrile Disorders
- FU ZI/REN SHEN/(SHEN FU TANG): Yang Qi Collapse
- LONG GU/FU ZI/REN SHEN: Devastated Yang, Collapsed Qi
- MAI MEN DONG/REN SHEN/WU WEI ZI: Severe Heart Lung Deficiency
- SHAN ZHU YU/LONG GU/MU LI/FU ZI/REN SHEN: Yang Devastated
- DA HUANG: Yang Ming Stage/Excess Heat In Intestine 542
- FU ZI: With Yang Fleeing 613

- REN SHEN: Collapsed Qi 767
- SHI GAO 477

SWEATING, PROMOTES

- XI HE LIU 451

SWEATING, REDUCES

- TIAN XIAN ZI 705

SWEATING, RESTING

- BAI SHAO 794
- MU LI 739
- WU BEI ZI 829

SWEATING, SEVERE, OIL-LIKE

- ROU GUI: Floating Yang 616

SWEATING, SPONTANEOUS

- BAI SHAO/GUI ZHI/(GUI ZHI TANG): Wind Cold w/Weakness, Deficiency
- BAI SHAO/LONG GU/MU LI/FU XIAO MAI: Yin And Blood Deficiency w/Yang Floating
- BAI ZHU/FANG FENG/HUANG QI/(YU PING FENG SAN): Qi Deficiency
- DONG CHONG XIA CAO/(with meat): Wei Qi Weakened
- FU XIAO MAI/HUANG QI/MU LI: Deficiency Induced
- FU XIAO MAI/MU LI/HUANG QI/MA HUANG GEN/(MU LI SAN): Body Weakness
- FU ZI/HUANG QI/GUI ZHI: Wei Qi Weakness
- GAN JIANG/FU ZI/(SI NI TANG): Collapsing Yang
- HUANG QI/REN SHEN: Qi Deficiency
- HUANG QI/FANG FENG: Wei Qi Deficient, Surface Deficient: Wei Qi Deficient
- HUANG QI/MU LI: Yang/Yin And Qi Deficient
- HUANG QI/MU LI/FU XIAO MAI/MA HUANG GEN/(MU LI SAN): Exterior Deficient
- LONG GU/HUANG QI/BAI SHAO: Surface Deficiency/Weak Wei Qi
- LONG GU/MU LI/WU WEI ZI
- MA HUANG GEN/HUANG QI/MU LI
- MA HUANG GEN/HUANG QI/DANG GUI
- MU LI/HUANG QI/FU XIAO MAI
- MU LI/HUANG QI/MA HUANG GEN/FU XIAO MAI/(MU LI SAN): Body Weakness
- REN SHEN/WU WEI ZI/MAI MEN DONG: Qi And Yin Deficiency
- SHAN ZHU YU/HUANG QI/DANG SHEN: Yang/Qi Deficient
- SUAN ZAO REN/WU WEI ZI/HUANG QI/MU LI
- SUAN ZAO REN/WU WEI ZI/REN SHEN: Bodily Weakness
- WU WEI ZI/HUANG QI: Yang Deficient
- WU WEI ZI/REN SHEN/MAI MEN DONG/(SHENG MAI SAN): Qi And Fluid Deficient
- BAI SHAO: Floating Yang 794
- BAI ZHU: Qi Deficient 760
- DONG CHONG XIA CAO 775
- FU XIAO MAI: Qi Deficient 820
- GOU QI ZI 798
- HUA QI SHEN 808
- HUANG QI: Deficient 765
- JING MI 767
- LONG GU 738

- AI YE (c): Fresh, Crushed Leaves, Numerous Times/Day, Warts Fell Off 3-10 Days 651
- BA DOU: Topical 550
- BU GU ZHI (c) 773
- CHAI HU (c): 60% Effective, IM Injection, 1 g Herb Equivalent For 20 Days, 0.5-1.0 ml 2.4 mm From Base Of Wart, 1x/2-3 Days, Injection Of Acupoints, Too, Needs 10 Treatments 457
- GU SUI BU (c): Repeated Tincture Application, Every 2 Hrs, 3 Days 778
- HONG HUA (c): Verruca Plana, Use Tea Of 9 g, 1x/Day For 10 Days, 92% Effective, May Cause Temporary Irritation 675
- SHUI NIU JIAO (c) 501
- WU MEI: Soften In Hot Water, Then Topical 830
- XU SUI ZI: Topical 556
- YA DAN ZI: Topical 538
- YA DAN ZI (c): Body, Hands, Genital, Causes Necrosis Of Cells, Topical Application Of Oil 538
- YI YI REN (c): 30% Cured, 10-30 g Decoction/Day, 1 Dose, 2-4 Weeks, *60 g Cooked With Husked Rice Given As Meal 1x/Day, Almost 50% Cured In 7-16 Days, Often Warts Will Become Enlarged, Red, Inflammed Before Disappearing 602

WARTS, FLAT FROM VIRUS(JUVENILLE VERRUCA PLANA)

- DI GU PI (c) 495

WARTS, MULTIPLE

- MA HUANG (c): Ma Xing Yi Gan Tang (Ma Huang, Xing Ren, Yi Yi Ren, Gan Cao) 448

WARTS, PLANTERS

- YA DAN ZI: Topical 538
- YI YI REN 602

WARTS, VARIOUS

- DI GU PI (c): 10% Injection, IM 495

WARTS, VIRAL

- BAN LAN GEN (c): Slow, 3-4 Week Course, 50% Herb Injection 2 ml IM, 1-2x/Day 515

WARTS/CORNS

- WU MEI: Soften In Hot Water, Then Topical 830

WIND HEAT RASH

- SHE TUI/CHAN TUI/SHENG DI HUANG/DANG GUI

YIN BOILS

- ROU GUI 616

YING WEI DISHARMONY

- DA ZAO/SHENG JIANG

End of Topic:
SKIN

SKIN CRACKED, BLEEDING OF HANDS, FEET

See: Skin Cracked, Bleeding Of Hands, Feet 355

SKIN RELATED TOPICS

See: Skin Skin Related Topics 368

SKIN, ABSORBED THROUGH

See: Skin Absorbed Through 350

SKIN, CANCER

See: Cancer/Tumors/Swellings/Lumps Skin, Cancer 71

SKIN, DRY, SCALY

See: Skin Dry, Scaly 356

SKIN, ERUPTIONS OF

See: Skin Eruptions Of/Skin, Eruptions 358

SLEEP DISORDERS WITH SCANTY URINE, IRRITABILITY, IN CHILDREN

See: Childhood Disorders Sleep Disorders With Scanty Urine, Irritability, Childhood 83

SLEEP RELATED TOPICS

See: Mental State/Neurological Disorders Sleep Related Topics 258

SMALL INTESTINE RELATED TOPICS

See: Abdomen/Gastrointestinal Topics Small Intestine Related Topics 37

SMOOTH MUSCLES

See: Musculoskeletal/Connective Tissue Smooth Muscles 275

SNAKE BITES

See: Trauma, Bites, Poisonings Snake Bites ... 413

SOMNOLENCE

See: Mental State/Neurological Disorders Somnolence 258

SORENESS RELATED TOPICS

See: Pain/Numbness/General Discomfort Soreness Related Topics 302

SORES AND RELATED TOPICS

See: Skin Sores And Related Topics 373

SORES, MOUTH

See: Oral Cavity Sores, Mouth 288

SPASM RELATED TOPICS

See: Musculoskeletal/Connective Tissue Spasm Related Topics 275

SPASTIC COLON

See: Bowel Related Disorders Spastic Colon ... 64

SPEECH RELATED TOPICS

See: Oral Cavity Speech Related Topics 288

SPERM RELATED TOPICS

SPERMATIC VARICOSITY

SPERMATORRHEA

SPERMICIDAL ACTION

SPIDER BITE

SPIRIT, CALMS

SPIROCHETTES, ANTI-

SPLANCHNOPTOSIS

End of Topic:
SPLANCHNOPTOSIS

SPLEEN :

DAMPNESS

EXTERNAL PATHOGEN W/SPLEEN DISORDERS

EXTERNAL PATHOGEN W/SPLEEN WEAKNESS

SPLEEN DAMPNESS

SPLEEN DAMPNESS CONGESTED

SPLEEN DAMPNESS W/EXTERNAL COLD

• XIANG RU/BAI ZHU: Vomiting, Diarrhea

SPLEEN DAMPNESS W/PAIN

SPLEEN DEFICIENCY

SPLEEN DEFICIENCY PATTERNS

SPLEEN DEFICIENCY W/DAMP OBSTRUCTION

• CHEN PI/BAI ZHU: Anorexia

SPLEEN DEFICIENCY W/DAMPNESS

SPLEEN DEFICIENCY W/DAMPNESS, DIARRHEA

SPLEEN DEFICIENCY W/DAMPNESS, EXCESS

• FU LING /DANG SHEN/BAI ZHU/(SI JUN ZI TANG):
Lassitude, Anorexia, Diarrhea

SPLEEN DEFICIENCY W/EXTERNAL PATH

SPLEEN DEFICIENCY W/QI/DAMPNESS OBSTRUCTION

• CAO DOU KOU/GAO LIANG JIANG: Anorexia, Abdominal
Pain, Distension

SPLEEN DEFICIENCY, COLD

SPLEEN DEFICIENCY, DAMP HEAT

• CHE QIAN ZI/CANG ZHU: Leukorrhea

SPLEEN DISORDERS W/EXTERNAL PATH

SPLEEN HEART DEFICIENCY

• FU LING /GAN CAO: Palpitations, Shortness Of Breath, Facial Edema

SPLEEN HEART YANG DEFICIENCY

• GUI ZHI/FU LING /BAI ZHU: Shortness Of Breath, Edema, Palpitations

SPLEEN KIDNEY DEFICIENCY

• SHAN YAO/DANG SHEN: Watery Stools, Fatigue, Weakness, Anorexia

SPLEEN KIDNEY DEFICIENCY, COLD

• PU HUANG/(quick fried ginger): Chronic Hemafecia
• ROU DOU KOU/BU GU ZHI: Daybreak Diarrhea
• WU YAO/WU ZHU YU: Abdominal Pain, Vomit, Diarrhea
• WU ZHU YU/WU WEI ZI/ROU DOU KOU/(SI SHEN WAN): Chronic Diarrhea
• YI ZHI REN/WU YAO/SHAN YAO/(SUO QUAN WAN): Urination Frequency/Incontinence

SPLEEN KIDNEY YANG DEFICIENCY

• FU ZI/GAN JIANG/GAN CAO/(SI NI TANG): Edema, Abdominal Distension
• FU ZI/BAI ZHU/FU LING /(ZHEN WU TANG): Dysuria, General Edema
• QIAN NIU ZI/CHEN XIANG/ROU GUI: Edema, Abdominal Distension
• ROU GUI/FU ZI: Cold Abdomen, Anorexia, Diarrhea
• ROU GUI/GAN JIANG/BAI ZHU/FU ZI/(GUI FU LI ZHONG WAN): Cold Epigastric Pain, Loose BM, Poor Appetite
• WU ZHU YU/WU WEI ZI: Early AM Diarrhea

SPLEEN LIVER DISHARMONY

SPLEEN LUNG DEFICIENCY QI

• DANG SHEN/HUANG QI

SPLEEN PAIN

SPLEEN QI DEFICIENCY

• DANG SHEN/BAI ZHU: Anorexia, Loose Stool, Vomiting
• HUANG QI/BAI ZHU: Weak, Lassitude

SPLEEN QI DEFICIENCY W/BLOOD DEFICIENCY

• TAI ZI SHEN/SUAN ZAO REN/WU WEI ZI: Palpitations, Insomnia, Sweating

SPLEEN QI DEFICIENCY W/HEART BLOOD DEFICIENCY

• SUAN ZAO REN/DANG SHEN/FU LING /LONG YAN ROU: Insomnia, Palpitations, Irritability

SPLEEN QI DEFICIENCY W/HEART BLOOD DEFICIENCY W/EMOTIONAL SYMPTOMS

• FU XIAO MAI/GAN CAO/DA ZAO

SPLEEN QI PROLAPSE

• HUANG QI/SHENG MA/CHAI HU: Spleen Qi Weak, Sunken

SPLEEN QI STAGNATION

• BAI DOU KOU/HOU PO/CANG ZHU/CHEN PI: Anorexia, Distention, Fullness

SPLEEN QI STAGNATION W/WEAKNESS

• SHA REN/CHEN PI/DANG SHEN/BAI ZHU/(XIANG SHA LIU JUN ZI WAN): Digestive Disorders

SPLEEN STOMACH DEFICIENCY

• HUO XIANG/BAI ZHU: Vomiting, Diarrhea
• MAI YA/GAN JIANG: Indigestion
• DA ZAO: Weakness, Lassitude, Shortness Of Breath

SPLEEN STOMACH DEFICIENCY QI

• REN SHEN/BAI ZHU

SPLEEN STOMACH DEFICIENCY W/ACCUMULATION OF TURBID DAMP

• BAI DOU KOU/CHEN PI

SPLEEN STOMACH DEFICIENCY W/HEAT

SPLEEN STOMACH DEFICIENCY, COLD

• BAI ZHU/GAN JIANG/REN SHEN/(LI ZHONG WAN): Pain, Cold, Diarrhea, Vomiting
• BAI ZHU/GAN JIANG: Vomiting, Abdominal Pain, Diarrhea
• CAO GUO/CANG ZHU/HOU PO/BAN XIA: Stomach, Cold Pain In
• CHEN XIANG/ZI SU YE: Hiccups, Vomiting
• FU LONG GAN/BAI ZHU/HUANG QI/ZHI GAN CAO: Diarrhea
• ROU DOU KOU/MU XIANG: Anorexia, Diarrhea, Cold Abdominal Pain
• ROU DOU KOU/DANG SHEN/BAI ZHU/GAN JIANG: Chronic Diarrhea
• ROU DOU KOU/BAN XIA/GAN JIANG: Vomiting, Diarrhea, Abdominal Distension, Anorexia
• ROU DOU KOU/BAN XIA/GAN JIANG/SHEN QU/SHA REN: Vomiting, Diarrhea, Abdominal Distension, Anorexia For Children
• XUAN FU HUA/DAI ZHE SHI/(XUAN FU DAI ZHE TANG): Vomit, Hiccups
• YI TANG/GUI ZHI/BAI SHAO/GAN CAO

SPLEEN STOMACH DISHARMONY

SPLEEN STOMACH DISHARMONY FROM DAMPNESS

- HOU PO/CANG ZHU/CHEN PI/(PING WEI SAN)

SPLEEN STOMACH QI OBSTRUCTING

- SHA REN/HOU PO: Abdominal, Epigastric Pain, Nausea, Vomiting

SPLEEN STOMACH QI STAGNATION

- CHEN PI/HOU PO/CANG ZHU/(PING WEI SAN): Nausea/Vomit, Fullness
- FO SHOU/MU XIANG/ZHI KE: Belching, Nausea, Anorexia, Distension
- MU XIANG/FU LING /ZHI KE/CHEN PI: Anorexia, Distension, Borborygmus, Diarrhea
- ZI SU YE/HUO XIANG: Cold

SPLEEN STOMACH QI STAGNATION FROM COLD, DEFICIENCY

- ROU DOU KOU/MU XIANG/SHENG JIANG/BAN XIA

SPLEEN STOMACH QI STAGNATION W/HEAT

- ZI SU YE/HUANG LIAN

SPLEEN STOMACH QI STAGNATION W/PHLEGM

- ZI SU YE/BAN XIA/HOU PO

SPLEEN STOMACH WEAKNESS W/LIVER QI RISING

- WU ZHU YU/REN SHEN/SHENG JIANG/(WU ZHU YU TANG): Headache, Vomiting

SPLEEN STOMACH WEAKNESS W/POOR APPETITE

- GU YA/DANG SHEN/BAI ZHU/CHEN PI

SPLEEN STOMACH WEAKNESS W/QI STAGNATION

- BAI ZHU/ZHI SHI/(ZHI ZHU WAN): Epigastric, Abdominal Fullness

SPLEEN STOMACH WEAKNESS, COLD

- GAN JIANG/BAI ZHU/FU LING /(LI ZHONG WAN): Distension, Vomiting, Nausea, Loose BM, Poor Appetite, Lassitude, Weak Pulse

SPLEEN STOMACH, COLD

SPLEEN STOMACH, COLD ATTACKING

- GAN JIANG/WU ZHU YU/BAN XIA: Pain, Vomiting, Diarrhea
- WU ZHU YU/GAN JIANG/MU XIANG

SPLEEN STOMACH, COLD, WEAK

- DING XIANG/SHA REN/BAI ZHU: Vomiting, Anorexia, Diarrhea

SPLEEN STOMACH, COLD, YANG DEFICIENCY

- CHUAN JIAO/GAN JIANG/DANG SHEN/YI TANG/(DA JIAN ZHONG TANG)

SPLEEN STOMACH, CONGESTION

SPLEEN STOMACH, DAMP HEAT INVADING

- XI GUA/(JUICE OF: FRESH DI HUANG,PEAR,SUGAR CANE)

SPLEEN STOMACH, DAMPNESS

- HUO XIANG/CANG ZHU/HOU PO/BAN XIA/(BU HUAN JIN ZHEN QI SAN): Epigastric, Abdominal Distension, Nausea, Anorexia

SPLEEN STOMACH, DAMPNESS BLOCKING

- BAI DOU KOU/HOU PO/CANG ZHU/CHEN PI: Anorexia, Distention, Fullness
- HOU PO/DA HUANG/ZHI SHI/(DA CHENG QI TANG): w/Abdominal Distension And Constipation
- PEI LAN/HUO XIANG/CANG ZHU/HOU PO/BAI DOU KOU
- SHA REN/BAI ZHU: Abdominal Pain, Diarrhea
- SHA REN/CANG ZHU/BAI DOU KOU/HOU PO

SPLEEN STOMACH, DAMPNESS BLOCKING, COLD

- CAO GUO/CANG ZHU/HOU PO/BAN XIA

SPLEEN STOMACH, DAMPNESS BLOCKING, SEVERE, COLD

- CAO DOU KOU/HOU PO/CANG ZHU/BAN XIA

SPLEEN STOMACH, DAMPNESS BLOCKING, TURBID W/VOMITING, DIARRHEA, CRAMPS

- CAN SHA/HUANG QIN/MU GUA/WU ZHU YU/(CAN SHI TANG)

SPLEEN STOMACH, DAMPNESS BLOCKING, VERY COLD

- CAO DOU KOU/ROU GUI/GAN JIANG

SPLEEN STOMACH, DAMPNESS STAGNATION

- CHEN PI/HOU PO/CANG ZHU/(PING WEI SAN): Stifling Sensation, Anorexia, Lassitude, Diarrhea, Tongue: White, Sticky

SPLEEN STOMACH, DAMPNESS, COLD

SPLEEN STOMACH, QI STAGNATION

SPLEEN WEAKNESS

- E ZHU/SAN LENG/SHAN ZHA/MU XIANG/ZHI SHI: Food Stagnation, Distension, Pain

SPLEEN WEAKNESS IN WATER METABOLISM

- BAI ZHU/REN SHEN/FU LING /(SI JUN ZI TANG): Anorexia, Lassitude, Loose Stools, Abdominal Distension

SPLEEN YANG WEAK

- FU ZI/REN SHEN/BAI ZHU/GAN JIANG/(FU ZI LI ZHONG WAN): Cold Epigastric Region

SPLEEN, BLOOD DEFICIENCY

- SHU DI HUANG/SHA REN

SPLEEN, DECREASES SIZE OF

SPLEEN, SWELLING OF

SPLEEN/STOMACH CONGESTED FIRE

SPLEEN/STOMACH QI SINKING

- CHAI HU/REN SHEN/HUANG QI/BAI ZHU/SHENG MA: Chronic Diarrhea, Organ Prolapse

SPLENOMEGALY

SPLENOMEGALY W/HEAT

- E ZHU/SAN LENG/SHAN ZHI ZI/SHENG DI HUANG

End of Topic:
SPLEEN

SPLEEN RELATED TOPICS

SPLEEN/STOMACH, ATTACKED BY LIVER

SPLENOMEGALY

SPLINTERS

SPONDYLITIS, HYPERTROPHIC

SPRAINS AND RELATED TOPICS

SPRAINS, ANALGESIC FOR

SPUTUM RELATED TOPICS

STAGNANT QI

STANDING, PROLONGED, IN ELDERLY

STARCH, DIGESTION

STEAMING BONE FEVER RELATED TOPICS

STERILITY

STERILITY, FEMALE

STIFFNESS

STIMULANT

STOMACH CANCER

STOMACH RELATED TOPICS

End of Topic:
STOMACH RELATED TOPICS

STOMACH/ DIGESTIVE DISORDERS :

ACID REGURGITATION

- GOU QI ZI/DANG GUI/SHU DI HUANG/BEI SHA SHEN/CHUAN LIAN ZI: Yin Deficiency And Liver Qi Stagnation
- HAI PIAO XIAO/ZHE BEI MU
- HAI PIAO XIAO/CHUAN BEI MU/(WU BEI SAN)
- HOU PO/CANG ZHU/FU LING : Stomach Excess
- LAI FU ZI/SHAN ZHA: Stagnant Stomach/Intestines
- WA LENG ZI/HAI PIAO XIAO
- WU ZHU YU/SHENG JIANG/BAN XIA: Cold In Stomach
- XIANG FU/CANG ZHU
- ZHE BEI MU/HAI PIAO XIAO

ACID REGURGITATION W/EPIGASTRIC PAIN

- MU LI/SHI JUE MING/(both calcined,in pwdr)

ACID REGURGITATION, FOOD STAGNATION, W/DIARRHEA, TENESMUS

- LAI FU ZI/SHAN ZHA/SHEN QU/CHEN PI/(BAO HE WAN)

AMYLASE INHIBITION

ANOREXIA

- BAI BIAN DOU/REN SHEN/BAI ZHU/FU LING /(SHEN LING BAI ZHU SAN): Spleen Deficient, Not Metabolizing Water
- BAI DOU KOU/HUO XIANG: Cold Damp/Food Stagnation
- BAI DOU KOU/HOU PO/CANG ZHU/CHEN PI: Spleen Stomach Dampness Or Qi Stagnation
- BAI DOU KOU/HUA SHI/YI YI REN/SHA REN/(SAN REN TANG): Damp Heat Febrile Disease, Early Stage
- BAI ZHU/REN SHEN/FU LING /(SI JUN ZI TANG): Spleen Weakness In Water Metabolism
- BEI SHA SHEN/MAI MEN DONG/SHENG DI HUANG/YU ZHU/(YI WEI TANG): Body Fluids Damaged By Febrile Disease
- CANG ZHU/HOU PO: Dampness Blocking Middle Jiao
- CAO DOU KOU/WU ZHU YU: Stomach Cold
- CAO DOU KOU/GAO LIANG JIANG: Spleen Deficient w/Qi/Dampness Obstruction
- CHAI HU/ZHI KE
- CHEN PI/BAI ZHU: Spleen Deficient w/Dampness
- CHEN PI/BAI ZHU/DANG SHEN
- DA ZAO/REN SHEN/BAI ZHU: Spleen Stomach Weakness
- DANG SHEN/HUANG QI: Lung Spleen Qi Deficient
- DANG SHEN/BAI ZHU: Spleen Qi Deficient
- DING XIANG/SHA REN/BAI ZHU: Spleen Stomach Cold And Weak
- FO SHOU/MU XIANG/QING PI
- FU LING /BAN XIA/CHEN PI: Congested Fluids
- FU LING /DANG SHEN/BAI ZHU/(SI JUN ZI TANG): Spleen Deficient w/Dampness
- GAN CAO/DANG SHEN: Spleen Deficient
- GU YA/DANG SHEN/BAI ZHU/CHEN PI: Spleen Stomach Weakness
- HUANG JING/REN SHEN: From Prolonged Sickness/Chronic Wasting
- HUANG JING/GOU QI ZI: General Debility
- HUANG JING/DANG SHEN/BAI ZHU: Spleen Stomach Qi Deficient
- HUANG JING/BEI SHA SHEN/MAI MEN DONG/GU YA: Spleen Stomach Yin Deficiency
- HUANG QI/REN SHEN: Qi Deficient
- HUANG QI/REN SHEN/BAI ZHU: Spleen Lung Qi Deficient
- HUO XIANG/BAN XIA: Dampness Blocking Middle Jiao

- HUO XIANG/CANG ZHU/HOU PO/BAN XIA/(BU HUAN JIN ZHEN QI SAN): Spleen Stomach Dampness
- LAI FU ZI/ZHI KE: Food Stagnation
- MU XIANG/SHA REN: Qi Blockage/Food Stagnation
- MU XIANG/FU LING /ZHI KE/CHEN PI: Spleen Stomach Qi Stagnation
- PEI LAN/HUO XIANG/CANG ZHU/HOU PO/BAI DOU KOU: Spleen Stomach, Dampness Blocking
- REN SHEN/BAI ZHU: Spleen Stomach Deficient Qi
- REN SHEN/FU LING /YUAN ZHI: Heart Spleen Deficiency
- REN SHEN/BAI ZHU/FU LING /GAN CAO/(SI JUN ZI TANG): Spleen Stomach Weakness
- ROU DOU KOU/MU XIANG: Spleen Stomach Deficiency Cold
- ROU DOU KOU/BAN XIA/GAN JIANG: Spleen Stomach Cold Deficient
- ROU GUI/FU ZI: Spleen Kidney Yang Deficiency
- SHAN YAO/DANG SHEN
- SHAN YAO/REN SHEN/BAI ZHU/FU LING /(SHEN LING BAI ZHU SAN): Spleen Stomach Weakness
- SHAN ZHA/MAI YA/SHEN QU: Food Stagnation
- TAI ZI SHEN/SHAN YAO/BAI BIAN DOU/GU YA/MAI YA: Spleen Deficiency
- TU SI ZI/SHAN YAO/FU LING /DANG SHEN: Kidney Spleen Deficient
- XIAO HUI XIANG/SHENG JIANG/HOU PO: Stomach Cold
- YI ZHI REN/DANG SHEN/BAN XIA/FU LING : Spleen Stomach Cold Deficiency
- YU JIN/YIN CHEN: Damp Heat Diseases

ANOREXIA, FOCAL DISTENTION

- GU YA/CHEN PI/SHA REN: Food Stagnation

ANOREXIA, IN CHILDREN

- ROU DOU KOU/BAN XIA/GAN JIANG/SHEN QU/SHA REN: Spleen Stomach Cold Deficient

ANOREXIA, INTERMITTENT FULLNESS, PAIN

- CHUAN LIAN ZI/YAN HU SUO/(JIN LING ZI SAN): Liver GB Fire/Stagnant Qi

ANOREXIA, LOOSE/MUSHY STOOL

- CHEN PI (c): Jian Pi Wan 621
- DANG SHEN (c): Best As 2: 1 Dang Shen, Gou Qi Zi ... 762

ANOREXIA, STOMACH/ABDOMINAL FULLNESS

- SHEN QU/ZHI KE: Cold Stagnation

ANOREXIA, STOMACH/ABDOMINAL PAIN

- MU XIANG/BAI ZHU

ANTIACID

See: Stomach/Digestive Disorders Indigestion
.... 393
- HAI PIAO XIAO (c): Contains Calcium Carbonate 821

ANTIEMETIC

- BAI DOU KOU (c) 577
- BAN XIA (c): Hot Water Soluble, Strong 710
- CHEN PI (c) 621
- DI YU (c): For Digitalis Induced But Not Apomorphine Induced Vomiting 656
- DING XIANG (c) 612

APPETITE SUPPRESSENT

APPETITE, INCREASES

APPETITE, LOSS OF

APPETITE, POOR

BELCHING

BELCHING, ACID REGURGITATION, PAIN

BELCHING, DISTASTEFUL

BELCHING, PUTRID ODOR

BELCHING, SOUR TASTE

CARMINATIVE

CRAMPS

DIGESTANT

- DAN SHEN/TAN XIANG/SHA REN/(DAN SHEN YIN): Qi/Blood Stagnation
- GAO LIANG JIANG/XIANG FU/(LIANG FU WAN): Cold, Qi Stagnation
- ROU DOU KOU/MU XIANG/SHENG JIANG/BAN XIA: Spleen Stomach Qi Stagnation w/Cold, Deficient
- SHA REN/HOU PO: Spleen Stomach Qi Obstructing
- SHENG JIANG/DA ZAO: Spleen Qi Weak
- WEI LING XIAN/SHA REN
- YANG JIN HUA/CHUAN XIONG/HAN FANG JI
- ZHE BEI MU/HAI PIAO XIAO
- CAO DOU KOU: Cold 579
- CAO GUO 580
- CHEN XIANG 622
- CHUAN LIAN ZI: Damp Heat Qi Stagnation 623
- DAN SHEN: Blood Stasis 672
- DANG GUI 795
- GAO LIANG JIANG: Cold 615
- HAI FENG TENG: Spleen/Stomach Cold 562
- JIANG HUANG: Stagnant Qi 678
- JIANG XIANG: Stagnant Qi 659
- LI ZHI HE: Spleen Stomach Qi Stagnation 626
- LU JIAO JIAO: Cold, Deficient 783
- LU LU TONG 681
- MEI GUI HUA: Liver Spleen/Stomach Disharmony 627
- MU HU DIE: Liver Qi Stagnation 702
- ROU GUI: Spleen Stomach Cold 616
- RU XIANG: Blood Stasis 685
- TAN XIANG 632
- WU LING ZHI 691
- WU YAO: Spleen Stomach Qi Stagnation 632
- XIANG FU 633
- XIANG FU (c): With AI Ye 633
- YAN HU SUO: Stagnant Qi 693
- YANG JIN HUA 714
- YING SU KE 832
- YU JIN 695

EPIGASTRIC PAIN W/ACID REGURGITATION
- MU LI/SHI JUE MING/(both calcined,in pwdr)

EPIGASTRIC PAIN, DISTENTION
- E ZHU/SAN LENG/SHAN ZHA/MU XIANG/ZHI SHI
- SAN LENG/E ZHU/QING PI/MAI YA
- SHI CHANG PU/HOU PO/CHEN PI: Turbid Damp In Middle Jiao
- XIAO HUI XIANG/GAN JIANG/MU XIANG: Stomach Cold
- E ZHU 673
- ROU DOU KOU 826

EPIGASTRIC PAIN, DISTENTION/FULLNESS IN CHEST
- MAI YA/CHAI HU/ZHI SHI/CHUAN LIAN ZI: Liver Stomach Qi Stagnation

EPIGASTRIC PAIN, FOOD STAGNATION W/DIARRHEA, TENESMUS, ACID REGURGITATION
- LAI FU ZI/SHAN ZHA/SHEN QU/CHEN PI/(BAO HE WAN)

EPIGASTRIC PAIN, NAUSEA
- WU ZHU YU: Liver Stomach Phlegm Disorder 618

EPIGASTRIC QI FORMATION
- ZHI KE 635

EPIGASTRIC REGION, STIFLING SENSATION
- CHEN PI/HOU PO/CANG ZHU/(PING WEI SAN)

EPIGASTRIC REGION, STIFLING, SENSATION
- GUA LOU REN/BAN XIA/HUANG LIAN/(XIAO XIAN XIONG TANG): Phlegm, Heat Accumulation

EPIGASTRIC, COLD
- FU ZI/REN SHEN/BAI ZHU/GAN JIANG/(FU ZI LI ZHONG WAN): Spleen Yang Weakness

EPIGASTRIC, FLANK PAIN
- CHAI HU: Liver Stomach Disharmony 457

FAT, IMPROVES DIGESTION OF
- NIU HUANG (c): Activates Pacreatic Enzymes 755

FOCAL DISTENTION
See: Pain/Numbness/General Discomfort Focal Distention 301
See: Stomach/Digestive Disorders Distention 388

FOCAL DISTENTION, STOMACH
- QING PI/SHAN ZHA/MAI YA/SHEN QU/(QING PI WAN)

FOCAL DISTENTION, STOMACH, ABDOMEN
- ZHI SHI/BAI ZHU/(ZHI ZHU WAN): Spleen/Stomach Deficient

FOOD ACCUMULATION
See: Stomach/Digestive Disorders Food Stagnation 391
See: Stomach/Digestive Disorders Food Congestion 391
See: Stomach/Digestive Disorders Indigestion 393
- HU JIAO 615

FOOD ACCUMULATION W/PALPABLE MASS
- DA HUANG 542
- ZHI SHI 635

FOOD ACCUMULATION, OVERNIGHT
- SHA REN 584
- XU SUI ZI 556

FOOD CONGESTION
See: Stomach/Digestive Disorders Food Accumulation 390

FOOD STAGNATION, QI OBSTRUCTION PAIN

• WU MEI/SHAN ZHA/HOU PO/SHA REN
• ZHI SHI/HOU PO
• ZHI SHI/DA HUANG

FOOD STAGNATION, SPLEEN DEFICIENCY

• SAN LENG/MU XIANG/BING LANG/QING PI/SHEN QU/DANG SHEN/BAI ZHU: Pain

FOOD STAGNATION, SPLEEN STOMACH DEFICIENCY

• JI NEI JIN/MAI YA/SHAN ZHA/BAI ZHU/DANG SHEN/SHAN YAO: Anorexia/Diarrhea

FOOD STAGNATION/QI BLOCKAGE

• MU XIANG/SHA REN: Tenesmus, Diarrhea, Pain, Anorexia

FOOD STAGNATION/RETENTION

• SHEN QU/SHAN ZHA/MAI YA: Fullness, No Appetite, Diarrhea

FOOD, AID TO DIGESTION

• BAI DOU KOU 577

GAS, DIGESTIVE, ELIMINATES

• ROU GUI PI (c) 617

GAS, DISTENTION, REDUCES

• MAI YA/(with tonifying herbs)

GAS, FOUL IN STOMACH/INTESTINES

• SU HE XIANG 758

GASTRALGIA

See: Stomach/Digestive Disorders Stomach,
Ache 397
• CHUAN JIAO: Cold With Vomiting, Diarrhea 610
• FO SHOU 624
• FU ZI: Cold 613
• GAO LIANG JIANG 615
• HOU PO 581
• PU HUANG 660
• WU ZHU YU 618
• XIANG FU 633
• YI ZHI REN 790

GASTRIC ACID, NEUTRALIZES

• ZHEN ZHU (c) 740

GASTRIC ATONY

• DONG CHONG XIA CAO (c) 775

GASTRIC CANCER

• BAN MAO (c): See Hepatic Cancer For More Details .. 837
• LU FENG FANG 841

GASTRIC PAIN

• MU DAN PI (c) 499

GASTRIC SECRETIONS

• LONG DAN CAO (c): Increases Before Meals, Decreases If After Meals 492

GASTRIC SECRETIONS, INCREASES

• JI NEI JIN (c): 30-37% 638
• SHENG JIANG (c) 450

GASTRIC SPASMS

• DONG CHONG XIA CAO (c) 775
• LUO LE 583
• XIANG FU (c): 120 g Herb, Gan Liang Jiang 90 g (Liang Fu Wan) , Grind To Fine pwdr, 3 g Each Morning, 80% Effective 633

GASTRIC TUMORS

• HUANG YAO ZI (c): Tincture 723

GASTRITIS

• HUA SHI (c): Protects Stomach From Nausea/Vomit .. 597
• JIU BI YING 625
• PI PA YE 703
• XIANG FU (c): Cold Stasis/Qi Stasis: 120 g Herb, Gan Liang Jiang 90 g (Liang Fu Wan) , Grind To Fine pwdr, 3 g Each Morning, 80% Effective 633

GASTRITIS, ACUTE

• FO SHOU (c): 50 g Boiled Take In 2 Doses When Cool For 3 Days 624

GASTRITIS, ACUTE, CHRONIC

• CANG ZHU (c): Ping Wei San, With Ginger Soup Or Boiled Water 578

GASTRITIS, ATROPHIC

• SANG YE (c) 466

GASTRITIS, CHRONIC

• MEI GUI HUA 627
• PU GONG YING (c): 15 g Decocted 2x With Tablespoon Rice Wine, Combined Decoction , 3 Doses, After Meals 529
• REN SHEN (c) 767
• YAN HU SUO (c): Reduces Secretion, 5-10 g Herb, Every Day, 76% Effective 693
• ZHU RU 729

GASTRITIS, CHRONIC, VOMITING

• BAN XIA (c): Xian Sha Liu Jun Zi Tang (Ban Xia, Chen Pi, Mu Xiang, Sha Ren, Fu Ling, Dang Shen, Bai Zhu, Gan Cao) 710

GASTRITIS, NEUROTIC

• MEI GUI HUA 627

GASTROPTOSIS

See: Stomach/Digestive Disorders Stomach,
Prolapse 399
• CHAI HU/REN SHEN/HUANG QI/BAI ZHU/SHENG MA: Spleen/Stomach Qi Sinking

INDIGESTION FROM CEREALS/CARBOHYDRATES

INDIGESTION FROM STARCHY FOODS

INDIGESTION IN INFANTS FROM IMPROPER NURSING

INDIGESTION W/ANOREXIA/DIARRHEA

- JI NEI JIN/MAI YA/SHAN ZHA/BAI ZHU/DANG SHEN/SHAN YAO: Spleen Stomach Deficiency

INDIGESTION W/DIARRHEA

INDIGESTION, ACUTE/CHRONIC

- SHA REN/MU XIANG

INDIGESTION, CHILDHOOD MILK STAGNATION

INDIGESTION, DISTENTION

- BAN XIA/HUANG LIAN: Hot And Cold Attacks Stomach

INDIGESTION, FOCAL DISTENTION/GAS

INDIGESTION, MILD

INDIGESTION, MILK IN INFANTS

MORNING SICKNESS

NAUSEA

- BAI DOU KOU/CHEN PI: Deficient Spleen Stomach w/Accumulation Of Dampness
- BAI MAO GEN/GE GEN: Warm Febrile Diseases
- CANG ZHU/HOU PO: Dampness Blocking Middle Jiao
- CAO GUO/CANG ZHU/HOU PO/BAN XIA: Spleen Stomach Cold Blockage
- CHEN PI/SHENG JIANG/ZHU RU
- CHUAN JIAO/GAN JIANG/DANG SHEN/YI TANG/(DA JIAN ZHONG TANG): Spleen Stomach Cold, Deficient
- FU LING /BAN XIA/CHEN PI: Congested Fluids
- GAN JIANG/HUANG LIAN
- GAN JIANG/BAI ZHU/FU LING /(LI ZHONG WAN): Spleen Stomach Weakness, Cold
- HOU PO/CANG ZHU/FU LING : Stomach Excess
- HUO XIANG/PEI LAN: Summer Heat Dampness
- HUO XIANG/CANG ZHU/HOU PO/BAN XIA/(BU HUAN JIN ZHEN QI SAN): Spleen Stomach Dampness
- HUO XIANG/ZI SU YE/BAN XIA/HOU PO/CHEN PI/(HUO XIAN ZHENG QI SAN): Digestion, Disturbance From Cold, Raw Food
- MU XIANG/SHA REN: Qi Blockage/Food Stagnation
- PI PA YE/ZHU RU/LU GEN: Stomach Heat
- SHA REN/HOU PO: Spleen Stomach Qi Obstructing
- SHA REN/CANG ZHU/BAI DOU KOU/HOU PO: Spleen Stomach, Dampness Blocking

NAUSEA, EXTERIOR CONDITION

NAUSEA, INDUCES MILD

NAUSEA/VOMITING

- BAI DOU KOU/CHEN PI: Spleen/Stomach Deficient w/Dampness
- BAN XIA/CHEN PI: Stomach Qi Disharmony
- BAN XIA/HUANG QIN: Rebellious Qi From Phlegm, Heat
- BAN XIA/SHENG JIANG/(XIAO BAN XIA TANG): Rebellious Stomach Qi, Cold Type
- BAN XIA/ZHU RU/PI PA YE: Rebellious Stomach Qi, Heat Type
- BAN XIA/SU GENG/SHA REN: Rebellious Stomach Qi, Pregnancy Type
- BAN XIA/REN SHEN/DA ZAO: Rebellious Stomach Qi, Stomach Weak Type

- HUO XIANG/BAN XIA: Dampness Blocking Middle Jiao
- LING YANG JIAO/SHI JUE MING/JU HUA/HUANG QIN:
Liver Fire Uprising
- PEI LAN/HUO XIANG/CANG ZHU/HOU PO/BAI DOU
KOU: Spleen Stomach, Dampness Blocking
- ROU DOU KOU/MU XIANG/SHENG JIANG/BAN XIA:
Spleen Stomach Qi Stagnation w/Cold, Deficient
- SHENG JIANG/DA ZAO: Spleen Qi Weak
- WU MEI/XI XIN/HUANG LIAN/(WU MEI WAN):
Roundworms In Biliary Tract
- XIANG FU/CANG ZHU
- ZHU RU/HUANG LIAN/CHEN PI/BAN XIA/SHENG JIANG:
Stomach Heat
- ZI SU YE/HUANG LIAN: Stomach Heat
- ZI SU YE/BAN XIA/HOU PO: Qi Stagnation w/Phlegm In
Spleen/Stomach
- BAI DOU KOU 577
- BAN XIA: Stomach Damp Phlegm 710
- BI BA: Stomach Cold 608
- CANG ZHU: Spleen Dampness 578
- CAO GUO: Spleen Stomach Cold, Deficient 580
- CHEN PI: Any Type 621
- FO SHOU 624
- GAN JIANG 614
- HOU PO 581
- HUA SHI (c): Protects Stomach In Gastritis 597
- HUANG LIAN 486
- HUO XIANG: Dampness From Spleen Transportation
Function Loss 582
- LAI FU ZI 639
- LIAN QIAO (c): Helps Reduce 525
- MU XIANG: Spleen Stomach Qi Stagnation 628
- PEI LAN: Dampness/Summer Heat 583
- SHA REN 584
- SHENG JIANG: Cold 450
- XIANG RU 453
- ZI SU YE 454

NAUSEA/VOMITING, INDUCES

- QIAN NIU ZI (c) 553

PAIN, EPIGASTRIC

- HUANG LIAN/WU ZHU YU
- SHENG JIANG/DA ZAO: Spleen Qi Weak

PEPTIC ULCER

See: Stomach/Digestive Disorders Ulcer 400

PEPTIC ULCER, BLEEDING

- BU GU ZHI (c): Hemostatic In 773

REBELLIOUS QI, VOMITING W/CLEAR FLUID

- GAO LIANG JIANG/BAN XIA/SHENG JIANG: Stomach Cold

REBELLIOUS STOMACH QI, COLD TYPE

- BAN XIA/SHENG JIANG/(XIAO BAN XIA TANG):
Nausea/Vomiting

REBELLIOUS STOMACH QI, HEAT TYPE

- BAN XIA/ZHU RU/PI PA YE

REBELLIOUS STOMACH QI, STOMACH WEAK TYPE

- BAN XIA/REN SHEN/DA ZAO: Nausea/Vomiting

REGURGITATION

- BAI JIE ZI 708
- CI WEI PI 819
- DAI ZHE SHI 735
- FU LONG GAN 657
- JI NEI JIN 638
- LU JIAO JIAO: Cold, Deficient 783
- LU JIAO SHUANG: Deficiency Cold 784
- QIAN DAN 845
- WU YAO 632

REGURGITATION OF FOOD

- DA FU PI: Food Stagnation 624

REGURGITATION OF SOUR FLUIDS

- WU ZHU YU/GAN JIANG: Cold Stomach
- WU ZHU YU/HUANG LIAN/(ZUO JIN WAN): Liver
Stomach Heat, Disharmony

REGURGITATION, ACIDIC

- HUANG LIAN/WU ZHU YU
- WU ZHU YU: Liver Stomach Disharmony 618

REGURGITATION, ACIDIC W/VOMITING, STABBING PAIN

- WA LENG ZI: Congealed Blood 690

RETCHING

- PI PA YE 703
- SHI HU: Dry Heaves 813

STARCH, DIGESTION

- GU YA (c): If Not Toasted Or Decocted 637

STOMACH

See: Stomach/Digestive Disorders Epigastric .. 389
- BAI SHAO (c): Inhibits Spasms Of 794
- CHI SHAO YAO (c): Smooth Muscle Inhibitor 668
- GAN CAO (c): Reduces Gastric Acid 763
- JI NEI JIN (c): Increase Peristalsis, Evacuation ... 638
- NIU XI (c): Inhibits Peristalsis 684
- SHAN ZHI ZI (c): Decreased Secretion, 1/10-1/5th Of
Atropine 476

STOMACH COLD

- BI BA/GAO LIANG JIANG: Abdomnl Pain, Vomiting
- CAO DOU KOU/WU ZHU YU: Abdominal Pain, Vomit,
Clear, Pale Lips, Tongue
- CHEN XIANG/ZI SU YE: Hiccups, Vomiting
- CHEN XIANG/DING XIANG/BAI DOU KOU: Belching,
Vomiting
- DING XIANG/WU ZHU YU: Abdominal Pain, Vomit
- GAN JIANG/GAO LIANG JIANG: Abdominal Pain,
Vomiting
- HU JIAO/GAO LIANG JIANG: Vomit, Diarrhea,
Abdominal Pain

STOMACH COLD, QI STAGNATION

STOMACH COLD/HEAT

STOMACH DEFICIENCY

STOMACH EXCESS

STOMACH EXCESS FIRE

STOMACH EXCESS HEAT

STOMACH EXCESS HEAT/TOXIC HEAT

STOMACH FIRE

STOMACH FIRE RISING

STOMACH HEART HEAT

STOMACH HEAT

STOMACH HEAT, INJURED YIN

STOMACH HEAT, THIRST

STOMACH INTESTINES DAMP STAGNATION

STOMACH INTESTINES HEAT ACCUMULATION

STOMACH INTESTINES STAGNATION

STOMACH LIVER ATTACKING

STOMACH PHLEGM FLUID

STOMACH QI DISHARMONY

STOMACH QI REFLUX

STOMACH QI, DEFICIENT W/HEAT

STOMACH QI, PROTECTS FROM OTHER HERBS

STOMACH REFLUX

STOMACH, DISTENTION, ANOREXIA

• SHEN QU/ZHI KE: Cold Stagnation

STOMACH, DISTENTION, PAIN

• GAN JIANG/HOU PO: Cold Congested Fluids

STOMACH, FIRM MASS

STOMACH, FLU

STOMACH, FOCAL DISTENTION

• ZHI SHI/HOU PO: Food Stagnation And Qi Obstruction

STOMACH, FULLNESS

• HOU PO/CANG ZHU/FU LING : Stomach Excess

STOMACH, FULLNESS, DISCOMFORT

• FO SHOU/MU XIANG/QING PI

STOMACH, FULLNESS, DISTENTION

• XIANG FU/SU GENG

STOMACH, FULLNESS, VOMITING

• HUANG LIAN/HUANG QIN/BAN XIA/GAN JIANG: Damp Heat In Middle

STOMACH, FULLNESS/DISCOMFORT

• CANG ZHU/HOU PO: Dampness Blocking Middle Jiao

STOMACH, FULLNESS/DISTENTION

• CHEN PI/HOU PO/CANG ZHU/(PING WEI SAN)

STOMACH, GAS

STOMACH, HYPERACIDITY

STOMACH, INCREASES SPUTUM IN

STOMACH, INDIGESTION

STOMACH, INDIGESTION, ACUTE/CHRONIC

• SHA REN/MU XIANG

STOMACH, INHIBITS SECRETIONS

STOMACH, INHIBITS SECRETIONS, PREVENTS STRESS ULCERS

STOMACH, MASSES

• TU BIE CHONG/BIE JIA/DA HUANG/MU DAN PI/TAO REN/(BIE JIA JIAN WAN): Tumors

STOMACH, PAIN

See: Stomach/Digestive Disorders Stomach, Ache 397
• CANG ZHU/XIANG FU: Blocked Qi, Dampness
• CAO DOU KOU/HOU PO/CANG ZHU/BAN XIA: Cold Very Damp Blockage
• CAO DOU KOU/ROU GUI/GAN JIANG: Very Cold Damp Blockage
• FO SHOU/MU XIANG/ZHI KE: Spleen Stomach Qi Stagnation
• GAN JIANG/GAN CAO: Stomach Spleen Cold Deficient
• GAO LIANG JIANG/XIANG FU/(LIANG FU WAN): Cold
• GOU QI ZI/DANG GUI/SHU DI HUANG/BEI SHA SHEN/CHUAN LIAN ZI: Yin Deficiency And Liver Qi Stagnation
• HAI PIAO XIAO/CHUAN BEI MU/(WU BEI SAN)
• LU HUI/LONG DAN CAO/HUANG QIN: Liver Channel Excess Heat
• MEI GUI HUA/XIANG FU/CHUAN LIAN ZI: Liver Qi Stagnation
• MEI GUI HUA/FO SHOU/XIANG FU/YU JIN: Liver, Stomach Qi Stagnation
• MO YAO/YAN HU SUO/WU LING ZHI/XIANG FU: Qi, Blood Stagnation
• MO YAO/CHUAN LIAN ZI/YAN HU SUO
• MU HU DIE/XIANG FU/CHUAN LIAN ZI: Stagnant Qi In Liver Stomach
• MU XIANG/SHA REN: Qi Blockage/Food Stagnation
• ROU GUI/GAN JIANG/BAI ZHU/FU ZI/(GUI FU LI ZHONG WAN): Spleen Kidney Yang Deficiency
• ROU GUI/GAN JIANG/WU ZHU YU/DANG GUI/CHUAN XIONG: Cold Stagnation
• RU XIANG/CHUAN LIAN ZI/YAN HU SUO
• TAN XIANG/SHA REN/DING XIANG/HUO XIANG: Stagnant Qi
• TAN XIANG/SHA REN/WU YAO: Cold, Qi Stagnation
• WA LENG ZI/HAI PIAO XIAO
• WU LING ZHI/(quick fried ginger): Deficient Cold, Blood Stasis
• WU LING ZHI/XIANG FU
• WU YAO/MU XIANG: Cold Stagnation, Qi Blockage
• WU ZHU YU/SHENG JIANG: Jue Yin/Shao Yin
• WU ZHU YU/HUANG LIAN/(ZUO JIN WAN): Liver Stomach Heat, Disharmony
• WU ZHU YU/GAN JIANG/MU XIANG: Cold Attacking Spleen, Stomach
• XIANG FU/MU XIANG: Liver Spleen Qi Blockage
• XIANG FU/MU XIANG/(XIANG YUAN-CITRON)/FO SHOU: Liver Attacking Stomach
• ZHE BEI MU/HAI PIAO XIAO

STOMACH, PAIN FROM SWELLING

STOMACH, PAIN W/ACID REGURGITATION

STOMACH, PAIN, DISTENTION

STOMACH, PAIN, DISTENTION IN PIT

STOMACH, PAIN, ESPECIALLY FROM CHRONIC HEPATITIS

STOMACH, PAIN, STABBING

STOMACH, PAIN, SWELLING

STOMACH, PAIN/DISTENTION

STOMACH, PAIN/PRESSURE/DISTENTION

STOMACH, PEPTIC ULCER, BLEEDING

STOMACH, POSTPARTUM DYSFUNCTION

STOMACH, PROBLEMS

STOMACH, PROLAPSE

STOMACH, PROLONGS TIME FOOD IN

STOMACH, PROTECTS LINING OF

STOMACH, REGULATES GASTRIC SECRETION

STOMACH, SPASMS

STOMACH, STAGNANT WATER IN

STOMACH, STUFFINESS, RIGIDITY

STOMACH, ULCERS, PAINFUL

STOMACH, UPSET

STOMACH, WEAK

STOMACHIC

STOMACHIC, AROMATIC BITTER

ULCER

ULCERS

ULCERS, GASTRIC

ULCERS, GASTRIC, PAINFUL

ULCERS, GASTRIC-INHIBITS FORMATION OF FROM NERVOUSNESS

ULCERS, GASTRIC/DUODENAL

ULCERS, GASTRIC/SKIN

ULCERS, GASTRIC/SMALL INTESTINE

ULCERS, PEPTIC

VOMITING, ABDOMINAL PAIN

- DING XIANG/WU ZHU YU: Stomach Cold

VOMITING, AFTER MEALS

- SHI CHANG PU/HUANG LIAN: Damp Heat Blocking Middle Jiao

VOMITING, BITTER, SOUR

VOMITING, BLOOD IN

- BAI JI/HAI PIAO XIAO/(WU JI SAN)
- CE BAI YE/DA JI/XIAO JI/BAI MAO GEN: Heat
- XIAN HE CAO/SHENG DI HUANG/MU DAN PI/SHAN ZHI ZI/CE BAI YE: Heat

VOMITING, CALF MUSCLE SPASMS

- MU GUA/HUO XIANG/SHA REN: Summer Heat

VOMITING, CAUSES

VOMITING, CHILDHOOD

- ROU DOU KOU/BAN XIA/GAN JIANG/SHEN QU/SHA REN: Spleen Stomach Cold Deficient

End of Topic:
TRANQUILIZING

TRAUMA, BITES, POISONINGS :

ACONITINE POISONING

See: Trauma, Bites, Poisonings Fu Zi Antidote
.... 410

ALCOHOLIC INTOXICATION

ALTITUDE SICKNESS, ACUTE

ALTITUDE SICKNESS, ACUTE, PREVENTION

ALTITUDE SICKNESS, IN MOUNTAINS

ANAPHYLACTIC SHOCK

ANTIDOTE, TOXICS

ANTIDOTE, TRIPTERGIUM WILFORDII POISONING

ANTIHISTAMINE

ANTIMONY POISONING ANTIDOTE

ANTIVENIN

BALLONFISH POISONING

BED BUGS

BITES, BUGS

BITES, CENTIPEDE

BITES, DOG

BITES, DOG, SNAKE, SPIDER

BITES, INSECT

BITES, INSECT, TOXIC

BITES, MOSQUITO

BITES, SCORPION

BITES, SNAKE

INFLAMMATORY, ANTI-, ENHANCES CORTICO STEROID LEVELS

INFLAMMATORY, ANTI-, REDUCES EDEMA

INJURIES

INJURIES, EXTERNAL

INJURIES, FROM COLD

INJURIES, PAIN

INJURIES, TRAUMATIC

INJURIES, TRAUMATIC, PAINFUL

INSECT BITES

INSECT BITES, TOXIC

INSECTICIDE

LACERATIONS

LACERATIONS, BLEEDING

LEAD POISONING

LIMB, SEVERED (FINGER)

MERCURY POISONING, NEUTRALIZES

MOSQUITO BITES

MOSQUITO REPELLANT

MOSQUITO REPELLENT

MOTION SICKNESS

MOUNTAIN SICKNESS

MUSCLES, TRAUMA TO

- GU SUI BU/XU DUAN
- GU SUI BU/XU DUAN/RU XIANG/MO YAO/ZI RAN TONG: Strong Combination

OPERATION, POST

PAIN, SWELLING, BRUISING

- SHUI ZHI/SAN QI

PAIN, TRAUMA

- ZE LAN/CHUAN XIONG

POISONING

POISONING W/FU ZI

- LU DOU/GAN CAO

POISONING, ACONITINE

POISONING, ANTIMONY

POISONING, ARSENIC, ANTIDOTE

POISONING, BALLONFISH, SLOWS ABSORBTION

POISONING, FISH

POISONING, FROM HYPNOTICS

POISONING, LEAD

POISONING, MERCURY, NEUTRALIZES

POISONING, PESTICIDES

POISONS, INHIBITS ABSORPTION IN GI

POST OPERATIVE PAIN

POST OPERATIVE RECOVERY, SPEEDS

- YI TANG/GUI ZHI/BAI SHAO/GAN CAO/HUANG QI

TOXINS, ANTIDOTE

TOXINS, ANTIDOTE FOR MANY SUBSTANCES

TOXINS, BENZENE POISONING CHRONIC

TOXINS, DETOXIFIES

TOXINS, FEBRILE

TOXINS, FISH, DOLPHIN

TOXINS, HELPS LIVER TO RECOVER FROM EXPOSURE

TOXINS, HELPS TO EXCRETE

TOXINS, LIVER

TOXINS, LIVER PROTECTING

TOXINS, NEUTRALIZES

TOXINS, SKIN/MUCOUS PROTECTING

TRAUMA

TRAUMA, BACK/LIMBS

TRAUMA, BLEEDING

TRAUMA, BLOOD STASIS

TRAUMA, BRUISES

TRAUMA, BY COLD

TRAUMA, CHEST/HYPOCHONDRIAC PAIN

TRAUMA, CONVALESCENT PHASE, TO REGAIN STRENGTH

TRAUMA, EXTERNAL

TRAUMA, FALLS

TRAUMA, HEAD INJURIES

TRAUMA, HEMORRHAGE OF

TRAUMA, INJURIES

TRAUMA, INJURIES, PAIN

TRAUMA, INJURIES, SWELLING

TRAUMA, INTERNAL

TRAUMA, INTERNAL, EXTERNAL

TRAUMA, INTERNAL/EXTERNAL

TRAUMA, LIGAMENTOUS INJURIES, ESPECIALLY

TRAUMA, MUSCULOSKELETAL

TRAUMA, PAIN

TRAUMA, PAIN LOWER BACK, LEGS

TRAUMA, PAIN, BLOOD STASIS

TRAUMA, PAIN, INJURIES, INTERNAL/EXTERNAL

TRAUMA, PAIN, MUSCLES, JOINTS

TRAUMA, PAIN, SWELLING

URINARY BLADDER :

ALBUMINURIA

• DANG SHEN (c): Dang Shen With Huang Qi, *Dang Shen
Gui LU Wan (Dang Shen, Gui Ban Jiao, LU Jiao Jiao, E
Jiao, Shu Di, Dang Gui) 762

BEDWETTING

See: Urinary Bladder Enuresis 421

BLADDER QI OBSTRUCTION

• ZHI MU/HUANG BAI/ROU GUI: Damp Heat In Lower
Burner

BLADDER STONES

See: Urinary Bladder Urinary Bladder Stones 422
• HUA SHI 597

BLADDER STONES, PREVENTS FORMATION OF

• ER CHA (c) 839

CHYLURIA

• BEI XIE 587
• GUAN ZHONG (c): Carbonized 521

- HUANG QI (c) 765
- MU TONG 599
- YU MI XU (c) 605

CYSTITIS

- LONG DAN CAO (c): Liver Gall Bladder Damp Heat, Use Modified Long Dan Xie Gan Tang 492
- QU MAI (c): With Bian Xu, Hai Jin Sha 600

DIURETIC

See: Kidneys Diuretic 198

DRIBBLING

- DENG XIN CAO 592
- SHI WEI 601

DRIBBLING W/PAIN

- BEI XIE 587

DYSURIA

See: Urinary Bladder Lin 421
See: Urinary Bladder Urination, Painful 427
See: Urinary Bladder Urination, Difficult 425
- BAI HUA SHE SHE CAO/BAI MAO GEN/CHE QIAN ZI/FU LING : Damp Heat
- BIAN XU/QU MAI/CHE QIAN ZI: Damp Heat In Lower Burner
- CHE QIAN ZI/ZE XIE: Ling Bing
- CHE QIAN ZI/MU TONG/SHAN ZHI ZI/HUA SHI/(BA ZHENG SAN)
- CHUAN NIU XI/TONG CAO/HUA SHI/QU MAI/(NIU XI TANG)
- DA DOU HUANG JUAN/HUA SHI/TONG CAO: Damp Heat, Damp Summer Heat, Damp Bi
- DI FU ZI/ZHU LING/TONG CAO/QU MAI: Damp Heat In Bladder
- DI FU ZI/HUA SHI/CHE QIAN ZI
- DI LONG/NIU XI/DONG KUI ZI/JIN QIAN CAO: Hot Lin
- DI LONG/CHE QIAN ZI/MU TONG: Urinary Bladder Heat Accumulation
- DONG KUI ZI/FU LING
- DONG KUI ZI/FU LING /BAI ZHU
- FU LING /ZHU LING/ZE XIE/BAI ZHU/(WU LING SAN)
- FU ZI/BAI ZHU/FU LING /(ZHEN WU TANG): Spleen Kidney Yang Deficient
- HAI GE KE/DONG KUI ZI/MU TONG
- HAI JIN SHA CAO/BIAN XU: Damp Heat
- HAI JIN SHA CAO/HUA SHI/JIN QIAN CAO/CHE QIAN ZI/HU PO: Damp Heat
- HU PO/HAI JIN SHA CAO/JIN QIAN CAO
- HUA SHI/MU TONG/CHE QIAN ZI/BIAN XU/SHAN ZHI ZI/(BA ZHENG SAN): Damp Heat In Urinary Bladder
- HUANG BAI/XI XIN
- KU SHEN/PU GONG YING/SHI WEI: Damp Heat
- PU HUANG/XIAO JI: Damp Heat In Bladder w/Hematuria
- QU MAI/HUA SHI: Hot
- SANG BAI PI/DA FU PI/FU LING PI/(WU PI YIN)
- SHI WEI/HUA SHI/HAI JIN SHA CAO/CHE QIAN ZI: Damp Heat
- TING LI ZI/HAN FANG JI/DA HUANG/(JI JIAO LI HUANG WAN)
- TONG CAO/HUA SHI/YI YI REN: Summer Heat Dampness

- TONG CAO/HUA SHI/CHE QIAN ZI: Urinary Bladder Damp Heat
- XIANG RU/BAI ZHU
- XIAO JI/OU JIE/HUA SHI/MU TONG/(XIAO JI YIN ZI)
- YI MU CAO/BAI MAO GEN
- YI YI REN/ZE XIE/BAI ZHU: Spleen Deficiency
- YIN CHEN/HUA SHI: Summer Heat/Fever, Hot
- YU CAO/CHE QIAN ZI/BAI MAO GEN: Damp Heat
- ZE XIE/FU LING /ZHU LING/BAI ZHU/(WU LING SAN)
- ZHU LING/FU LING /ZE XIE/(SI LING SAN)
- BAI HUA SHE SHE CAO: Damp Heat 511
- BI ZI CAO 587
- BIAN XU 588
- CHE QIAN CAO (c): 15-30 g 589
- CHE QIAN ZI 590
- CHE QIAN ZI (c): 3-10 g 590
- CHI XIAO DOU 591
- DA DOU HUANG JUAN 506
- DAN ZHU YE: Small Intestine Heat 470
- DENG XIN CAO 592
- DI FU ZI: Damp Heat In UB 592
- DI LONG 744
- DONG KUI ZI 594
- FENG WEI CAO 496
- GAN SUI 551
- GUI ZHI 445
- HAI JIN SHA 522
- HAI JIN SHA CAO: Damp Heat 522
- HAN FANG JI 596
- HAN SHUI SHI 471
- HU PO 737
- HUA SHI: Hot 597
- HUANG QIN: Damp Heat 489
- JIN QIAN CAO 598
- JIN YIN HUA 524
- KU SHEN 491
- LU LU TONG 681
- LU XIAN CAO 566
- LUO BU MA 748
- MU TONG: Damp Heat, With Concentrated Urine ... 599
- NIU XI: Auxillary Herb 684
- QU MAI 600
- SANG BAI PI: Lung Heat 703
- SHAN ZHI ZI 476
- SHANG LU 554
- SHI SHANG BAI: Damp Heat 534
- SHI WEI 601
- SHU FU 687
- TONG CAO: Damp Heat 601
- WU JIA PI 574
- WU JIA SHEN 771
- XI GUA 509
- XIANG RU: Especially As External Pattern ... 453
- XU SUI ZI 556
- YI MU CAO 694
- YIN CHEN 603
- YU MI XU (c) 605
- YU XING CAO: Damp Heat 539
- ZE XIE 605
- ZHI MU 480

- ZHU LING: Dampness 606
- ZHU LING (c): 6-12 g/Day 606
- ZHU MA GEN 607

DYSURIA W/EDEMA

- ZE XIE/MU DAN PI/(tonify SP & QI)
- BAI MAO GEN 653

DYSURIA W/HEMATURIA

- TONG CAO/QU MAI: Heat
- BA JIAO GEN 510
- HE YE 507
- RONG SHU XU 570
- XUE YU TAN 666
- XUE YU TAN (c): w/Hua Shi 666

DYSURIA W/SCANTY URINE, EDEMA

- ZE XIE/MU TONG
- ZE XIE/SHA REN

DYSURIA W/STONES

- PENG SHA 844

DYSURIA, DRIBBLING

- CHE QIAN ZI/HAI JIN SHA CAO: Heat In Lower Burner

DYSURIA, HOT

- JIN QIAN CAO/BIAN XU

DYSURIA, INFECTION

- HU PO 737

DYSURIA, PAINFUL

- ZHU LING/FU LING
- ZHU LING/MU TONG/HUA SHI: Heat

DYSURIA, SHORT STABBING

- SHI WEI/QU MAI/HUA SHI: Damp Heat In Lower Burner

ENURESIS

See: Urinary Bladder Urinary Incontinence 423
- SHA YUAN ZI/FU PEN ZI: Liver Kidney Deficiency
- WU YAO/YI ZHI REN/SHAN YAO/(SUO QUAN WAN):
  Cold Deficient Kidneys
- YI ZHI REN/WU YAO/SHAN YAO/(SUO QUAN WAN):
  Spleen Kidney Cold, Deficient
- BU GU ZHI 773
- CAO MIAN HUA ZI 850
- DANG GUI (c) 795
- DU ZHONG 775
- FU PEN ZI: Kidney Yang Deficient 820
- GOU JI 778
- JI NEI JIN 638
- JIANG CAN (c) 746
- JIN YING ZI 823
- JIU CAI ZI 782
- QIAN SHI 826
- SHA YUAN ZI 786
- SHAN YAO 769
- SHI DI 630
- TU SI ZI 787

- WU YAO 632
- WU YAO (c): Suo Chuan Pill 632
- YI ZHI REN 790

ENURESIS, CHILDHOOD

See: Childhood Disorders Enuresis, Childhood . 81
- SANG PIAO XIAO/YUAN ZHI/FU SHEN/DANG
  SHEN/DANG GUI
- BU GU ZHI (c): Herb Powder 773
- FU XIAO MAI 820
- JI NEI JIN (c): 9 g Roasted, Powdered Mixed With Water
  And Drunk With Sang Piao Xiao, 9 g, Duan Long Gu, 12
  g, Duan Mu LI, 12 g, Wheat/Barley, Zhi Gan Cao 638
- MA HUANG (c): May Cause Urinary Retention By
  Bladder 448
- SANG PIAO XIAO: Kidney Yang Deficient 827

ENURESIS, CHILDHOOD NOCTURNAL

- FU XIAO MAI/SANG PIAO XIAO/YI ZHI REN

ENURESIS, NOCTURNAL

See: Urinary Bladder Nocturia 422
- JIN YING ZI/QIAN SHI/TU SI ZI: Kidney Deficient
- SANG PIAO XIAO/LONG GU/MU LI/TU SI ZI/BU GU ZHI:
  Kidney Yang Deficient

EXCRETION

- CANG ZHU (c): Increases Salts Excretion, Not Diuretic:
  Increase Ion Output, Not So Much Fluids 578

GLUCOSURIA

- WEI LING XIAN (c): Controlled 572

HEMATURIA

See: Hemorrhagic Disorders Hematuria 169

INCONTINENCE

- JIU CAI ZI 782
- LIAN XU: Kidney Deficient 823
- SHAN ZHU YU 827

LI, HOT

- BAI MAO GEN/CHE QIAN ZI/JIN QIAN CAO

LI, W/STONES

- PENG SHA 844

LIN

See: Urinary Bladder Urinary Painful Obstruction
.... 424
See: Urinary Bladder Dysuria 420

LIN DISEASE, PAINFUL URINATION SYNDROME

- SHU YANG QUAN 535

LIN, HEAT TYPE

- SHAN ZHI ZI/HUA SHI: Damp Heat In Bladder

LIN, HOT, PAINFUL W/STONES

- DI LONG/NIU XI/DONG KUI ZI/JIN QIAN CAO

NOCTURIA

See: **Urinary Bladder** Enuresis, Nocturnal 421
* JIU CAI ZI/LONG GU/SANG PIAO XIAO: Kidney Yang Deficient
* SANG PIAO XIAO/SHAN ZHU YU/HUANG QI: Kidney Deficient
* SANG PIAO XIAO: In Children 827
* SHI DI 630
* YI ZHI REN 790

OLIGURIA

See: **Urinary Bladder** Urination, Scanty 428
* CHE QIAN CAO 589
* CHE QIAN ZI 590
* CHI FU LING 483
* DAN ZHU YE 470
* DONG GUA PI 593
* DONG KUI ZI 594
* FU LING 594
* HAN FANG JI 596
* JING MI 767
* LUO BU MA 748
* ZHU LING 606

PAINFUL URINARY DYSFUNCTION

* HAI FU SHI: Hot 720

POLYURIA

* FU PEN ZI 820
* YING SU KE 832

PROTEINURIA, REDUCES

* HUANG QI (c): Needs High Doses 765

URETHRITIS

* BIAN XU 588
* CHUAN XIN LIAN 518
* LONG DAN CAO (c): Liver Gall Bladder Damp Heat, Use Modified Long Dan Xie Gan Tang 492
* PU HUANG (c): Pu Huang San (Pu Huang, Semen Malval Verticillatae, Sheng Di, Equal Amounts) 660

URETHRITIS, ACUTE

* HAI JIN SHA 522
* HAI JIN SHA CAO 522
* JIN QIAN CAO 598

URINARY BLADDER CANCER

* SHAN DOU GEN 532

URINARY BLADDER COLD DAMP W/TURBID URINE

* BEI XIE/YI ZHI REN/SHI CHANG PU/WU YAO/(BI XIE FEN QING YIN)

URINARY BLADDER DAMP HEAT

* DI FU ZI/ZHU LING/TONG CAO/QU MAI: Dysuria
* PU HUANG/XIAO JI
* CHI FU LING 483
* SHI SHANG BAI 534

URINARY BLADDER DYSFUNCTION

* MU TONG 599

URINARY BLADDER STIMULANT

* HUANG LIAN (c): Stimulates Smooth Muscles 486

URINARY BLADDER STONES

See: **Urinary Bladder** Bladder Stones 419
* JIN QIAN CAO/HAI JIN SHA CAO/JI NEI JIN/(SAN JIN TANG)
* JIN QIAN CAO 598
* JIN QIAN CAO (c): Urine Becomes Acidic Which Dissolves Alkaline Induced Stones 598
* QIAN CAO GEN (c): Helps Passage Of, Helps To Prevent Formation Of, Especially Calcium Carbonate Stones, But Removes By Stimulation Of Muscles In Bladder ... 662
* ZHI XUE CAO 697

URINARY BLADDER STONES W/DYSURIA

* PENG SHA 844

URINARY BLADDER, ACUTE BACTERIAL CYSTITIS

* SHAN ZHI ZI (c) 476

URINARY BLADDER, DAMP HEAT

* BIAN XU/QU MAI/MU TONG/HUA SHI/(BA ZHEN SAN)
* DI FU ZI/HUA SHI/CHE QIAN ZI
* HAI JIN SHA CAO/HUA SHI/JIN QIAN CAO/CHE QIAN ZI/HU PO: All Types Of Manifestations
* HUA SHI/MU TONG/CHE QIAN ZI/BIAN XU/SHAN ZHI ZI/(BA ZHENG SAN)
* JIN QIAN CAO/HAI JIN SHA CAO/JI NEI JIN/(SAN JIN TANG): Hot Painful Urination
* SHI WEI/HUA SHI/HAI JIN SHA CAO/CHE QIAN ZI: All Manifestations
* TONG CAO/HUA SHI/CHE QIAN ZI

URINARY BLADDER, DAMP HEAT FLOWING INTO

* CHE QIAN ZI/MU TONG/SHAN ZHI ZI/HUA SHI/(BA ZHENG SAN)

URINARY BLADDER, INCREASES TONE

* MA HUANG (c): Reduces Urination 448

URINARY DIFFICULTY

* DONG KUI ZI/MU TONG
* SHANG LU/CHI XIAO DOU

URINARY DIFFICULTY W/EXCESS EDEMA

* SHANG LU/BING LANG

URINARY DISCOMFORT

* DA DOU HUANG JUAN/HUA SHI/TONG CAO: Damp Heat, Damp Summer Heat, Damp Bi
* DONG KUI ZI/FU LING
* HUA SHI/DONG KUI ZI
* ROU GUI/HUANG BAI/ZHI MU: Kidney Deficient
* ZE XIE/SHA REN

URINARY DISORDERS

URINARY DISORDERS, THIRST OF

URINARY DRIBBLING, WHITE

URINARY DYSFUNCTION

• BAI WEI/DAN ZHU YE: Yin Deficient, Blood Heat
• FU LING /CHE QIAN ZI
• HUA SHI/DONG KUI ZI: Damp Heat In Urinary Bladder
• HUA SHI/GAN CAO/(LIU YI SAN): Summer Heat
• JING DA JI/GAN JIANG

URINARY DYSFUNCTION, PAINFUL

• HAI GE KE/DONG KUI ZI/MU TONG
• MU TONG/CHE QIAN ZI: Heat In Heart Small Intestine Channel
• TONG CAO/HUA SHI/YI YI REN: Summer Heat Dampness
• TONG CAO/QU MAI: Heat w/Blood

URINARY DYSFUNCTION, PAINFUL W/IRRITABILITY

• FU LING /ZE XIE/GUI ZHI/BAI ZHU: Dampness Obstruction

URINARY DYSFUNCTION, PAINFUL W/LINGERING DAMPNESS

• FU LING /ZE XIE

URINARY DYSFUNCTION, PAINFUL W/STONES

• JI NEI JIN/JIN QIAN CAO
• YU JIN/JIN QIAN CAO

URINARY DYSFUNCTION, PAINFUL, HOT

• HU PO/HAI JIN SHA CAO/JIN QIAN CAO
• JIN QIAN CAO/BIAN XU
• NIU XI/DANG GUI/HUANG QIN
• SHAN ZHI ZI/HUA SHI: Damp Heat In Urinary Bladder

URINARY DYSFUNCTION, PAINFUL, TURBID

• FU LING /CHE QIAN ZI

URINARY FREQUENCY

See: **Urinary Bladder** Urination, Frequent 426
• BA JI TIAN/BU GU ZHI/FU PEN ZI: Kidney Yang Deficient
• BEI XIE/YI ZHI REN/WU YAO: Especially Yang Deficient
• DONG KUI ZI/MU TONG
• FU PEN ZI/SANG PIAO XIAO/YI ZHI REN: Deficient Lower Jiao
• FU ZI/ROU GUI: Kidney Yang Deficiency

• HAI MA/GOU QI ZI/DA ZAO: Kidney Yang Deficient
• JIU CAI ZI/LONG GU/SANG PIAO XIAO: Kidney Yang Deficient
• SANG PIAO XIAO/SHAN ZHU YU/HUANG QI: Kidney Deficiency
• WU YAO/YI YI REN/SHAN YAO/(SUO QUAN WAN): Cold Deficient Kidneys

URINARY FREQUENCY IN ADULTS

• JI NEI JIN/SANG PIAO XIAO/LONG GU/MU LI

URINARY FREQUENCY, NIGHT/DAY

• BU GU ZHI/TU SI ZI/YI ZHI REN: Kidney Yang Deficient

URINARY FREQUENCY, NIGHTS

See: **Urinary Bladder** Urination, Nigh Frequency
.... 427

URINARY FREQUENCY, PAIN, URGENCY

• HUA SHI/DONG KUI ZI
• HUANG BAI/XI XIN

URINARY INCONTINENCE

See: **Urinary Bladder** Enuresis 421
• BA JI TIAN/BU GU ZHI/FU PEN ZI: Kidney Yang Deficient
• BAI GUO/SANG PIAO XIAO/YI ZHI REN
• BEI XIE/YI ZHI REN/WU YAO: Especially Yang Deficient
• FU PEN ZI/SANG PIAO XIAO/YI ZHI REN: Deficient Lower Jiao
• LU FENG FANG/SANG PIAO XIAO
• SANG PIAO XIAO/SHAN ZHU YU/HUANG QI: Kidney Deficiency
• SHUI ZHI/MANG XIAO/DA HUANG: Blood Stasis/Ecchymosis From Heat Invasion
• SUO YANG/SANG PIAO XIAO: Kidney Yang Deficient

URINARY INCONTINENCE, CHILDHOOD

- FU XIAO MAI/SANG PIAO XIAO/YI ZHI REN
- JI NEI JIN/SANG PIAO XIAO/LONG GU/MU LI
- YI ZHI REN/WU YAO/SHAN YAO/(SUO QUAN WAN): Spleen Kidney Cold, Deficient
- SANG PIAO XIAO 827

URINARY INCONTINENCE, PRENATAL/POSTPARTUM

- BAI WEI/BAI SHAO/(IN WINE)

URINARY INFECTIONS

- SHAN ZI CAO 664

URINARY INFECTIONS, ACUTE

- SHI WEI 601

URINARY OBSTRUCTION

- DAI MAO 743
- QU MAI 600

URINARY OBSTRUCTION, PARTIAL

- DI LONG 744

URINARY PAINFUL OBSTRUCTION

See: Urinary Bladder Lin 421
- NIU XI/JIN QIAN CAO: Especially w/Stones And Hematuria

URINARY RETENTION

- DI LONG/NIU XI/DONG KUI ZI/JIN QIAN CAO: Hot Lin
- HU PO/HAI JIN SHA CAO/JIN QIAN CAO: Urinary Bladder/Kidney Stones
- DENG XIN CAO 592
- WU JIU GEN PI 555
- XU SUI ZI 556

URINARY RETENTION W/AFTERNOON FEVERS

- ZHI MU/HUANG BAI/ROU GUI: Damp Heat In Lower Burner

URINARY RETENTION, POSTPARTUM

- HUANG QI (c) 765
- YI MU CAO (c): With Acupuncture 694

URINARY STONES

- BIAN XU/QU MAI/CHE QIAN ZI
- DI LONG/NIU XI/DONG KUI ZI/JIN QIAN CAO: Hot Lin
- DONG KUI ZI/CHE QIAN ZI/HAI JIN SHA CAO
- HU PO/HAI JIN SHA CAO/JIN QIAN CAO: Urine Retention From
- JI NEI JIN/JIN QIAN CAO
- NIU XI/JIN QIAN CAO
- QU MAI/HAI JIN SHA CAO
- YU JIN/JIN QIAN CAO
- DAN ZHU YE (c): Dao Chi San (Dan Zhu Ye, Sheng Di, Tian Xian Teng, Gan Cao) 470
- HAI FU SHI 720
- HAI JIN SHA 522

- HAI JIN SHA CAO: Damp Heat 522
- HUA SHI 597
- JI NEI JIN 638
- MU TONG 599
- NIU XI (c): Niu Xi-Ru Xiang Powder 684
- YU MI XU (c) 605

URINARY STONES, CAUSING BLEEDING

- ZI ZHU CAO/JIN QIAN CAO

URINARY STONES, EXPULSION

- HU TAO REN (c): Use Paste, In Few Days As Milky Urine 782

URINARY STONES, W/HEAMTURIA, LOWER BACK PAIN

- NIU XI: Raw 684

URINARY SYSTEM, ACUTE INFECTION

- CHE QIAN CAO 589

URINARY TRACT BLEEDING

- HUANG BAI (c) 485

URINARY TRACT DISORDERS

- HU PO/JIN QIAN CAO/MU TONG/BAI MAO GEN

URINARY TRACT DYSFUNCTION

- KU SHEN/FU LING : Damp Hot Edema

URINARY TRACT INFECTIONS

- HAI JIN SHA CAO/BIAN XU
- YU XING CAO/CHE QIAN ZI/BAI MAO GEN
- BAI HUA SHE SHE CAO 511
- BAI HUA SHE SHE CAO (c) 511
- BEI XIE: With Milky Urine 587
- BI CHENG QIE (c): Volatile Oil Prevents 609
- BIAN XU 588
- CHE QIAN ZI 590
- CHUAN XIN LIAN: Acute 518
- DAN ZHU YE 470
- DAN ZHU YE (c): Dao Chi San (Dan Zhu Ye, Sheng Di, Tian Xian Teng, Gan Cao) 470
- DENG XIN CAO 592
- DI LONG: Hot 744
- HAI FU SHI 720
- HAI JIN SHA CAO: Damp Heat 522
- HU HUANG LIAN (c) 484
- LIAN QIAO 525
- LU XIAN CAO (c): Controls Acute Symptoms, Did Not Eliminate Infection 566
- NIU XI: Auxillary Herb 684
- TU FU LING 536
- YU XING CAO 539
- ZE XIE 605
- ZHU LING (c): 6-12 g/Day 606

URINARY TRACT INFECTIONS, ACUTE

- BAI WEI: Damp Heat 495
- DI FU ZI 592
- DONG KUI ZI 594

URINATION, DRIBBLING W/BLOOD

URINATION, DRIBBLING W/TURBID DISCHARGE

URINATION, DRIBBLING, CONCENTRATED, RED/YELLOW/TURBID

URINATION, DYSFUNCTION

URINATION, EXCESS

URINATION, EXCESS AT NIGHT

URINATION, EXCESS/FREQUENT

URINATION, FREQUENT

URINATION, FREQUENT W/SCANTY AMOUNT

URINATION, PAINFUL, BURNING, DRIBBLING
• QU MAI/SHAN ZHI ZI: Damp Heat In Lower Jiao

URINATION, PAINFUL, CHILDHOOD
• DONG KUI ZI/MU TONG

URINATION, PAINFUL, DARK
• DENG XIN CAO/DAN ZHU YE: Heart Fire

URINATION, PAINFUL, DRIBBLING

URINATION, PAINFUL, DRIBBLING, CONCENTRATED, RED/YELLOW/TURBID

URINATION, PAINFUL, HOT
• QU MAI/HUA SHI

URINATION, PAINFUL, INCOMPLETE W/IRRITABILITY
• DENG XIN CAO/HUA SHI: Damp Heat In Heart, Urinary Bladder, Lung

URINATION, PAINFUL, LI

URINATION, PAINFUL, TURBID

URINATION, PAINFUL, W/BLOOD

URINATION, PAINFUL, W/STONES

URINATION, POST-URINE DRIPS

URINATION, PROMOTES

URINATION, REDUCED
• HUANG QI/HAN FANG JI: Wind Edema
• YU JIN/YIN CHEN: Damp Heat Diseases

URINATION, REDUCES PROTEINURIA

URINATION, RETENTION
• ROU GUI/HUANG BAI/ZHI MU: Kidney Deficient

URINATION, SANDY

URINATION, SCANTY
• HUANG QI/HAN FANG JI/BAI ZHU/(FANG JI HUANG QI TANG): Spleen Deficient w/Poor Water Metabolism
• ZE XIE/SHA REN
• ZHU LING/FU LING

WIND COLD BI, IN ELDERLY

WIND DAMP

WIND DAMP BI, IN ELDERLY

WIND DAMP COLD BI, IN ELDERLY

WIND DAMP LATERAL HEADACHE

End of Topic:
WIND DAMP LATERAL HEADACHE

WIND DISORDERS :

AVERSION TO WIND

• BAI SHAO/GUI ZHI/(GUI ZHI TANG): Wind Cold
w/Weakness, Deficiency

CONVULSIONS

DIZZINESS

EXTERNAL WIND

• JING JIE/BO HE: Cause Sweating

SPASMS

VERTIGO

See Also: Vertigo (Topics: Ears, Phlegm)

WIND

• QUAN XIE/WU GONG/(ZI JING SAN): Spasms,
Convulsions, Cramping

WIND BI

WIND COLD

• CHUAN XIONG/FANG FENG/JING JIE: Headache
• DOU CHI JIANG/JING JIE/ZI SU YE
• DU HUO/MA HUANG: Body Aches, No Sweat
• DU HUO/FANG FENG/BAI ZHI: Toothache
• FU ZI/MA HUANG/XI XIN/(MA HUANG FU ZI XI XIN
TANG): Common Cold w/Deficient Yang
• GE GEN/MA HUANG/GUI ZHI/BAI SHAO: Stiffness Upper
Back/Neck
• GUI ZHI/MA HUANG: Excess

• JIE GENG/ZI SU YE: Productive Cough
• JIE GENG/BAN XIA: Cough
• SHENG JIANG/DA ZAO
• XI XIN/QIANG HUO/FANG FENG/(JIU WEI QIANG HUO
TANG): Chills, Fever, General Pain
• XING REN/ZI SU YE: Dry Cough

WIND COLD ASTHMA W/CHEST CONSTRICTION FROM PHLEGM

• SHE GAN/MA HUANG/XI XIN/SHENG JIANG

WIND COLD BI

• JING JIE/BO HE/FANG FENG/QIANG HUO

WIND COLD COUGH, WHEEZING

• MA HUANG/XING REN

WIND COLD DAMP

• DU HUO/QIANG HUO/GAO BEN/MAN JING ZI:
Headaches
• GAO BEN/XI XIN: Headache
• HAI TONG PI/NIU XI/QIANG HUO: Joint Pain, Low Back,
Legs
• HAI TONG PI/KUAN JIN TENG/GUI ZHI/(external wash
for 1 month): Muscle Spasm, Joint Pain, Trauma/Bi

WIND COLD DAMP BI

• MA HUANG/GUI ZHI

WIND COLD DAMP ITCHING

• BAI XIAN PI/KU SHEN/SHE CHUANG ZI

WIND COLD DAMP, EXTERIOR INVASION

• CANG ZHU/FANG FENG/XI XIN

WIND COLD EXTERIOR EXCESS PATTERNS

WIND COLD EXTERIOR EXCESS WITHOUT SWEAT

• MA HUANG/GUI ZHI

WIND COLD EXTERIOR SYNDROME

• DAN DOU CHI/CONG BAI
• DU HUO/QIANG HUO/(QIANG HUO SHENG SHI TANG)
• JING JIE/BO HE/FANG FENG/QIANG HUO

WIND COLD EXTERIOR W/GENERAL PAIN

• FANG FENG/JING JIE/QIANG HUO

WIND COLD EXTERIOR W/HEADACHE, SEVERE GENERAL PAIN

• QIANG HUO/FANG FENG/BAI ZHI/CANG ZHU

WIND COLD EXTERIOR W/SUPRAORBITAL PAIN, NASAL OBSTRUCTION

- BAI ZHI/CONG BAI/DAN DOU CHI/SHENG JIANG

WIND COLD IN SUMMER

- HUO XIANG/ZI SU YE/BAN XIA/HOU PO/CHEN PI/(HUO XIAN ZHENG QI SAN): Chills, Fever, Headache, Nausea, Diarrhea
- XIANG RU/BAI BIAN DOU: Vomiting, Diarrea
- XIANG RU 453

WIND COLD PATTERNS

- GAO BEN 444

WIND COLD PHLEGM

- XI XIN/MA HUANG: Cough, Wheezing

WIND COLD W/CHRONIC ILLNESS

- YI TANG/GUI ZHI/BAI SHAO/GAN CAO
- YI TANG/GUI ZHI/BAI SHAO/GAN CAO/HUANG QI: Severely Weak

WIND COLD W/DAMP OBSTRUCTION IN MIDDLE JIAO

- HUO XIANG/ZI SU YE

WIND COLD W/DAMPNESS

- ZI SU YE/HUO XIANG: Vomiting, Diarrhea, Abdominal Pain

WIND COLD W/DEFICIENT QI

- REN SHEN/ZI SU YE

WIND COLD W/PHLEGM

- BAI QIAN/JIE GENG: Cough

WIND COLD W/SURFACE DEFICIENCY

- BAI SHAO/GUI ZHI/(GUI ZHI TANG)

WIND COLD W/YING-WEI DISHARMONY

- GUI ZHI/BAI SHAO: Surface Deficient

WIND COLD, COMMON COLD W/HEADACHE, NASAL OBSTRUCTION, COUGH

- ZI SU YE/SHENG JIANG/CHEN PI/XIANG FU/XING REN

WIND COLD, INITIAL STAGE

- CONG BAI/DAN DOU CHI
- CONG BAI/DAN DOU CHI/SHENG JIANG
- CONG BAI 442

WIND COLD, MILD

- FANG FENG 444

WIND DAMP

See: Pain/Numbness/General Discomfort Bi Disorders 297
- BEI XIE/NIU XI: Cold Back Pain

- CAN SHA/DU HUO/NIU XI: Pain In Extremities
- CANG ZHU/HUANG BAI/NIU XI/(SAN MIAO WAN): Skin Lesions
- MAN JING ZI/CHUAN XIONG/FANG FENG: General Pain
- QIANG HUO/DU HUO: Surface And Deep
- YI YI REN/MA HUANG/XING REN/GAN CAO: General Pain

WIND DAMP BI

- DU HUO/QIN JIAO/FANG FENG/SANG JI SHENG/(DU HUO JI SHENG TANG)
- HAN FANG JI/YI YI REN/HUA SHI/CAN SHA/MU GUA
- WEI LING XIAN/DU HUO/SANG JI SHENG/DANG GUI
- JI XUE TENG: Sore Joints 677

WIND DAMP BI OF JOINTS

- DI LONG/TIAN NAN XING/CHUAN WU/(XIAO HUO LU DAN)
- LU LU TONG/QIANG HUO/DU HUO/JI XUE TENG

WIND DAMP BI W/COLD SIGNS

- QIN JIAO/QIANG HUO/DU HUO/GUI ZHI/FU ZI

WIND DAMP BI W/HEAT SIGNS

- QIN JIAO/HAN FANG JI/REN DONG TENG

WIND DAMP LATERAL HEADACHE

- CHUAN XIONG/QIANG HUO/JIANG CAN

WIND DAMP PAIN IN JOINTS, SHOULDER, BACK

- GUANG FANG JI/WEI LING XIAN

WIND DAMP PAIN W/DEFICIENT BLOOD

- FANG FENG/QIN JIAO

WIND DAMP PAIN, SWELLIING

- CHUAN SHAN JIA/DANG GUI/CHUAN XIONG/QIANG HUO/FANG FENG: Joints

WIND DAMP, CHRONIC

- BAI HUA SHE 558

WIND DAMP, EXTERNAL CONDITIONS

- JING JIE/BO HE/HUO XIANG/PEI LAN

WIND DAMP, JOINTS

See: Musculoskeletal/Connective Tissue Joints, Pain 268

WIND DAMP, PAIN OF

- QIANG HUO/FANG FENG

WIND DAMP, STAGNANT QI BLOCKING BLOOD CHANNELS

- CHUAN XIONG/DANG GUI: Pain, Numb, Paralysis

WIND DISEASES

- SHI CHANG PU 757

WIND DISORDERS

See: Mental State/Neurological Disorders Neurological Disorders w/Shaking 255

WIND EDEMA

- HUANG QI/HAN FANG JI: Nubness, Pain, Swelling, Reduced Urination
- HAN FANG JI 596

WIND EVIL

- XI XIAN CAO 575

WIND HEAT

See: **Infectious Diseases** Common Cold 182
See: **Infectious Diseases** Influenza 188
- BO HE/NIU BANG ZI: Sores
- DI FU ZI/SHENG DI HUANG/BAI XIAN PI: Itch
- FU PING/JING JIE/BO HE/LIAN QIAO
- GE GEN/CHAI HU
- GE GEN/CHAI HU/HUANG QIN: Painful Eyes, Dry Throat
- GUA LOU/ZHE BEI MU/JIE GENG/CHEN PI: Cough, Thick Sputum, Dry Throat
- JIE GENG/GAN CAO: Hoarseness, Sore Throat
- JIN YIN HUA/LIAN QIAO/JING JIE
- JIN YIN HUA/LIAN QIAO/NIU BANG ZI: Common Cold
- JING JIE/BO HE/SANG YE/JU HUA: Common Cold
- JING JIE/BO HE/HUANG QIN/JU HUA: Eye Inflammations
- JING JIE/LIAN QIAO/BO HE/JIE GENG
- JUE MING ZI/JU HUA: Eye Pain
- JUE MING ZI/CHUAN XIONG/MAN JING ZI: Headache, Temporal
- LIAN QIAO/BAN LAN GEN/JING JIE/BO HE: Colds, Flu
- LIAN QIAO/NIU BANG ZI/BO HE: Common Colds
- MAN JING ZI/JU HUA: Headache, Dizzy
- MI MENG HUA/MU ZEI/GU JING CAO: Excess Tearing
- NIU BANG ZI/JIE GENG: Productive Cough, Sore Throat
- NIU BANG ZI/JIE GENG/BO HE: Productive Cough, Sore Throat
- QIAN HU/JIE GENG: Cough, Runny Nose, Headache
- QIAN HU/BO HE/NIU BANG ZI/JIE GENG: Cough
- SANG YE/JU HUA: Cough, Eye Redness, Pain
- SANG YE/JU HUA/BO HE/JING JIE: Common Cold
- SANG YE/JU HUA/JIE GENG/XING REN/BEI SHA SHEN: Cough
- SHENG MA/XUAN SHEN/JIE GENG/NIU BANG ZI: Sore Throat
- XING REN/SANG YE: Dry Cough
- XUAN SHEN/NIU BANG ZI: Sore Throat, Purpuric Rashes
- ZHE BEI MU/LIAN QIAO/NIU BANG ZI: Cough, Acute
- BAI WEI 495
- BO HE: Fever, Headache, Cough 456
- DAI MAO: Red Eyes 743
- DAN ZHU YE 470
- FU PING: Aches in Head/Body 460
- GOU TENG: Headache, Fever, Red Eyes 745
- JING JIE 447
- LA MEI HUA: Eye Irritation 680
- LIAN QIAO: Common Cold 525
- NIU BANG ZI: Fever, Cough, Sore, Red, Swollen Throat
  465
- SANG YE: Fever, Headache, Cough 466

WIND HEAT EXTERIOR SYNDROME

- DAN DOU CHI/NIU BANG ZI/LIAN QIAO

WIND HEAT EXTERIOR W/HEADACHE, RED EYES

- FANG FENG/JING JIE/HUANG QIN/BO HE/LIAN QIAO

WIND HEAT EXTERIOR W/SORE THROAT, COUGH

- SANG YE/JU HUA/JIE GENG/BO HE/LIAN QIAO

WIND HEAT EXTERIOR, WITH RED, SORE EYES

- BO HE/JIE GENG/NIU BANG ZI/JU HUA

WIND HEAT FEVER W/DYSPNEA, COUGH

- SHI GAO (c) 477

WIND HEAT IN LIVER CHANNEL

- CHAN TUI/JU HUA/MU ZEI: Eyes Red, Watery
- BAI JI LI: Headache, Dizziness, Red, Swollen Eyes 743
- GE GEN 460
- GU JING CAO 461

WIND HEAT IN LUNGS

- PANG DA HAI/SHI CHANG PU/BO HE: Hoarseness

WIND HEAT PHLEGM

- ZHU LI/BAN XIA

WIND HEAT W/EYE PROBLEMS

- MU ZEI/CHAN TUI/GU JING CAO/XIA KU CAO/BAI JI LI

WIND HEAT W/HOARSE VOICE, SORE THROAT

- CHAN TUI/PANG DA HAI/NIU BANG ZI/JIE GENG

WIND HEAT, DAMPNESS

- GU JING CAO/FANG FENG

WIND HEAT, EARLY STAGE

- JIN YIN HUA 524

WIND HEAT, EARLY STAGE W/SORE THROAT

- CHUAN XIN LIAN/JIN YIN HUA/JIE GENG/NIU BANG ZI

WIND HEAT, HOT PHLEGM

- HOU ZAO/SHE XIANG/SHI CHANG PU: Respiratory Disorders

WIND HEAT, YIN DEFICIENCY

- YU ZHU/BAI WEI/(herbs to clear Wind Heat)
- YU ZHU 815

WIND HEAT/COLD W/COPIOUS SPUTUM

- QIAN HU 725

WIND IN THE HEAD, RELEASES

- JING JIE/BO HE

WIND IN YANG MING

- BAI ZHI 441

WIND PHLEGM

- TIAN NAN XING/TIAN MA: Dizzy, Seizures, Muscle Spasms
- TIAN NAN XING/BAN XIA/TIAN MA/BAI FU ZI: Dizziness, Vertigo, Facial Paralysis, etc
- ZHU SHA/HAI GE KE: Dizziness
- BAN XIA: Vertigo 710
- SU HE XIANG 758

WIND PHLEGM DIZZINESS

- TIAN MA 750
- ZHU SHA 741

WIND PHLEGM HEAT SEIZURES

- JIANG CAN 746

WIND PHLEGM OBSTRUCTION OF CHANNELS

- TIAN NAN XING/BAI FU ZI: Spasms, Paralysis

WIND PHLEGM RISING HEADACHE

- BAI FU ZI/BAI ZHI/TIAN MA/TIAN NAN XING

WIND PHLEGM W/PERICARDIUM ENVOLVEMNT

- BAI FAN: Irritability, Delirium, Convulsions 836

WIND RASH

- See: Skin Rashes 365
- CANG ER ZI/BAI JI LI
- CHAN TUI/BO HE
- CHAN TUI/BO HE/JU HUA/SANG YE
- FU PING/BO HE/CHAN TUI/SHENG MA
- HE SHOU WU/KU SHEN/BAI XIAN PI/JING JIE: Blood Deficient
- JIANG CAN/CHAN TUI/FANG FENG/MU DAN PI
- JING JIE/BO HE
- LU FENG FANG/CHAN TUI/(tincture)
- LU LU TONG/CHAN TUI/BAI XIAN PI
- WU WEI ZI/(in rice wine,160 proof): Skin Itch
- FU PING 460
- HE SHOU WU: Deficient Blood 799
- JIANG CAN: Skin Lesions 746
- ZHI XUE CAO 697

WIND RASH, CHRONIC

- WU SHAO SHE/CHAN TUI/JING JIE/CHI SHAO YAO: Wind Heat In Skin

WIND STROKE

- See: Circulation Disorders Stroke 87
- BAI HUA SHE/QUAN XIE/DANG GUI/(in wine): Hemiplegia

WIND STROKE W/PHLEGM OBSTRUCTION

- TIAN ZHU HUANG 726

WIND STROKE, PHLEGM BLOCKING CHANNELS

- BAI FU ZI/JIANG CAN/QUAN XIE: Facial Paralysis, Hemiplegia

WIND, EPIDEMIC

- ZAO JIAO CI 716

WIND, EXTERNAL

- DAN DOU CHI/CONG BAI: Initial Stage
- JING JIE/BO HE
- JING JIE/BO HE/DANG GUI/CHUAN XIONG: During Postpartum

WIND, EXTERNAL, EXCESS CONDITION

- JING JIE/FANG FENG

WIND, HEAT, PHLEGM

- TIAN ZHU HUANG/JIANG CAN: Cough, Mental Disorders

WIND, INTERNAL

- ZHU SHA/XI JIAO/NIU HUANG: Convulsions, High Fever, Unconsciousness

WIND, INTERNAL W/YIN DEFICIENCY

- BIE JIA/LONG GU/BAI SHAO/E JIAO

WIND, PHLEGM OBSTRUCTING CHANNEL

- FANG FENG/TIAN NAN XING/(Zhen Yu San)

WIND, SENSITIVITY TO

- HUANG QI/HAN FANG JI: Wind Edema

WINDSTROKE

- DI LONG/HUANG QI/DANG GUI/CHI SHAO YAO: Hemiplegia
- JI XUE TENG/DAN SHEN/DU ZHONG: Stabilized
- QUAN XIE/JIANG CAN/GOU TENG/TIAN MA: Facial Paralysis
- RU XIANG/DI LONG/CHUAN WU: Spasm, Rigidity
- SHE XIANG/SU HE XIANG/DING XIANG/(SU HE XIANG WAN): Unconsciousness
- BAI FU ZI: Wind Phlegm 708
- JI XUE TENG: Paralysis, Vertigo 677
- NIU HUANG 755
- QUAN XIE 749
- TIAN MA: Liver Wind/Wind Phlegm 750

WINDSTROKE FROM PHLEGM OBSTRUCTION

- SHE XIANG/XI JIAO/NIU HUANG/(SHI BAO DAN): Coma

WINDSTROKE OF FACE

- QUAN XIE/BAI FU ZI/JIANG CAN/(QIAN ZHEN SAN)

WINDSTROKE, PHLEGM OBSTRUCTION

- SHENG JIANG/ZHU LI: Aphasia, Numbness
- TIAN ZHU HUANG/SHI CHANG PU: Coma

WINDSTROKE, PHLEGM OBSTRUCTION OF HEART

• ZHU LI/SHENG JIANG/(large amounts juice): Coma

WINDSTROKE, STIFFNESS

WINDSTROKE, UNCONSCIOUSNESS

• SU HE XIANG/SHE XIANG/DING XIANG/AN XI XIANG/(SU HE XIANG WAN)

End of Topic:
WIND DISORDERS

WIND HEAT

WIND HEAT RASH

WIND IN THE HEAD, RELEASES

WIND PHLEGM

WIND RASH

WIND RELATED TOPICS

WIND STROKE

WIND, LIVER

WINDPIPE, RATTLING SOUND

WINDSTROKE

WITHDRAWAL, EMOTIONAL

WOMEN'S DISEASES

WORM POISONING

WORMS AND RELATED TOPICS

WORRIES, CONGESTED

WOUNDS AND RELATED TOPICS

XUE LEVEL HEAT

YANG COLLAPSE

YANG DEFICIENCY

YANG FLOATING

YANG MING STAGE DISEASE

YANG QI COLLAPSE SYNDROME

End of Topic:
YANG QI COLLAPSE SYNDROME

YANG RELATED DISORDERS/ TOPICS :

YANG COLLAPSE

• GAN JIANG/FU ZI/(SI NI TANG): Cold Sweats, Cold Extremities, Spontaneous Sweating, Listless, Fading Pulse

YANG COLLAPSE SYNDROME

• FU ZI/GAN JIANG/GAN CAO/(SI NI TANG)

YANG DEFICIENCY

• BEI XIE/YI ZHI REN/WU YAO: Urinary Frequency/Incontinence
• FU ZI/HUANG QI: Spontaneous Sweating, Chills
• HUANG QI/FU ZI: Spontaneous Sweating

YANG DEFICIENCY W/COLD LIMBS, WEAK PULSE

YANG DEFICIENCY W/EXCESS COLD DAMPNESS

• FU ZI/BAI ZHU: Edema, Diarrhea, Stomach Pain

YANG DEPLETION

YANG DEVASTATION

• REN SHEN/FU ZI/(SHEN FU TANG)

YIN RELATED DISORDERS/ TOPICS :

YIN DEFICIENCY W/FIRE

- **SHENG DI HUANG/XUAN SHEN:** Dry Throat, Irritability

YIN DEFICIENCY W/FIRE RISING

- **SHU DI HUANG/GUI BAN/HUANG BAI/ZHI MU/(ZHI BAI DI HUANG WAN):** Afternoon Fever, Palms Hot, Sweaty, Night Sweating, Red Tongue, Scanty Coating
- TIAN MEN DONG 814

YIN DEFICIENCY W/HEAT

- **HUANG BAI/ZHI MU/SHENG DI HUANG:** Nocturnal Emissions, Night Sweats
- **NIU XI/SHENG DI HUANG/DAI ZHE SHI:** Gums, Painful And Swollen
- NU ZHEN ZI/DI GU PI/MU DAN PI/SHENG DI HUANG
- HU HUANG LIAN 484
- HUA QI SHEN 808
- MAI MEN DONG 810
- MU LI 739
- NU ZHEN ZI 812
- SHENG DI HUANG 500
- TIAN MEN DONG 814

YIN DEFICIENCY W/HEAT, BLOOD DEFICIENCY

- **SHENG DI HUANG/SHU DI HUANG**

YIN DEFICIENCY W/INTERNAL HEAT

- **BIE JIA/YIN CHAI HU/DI GU PI/(QING GU SAN):** Afternoon Fever, Night Sweats
- **SHI HU/SHENG DI HUANG/BAI WEI/TIAN MEN DONG:** Afternoon Fevers

YIN DEFICIENCY W/INTERNAL WIND

- **BIE JIA/LONG GU/BAI SHAO/E JIAO**

YIN DEFICIENCY W/RISING YANG

- BAI MU ER 803

YIN DEFICIENCY W/YANG RISING

- **CI SHI/NIU XI/DU ZHONG/SHI JUE MING:** Dizzy, Flushed Face, Heavy Headed, Palpitations
- **CI SHI/LONG GU/MU LI:** Dizzy, Vertigo
- **GUI BAN/BIE JIA:** Afternoon Fever, Night Sweats
- **LONG GU/MU LI/NIU XI/DAI ZHE SHI:** Insomnia, Irritability, Blurred Vision, Dizziness
- **MU LI/LONG GU:** Headache, Dizzy, Tinnitus
- **NIU XI/DAI ZHE SHI/MU LI/LONG GU/(ZHEN GAN XI FENG TANG):** Liver Wind Rising
- MU LI 739

YIN DEFICIENCY WIND

- YU ZHU 815

YIN DEFICIENCY, FIRE RISING

- **SHI GAO/SHU DI HUANG:** Headache, Toothache, Thirst

YIN DEFICIENCY, HEAT

See: **Heat** Deficient Fire 161

YIN DEFICIENCY, LIVER QI STAGNATION

- **GOU QI ZI/DANG GUI/SHU DI HUANG/BEI SHA SHEN/CHUAN LIAN ZI:** Stomach/Flank Pain w/Dry Throat, Regurgitation, Bitterness

YIN SEPARATING FROM YANG

- FU ZI 613

YIN TONIFICATION

- **HAI LONG/E JIAO**

YIN, BLOOD DEFICIENCY

- **GOU QI ZI/SHU DI HUANG/TU SI ZI/DU ZHONG:** Dizziness, Impotence, Spermatorrhea, Tinnitus
- **SANG SHEN ZI/SHENG DI HUANG/SHU DI HUANG:** Insomnia, Blurred Vision, Dizziness

YIN, QI DEFICIENCY

- **REN SHEN/WU WEI ZI/MAI MEN DONG:** Diabetes

YIN, YANG DEFICIENCY

- **LU JIAO JIAO/GUI BAN**

YIN/BLOOD DEFICIENCY

- SANG SHEN ZI 801

YIN/YANG SEPARATION

- ROU GUI 616
- ROU GUI PI 617

End of Topic:
YIN RELATED DISORDERS/TOPICS

YIN RELATED TOPICS

See: **Yin Related Disorders/Topics** Yin Related Topics 437

YIN SEPARATING FROM YANG

See: **Yin Related Disorders/Topics** Yin Separating From Yang 438

YING & BLOOD STAGE HEAT DISORDERS

See: **Heat** Ying & Blood Stage Heat Disorders 164

YING STAGE HEAT

See: **Heat** Ying Stage Heat 164

YING WEI DISHARMONY

See: **Skin** Ying Wei Disharmony 380

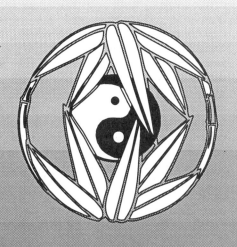

PART II
Herb
Synopsis

Read Important Note, Next Page! ⟶

From *How to Use This Book*:

In order to give the appearance of a free-flowing, multi-columned text describing the uses, clinical applications and clinical notes or precautions, I had to use the particular desktop publishing software's "table format." This works well in most cases, except where a table "breaks" at the end of a page and carries over to the next page. Notice (see example in Figure 8) that unlike normal multi-column text which snakes from the bottom of one column to the top of another and finally the last text in the last column on the right continues to the top of the next page on the left, **this book's "text columns" do not snake from column to column when there is a break across a page. Rather, the left column ends at the bottom of the page and then continues on the next page in the left column.** This is important to know about this book's layout. Without this tidbit of information, you may think you're missing something or not know to turn the page. To help matters, I've included a footer which lets you know that the table continues on the next page.

Figure 8: PLEASE NOTE: Table columns continue each column to the next page, not across columns.

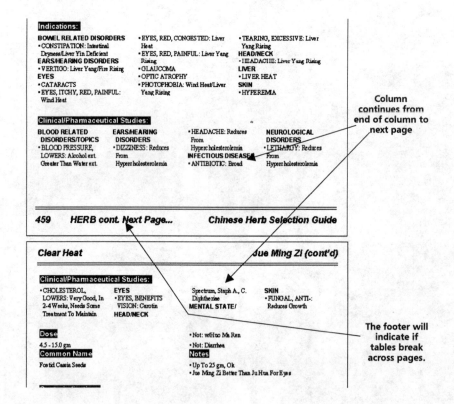

Release Exterior Conditions: Spicy, Warm

BAI ZHI 白芷 *RADIX ANGELICAE*

Traditional Functions:

1. Expels Wind from the Yang Ming channel and reduces pain
2. Reduces swelling and promotes discharge of pus
3. Dries Dampness and controls discharge
4. Opens up the nasal passages

Traditional Properties:

Enters: LU, ST,

Properties: SP, W

Indications:

ABDOMEN/ GASTROINTESTINAL TOPICS
• INTESTINAL WIND
BOWEL RELATED DISORDERS
• FISTULA
• HEMORRHOIDS
CANCER/TUMORS/SWELLINGS/ LUMPS
• SWELLINGS, REDUCES LOCAL
EARS/HEARING DISORDERS
• DIZZINESS
EYES
• EYES, IRRITATION
• SUPRAORBITAL PAIN
FLUID DISORDERS
• DAMPNESS, EXTERNAL– SURFACE COMPLEX
HEAD/NECK

• HEADACHE, FRONTAL
HEMORRHAGIC DISORDERS
• HEMAFECIA: Fresh
INFECTIOUS DISEASES
• COMMON COLD: Wind Cold
• INFECTIONS W/PUS
MUSCULOSKELETAL/ CONNECTIVE TISSUE
• ARTHRITIS: Wind Damp Cold Bi
NOSE
• SINUS CONGESTION
• SINUSITIS W/HEADACHE
ORAL CAVITY
• TOOTHACHE
SEXUALITY, FEMALE: GYNECOLOGICAL
• BREASTS, SWOLLEN, PAINFUL, ABSCESS

• LEUKORRHEA, PINK/WHITE DISCHARGE: Cold Damp In Lower Jiao
SKIN
• ABSCESS, HELPS TO DRAIN
• CARBUNCLES, INITIAL STAGE
• DRYNESS
• PRURITUS, DRY
• PUS, HELPS TO DISCHARGE
• SKIN, DISORDERS
• SKIN, SORES, SWOLLEN, TOXIC: Relieves Surface Complex
• SORES, INITIAL STAGE
URINARY BLADDER
• URINATION, PAINFUL, DRIBBLING: With Deficiency Cold
WIND DISORDERS
• WIND IN YANG MING

Clinical/Pharmaceutical Studies:

FEVERS
• ANTIPYRETIC
HEAD/NECK
• HEADACHE: w/Bing Pian And Inhaled Through Nostrils
INFECTIOUS DISEASES
• ANTIBIOTIC: Gram Positive, Typhi, TB, Shigella, Salmonella,

Staph
MENTAL STATE/ NEUROLOGICAL DISORDERS
• TRIGEMINAL NEURALGIA: w/ Bing Pian And Inhaled Through Nostrils
ORAL CAVITY
• TOOTHACHE: w/Bing Pian And

Inhaled Through Nostrils
PAIN/NUMBNESS/GENERAL DISCOMFORT
• ANALGESIC: Local
SKIN
• FUNGAL, ANTI-: Skin Fungi
TRAUMA, BITES, POISONINGS
• TOXIC, ANTI-: Snakebite

Dose

3 - 9 gm

Common Name

Angelica

Contraindications

Not: Yin Deficiency

Notes

Warming And Very Drying

CHUAN SHAN LONG

川山龍
（川山龙）

RHIZOMA DIOSCOREAE NIPPONICAE

Traditional Functions:

1. Vitalizes Blood and relaxes the Luo and tendons
2. Dispels Wind, Cold and Damp Bi
3. Stops cough and wheezing and disperses Phlegm
4. Promotes water metabolism
5. Clears food stagnation

Traditional Properties:

Enters: SP, LV,

Properties: BIT, N

Indications:

EXTREMITIES
• EXTREMITIES, NUMB
LUNGS
• BRONCHITIS, CHRONIC
**MUSCULOSKELETAL/
CONNECTIVE TISSUE**
• ARTHRITIS: For Opening The Luo

Channels/Wind, Cold, Damp Bi
**PAIN/NUMBNESS/GENERAL
DISCOMFORT**
• BI, WIND DAMP, CHRONIC:
Open Luo, Arrest Pain
SKIN

• BOILS
**STOMACH/DIGESTIVE
DISORDERS**
• INDIGESTION
TRAUMA, BITES, POISONINGS
• SPRAINS

Clinical/Pharmaceutical Studies:

**BLOOD RELATED
DISORDERS/TOPICS**
• ANTICOAGULANT
• BLOOD PRESSURE,
LOWERS
• CHOLESTEROL,
LOWERS: Take For 10
Weeks
**CANCER/TUMORS/
SWELLINGS/LUMPS**
• THYROID ADENOMA
**CIRCULATION
DISORDERS**
• ATHEROSCLEROSIS
• CEREBRAL
ARTERIOSCLEROSIS: 2-
3 Months Of Taking
Saponin Extract, 0.02-0.2 g/
Day Improved Many
Symptoms
• HYPERTENSION W/

ARTERIOSCLEROSIS
**ENDOCRINE RELATED
DISORDERS**
• HYPERTHYROIDISM
• THYROID, ADENOMA
HEART
• ANGINA PECTORIS
• CARDIOTONIC
• HEART DISEASE: Tabs,
160 mg Each, 2 Tabs 3x/
Day, 92% Remission From
Angina, *With Huai Hua
Mi, Rz Hemsleya
Macrosperma
• HEART FAILURE
• HEART, AFFECTS RATE:
Decreases Rate, Greater
Coronary Circulation
• MYOCARDIAL
INFARCTION

INFECTIOUS DISEASES
• BRUCELLOSIS,
CHRONIC: Decoction
Helped
KIDNEYS
• DIURETIC
LUNGS
• ANTITUSSIVE: Oral
• ASTHMA: Suppressed In
70%, 100% Cases, 0.15,
0.25 g/kg, Respectively
• BRONCHITIS,
CHRONIC: Decoction/
Tablet With Herb, Huang
Qin, Jie Geng, Zi Wan, Bai
Bu, Wu Wei Zi, *Tablet/
Decoction Of Herb, Huang
Qin, Chuan Bei Mu
• EXPECTORANT: Oral
MUSCULOSKELETAL/

CONNECTIVE TISSUE
• ARTHRITIS,
RHEUMATIC: Medicinal
Wine Of/Herb With Dog
Bones
**NUTRITIONAL/
METABOLIC
DISORDERS/TOPICS**
• HYPOXIA, TOLERANCE
TO: Oral Dose Decreased
Oxygen Consumption
**SEXUALITY, FEMALE:
GYNECOLOGICAL**
• UTERUS, STIMULATES:
Low Doses, High Doses
Inhibits
**TRAUMA, BITES,
POISONINGS**
• RADIATION,
PROTECTION

Dose

15 - 30 gm

Notes

Side Effects: Mild, Disappear Spontaneously,
Commonly Diarrhea

CONG BAI

蔥白
（葱白）

HERBA ALLII FISTULOSI

Traditional Functions:

1. Relieves the Surface and causes sweating.
2. Disperses Cold and promotes the circulation of Yang and Blood

Traditional Properties:

Enters: LU, ST,

Properties: SP, W

Indications:

ABDOMEN/
GASTROINTESTINAL TOPICS
• ABDOMEN, PAIN OF/
DISTENTION: Cold
BOWEL RELATED DISORDERS
• DIARRHEA
EXTERIOR CONDITIONS
• EXTERIOR PATHOGENS
EYES

• EYES, DISORDERS
INFECTIOUS DISEASES
• COMMON COLD: Wind Cold
• FEBRILE DISEASES
MUSCULOSKELETAL/
CONNECTIVE TISSUE
• ARTHRITIS, PAIN: Cramping-Like
NOSE
• NASAL CONGESTION: Yang Qi

Blocked By Cold
ORAL CAVITY
• THROAT, SORE
SEXUALITY, FEMALE:
GYNECOLOGICAL
• MISCARRIAGE: Habitual, Stops
WIND DISORDERS
• WIND COLD, INITIAL STAGE

Clinical/Pharmaceutical Studies:

FEVERS
• ANTIPYRETIC
INFECTIOUS DISEASES
• ANTIBIOTIC: (Oil) Diphtheria,
Staph, Strep, Shigella
KIDNEYS
• DIURETIC
LUNGS

• EXPECTORANT
SEXUALITY, FEMALE:
GYNECOLOGICAL
• MASTITIS: w/Ban Xia, Ginger
Juice Via Enema, 97% Effective
• TRICHOMONAS, VAGINAL:
Inhibits

SKIN
• FUNGAL, ANTI-: White
Ringworm
• SUDORIFIC
STOMACH/DIGESTIVE
DISORDERS
• STOMACHIC

Dose

6 - 15 gm

Common Name

Scallion/Chinese Chive

Contraindications

Not: Taken With Honey

DI JIAO　　　地椒　　　*HERBA*
THYMI SERPYLLI

Traditional Functions:

1. Warms the Middle Jiao and disperses Cold
2. Expels Wind and controls pain

Traditional Properties:

Enters:

Properties: SP, W

Indications:

ABDOMEN/
GASTROINTESTINAL TOPICS
• ABDOMEN, PAIN OF
BOWEL RELATED DISORDERS
• DIARRHEA
• FLATULENCE FROM POOR DIET
LUNGS

• COUGH: Wind Cold
ORAL CAVITY
• THROAT, SWOLLEN
• TOOTHACHE
PAIN/NUMBNESS/GENERAL
DISCOMFORT

• ACHING, GENERALIZED
SKIN
• PRURITUS
STOMACH/DIGESTIVE
DISORDERS
• VOMITING

Clinical/Pharmaceutical Studies:

LUNGS
• BRONCHITIS: Contains Thymol
• COUGH
• EXPECTORANT
• RESPIRATORY TRACT,
RELAXES
PAIN/NUMBNESS/GENERAL

DISCOMFORT
• ANALGESIC: Thymol
SEXUALITY, FEMALE:
GYNECOLOGICAL
• DYSMENORRHEA: Reduces
Cramps, Small Amounts
• UTERUS, STIMULATES: Large

Amounts
SKIN
• FUNGAL, ANTI-: Oil Of
STOMACH/DIGESTIVE
DISORDERS
• INDIGESTION: Antispasmodic

Dose

3 - 6 gm

Common Name

Thyme

Notes

Oil Can Be Toxic In Small Quantities
Possible Rash From Oil
May Suppress Thyroid

FANG FENG

防風
(防风)

RADIX SILERIS
(LEDEBOURIELLAE SESLOIDIS)

Traditional Functions:

1. Relieves the Surface and dispels Wind
2. Dissipates Wind Damp Bi
3. Expels Liver Wind and intestinal Wind

Traditional Properties:

Enters: SP, UB, LV,

Properties: SP, SW, <W

Indications:

ABDOMEN/ GASTROINTESTINAL TOPICS
• INTESTINAL WIND
BOWEL RELATED DISORDERS
• DIARRHEA, PAINFUL W/ BRIGHT BLOOD IN BM
• HEMORRHOIDS, BLOODY STOOL: (Charred)
COLD
• CHILLS: Wind Cold
EARS/HEARING DISORDERS
• VERTIGO
EXTREMITIES
• FEET, TREMORS
• HANDS, TREMORS
FLUID DISORDERS
• DAMPNESS: Moves But Not Drying

• DAMPNESS, EXTERNAL: Surface Complex
HEAD/NECK
• HEADACHE: Wind Cold
• MIGRAINE
HEMORRHAGIC DISORDERS
• HEMORRHAGE: Raise The Yang To Stop
INFECTIOUS DISEASES
• COMMON COLD W/HEADACHE, BODYACHE, STIFF NECK: Wind Cold
• TETANUS
MENTAL STATE/ NEUROLOGICAL DISORDERS
• CONVULSIONS
MUSCULOSKELETAL/

CONNECTIVE TISSUE
• ARTHRITIS: Wind Damp Cold Bi
• OSTEALGIA
• SPASMS
PAIN/NUMBNESS/GENERAL DISCOMFORT
• BI, WIND DAMP COLD
• BODY ACHES: Wind Cold
SKIN
• RASHES, PRURITIC: Wind Damp
• SKIN, SORES, SWOLLEN, TOXIC: Relieves Surface Complex
SPLEEN
• SPLEEN LIVER DISHARMONY
WIND DISORDERS
• WIND BI
• WIND COLD, MILD

Clinical/Pharmaceutical Studies:

FEVERS
• ANTIPYRETIC: Mild Within 30 Minutes, Decoction Stronger Than Extract, Lasts 2.5+Hrs
INFECTIOUS DISEASES
• ANTIBIOTIC: Salmonella, Echo Viruses, Shegella, Pseudomonas, Staph Aureus
• COMMON COLD: Granular Infusion Of Fang Feng, 15 g, Jing Jie, 15 g, Zi Su Ye, 10 g, Each Gram= 8-12g Crude Herb, 3 Doses/

Day
• VIRAL, ANTI-: Some Flu, et al
MENTAL STATE/ NEUROLOGICAL DISORDERS
• CONVULSIVE, ANTI-: Less Than Pentobarbital
PAIN/NUMBNESS/ GENERAL DISCOMFORT
• ANALGESIC: Significant, In Enema/Subcutaneous Injection, Oral ETOH Extract

SKIN
• FUNGAL, ANTI-
• ROSACEA: Fang Feng, Shan Zhi Zi, Chen Pi, Chuan Xiong, Huang Qin, Lian Qiao, Du Huo, Jie Geng, All 9 g, Jing Jie, Huang Lian, Gan Cao, Each 6 g, Decoct Take As 2 Doses In One Day, 3 Treatments/2 Days, Plus Topical Ointment Of Da Feng Zi, Mercury, Xing Ren 1x/Day, 100% Cure

Rate
TRAUMA, BITES, POISONINGS
• ANTIDOTE, TOXICS: Arsenic Poisoning--Fang Feng, 12 g, LU Dou, Brown Sugar, 9g Each, Gan Cao, 3 g, Decoct, Take In 2 Doses/Day For 14 Days For 1 Course, Similar To IM Injection Of 100 mg Dimercaprol
• INFLAMMATORY, ANTI- : Decoction/ETOH Extract

Dose

3 - 9 gm

Contraindications

Not: Def Yin With Heat

Precautions

Watch: Spasms From Blood Def

GAO BEN

藁本

RADIX LIGUSTICI SINENSIS

Traditional Functions:

1. Dispels Wind Cold and Cold Damp and reduces pain

Traditional Properties:

Enters: UB,

Properties: SP, W

Indications:

ABDOMEN/
GASTROINTESTINAL TOPICS
• ABDOMEN, PAIN OF,
  DIARRHEA
• HERNIA: Cold, Damp
BOWEL RELATED DISORDERS
• DIARRHEA
CANCER/TUMORS/SWELLINGS/
LUMPS
• MASSES: Cold, Damp
EARS/HEARING DISORDERS
• DIZZINESS
FLUID DISORDERS

• DAMPNESS, EXTERNAL--
  SURFACE COMPLEX
HEAD/NECK
• HEADACHE: Vertex Pain/Wind
  Cold
• MIGRAINE
INFECTIOUS DISEASES
• COMMON COLD: Wind Cold
MUSCULOSKELETAL/
CONNECTIVE TISSUE
• ARTHRITIS: Wind Damp Cold Bi
• BACK, LOWER PAIN, ACUTE:

Wind Cold
• JOINTS, PAIN
PAIN/NUMBNESS/GENERAL
DISCOMFORT
• BI, WIND DAMP: Shoulders,
  Extremities
• PAIN: Vertex To Teeth
SKIN
• SCABIES: Topical
• TINEA FUNGUS: Topical
WIND DISORDERS
• WIND COLD PATTERNS

Clinical/Pharmaceutical Studies:

INFECTIOUS DISEASES
• VIRAL, ANTI-: Flu
MUSCULOSKELETAL/
CONNECTIVE TISSUE
• ANTISPASMODIC
PAIN/NUMBNESS/

GENERAL
DISCOMFORT
• ANALGESIC
SEXUALITY, FEMALE:
GYNECOLOGICAL

• MENSTRUATION,
  DISORDERS OF
SKIN
• FUNGAL, ANTI-:
  Dermatomycoses,

Aqueous Extract Very
Effective
TRAUMA, BITES,
POISONINGS
• INFLAMMATORY, ANTI-

Dose

3 - 9 gm

Common Name

Chinese Lovage Root

Contraindications

Not: Headache From Def Blood, Def. Yin Patterns-Very
Drying, Warming

GUI ZHI

桂枝

RAMULUS CINNAMOMI CASSIAE

Traditional Functions:

1. Harmonizes the Ying and Wei Qi levels
2. Warms and promotes the flow of Qi in the channels
3. Relieves muscles promoting the flow of Qi
4. Moves the Yang, opens Qi obstruction and transforms Qi
5. Strengthens the Heart Yang

Traditional Properties:

Enters: LU, HT, UB,

Properties: SP, SW, W

Indications:

ABDOMEN/
GASTROINTESTINAL TOPICS
• ABDOMEN, PAIN OF: Cold
CHEST
• CHEST, PAIN
EXTREMITIES
• ARMS, PAIN, SORE
• LIMBS, PAIN: Wind Cold Damp
FLUID DISORDERS
• EDEMA: Cold Phlegm/Yang
  Deficiency
HEART
• ANGINA PECTORIS: Chest Bi
  Strangulating Pain
• PALPITATIONS: Deficiency

Patterns
INFECTIOUS DISEASES
• COMMON COLD: Wind Cold
LIVER
• JAUNDICE, YIN
LUNGS
• COUGH: Cold Phlegm
• LUNGS, DYSPNEA: Cold Phlegm
MUSCULOSKELETAL/
CONNECTIVE TISSUE
• ARTHRITIS: Wind Damp Cold Bi
• JOINTS, PAIN: Wind Cold Damp
• SHOULDERS, JOINT PAIN
PAIN/NUMBNESS/GENERAL
DISCOMFORT

• ACHES, PAINS, GENERAL
• BI, WIND DAMP COLD
SEXUALITY, FEMALE:
GYNECOLOGICAL
• AMENORRHEA
• DYSMENORRHEA: Cold
  Stagnating The Blood
SKIN
• SURFACE DEFICIENCY
  PATTERN: Wind Cold
URINARY BLADDER
• DYSURIA
• URINATION, PAINFUL,
  DRIBBLING: With Deficiency Cold

Clinical/Pharmaceutical Studies:

ABDOMEN/ GASTROINTESTINAL TOPICS
• ABDOMEN, PAIN OF: Smooth Muscle Spasms
FEVERS
• ANTIPYRETIC: Mild, Stimulates Blood Circulation To Skin
FLUID DISORDERS
• EDEMA, CARDIAC/ RENAL: Wu Ling San
HEAD/NECK
• HEADACHE: From Blood Vessel Spasms
HEART
• CARDIOTONIC
IMMUNE SYSTEM RELATED DISORDERS/ TOPICS
• ALLERGIC, ANTI-: Strong
INFECTIOUS DISEASES
• ANTIBIOTIC: Potent

Inhibitor Of Salmonella, Echo Viruses, E.Coli, B. Subtillis, Staph.Aureus
• COMMON COLD: Wind Cold Type:3-9 g
• INFLUENZA: Prophylaxis, Use Aerosol Of Gui Zhi, Xiang Ru, 12.5 g Each, Grind For 150 Applications Into Throat, 2x/Day To Prevent Flu, Will Decrease Symptoms, Reduce Incidence
• VIRAL, ANTI-: Asian Flu A, Marked
KIDNEYS
• DIURETIC, STRONG
• NEPHRITIS, ALLERGIC: Wu Ling San
LUNGS
• ANTITUSSIVE: Excretion In Lungs Of Absorbed Oil Thinned Bronchial Secretions

MENTAL STATE/ NEUROLOGICAL DISORDERS
• CONVULSIVE, ANTI-: Chai Hu Gui Zhi Tang (Gui Zhi, Chai Hu, Bai Shao, Sheng Jiang) , Antagonized Audiogenic Seizures
• HYPNOTIC
• SEDATIVE: Cinnamic Aldehyde 250-500 mg/kg Could Antagonize Methamphetamine
• TRANQUILIZING: To CNS
PAIN/NUMBNESS/ GENERAL DISCOMFORT
• ANALGESIC: Raises Cerebral Pain Threshold
SEXUALITY, FEMALE: GYNECOLOGICAL

• ABORTIFACIENT: Oil Of, Used Since Ancient Times
• UTERUS, MYOMA: Modified Gui Zhi Fu Ling Wan, 60 Doses
SKIN
• DERMATITIS, ALLERGIC: Chai Hu Gui Zhi Tang
• FUNGAL, ANTI-: White Ringworm, et al.
• URTICARIA, ALLERGIC: Chai Hu Gui Zhi Tang
STOMACH/DIGESTIVE DISORDERS
• STOMACHIC: Improves Digestion, Increases Gastric Secretions
TRAUMA, BITES, POISONINGS
• FROSTBITE: With Dang Gui

Dose

3 - 6 gm

Common Name

Saigon Cinnamon Twigs

Precautions

Watch: Pregnancy

Notes

Do Not Give If Excess/Def Heat Present

HU SUI
(YUAN SUI ZI)

胡荽

HERBA /FRUCTUS CORIANDRI

Traditional Functions:

1. Relieves the Surface, expels Wind
2. Promotes the eruption of rashes
3. Strengthens the Stomach and regulates Qi
4. Resolves Phlegm

Traditional Properties:

Enters: LU, ST

Properties: SP, W

Indications:

BOWEL RELATED DISORDERS
• HEMORRHOIDS, EXTERNAL BY EXPOSURE TO FUMES

• RECTAL PROLAPSE: External Application Of Decoction With A Sponge
INFECTIOUS DISEASES
• MEASLES, EARLY

STAGE: Wind Cold, No Rash Yet
SKIN
• RASHES, INCOMPLETE EXPRESSION OF: With

Wind Cold Complex
STOMACH/DIGESTIVE DISORDERS
• INDIGESTION

Clinical/Pharmaceutical Studies:

• AROMATIC
STOMACH/DIGESTIVE

DISORDERS
• CARMINATIVE

• STOMACHIC

Dose

6 - 9 gm

Common Name

Coriander /Chinese Parsley

Contraindications

Not: Measles w/o Rash From Excess Toxic Heat In Interior

JING JIE 荆芥 FLOS SCHIZONEPETAE TENUIFOLIAE

Traditional Functions:

1. Relieves the Surface and dispels Wind
2. Promotes rashes to surface and reduces itching
3. Controls bleeding when charred

Traditional Properties:

Enters: LU, LV,

Properties: SP, <W

Indications:

CANCER/TUMORS/SWELLINGS/ LUMPS
• TUMORS
CIRCULATION DISORDERS
• STROKE, MOUTH TIGHTNESS
FEVERS
• FEVER: Common Cold
HEAD/NECK
• HEADACHE
HEMORRHAGIC DISORDERS
• EPISTAXIS
• HEMAFECIA
• HEMATEMESIS
• HEMORRHAGE, AS AUXILLIARY HERB
• HEMOSTATIC: Mild
INFECTIOUS DISEASES
• COMMON COLD W/HEADACHE,

SORE THROAT: Wind Heat
• MEASLES, EARLY STAGE
• TETANUS
ORAL CAVITY
• LARYNGITIS
• MOUTH, TIGHTNESS: Wind Struck
• THROAT, SORE, SWOLLEN
SEXUALITY, FEMALE: GYNECOLOGICAL
• MENORRHAGIA
• POSTPARTUM, SYNCOPE: Blood Disorders
• PRURITUS, VAGINAL
• UTERINE BLEEDING
SKIN
• ABSCESS
• BOILS, INITIAL STAGE:

Especially If With Chills/Fever
• ITCHING, GENERAL
• RASHES, INCOMPLETE EXPRESSION OF: Early Stage/ With Wind Cold Complex
• RASHES, W/PRURITUS: Blood Heat, Wind (Raw) , Clears Wind
• SCABIES
• SKIN, ERUPTIONS, BRINGS TO SURFACE
• SKIN, SORES, SWOLLEN, TOXIC: Relieves Surface Complex
• SORES
• URTICARIA
WIND DISORDERS
• WIND COLD
• WIND HEAT

Clinical/Pharmaceutical Studies:

CANCER/TUMORS/ SWELLINGS/LUMPS
• CANCER: Weakly Inhibits
CIRCULATION DISORDERS
• BLOOD CIRCULATION, INCREASES SUBCUTANEOUS
FEVERS
• ANTIPYRETIC: Possible, Very Weak
HEMORRHAGIC DISORDERS
• HEMOSTATIC: Shortens Coagulation Time (Only When Charred)
INFECTIOUS DISEASES
• BACTERIAL, ANTI-: TB, Strong Against Staph Aureus, Diphteriae, Active

Against B.Anthracis, Beta Strep, Salmonell, Shigella
• COMMON COLD: Jing Fang Bai Du San (Herb, Fang Feng, Qiang Huo, Du Huo, Chai Hu, Chuan Xiong, Jie Geng, Bo He, Qian Hu, Zhi Ke, Sheng Jiang, Gan Cao) , *Yin Qiao San, *Biao LI Shuang Jie Tang (Diaphoretic-Purgative Decoction) , Symptoms Gone In 1-2 Days, Cure In 4-6 Days
• VIRAL, ANTI-: None Noted Against Flu
LUNGS
• TUBERCULOSIS: In High Concentrations
MUSCULOSKELETAL/

CONNECTIVE TISSUE
• ANTISPASMODIC
SKIN
• ABSCESS: Incrase Healing Process
• ALLERGIC DERMATITIS: Jing Fang Bai Du Tang/Wu Wei Xiao Du Yin, Modified Helped
• DIAPHORETIC, VERY WEAK
• ECZEMA: Jing Fang Bai Du Tang/Wu Wei Xiao Du Yin, Modified Helped
• EXANTHEMA DESQUAMATIVUM: Jing Fang Bai Du Tang/Wu Wei Xiao Du Yin, Modified Helped
• PSORIASIS: Jing Fang

Bai Du Tang/Wu Wei Xiao Du Yin, Modified Helped
• SKIN, DISORDERS: Fine Powder Applied Evenly To Skin And Rubbed Until Skin Felt Hot
• URTICARIA: Jing Fang Bai Du Tang/Wu Wei Xiao Du Yin, Modified Helped
• URTICARIA, MILD: Fine Powder Applied Evenly To Skin And Rubbed Until Skin Felt Hot, 1-2 Applications Cured, More Severe Cases, Up To 4 Application
TRAUMA, BITES, POISONINGS
• INFLAMMATORY, ANTI-

Dose

3 - 9 gm

Contraindications

Not: Liver Wind

Not: Open Sores Or Measles
Not: w/Spontaneous Sweating

Notes

Carbonize For Bleeding

MA HUANG

麻黃
（麻黃）

HERBA EPHEDRAE

Traditional Functions:

1. Relieves the Surface and dissipates Cold
2. Circulates Lung Qi and relieves asthma
3. Regulates water circulation by inducing urination and reduces edema

Traditional Properties:

Enters: LU, UB,

Properties: SP, <BIT, W

Indications:

CANCER/TUMORS/ SWELLINGS/LUMPS
- SWELLINGS: Wind
- SWELLINGS, INFLAMMED

COLD
- CHILLS: Wind Cold Exterior Excess Patterns

EXTERIOR CONDITIONS
- EXTERIOR, RELEASES: Very Good

FEVERS
- FEVER: Wind Cold Exterior Excess Patterns

FLUID DISORDERS

- EDEMA: Especially From External Pathogen, Smooths Lung Qi Circulation To Remove/ Wind Fluid
- EDEMA, ACUTE NEPHRITIC

HEAD/NECK
- HEADACHE: Wind Cold Exterior Excess Patterns

INFECTIOUS DISEASES
- COMMON COLD: Wind Cold

LUNGS
- COUGH: Cold Phlegm/ Lung Heat/Wind Cold

- COUGH IN CHILDREN
- COUGH, WHEEZING
- DYSPNEA
- LUNGS, DYSPNEA: Cold Phlegm/Lung Heat
- WHEEZING

MUSCULOSKELETAL/ CONNECTIVE TISSUE
- ARTHRITIS: Wind Damp Cold Bi
- OSTEALGIA

SIX STAGES/ CHANNELS
- TAI YANG STAGE DISEASE

SKIN
- ABSCESS, YIN, INTERNAL SINKING OF
- ADIAPHORESIS: Wind Cold Exterior Excess Patterns
- RASHES, INCOMPLETE EXPRESSION OF, W/ COUGH, DYSPNEA
- SKIN, ERUPTIONS, BRINGS TO SURFACE
- URTICARIA

WIND DISORDERS
- WIND COLD EXTERIOR EXCESS PATTERNS

Clinical/Pharmaceutical Studies:

ABDOMEN/ GASTROINTESTINAL TOPICS
- GASTROINTESTINAL TRACT, RELAXES, INHIBITS PERISTALSIS

CIRCULATION DISORDERS
- BLOOD VESSELS: Vasodilates, Reduces Blood Flow In Heart, Brain, Muscles
- HYPOTENSION: From Anesthesia, Injection IM
- VASOCONSTRICTOR

ENDOCRINE RELATED DISORDERS
- MYASTHENIA GRAVIS

EYES
- PUPILS, DILATES: When Instilled Directly, More So In More Pigmented Irises

FEVERS
- ANTIPYRETIC: Essential Oil

HEART
- CARDIAC BLOOD FLOW, INCREASES

IMMUNE SYSTEM RELATED DISORDERS/ TOPICS
- ALLERGIC, ANTI-: Release Of Mediators

- ASTHMA, BRONCHIAL: Oral Can Alleviate Attack, Decoction Of Roasted Herb, Sugar, 30 g Each
- ASTHMA, IN CHILDREN: In Ma Xing Shi Gan Tang
- BRONCHITIS, CHRONIC ASTHMATIC: San Ao Tang (Herb, Xing Ren, Gan Cao, Zi Su Zi, Di Long) Modified
- BRONCHITIS, CHRONIC, GERIATRIC: Ma Xing She Gan Tang
- BRONCHODILATORY: Mild, Prolonged, Less Than Epinephrine
- PNEUMONIA, CHILDHOOD: Concentrated Crude ETOH Extract Of Fei Qing Tang (Ma Huang, Lian Qiao, Xing Ren, Shi Gao, Jin Yin Hua, Huang Qin, Da Qing Ye, Ting LI Zi, Bai Qian, Ma Dou Ling, Zi Su Zi, Gan Cao) , All Recovered Fine Without Antibiotics, * Ma Xing Shi Gan Tang Also Effective
- WHOOPING COUGH: 3-5 Years Old, Ma Xing Shi Gan Tang With Bai Bu,

- NASAL MUCOSA, CLEARS: As In Asthma
- NOSE: Vasoconstricts Mucosa, Longer, Stronger Than Pseudoephedrine
- RHINITIS: As Nose Drops, 100% Decoction

NUTRITIONAL/ METABOLIC DISORDERS/TOPICS
- BODY TEMPERATURE, LOWERS

SEXUALITY, FEMALE: GYNECOLOGICAL
- UTERUS, INCREASES TONICITY

SKIN
- DIAPHORETIC: Mild
- ECZEMA: Ma Huang Chan Tui Tang, Modified (Ma Huang, Chan Tui, Huai Hua, Huang Lian, Fu Ping, Gan Cao) Or Ma Huang Lian Qiao Chi Xiao Dou Tang (Ma Huang, Lian Qiao, Chi Xiao Dou, Xing Ren, Gan Cao, Sheng Jiang, Da Zao, Zi Bai Pi (Cortex Catalpae Radicis))
- RASHES, DRUG INDUCED: Ma Huang Chan Tui Tang, Modified (Ma Huang, Chan Tui, Huai Hua, Huang Lian, Fu Ping,

Catalpae Radicis))
- SKIN, PITYRIASIS ROSEA: Ma Huang Chan Tui Tang, Modified (Ma Huang, Chan Tui, Huai Hua, Huang Lian, Fu Ping, Gan Cao) Or Ma Huang Lian Qiao Chi Xiao Dou Tang (Ma Huang, Lian Qiao, Chi Xiao Dou, Xing Ren, Gan Cao, Sheng Jiang, Da Zao, Zi Bai Pi (Cortex Catalpae Radicis))
- SKIN, VARICELLA: Ma Huang Chan Tui Tang, Modified (Ma Huang, Chan Tui, Huai Hua, Huang Lian, Fu Ping, Gan Cao) Or Ma Huang Lian Qiao Chi Xiao Dou Tang (Ma Huang, Lian Qiao, Chi Xiao Dou, Xing Ren, Gan Cao, Sheng Jiang, Da Zao, Zi Bai Pi (Cortex Catalpae Radicis))
- URTICARIA: Ma Huang Chan Tui Tang, Modified (Ma Huang, Chan Tui, Huai Hua, Huang Lian, Fu Ping, Gan Cao) Or Ma Huang Lian Qiao Chi Xiao Dou Tang (Ma Huang, Lian Qiao, Chi Xiao Dou, Xing Ren, Gan Cao, Sheng Jiang,

Clinical/Pharmaceutical Studies:

Suppressed By ETOH/ Aqueous Extract

INFECTIOUS DISEASES
- COMMON COLD: Ma Huang Tang
- INFLUENZA: Ma Huang Tang, Or Volatile Oil
- VIRAL, ANTI-: Essential Oil, Influenza, Therapeutic Effect

KIDNEYS
- DIURETIC: Marked
- NEPHRITIS, CHILDHOOD: Ma Huang, Bai Zhu Decoction

LUNGS
- ANTITUSSIVE: Oral, Aqueous Extract

Ting LI Zi, Da Zao, Maltose, Effective In Catarrhal, Spastic Stages, * Wen Fei Huay Yin Tang (AKA, Xiao Qing Long Tang)

MENTAL STATE/ NEUROLOGICAL DISORDERS
- LETHARGY: Ma Huang Fu Zi Xi Xin Tang
- STIMULANT, CNS

MUSCULOSKELETAL/ CONNECTIVE TISSUE
- ARTHRITIS, RHEUMATOID: Yang Harmonizing Decoction

NOSE

Gan Cao) Or Ma Huang Lian Qiao Chi Xiao Dou Tang (Ma Huang, Lian Qiao, Chi Xiao Dou, Xing Ren, Gan Cao, Sheng Jiang, Da Zao, Zi Bai Pi (Cortex Catalpae Radicis))
- SKIN, PAINT ALLERGY RASH: Ma Huang Chan Tui Tang, Modified (Ma Huang, Chan Tui, Huai Hua, Huang Lian, Fu Ping, Gan Cao) Or Ma Huang Lian Qiao Chi Xiao Dou Tang (Ma Huang, Lian Qiao, Chi Xiao Dou, Xing Ren, Gan Cao, Sheng Jiang, Da Zao, Zi Bai Pi (Cortex

Da Zao, Zi Bai Pi (Cortex Catalpae Radicis))
- WARTS, MULTIPLE: Ma Xing Yi Gan Tang (Ma Huang, Xing Ren, Yi Yi Ren, Gan Cao)

TRAUMA, BITES, POISONINGS
- TOXIC, ANTI-: Morphine, Barbitol Poisoning

URINARY BLADDER
- ENURESIS, CHILDHOOD: May Cause Urinary Retention By Bladder
- URINARY BLADDER, INCREASES TONE: Reduces Urination

Dose

1.5 - 9.0 gm

Contraindications

Not: Insomnia/Spontaneous Sweating

Precautions

Watch: Deficiency/Asthma/Cough From Kidney Weakness

Notes

Can Raise BP

Can Cause Heavy Sweating

Bake w/Honey For Asthma

Asthma: 9-12 g

Acute Toxic Reaction: Headache, Restlessness, Insomnia, Drippy Nose, Dry Mouth, Tearing, Palpitation, Fever, Sweating, Nausea, Vomiting, Tinnitus, Raised Body Temperature

Treatment: Induce Vomiting, Purge To Reduce Absorption, Babituates Will Reduce Severe Nervousness, Fluid Replenishment

Plant Has 1-2% Alkaloids, 40-90% Is Ephedrine

The Volatile Oil Has A Sedative Effect

Body Quickly Adapts To Ephedrine, Effect Restored In Few Hours

---

QIANG HUO   羌活   *RADIX NOTOPTERYGII*

Traditional Functions:

1. Relieves the Surface and dissipates Cold and Damp
2. Expels Wind Damp Bi in the upper body
3. Guides Qi to the Tai Yang and Du channels

Traditional Properties:

Enters: KI, UB,

Properties: SP, BIT, ARO, W

Indications:

CANCER/TUMORS/ SWELLINGS/LUMPS
- SWELLINGS, PAIN

COLD
- COLD, AVERSION TO

FEVERS
- FEVER

FLUID DISORDERS
- DAMPNESS, EXTERNAL: Surface Complex

HEAD/NECK
- HEADACHE, OCCIPITAL PAIN: In Wind Cold Damp

- NECK, PAIN

HERBAL FUNCTIONS
- GUIDING HERB: Qi To Tai Yang And Du Ch's

INFECTIOUS DISEASES
- COMMON COLD W/ FEVER, HEADACHE, HEAVY SENSATION: Wind Cold

MENTAL STATE/ NEUROLOGICAL DISORDERS
- SLEEPINESS: In Wind Cold Damp

MUSCULOSKELETAL/

CONNECTIVE TISSUE
- ARTHRITIS: Wind Damp Cold Bi
- ARTHRITIS, JOINT PAIN
- BACK, PAIN
- JOINTS, PAIN: Upper Limbs & Head, Neck, Back, Wind Damp Cold Bi
- SHOULDERS, PAIN

PAIN/NUMBNESS/ GENERAL DISCOMFORT
- ANALGESIC: Stomach, Muscles, Joints

- BI, WIND DAMP: Shoulders, Extremities
- BODY ACHES
- HEAVINESS SENSATION: In Wind Cold Damp

SKIN
- BOILS
- SWEATING, LACK OF

WIND DISORDERS
- WIND COLD DAMP: Joint Pain, Heaviness Feeling, Sleepiness, Occipital Pain

Clinical/Pharmaceutical Studies:

FEVERS
• ANTIPYRETIC

LUNGS
• TUBERCULOSIS: Ethanol Extract
Inhibits

MUSCULOSKELETAL/
CONNECTIVE TISSUE
• ANTISPASMODIC
• ARTHRITIS, RHEUMATIC

PAIN/NUMBNESS/GENERAL

DISCOMFORT
• ANALGESIC

SKIN
• DIAPHORETIC
• FUNGAL, ANTI-: Inhibits

Dose

3 - 9 gm

Contraindications

Not: Joint Pain From Def Blood
Not: Headache From Def Yin

SHENG JIANG   生姜   RHIZOMA ZINGIBERIS OFFICINALIS RECENS

Traditional Functions:

1. Relieves the Surface and dissipates Cold
2. Warms the Middle Jiao and controls vomiting
3. Disperses Cold, transforms Phlegm and reduces coughing
4. Removes toxic effect of other herbs and substances
5. Harmonizes the Ying and Wei Qi levels

Traditional Properties:

Enters: LU, ST, SP

Properties: SP, H

Indications:

ABDOMEN/
GASTROINTESTINAL TOPICS
• ABDOMEN, FULLNESS OF, PAIN

BOWEL RELATED DISORDERS
• DIARRHEA

CHEST
• CHEST, PAIN, SWELLING

COLD
• COLD, EXTERNAL

EXTERIOR CONDITIONS
• EXTERIOR PATHOGEN: Relieves
Very Little

HEAD/NECK
• ALOPECIA: Topical Application

INFECTIOUS DISEASES
• COMMON COLD: Wind Cold

LUNGS
• COUGH: Wind Cold, Acute/Lung
Disorders With Phlegm
• LUNG SPUTUM, CHRONIC
• WHEEZING

PHLEGM
• PHLEGM FLUID
• PHLEGM RETENTION

SEXUALITY, FEMALE/
GYNECOLOGICAL
• MORNING SICKNESS:
Gestational Foul Obstruction--Cold

SKIN
• DIAPHORETIC, WEAK
• SWEATING W/SURFACE
DEFICIENCY

STOMACH/DIGESTIVE
DISORDERS
• HICCUPS: Qi Deficiency-Cold
• NAUSEA/VOMITING: Cold
• VOMITING: Qi Deficiency-Cold

TRAUMA, BITES, POISONINGS
• DETOXIFIES OTHER HERBS

WIND DISORDERS
• WIND COLD

Clinical/Pharmaceutical Studies:

ABDOMEN/
GASTROINTESTINAL TOPICS
• INTESTINES, OBSTRUCTION
DUE TO ROUNDWORMS: Ginger
Honey Mixture

BLOOD RELATED DISORDERS/
TOPICS
• BLOOD PRESSURE, RAISES

BOWEL RELATED DISORDERS
• DYSENTERY, BACILLARY: With
Brown Sugar, As Paste, Pain,
Tenesmus Gone In 5-6 Days

EXTREMITIES
• LEGS, PAIN JOINTS: Injections Of
5-10% Solution Into Painful Points,
Ashi Points/Trigger Points/Nodules

HEART
• HEART, STIMULATES: Alcohol
Extract

INFECTIOUS DISEASES
• BACTERIAL, ANTI-: Juice Kills

RESPIRATORY CENTER: Alcohol
Extract

MUSCULOSKELETAL/
CONNECTIVE TISSUE
• BACK, LOWER PAIN: Injections
Of 5-10% Solution Into Painful
Points, Ashi Points/Trigger Points/
Nodules
• JOINTS, PAIN: Injections Of 5-10%
Solution Into Painful Points, Ashi
Points/Trigger Points/Nodules

PAIN/NUMBNESS/GENERAL
DISCOMFORT
• ANALGESIC

PARASITES
• INTESTINAL OBSTRUCTION
DUE TO ROUNDWORMS: Ginger
Honey Mixture

SEXUALITY, MALE/
UROLOGICAL TOPICS
• ORCHITIS, ACUTE: External

• DIAPHORETIC: Essential Oil
Which Stimulate Capillary Blood
Circulation
• FUNGAL, ANTI-: Trichomonas,
2.5, 5, 25% Aqueous Extract Kills

STOMACH/DIGESTIVE
DISORDERS
• CARMINATIVE
• GASTRIC SECRETIONS,
INCREASES
• STOMACHIC: Essential Oil
• ULCERS, GASTRIC/DUODENAL:
50 gm Washed, Minced, Decocted
With 300 ml Water, 30 Min, Take 2
Days, 3x/Day, Symptoms Improved,
No Radical Cure
• VOMITING: Stomach Cold:Ginger
Or With Ban Xia (Xiao Ban Xia
Tang) Plus Huang Lian, Zhu Ru If
Heat Present
• VOMITING, INHIBITS: 30 ml Of

Clinical/Pharmaceutical Studies:

Typhi, Cholera
LUNGS
• LUNG STIMULATES

Application Of 6-10 Slices Over
Testes, Change Daily (Not If Sores!)
SKIN

10-50% Solution
TRAUMA, BITES, POISONINGS
• INFLAMMATORY, ANTI-

Dose
3 - 9 gm

Common Name
Fresh Ginger Rhizome

Contraindications
Not: LU Heat

Not: ST Heat w/Vomiting

Not: Yin Def Heat

Notes
Very Safe

SU GENG
(ZI SU GENG)

蘇梗
（苏梗）

CAULIS
PERILLAE ACUTAE

Traditional Functions:

1. Promotes and circulates Qi of the chest
2. Calms restless fetus

Traditional Properties:

Enters: LU, SP, ST

Properties: SP, W, SW

Indications:

ABDOMEN/
GASTROINTESTINAL TOPICS
• ABDOMEN, PAIN OF,
  DISTENTION
CHEST
• CHEST, PAIN, DISTENTION

• COSTAL REGION, PAIN,
  DISTENTION
SEXUALITY, FEMALE:
GYNECOLOGICAL
• FETUS, RESTLESS: Qi Stagnation
• MORNING SICKNESS:

Gestational Foul Obstruction--Cold
• POSTPARTUM, PAIN
STOMACH/DIGESTIVE
DISORDERS
• HICCUPS

Dose
6 - 9 gm

Common Name
Purple Perilla Stalk

Contraindications
Not: Boil For A Long Time

XI HE LIU
(CHUI SI LIU/CHENG LIU)

西河柳

CACUMEN
TAMARICIS

Traditional Functions:

1. Clears the Surface and promotes diaphoresis
2. Promotes the eruption of rashes

Traditional Properties:

Enters: LU, ST, HT,

Properties: SP, W

Indications:

INFECTIOUS DISEASES
• MEASLES, EARLY
  STAGE: Wind-Cold, w/o

Rash
LUNGS
• BRONCHITIS,

CHRONIC
• COUGH: Wind Pathogen
SKIN

• RASHES, INCOMPLETE
  EXPRESSION OF: With
  Wind Cold Complex

Clinical/Pharmaceutical Studies:

CIRCULATION DISORDERS
• CAPILLARIES, SUBCUTANEOUS,
  DILATES
FEVERS
• ANTIPYRETIC

INFECTIOUS DISEASES
• BACTERIAL, ANTI-: Inhibits
  Pneumococcus, Strep, Staph
• VIRAL, ANTI-: Flu

LUNGS
• ANTITUSSIVE: On Injection
SKIN
• SUDORIFIC

Dose
3 - 15 gm

Common Name
Tamarisk Tops

Contraindications
Not: Measles w/Rash

Notes
Large Dose May Cause Restlessness
External Application: 90-150 gm

XI XIN

細辛
(细辛)

HERBA
ASARI CUM RADICE

Traditional Functions:

1. Eliminates Cold from the Surface
2. Disperses Wind and stops pain of Wind Cold
3. Warms the Lungs and transforms Phlegm
4. Opens up areas of stagnation

Traditional Properties:

Enters: LU, HT, KI,

Properties: SP, W

Indications:

COLD
• EXTERNAL COLD W/
  YANG DEFICIENCY
EXTERIOR
  CONDITIONS
• EXTERIOR COLD W/
  YANG DEFICIENCY
HEAD/NECK
• HEAD/BODY ACHES:
  Very Good
• HEADACHE: Wind Cold
HEART
• ANGINA PECTORIS:
  Chest Bi Strangulating
  Pain
INFECTIOUS DISEASES
• COMMON COLD W/

MAINLY HEAD, BODY
ACHES
LUNGS
• BRONCHITIS,
  CHRONIC W/THIN,
  COPIUS PHLEGM
• COUGH: Cold Phlegm/
  Wind Cold
• COUGH/WHEEZING:
  Phlegm Fluid
• LUNGS, DYSPNEA:
  Cold Phlegm
MENTAL STATE/
NEUROLOGICAL
DISORDERS
• MENTAL CLOUDINESS:

Excess (Shut-In Complex)
• UNCONSCIOUSNESS:
  (Mental Cloudiness) Excess
  (Shut-In Complex)
MUSCULOSKELETAL/
CONNECTIVE TISSUE
• ARTHRITIS: For
  Expelling Cold, Dampness/
  Wind Damp Cold Bi
• JOINTS, PAIN: Wind
  Damp Bi
NOSE
• SINUSITIS
• SINUSITIS W/
  HEADACHE
ORAL CAVITY

• TOOTHACHE, SEVERE
PAIN/NUMBNESS/
GENERAL
DISCOMFORT
• BI, WIND DAMP,
  CHRONIC: Open Luo,
  Arrest Pain
• HEAD/BODY ACHES:
  Very Good
• PAIN RELIEF FROM
  STAGNANT QI
PHLEGM
• PHLEGM FLUID
QI RELATED
DISORDERS/TOPICS
• QI STAGNATION

Clinical/Pharmaceutical Studies:

CIRCULATION
DISORDERS
• HYPERTENSION, ANTI-
• VASODILATOR
FEVERS
• ANTIPYRETIC: Volatile
  Oil
HEAD/NECK
• HEADACHE: 1-3 g In
  Decoction
HEART
• CARDIOTONIC
IMMUNE SYSTEM
RELATED DISORDERS/
TOPICS
• ALLERGIC, ANTI-:
  Aqueous/ETOH Extract
INFECTIOUS DISEASES
• ANTIBIOTIC: Potent
  Gram + Inhibitor (Volatile

Oil) , Shigella, Strep,
Salmonella Typhi
• COMMON COLD: 1-3 g
  In Decoction
KIDNEYS
• DIURETIC
LUNGS
• ANTITUSSIVE
• COUGH: 1-3 g In
  Decoction
MENTAL STATE/
NEUROLOGICAL
DISORDERS
• TRANQUILIZING:
  Essential Oil, Starts With
  Extreme Stimulation
MUSCULOSKELETAL/
CONNECTIVE TISSUE
• MUSCLES, SMOOTH
  RELAXES

ORAL CAVITY
• GINGIVITIS: Patent,
  Yatonshui (Toothache
  Liquid--Xi Xin, Bing Pian,
  Bi Ba, Gao Liang Jiang)
  Apply With Cotton Ball
• MOUTH, APHTHOUS
  STOMATITIS: Plaster Of
  Herb Powder, 9-15 g,
  Water, Small Amount
  Glycerin/Honey Put On
  Navel With Gauze, Fix
  With Tape, Retain 3 Days
  Or More, May Need 2
  Applications, 94%
  Effective
• MOUTH, SMALL
  ULCERS, SPEEDS
  HEALING: Mix With
  Water, Glycerin Place On

Navel For At Least 3 Days
• TOOTH EXTRACTION:
  Local Injection, With
  Uncured Tian Nan Xing
• TOOTHACHE: Patent,
  Yatonshui (Toothache
  Liquid--Xi Xin, Bing Pian,
  Bi Ba, Gao Liang Jiang)
  Apply With Cotton Ball
PAIN/NUMBNESS/
GENERAL
DISCOMFORT
• ANALGESIC: Dental,
  Oral Pain, Inflammation,
  Decoction, Volatile Oil
• ANESTHETIC, LOCAL:
  Injection Of 3% Volatile
  Oil, Adding 0.1%
  Epinephrine Prolonged
  Duration

Dose
1.5 - 4.5 gm
Common Name
Chinese Wild Ginger
Contraindications
Not: Headache From Def Yin And Yang Rising

Not: Cough From LU Heat

Notes
May Cause Numbing Of Tongue

Large Doses Of Essential Oil Can Cause Respiratory Paralysis

Toxic To Kidneys In Large Doses, Watch Patients With Renal Insufficiency

---

XIANG RU

香薷

HERBA ELSHOLTZIAE SPLENDENTIS

Traditional Functions:

1. Relieves the Surface, dispels Summer Heat and transforms Phelgm and Dampness
2. Regulates water circulation by inducing urination and reduces edema

Traditional Properties:

Enters: LU, ST,

Properties: SP, ARO, <W

Indications:

ABDOMEN/
  GASTROINTESTINAL TOPICS
• ABDOMEN, PAIN OF
BOWEL RELATED DISORDERS
• DIARRHEA: Summer Heat
COLD
• COLD, AVERSION TO
FEVERS
• CHILLS, FEVER: Summer Heat/
  Damp
• FEVER
FLUID DISORDERS
• EDEMA, BODY, LEGS: Especially
  As External Pattern
HEAD/NECK

• HEADACHE: Summer Heat/Damp
HEAT
• SUMMER HEAT: From Too Many/
  Much Cold Beverages
• SUMMER HEAT DAMPNESS
INFECTIOUS DISEASES
• COMMON COLD, IN SUMMER
  W/DAMPNESS
KIDNEYS
• DIURETIC, MILD
NUTRITIONAL/METABOLIC
  DISORDERS/TOPICS
• BERIBERI
PAIN/NUMBNESS/GENERAL
  DISCOMFORT

• BODY ACHES: Summer Heat/
  Damp
SKIN
• ADIAPHORESIS: Summer Heat/
  Damp
STOMACH/DIGESTIVE
  DISORDERS
• NAUSEA/VOMITING
URINARY BLADDER
• DYSURIA: Especially As External
  Pattern
• URINATION, SCANTY
WIND DISORDERS
• WIND COLD IN SUMMER

Clinical/Pharmaceutical Studies:

FEVERS
• ANTIPYRETIC
INFECTIOUS DISEASES
• BACTERIAL, ANTI-: Broad
  Spectrum

• VIRAL, ANTI-
KIDNEYS
• DIURETIC: Essential Oil
SKIN
• DIAPHORETIC

STOMACH/DIGESTIVE
  DISORDERS
• STOMACHIC: Stimulates Gastric
  Secretion, Peristalsis

Dose
3 - 9 gm
Common Name
Aromatic Madder
Contraindications
Not: Def Exterior Patterns With Sweating

XIN YI HUA

辛夷花

FLOS MAGNOLIAE LILIFLORAE

Traditional Functions:

1. Disperses Wind and opens the nasal passages and sinuses

Traditional Properties:

Enters: LU, ST,

Properties: SP, <W

Indications:

NOSE
- NASAL CONGESTION: Cold

- NASAL OBSTRUCTIONS, ANY
- NASAL SECRETIONS, RUNNY

- SINUSITIS W/HEADACHE

Clinical/Pharmaceutical Studies:

BLOOD RELATED DISORDERS/TOPICS
- BLOOD PRESSURE, LOWERS: Injected/Oral, Not Essential Oil

INFECTIOUS DISEASES
- COMMON COLD: Nose Drops Decreases Incidence, Does Not Treat, Though
- INFLUENZA W/ HEADACHE: With Zi Su Ye As Tea

MENTAL STATE/ NEUROLOGICAL DISORDERS
- SEDATIVE: Essential Oil

MUSCULOSKELETAL/ CONNECTIVE TISSUE
- MUSCLES, STRIATED, CURARE-LIKE ACTION: When Injected, Or Other Parts Of Plant

NOSE
- NASAL SECRETIONS, DECREASES: Topical, Essential Oil

- RHINITIS, ALLERGIC/ SIMPLE: Nose Drops Of Water Distillate Of Xin Yi Hua, Extract Of Huang Qin, 2-3x/Day In Nose For 2-3 Weeks, 80% Effective
- RHINITIS, ATROPHIC: Topical Application Of Ointment From Herb, Chan Su, She Xiang, Bing Pian, Glycerin
- RHINITIS, CHRONIC W/ HEADACHE
- RHINITIS, CHRONIC/ ACUTE/ALLERGIC: Xin Yi Hua, Cang Er Zi, Yu Xing Cao, Qian LI Guang (Herba Senecionis) , 150 g Each, Plus Few Drops Menthol, Boiled In Water, Filtered Then Concentrated To 500 ml, 80-90% Effective
- RHINITIS, HYPERTROPHIC/ ACUTE: Volatile Oil

Emulsion, "Ointment Of Alcohol Extract Apply In Nasal Cavity With Gauze, Retain 2-3 Hrs, 1x/Day Or 2, 10 Applications, 4-5 Applications To Show Improvement
- SINUSITIS: Xin Yi Hua Repeatedly Soaked In Banana Stump Juice Then Sun Dried Added To Musk, Bing Pian
- SINUSITIS, PARANASAL: With Cang Er Zi, Du Huo, Bo He Or Xi Xin (Cang Er Zi San) , " With Jing Jie, Huang Qin (Xin Yi Jing Jie San) , " Paste Made With Xin Yi Hua, Hai Er Cha, Ru Xiang, Bing Pian, Glycerin, 2-8 Days

PAIN/NUMBNESS/ GENERAL DISCOMFORT

- ANALGESIC: Essential Oil

SEXUALITY, FEMALE: GYNECOLOGICAL
- UTERUS, STIMULATES: Non-Essential Oil, Water/ ETOH Soluble, Starts 20-60 Min After Ingestion, Lasts 8-24 Hours

SKIN
- ECZEMA: Topical Application Of Ju Hua Powder (Xin Yi Hua, Ju Hua, Hua Shi, Bing Pian, Amylum)
- FUNGAL, ANTI-: 15-30% Decoction, Dermatomycoses, Very Strong, Candida, Needs High Concentration
- SKIN, PRICKLY HEAT: Topical Application Of Ju Hua Powder (Xin Yi Hua, Ju Hua, Hua Shi, Bing Pian, Amylum)

Dose
3 - 9 gm

Contraindications
Not: Yin Deficiency Fire

Notes
Overdosing: Redness Of Eyes, Dizziness

Intranasal Application May Cause Irritation

Oral Much Less Toxic

ZI SU YE
(*SU YE*)

紫蘇葉
(紫苏叶)

FOLIUM PERILLAE FRUTESCENTIS

Traditional Functions:

1. Relieves the Surface and dissipates Cold
2. Circulates Qi and harmonizes and strengthens the Middle Jiao
3. Calms restless fetus
4. Reduces fish and crab poisoning ·

Traditional Properties:

Enters: LU, SP,

Properties: SP, ARO, W

Indications:

ABDOMEN/ GASTROINTESTINAL TOPICS
- ABDOMEN, FULLNESS OF/ DISTENTION
- ABDOMEN, PAIN OF

CHEST
- CHEST, DISCOMFORT, STUFFY

COLD
- CHILLS: Wind Cold

INFECTIOUS DISEASES
- COMMON COLD W/O SWEAT: Wind Cold

LUNGS
- COUGH: Wind Cold
- COUGH, WHEEZING

NOSE
- NASAL CONGESTION: Wind Cold

- MORNING SICKNESS

STOMACH/DIGESTIVE DISORDERS
- ANOREXIA
- DIGESTIVE DISTURBANCE
- NAUSEA/VOMITING
- VOMITING

TRAUMA, BITES, POISONINGS
- SEAFOOD POISONING,

Indications:

FEVERS
• FEVER: Wind Cold
HEAD/NECK
• HEADACHE: Wind Cold

SEXUALITY, FEMALE:
  GYNECOLOGICAL
• FETUS, RESTLESS, CALMS

VOMITING OF: Fish/Crabs
WIND DISORDERS
• WIND COLD

Clinical/Pharmaceutical Studies:

BLOOD RELATED DISORDERS/
  TOPICS
• BLOOD GLUCOSE, INCREASES
FEVERS
• ANTIPYRETIC: Mild
INFECTIOUS DISEASES
• ANTIBIOTIC: Bacteriostatic, Staph

Aureus
LUNGS
• ANTITUSSIVE
• PULMONARY DISEASE
  TREATMENT
MENTAL STATE/
  NEUROLOGICAL DISORDERS

• HYPNOTIC: Extract Increases
  Length Of Sleep
MUSCULOSKELETAL/
  CONNECTIVE TISSUE
• ANTISPASMODIC
SKIN
• DIAPHORETIC

Dose

3 - 9 gm

Common Name

Perilla Leaf

Precautions

Watch: Surface Deficiency With Febrile Disease

Notes

Do Not Boil Long Term

Release Exterior Conditions: Spicy, Cool

BO HE   薄荷   HERBA MENTHAE

Traditional Functions:

1. Disperses Wind Heat
2. Clears the head and eyes and cleanses the throat
3. Promotes the eruption of measles
4. Circulates the Liver Qi, relieving Liver Qi stagnation

Traditional Properties:

Enters: LU, LV,

Properties: SP, ARO, CL

Indications:

CHEST
- CHEST, LATERAL, PRESSURE IN: Liver Qi Stagnation

EYES
- CONJUNCTIVITIS
- EYES, RED: Wind Heat
- EYES, RED, CONGESTED: Liver Heat

FEVERS
- FEVER: Wind Heat

HEAD/NECK
- HEADACHE, SORE THROAT

IMMUNE SYSTEM RELATED DISORDERS/TOPICS
- LYMPH NODES, SWELLING

INFECTIOUS DISEASES
- COMMON COLD: Wind Heat

- MEASLES, EARLY STAGE

LIVER
- LIVER QI CONGESTION W/ SUBCOSTAL PAIN

LUNGS
- COUGH, SPUTUM

MENTAL STATE/ NEUROLOGICAL DISORDERS
- EMOTIONAL INSTABILITY: Liver Qi Stagnation

ORAL CAVITY
- BREATH, FOUL
- MOUTH, SORES
- THROAT, PAIN, SWOLLEN
- THROAT, SORE, HEADACHE: Wind Heat
- TOOTHACHE

SEXUALITY, FEMALE:

GYNECOLOGICAL
- MENSTRUATION, DISORDERS OF: Liver Qi Stagnation

SKIN
- HYPEREMIA
- RASHES
- RASHES, INCOMPLETE EXPRESSION OF: Early Stage
- RASHES, W/PRURITUS: Clears Wind
- SCABIES
- SKIN, SORES/LESIONS

WIND DISORDERS
- WIND HEAT: Fever, Headache, Cough

Clinical/Pharmaceutical Studies:

ABDOMEN/ GASTROINTESTINAL TOPICS
- INTESTINES, INHIBITS: Oil Of

CANCER/TUMORS/ SWELLINGS/LUMPS
- CERVICAL CANCER: Infusion Inhibited

FEVERS
- ANTIPYRETIC: Orally, Small Amounts By Dilation Of Skin Capillaries

HEAD/NECK
- HEADACHE: Topically As Menthol

IMMUNE SYSTEM RELATED DISORDERS/ TOPICS
- ALLERGIC DERMATITIS: Modify

Proteus Vulgaris
- COMMON COLD: Yin Qiao San, Jing Fang Bai Du San, Sang Ju Yin All Have Bo He, *Fumigation Of Home With Rice Vinegar And Herb In Water Helped Prevent
- ENCEPHALITIS B, EPIDEMIC: Fresh Herbs Da Qing Ye, Bo He, Qing Hao Can Help
- VIRAL, ANTI-: Some Against Herpes Simplex, Variola, Semliki Forest, Mumps, Not Flu

LUNGS
- EXPECTORANT

MUSCULOSKELETAL/ CONNECTIVE TISSUE
- ANTISPASMODIC
- MUSCLES, SMOOTH,

Helping Symptoms
- THROAT, SORE: Cured With "Modified Solidaga Decurrens Decoction" (Herba Solidago, Bo He, She Gan, Herba Rhodeae, Herba Peristrophis, Zou Ma Tai (Radix Ardisiae), Gan Cao), 1-3 Doses Effective, Any Of Herbs May Be Used Singly, Too

PAIN/NUMBNESS/ GENERAL DISCOMFORT
- ANALGESIC: Local Application
- NEURALGIA: Topically As Menthol

PARASITES
- ASCARIASIS: Oil Is Effective

SEXUALITY, FEMALE:

g), Applied With Towel As Hot Compress Over Area, Morning, Evening, All Had Good Results

SKIN
- ALLERGIC DERMATITIS: Modify Jing Feng Bai Du Tang
- BURNS: Reduces Inflammation
- DIAPHORETIC: Orally, Small Amounts By Dilation Of Skin Capillaries
- ECZEMA
- PRURITUS: Topically As Menthol
- PSORIASIS
- SKIN, IRRITATES
- URTICARIA

STOMACH/DIGESTIVE DISORDERS

Clinical/Pharmaceutical Studies:

Jing Feng Bai Du Tang
INFECTIOUS DISEASES
- **ANTIBIOTIC:**
Solmonella, Echo Viruses,
Staph Aureus, Strep,
Neisseria, Shigella, B.
Anthracis, C.Diphtheriae,
E.Coli, Candida Albicans,

INHIBITS
NOSE
- **RHINITIS:** Menthol
Dilutes Thick Mucus,
Helping Symptoms
ORAL CAVITY
- **LARYNGITIS:** Menthol
Dilutes Thick Mucus,

GYNECOLOGICAL
- **ABORTIFACIENT:** Early
Pregnancy, (In Mice)
- **CERVIX, CANCINOMA:**
Infusion Inhibited
- **MASTITIS, ACUTE:**
Filtered Decoction, 60 g
And Leaf Of Jie Geng (60

- **STOMACHIC**
- **ULCERS, GASTRIC:**
Agent In Oil Has Some
Effect
**TRAUMA, BITES,
POISONINGS**
- **INFLAMMATORY, ANTI-**
: Local Application

Not: Def Yin w/Heat

Dose

2.4 - 9.0 gm

Common Name

Peppermint

Contraindications

Not: Def Surface

Notes

Add Last To Cooking Formula, Do Not Cook Long
Term

Will Gradually Penetrate Skin

Side Effects Very Rare

CHAI HU   柴胡   *RADIX BUPLEURI*

Traditional Functions:

1. Clears Shao Yang Heat patterns
2. Relieves Liver Qi stagnation
3. Raises the Yang Qi in patterns of Spleen or Stomach deficiency
4. Disperses Wind Heat

Traditional Properties:

Enters: PC, SJ, LV, GB,

Properties: BIT, <SP, CL

Indications:

- **PROLAPSE OF ORGANS:** Sinking
Of Central Qi
**ABDOMEN/
GASTROINTESTINAL TOPICS**
- **ABDOMEN, BLOATING:** Liver
Stomach Disharmony
- **FLANK PAIN:** Shao Yang Disorder
- **SUBCOSTAL PAIN**
BOWEL RELATED DISORDERS
- **ANAL PROLAPSE**
- **DIARRHEA:** Spleen Deficient With
Sinking Of Qi
- **HEMORRHOIDS**
- **RECTAL PROLAPSE**
CHEST
- **CHEST, CONSTRICTION:** Liver
Stomach Disharmony/Shao Yang
Disorder
- **CHEST/FLANK PAIN:** Liver Qi
Stagnation
EARS/HEARING DISORDERS

- **DEAFNESS**
- **DIZZINESS:** Liver Qi Stagnation
- **EARS, HEARING, POOR**
- **VERTIGO:** Liver Qi Stagnation
FEVERS
- **CHILLS, FEVER:** Shao Yang
Disorder
INFECTIOUS DISEASES
- **COMMON COLD:** Wind Heat
- **MALARIA**
- **MALARIA, CHILLS, FEVER OF**
LIVER
- **JAUNDICE**
- **LIVER QI CONGESTION W/
SUBCOSTAL PAIN**
- **LIVER SPLEEN DISHARMONY**
**MENTAL STATE/
NEUROLOGICAL DISORDERS**
- **EMOTIONAL INSTABILITY:**
Liver Qi Stagnation
- **IRRITABILITY:** Shao Yang

Disorder
ORAL CAVITY
- **MOUTH, BITTER TASTE:** Shao
Yang Disorder
**SEXUALITY, FEMALE:
GYNECOLOGICAL**
- **LACTATION, INSUFFICIENT:** w/
Liver Qi Congestion Add
- **MENSTRUATION, DISORDERS
OF:** Liver Qi Stagnation
- **MENSTRUATION, IRREGULAR**
- **UTERUS, PROLAPSE**
**STOMACH/DIGESTIVE
DISORDERS**
- **EPIGASTRIC, FLANK PAIN:**
Liver Stomach Disharmony
- **INDIGESTION:** Liver Stomach
Disharmony
- **NAUSEA:** Liver Stomach
Disharmony
- **VOMITING:** Shao Yang Disorder

Clinical/Pharmaceutical Studies:

**ABDOMEN/
GASTROINTESTINAL
TOPICS**
- **INTESTINES,
STIMULATES**
- **PANCREATITIS, ACUTE:**
Da Chai Hu Tang,
Modified
BLOOD RELATED

Capillary Permeability,
Other Antibody Formation
INFECTIOUS DISEASES
- **ANTIBIOTIC:** TB, Flu,
Polio
- **COMMON COLD,**
FEVER OF: Within 24
Hrs, e.g. Xiao Chai Hu
Tang

Glucose For IV Infusion,
1x/Day, 10 Courses
- **LIVER, HELPS
RECOVER FROM
ALCOHOL, TYPHOID,
ORGANIC PHOSPHATES**
- **LIVER, PROTECTANT:**
Decoction Increases Bile,
Reduces Damage From

Injection IP Of Flavones
- **METABOLISM,
INCREASE PROTEIN
SYNTHESIS**
ORAL CAVITY
- **CANDIDIASIS, ORAL:**
Even Not Responsive To
Nystatin, Trichomycin,
Amphotericin Effectively

Clinical/Pharmaceutical Studies:

DISORDERS/TOPICS
- BLOOD GLUCOSE: Increases From Oral
- BLOOD PRESSURE, LOWERS SLIGHTLY, AQUEOUS EXTRACT

CHEST
- INTERCOSTAL NEURALGIA

FEVERS
- ANTIPYRETIC: Slight, Oral

GALL BLADDER
- BILIARY TRACT INFECTION: Da Chai Hu Tang, Modified
- GALL BLADDER, CHOLAGOGUE: Increase Secretion Of Bile By Liver

IMMUNE SYSTEM RELATED DISORDERS/ TOPICS
- IMMUNE SYSTEM, STRENGTHENS: Inhibits Effect Of Histamine On

- INFLUENZA, FEVER OF: Within 24 Hrs, e.g. Xiao Chai Hu Tang
- MALARIA: Antiplasmodial Action
- MALARIA, FEVER OF: Within 24 Hrs, e.g. Xiao Chai Hu Tang
- VIRAL, ANTI-: Flu

KIDNEYS
- DIURETIC: Oral Small Doses, Large Doses May Cause Edema

LIVER
- HEPATITIS, CHRONIC W/HEPATOMEGALY: Chai Hu With Dan Shen Injection Solution, Vit C, B Orally Helped, Too, 10 Day Courses
- HEPATITIS, INFECTIOUS: Injection, 1:2, 10-20 ml In 50% Glucose, IV, 1-2x/Day/20-30 ml In 250-500 ml 10%

Toxins, Bacteria, Used With Gan Cao
- LIVER, REDUCES ENZYMES: Reduces SGOT/SGPT

LUNGS
- ANTITUSSIVE: Strong, Similar To Codeine
- PNEUMONIA, FEVER OF: Within 24 Hrs, e.g. Xiao Chai Hu Tang

MENTAL STATE/ NEUROLOGICAL DISORDERS
- SEDATIVE: Significant, Oral, Resembling Meprobamate, Antagonized Caffeine, Methamphetamine
- TRANQUILIZING

NUTRITIONAL/ METABOLIC DISORDERS/TOPICS
- METABOLISM, HYPOXIA TOLERANCE:

Treated With Chai Hu Qing Gan Tang

PAIN/NUMBNESS/ GENERAL DISCOMFORT
- ANALGESIC: Moderate, Oral

SKIN
- WARTS: 60% Effective, IM Injection, 1 g Herb Equivalent For 20 Days, 0.5-1.0 ml 2.4 mm From Base Of Wart, 1x/2-3 Days, Injection Of Acupoints, Too, Needs 10 Treatments

STOMACH/DIGESTIVE DISORDERS
- ULCERS, GASTRIC: Small Doses Help

TRAUMA, BITES, POISONINGS
- INFLAMMATORY, ANTI-: Saponin When Given Orally To Some Types Of Inflammation

Dose

3 - 18 gm

Common Name

Hare's Ear Root

Contraindications

Not: Liver Yang Rising/Yin Def

Precautions

Watch: Menstruation-Dizziness Possible
Watch: Drying In Yin Def

Notes

Raw: For External Pathogens

Stir-Bake: Reduce Diaphoretic Action

May Cause Mild Lassitude, Sedation, Drowsiness In

Small Doses, Large Doses May Cause Deep Sedation

With Poor Sleep, Gastric Symptoms Can Be Relieved

With Gan Cao Addition

Some Strains Of Herb Can Be More Toxic Than Others

Herb Seems To Accumulates In Body, Thus Necessitating A Reduction In Dose After The Acute Phase Of Treatment

---

CHAN TUI

蟬 蛻
(蝉 蜕)

PERIOSTRACUM CICADAE

Traditional Functions:

1. Disperses Wind Heat
2. Promotes the eruption of measles
3. Clears the eyes and removes superficial visual obstruction
4. Stabilizes spasms
5. Moistens the throat and opens the voice
6. Pacifies infants
7. Reduces itching

Traditional Properties:

Enters: LU, LV,

Properties: SW, SA, <C

Indications:

CHILDHOOD DISORDERS
- FEAR SPASMS, CHILDHOOD

EYES
- EYES, INFECTIONS
- EYES, RED, CONGESTED: Liver

EXPRESSION OF RASH
- TETANUS: Auxillary Herb

LUNGS
- RESPIRATORY TRACT INFECTION

- SPASMS, W/FEVER, ACUTE

NOSE
- RHINITIS

ORAL CAVITY
- HOARSENESS

Indications:

Heat
- VISION, BLURRED: Wind Heat
- VISUAL OPACITY

INFECTIOUS DISEASES
- COMMON COLD W/FEVER, HOARSENESS
- FEBRILE DISEASES, CHILDHOOD: Wind Convulsions, Spasms, Night Terrors, Delirium
- MEASLES, INCOMPLETE

MENTAL STATE/ NEUROLOGICAL DISORDERS
- CONVULSIONS, CHILDHOOD: Febrile Disease Wind
- DELIRIUM, CHILDHOOD: Febrile Disease Wind

MUSCULOSKELETAL/ CONNECTIVE TISSUE
- SPASMS, CHILDHOOD: Febrile Disease Wind

- LARYNGITIS
- THROAT, SORE, SWOLLEN: Wind Heat

SKIN
- RASHES, INCOMPLETE EXPRESSION OF: Early Stage
- RASHES, INITIAL STAGE: Wind
- RASHES, W/PRURITUS: Clears Wind

Clinical/Pharmaceutical Studies:

CANCER/TUMORS/ SWELLINGS/LUMPS
- CANCER: Inhibits Growth Without Affecting Normal Cells

EYES
- CATARACTS: 9 g PO/ Day Effective Treatment
- CORNEAL OPACITY: Injection/Eye Drops, 76% Effective, Make Drops With Snake Slough

FEVERS
- ANTIPYRETIC: At 1 g/ kg PO, Decoction, Head, Limbs Most Potent

IMMUNE SYSTEM RELATED DISORDERS/ TOPICS
- ALLERGIC REACTIONS

INFECTIOUS DISEASES
- INFLUENZA, HIGH

FEVER OF: Chan Tui, Jiang Can
- TETANUS: Spasms, Promoted Recovery, With Other Herbs, Wu Zhui Feng San (Chan Tui 30g, Tian Nan Xing 6g, Tian Ma 6 g, Quan Xie With Tails 7 Pieces, Jiang Can 7 Pcs), Given Orally With 1.5 g Zhu Sha And Yellow Wine, Confirmed Effective, 0.5-3 Days Treatment, May Use Chan Tui Alone, 9-15 g/Dose PO With Yellow Wine 3x/Day

KIDNEYS
- NEPHRITIS, ACUTE: 80% Cured By Chan Tui Fu Ping Tang, Modified

MENTAL STATE/ NEUROLOGICAL

DISORDERS
- BELL'S PALSY: Feng Chan San (Xiaon Feng Chan 3 Pieces, Shi Gao 3g Grind Into Fine Powder) PO With Hot Yellow Wine At Bed, 90% Cure, *Qian Zheng San Also Helped
- NICOTINE, DECREASES MUSCULAR TREMORS FROM
- SEDATIVE: As Herb Decoction Or Wu Zhui Feng San

MUSCULOSKELETAL/ CONNECTIVE TISSUE
- SPASMS: Decreased From Tetanus/Other Drugs, Add With Other Herbs

PAIN/NUMBNESS/ GENERAL

DISCOMFORT
- ANALGESIC

SKIN
- ALLERGIC REACTIONS
- ECZEMA: Decoction Of Chan Tui, Ma Huang, etc, High Cure Rate
- RASHES, DRUG INDUCED: Decoction Of Chan Tui, Ma Huang, etc, High Cure Rate
- SKIN, PAINT ALLERGY RASH
- URTICARIA: 3 g, Glutinous Rice Wine 50 g Cured, No Relapse, Chronic Treated With Honeyed Pills Or With Bai Ji LI, *Decoction Of Chan Tui, Ma Huang, etc, High Cure Rate

Dose

3 - 15 gm

Common Name

Cicada Moulting

Contraindications

Not: Def External Pattern

Precautions

Watch: Pregnancy

Notes

15-30 gm For Chronic Nephritis, Tetanus

DAN DOU CHI   淡豆豉   *SEMEN SOJAE PRAEPARATUM*

Traditional Functions:

1. Relieves the surface: Wind Cold or Heat
2. Removes restlessness from Yin deficiency or resolution of exterior Heat

Traditional Properties:

Enters: LU, ST

Properties: SP, <BIT, C

Indications:

EXTERIOR CONDITIONS
- EXTERIOR HOT/COLD

HEAD/NECK
- HEADACHE: Wind Heat

INFECTIOUS DISEASES
- COMMON COLD

MENTAL STATE/ NEUROLOGICAL DISORDERS
- INSOMNIA: Post Exterior Heat Illness
- IRRITABILITY: Post Exterior Heat

Illness
YIN RELATED DISORDERS/ TOPICS
- YIN DEFICIENCY W/EXTERNAL PATHOGEN

Clinical/Pharmaceutical Studies:

SKIN
- DIAPHORETIC, VERY WEAK

STOMACH/DIGESTIVE DISORDERS

- STOMACHIC: Enzyme-Like, Tonifies Stomach

Dose

9 - 15 gm

Common Name

Prepared Soybean

Contraindications

Not: Nursing Mothers-Restrains Lactation

FU PING

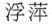 浮萍

HERBA LEMNAE SEU SPIRODELAE

Traditional Functions:

1. Relieves the surface
2. Promotes rashes to surface
3. Circulates fluids and reduces swelling
4. Dissipates Wind Damp

Traditional Properties:

Enters: LU,

Properties: SP, C

Indications:

EXTERIOR CONDITIONS
- EXTERIOR PATHOGEN: Heat w/ Head & Body Aches

FLUID DISORDERS
- EDEMA: Wind-Fluid
- EDEMA, HOT SUPERFICIAL: Upper Body With Dysuria

HEAD/NECK
- FACE, BLISTERS OF: Topical
- HEADACHE: Exterior Heat

INFECTIOUS DISEASES
- COMMON COLD: Wind Heat
- MEASLES, EXPRESSION OF

MENTAL STATE/ NEUROLOGICAL DISORDERS
- EPILEPSY
- PARALYSIS: Wind Damp

MUSCULOSKELETAL/ CONNECTIVE TISSUE
- ARTHRITIS, PAIN: Wind Damp Bi

PAIN/NUMBNESS/GENERAL DISCOMFORT
- BODY ACHES: Exterior Heat

SKIN
- ACNE
- ALBINISM: Topical

- ERYSIPELAS: Topical
- EXANTHEMA, EXPRESSION OF
- FUNGAL INFECTIONS: Topical
- RASHES: Wind Heat
- RASHES, INCOMPLETE EXPRESSION OF: Early Stage
- RASHES, W/PRURITUS: Clears Wind
- SORES: Topical

URINARY BLADDER
- URINATION, PAINFUL

WIND DISORDERS
- WIND RASH

Clinical/Pharmaceutical Studies:

BLOOD RELATED DISORDERS/ TOPICS
- BLOOD PRESSURE, RAISES

FEVERS

- ANTIPYRETIC: Weak, Oral

HEART
- CARDIOTONIC

KIDNEYS

- DIURETIC

SKIN
- PRURITUS

Dose

3 - 6 gm

Common Name

Duckweed

Contraindications

Not: w/Profuse Sweating-Excess/Def

GE GEN

葛根

RADIX PUERARIAE

Traditional Functions:

1. Relieves the surface
2. Clears Exterior Heat and relieves muscles of neck and back
3. Helps generate fluids and allays thirst
4. Promotes the eruption of measles
5. Stops diarrhea

Traditional Properties:

Enters: SP, ST,

Properties: SW, SP, CL

Indications:

BLOOD RELATED DISORDERS/ TOPICS
• BLOOD PRESSURE, LOWERS
BOWEL RELATED DISORDERS
• DIARRHEA: Heat/Spleen Deficient/ Spleen Deficient With Sinking Of Qi/ Damp Heat
• DYSENTERY
ENDOCRINE RELATED DISORDERS
• DIABETES: Internal Heat With Exhaustion Thirst
FEVERS
• FEVER: External Heat
FLUID DISORDERS

• THIRST: External Heat/Fluid Injury/ Stomach Heat
HEAD/NECK
• HEADACHE: External Heat/ Hypertension
• NECK, SPASMS, STIFF
INFECTIOUS DISEASES
• COMMON COLD: Wind Heat
• MEASLES, EXPRESSION OF
MENTAL STATE/ NEUROLOGICAL DISORDERS
• RESTLESSNESS
MUSCULOSKELETAL/ CONNECTIVE TISSUE

• BACK, UPPER: Stiff, Tight
SKIN
• DIAPHORETIC, WEAK
• RASHES, INCOMPLETE EXPRESSION OF: Early Stage
• SKIN, ERUPTIONS
STOMACH/DIGESTIVE DISORDERS
• STOMACH HEAT, THIRST: Diabetes
WIND DISORDERS
• WIND COLD
• WIND HEAT IN LIVER CHANNEL

Clinical/Pharmaceutical Studies:

BLOOD RELATED DISORDERS/TOPICS
• BLOOD GLUCOSE, REDUCES
• BLOOD PRESSURE, LOWERS: Mild, 20 g/Day For 14 Days
CIRCULATION DISORDERS
• BLOOD CIRCULATION, INCREASES IN HEART/ BRAIN, LESS THAN PAPAVERINE
• HYPERTENSION: Reduces Pain, Slight BP Drop, *Decoction 10-15 g In 2 Doses, 2-8 Weeks, Neck Pain, Stiffness, 85% Had Relief Of Neck Symptoms, Relief Started 1 Week After Treatment,

Persisting 1-2 Weeks, Some Had No Symptom Relapse For 3-9 Months, Other Symptoms Relieved, Too, BP Not Lowered
EARS/HEARING DISORDERS
• DEAFNESS, SUDDEN: w/Vit B's
• DIZZINESS: Hypertension, Reduces
• EARS, DEAFNESS, SUDDEN, EARLY STAGE: ETOH Extract Tablet, Each = 1.5 g Of Herb, 1-2 Tabs, 3x/Day, Some Injected, Too, With Vit B Complex, 1-2 Months, Hearing Improved In 80% Cases
ENDOCRINE RELATED

DISORDERS
• HORMONES: Estrogen-Like (Weaker Than Diethystilbesterol), Follicular
FEVERS
• ANTIPYRETIC: Aqueous Extract, Slight, ETOH Extract, Marked, Oral Dose
HEAD/NECK
• HEADACHE: Hypertension, Reduces
• MIGRAINE
• NECK, STIFFNESS/PAIN: From Common Cold/ Hypertension
HEART
• ANGINA PECTORIS: Helps Increase Blood Flow, Reduces Platelet

Aggregation, 3-4 Tabs, 3x/ Day (10 mg Of Flavones), Helped Pain, *Xin Xue Ning Tablet (Ge Gen, Shan Zha Extract, 6:1), 90% Had Relief, 43% Marked
• HEART ATTACK: Increases Blood Flow, Helps Metabolism Of Myocardium, Reduces Platelet Aggregation
• HEART, BETA-BLOCKER: Wide Spectrum, B1 Primarily
MUSCULOSKELETAL/ CONNECTIVE TISSUE
• ANTISPASMODIC IN SMOOTH MUSCLE: Action Similar To And 1/3 Of Papaverine

Dose
9 - 24 gm
Common Name
Common Kudzu Root

Contraindications
Not: Excess Sweat, Stomach Cold
Notes
Bake For Diarrhea
No Toxic Effects

GU JING CAO　谷精草　*SCAPUS ERIOCAULONIS BUERGERIANI*

Traditional Functions:
1. Disperses Wind Heat
2. Brightens the eyes, and removes visual opacity

Traditional Properties:
Enters: ST, LV,

Properties: SP, SW, N

Indications:

EYES
- CORNEAL OPACITY
- EYES, BRIGHTENS
- EYES, RED, SWOLLEN: Wind Heat In Liver Channel
- EYES, SPOTS IN FRONT OF

- PTERYGIUM

HEAD/NECK
- HEADACHE, SEVERE INTERMITTENT: Wind

ORAL CAVITY

- LARYNGITIS
- TOOTHACHE

WIND DISORDERS
- WIND HEAT IN LIVER CHANNEL

Clinical/Pharmaceutical Studies:

INFECTIOUS DISEASES
- ANTIBIOTIC: Pseud Aeruginosa

SKIN

- FUNGAL, ANTI-: Many

Dose

9 - 15 gm

Common Name

Pipewort Scapus

Contraindications

Not: Def Blood

Notes

Avoid Contact w/Iron

GUI ZHEN CAO
(XIAN FENG CAO/NIAN SHEN CAO)

鬼針草
（鬼针草）

HERBA
BIDENTIS BIPINNATAE

Traditional Functions:

1. Releases the exterior and relieves the surface
2. Clears Heat and removes toxins
3. Moves stagnancy
4. Dispels Wind Damp
5. Vitalizes the Blood dispersing stagnant Blood

Traditional Properties:

Enters: LU, LI

Properties: BIT, N

Indications:

ABDOMEN/ GASTROINTESTINAL TOPICS
- APPENDICITIS
- ENTERITIS

BOWEL RELATED DISORDERS
- DIARRHEA
- DYSENTERY
- HEMORRHOIDS

CHILDHOOD DISORDERS
- MALNUTRITION, CHILDHOOD

INFECTIOUS DISEASES

- INFLUENZA

KIDNEYS
- NEPHRITIS, ACUTE

LIVER
- HEPATITIS
- JAUNDICE

MENTAL STATE/ NEUROLOGICAL DISORDERS
- EPILEPSY, CHILDHOOD

MUSCULOSKELETAL/ CONNECTIVE TISSUE

- ARTHRITIS
- ARTHRITIS, RHEUMATOID

ORAL CAVITY
- THROAT, SORE, SWOLLEN

STOMACH/DIGESTIVE DISORDERS
- STOMACH, ACHE

TRAUMA, BITES, POISONINGS
- INSECT BITES
- SCORPION BITE
- SPRAINS

Clinical/Pharmaceutical Studies:

ABDOMEN/ GASTROINTESTINAL TOPICS
- INTESTINES, BACTERIA, INHIBITS

PATHOGENIC BLOOD RELATED DISORDERS/TOPICS
- BLOOD PRESSURE, LOWERS

INFECTIOUS DISEASES
- BACTERIAL, ANTI-: Gram Positive Bacteria From Alcohol Extract

TRAUMA, BITES,

POISONINGS
- INFLAMMATORY, ANTI-: Synergistic With Xi Xian Cao/Chou Wu Tong

Dose

15 - 60 gm

Common Name

Bidens/Hairy Beggar-Ticks

JU HUA 　　　　　　　　菊花 　　　　　　　*FLOS CHRYSANTHEMI MORIFOLII*

Traditional Functions:

1. Disperses Wind Heat
2. Clears Liver channel eye problems
3. Subdues Liver Wind and Liver Yang rising
4. Neutralizes toxins
5. White used more to pacify Liver, expel Wind and brighten eyes
6. Yellow used more to clear Wind Heat

Traditional Properties:

Enters: LU, LV,

Properties: SW, <BIT, <C

Indications:

CANCER/TUMORS/SWELLINGS/ LUMPS
- SWELLINGS, TOXIC
- TUMORS

CIRCULATION DISORDERS
- HYPERTENSION

EARS/HEARING DISORDERS
- DEAFNESS: Liver Yang Rising
- DIZZINESS: Liver Yang Rising
- VERTIGO: Liver Yang/Fire Rising

EYES
- EYES, PAIN, RED, DRY: Wind Heat
- EYES, RED, CONGESTED: Liver

Heat
- EYES, SPOTS, BLURRY, DIZZINESS: Wind Heat/Kidney Liver Yin Deficient
- TEARING, EXCESSIVE: Wind Heat

FEVERS
- FEVER: Wind Heat

HEAD/NECK
- HEADACHE: Liver Yang Rising/ Wind Heat

INFECTIOUS DISEASES
- COMMON COLD W/FEVER: Wind Heat

LIVER
- LIVER YANG RISING: Dizziness, Headache, Deafness

LUNGS
- COUGH: Wind Heat

MUSCULOSKELETAL/ CONNECTIVE TISSUE
- SPASMS, CONVULSIONS: Internal Deficiency Wind

SKIN
- FURUNCLES: Deep-Rooted, Nail-Like
- SKIN, SORES, SWOLLEN, TOXIC: Relieves Surface Complex

Clinical/Pharmaceutical Studies:

BLOOD RELATED DISORDERS/TOPICS
- BLOOD COAGULATION: Shortened Time With Oral Powder

CIRCULATION DISORDERS
- ATHEROSCLEROSIS, LOWERS BLOOD PRESSURE: With Jin Yin Hua, Huai Hua, Shan Zha, With Shan Zha For Best Effect
- CEREBRAL ARTERIOSCLEROSIS: Ju Hua, Jin Yin Hua, Huai Hua, Shan Zha
- HYPERTENSION: Lowers BP, With Jin Yin Hua, Huai Hua, Shan Zha, Best Action With Jin Yin Hua, 10-30 Days Treatment

EYES
- CENTRAL RETINITIS: Gou Qi Zi, Ju Hua Shu Di Tang/Wan, Modified
- CONJUNCTIVITIS: With Xia Ku Cao, Jue Ming Zi,

Bai Ji LI, Chan Tui Or With Bai Ji LI, Mu Zei, etc For Steam Therapy Of Eyes
- OPTIC NEURITIS: Gou Qi Zi, Ju Hua Shu Di Tang/ Wan, Modified

FEVERS
- ANTIPYRETIC: Probably Needs Large Doses

HEART
- ANGINA PECTORIS: Concentrated Decoction, 80% Marked Effects, 20 Days Of Treatment
- HEART, INCREASES CORONARY BLOOD FLOW: Increases Coronary Artery Flow, Markedly Dilated Arteries

INFECTIOUS DISEASES
- ANTIBIOTIC: Staph A., Strep, Shigella, Spirochttes, Diplococcus Pneumoniae
- VIRAL, ANTI-: Flu

LIVER
- HEPATITIS, ACUTE,

VIRAL: 80% Effective As IM Injection Of Distillate Of Fresh Plant, As Volatile Oil, 4-8 mg/2 ml

LUNGS
- BRONCHITIS, ACUTE: 80% Effective As IM Injection Of Distillate Of Fresh Plant, As Volatile Oil, 4-8 mg/2 ml
- RESPIRATORY TRACT INFECTION, UPPER

MENTAL STATE/ NEUROLOGICAL DISORDERS
- SEDATIVE

ORAL CAVITY
- MOUTH, ULCERS: Juice Of Bai Ju Hua Leaves, Flesh Of Few Live Clams, Small Amount Of Bing Pian Apply Several Times/ Day, Cure In Few Days
- THROAT, SORE: Sang Ju Yin, Two Flowers Decoction (Ju Hua, Jin Yin Hua, Gan Cao, Pang Da Hai)

- TONSILLITIS: 80% Effective As IM Injection Of Distillate Of Fresh Plant, As Volatile Oil, 4-8 mg/2 ml

SKIN
- BURNS, SMALL AREA: Distillates Of Fresh Ju Hua, Luo Le (Sweet Basil) To Prevent/Treat
- FUNGAL, ANTI-
- SKIN, LOCAL INFECTIONS: Crushed Fresh Leaf
- ULCERS: Distillates Of Fresh Ju Hua, Luo Le (Sweet Basil) To Prevent/ Treat

TRAUMA, BITES, POISONINGS
- ANTIHISTAMINE: About 1/4 Strength Of Rutin
- INFLAMMATORY, ANTI-
- WOUNDS, INFECTED: Distillates Of Fresh Ju Hua, Luo Le (Sweet Basil) To Prevent/Treat

Dose

9 - 18 gm

Common Name

Chrysanthemum Flower

Precautions

Watch: Low BP

Notes

Use For Short Periods-May Weaken LV

Yellow: Used More For Wind Heat Conditions

White: Used More To Pacify Liver And Deficient

Conditions, More Glycosides Then Yellow

Very Low Toxicity

May Cause Diarrhea, Upper Abdominal Pain

MAN JING ZI

蔓荊子

FRUCTUS VITICIS

Traditional Functions:

1. Disperses Wind Heat
2. Clears Heat and benfits the head and eyes
3. Helps drain Dampness

Traditional Properties:

Enters: ST, UB, LV,

Properties: BIT, SP, CL

Indications:

CANCER/TUMORS/SWELLINGS/
LUMPS
• BREAST CANCER
EYES
• CATARACTS
• EYES, PAIN, INTERNALLY
• EYES, PAIN, RED, SWOLLEN:
Wind Heat In Liver Channel
• EYES, SPOTS IN FRONT OF:
Wind Heat In Liver Channel
• NIGHT BLINDNESS
• TEARING, EXCESSIVE: Wind
Heat In Liver Channel
HEAD/NECK

• HEAD, HEAVY
• HEADACHE: Good For Yang
Rising Pattern
INFECTIOUS DISEASES
• COMMON COLD W/MIGRAINE
HEADACHE
MENTAL STATE/
NEUROLOGICAL DISORDERS
• MENTAL DULLNESS
MUSCULOSKELETAL/
CONNECTIVE TISSUE
• ARTHRITIS: Wind Damp Cold Bi
• CRAMPS: Wind Damp, Auxillary
Herb

• STIFFNESS: Wind Damp,
Auxillary Herb
PAIN/NUMBNESS/GENERAL
DISCOMFORT
• BI, WIND DAMP, EXTREMITIES:
Auxillary Herb:Stiffness, Numbness,
Cramping, Heaviness
• HEAVINESS SENSATION: Wind
Damp, Auxillary Herb
• NUMBNESS: Wind Damp,
Auxillary Herb
SEXUALITY, FEMALE:
GYNECOLOGICAL
• BREASTS, CANCER

Clinical/Pharmaceutical Studies:

FEVERS
• ANTIPYRETIC
HEAD/NECK
• HAIR GROWTH: Promotes Beard

Growth
MENTAL STATE/
NEUROLOGICAL DISORDERS
• SEDATIVE

PAIN/NUMBNESS/GENERAL
DISCOMFORT
• ANALGESIC

Dose

3 - 9 gm

Precautions

Watch: Def Yin/Blood Headaches, Eye Problems
Watch: Def ST Qi

MU ZEI

木賊

HERBA EQUISETI HIEMALIS

Traditional Functions:

1. Disperses Wind Heat and removes visual opacity

Traditional Properties:

Enters: LU, LV,

Properties: SW, BIT, N

Indications:

BOWEL RELATED DISORDERS
• HEMORRHOIDS
• HEMORRHOIDS, BLOODY
STOOL
• RECTAL PROLAPSE: Topical

• EYES, RED, CONGESTED: Liver
Heat
• EYES, RED, SWOLLEN, PAIN,
CLOUDINESS: Wind Heat
• PTERYGIUM: Wind Heat

• HEADACHE
HEMORRHAGIC DISORDERS
• HEMAFECIA
SEXUALITY, FEMALE:
GYNECOLOGICAL

Indications:

EYES
- CATARACTS
- CONJUNCTIVITIS
- CORNEAL OPACITY

- TEARING, EXCESSIVE: Wind Heat
- VISION, BLURRED: Wind Heat

HEAD/NECK

- UTERINE BLEEDING

SKIN
- HYPEREMIA

Clinical/Pharmaceutical Studies:

- ASTRINGENT

**CANCER/TUMORS/
SWELLINGS/LUMPS**
- LIVER CANCER
- STOMACH CANCER

- TONGUE CANCER

KIDNEYS
- DIURETIC

LUNGS
- SILICOSIS: Helps

Coughing But No
Objective Signs Of
Improvement

**STOMACH/DIGESTIVE
DISORDERS**

- APPETITE, INCREASES

**TRAUMA, BITES,
POISONINGS**
- INFLAMMATORY, ANTI-

Dose

3 - 9 gm

Common Name

Scouring Rush

Precautions

Watch: Chronic Application

Watch: During Pregnancy

Watch: Qi, Blood Deficiency

Notes

Somewhat Drying

NIU BANG ZI   牛蒡子   FRUCTUS ARCTII LAPPAE

Traditional Functions:

1. Disperses Wind Heat and cleanses the throat
2. Reduces swellings and neutralizes toxins
3. Promotes the eruption of measles
4. Moistens intestines, promoting passage of stool

Traditional Properties:

Enters: LU, ST,

Properties: SP, <BIT, <C

Indications:

BOWEL RELATED DISORDERS
- CONSTIPATION: Wind Heat

**CANCER/TUMORS/SWELLINGS/
LUMPS**
- SWELLINGS, RED

INFECTIOUS DISEASES
- COMMON COLD W/SORE
THROAT, COUGH
- MEASLES, INCOMPLETE
EXPRESSION OF RASH
- MUMPS

LUNGS

- COUGH: Lung Heat/Wind Heat
- LUNGS, DYSPNEA: Lung Heat

ORAL CAVITY
- THROAT, SWOLLEN, SORE, RED:
Wind Heat

**SEXUALITY, FEMALE:
GYNECOLOGICAL**
- BREASTS, SWOLLEN, PAINFUL,
ABSCESS

SKIN
- ABSCESS: Topical
- ERYTHEMA, UNERUPTED

- RASHES, ACUTE FEBRILE
MACULOPAPULAR
- RASHES, INCOMPLETE
EXPRESSION OF: Early Stage
- RASHES, W/PRURITUS: Clears
Wind
- SKIN, SORES, SWOLLEN, TOXIC:
Relieves Surface Complex

WIND DISORDERS
- WIND HEAT: Fever, Cough, Sore,
Red, Swollen Throat

Clinical/Pharmaceutical Studies:

**ABDOMEN/
GASTROINTESTINAL TOPICS**
- INTESTINES, PERISTALSIS,
INHIBITS

**BLOOD RELATED DISORDERS/
TOPICS**
- BLOOD GLUCOSE, REDUCES

BOWEL RELATED DISORDERS

- PURGATIVE

INFECTIOUS DISEASES
- ANTIBIOTIC: Strep., Pneumonia

KIDNEYS
- DIURETIC

**MENTAL STATE/
NEUROLOGICAL DISORDERS**
- CNS, STIMULANT: Large Doses

Could Produce Convulsions, Then
Paralysis

**SEXUALITY, FEMALE:
GYNECOLOGICAL**
- UTERUS, INHIBITS
CONTRACTION

SKIN
- FUNGAL, ANTI-

Dose

3 - 9 gm

Common Name

Great Burdock Fruit

Contraindications

Not: Def SP Qi w/Diarrhea

Not: w/Open Sores And Boils

SANG YE

桑葉
（桑叶）

FOLIUM MORI ALBAE

Traditional Functions:

1. Disperses Wind Heat with cough
2. Clears Heat from the Lungs
3. Clears Liver channel eye problems

Traditional Properties:

Enters: LU, LV,

Properties: SW, <BIT, <C

Indications:

EARS/HEARING DISORDERS
• VERTIGO: Liver Yang/Fire Rising
EYES
• CONJUNCTIVITIS, ACUTE
• EYES, PROBLEMS: Wind Heat Or Deficient Yin:Red, Sore, Dry, Painful Eyes
• EYES, RED, CONGESTED: Liver Heat
FEVERS
• FEVER: From Exertion/Wind Heat
FLUID DISORDERS
• THIRST

HEAD/NECK
• HEADACHE: Wind Heat
HEMORRHAGIC DISORDERS
• HEMATEMESIS
• HEMORRHAGE: Cool Blood To Stop
INFECTIOUS DISEASES
• COMMON COLD W/FEVER, HEADACHE, SORE THROAT
LUNGS
• COUGH: Lung Dryness/Lung Heat/ Wind Heat

• COUGH, LUNG EXHAUSTION: Tuberculosis
• LUNG HEAT W/THICK YELLOW SPUTUM
• LUNGS, DYSPNEA: Lung Heat
ORAL CAVITY
• MOUTH, DRY: Lung Dry/Heat
SKIN
• HYPEREMIA
WIND DISORDERS
• WIND HEAT: Fever, Headache, Cough

Clinical/Pharmaceutical Studies:

ABDOMEN/ GASTROINTESTINAL TOPICS
• INTESTINES, INHIBITS
BOWEL RELATED DISORDERS
• CONSTIPATION: Body Fluid Depletion, San Ma Wan (Sang Ye, Hu Ma Ren)
• FISTULA, PRURULENT: Injected
EARS/HEARING DISORDERS
• VERTIGO: San Ma Wan (Sang Ye, Hu Ma Ren)
ENDOCRINE RELATED DISORDERS
• DIABETES
• ENDOCRINE: Hypoglycemic
EYES
• CORNEAL ULCERS
• KERATITIS, DEEP: Ming Mu Xiao Yan Wan (Includes 18 Herb With Sang Ye)
• VISION, BLURRED: San Ma Wan (Sang Ye, Hu Ma Ren)
GALL BLADDER
• CHOLECYSTITIS, CHRONIC
IMMUNE SYSTEM RELATED DISORDERS/TOPICS
• IMMUNE SYSTEM ENHANCEMENT: Increased

Phagocytosis, Sang Ju Yin
INFECTIOUS DISEASES
• BACTERIAL, ANTI-: Strong Action, B.Typhi, Staph., Strep, Diphteriae, B.Antracis
• COMMON COLD: Sang Ju Yin (Sang Ye, Ju Hua, Jie Geng, Xing Ren, LU Ren, Lian Qiao, Bo He, Gan Cao), Early Stage, With Cough, Mild Fever, Headache, Nasal Congestion
• ELEPHANTIASIS, LOWER EXTREMITIES: Injected, 10% Extract, 5 ml, 1-2x/Day 15-21 Days, Bind Limb 3 Days After Medication, Softened Skin, Reduced Limb Size
• MEASLES, EARLY STAGE: Sang Ju Yin, (Sang Ye, Ju Hua, Jie Geng, Xing Ren, LU Ren, Lian Qiao, Bo He, Gan Cao)
• SPIROCHETTES, ANTI-: High Doses, Concentration--30 mg/ml
LUNGS
• BRONCHIECTASIS, W/ HEMOPTYSIS
• COUGH, CHRONIC: San Ma Wan (Sang Ye, Hu Ma Ren)
• RESPIRATORY TRACT

INFECTION, UPPER, CHILDREN: Acute Fever, Cough–Qing Wen Tang Yi Hao (Sang Ye, LU Ren, Shi Gao, Da Qing Ye, Gan Cao, Bai Mao Gen)
• WHOOPING COUGH: Sang Xing Tang (Sang Ye, Xing Ren, Chuan Bei Mu, Nan Sha Shen, Dan Dou Chi, Cortex Gardeniae (Shan Zhi Zi?), Pericarium Pyri), Helped With 1 Dose, 3 Doses To Stop Cough In Most Cases
NUTRITIONAL/METABOLIC DISORDERS/TOPICS
• METABOLISM: Promotes Anabolism
ORAL CAVITY
• THROAT, SORE, ESOPHAGITIS
• VOICE LOSS
SKIN
• DIAPHORETIC
• SKIN, PROMOTES CELL GROWTH
• SKIN, ROUGH, DRY: San Ma Wan (Sang Ye, Hu Ma Ren)
STOMACH/DIGESTIVE DISORDERS
• GASTRITIS, ATROPHIC

Dose

3 - 12 gm

Common Name

White Mulberry Leaf

Contraindications

Not: LU Def/Cold

Notes

Toxic To LV & KI, If Taken In Large Doses For Long Term

SHENG MA

升麻
（升麻）

RHIZOMA CIMICIFUGAE

Traditional Functions:

1. Relieves the surface, disperses Wind Heat
2. Promotes the eruption of measles
3. Raises the Yang Qi in patterns of Spleen or Stomach deficiency
4. Neutralizes toxic Heat in the Stomach

Traditional Properties:

Enters: LU, SP, ST,

Properties: SW, SP, <BIT, CL

Indications:

- PROLAPSE OF ORGANS: Sinking Of Central Qi
BOWEL RELATED DISORDERS
- DIARRHEA: Spleen Deficient With Sinking Of Qi
- DIARRHEA, CHRONIC
- DYSENTERY, CHRONIC
- HEMORRHOIDS, BLOODY STOOL: Use Charred
- RECTAL PROLAPSE: From Chronic Diarrhea
FEVERS
- CHILLS/FEVER
HEMORRHAGIC DISORDERS
- HEMORRHAGE: Raise The Yang To Stop
HERBAL FUNCTIONS

- GUIDING HERB TO HEAD/FACE
INFECTIOUS DISEASES
- COMMON COLD: Wind Heat
- COMMON COLD W/HEADACHE, SORE THROAT
- INFECTIONS, EPIDEMIC
- MEASLES, EARLY STAGE
- MUMPS
ORAL CAVITY
- CANKERS
- GUMS, PAIN, SWELLING
- GUMS, ULCERS
- LIPS, ULCERS
- ORAL INFECTIONS
- ORAL ULCERS
- STOMATITIS
- TEETH, SORE

- THROAT, SORE, SWOLLEN
SEXUALITY, FEMALE: GYNECOLOGICAL
- MENORRHAGIA
- MENSTRUATION, DISORDERS OF: Dredge, Regulate Chong, Ren
- UTERUS, PROLAPSE
SKIN
- BOILS, TOXIC: Heat, Toxins, Swellings
- RASHES, INCOMPLETE EXPRESSION OF: Early Stage
- SKIN, ERUPTIONS, LATENT
- SKIN, SORES, SWOLLEN: Heat, Toxins, Swelling, Relieves Surface Complex

Clinical/Pharmaceutical Studies:

BLOOD RELATED DISORDERS/ TOPICS
- BLOOD PRESSURE, LOWERS
- THROMBOCYTOPENIA: Sheng Ma Bie Jia Tang
BOWEL RELATED DISORDERS
- RECTAL PROLAPSE: Bu Zhong Yi Qi Tang
CANCER/TUMORS/SWELLINGS/ LUMPS
- CERVICAL CANCER: 90% Inhibition Against, Hot Aqueous Extract, Also Bu Zhong Yi Qi Tang
ENDOCRINE RELATED DISORDERS
- HORMONE-LIKE: Wild Herb, Female Organs Increased Weight, Estrus Affected In Immature Or Climacteric Rats
FEVERS
- ANTIPYRETIC: MEOH/ETOH Extracts
INFECTIOUS DISEASES
- ANTIBIOTIC: TB
- INFLUENZA

- MEASLES W/PNEUMONIA
- MUMPS
- SYPHILIS, CONGENITAL
- VIRAL, ANTI-
KIDNEYS
- NEPHRITIS W/HEMATURIA: Sheng Ma Bie Jia Tang
MENTAL STATE/ NEUROLOGICAL DISORDERS
- CONVULSIVE, ANTI-: 1/10-1/3 Of Papaverine
- SEDATIVE: Tincture
MUSCULOSKELETAL/ CONNECTIVE TISSUE
- RHEUMATISM, CHRONIC
ORAL CAVITY
- HALITOSIS: Water-Alcohol Extract
- MOUTH, DISEASES OF: Water-Alcohol Extract
- MOUTH, PERIODONTITIS: Qing Wei San--Sheng Ma, Huang Lian, Sheng Di, Dan Shen, Dang Gui
- THROAT, SORE, ACUTE: Qing Wei San--Sheng Ma, Huang Lian,

Sheng Di, Dan Shen, Dang Gui
- TONSILLITIS
PAIN/NUMBNESS/GENERAL DISCOMFORT
- ANALGESIC: Headache
SEXUALITY, FEMALE: GYNECOLOGICAL
- CERVIX, CANCINOMA: 90% Inhibition Against, Hot Aqueous Extract, Also Bu Zhong Yi Qi Tang
- UTERUS, PROLAPSE: Bu Zhong Yi Qi Tang
SKIN
- FUNGAL, ANTI-: Strong
- SKIN, PROTECTION OF: Alcohol Extract Of
- ULCERS: Methanol, Aqueous Extracts Can Prevent/Help
STOMACH/DIGESTIVE DISORDERS
- GASTROPTOSIS: Bu Zhong Yi Qi Tang
TRAUMA, BITES, POISONINGS
- INFLAMMATORY, ANTI-
- TOXIC, ANTI-

Dose

3 - 9 gm

Common Name

Black Cohosh Rhizome

Contraindications

Not: Def Yin w/Heat
Not: Erupted Measles
Not: w/Dyspnea

Not: Excess Upper, Def Lower

Notes

Toxic In Overdose

Side Effects May Include: Vomiting Common, Gastric
Irritation

Overdose: Lassitude, Vertigo, Tremor, Severe Headache,
Collapse

YE JU HUA   野菊花   FLOS CHRYSANTHEMI INDICI

Traditional Functions:

1. Subdues Fire and neutralizes toxins
2. Calms rising Liver Yang

Traditional Properties:

Enters: LU, LV,

Properties: BIT, SP, CL

Indications:

CANCER/TUMORS/SWELLINGS/
  LUMPS
• TUMORS
CIRCULATION DISORDERS
• HYPERTENSION: Liver Heat
EARS/HEARING DISORDERS
• DIZZINESS
EYES
• EYES, INFLAMMATION

HEAD/NECK
• HEADACHE
ORAL CAVITY
• THROAT, INFLAMMATION
SEXUALITY, FEMALE:
  GYNECOLOGICAL
• BREASTS, SWOLLEN, PAINFUL,
  ABSCESS

• CERVIX, INFLAMMATION
SKIN
• CARBUNCLES
• ECZEMA
• FURUNCLES: Deep-Rooted, Nail-
  Like
• SKIN, ITCHING
• SORES

Clinical/Pharmaceutical Studies:

ABDOMEN/
  GASTROINTESTINAL
  TOPICS
• APPENDICITIS: With Pu
  Gong Ying, Wei Ling Xian,
  Hai Jin Sha, Bai Mao Gen,
  Jin Yin Hua
• ENTERITIS: (Intestinal
  Inflammation, Especially
  The Mucous Lining) With
  Pu Gong Ying, Wei Ling
  Xian, Hai Jin Sha, Bai Mao
  Gen, Jin Yin Hua
CIRCULATION
  DISORDERS
• HYPERTENSION: ETOH
  Extract, Slow Onset,
  Prolonged Effect, Acute
  Lowering Of BP By
  Peripheral Vessel Dilation, *
  2 ml Fluid Extract (4 g
  Herb) , 3x/Day PO,
  Improved Symptoms, *
  Decoction Of Ye Ju Hua,
  Gou Teng, Xia Ku Cao,
  Jue Ming Zi, Che Qian
  Cao, Used In Stage I, II
  Hypertension
EYES
• CONJUNCTIVITIS,

• HEART, INCREASES
  CORONARY BLOOD
  FLOW: Lasts 10 Minutes
IMMUNE SYSTEM
  RELATED DISORDERS/
  TOPICS
• IMMUNE SYSTEM
  ENHANCEMENT:
  Increased Phagocytic
  Function Of WBC
INFECTIOUS DISEASES
• BACTERIAL, ANTI-: 1:5
  Decoction Staph Aureus,
  Shigella, Many Others,
  Fresh More Potent, Heat
  Reduced Effect
• COMMON COLD,
  REDUCES FREQUENCY
  OF: Take Oral 1-4x/Month
  Depending On Past Cold
  Frequency, *As Compound
  Decoction Reduces
  Symptoms, With Bai Mao
  Gen/Nian Shen Cao Or Bo
  He, Jie Geng, *As
  Ointment For External Use
  In Nasal Passages
• INFLUENZA: As
  Compound Decoction
  Reduces Symptoms, With

• MENINGITIS,
  EPIDEMIC
  CEREBROSPINAL:
  Spray Throat With 2 ml 50%
  Decoction, Cleared 82%
  Of Bacteria In 3 Days, 1-2
  Sprayings
• PAROTITIS: With Pu
  Gong Ying, Wei Ling Xian,
  Hai Jin Sha, Bai Mao Gen,
  Jin Yin Hua
• SCARLET FEVER,
  PREVENTATIVE: Spray
  Throat With 2 ml, 50%
  Decoction For 3 Days
• VIRAL, ANTI-: Echo,
  Herpes, Some Influenza,
  Not Some Cold
LUNGS
• BRONCHITIS, ACUTE:
  Injection Of Volatile
  Distillate Less ETOH
  Insoluble Portion, 88%
  Effective
• BRONCHITIS,
  CHRONIC: Reduces
  Acute Attacks
• BRONCHITIS,
  CHRONIC, GERIATRIC:
  With SI Gua Luo

SEXUALITY, FEMALE:
  GYNECOLOGICAL
• CERVICITIS, CHRONIC:
  Topical
• CERVIX, EROSION OF:
  With Pu Gong Ying, Wei
  Ling Xian, Hai Jin Sha,
  Bai Mao Gen, Jin Yin Hua
• MASTITIS: With Pu
  Gong Ying, Wei Ling Xian,
  Hai Jin Sha, Bai Mao Gen,
  Jin Yin Hua
• PELVIC INFECTIONS:
  As Suppository
SKIN
• ABSCESS: Herb/Wu Wei
  Xiao Du Tang (Ye Ju Hua,
  Jin Yin Hua, Pu Gong Ying,
  Zi Hua Di Ding, Tian Kui
  Zi (Semen Semiaquilegiae)
  , *Herb, Fu Ling, Shan Zhi
  Zi, Browned, Sang Ye, Che
  Qian Cao
• ECZEMA: Herb Decocted
  With Flos Sesamum
  Indicum, Alum (Calcined) ,
  Externally As Wash/Hot
  Compress
• FURUNCLES: Calcinated
  Root With Small Amount

Clinical/Pharmaceutical Studies:

EPIDEMIC: With Pu Gong Ying, Wei Ling Xian, Hai Jin Sha, Bai Mao Gen, Jin Yin Hua

- HORDEOLUM: With Pu Gong Ying, Wei Ling Xian, Hai Jin Sha, Bai Mao Gen, Jin Yin Hua

HEART

Bai Mao Gen/Nian Shen Cao Or Bo He, Jie Geng, * Spray Throat With 2 ml, 50% Decoction For 3 Days, Preventative

- MEASLES, PREVENTATIVE: Spray Throat With 2 ml, 50% Decoction For 3 Days

ORAL CAVITY

- STOMATITIS: With Pu Gong Ying, Wei Ling Xian, Hai Jin Sha, Bai Mao Gen, Jin Yin Hua
- TONSILLITIS: With Pu Gong Ying, Wei Ling Xian, Hai Jin Sha, Bai Mao Gen, Jin Yin Hua

Bing Pian, Tea Oil, Apply Topically To Face

TRAUMA, BITES, POISONINGS

- SNAKE BITES: Injection, Reduces Mortality Of Cobra, Krait
- WOUNDS: 20% Oil

Dose

6 - 18 gm

Common Name

Wild Chrysanthemum Flower

Notes

Occasional Nausea And Vomiting, Low Toxicity

Oral Side Effects: Possible Anorexia, Borborygmus, Mushy Stool

Clear Heat, Subdues Fire

DAN ZHU YE

淡竹葉
(淡竹叶)

HERBA LOPHATHERI GRACILIS

Traditional Functions:

1. Clears Heat and reduces restlessness
2. Clears Stomach or Heart fire
3. Promotes urination and clears Damp Heat
4. Disperses Wind Heat
5. Clears blazing Stomach or Heart fire

Traditional Properties:

Enters: ST, HT, SI,

Properties: SW, BL, C

Indications:

ABDOMEN/ GASTROINTESTINAL TOPICS
• HEAT IN SMALL INTESTINE CHANNEL
FEVERS
• FEVER, RESTLESSNESS, THIRST
FLUID DISORDERS
• THIRST: Heat
HEAT
• HEAT IN SMALL INTESTINE CHANNEL
MENTAL STATE/

NEUROLOGICAL DISORDERS
• IRRITABILITY
ORAL CAVITY
• GUMS, PAIN, SWELLING: Heart/ Stomach Heat
• MOUTH, SORES: Heart/Stomach Heat
• TONGUE, SORES
SIX STAGES/CHANNELS
• TAI YANG STAGE DISEASE
STOMACH/DIGESTIVE

DISORDERS
• STOMACH HEART HEAT
URINARY BLADDER
• DYSURIA: Small Intestine Heat
• URINARY TRACT INFECTIONS
• URINATION, PAINFUL, DRIBBLING, CONCENTRATED, RED/YELLOW/TURBID
• URINATION, SCANTY
WIND DISORDERS
• WIND HEAT

Clinical/Pharmaceutical Studies:

BLOOD RELATED DISORDERS/ TOPICS
• BLOOD GLUCOSE, INCREASES
CANCER/TUMORS/SWELLINGS/ LUMPS
• CANCER, ANTI-: Extract Restrains Ehrlich Carcinoma, Sarcoma-180, 100 g/kg Needed
EYES
• CORNEAL ULCERS, SERPIGINOUS: Topical Application Of Juice, 95%
• HORDEOLUM: Topical

Application Of Juice, 95%
FEVERS
• FEVER, FROM ACUTE INFECTIONS: 3-9 g Decoction, Best As Formula, e.g. Zhu Ye Liu Bang Tang/Zhu Ye Shi Gao Tang
• FEVER, REDUCES: Orally, (Water Extract, Only)
INFECTIOUS DISEASES
• BACTERIAL, ANTI-: Staph. Aureus, Pseudomonas
KIDNEYS
• DIURETIC, WEAK: Less Than Mu

Tong, Zhu Ling
URINARY BLADDER
• URINARY STONES: Dao Chi San (Dan Zhu Ye, Sheng Di, Tian Xian Teng, Gan Cao)
• URINARY TRACT INFECTIONS: Dao Chi San (Dan Zhu Ye, Sheng Di, Tian Xian Teng, Gan Cao)
• URINATION, SCANTY: From Acute Infection:3-9 g Decoction, Best As Formula, e.g. Zhu Ye Liu Bang Tang/Zhu Ye Shi Gao Tang

Dose

9 - 18 gm

Common Name

Bamboo Leaves

Precautions

Watch: Pregnancy

HAN SHUI SHI

寒水石
(寒水石)

CALCITUM

Traditional Functions:

1. Subdues fire and clears summer Heat
3. Cools scalding burns when used topically

Traditional Properties:

Enters: ST, HT, KI,

Properties: SP, SA, C

Indications:

FEVERS
- FEVER, HIGH: Summer Heat

FLUID DISORDERS
- THIRST: Summer Heat

HEAT
- HEAT DISEASES: Strong Heat, Restless Thirst

- SUMMER HEAT

MENTAL STATE/ NEUROLOGICAL DISORDERS
- IRRITABILITY: Summer Heat
- RESTLESSNESS

ORAL CAVITY
- MOUTH, DRYNESS

- TOOTHACHE

SKIN
- ERYSIPELAS
- SCALDS, TOPICAL FOR

URINARY BLADDER
- DYSURIA

Clinical/Pharmaceutical Studies:

FEVERS
- ANTIPYRETIC

TRAUMA, BITES, POISONINGS

- INFLAMMATORY, ANTI-

Dose

9 - 30 gm

Common Name

Calcite

Contraindications

Not: w/Cold Def SP/ST

JUE MING ZI
(CAO JUE MING)

決明子

SEMEN CASSIAE TORAE

Traditional Functions:

1. Dissipates Wind Heat eye symptoms
2. Clears Liver Fire and clears the eyes
3. Moistens and lubricates the intestines

Traditional Properties:

Enters: KI, LV, GB,

Properties: BIT, SW, SA, C

Indications:

BOWEL RELATED DISORDERS
- CONSTIPATION: Intestinal Dryness/Liver Yin Deficient

EARS/HEARING DISORDERS
- VERTIGO: Liver Yang/Fire Rising

EYES
- CATARACTS
- EYES, ITCHY, RED, PAINFUL: Wind Heat

- EYES, RED, CONGESTED: Liver Heat
- EYES, RED, PAINFUL: Liver Yang Rising
- GLAUCOMA
- OPTIC ATROPHY
- PHOTOPHOBIA: Wind Heat/Liver Yang Rising

- TEARING, EXCESSIVE: Liver Yang Rising

HEAD/NECK
- HEADACHE: Liver Yang Rising

LIVER
- LIVER HEAT

SKIN
- HYPEREMIA

Clinical/Pharmaceutical Studies:

BLOOD RELATED DISORDERS/TOPICS
- BLOOD PRESSURE, LOWERS: Alcohol ext. Greater Than Water ext.
- CHOLESTEROL, LOWERS: Very Good, In 2-4 Weeks, Needs Some Treatment To Maintain

EARS/HEARING DISORDERS
- DIZZINESS: Reduces From Hypercholesterolemia

EYES
- EYES, BENEFITS VISION: Carotin

HEAD/NECK

- HEADACHE: Reduces From Hypercholesterolemia

INFECTIOUS DISEASES
- ANTIBIOTIC: Broad Spectrum, Staph A., C. Diphtheriae

MENTAL STATE/

NEUROLOGICAL DISORDERS
- LETHARGY: Reduces From Hypercholesterolemia

SKIN
- FUNGAL, ANTI-: Reduces Growth

Dose

4.5 - 15.0 gm

Common Name

Foetid Cassia Seeds

Contraindications

Not: w/Huo Ma Ren

Not: Diarrhea

Notes

Up To 25 gm, Ok

Jue Ming Zi Better Than Ju Hua For Eyes

LIAN ZI XIN
(LIAN XIN)

蓮 子 心
（莲子心）

PLUMULA
NELUMBINIS NUCIFERAE

Traditional Functions:

1. Subdues Heart Fire

Traditional Properties:

Enters: HT

Properties: BIT, C

Indications:

CIRCULATION DISORDERS
• HYPERTENSION
FEVERS
• THIRST IN FEBRILE DISEASES
HEART
• PERICARDIUM, HEAT IN

HEMORRHAGIC DISORDERS
• HEMATEMESIS
• HEMOPTYSIS
MENTAL STATE/
NEUROLOGICAL DISORDERS

• DELIRIUM: Heat In Pericardium
• INSOMNIA: Excess Heart Fire
• IRRITABILITY: Excess Heart Fire
• MENTAL CONFUSION: Heat In
  Pericardium

Clinical/Pharmaceutical Studies:

BLOOD RELATED DISORDERS/
  TOPICS
• BLOOD PRESSURE, LOWERS:
  Releases Histamines, Which Dilate
  Peripheral Blood Vessels
CIRCULATION DISORDERS

• VASODILATOR, LOWERS
  BLOOD PRESSURE: From Release
  Of Histamine
HEART
• CORONARY ARTERIES,

DILATES
SEXUALITY, FEMALE:
GYNECOLOGICAL
• UTERUS, INHIBITS: Relaxes
  Smooth Muscle, Strongly

Dose

1.5 - 6.0 gm

Common Name

Lotus Plumule

Contraindications

Not: w/Masses In Abdomen & Constipation

LU GEN

蘆 根
（芦根）

RHIZOMA
PHRAGMITIS COMMUNIS

Traditional Functions:

1. Clears Heat and generates fluids
2. Clears Lung Heat
3. Clears Stomach Heat with reflux
4. Promotes urination in Heat patterns
5. Promotes rashes to surface

Traditional Properties:

Enters: LU, ST,

Properties: SW, C

Indications:

ENDOCRINE RELATED
  DISORDERS
• DIABETES: Internal Heat With
  Exhaustion Thirst
FEVERS
• FEVER, HIGH W/THIRST,

• COUGH: Lung Dryness/Lung Heat,
  Acute/Wind Heat
• LUNG ATROPHY
• LUNG HEAT, ACUTE: Cough w/
  Thick Sputum
• LUNGS, ABSCESS

• RASHES, INCOMPLETE
  EXPRESSION OF: Early Stage
STOMACH/DIGESTIVE
  DISORDERS
• BELCHING: Stomach Heat
• HICCUPS: Qi Deficiency–Heat

Indications:

RESTLESSNESS
- FEVER, UNCONTROLLED
FLUID DISORDERS
- THIRST: Fluid Injury/Heat
GALL BLADDER
- GALL BLADDER, STONES
HEAT
- HEAT: In Yang Ming, Qi Level
- HEAT, INTERNAL
HEMORRHAGIC DISORDERS
- HEMATURIA: Heat
INFECTIOUS DISEASES
- COMMON COLD: Wind Heat
LUNGS

- LUNGS, ABSCESS W/PURULENT
  VOMIT
- LUNGS, DYSPNEA: Lung Heat
MENTAL STATE/
NEUROLOGICAL DISORDERS
- RESTLESSNESS
ORAL CAVITY
- MOUTH, DRY
- THROAT, DRY
SEXUALITY, FEMALE:
GYNECOLOGICAL
- MORNING SICKNESS:
  Gestational Foul Obstruction--Heat
SKIN

- STOMACH REFLUX
- VOMITING: Qi Deficiency--Heat/
  Stomach Heat
TRAUMA, BITES, POISONINGS
- FISH TOXINS
- POISONING, FISH
URINARY BLADDER
- URINARY TRACT STONES
- URINATION, PAINFUL,
  DRIBBLING, CONCENTRATED,
  RED/YELLOW/TURBID
- URINATION, SCANTY: Heat
- URINATION, SCANTY/LACK OF:
  Brownish

Clinical/Pharmaceutical Studies:

GALL BLADDER
- GALL BLADDER, STONES:
  Helps To Dissolve
INFECTIOUS DISEASES
- ANTIBIOTIC: B-Hemolytic Strep
KIDNEYS
- DIURETIC

LUNGS
- BRONCHITIS: L-Asparagine
  Ingredient
- PULMONARY ABSCESSES
STOMACH/DIGESTIVE
DISORDERS
- FOOD POISONING: Fish/Crab

Meat
URINARY BLADDER
- URINARY TRACT INFECTIONS,
  ACUTE
- URINATION, FREQUENT W/
  SCANTY FLOW, PAIN

Dose

15 - 60 gm

Common Name

Reed Phizome

Precautions

Watch: Cold, Def SP/ST

LU JING
(WEI JING)

蘆莖/葦莖
(芦茎/苇茎)

RAMULUS
PHRAGMITIS

Traditional Functions:

1. Clears Heat and generates fluids
2. Clears Heat from Lungs
3. Clears Stomach Heat
4. Promotes urination in Heat patterns
5. Encourages rashes to surface

Traditional Properties:

Enters: LU, ST,

Properties: SW, C

Indications:

FEVERS
- FEVER, UNCONTROLLED
HEMORRHAGIC DISORDERS
- HEMATURIA
LUNGS
- LUNG HEAT, ACUTE: Cough w/

Thick Sputm
SKIN
- RASHES, ENCOURAGES
  EXPRESSION OF
STOMACH/DIGESTIVE

DISORDERS
- BELCHING
- VOMITING
URINARY BLADDER
- URINATION, SCANTY

Clinical/Pharmaceutical Studies:

INFECTIOUS DISEASES
- ANTIBIOTIC: B-Hemolytic Strep

LUNGS

- PULMONARY ABSCESSES

Dose

15 - 30 gm

Common Name

Reed Stem

Contraindications

Not: Cold, Def SP/ST

MI MENG HUA

密蒙花

FLOS BUDDLEIAE OFFICINALIS

Traditional Functions:

1. Clears Liver Heat and benefits the eyes
2. Moistens deficient Liver and clears eyes

Traditional Properties:

Enters: LV,

Properties: SW, CL

Indications:

EYES
- CATARACTS
- CORNEAL OPACITY
- EYES, DISEASES OF
- EYES, PAIN, RED, SWOLLEN
- EYES, RED, CONGESTED: Liver Heat
- EYESIGHT, IMPROVES FROM INTERNAL PROBLEMS
- NEBULA
- OPTIC ATROPHY
- PHOTOPHOBIA
- TEARING, EXCESSIVE, EXCRETION
- VISION, OBSTRUCTIONS

LIVER
- LIVER HEAT, MILD CLEARING
- LIVER YIN DEFICIENCY W/ YANG RISING

SKIN
- HYPEREMIA

Clinical/Pharmaceutical Studies:

GALL BLADDER
- GALL BLADDER DUCT, SMOOTH MUSCLE, ANTISPASMATIC, NOTED
- GALL BLADDER, BILE SECRETION, INCREASES: Slightly, Temporarily

KIDNEYS
- DIURETIC: Slightly

MUSCULOSKELETAL/ CONNECTIVE TISSUE
- SMOOTH MUSCLE, ANTISPASMATIC, NOTED ON GB

DUCT
NUTRITIONAL/METABOLIC DISORDERS/TOPICS
- VITAMIN P-LIKE: Reduces Permeability Of Skin, Small Intestine Blood Vessels

Dose

6 - 9 gm

Notes

Milder Than Jue Ming Zi

QIAN LI GUANG
(JIU LI MING)

千里光

HERBA SENECIONIS

Traditional Functions:

1. Clears Heat and bightens the eyes
2. Kills intestinal parasites

Traditional Properties:

Enters: LV, LI

Properties: BIT, C

Indications:

- INFLAMMATORY DISEASES, ACUTE

BLOOD RELATED DISORDERS/ TOPICS
- SEPTICEMIA

BOWEL RELATED DISORDERS
- DYSENTERY: Intestinal Inflammation

EYES
- HYPEREMIA: Wind Fire
- NEBULA

INFECTIOUS DISEASES
- INFLUENZA

LIVER
- JAUNDICE

SKIN
- CARBUNCLES
- ECZEMA
- FUNGAL INFECTIONS: Moist
- PIMPLES
- PRURITUS
- SKIN, LESIONS

TRAUMA, BITES, POISONINGS
- DOG BITES: Topical Dressing
- INSECT BITES: Topical Dressing
- POISONING, LEAD
- SNAKE BITES: Topical Dressing

Clinical/Pharmaceutical Studies:

ABDOMEN/ GASTROINTESTINAL TOPICS
- APPENDICITIS, ACUTE: Very Good, 4.5 g Of Crude Herb 4x/Day
- ENTERITIS, ACUTE: Very Good, 4.5 g Of Crude Herb 4x/Day

Drops, 50% Solution
- CORNEAL ULCERS: Similar To Chloramphenicol, As Eye Drops, 50% Solution
- KERATITIS: Similar To Chloramphenicol, As Eye Drops, 50% Solution
- TRACHOMA: Similar To

- MENINGITIS, EPIDEMIC: Controls Spread Of, Can Eliminate In Carriers
- SURGICAL INFECTIONS: Local Application Of Mashed Fresh Leaves

LUNGS
- ANESTHETIC

SEXUALITY, FEMALE: GYNECOLOGICAL
- CERVICITIS, CHRONIC
- TRICHOMONAS, VAGINAL: Alone Or w/ Peel Of Hua Jiao (3:1) In Vagina, Then Pack Vagina With Cotton Balls Soaked

Clinical/Pharmaceutical Studies:

BOWEL RELATED DISORDERS
• DYSENTERY, BACILLARY, ACUTE: Very Good, 4.5 g Of Crude Herb 4x/Day

CHILDHOOD DISORDERS
• DIAPER RASH

EXTREMITIES
• LEGS, ULCERS: Topical
• ULCERS, LEGS: Topical

EYES
• CONJUNCTIVITIS, ACUTE/SUBACUTE: Similar To Chloramphenicol, As Eye

Chloramphenicol, As Eye Drops, 50% Solution

HEART
• CARDIOTONIC: Similar To Digitalis

INFECTIOUS DISEASES
• BACTERIAL, ANTI-: 50% Aqueous Decoction: Shigella, Staph Aureous– Very Strong
• CELLULITIS: Topical
• LEPTOSPIROSIS: Use Qian LI Guang + Jin Yin Hua Powder In Caps, High Cure Rate, 1-2 Days, Can Be Used Preventatively, Equal To Vaccine

• BRONCHITIS, CHRONIC, GERIATRIC
• PNEUMONIA, LOBAR: Very Good, 4.5 g Of Crude Herb 4x/Day
• RESPIRATORY TRACT, UPPER INFECTION: Very Good, 4.5 g Of Crude Herb 4x/Day

ORAL CAVITY
• TONSILLITIS: Very Good, 4.5 g Of Crude Herb 4x/Day

PAIN/NUMBNESS/GENERAL DISCOMFORT

In Decoction 12-24 Hours, 1/Day, 5 Days For Course
• UTERUS, STIMULATES

SKIN
• ABSCESS: Topical
• BURNS, W/INFECTION: Topical
• ERYSIPELAS: Very Good, 4.5 g Of Crude Herb 4x/Day

TRAUMA, BITES, POISONINGS
• SURGERY, INFECTIONS FROM: Local Application Of Mashed Fresh Leaves
• WOUNDS: Topical

Dose

9 - 15 gm

Notes

Leaves/Flowers Strongest, When Harvested In Month Of May

Heat Stable

May Cause Nausea, Increased BM, Rarely, Drug Rash

QING XIANG ZI   青葙子   SEMEN CELOSIAE ARGENTEAE

Traditional Functions:

1. Dissipates Wind Heat eye symptoms
2. Clears Liver Fire and clears the eyes

Traditional Properties:

Enters: LV,

Properties: BIT, <C

Indications:

CIRCULATION DISORDERS
• HYPERTENSION

EYES
• CATARACTS: Wind Heat/Deficient Yin

• CORNEAL OPACITY
• EYES, PAIN, RED, SWOLLEN
• EYES, RED, CONGESTED: Liver Heat
• EYES, RED, SORE, DRY,

PAINFUL: Wind Heat/Deficient Yin
• VISION, SUPERFICIAL OBSTRUCTIONS: Wind Heat/Deficient Yin

INFECTIOUS DISEASES

• LEPROSY

SKIN
• HYPEREMIA
• PRURITUS: Wind Heat
• SCABIES

Clinical/Pharmaceutical Studies:

BLOOD RELATED DISORDERS/TOPICS
• BLOOD PRESSURE, LOWERS: 1 Month Treatment

CIRCULATION DISORDERS
• HYPERTENSION: 1 Month Treatment

EYES

• PUPILS, DILATES: Therefore Contraindicated For Glaucoma

INFECTIOUS DISEASES
• BACTERIAL, ANTI-: Psudomonas

Dose

4.5 - 15.0 gm

Contraindications

Not: w/Dilated Eyes From Def LV/KI
Not: Glaucoma, Dilates Eyes

SHAN ZHI ZI
(ZHI ZI)

山栀子
（山栀子）

FRUCTUS GARDENIAE JASMINOIDIS

Traditional Functions:

1. Clears Heat and relieves restlessness
2. Drains Damp Heat in any of the three Jiao (Burners)
3. Cools the Blood and stops bleeding
4. Topical use for traumatic swelling with congealed Blood

Traditional Properties:

Enters: LU, ST, HT, SJ, LV,

Properties: BIT, C

Indications:

ABDOMEN/ GASTROINTESTINAL TOPICS
- ABDOMEN, DISTENTION OF: Damp Heat

BOWEL RELATED DISORDERS
- DIARRHEA, BLOODY
- HEMORRHOIDS, BLOODY STOOL

CANCER/TUMORS/ SWELLINGS/LUMPS
- TUMORS

CHEST
- CHEST, PAIN

ENDOCRINE RELATED DISORDERS
- DIABETES

EYES
- CORNEA, INFLAMMATION
- EYES, RED
- EYES, SORES: Damp Heat Of Gall Bladder/San Jiao Channels

FEVERS
- FEVER, HIGH W/ RESTLESSNESS,

INSOMNIA

FLUID DISORDERS
- THIRST

HEAD/NECK
- FACE, SORES: Damp Heat Of Gall Bladder/San Jiao Channels

HEAT
- HEAT: In Yang Ming, Qi Level

HEMORRHAGIC DISORDERS
- BLEEDING: Heat
- EPISTAXIS: Blood Heat
- HEMAFECIA: Blood Heat
- HEMATEMESIS: Blood Heat
- HEMATURIA: Blood Heat
- HEMORRHAGE: Cool Blood To Stop

LIVER
- HEPATITIS, ACUTE, ICTERIC
- JAUNDICE: Damp Heat With Liver Gall Bladder Qi Stagnation

- LIVER GALL BLADDER DAMP HEAT

LUNGS
- COUGH: Lung Heat
- LUNGS, DYSPNEA: Lung Heat

MENTAL STATE/ NEUROLOGICAL DISORDERS
- DELIRIUM: Heat
- INSOMNIA: Deficiency Restlessness/Heat
- IRRITABILITY: Heat
- RESTLESSNESS: Heat
- UNCONSCIOUSNESS: (Mental Cloudiness) Use w/ Heat Shut-In Herbs

NOSE
- NOSE, SORES: Damp Heat Of Gall Bladder/San Jiao Channels

ORAL CAVITY
- ESOPHAGITIS
- MOUTH, SORES: Damp Heat Of Gall Bladder/San Jiao Channels
- TONSILLITIS

SEXUALITY, FEMALE:

GYNECOLOGICAL
- MASTITIS
- MENSTRUATION, DISORDERS OF: Clear Chong, Ren

SKIN
- BOILS, TOXIC: Heat, Toxins, Swellings
- ECZEMA: Damp Heat
- HYPEREMIA
- SKIN, SORES: Damp Heat
- SKIN, SORES, SWOLLEN: Heat, Toxins, Swelling, Topical

STOMACH/DIGESTIVE DISORDERS
- STOMACH, ACHE

TRAUMA, BITES, POISONINGS
- INFLAMMATION
- SWELLING, TRAUMA: Topical With Egg White

URINARY BLADDER
- URINATION, PAINFUL, DRIBBLING, CONCENTRATED, RED/ YELLOW/TURBID

Clinical/Pharmaceutical Studies:

BLOOD RELATED DISORDERS/TOPICS
- BLOOD PRESSURE, LOWERS: Long Lasting, Decoction/ETOH Extract

BOWEL RELATED DISORDERS
- DIARRHEA: Orally

CANCER/TUMORS/ SWELLINGS/LUMPS
- ANTINEOPLASTIC: Inhibits Ascitic Carcinoma, Orally
- SWELLINGS: w/Egg White & pwdr

FEVERS
- ANTIPYRETIC: Inhibits Thermoregulatory Center, Similar To Huang Lian/Qin

GALL BLADDER

Orally, Similar To Sodium Hexahydrocholate, Strongest When Combined With Yin Chen, Da Huang And Herb
- GALL BLADDER, STIMULATES CONTRACTION: Oral, Aqueous Extract, 20-40 Min After Intake

HEMORRHAGIC DISORDERS
- BLEEDING, LOCAL: Powder

INFECTIOUS DISEASES
- BACTERIAL, ANTI-: Hemolytic Strep., Spirochetes, Staph.Aureus, Diplococcus Meningitidis

LIVER

NEUROLOGICAL DISORDERS
- CNS, RELAXANT
- TRANQUILIZING: Aqueous Extract

PAIN/NUMBNESS/ GENERAL DISCOMFORT
- ANALGESIC: Aqueous Extract

PARASITES
- SCHISTOSOMIASIS: Stops Movement Of

SKIN
- FUNGAL, ANTI-: Tinea, And Others (Aqueous Extract)
- SKIN, INFECTIONS: And Mucous Membranes

STOMACH/DIGESTIVE

Hemostatic, 3-6 g, 3x/Day PO

TRAUMA, BITES, POISONINGS
- BRUISES: Speeds Healing Of, Dressing Made Of Powder, Alcohol Helped Reduce Swelling, Pain
- SPRAINS, ACUTE: As Paste With Water, Alcohol, Reduces Pain, Swelling-- Takes A Couple Of Days, * (Another Source, Says) Dressing Made Of Powder, Alcohol Helped Reduce Swelling, Pain, Functions Returned In 5 Days
- TRAUMA, EXTERNAL: Speeds Healing Of Soft

Clinical/Pharmaceutical Studies:

- BILE SECRETION, INCREASES: (Injected, Not With Oral/Other Study Shows It Does When Degraded In Intestine), ETOH Extract Works
- HEPATITIS, ICTERIC: 30 Days Of Treatment
- LIVER, PROTECTANT: Reduces Damage From Carbon Tetrachloride

MENTAL STATE/

DISORDERS
- STOMACH: Decreased Secretion, 1/10-1/5th Of Atropine
- STOMACH, BLEEDING: Sterilized Powder Used As

Tissue
URINARY BLADDER
- URINARY BLADDER, ACUTE BACTERIAL CYSTITIS

Dose

3 - 9 gm

Common Name

Cape Jasmine/Gardenia Ft.

Contraindications

Not: SP Def Cold, Loose Diarrhea

Notes

Can Induce Diarrhea

SHI GAO   石膏   GYPSUM

Traditional Functions:

1. Clears Heat and subdues Fire: Yang Ming stage or Qi stage level
2. Clears excess Lung Heat
3. Clears Stomach or Heart Fire
4. Topical astringent for eczema, burns and ulcerated sores
5. Reinforces fluids, relieves thirst

Traditional Properties:

Enters: LU, ST,

Properties: SW, SP, >C

Indications:

CIRCULATION DISORDERS
- STROKE, HEAT W/ PERSPIRATION
- TIDAL PULSE

FEVERS
- ANTIPYRETIC
- FEVER, WITHOUT CHILLS

FLUID DISORDERS
- THIRST: Fluid Injury

HEAD/NECK
- HEADACHE: Stomach Fire

HEAT
- HEAT: In Yang Ming, Qi Level

- HEAT STROKE
- QI LEVEL HEAT, EXCESS: Profuse Sweat, Tidal Pulse, High Fever, Irritability, Thirst, Red Tongue With Yellow Coating

LUNGS
- ASTHMA: Lung Heat
- COUGH: Lung Heat
- DYSPNEA: Lung Heat

MENTAL STATE/ NEUROLOGICAL DISORDERS
- AGITATION
- CONSCIOUSNESS,

LOSS OF
- DELIRIUM
- IRRITABILITY
- MANIA
- MENTAL DULLNESS

NOSE
- SINUSITIS: Heat, Needs Sinusitis Herbs, Too

ORAL CAVITY
- GINGIVITIS
- GUMS, PAIN, SWELLING: Stomach Fire
- THROAT, DRY
- TOOTHACHE, ACUTE: Stomach Fire

SIX STAGES/ CHANNELS
- YANG MING STAGE DISEASE

SKIN
- ABSCESS
- BURNS: Topical/Internal
- ECZEMA: Topical/Internal
- ERUPTIONS OF
- RASHES, INCOMPLETE EXPRESSION OF, W/ COUGH, DYSPNEA
- SORES: Topical/Internal
- SWEAT: Inhibits Secretion Of

Clinical/Pharmaceutical Studies:

- HETRAZAN, REACTION TO: Shi Gao, Man Jing Zi

ABDOMEN/ GASTROINTESTINAL TOPICS
- SMALL INTESTINE: Inhibits Transportation

BLOOD RELATED DISORDERS/ TOPICS
- BLOOD PRESSURE, LOWERS: Dilates Blood Vessels, Reduces High BP From Neck Artery Obstruction

BOWEL RELATED DISORDERS
- DIARRHEA, SUMMER

ENDOCRINE RELATED DISORDERS
- DIABETES MELLITUS: Bai Hu Tang

Sulfate
FLUID DISORDERS
- THIRST: Reduces From Many Types Of Induced Thirst

GALL BLADDER
- GALL BLADDER: Decreases Bile Secretion

HEAT
- HEATSTROKE

INFECTIOUS DISEASES
- ENCEPHALITIS B
- MEASLES

LUNGS
- PNEUMONIA, LOBAR: Shi Gao With Zhi Mu

MENTAL STATE/ NEUROLOGICAL DISORDERS

Content
NUTRITIONAL/METABOLIC DISORDERS/TOPICS
- CALCIUM REDUCES, IN SOME GLANDS: (Pitutary, Pancreas, Adrenals)
- CALCIUM, INCREASES IN SPLEEN

ORAL CAVITY
- MOUTH, SORES: Stomatitis

SEXUALITY, FEMALE: GYNECOLOGICAL
- UTERUS, STIMULATES

SKIN
- BURNS: Local Application As Fine Powder
- SCABIES: Fu Ping Shi Gao

Clinical/Pharmaceutical Studies:

EYES
• CONJUNCTIVITIS, ACUTE
FEVERS
• ANTIPYRETIC: Strong, Fast, Short Acting, More So Than Pure Calcium

• CONVULSIVE, ANTI-: Inhibits Muscles
• SEDATIVE: Inhibits Muscles
• TRANQUILIZING: Calcium

Decoction
WIND DISORDERS
• WIND HEAT FEVER W/ DYSPNEA, COUGH

Dose

15 - 60 gm

Contraindications

Not: Weak ST
Not: Minute Pulse

Not: Def Yang

Notes

Needs Clear Heat And Toxins Herbs For Pathogens
For Fever: 60-120 gm

XIA KU CAO

夏枯草

SPICA PRUNELLAE VULGARIS

Traditional Functions:

1. Clears Liver Fire and cleanses the eyes
2. Clears Phlegm Fire nodules and entanglements

Traditional Properties:

Enters: LV, GB,

Properties: SP, <BIT, C

Indications:

CANCER/TUMORS/SWELLINGS/ LUMPS
• INGUINAL CANAL NODULES: Phlegm Fire
• LIPOMA: Phlegm Fire
• THYROID TUMORS
CIRCULATION DISORDERS
• HYPERTENSION
EARS/HEARING DISORDERS
• DIZZINESS: Liver Fire
• VERTIGO: Liver Yang/Fire Rising
ENDOCRINE RELATED DISORDERS
• GOITER: Phlegm Fire
• THYROID, ENLARGEMENT
• THYROID, TUMORS
EYES
• EYEBALL PAIN: Liver Fire

• EYES, PAIN W/O REDNESS/ SWOLLEN: Liver Deficient
• EYES, RED, CONGESTED: Liver Heat
• EYES, SWOLLEN: Liver Fire
• TEARING, EXCESSIVE
HEAD/NECK
• HEADACHE: Liver Fire
IMMUNE SYSTEM RELATED DISORDERS/TOPICS
• GLANDS, SWOLLEN: Phlegm Fire
• LYMPH GLANDS, ENLARGEMENT, CHRONIC: Phlegm Nodules
• LYMPH NODES, SWELLING IN NECK: Phlegm Fire

INFECTIOUS DISEASES
• MUMPS
• SCROFULA: Phlegm Fire
LIVER
• LIVER DEFICIENCY EYE PAIN: No Red, Pain More Afternoon
• LIVER FIRE BLAZING
SEXUALITY, FEMALE: GYNECOLOGICAL
• BREASTS, ABSCESS OF
• LEUKORRHEA, PINKISH W/ WHITE MATTER
• MASTITIS, ACUTE
SKIN
• BOILS
TRAUMA, BITES, POISONINGS
• WOUNDS, INFECTED

Clinical/Pharmaceutical Studies:

CANCER/TUMORS/ SWELLINGS/LUMPS
• THYROID ADENOMA: Cooked With Golden Carp In A Bain-Marie, Nodule Disappeared In 2 Months
CIRCULATION DISORDERS
• HYPERTENSION: Moderate Over 2 Weeks, Vasodilates, Aqueous/30% ETOH Extract, Whole Plant Stronger Than Spikes, *30 g As Decoction, May Add Jue Ming Zi, 30 g,

Best In 1ST/2ng Stage
• VASODILATOR: Renal In Hypertension
INFECTIOUS DISEASES
• ANTIBIOTIC: Inhibits Broad Spectrum— Pseudomonas, B.Typhi, E. Coli, Mycobacterium, etc
KIDNEYS
• DIURETIC
LIVER
• HEPATITIS, ACUTE, ICTERIC
LUNGS
• TUBERCULOSIS,

CERVICAL LYMPH NODES: Bai Tou Weng Xia Ku Cao Tang (Bai Tou Weng, Herb) , 2-4 Weeks Shrunk Nodes, Healed Ulcerations
• TUBERCULOSIS, PULMONARY: Infiltrative, With Qing Hao, Gui Ban, Help Absorb Lesions, *With LU Cao (Herba Humuli) , 30 g Each, Especially Help Cough, Anorexia In TB
MUSCULOSKELETAL/

CONNECTIVE TISSUE
• MUSCLES, SMOOTH STIMULATES
SEXUALITY, FEMALE: GYNECOLOGICAL
• UTERUS, STIMULATES: Strong Contraction Of Smooth Muscle
SKIN
• FUNGAL, ANTI-: Inhibits Some Skin
• SKIN, INFECTIONS, SWOLLEN: Inhibits Transplanted Skin Infections

Dose

4.5 - 30.0 gm

Common Name

Selfheal

Precautions

Watch: Def SP/ST

XIONG DAN   熊膽   *FEL*
                 （熊胆）   *URSI*

Traditional Functions:

1. Clears Heat and subdues Fire
2. Clears Liver Fire and clears eyes
3. Clears Heat and neutralizes toxic Heat of the skin
4. Clears Heat and relieves spasms
5. Reduces swelling and relieves pain
6. Kills worms

Traditional Properties:

Enters: SP, ST, HT, LV, GB,

Properties: BIT, C

Indications:

**ABDOMEN/
GASTROINTESTINAL TOPICS**
• ABDOMEN, PAIN OF,
ASCARIASIS
BOWEL RELATED DISORDERS
• DIARRHEA, CHRONIC
• DYSENTERY, CHRONIC
SUMMER
• FISTULA: Topical
• HEMORRHOIDS, PAIN,
SWELLING: Intestinal Wind,
Topical
CHILDHOOD DISORDERS
• INFANTILE CONVULSIONS
• MALNUTRITION, CHILDHOOD
EYES
• CONJUNCTIVITIS, ACUTE
• CORNEAL OPACITY: Topical
• EYES, RED, CONGESTED: Liver
Heat

• EYES, RED, SWOLLEN–SEVERE:
Liver Fire:Topical
• EYES, SUPERFICIAL
OBSTRUCTION
• NEBULA
FEVERS
• FEVER
HEAD/NECK
• TICS
HEAT
• HEAT, FEVER, HIGH &
CONVULSIONS
LIVER
• JAUNDICE, ICTERIC: Heat
Dominant
**MENTAL STATE/
NEUROLOGICAL DISORDERS**
• CONVULSIONS, FEVER, ACUTE
• CONVULSIONS, INFANTILE
• DELIRIUM, BURNS, FROM

EXTENSIVE
**MUSCULOSKELETAL/
CONNECTIVE TISSUE**
• SPASMS, W/FEVER, ACUTE
ORAL CAVITY
• THROAT, SORE
• TOOTHACHE: Wind
PARASITES
• ROUNDWORMS, PAIN
• TAPEWORMS
SKIN
• BOILS
• FURUNCLES, MALIGNANT
• HYPEREMIA
• SKIN, LESIONS: Hot:Topical
TRAUMA, BITES, POISONINGS
• FRACTURES
• SPRAINS
• TRAUMA, PAIN, SWELLING

Clinical/Pharmaceutical Studies:

**BLOOD RELATED
DISORDERS/TOPICS**
• BLOOD PRESSURE,
LOWERS: When A
Sequelae To Acute
Nephritis In Childhood
**BOWEL RELATED
DISORDERS**
• HEMORRHOIDS: Mix
With Borneol, Pig Bile,
Topical Application
**CIRCULATION
DISORDERS**
• HYPERTENSION,
RENAL, ACUTE: 0.5 g,
2x/Day To Children,
BP Lowered To Normal In 4-5
Days
EYES
• FUNDAL

• OPTIC NEURITIS:
Subconjunctival Injection,
20% Bile , 0.2 ml/Dose
FEVERS
• ANTIPYRETIC
GALL BLADDER
• BILIARY TRACT
INFECTION: With Jiang
Huang, Yin Chen
• CHOLELITHIASIS: With
Jiang Huang, Yin Chen,
May Be Used For
Cholesterol Stones,
Chenodeoxycholic Acid,
0.75-1.0 g Divided In 3-4
Doses/Day, 3-18 Months,
40% Effective
• GALL BLADDER, BILE
SECRETION,
STIMULATES

KIDNEYS
• HYPERTENSION,
ACUTE RENAL: 0.5 g,
2x/Day To Children, BP
Lowered To Normal In 4-5
Days
LIVER
• JAUNDICE: With Jiang
Huang, Yin Chen
LUNGS
• ANTITUSSIVE
• EXPECTORANT
**MENTAL STATE/
NEUROLOGICAL
DISORDERS**
• COMA: From Trauma
• CONVULSIONS,
YOUNG CHILDREN/
INFANTS
• CONVULSIVE, ANTI-:

REDUCES SPASMS:
Action Similar To
Papaverine
**NUTRITIONAL/
METABOLIC
DISORDERS/TOPICS**
• VITAMIN D, CALCIUM:
Stimulates Absorption Of
ORAL CAVITY
• TOOTHACHE: From
Dental Carries, Mix With
Borneol, Pig Bile, Topical
Application
**PAIN/NUMBNESS/
GENERAL
DISCOMFORT**
• ANALGESIC
**STOMACH/DIGESTIVE
DISORDERS**
• INDIGESTION

Clinical/Pharmaceutical Studies:

HEMORRHAGE:
Subconjunctival Injection,
20% Bile , 0.2 ml/Dose
• LENS OPACITY:
Subconjunctival Injection,
20% Bile , 0.2 ml/Dose,
Better With Small Amount
Of Musk

IMMUNE SYSTEM
RELATED DISORDERS/
TOPICS
• ALLERGIC, ANTI-
INFECTIOUS DISEASES
• BACTERIOSTATIC
• PERTUSSIS, COUGH
PAROXYSMS

Can Counteract Strychnine
• SEDATIVE
• TRANQUILIZING
MUSCULOSKELETAL/
CONNECTIVE TISSUE
• ANTISPASMODIC:
Similar To Papaverine
• MUSCLES, SMOOTH,

• STOMACH, ACHE:
Neurotic
TRAUMA, BITES,
POISONINGS
• ANTIDOTE, TOXICS:
Strychnine
• INFLAMMATORY, ANTI-
• TOXINS, ANTIDOTE

Not: Pregnancy, Liver Diseases, Intestinal Disturbances

Dose

0.15 - 1.50 gm

Common Name

Bear Gall Bladder

Contraindications

Not: w/Sheng Di

Not: w/Han Fang Ji

Notes

Usually Pill/Capsule Form

Use Cow Gall Bladder As Substitute

Oral For Pain/Inflammation: 0.6-2.5 gm

Common To Get Diarrhea

YE MING SHA   夜明砂   EXCREMENTUM VESPERTILII MURINI

Traditional Functions:

1. Clears Liver Heat and clears the eyes
2. Vitalizes the Blood
3. Supports treatment of childhood nutritional impairment

Traditional Properties:

Enters: LV,

Properties: SP, C

Indications:

CHILDHOOD DISORDERS
• CONVULSIONS, CHILDHOOD
• NUTRITIONAL IMPAIRMENT,
CHILDHOOD

EYES
• CATARACTS
• EYES, RED, CONGESTED: Liver
Heat

• EYES, SUPERFICIAL VISUAL
OBSTRUCTION
• NEBULA
• NIGHT BLINDNESS

Clinical/Pharmaceutical Studies:

EYES
• EYES, IMPROVES VISION:

Possibly Helps Because Rich In Vit   A

Dose

3 - 9 gm

Common Name

Bat Feces

Precautions

Watch: Pregnancy

ZHI MU   知母   RADIX ANEMARRHENAE ASPHODELOIDIS

Traditional Functions:

1. Clears Heat and subdues Fire in Qi stage
2. Nourishes Kidney/Lung Yin and moistens dryness
3. Drains Heat in painful urination
4. Clears Heat from Lung and Stomach and generates fluids

Traditional Properties:

Enters: LU, ST, KI,

Properties: BIT, C

Indications:

BOWEL RELATED DISORDERS
- CONSTIPATION: Intestinal Dryness
- CONSTIPATION W/ DEFICIENT BLOOD
- TENESMUS

ENDOCRINE RELATED DISORDERS
- DIABETES: Internal Heat With Exhaustion Thirst

ENERGETIC STATE
- DEFICIENCY

FEVERS
- FEVER, AFTERNOON/ LOW GRADE
- FEVER, HIGH: Lung Stomach Excess Heat
- FEVER, HIGH W/ THIRST, RESTLESSNESS: Acute Infectious Disease
- FEVER, IRRITABILITY, RESTLESSNESS
- STEAMING BONE FEVER: Yin Deficient Heat

- STEAMING BONE FEVER W/SWEAT

FLUID DISORDERS
- DRYNESS, HEAT
- THIRST: Fluid Injury/ Lung Stomach Excess Heat

HEAT
- DRYNESS, HEAT
- HEAT: In Yang Ming, Qi Level
- HEAT IN FIVE CENTERS
- HEAT, RESTLESS W/ CONSUMPTION THIRST

INFECTIOUS DISEASES
- MALARIA, CHILLS, FEVER OF

KIDNEYS
- KIDNEY HEAT

LUNGS
- BRONCHITIS, CHRONIC
- COUGH: Lung Dryness/ Lung Heat
- COUGH, CHRONIC
- COUGH, EXHAUSTION W/STEAMING BONE

FEVER
- COUGH, FROM FATIGUE
- COUGH, LUNG EXHAUSTION: Tuberculosis
- LUNG STOMACH EXCESS HEAT: High Fever, Irritability, Thirst, Rapid, Flooding Pulse
- TUBERCULOSIS

MENTAL STATE/ NEUROLOGICAL DISORDERS
- IRRITABILITY: Lung Stomach Excess Heat/Yin Deficiency With Heat

MUSCULOSKELETAL/ CONNECTIVE TISSUE
- BACK, LOWER PAIN

ORAL CAVITY
- GUMS, BLEEDING: Yin Deficiency With Heat
- ORAL INFLAMMATION: Yin Deficiency

SEXUALITY, EITHER SEX

- SEXUAL DRIVE, INCREASED ABNORMALLY: Kidney Heat

SEXUALITY, MALE: UROLOGICAL TOPICS
- NOCTURNAL EMISSIONS: Kidney Heat
- SPERMATORRHEA: Kidney Heat

SIX STAGES/ CHANNELS
- YANG MING STAGE DISEASE: (ST/LI)

SKIN
- NIGHT SWEATS: Yin Deficiency With Heat

URINARY BLADDER
- DYSURIA
- URINATION, PAINFUL: Heat

YIN RELATED DISORDERS/TOPICS
- YIN DEFICIENCY W/ DEFICIENT FIRE

Clinical/Pharmaceutical Studies:

BLOOD RELATED DISORDERS/ TOPICS
- BLOOD GLUCOSE, REDUCES: Aqueous Extract, Not ETOH
- BLOOD PRESSURE, LOWERS

ENDOCRINE RELATED DISORDERS
- DIABETES MELLITUS: Decoction Of Herb, Tian Hua Fen, Mai Dong 12 g Each, Huang Lian, 4.5 g

FEVERS
- ANTIPYRETIC: No Fever Response When Given With Pathogenic Bacteria, Some When Injected, Prolonged
- FEVER, EPIDEMIC HEMORRHAGIC: Bai Hu Tang, Marked Reduction Of Fever

- FEVER, HIGH W/PROLONG SWEATING, THIRST: Bai Hu Tang (Zhi Mu 15 g, Shi Gao, 30 g, Gan Cao 6g)

INFECTIOUS DISEASES
- ANTIBIOTIC: Strongly Inhibits– Staph A., Salmonella Typhi, E.Coli, B.Subtilis, V.Choerae, Hemolytic Streptococcus, Pertussis
- ENCEPHALITIS B: Encephalitis Injection (Ban Lan Gen, Da Qing Ye, Lian Qiao, LU Gen, Shi Gao, Zhi Mu, Sheng Di, Berberine (Huang Lian) , Yu Jin)

KIDNEYS
- DIURETIC

LUNGS
- BRONCHITIS, CHRONIC: Heat,

Decoction Herb, Huang Qin, Sang Bai Pi, Fu Ling, Mai Dong 9 g Each, Jie Geng, Gan Cao, 3 g Each
- EXPECTORANT
- TUBERCULOSIS: Decreases Active Sites In Lungs (2.5% Powder, If Greater, Increased Mortalitiy)
- TUBERCULOSIS, PULMONARY W/HECTIC FEVER: 6-15 g/Day As Decoction

SKIN
- FUNGAL, ANTI-: Skin Fungi/ Candida Albicans, 100% Decoction Inhibited

TRAUMA, BITES, POISONINGS
- INFLAMMATORY, ANTI-, ENHANCES CORTICO STEROID LEVELS: With Shu Di, Gan Cao

Dose

3 - 24 gm

Contraindications

Not: Def SP Diarrhea

Notes

w/Huang Bai For Def Heat

w/Shi Gao For Excess Heat

Bake To Reduce Coldness

w/Wine To Increase Ascending Nature

ZHU YE

竹葉
（竹叶）

FOLIUM BAMBUSAE

Traditional Functions:

1. Clears Heat and reduces irritability
2. Promotes urination

Traditional Properties:

Enters: HT, LU, ST

Properties: SW, C

Indications:

CHILDHOOD DISORDERS
• CONVULSIONS, CHILDHOOD

FEVERS
• THIRST, FEBRILE DISEASES

FLUID DISORDERS
• THIRST: Febrile Diseases
• THIRST, FEBRILE DISEASES

HEART
• HEART FIRE FLARING: Mouth, Tongue Ulcers

HEAT
• HEAT: In Yang Ming, Qi Level

HEMORRHAGIC DISORDERS
• EPISTAXIS

ORAL CAVITY
• MOUTH, ULCERS
• TONGUE, ULCERS

STOMACH/DIGESTIVE DISORDERS
• VOMITING

Dose

9 - 15 gm

Common Name

Bamboo Leaf

Precautions

Watch: Diarrhea

Clear Heat And Dry Dampness

CHI FU LING

赤茯苓
（赤茯苓）

SCLEROTIUM PORIAE COCOS RUBRAE

Traditional Functions:

1. Promotes urination and filters out Dampness
2. Clears Heat and cools the Blood

Traditional Properties:

Enters: LU, SP, HT,

Properties: SW, BL, <C

Indications:

ABDOMEN/
 GASTROINTESTINAL TOPICS
• SMALL INTESTINE, DAMP HEAT
BOWEL RELATED DISORDERS
• DIARRHEA
• DYSENTERY
FLUID DISORDERS

• THIRST, DEFICIENT YIN
HEMORRHAGIC DISORDERS
• BLEEDING: Deficient
INFECTIOUS DISEASES
• GONORRHEA
KIDNEYS
• DIURETIC, MILD

SKIN
• SKIN, RASHES
URINARY BLADDER
• URINARY BLADDER DAMP
 HEAT
• URINATION, SCANTY
• URINATION, TURBID

Dose

6 gm

Common Name

Red Tuckahoe

Contraindications

Not: Spermatorrhea, Polyuria, Prolapse Of Urogenital
Organs

CHUN PI
(CHUN BAI PI)

椿皮

CORTEX AILANTHI

Traditional Functions:

1. Clears Heat and dries Dampness
2. Expels Dampness, controls leukorrhea

Traditional Properties:

Enters: LI, LV,

Properties: BIT, A, C

Indications:

BOWEL RELATED DISORDERS
• DIARRHEA FROM SUMMER
 HEAT
• DYSENTERY, CHRONIC MUCUS/
 BLOOD STOOL

• HEMORRHOIDS
• STOOLS, BLOODY
HEMORRHAGIC DISORDERS
• HEMORRHAGE: Astringe To Stop

SEXUALITY, FEMALE:
 GYNECOLOGICAL
• LEUKORRHEA: Damp Heat
• MENORRHAGIA

Clinical/Pharmaceutical Studies:

INFECTIOUS DISEASES
• ANTIBIOTIC: Typhoid, Bacillus

Dysenteriae
PARASITES

• ANTIPARASITIC: Trichomonas
 Vaginalis

Dose

3 - 9 gm

Common Name

Tree Of Heaven Bark

Contraindications

Not: Cold, Def SP/ST

GAN LAN

橄欖
（橄榄）

FRUCTUS CANARII

Traditional Functions:

1. Clears Heat from the Lungs and relieves toxins
2. Moistens the throat and promotes the secretion of body fluids

Traditional Properties:

Enters: LU, ST

Properties: SW, A, SO, N

Indications:

BOWEL RELATED DISORDERS
• DYSENTERY: Bacterial
FLUID DISORDERS
• THIRST
HEMORRHAGIC DISORDERS
• HEMOPTYSIS

LUNGS
• COUGH
MENTAL STATE/ NEUROLOGICAL DISORDERS
• EPILEPSY
• RESTLESSNESS

ORAL CAVITY
• THROAT, SWOLLEN, SORE
TRAUMA, BITES, POISONINGS
• ALCOHOLIC INTOXICATION
• FISH TOXINS

Dose

4.5 - 9.0 gm

Common Name

Chinese Olive

HU HUANG LIAN

胡黃連
（胡黄连）

RHIZOMA PICRORRHIZAE

Traditional Functions:

1. Clears Heat and dries Dampness
2. Clears deficiency Heat
3. Reduces fever of chronic childhood nutritional impairment with abdominal distension
4. Kills intestinal parasites

Traditional Properties:

Enters: LI, ST, LV,

Properties: BIT, C

Indications:

ABDOMEN/ GASTROINTESTINAL TOPICS
• ABDOMEN, DISTENTION OF: Chronic Childhood Malnutrition/ Damp Heat
BOWEL RELATED DISORDERS
• DIARRHEA: Damp Heat
• DYSENTERY: Blood Heat/Damp Heat
• HEMORRHOIDS
CHILDHOOD DISORDERS
• MALNUTRITION SYNDROME, CHRONIC, CHILDHOOD: With Abdominal Distension/Afternoon

Fevers
EYES
• EYES, RED
FEVERS
• FEVER, AFTERNOON: Chronic Childhood Malnutrition
• FEVER, LOW GRADE, CHRONIC
• STEAMING BONE FEVER: Yin Deficient Heat/Overexertion, Hectic Fever
HEART
• HEART, RESTLESS
HEAT
• DAMP HEAT SORES

LIVER
• JAUNDICE
MENTAL STATE/ NEUROLOGICAL DISORDERS
• CONVULSIONS, INFANTILE
• EPILEPSY, CHILDHOOD
• RESTLESSNESS
SKIN
• BOILS
• HYPEREMIA
YIN RELATED DISORDERS/ TOPICS
• YIN DEFICIENCY W/HEAT

Clinical/Pharmaceutical Studies:

GALL BLADDER
• CHOLAGOGUE
INFECTIOUS DISEASES
• ANTIBIOTIC: General
LIVER

• HEPATITIS
SKIN
• FUNGAL, ANTI-
STOMACH/DIGESTIVE

DISORDERS
• STOMACHIC
URINARY BLADDER
• URINARY TRACT INFECTIONS

Dose
1.5 - 9.0 gm

Precautions
Watch: Def SP/ST

HUANG BAI
(HUANG BO)

黃柏
(黄柏)

CORTEX
PHELLODENDRI

Traditional Functions:

1. Clear Heat, dries Dampness, mainly of the lower burner
2. Reduces ascending Kidney deficient Fire
3. Sedates Fire and eliminates toxins

Traditional Properties:

Enters: LI, KI, UB,

Properties: BIT, C

Indications:

• ASTRINGENT
ABDOMEN/
GASTROINTESTINAL TOPICS
• ABDOMEN, DISTENTION OF:
Damp Heat
• APPENDICITIS W/PAIN
BOWEL RELATED DISORDERS
• DIARRHEA: Damp Heat
• DYSENTERY: Blood Heat/Damp
Heat
• HEMORRHOIDS
EARS/HEARING DISORDERS
• TINNITUS: Use With Wine
EXTREMITIES
• LEG QI, HOT
• LIMBS, ATROPHY
EYES
• EYES, RED: With Wine
FEVERS
• FEVER, AFTERNOON
• FEVER, TIDAL, CHRONIC: With
Night Sweats, Seminal Emission
• STEAMING BONE FEVER: Yin
Deficient Heat
• STEAMING BONE FEVER W/
SWEAT
FLUID DISORDERS
• THIRST: From Urinary Disturbance
HEAT

• DEFICIENT FIRE RISING
• HEAT: Mild Fluid Damage/Absence
Of Fluids
HEMORRHAGIC DISORDERS
• HEMAFECIA
• HEMORRHAGE: Cool Blood To
Stop
KIDNEYS
• KIDNEY FIRE
• PREMIERE FIRE, PURGES
LIVER
• JAUNDICE: Damp Heat
MENTAL STATE/
NEUROLOGICAL DISORDERS
• PARALYSIS
MUSCULOSKELETAL/
CONNECTIVE TISSUE
• JOINTS, PAIN, SWELLING, RED:
Hot Bi
ORAL CAVITY
• ULCERS, ORAL
SEXUALITY, FEMALE:
GYNECOLOGICAL
• LEUKORRHEA, PINKISH W/
WHITE MATTER: Damp Heat
• MENSTRUATION, DISORDERS
OF: Clear Chong, Ren
SEXUALITY, MALE:

UROLOGICAL TOPICS
• SEMINAL EMISSIONS
SKIN
• ABSCESS
• BOILS, TOXIC: Heat, Toxins,
Swellings
• ECZEMA: Damp Heat
• FURUNCLES
• NIGHT SWEATS: Yin Deficient
• SKIN, SORES, SWOLLEN: Heat,
Toxins, Swelling/Damp Heat
• SKIN, ULCERS
• SWEATING, AFTERNOON
STOMACH/DIGESTIVE
DISORDERS
• STOMACHIC
TRAUMA, BITES, POISONINGS
• INFLAMMATORY, ANTI-
URINARY BLADDER
• URINARY DISORDERS, THIRST
OF
• URINARY TRACT INFECTIONS,
ACUTE
• URINATION, DRIBBLING W/
TURBID DISCHARGE
• URINATION, PAINFUL,
DRIBBLING, CONCENTRATED,
RED/YELLOW/TURBID

Clinical/Pharmaceutical Studies:

• ASTRINGENT
ABDOMEN/
GASTROINTESTINAL TOPICS
• ENTERITIS, ACUTE: Bai Tou
Weng Tang
• INTESTINES, PERISTALSIS,
INCREASES FREQUENCY OF
• PANCREAS, INCREASES
SECRETIONS

ENHANCEMENT: Markedly
Increases Antibody Formation
INFECTIOUS DISEASES
• ANTIBIOTIC: Berberine Less Than
Huang Lian
• BACTERIAL, ANTI-: Staph, Strep,
Typhoid, Cholera
• ELEPHANTIASIS
• MENINGITIS, CEREBROSPINAL:

SEXUALITY, FEMALE:
GYNECOLOGICAL
• CERVICITIS: Trichomonas
Infections
• CERVIX, EROSION OF
• VAGINITIS: Candidial/
Trichomonal
SEXUALITY, MALE:
UROLOGICAL TOPICS

Clinical/Pharmaceutical Studies:

BLOOD RELATED DISORDERS/ TOPICS
- BLOOD GLUCOSE, REDUCES
- BLOOD PRESSURE, LOWERS: Prolonged, Marked CNS Response
- BLOOD, PLATELETS, PROTECTANT

BOWEL RELATED DISORDERS
- ANAL FISSURES: 10% Solution, Apply Repeatedly With Cotton With Pressure
- DYSENTERY, BACILLARY, ACUTE/CHRONIC: Fluid Extract, 3-4 Days, Pills Of Powder And 10% Alcohol, 4 g 2x/Day For 7 Days

EARS/HEARING DISORDERS
- EARS, CHRONIC SUPPURATIVE OTITIS MEDIA

EYES
- CONJUNCTIVITIS: Best Results From Best Grade

FEVERS
- ANTIPYRETIC

GALL BLADDER
- CHOLAGOGUE

IMMUNE SYSTEM RELATED DISORDERS/TOPICS
- IMMUNE SYSTEM

Fluid Extract Cured, *Retention Enema With Gan Cao, *Throat Spray Of 50% Decoction To Act As Preventative
- SURGICAL INFECTIONS

KIDNEYS
- DIURETIC

LIVER
- HEPATITIS B: Selectively Inhibits Surface Antigen, Not From Known Active Ingredients

LUNGS
- TUBERCULOSIS: Powder Reduced Fever, Cough Abated, Appetite Increased

MENTAL STATE/ NEUROLOGICAL DISORDERS
- CNS, INHIBITOR: Milder Than Curare

MUSCULOSKELETAL/ CONNECTIVE TISSUE
- OSTEOMYELITIS, CHRONIC: With Fistulation

NOSE
- SINUSITIS, MAXILLARY, CHRONIC

SEXUALITY, EITHER SEX
- GENITALS, ECZEMA

- PENIS, EDEMA IN PREPUCE, CHILDHOOD

SKIN
- ECZEMA: Ears, Very Effective, * Exudative Type, Er Miao San (Huang Bai, Cang Zhu), *Scrotal And Others
- ECZEMA, CHILDHOOD/ INFANTS
- IMPETIGO
- RASHES, DIAPER
- SKIN, DISORDERS: Topical Antiseptic, Instead Of Ethacridine

STOMACH/DIGESTIVE DISORDERS
- STOMACHIC

TRAUMA, BITES, POISONINGS
- FRACTURES: Used In Fixation Of
- INFLAMMATORY, ANTI-: Quite Strong--Berberine
- SPRAINS
- SURGERY, INFECTIONS FROM
- WOUNDS, PROMOTES HEALING

URINARY BLADDER
- URINARY TRACT BLEEDING
- URINARY TRACT INFECTIONS, ACUTE

Dose
4.5 - 9.0 gm

Common Name
Amur Cork-Tree Bark

Contraindications
Not: Def, Cold Spleen

Notes
Fry w/Salt To Nourish Essence

Fry w/Wine To Clear Heat In Upper Jiao

1 Report Of Allergic Skin Rash With Huang Bai Use

See More In Huang Lian Entry

HUANG LIAN

黄連
(黄连)

RHIZOMA COPTIDIS

Traditional Functions:

1. Sedates Fire and eliminates toxins
2. Clears Heat, dries Dampness, especially in Stomach and Small Intestines
3. Sedates Heart Fire in Heart-Kidney disharmony
4. Clears Heat and stops bleeding
5. Clears Stomach Fire
6. Topically clears Heat from eyes, tongue or mouth
7. Used for boils, carbuncles and abscesses

Traditional Properties:

Enters: LI, ST, HT, LV,

Properties: BIT, C

Indications:

ABDOMEN/ GASTROINTESTINAL TOPICS
- ABDOMEN, DISTENTION OF: Damp Heat
- ABDOMEN, LUMPS W/ DISTENTION

- EARS, OTITIS MEDIA

EYES
- EYES, RED, CONGESTED: Liver Heat

FEVERS
- FEVER, HIGH

FLUID DISORDERS
- THIRST

- COMA: Heat In Pericardium
- CONVULSIONS, FEVER, ACUTE
- DISORIENTATION: Heat In Pericardium
- HYSTERIA
- INSOMNIA: Heart

- ULCERS, ORAL: Tongue/ Mouth (Topically)

SKIN
- ABSCESS
- BOILS, TOXIC: Heat, Toxins, Swellings
- ECZEMA: Damp Heat
- SCABIES

Indications:

- APPENDICITIS W/PAIN
- GASTROINTESTINAL DAMP HEAT

BOWEL RELATED DISORDERS
- DIARRHEA: Damp Heat
- DYSENTERY: Blood Heat
- DYSENTERY, HEAT W/ ABDOMINAL PAIN
- HEMORRHOIDS
- TENESMUS

CANCER/TUMORS/ SWELLINGS/LUMPS
- LEUKEMIA
- TUMORS

CHEST
- CHEST, FULLNESS

EARS/HEARING DISORDERS

HEART
- HEART RESTLESSNESS

HEAT
- HEAT: Throat, Sore, Red Eyes
- HEAT, EXCESS

HEMORRHAGIC DISORDERS
- HEMAFECIA
- HEMATEMESIS
- HEMATURIA
- HEMOPTYSIS
- HEMORRHAGE: Cool Blood To Stop

LIVER
- JAUNDICE: Damp Heat

MENTAL STATE/ NEUROLOGICAL DISORDERS

Kidney Discommunication
- IRRITABILITY: Heat In Pericardium/Heart Kidney Discommunication
- MANIC BEHAVIOR
- MENTAL CLOUDINESS: Use w/Heat Shut-In Herbs

MUSCULOSKELETAL/ CONNECTIVE TISSUE
- SPASMS, W/FEVER, ACUTE

NOSE
- NOSEBLEED

ORAL CAVITY
- HALITOSIS
- MOUTH, INFLAMMATION
- TONGUE, INFLAMMATION OF

- SKIN, SORES: Damp Heat
- SKIN, SORES, SWOLLEN: Heat, Toxins, Swelling

STOMACH/DIGESTIVE DISORDERS
- ACID REGURGITATION: Stomach Heat
- BELCHING, PUTRID ODOR: Stomach Fire
- HICCUPS: Qi Deficiency--Heat
- NAUSEA/VOMITING
- STOMACH HEAT: Acid Regurgitation/Vomiting
- VOMITING: Qi Deficiency, Heat/Stomach Heat

Clinical/Pharmaceutical Studies:

ABDOMEN/ GASTROINTESTINAL TOPICS
- GASTROENTERITIS, ACUTE: Oral Powder, 100% Cure
- INFLAMMATORY BOWEL DISEASE: Local Application
- INTESTINES, INDUCES SPASMS: In Mice
- INTESTINES, STIMULATES: Stimulates Smooth Muscles
- PERITONITIS: Topical 20% Vaseline Dressing, 3% Solution With Oral Powder

BLOOD RELATED DISORDERS/TOPICS
- BLOOD CELLS, WHITE: Increases Phagocytosis
- BLOOD PRESSURE, LOWERS: Short Lived, Injection
- CHOLESTEROL, LOWERS: Oral/Injected
- PYEMIA: Staph Aureus
- SEPTICEMIA

BOWEL RELATED DISORDERS
- ANAL FISSURES: 10% Solution, Apply Repeatedly With Cotton With Pressure
- COLON, BALANTIDIASIS OF: Protozoan Infection Of GI Tract, With Vomiting Abdominal Pain, Weight

- CONJUNCTIVITIS, ACUTE: Eye Drops With Extract, Borax Or As Ointment, *Washing Eyes With 5% Decoction Several Times, 95% Cured
- CORNEAL: Bathing Eyes With 10% In 3% Boric Acid Solution, Markedly Improved
- EYES, BLEPHARITIS MARGINALIS: Bathing Eyes With 10% In 3% Boric Acid Solution, Markedly Improved
- HORDEOLUM: Bathing Eyes With 10% In 3% Boric Acid Solution, Markedly Improved
- KERATITIS: Bathing Eyes With 10% In 3% Boric Acid Solution, Markedly Improved
- KERATITIS, HERPES SIMPLEX: Bathing Eyes With 10% In 3% Boric Acid Solution, Markedly Improved
- KERATITIS, SUPERFICIAL: 5-10% Solution
- TRACHOMA: Bathing Eyes With 10% In 3% Boric Acid Solution, Markedly Improved
- ULCERS: Bathing Eyes With 10% In 3% Boric Acid Solution, Markedly Improved

FEVERS
- ANTIPYRETIC

- MEASLES: Prophylactic/ Therapeutic
- SCARLET FEVER: 10% Solution, Equal To Penicillin/Sulfa
- TYPHOID FEVER: Caps 2g/4 Hrs PO Until 3-5 Days After Fever Recovery, May Use Mu Xiang Huang Lian Pian
- VIRAL, ANTI-: Flu, Newcastle

LIVER
- HEPATITIS, TOXIC: From Industrial Toxins

LUNGS
- BRONCHI, SMOOTH MUSCLES STIMULANT
- BRONCHITIS, CHRONIC/ACUTE: Orally And Also As Aerosol
- LUNGS, ABSCESS: Powder PO
- LUNGS, BRONCHIOLES, CONTRACTS
- LUNGS, CANDIDIASIS OF
- PNEUMONIA: Powder PO
- TUBERCULOSIS, PULMONARY: Oral, As Berberine, 0.3 g 3x/Day For 3 Months
- TUBERCULOUS PLEURISY, EXUDATIVE: PO As Berberine 0.2-0.3 g 3x/Day, Cure Rate 93%, Fluid Absorbed In 11-20 Days, Good For Patients Allergic To Streptomycin,

Borax, Bing Pian, Calomelas, Hai Piao Xiao, Long Gu, Gan Cao, Shan Zhi Zi, Bai Ji)
- TONSILLITIS, ACUTE: Prompt Effect With Oral Dose/Aerosol
- TONSILLITIS, CHRONIC: Injection Into Tonsils

PAIN/NUMBNESS/ GENERAL DISCOMFORT
- ANALGESIC
- ANESTHETIC, LOCAL

PARASITES
- TRICHOMONAS: 20% Solution, Topical

SEXUALITY, FEMALE: GYNECOLOGICAL
- CERVIX, EROSION OF
- GYNECOLOGICAL INFLAMMATORY DISEASES
- MASTITIS: Topical 20% Vaseline Dressing, 3% Solution With Oral Powder
- UTERUS, STIMULATES
- VAGINITIS

SKIN
- ABSCESS: Topical 20% Vaseline Dressing, 3% Solution With Oral Powder
- BOILS, MULTIPLE: Topical Jin Huang San, Oral Detoxican Decoction Of Huang Qin, Huang Lian (Huang Lian, Huang Qin, Mu Dan Pi, Chi Shao, Jin Yin Hua, Lian Qiao, Gan Cao, Shan Zhi Zi)

Clinical/Pharmaceutical Studies:

Loss
- DIARRHEA
- DYSENTERY, AMOEBIC: Use With Mu Xiang, Wu Mei To Be Effective
- DYSENTERY, BACILLARY: Equal To Sulfa/Chloramphenicol, No Side Efects, Use As Powder, Syrup, Decoction, Dried Fluid Extract, By Mouth/Enema, Use With Other Herbs, e.g. Mu Xiang
- ULCERATIVE COLITIS: Local Application

CANCER/TUMORS/ SWELLINGS/LUMPS
- ANTINEOPLASTIC: Slight
- GRANULOMA: Shrinks

CIRCULATION DISORDERS
- ATHEROSCLEROSIS, PREVENTS
- BLOOD VESSELS, RELAXES
- HYPERTENSION: Daily 0.74-4.0 g As Berberine, Better If Used With Reserpine, More Effective For Early Or Second Stages, 70-93% Effective

EARS/HEARING DISORDERS
- EARS, OTITIS EXTERNA, DIFFUSE: 10% Extract Plus 3% Boric Acid
- EARS, OTITIS MEDIA, CHRONIC/ SUPPURATIVE: 10% Extract Plus 3% Boric Acid As Ear Drops

ENDOCRINE RELATED DISORDERS
- ANTIADRENALINE: Counters Blood Pressure Raise, Arrhythmic Effect

EXTREMITIES
- HANDS, NAILS, PARONYCHIA: Topical 20% Vaseline Dressing, 3% Solution With Oral Powder

EYES

FLUID DISORDERS
- ANTIDIURETIC

GALL BLADDER
- BILE SECRETION, INCREASES
- CHOLECYSTITIS, CHRONIC: Decrease Viscosity And Increases Volume Of Bile, Very Effective, *Symptom Relief 1-2 Days After Oral 3x/Day, As 5-20 mg Berberine

HEART
- HEART, INCREASES CORONARY BLOOD FLOW: Increases Blood Flow To Coronary Artery

IMMUNE SYSTEM RELATED DISORDERS/ TOPICS
- IMMUNE SYSTEM: Increases WBC Phagocytosis
- LYMPHADENITIS: Topical 20% Vaseline Dressing, 3% Solution With Oral Powder

INFECTIOUS DISEASES
- ANTIBIOTIC: Broad Spectrum, Greater Than Sulfa, Less Than Streptomycin
- BRUCELLOSIS
- CELLULITIS: Topical 20% Vaseline Dressing, 3% Solution With Oral Powder
- CHOLERA: Controls Diarrhea In Mild Cases, In Early Stage Helped Disease, Too
- DIPHTHERIA, MILD: Powder 0.6 g, 4-6x/Day, Plus Gargle Of 1% Solution Of Same, 1-3 Days Fever Gone, Pseudomembrane Gone In 3 Days, Negative Culture In 2-8 Days
- INFECTIONS, SUPPURATIVE: Topical 20% Vaseline Dressing, 3% Solution With Oral Powder
- LEPROSY

Isoniazid Or Drug Resistent Bacteria
- WHOOPING COUGH: 100% Decoction, 33% Cured, Marked Effect 27%, About 2 Days To Marked Effect

MENTAL STATE/ NEUROLOGICAL DISORDERS
- CNS, PROLONGS SLEEPING
- CNS, STIMULANT, CEREBRAL CORTEX, SMALL DOSES
- CURARE, ANTI-

MUSCULOSKELETAL/ CONNECTIVE TISSUE
- MUSCLES, RELAXANT: 3x Potent As Meprobamate
- SMOOTH MUSCLE, CONTRACTS (EXCEPT VESSELS)

NOSE
- RHINITIS, CHRONIC: Nasal Inserts Of Gauze Soaked With 10% Solution, 1x/Day For 7-10 Days, Recovers Sense Of Smell, Reduces Secretions
- SINUSITIS, MAXILLARY: Injection Into Sinus With 2 ml 10% Decotion In 3% Boric Acid, Equally Effective As Penicillin
- SINUSITIS, MAXILLARY, CHRONIC: Injection Into Sinus With 2 ml 30% Decotion

ORAL CAVITY
- MOUTH, GINGIVITIS, VINCENT'S (TRENCH MOUTH) : 10% In Boric Acid Solution Topically Or Decociton And Gargle, Rapidly Cured
- MOUTH, HERPETIC STOMATITIS: Apply Huang Lian San (See Mouth, Ulcers For Rx)
- MOUTH, ULCERS: Apply Huang Lian San (Huang Lian, Qing Dai,

- BURNS: Promotes Healing, 1ST/2nd Degree, Topical, *With Di Yu As Powder
- CARBUNCLES: Topical 20% Vaseline Dressing, 3% Solution With Oral Powder
- ECZEMA: Satisfactory Results From Short Courses Of Herb With Castor Oil, With Vit C, Better Than Zinc Oxide Ointment
- ERYTHEMA MULTIFORME, EXUDATIVE: (Usually On Extremities) Local, Oral
- FUNGAL, ANTI-: Strongly Inhibits
- FURUNCLES: Topical 20% Vaseline Dressing, 3% Solution With Oral Powder
- SKIN, PIMPLES, INFLAMMED HAIR FOLLICULES: Topical Jin Huang San, Oral Detoxican Decoction Of Huang Qin, Huang Lian (Huang Lian, Huang Qin, Mu Dan Pi, Chi Shao, Jin Yin Hua, Lian Qiao, Gan Cao, Shan Zhi Zi)

STOMACH/DIGESTIVE DISORDERS
- DIGESTION: Increases Secretion Of Bile, Pancreatic Juice, Saliva
- ULCERS, GASTRIC-INHIBITS FORMATION OF FROM NERVOUSNESS

TRAUMA, BITES, POISONINGS
- INFLAMMATION, SUPERFICIAL/DEEP
- INFLAMMATORY, ANTI- : MEOH Extract
- WOUNDS: Oral, External Use

URINARY BLADDER
- URINARY BLADDER STIMULANT: Stimulates Smooth Muscles

Dose

1.5 - 9.0 gm

Common Name

Golden Thread/Coptis Rz

Contraindications

Not: Def Yin
Not: Cold Def ST
Not: Def SP/KI

Precautions

Watch: Large Doses Can Damage SP

Notes

Give Every 4 Hours For Maximum Effect
Safe Up To 100 Gms/Dose
Stir Bake To Reduce Cold Property

Add Wine To Direct Effects To Head And Eyes
Prepare With Ginger To Clear Stomach Heat, Reduce
Vomiting
w/Salt To Clear Heat In Large Intestine, UB
w/Vinegar To Clear Liver/Gall Bladder Fire
Carbonize To Act As Hemostatic
May Produce Transient Diarrhea, Abdominal Distention,
Borborygmus, Frequent Urination, Anorexia, Vomiting
No Side Effects For 12g/Day For 3 Weeks
IV Infusion May Cause Sudden Circulatory, Respiratory
Arrest, Especially In Women With Low Calcium Levels
Berberine, Main Active Ingredient, Is Slowly Absorbed
Orally, Peaking In Blood 8 Hrs After Ingestion

HUANG QIN

黄芩
(黃芩)

RADIX SCUTELLARIAE BAICALENSIS

Traditional Functions:

1. Clears Heat and relieves toxins, particularly in the Upper Burner--Lungs
2. Clears Heat and dries Dampness, especially in the Stomach and intestines
3. Brings down rising Liver Yang
4. Stops bleeding and calms the fetus

Traditional Properties:

Enters: LU, LI, HT, GB,

Properties: BIT, C

Indications:

ABDOMEN/
GASTROINTESTINAL TOPICS
• ABDOMEN, DISTENTION OF:
Damp Heat
• APPENDICITIS W/PAIN
• ENTERITIS
• GASTROENTERITIS
• HYPOCHONDRIAC REGION,
FULLNESS FEELING OF
BOWEL RELATED DISORDERS
• DIARRHEA: Damp Heat
• DYSENTERY
• HEMORRHOIDS, BLOODY
STOOL
• HEMORRHOIDS, PAIN,
SWELLING
CHEST
• CHEST, DISCOMFORT,
HEAVINESS: Damp Heat
CIRCULATION DISORDERS
• HYPERTENSION
FEVERS
• FEVER: Damp Heat
• FEVER, HIGH
FLUID DISORDERS
• THIRST, INABILITY TO DRINK:
Damp Heat
• THIRST, RESTLESS: Heat Disease
• WATER RETENTION
HEAD/NECK

• FACE, FLUSHED: Liver Yang
Rising
• HEADACHE, RED EYES,
IRRITABILITY: Liver Yang Rising
HEAT
• DAMP HEAT DISORDERS
• HEAT: Mild Fluid Damage/Absence
Of Fluids
HEMORRHAGIC DISORDERS
• HEMATEMESIS: Heat
Accumulation
• HEMORRHAGE: Cool Blood To
Stop
INFECTIOUS DISEASES
• FEBRILE DISEASES, ALL
• MALARIA, CHILLS, FEVER OF
LIVER
• JAUNDICE: Damp Heat, Auxillary
Herb
• LIVER YANG RISING
LUNGS
• COUGH: Lung Heat
• LUNGS, DYSPNEA: Lung Heat
MENTAL STATE/
NEUROLOGICAL DISORDERS
• INSOMNIA
• IRRITABILITY: Heat/Liver Yang
Rising
NOSE
• SINUSITIS: Heat, Needs Sinusitis

Herbs Added
SEXUALITY, FEMALE:
GYNECOLOGICAL
• FETUS, RESTLESS: Damp Heat/
Gestational Heat
• MENSTRUATION, DISORDERS
OF: Clear Chong, Ren
• MISCARRIAGE, THREATENED
• MORNING SICKNESS:
Gestational Foul Obstruction--Heat
SKIN
• BOILS, TOXIC: Heat, Toxins,
Swellings
• ECZEMA: Damp Heat
• FURUNCLES
• SKIN, SORES: Damp Heat
• SKIN, SORES, SWOLLEN: Heat,
Toxins, Swelling, Topical/Internal
STOMACH/DIGESTIVE
DISORDERS
• ANOREXIA
• VOMITING
TRAUMA, BITES, POISONINGS
• INFLAMMATION
URINARY BLADDER
• DYSURIA: Damp Heat
• URINARY TRACT INFECTIONS,
ACUTE
• URINATION, DRIBBLING

Clinical/Pharmaceutical Studies:

ABDOMEN/ GASTROINTESTINAL TOPICS
- INTESTINES, PERISTALSIS, INHIBITS: Antispasmodic
- PANCREATITIS, RETROGRADE: IV Infusion

BLOOD RELATED DISORDERS/TOPICS
- BLOOD GLUCOSE, INCREASES
- BLOOD PRESSURE, LOWERS: 1 g/kg Of Extract Markedly Lowers, Give Extract PO 3x/Day For 4 Weeks, Neurogenic Hypertension, Vasodilator
- BLOOD, WBC: Marked Increase Of
- CHOLESTEROL, LOWERS: In Those With High Cholesterol Diets Or Disfunctional/Removed Thyroid

BOWEL RELATED DISORDERS
- DYSENTERY, BACILLARY: Herb With He Zi, Equal Amounts, Powder By Alum Precipitation, 5 Days To Cure, *Tablet, Decoction, Capsule, Extract 96% Cured, Symptoms Rapidly Disappeared

EYES
- EYES, DISEASES OF: (Corneal Ulcer, Cleritis, Papilitis, Optic Neuritis) Alcohol Precipitated Decoction Of Herb With Jin Yin Hua, Subconjunctival Injection

FEVERS
- ANTIPYRETIC:

Decoction, 2 g/kg PO, Varies With Crop, Not With Normal Temperature

GALL BLADDER
- BILE SECRETION, INCREASES: Decoction/ Tincture
- BILIARY TRACT INFECTION: IV Infusion
- CHOLECYSTITIS W/ STONES: IV Infusion
- CHOLECYSTITIS, ACUTE: IV Infusion

IMMUNE SYSTEM RELATED DISORDERS/ TOPICS
- ALLERGIC DISORDERS: Oral, Inhibits Mast Cells' Release Of Enzymes
- ALLERGIC, ANTI-: Skin
- TRACHEAL CONSTRICTION, ALLERGIC

INFECTIOUS DISEASES
- ANTIBIOTIC: Decoction Broad Spectrum--Staph A., C.Diphtheriae, Pseudomonas A., Streptococcus, Pneumoniae, N. Menignitidis, Leptospirosis (Need High Doses), Neisseria Meningitidis, Vibrio Cholerae, Can Treat Against Penicillian Resistant Bacteria
- LEPTOSPIROSIS: Tabs Of Herb, Jin Yin Hua, Lian Qiao, .3.7 g Crude Drug Extracted To 0.5 g, 10-15 Tabs/6 Hrs, Best In Moderate Cases
- MENINGITIS, CEREBROSPINAL, CARRIERS OF: Spray 20% Decoction 2 ml To Throat
- SCARLET FEVER: Oral

Decoction, Markedly Reduced Incidence
- VIRAL, ANTI-: Extract, Decoction Inhibited Some Flu

KIDNEYS
- DIURETIC: Orally Given ETOH Extract

LIVER
- HEPATITIS, CHRONIC: May Need Long Term Therapy With, 1 Year
- HEPATITIS, INFECTIOUS: Icteric/ Non-Icteric, Improved Symptoms, Restored Liver Functions
- LIVER, CIRRHOSIS W/ BILARY TRACT INFECTION: IV Infusion

LUNGS
- ASTHMA, ALLERGIC
- BRONCHITIS, ACUTE, CHILDHOOD: 50% Decoction, Less Than 1 Yr 6 ml, Greater Than 1 8-10 ml, Increase If Greater Than 5 Yrs, 3x/Day, Body Temperature Normal In 3 Days
- BRONCHITIS, CHRONIC: Huang Qin, Gan Cao, Lime Water (Calcium Hydroxide Solution), Good Response In Simple Disease
- BRONCHODILATORY, ASTHMA: Similar To Ephedrine
- LUNGS, REDUCES BLEEDING CAUSED BY LOW PRESSURE
- RESPIRATORY TRACT INFECTION, ACUTE, CHILDHOOD: 50% Decoction, Less Greater

Than 5 Yrs, 3x/Day, Body Temperature Normal In 3 Days
- TRACHEA, CONSTRICTION, ALLERGIC

MENTAL STATE/ NEUROLOGICAL DISORDERS
- CNS, INHIBITOR
- PARALYSIS, CEREBROVASCULAR HEMORRAGE/ OCCULSION: Scutellarin Component
- REFLEXES, REDUCES
- SEDATIVE: Insomnia In Hypertension/Increase Excitablity, Injection Gives Mild Effects

ORAL CAVITY
- TONSILLITIS, ACUTE, CHILDHOOD: 50% Decoction, Less Than 1 Yr 6 ml, Greater Than 1 8-10 ml, Increase If Greater Than 5 Yrs, 3x/Day, Body Temperature Normal In 3 Days

PARASITES
- ASCARIASIS, W/ CHOLECYSTITIS: IV Infusion

SKIN
- DERMATITIS, ALLERGIC
- FUNGAL, ANTI-: Decoction 9 Kinds Of Skin, Extract Stronger, More Fungi

TRAUMA, BITES, POISONINGS
- DETOXIFIES: Antagonizes Strychnine, Probably Due To Glucuronic Acid

Dose

3 - 15 gm

Common Name

Baical Skullcap Root

Contraindications

Not: Def Lung Heat Or Cold Spleen

Notes

Loosens Stools

Tongue Enlarges Soon w/Ingestion, Because Of Cold Nature

Weakens KI

Raw: Calms Fetus

Prepare w/Wine For Upper Jiao Heat

Carbonize To Act As Hemostatic And Clear Blood Heat

KU SHEN   苦参   RADIX SOPHORAE FLAVESCENTIS

Traditional Functions:

1. Clears Heat and dries Dampness
2. Disperses Wind and stops itching
3. Clears Heat and promotes urination
4. Kills intestinal parasites

Traditional Properties:

Enters: LI, ST, HT, SI, UB, LV,

Properties: BIT, C

Indications:

ABDOMEN/
GASTROINTESTINAL TOPICS
• SMALL INTESTINE, DAMP HEAT
BOWEL RELATED DISORDERS
• DIARRHEA: Damp Heat
• DYSENTERY: Blood Heat
• DYSENTERY, ACUTE
• DYSENTERY, BLOODY STOOL
• DYSENTERY, CHRONIC: Damp Heat
• HEMORRHOIDS, BLOODY STOOL
• HEMORRHOIDS, PAIN, SWELLING
FLUID DISORDERS
• EDEMA: Hot
HEAT
• DAMP HEAT
• DAMP HEAT SORES

HEMORRHAGIC DISORDERS
• HEMAFECIA
INFECTIOUS DISEASES
• LEPROSY
• SYPHILIS
LIVER
• JAUNDICE: Damp Heat
NUTRITIONAL/METABOLIC DISORDERS/TOPICS
• MALNUTRITION ACCUMULATION
SEXUALITY, EITHER SEX
• GENITALS, PRURITUS
SEXUALITY, FEMALE: GYNECOLOGICAL
• LEUKORRHEA: Damp Heat
• VAGINITIS
SKIN

• ECZEMA: Damp Heat
• ITCHING, GENERAL
• RASHES, PRURITIC: Wind Damp, External Application
• RINGWORM
• SCABIES
• SKIN, LESIONS W/CHRONIC ITCHING/SEEPAGE/BLEEDING
• SKIN, SORES: Damp Heat
• SKIN, SORES, INTRACTABLE
URINARY BLADDER
• URINARY TRACT INFECTIONS, ACUTE
• URINATION, CONCENTRATED URINE
• URINATION, PAINFUL, DRIBBLING, CONCENTRATED, RED/YELLOW/TURBID

Clinical/Pharmaceutical Studies:

BLOOD RELATED DISORDERS/TOPICS
• LEUKOPENIA: 10% Total Alkaloid Injection, 200-400 mg Per Day IM In 2 Doses, Increased By 2nd Day
BOWEL RELATED DISORDERS
• DYSENTERY: Intestinal Trichomoniasis
• DYSENTERY, BACILLARY, ACUTE: Tablet, 4 Days To Reduce Frequency, 5 Days To Have Normal Stool
CANCER/TUMORS/ SWELLINGS/LUMPS
• ANTINEOPLASTIC
• CERVICAL CANCER: Matrine Ingredient
• LIVER CANCER: Matrine Ingredient

CHILDHOOD DISORDERS
• INSOMNIA, CHILDHOOD
FEVERS
• ANTIPYRETIC
FLUID DISORDERS
• EDEMA, ANY TYPE: Martrine Ingredient
HEART
• ARRHYTHMIAS: Premature Beats, Sinus Tachycardia, Atrial Fibrillation, Use Tablet Or Herb Injection
• HEART RATE, REDUCES
INFECTIOUS DISEASES
• BACTERIAL, ANTI-: TB, E.Coli, Shigella, Proteus, Streptococcus, Staph
KIDNEYS
• DIURETIC

LIVER
• HEPATITIS, ACUTE
• LIVER, CANCER: Matrine Ingredient
LUNGS
• ANTIASTHMATIC: Total Alkaloids Treated With Acetone, Crystallized Similar To Equal Amount Of Aminophylline, Orally, Lasts 2 Hours
• BRONCHITIS, CHRONIC ASTHMATIC
MENTAL STATE/ NEUROLOGICAL DISORDERS
• INSOMNIA: Root Syrup, 0.5 g/ml, 20 ml Oral, Good Hypnotic Effect For Infection/Neurosis
SEXUALITY, FEMALE: GYNECOLOGICAL
• TRICHOMONAS,

VAGINAL: Alcohol Extract, Less Than Huang Lian, Equal To She Chuang Zi
SKIN
• ECZEMA: Injection Or Tablet, 0.3 g, 5 Tabs/Day
• ECZEMA, PERINEUM: Injection Or Tablet, 0.3 g, 5 Tabs/Day
• FUNGAL, ANTI-: Many Common, Use 8% Extract
• PSORIASIS: Purified Alkaloids, Definite Effect
• SKIN, SEBORRHEIC DERMATITIS: Injection Or Tablet, 0.3 g, 5 Tabs/ Day
• ULCERS: Prevents Formation
• URTICARIA: Matrine Ingredient

Dose
4.5 - 15.0 gm

Contraindications
Not: w/LI, LU

Not: Cold, Def SP/ST

Notes
Do Not Inject

Large Dose: May Cause Paralysis, Spasms, Repiratory Paralysis

Active Components Similar To Shan Dou Gen

May Have Nausea, Vomiting, Constipation, Mild Dizziness

LONG DAN CAO

龍膽草
（龙胆草）

RADIX GENTIANAE SCABRAE

Traditional Functions:

1. Clears Heat, dries Dampness from the Liver and Gall Bladder channels
2. Sedates and clears excessive Liver Fire

Traditional Properties:

Enters: UB, LV, GB,

Properties: BIT, C

Indications:

ABDOMEN/ GASTROINTESTINAL TOPICS
• FLANK PAIN: Liver Wind Heat
CIRCULATION DISORDERS
• HYPERTENSION W/DIZZINESS, TINNITUS
EARS/HEARING DISORDERS
• DEAFNESS, SUDDEN: Damp Heat In Gall Bladder
• EARS, PAINFUL, SWOLLEN: Damp Heat In Gall Bladder
• VERTIGO: Liver Yang/Fire Rising
EYES
• EYES, CONGESTED: Damp Heat In Gall Bladder
• EYES, RED, CONGESTED: Liver Heat
FEVERS
• FEVER: Liver Wind Heat
HEAD/NECK
• HEADACHE: Liver Fire

LIVER
• JAUNDICE: Liver/Gall Bladder Damp Heat
• LIVER FIRE BLAZING
• LIVER WIND HEAT: Fever, Spasms, Convulsions, Flank Pain
MENTAL STATE/ NEUROLOGICAL DISORDERS
• CONVULSIONS, FRIGHT: Liver Wind Heat
• EPILEPSY
MUSCULOSKELETAL/ CONNECTIVE TISSUE
• SPASMS: Liver Wind Heat
ORAL CAVITY
• MOUTH, BITTER TASTE
• THROAT, SWOLLEN, SORE: Damp Heat In Gall Bladder
SEXUALITY, EITHER SEX
• GENITAL AREA DAMPNESS,

PAIN, SWELLING: Liver/Gall Bladder Damp Heat
• GENITALS, PRURITUS: Liver/ Gall Bladder Damp Heat
SEXUALITY, FEMALE: GYNECOLOGICAL
• LEUKORRHEA: Smelly:Liver/Gall Bladder Damp Heat
SEXUALITY, MALE: UROLOGICAL TOPICS
• SCROTUM, SWELLING, SORE
SKIN
• ECZEMA: Damp Heat
• SKIN, SORES: Damp Heat
URINARY BLADDER
• URINARY TRACT INFECTIONS, ACUTE
• URINATION, PAINFUL, DRIBBLING, CONCENTRATED, RED/YELLOW/TURBID

Clinical/Pharmaceutical Studies:

BLOOD RELATED DISORDERS/TOPICS,
• BLOOD PRESSURE, LOWERS: Injection Of 20% Tincture, Lasts 15 Minutes
EARS/HEARING DISORDERS
• EARS, OTITIS MEDIA: Liver Gall Bladder Damp Heat, Use Modified Long Dan Xie Gan Tang
EYES
• CONJUNCTIVITIS: Liver Gall Bladder Damp Heat, Use Modified Long Dan Xie Gan Tang
• CORNEAL ULCERS: Liver Gall Bladder Damp Heat, Use Modified Long

Increases Bile Flow, Injection
IMMUNE SYSTEM RELATED DISORDERS/ TOPICS
• ALLERGIES, ANTIANAPHYLACTIC, ANTIHISTAMINE: Gentianine
• IMMUNE SYSTEM: Suppressed Antibody Formation
INFECTIOUS DISEASES
• ANTIBIOTIC: Many Fungi, Leptospirosis (Need High Doses)
• ENCEPHALITIS B: 20% Syrup, 10-15 3x/Day Orally For Mild Cases, If

Xie Gan Tang (Long Dan Cao, Shan Zhi Zi, Huang Qin, Chai Hu, Dang Gui, Sheng Di, Ze Xie, Gan Cao, Che Qian Zi, Mu Tong), 62 Doses
• LIVER, PROTECTANT: Injection
• LIVER, REDUCES ENZYMES: Lowers SGPT:Long Dan Xie Gan Tang, 1-5 Months
MENTAL STATE/ NEUROLOGICAL DISORDERS
• CNS, STIMULANT: At Low Doses, High Doses Anesthetic
MUSCULOSKELETAL/

GYNECOLOGICAL
• PELVIC INFECTIONS, ACUTE: Liver Gall Bladder Damp Heat, Use Modified Long Dan Xie Gan Tang
SKIN
• ECZEMA: Liver Gall Bladder Damp Heat, Use Modified Long Dan Xie Gan Tang
• RASHES, DRUG INDUCED): Liver Gall Bladder Damp Heat, Use Modified Long Dan Xie Gan Tang
STOMACH/DIGESTIVE DISORDERS
• GASTRIC SECRETIONS:

Clinical/Pharmaceutical Studies:

Dan Xie Gan Tang
- KERATITIS: Liver Gall Bladder Damp Heat, Use Modified Long Dan Xie Gan Tang

FEVERS
- ANTIPYRETIC

GALL BLADDER
- CHOLECYSTITIS, ACUTE/CHRONIC: Liver Gall Bladder Damp Heat, Use Modified Long Dan Xie Gan Tang
- GALL BLADDER, CHOLAGOGUE:

Coma/Vomiting 2:1 Injection, 2-4 ml IM 3-4x/ Day Up To 3 Days After Fever Subsides, More Serious Cases Needed Western Medicine, Too

KIDNEYS
- DIURETIC
- PYELONEPHRITIS, ACUTE: Liver Gall Bladder Damp Heat, Use Modified Long Dan Xie Gan Tang

LIVER
- HEPATITIS: Long Dan

CONNECTIVE TISSUE
- MUSCLES, SKELETAL: Relaxed

PAIN/NUMBNESS/ GENERAL DISCOMFORT
- ANALGESIC, SYNERGISTIC: No Action By Itself

PARASITES
- ASCARIASIS, SWINE: Decoction Paralyzing, Lethal To
- PARASITES, MALARIA

SEXUALITY, FEMALE:

Increases Before Meals, Decreases If After Meals

TRAUMA, BITES, POISONINGS
- INFLAMMATORY, ANTI-: Gentianine

URINARY BLADDER
- CYSTITIS: Liver Gall Bladder Damp Heat, Use Modified Long Dan Xie Gan Tang
- URETHRITIS: Liver Gall Bladder Damp Heat, Use Modified Long Dan Xie Gan Tang

Dose

3 - 9 gm

Common Name

Chinese Gentian Root

Contraindications

Not: Def, Cold SP/ST w/Diarrhea

Notes

Raw: For Descending Action

With Wine: Ascending Action

With Bile: For Fire

With Honey: SP/ST Area

Overdose: May Cause Headache, Vertigo, Facial Flushing

QIN PI   秦皮   CORTEX FRAXINI

Traditional Functions:

1. Clears Heat and dries Dampness, especially in the Stomach and intestines
2. Clears Liver Fire and brightens the eyes
3. Disperses Wind Damp Hot Bi
4. Stops cough and relieves asthma

Traditional Properties:

Enters: LI, ST, LV,

Properties: BIT, C

Indications:

ABDOMEN/ GASTROINTESTINAL TOPICS
- INTESTINES, BLEEDING IN WOMEN

BOWEL RELATED DISORDERS
- DIARRHEA: Heat/Damp Heat
- DYSENTERY: Blood Heat/Damp Heat

EYES
- CATARACTS

- EYES, PAIN, REDNESS: Liver Fire
- TEARING, EXCESSIVE
- VISION, SUPERFICIAL OBSTRUCTIONS: Liver Fire

HEMORRHAGIC DISORDERS
- INTESTINAL BLEEDING IN WOMEN

LUNGS

- ASTHMA
- COUGH

PAIN/NUMBNESS/GENERAL DISCOMFORT
- BI PAIN: Hot, Primarily

SKIN
- ECZEMA: Damp Heat
- HYPEREMIA
- SKIN, SORES: Damp Heat

Clinical/Pharmaceutical Studies:

BLOOD RELATED DISORDERS/TOPICS
- ANTICOAGULANT
- BLOOD PRESSURE, RAISES

BOWEL RELATED DISORDERS
- DYSENTERY, BACILLARY, CHILDREN: Decoction 18 g/40 ml, Less Than 1yr, 8-10 ml/Day, 1-3 Yrs, 10

- CONJUNCTIVITIS: Eye Wash From Decoction 5-15 g, Mu Zei, Jue Ming Zi Or Oral Decoction Of Qin Pi, Huang Lian, Dan Zhu Ye

INFECTIOUS DISEASES
- BACTERIAL, ANTI-: Inhibits Staph.Aureus, E. Coli, B.Dysenteriae, N. Gonorrhoeae

KIDNEYS

CHRONIC: 1:1 Aerosol, 2 ml Each Time For 10x, Generally 2 Courses, Extract Tablet, 0.3 g Or Extract/Tab, 2 Tabs, 3x/ Day For 3 Course, 10 Days/ Course, Both Treatments Very Effective For Short-Term Control Of Dyspnea
- EXPECTORANT

MENTAL STATE/ NEUROLOGICAL

SWELLINGS

PAIN/NUMBNESS/ GENERAL DISCOMFORT
- ANALGESIC, MILD: Stronger Than Aspirin, Less Than Codeine, Injection

SKIN
- SKIN, PROTECTS FROM SUN/UV EXPOSURE

TRAUMA, BITES,

Clinical/Pharmaceutical Studies:

ml/Day, Greater Than 3 Yrs, 15 ml/Day, Divided Into 4 Doses/PO For 7-14 Days, Negative Stools In 3 Days, Cure Rate--80%

EYES

- DIURETIC: Short Term

LUNGS
- ANTITUSSIVE: Significant
- ASTHMA
- BRONCHITIS,

DISORDERS
- CONVULSIVE, ANTI-
- SEDATIVE

MUSCULOSKELETAL/ CONNECTIVE TISSUE
- ANKLE JOINT

POISONINGS
- INFLAMMATORY, ANTI- : Arthritis, Granulomas, Erythemotous, Stronger Than Aspirin

Dose

4.5 - 9.0 gm

Common Name

Bark Of Korean Ash

Contraindications

Not: Cold Def. SP

Notes

Possible Vomiting, Low Toxicity

Clear Heat, Cools The Blood

BAI WEI   白薇   RADIX CYNANCHI ATRATI

Traditional Functions:

1. Clears Heat and cools the Blood
2. Clears deficient Yin fever

Traditional Properties:

Enters: LU, ST, KI, LV,

Properties: BIT, SA, C

Indications:

BLOOD RELATED DISORDERS/ TOPICS
• BLOOD HEAT
CIRCULATION DISORDERS
• SYNCOPE: Blood Heat
FEVERS
• FEVER, POSTPARTUM
• FEVER, SUMMER IN CHILDREN
• FEVER, TIDAL
• STEAMING BONE FEVER: Yin Deficient Heat
HEAT
• HEAT, EXHAUSTION W/ SURFACE COMPLEX
HEMORRHAGIC DISORDERS

• HEMATURIA
• HEMORRHAGE: Cool Blood To Stop
INFECTIOUS DISEASES
• FEBRILE DISEASES, SEQUELAE OF
LUNGS
• COUGH: Yin Deficient Fever
ORAL CAVITY
• PHARYNGITIS
SEXUALITY, FEMALE: GYNECOLOGICAL
• POSTPARTUM, DEFICIENCY RESTLESSNESS

SKIN
• ABSCESS
TRAUMA, BITES, POISONINGS
• SNAKE BITES
URINARY BLADDER
• URINARY TRACT INFECTIONS, ACUTE: Damp Heat
• URINATION, FREQUENT W/ SCANTY AMOUNT
• URINATION, PAINFUL, DRIBBLING, CONCENTRATED, RED/YELLOW/TURBID
WIND DISORDERS
• WIND HEAT

Clinical/Pharmaceutical Studies:

HEART
• CARDIOGLYCOSIDE-LIKE

KIDNEYS

• DIURETIC

Dose

4.5 - 9.0 gm

DI GU PI   地骨皮   CORTEX LYCII CHINENSIS RADICIS

Traditional Functions:

1. Clears Heat and cools the Blood
2. Clears deficient Fire
3. Clears Lung Heat and reduces cough

Traditional Properties:

Enters: LU, KI,

Properties: SW, C

Indications:

CIRCULATION DISORDERS
• HYPERTENSION
ENDOCRINE RELATED DISORDERS
• DIABETES: Internal Heat With Exhaustion Thirst

Deficient Heat
• STEAMING BONE SYNDROME W/SWEATING
FLUID DISORDERS
• THIRST: Fluid Injury
HEMORRHAGIC DISORDERS

• HEMOPTYSIS
LUNGS
• ASTHMA
• COUGH: Lung Heat w/Difficult Sputum
• LUNGS, DYSPNEA: Lung Heat

Indications:

- DIABETES MELLITUS
FEVERS
- FEVER, LOW GRADE, CHRONIC
- STEAMING BONE FEVER: Yin

- BLEEDING: Blood Heat
- EPISTAXIS
- HEMATEMESIS
- HEMATURIA

- TUBERCULOSIS
SKIN
- NIGHT SWEATS
- PERSPIRATION W/THIRST

Clinical/Pharmaceutical Studies:

BLOOD RELATED DISORDERS/ TOPICS
- BLOOD GLUCOSE, REDUCES: Slowly, 4-5 Hours
- CHOLESTEROL, LOWERS: Large Doses For 3 Weeks
CIRCULATION DISORDERS
- HYPERTENSION: Water/Alcohol Extract, Vasodilator
ENDOCRINE RELATED DISORDERS
- DIABETES MELLITUS
FEVERS
- ANTIPYRETIC: Slightly Less Than Aspirin, ETOH/Aqueous Extract
- FEVER: Yin Deficient Type, Use With Tian Men Dong, Sheng Di, Chuan Bei Mu, Zhi Mu, E Jiao, Pi Pa Ye, Chai Hu, Nan Sha Shen
GALL BLADDER
- CHOLECYSTITIS, CHRONIC: With Yin Chen Hao, Huang Lian, Qing Hao
HEART
- HEART RATE, REDUCES
IMMUNE SYSTEM RELATED DISORDERS/TOPICS
- ALLERGIC, ANTI-: No Side

Effects, More For Skin, Mucous Membranes Than Internal Organs
- ANAPHYLACTIC PURPURA: Di Gu Pi, 50 g, Xu Chang Qing (Radix/ Herba Cynanchu Paniculatum) , 25 g)
INFECTIOUS DISEASES
- BACTERIAL, ANTI-: Staph
- MALARIA: With Tea Leaves 2-3 Hours Before Fever, Reduces Fever
- VIRAL, ANTI-: Asian Flu Inhibited By Decoction
LUNGS
- COUGH: Lung Heat--With Qian Yi Xie Bai Powder (Sang Bai Pi, Gan Cao, Jing Mi) Then Add Huang Qin, Shi Gao, Chuan Bei Mu For Better Effect
NUTRITIONAL/METABOLIC DISORDERS/TOPICS
- WEIGHT, INCREASES: Used With Farm Animals
ORAL CAVITY
- ANALGESIC, DENTAL: w/Conc. Decoc., 1 Min To Analgesia
- TEETH, PULPITIS: 30 g Into 500 ml Water, Decoct To 50 ml, Filter, Fill Tooth Cavity With Cotton Soaked, Prompt Analgesia Which

Lasted A Few Days
SEXUALITY, FEMALE: GYNECOLOGICAL
- UTERUS, STIMULATES
SKIN
- ANAPHYLACTIC PURPURA: Di Gu Pi, 50 g, Xu Chang Qing (Radix/ Herba Cynanchu Paniculatum) , 25 g)
- DERMATITIS, CONTACT: Di Gu Pi, 50 g, Xu Chang Qing (Radix/ Herba Cynanchu Paniculatum) , 25 g)
- ECZEMA: 10% Injection, IM
- ERYSIPELAS
- FUNGAL INFECTIONS, HANDS: 30 g Decocted With Gan Cao, 15 g, Use As Wash
- RASHES, DRUG INDUCED: Di Gu Pi, 50 g, Xu Chang Qing (Radix/ Herba Cynanchu Paniculatum) , 25 g)
- TINEA MANUUM: 30 g Decocted With Gan Cao, 15 g, Use As Wash
- URTICARIA, CHRONIC: Di Gu Pi, 50 g, Xu Chang Qing (Radix/Herba Cynanchu Paniculatum) , 25 g)
- WARTS, FLAT FROM VIRUS (JUVENILLE VERRUCA PLANA)
- WARTS, VARIOUS: 10% Injection, IM

Dose
9 - 15 gm
Common Name
Matrimony-Vine/Wolfberry

Contraindications
Not: Def Cold SP With Diarrhea
Not: For Exterior Conditions
Notes
Low Toxicity

FENG WEI CAO

鳳尾草
（凤尾草）

HERBA PTERIS

Traditional Functions:
1. Clears Heat and cools Blood
2. Promotes diuresis
3. Astringes diarrhea

Traditional Properties:
Enters: LU, LI

Properties: SW, BIT, C

Indications:

BOWEL RELATED DISORDERS
- DIARRHEA
- DYSENTERY

INFECTIOUS DISEASES
- GONORRHEA
ORAL CAVITY

- THROAT, SORE
URINARY BLADDER
- URINATION, PAINFUL

Clinical/Pharmaceutical Studies:

INFECTIOUS DISEASES

- BACTERIAL, ANTI-: Shigella

Dose
9 - 18 gm

Common Name
Phoenix-Tail Fern

HONG TENG
(DA XUE TENG)

紅藤
(红藤)

CAULIS SARGENTODOXAE

Traditional Functions:

1. Clears Blood Heat
2. Vitalizes the Blood and dispels stasis
3. Opens the channels and dispels Wind
4. Kills parasites

Traditional Properties:

Enters: LI, LV

Properties: BIT, N

Indications:

**ABDOMEN/
GASTROINTESTINAL TOPICS**
• APPENDICITIS, ACUTE/
CHRONIC
BOWEL RELATED DISORDERS
• DYSENTERY
**CANCER/TUMORS/SWELLINGS/
LUMPS**
• TUMORS: Blood Stasis, Herbs
Used Other Than Vitalize Blood
CHILDHOOD DISORDERS

• MALNUTRITION, CHILDHOOD
HEMORRHAGIC DISORDERS
• HEMATURIA
**MUSCULOSKELETAL/
CONNECTIVE TISSUE**
• ARTHRITIS, PAIN: Wind Damp
PARASITES
• PARASITES, INTESTINAL PAIN
OF
SEXUALITY, FEMALE:

GYNECOLOGICAL
• AMENORRHEA: Blood Stasis, In
Addition To Vitalize Blood Herbs
• MENORRHALGIA
• MENSTRUATION, DISORDERS
OF
• POSTPARTUM, ABDOMINAL
PAIN: Blood Stasis
TRAUMA, BITES, POISONINGS
• TRAUMA, INJURIES: Die Da

Clinical/Pharmaceutical Studies:

**ABDOMEN/
GASTROINTESTINAL TOPICS**
• APPENDICITIS, ACUTE
INFECTIOUS DISEASES
• BACTERIAL, ANTI-: Staph,

Streptococci, Pseudomonas, E.Coli,
etc
**MUSCULOSKELETAL/
CONNECTIVE TISSUE**
• ARTHRITIS, RHEUMATIC

PARASITES
• ASCARIASIS, BILIARY
SKIN
• BURNS

Dose
9 - 30 gm

Common Name
Sargentodoxa

Contraindications
Not: Pregnancy

HU ZHANG
(HU CHANG)

虎杖
(虎杖)

RHIZOMA POLYGONI CUSPIDATI

Traditional Functions:

1. Clears Heat, removes toxins and disperses Dampness
2. Vitalizes Blood and disperses swellings
3. Cause rebellious Lung Qi to descend

Traditional Properties:

Enters: LU, LV, GB

Properties: BIT, C, SO, <SP

Indications:

**BLOOD RELATED DISORDERS/
TOPICS**
• BLOOD HEAT
BOWEL RELATED DISORDERS
• CONSTIPATION: Heat
Entanglement
• DYSENTERY
• HEMORRHOIDS, PAIN,

• ANGINA PECTORIS: Chest Bi
Strangulating Pain
LIVER
• HEPATITIS
• JAUNDICE: Damp Heat
LUNGS
• BRONCHITIS, CHRONIC/ACUTE
• PNEUMONIA

• AMENORRHEA
• DYSMENORRHEA
• LEUKORRHEA
• MASTITIS
• UTERINE BLEEDING
SKIN
• BURNS
• FURUNCLES

Indications:

SWELLING
GALL BLADDER
• CHOLECYSTITIS
• GALL BLADDER, STONES
HEAD/NECK
• HEADACHE
HEART

MUSCULOSKELETAL/
CONNECTIVE TISSUE
• ARTHRITIS
• JOINTS, PAIN, SWELLING, RED:
  Hot Bi
SEXUALITY, FEMALE:
  GYNECOLOGICAL

TRAUMA, BITES, POISONINGS
• INSECT BITES
• SNAKE BITES
• TRAUMA, EXTERNAL
URINARY BLADDER
• URINARY TRACT STONES

Clinical/Pharmaceutical Studies:

ABDOMEN/
GASTROINTESTINAL
TOPICS
• APPENDICEAL
  ABSCESS
• APPENDICITIS W/
  DIFFUSE PERITONITIS:
  Appendicitis Syrup (Hu
  Zhang, Pu Gong Ying, Da
  Huang, Bai Hua She She
  Cao)
BLOOD RELATED
DISORDERS/TOPICS
• CHOLESTEROL,
  TRIGLYCERIDES,
  LOWERS
• HYPERLIPIDEMIA
• LEUKOPENIA,
  RADIATION/
  CHEMOTHERAPY
  INDUCED: Significantly
  Increased WBC
BOWEL RELATED
DISORDERS
• PURGATIVE
GALL BLADDER
• GALL BLADDER,
  STONES
HEART

• CARDIOTONIC: Similar
  To Aminophylline, But
  Slower
INFECTIOUS DISEASES
• BACTERIAL, ANTI-:
  Staph Aureus, Strep, E.
  Coli, Pseudo.A., Proteus,
  Salmonella, At Higher
  Concentrations-
  Spirochetes
• HERPES ZOSTER
• VIRAL, ANTI-: Echo11,
  Herpes Simplex, (Both By
  Decoction) , 10% Inhibits
  Flu, Asian A, 2%
  Adenovirus, Poliomyelitis,
  Coxsackie, Encephalitis B,
  20% Solution, Hepatitis B
LIVER
• HEPATITIS: Better For
  Acute, Icteric Viral, Some
  What Effective In Chronic
  Persistent, Ineffective In
  Chronic Hepatitis, Use
  Herb, Syrup, Or
  Compound–With Yin
  Chen, Tian Ji Huang, et al
• JAUNDICE, NEONATAL:
  50% Syrup Can Be Used

With Steroids To Hasten
Recovery
LUNGS
• ANTITUSSIVE
• ASTHMA: Large Dose,
  Oral, Compound Yin Yang
  Lian Tang (Hu Zhang, Pi
  Pa Ye, Shi Da Cong Lao Ye
  (Mahonia Bealei))
• BRONCHITIS,
  CHRONIC: Singly Or
  With Yu Xing Cao, Folium
  Elaeagnus Pungens
• BRONCHODILATORY
• EXPECTORANT
• LUNG INFECTION
• PNEUMONIA: By Itself/
  Hu Zhang Tang (Hu Zhang,
  Yu Xing Cao, Ban Zhi
  Lian, Ya Zhi Cao (Herba
  Commelinae) , Rhizoma
  Fagopyri Cymosi) , Body
  Temp Normal In 1-1.5
  Days
• RALES, DRY/MOIST
MUSCULOSKELETAL/
CONNECTIVE TISSUE
• ARTHRITIS: ETOH
  Tincture/Extract

• ARTHRITIS,
  RHEUMATIC/
  RHEUMATOID: Singly
  Or With Rhizoma
  Fagopyrum Cymosum,
  Ficus Pandurata
• BACK, LOWER PAIN:
  Lumbar Hypertrophy
• OSTEOARTHRITIS
• OSTEOMYELITIS,
  CHRONIC
ORAL CAVITY
• TONSILLITIS
SEXUALITY, FEMALE:
GYNECOLOGICAL
• CERVIX, EROSION OF
• VAGINAL
  CANDIDIASIS
SKIN
• BURNS: 2nd Degree,
  Ointment, Powder,
  Dressing From
  Concentrated Decoction
• PSORIASIS
• SCALDS
TRAUMA, BITES,
POISONINGS
• SNAKE BITES

Dose

9 - 30 gm

Common Name

Bushy Knotweed/Giant Knot

Contraindications

Not: Pregnancy

Notes

Mild Side Effects, Possible Digestive Symptoms
Has Similar Ingredients As Da Huang

HUO TAN MU CAO

火炭母草

HERBA
POLYGONI CHINESE

Traditional Functions:

1. Reduces Heat, dries Dampness and removes toxin
2. Clear Heat and cools Blood

Traditional Properties:

Enters: LU

Properties: SO, CL

Indications:

BOWEL RELATED DISORDERS
• DIARRHEA
• DYSENTERY, RED
FEVERS

LIVER
• JAUNDICE
LUNGS
• LUNG DISEASES

SEXUALITY, FEMALE:
GYNECOLOGICAL
• LEUKORRHEA
SKIN

Indications:

- FEVER, SPASMS OF **HEAD/NECK**
- HEADACHE: From General Debility

ORAL CAVITY
- PHARYNGOLARYNGITIS
- THROAT, SORE

- SORES, SUPPURATIVE
TRAUMA, BITES, POISONINGS
- TRAUMA

Clinical/Pharmaceutical Studies:

ABDOMEN/ GASTROINTESTINAL TOPICS
- SMALL INTESTINE, ILEUM,

INDUCES CONTRACTIONS
- SMALL INTESTINE, JEJUNUM, INCREASES ELASTICITY

SEXUALITY, FEMALE: GYNECOLOGICAL
- UTERUS, INHIBITS FUNCTION

Dose

15 - 30 gm

Common Name

Chinese Smartweed

MU DAN PI

牡丹皮

CORTEX MOUTAN RADICIS

Traditional Functions:

1. Clears Heat and cools the Blood
2. Clears deficiency Fire
3. Vitalizes Blood and removes congealed Blood
4. Clears Liver Fire rising
5. Reduces swelling and promotes discharge of pus

Traditional Properties:

Enters: HT, KI, LV,

Properties: SP, BIT, CL

Indications:

ABDOMEN/ GASTROINTESTINAL TOPICS
- ABDOMEN, PAIN OF
- APPENDICITIS W/PAIN
- FLANK PAIN: Liver Fire
- INTESTINES, ABSCESS
CANCER/TUMORS/SWELLINGS/ LUMPS
- LUMPS: Liver Blood Stagnation
- MASSES, HARD
- TUMORS: Blood Stasis, Herbs Used Other Than Vitalize Blood
EYES
- EYES, PAIN: Liver Fire
FEVERS
- BONE STEAMING FEVER: From Extreme Fatigue, Fever
- FEVER, HIGH
- STEAMING BONE FEVER: Yin Deficient Heat
HEAD/NECK
- ALOPECIA: Blood Heat Complex
- FLUSHING: Liver Fire

- HAIR, PREMATURE WHITENING: Blood Heat
- HEADACHE: Liver Fire
HEART
- ANGINA PECTORIS: Chest Bi Strangulating Pain
HEMORRHAGIC DISORDERS
- EPISTAXIS
- HEMATEMESIS
- HEMOPTYSIS
MENTAL STATE/ NEUROLOGICAL DISORDERS
- CONVULSIONS
MUSCULOSKELETAL/ CONNECTIVE TISSUE
- JOINTS, PAIN, SWELLING, RED: Hot Bi, Toxic Heat With Stasis
ORAL CAVITY
- THROAT, PAIN, SWOLLEN
SEXUALITY, FEMALE: GYNECOLOGICAL
- AMENORRHEA: Blood Stasis, In Addition To Vitalize Blood Herbs

- BREASTS, SWOLLEN, PAINFUL, ABSCESS
- DYSMENORRHEA: Liver Fire
- MENSTRUATION, DISORDERS OF: Clear Chong, Ren
- POSTPARTUM, ABDOMINAL PAIN: Blood Stasis
SKIN
- BOILS
- CARBUNCLES
- ECZEMA: Damp Heat
- RASHES, W/PRURITUS: Blood Heat, Wind
- SKIN, SORES: Damp Heat
- SKIN, SORES, SWOLLEN, TOXIC: Blood Stasis, Swelling
- SKIN, SUBCUTANEOUS BLEEDING
- SORES, NON-DRAINING: Topical
TRAUMA, BITES, POISONINGS
- BRUISES: Trauma
- TRAUMA, INJURIES: Die Da

Clinical/Pharmaceutical Studies:

ABDOMEN/ GASTROINTESTINAL TOPICS
- APPENDICITIS, ACUTE/ CHRONIC: Da Huang Mu Dan Pi Tang, 2x/Day, 10 Days
BLOOD RELATED DISORDERS/TOPICS
- BLOOD PRESSURE,

CIRCULATION DISORDERS
- HYPERTENSION
EARS/HEARING DISORDERS
- EARS, OTITIS MEDIA: 10% Decoction, 50 ml Before Bed For 10 Days
FEVERS
- ANTIPYRETIC: Less

DISORDERS
- HYPNOTIC: Orally, Synergizes Chloral Hydrate, Barbituates
- TRANQUILIZING: Oral/ IP Injection, Antagonized Caffeine
MUSCULOSKELETAL/ CONNECTIVE TISSUE
- ARTHRITIS, PAIN

GENERAL DISCOMFORT
- ANALGESIC: Oral/IP Injection
SEXUALITY, FEMALE: GYNECOLOGICAL
- UTERUS: Congests Blood In
- UTERUS, BLOOD STASIS

Clinical/Pharmaceutical Studies:

LOWERS: Gradual:15-18 g/Day In 3 Doses As Decoction, Increased To 50 g/Day If No Side Effects, 3-5 Days For Significant Lowering Of Pressure, 6-33 Days Treatment

BOWEL RELATED DISORDERS
• DYSENTERY, BACILLARY: 50% Decoction To Cured

Than Aspirin
FLUID DISORDERS
• EDEMA, FEET, LEGS
INFECTIOUS DISEASES
• BACTERIAL, ANTI-: Strong (Many) –Staph A., Bac.Subtl., Salmonella
• VIRAL, ANTI-: Flu: Decoction Inhibited, Inconsistent, Though
MENTAL STATE/ NEUROLOGICAL

NOSE
• RHINITIS, ALLERGIC: Symptom Removal (ETOH ext) , *10% Decoction, 50 ml Before Bed For 10 Days
NUTRITIONAL/ METABOLIC DISORDERS/TOPICS
• HYPOTHERMIA
PAIN/NUMBNESS/

SKIN
• FUNGAL, ANTI-
• SKIN, ITCHING
STOMACH/DIGESTIVE DISORDERS
• GASTRIC PAIN
• STOMACH, INHIBITS SECRETIONS
TRAUMA, BITES, POISONINGS
• INFLAMMATORY, ANTI-

Not: Diarrhea

Dose

4.5 - 12.0 gm

Common Name

Cortex Of Tree Peony Root

Contraindications

Not: Cold

Precautions

Watch: Pregnancy/Excess Menstruation

Notes

w/Zhi Zi&San Yao San For Menstrual Problems

May Cause Nausea, Dizziness Which Disappear

SHENG DI HUANG
(SHENG DI)

生地黄
（生地黄）

RADIX REHMANNIAE GLUTINOSAE

Traditional Functions:

1. Clears Heat and cools the Blood
2. Nourishes the Yin and Blood and generates fluids
3. Cools Heart Fire rising

Traditional Properties:

Enters: HT, KI, LV,

Properties: SW, BIT, C

Indications:

BLOOD RELATED DISORDERS/TOPICS
• BLOOD HEAT LEVEL
BOWEL RELATED DISORDERS
• STOOLS, DRY
ENDOCRINE RELATED DISORDERS
• DIABETES: Internal Heat With Exhaustion Thirst
• WASTING & THIRSTING SYNDROME
FEVERS
• FEVER, AFTERNOON
• FEVER, LOW GRADE, CONTINUOUS
• FEVER, VERY HIGH
• FEVER, YIN DEFICIENCY
• STEAMING BONE FEVER: Yin Deficient Heat

FLUID DISORDERS
• THIRST: Fluid Injury
HEAD/NECK
• ALOPECIA: Blood Heat Complex
• HAIR, PREMATURE WHITENING: Blood Heat
• MALAR FLUSH
HEAT
• BLOOD HEAT LEVEL
• YING STAGE HEAT
HEMORRHAGIC DISORDERS
• EPISTAXIS
• HEMAFECIA
• HEMATEMESIS
• HEMATURIA
• HEMOPTYSIS
• HEMORRHAGE: Blood Heat/Cool Blood To Stop/ Deficiency Caused
INFECTIOUS DISEASES

• FEBRILE DISEASES
LUNGS
• COUGH: Lung Dryness
• COUGH, LUNG EXHAUSTION: Tuberculosis
MENTAL STATE/ NEUROLOGICAL DISORDERS
• INSOMNIA
• IRRITABILITY
MUSCULOSKELETAL/ CONNECTIVE TISSUE
• SPASMS, CONVULSIONS: Deficiency Wind–Liver Kidney
ORAL CAVITY
• LIPS, DRY
• MOUTH, DRY: Injured Fluids
• MOUTH, SORES: Heart Fire Flaring

• THROAT, SORE: Yin Deficient
• TONGUE, RED FROM FEVER
• TONGUE, SORES: Heart Fire Flaring
SEXUALITY, FEMALE: GYNECOLOGICAL
• MENORRHAGIA
• MENSTRUATION, DISORDERS OF: Clear Chong, Ren
SKIN
• EXANTHEMA
• MACULA
• MALAR FLUSH
• RASHES, W/PRURITUS: Blood Heat, Wind
• SKIN, ERUPTIONS
YIN RELATED DISORDERS/TOPICS
• YIN DEFICIENCY W/ HEAT

Clinical/Pharmaceutical Studies:

**BLOOD RELATED DISORDERS/
TOPICS**
• BLOOD PRESSURE, RAISES
• HYPERGLYCEMIA, REDUCES
BOWEL RELATED DISORDERS
• LAXATIVE
CIRCULATION DISORDERS
• HYPERTENSION: 30-50 g/Day
For 2 Weeks
HEART
• CARDIOTONIC: In Moderate Dose
HEMORRHAGIC DISORDERS
• HEMOSTATIC
**IMMUNE SYSTEM RELATED
DISORDERS/TOPICS**
• IMMUNOLOGICAL DISEASE
INFECTIOUS DISEASES
• BACTERIAL, ANTI-

KIDNEYS
• DIURETIC
LIVER
• HEPATITIS, ANICTERIC
• HEPATITIS, INFECTIOUS: IM
Injection, 12 g Of Herb With 6 g Gan
Cao, 10 Day Course, SGPT
Lowering, Or Decoction Of Same
Works
• LIVER, PROTECTANT
• LIVER, REDUCES DEPLETION
GLYCOGEN
LUNGS
• BRONCHIAL ASTHMA:
Decoction Improves Symptoms
**MUSCULOSKELETAL/
CONNECTIVE TISSUE**
• ARTHRITIS, RHEUMATIC/

RHEUMATOID: Decoction,
Reduces Joint Pain, Swelling, Better
Movement
SKIN
• ECZEMA: Intermittent Decoction,
90 g/Day
• FUNGAL, ANTI-: Aqueous Extract,
*Many
• NEURODERMATITIS: Intermittent
Decoction, 90 g/Day
• URTICARIA: Decoction Improves
Symptoms.
TRAUMA, BITES, POISONINGS
• INFLAMMATORY, ANTI-: Only
Decoction
• RADIATION, ANTI-: 100%
Preparation Injection, 1 ml IP, 6
Days, Reduced Platelet Damage

Dose
9 - 30 gm

Common Name
Chinese Foxglove Root

Contraindications
Not: Damp Phlegm/Def SP w/Damp/Diarrhea

Not: Def Yang

Not: Pregnancy w/Def Blood

Notes
Greasy

Mild Side Effects: Diarrhea, Abdominal Pain, Fatigue
Which Disappear In Few Days

SHUI NIU JIAO 水牛角 CORNU BUBALI

Traditional Functions:

1. Clears Heat and cools the Blood
2. Neutralizes toxic Heat in Ying and Xue levels
3. Clears Blood Heat and sedates tremors

Traditional Properties:

Enters: HT, LV, ST,

Properties: BIT, SA, C

Indications:

**CANCER/TUMORS/SWELLINGS/
LUMPS**
• CANCER
CIRCULATION DISORDERS
• SYNCOPE: Ying/Xue Heat
FEVERS
• FEVER, VERY HIGH: Ying/Xue
Level
HEMORRHAGIC DISORDERS

• HEMATEMESIS
LIVER
• LIVER HEART SPASMS
**MENTAL STATE/
NEUROLOGICAL DISORDERS**
• AGITATION
• CONVULSIONS
• DELIRIUM

• MANIA
• RESTLESSNESS
NOSE
• NOSEBLEED
SKIN
• ERYTHEMA
• MACULATION
• PURPURA

Clinical/Pharmaceutical Studies:

**BLOOD RELATED
DISORDERS/TOPICS**
• BLOOD CLOTTING
TIME, SHORTENS
FEVERS
• ANTIPYRETIC: Not
Shown In Animals, In
Humans, Though
HEART
• CARDIOTONIC
• HEART, TONIFIES
IMMUNE SYSTEM

Nodes
INFECTIOUS DISEASES
• ENCEPHALITIS B:
Angong Niu Huang San,
Using Shui Niu Jiao
Instead Of Xi Jiao, Equally
Effective
• INFLUENZA, VIRAL,
FEVER OF
LIVER
• HEPATITIS
LUNGS

• SCHIZOPHRENIA,
ACUTE: 3 Tabs, 3x/Day
For 1 Month, May Be
Increased To 5 Tabs, 3x/
Day If No Adverse Effects
• TRANQUILIZING
**MUSCULOSKELETAL/
CONNECTIVE TISSUE**
• ARTHRITIS,
RHEUMATIC,
RHEUMATOID: More
Effective In Younger

(Mouth, Genital Ulcers,
Iritis, Joint Pain, Unknown
Origin)
ORAL CAVITY
• TONSILLITIS, ACUTE,
FEVER OF
SKIN
• PSORIASIS
• PURPURA
THROBOPENIC
HEMORRHAGICA: 1 g/
Tab, 5-8 Tabs, 3x/Day, 1

Clinical/Pharmaceutical Studies:

**RELATED DISORDERS/
TOPICS**
• **IMMUNE RESPONSE:**
Raises White Blood Cell
Count, Increase Tissue
Activity In Spleen, Lymph

• RESPIRATORY TRACT,
UPPER INFECTION,
FEVER OF
**MENTAL STATE/
NEUROLOGICAL
DISORDERS**

Patients With Fever, 5 Tabs,
3x/Day Plus Other Herbs,
If No Improvement In 1
Month, 8 Tabs/Day
• BEHCET'S SYNDROME:

Month Shortest, Usually 3-
6 Months Course, If Less
Than 2 Yrs, 3-4 Tabs, 3x/
Day
• WARTS

Dose

30 - 120 gm

Common Name

Water Buffalo Horn

Notes

Substitute For Xi Jiao

Mild Side Effects: GI Discomfort, Nausea, Diarrhea,
Insomnia In Only Few Patients

XI JIAO

犀角
（犀角）

CORNU RHINOCERI

Traditional Functions:

1. Clears Heat and cools the Blood
2. Neutralizes toxic Heat in Ying and Xue levels
3. Clears Blood Heat and sedates tremors

Traditional Properties:

Enters: ST, HT, LV,

Properties: BIT, SO, SA, C

Indications:

**CANCER/TUMORS/
SWELLINGS/LUMPS**
• CANCER
**CIRCULATION
DISORDERS**
• SYNCOPE: Ying/Xue
Heat
FEVERS
• FEVER, VERY HIGH:
Ying/Xue Level~
Endangered Species!
HEAT
• HEAT, TOXIC
• XUE LEVEL HEAT:
High Fever

• YING STAGE HEAT:
High Fever
**HEMORRHAGIC
DISORDERS**
• EPISTAXIS
• HEMAFECIA
• HEMATEMESIS
• HEMOPTYSIS
INFECTIOUS DISEASES
• EPIDEMICS,
SEASONAL
LIVER
• JAUNDICE
• LIVER HEART SPASMS
MENTAL STATE/

**NEUROLOGICAL
DISORDERS**
• AGITATION
• CONVULSIONS
• DELIRIOUS SPEECH
• DELIRIUM
• MANIA
• MENTAL CLOUDINESS
• RESTLESSNESS
• UNCONSCIOUSNESS:
(Mental Cloudiness) , Use
w/Heat Shut-In Herbs
SKIN
• ABSCESS, W/MENTAL
DULLNESS, HIGH

FEVER, SPASMS: Blood
Heat
• ERUPTIONS OF
• ERYTHEMA
• MACULA
• PURPURA
• RASHES, INCOMPLETE
EXPRESSION OF: Blood
Heat, Wind
• SORES, TOXIC HEAT
• SORES, W/MENTAL
DULLNESS, HIGH
FEVER, SPASMS: Blood
Heat

Clinical/Pharmaceutical Studies:

**BLOOD RELATED DISORDERS/
TOPICS**
• **BLOOD HEAT:** With Sheng Di, Chi
Shao (e.g. Xi Jiao Shu Di Tang)
• BLOOD PRESSURE, RAISES
• LYMPHOCYTES, INCREASES
• THROMBOCYTOPENIC
PURPURA: With Epistaxis, Gum
Bleeding, Hemafecia, Hematemesis,
Xi Jiao Sheng Di Tang, 3+ Doses To
Cure

FEVERS
• ANTIPYRETIC: IV Injection, Not
For Oral, Not Shown In Animals, In
Humans, Though
HEART
• CARDIOTONIC: Only In
Dysfunctioning Hearts
• HEART, TONIFIES
HEMORRHAGIC DISORDERS
• BLEEDING: Blood Heat Types,
With Sheng Di, Chi Shao (e.g. Xi

Jiao Sheng Di Tang)
INFECTIOUS DISEASES
• ENCEPHALITIS B W/
PERSISTENT HIGH FEVER: With
Shi Gao, Mang Xiao, etc
**MENTAL STATE/
NEUROLOGICAL DISORDERS**
• CONVULSIVE, ANTI-:
Antagonizes Strycnine
• TRANQUILIZING

Dose

0.9 - 9.0 gm

Common Name

Rhinoceros Horn

Contraindications

Not: w/Fu Zi/Cho Wu/Chuan Wu

Precautions

Watch: Pregnancy

Notes

Drink In Slurry

Substitute Shui Niu Jiao, Research Shows Same

Excess Cases Only

Endangered Species! Do Not Use.

XUAN SHEN

玄參
（玄参）

RADIX SCROPHULARIAE NINGPOENSIS

Traditional Functions:

1. Clears Heat and cools the Blood
2. Moistens the Yin
3. Softens firm mass and disperses entanglement
4. Subdues Fire and neutralizes toxic Heat

Traditional Properties:

Enters: LU, ST, KI,

Properties: SA, <BIT, C

Indications:

• ORGAN PROLAPSE
BOWEL RELATED DISORDERS
• CONSTIPATION: From Dehydration/Intestinal Dryness
CIRCULATION DISORDERS
• VASCULITIS: 30-90 gm
ENDOCRINE RELATED DISORDERS
• DIABETES: Internal Heat With Exhaustion Thirst
• GOITER: Phlegm Fire
• THYROID, ENLARGEMENT
EYES
• EYES, RED
• EYES, SWOLLEN
FEVERS
• FEVER: 18-30 gm
• STEAMING BONE FEVER: Yin Deficient Heat
FLUID DISORDERS
• THIRST: Fluid Injury

HEAD/NECK
• NECK, LYMPH GLANDS SWOLLEN: Phlegm Fire
HEAT
• YING & BLOOD STAGE HEAT DISORDERS
HEMORRHAGIC DISORDERS
• HEMOPTYSIS
• HEMORRHAGE: Blood Heat
IMMUNE SYSTEM RELATED DISORDERS/TOPICS
• LYMPH GLANDS, ENLARGEMENT, CHRONIC: Phlegm Nodules
• LYMPH TUBERCULOSIS: 30-90gm
INFECTIOUS DISEASES
• FEBRILE DISEASES, SEQUELAE OF
• SCROFULA
LUNGS

• COUGH: Lung Dryness
MENTAL STATE/ NEUROLOGICAL DISORDERS
• INSOMNIA, RESTLESS: From Heat
• IRRITABILITY: 18-30 gm
MUSCULOSKELETAL/ CONNECTIVE TISSUE
• SPASMS, CONVULSIONS: Deficiency Wind–Liver Kidney
ORAL CAVITY
• THROAT, SORE, SWOLLEN, ACUTE
SEXUALITY, FEMALE: GYNECOLOGICAL
• BREASTS, SWOLLEN, PAINFUL, ABSCESS
SKIN
• BOILS
• MACULA
• SKIN, ERUPTIONS

Clinical/Pharmaceutical Studies:

BLOOD RELATED DISORDERS/TOPICS
• BLOOD GLUCOSE, REDUCES
• BLOOD PRESSURE, LOWERS: Vasodilation, Especially Effective In Renal Hypertension
• HEMOLYTIC
CIRCULATION DISORDERS
• BLOOD VESSELS, DILATES
• VASODILATOR: Renal In Hypertension
FEVERS

• ANTIPYRETIC
• FEVER, HECTIC/ DEFICIENCY: Yin Def-- Yang Ying Qing Fei Tang (Xuan Shen, Sheng Di, Mai Dong, Bai Shao, Mu Dan Pi, Gan Cao, Bo He)
• FEVER, YIN IMPAIRMENT, IRRITABILITY, INSOMNIA, THIRST: Qing Yin Tang (Xuan Shen With Sheng Di, Mai Dong, Dan Shen, Jin Yin Hua, Lian Qiao, Dan Zhu Ye)
HEART

• CARDIOTONIC
INFECTIOUS DISEASES
• BACTERIAL, ANTI-: Pseud.Aeruginosa
• DIPHTHERIA: Yang Ying Qing Fei Tang (Xuan Shen, Sheng Di, Mai Dong, Bai Shao, Mu Dan Pi, Gan Cao, Bo He)
• FEBRILE DISEASES, SEASONAL W/ DEPLETION OF BODILY FLUIDS: Zeng Ye Tang (Xuan Shen, Sheng Di, Mai Dong), Has Laxative Effect, Too, 9-15 g, Max

30 g/Dose
LUNGS
• COUGH, HEMOPTYSIS: Yang Ying Qing Fei Tang (Xuan Shen, Sheng Di, Mai Dong, Bai Shao, Mu Dan Pi, Gan Cao, Bo He)
ORAL CAVITY
• THROAT, SORE: Yin Def Heat–Yang Ying Qing Fei Tang (Xuan Shen, Sheng Di, Mai Dong, Bai Shao, Mu Dan Pi, Gan Cao, Bo He)
SKIN
• FUNGAL, ANTI-

Dose

9 - 12 gm

Common Name

Ningpo Figwort Root

Contraindications

Not: w/LI LU

Precautions

Watch: Def SP Diarrhea

Watch: In Damp SP

Notes

For Fevers, Vexation: 18-30gm

For Vasculitis, Lymph TB: 30-90gm

Used With Other Herbs

YIN CHAI HU

銀柴胡
(银柴胡)

RADIX STELLARIAE DICHOTOMAE

Traditional Functions:

1. Clears deficient Yin fever
2. Clear Heat, cools Blood and controls bleeding
3. Reduces Heat from some forms of childhood nutritional impairment

Traditional Properties:

Enters: ST, KI, LV,

Properties: SW, <C

Indications:

ENERGETIC STATE
• DEBILITY, GENERAL
FEVERS
• FEVER, CHILDHOOD MALNUTRITION
• FEVER, LOW GRADE
• FEVER, YIN DEFICIENCY

• STEAMING BONE FEVER: Yin Deficient Heat
HEMORRHAGIC DISORDERS
• EPISTAXIS: Blood Heat
• HEMATURIA: Blood Heat
• HEMOPTYSIS: Blood Heat
INFECTIOUS DISEASES

• MALARIA, CHRONIC: Yin Deficient
SEXUALITY, FEMALE: GYNECOLOGICAL
• UTERINE BLEEDING: Blood Heat
SKIN
• PERSPIRATION, NIGHT TIME

Clinical/Pharmaceutical Studies:

CIRCULATION DISORDERS

• ATHEROSCLEROSIS

Dose

3 - 9 gm

Contraindications

Not: Wind Cold Fever

Not: Fever From Def Blood With No Heat Signs

ZI CAO

紫草

RADIX LITHOSPERMI SEU ARNEBIAE

Traditional Functions:

1. Clears Heat and cools and vitalizes the Blood
2. Clears Damp Heat skin lesions when used topically
3. Promotes rashes to surface and clears toxic Heat
4. Moistens the intestines and facilitates passage of stool

Traditional Properties:

Enters: HT, PC, LV,

Properties: SA, SW, C

Indications:

BOWEL RELATED DISORDERS
• CONSTIPATION W/BLOOD HEAT: Mild
CANCER/TUMORS/SWELLINGS/ LUMPS
• SWELLINGS
• TUMORS
INFECTIOUS DISEASES
• CHICKEN POX

• VAGINAL PRURITUS
SKIN
• ABSCESS, W/MENTAL DULLNESS, HIGH FEVER, SPASMS: Blood Heat
• BURNS
• CARBUNCLES
• DERMATITIS
• ECZEMA: External

Wind
• RASHES, VERY DARK PURPLE
• RASHES, W/PRURITUS: Blood Heat, Wind
• SKIN, ERUPTIONS
• SKIN, LESIONS
• SKIN, SORE W/MENTAL DULLNESS, HIGH FEVER, SPASMS: Blood Heat

---

Indications:

- MEASLES
SEXUALITY, FEMALE:
  GYNECOLOGICAL

- MACULA
- RASHES, INCOMPLETE
  EXPRESSION OF: Blood Heat,

- ULCERS, SKIN: Topical
TRAUMA, BITES, POISONINGS
- FROSTBITE

Clinical/Pharmaceutical Studies:

**CANCER/TUMORS/SWELLINGS/
  LUMPS**
- ANTINEOPLASTIC:
  Chorionepithelioma, Chorioadenoma,
  Acute Lymphocytic Leukemia,
  Breast Cancer
CHILDHOOD DISORDERS
- INFANTILE DERMATITIS
**ENDOCRINE RELATED
  DISORDERS**
- ESTRUS, INHIBITS
FEVERS
- ANTIPYRETIC
HEART
- HEART, STIMULATES

.**INFECTIOUS DISEASES**
- ANTIBIOTIC: Inhibits Gram +/-,
  Staph A.
- MEASLES, BUT NOT LATENT
  PERIOD
**SEXUALITY, FEMALE:
  GYNECOLOGICAL**
- CERVICITIS
- CONTRACEPTIVE, IN FEMALE
  RATS: Aqeous Extract, Orally
  200mg/100g, Very Marked/30% Of
  Food
- ESTRUS, INHIBITS
- OVULATION, REDUCES
- VAGINITIS

SKIN
- BURNS: Cream Of The Extract On
  Cloth
- DERMATITIS: Cream Of The
  Extract On Cloth
- ECZEMA
- FUNGAL, ANTI-
- PITYRIASIS ROSEA
- PSORIASIS
- RASHES, POX
TRAUMA, BITES, POISONINGS
- TOXINS, HELPS TO EXCRETE
- WOUNDS, PROMOTES
  HEALING

Dose

4.5 - 9.0 gm

Common Name

Groomwell Root

Contraindications

Not: Normal Measles

Precautions

Watch: Def SP/ST w/Diarrhea

Notes

Large Doses: Hematuria, Pyuria, Diarrhea

Clear And Relieve Summer Heat

BAI BIAN DOU
(BIAN DOU)

白扁豆
（白扁豆）

SEMEN
DOLICHORIS LABLAB

Traditional Functions:

1. Clears Summer Heat and Dampness
2. Tonifies the Spleen, removes Dampness

Traditional Properties:

Enters: SP, ST,

Properties: SW, N

Indications:

**BOWEL RELATED
DISORDERS**
• DIARRHEA: Spleen
Deficiency/Summer Heat
• DIARRHEA, CHRONIC
W/STOMACH
GROWLING: Spleen
Deficient
**CHILDHOOD
DISORDERS**
• INFANTILE

MALNUTRITION
ENERGETIC STATE
• WEAKNESS: Qi
Deficiency
FLUID DISORDERS
• THIRST
HEAT
• SUMMER HEAT:
Especially With Vomiting/
Diarrhea

• SUNSTROKE W/FEVER,
THIRST
**SEXUALITY, FEMALE:
GYNECOLOGICAL**
• LEUKORRHEA: Spleen
Deficient
SPLEEN
• SPLEEN STOMACH
DEFICIENCY W/HEAT
STOMACH/DIGESTIVE

DISORDERS
• VOMITING: Summer
Heat
**TRAUMA, BITES,
POISONINGS**
• ALCOHOLIC
INTOXICATION
• BALLONFISH
POISONING: Slows
Absorption

Clinical/Pharmaceutical Studies:

**BLOOD RELATED DISORDERS/
TOPICS**
• BLOOD: Lengthens Coagulation
Time
• BLOOD GLUCOSE, REDUCES

• BLOOD, RBC: Accumulation
Affect
• CHOLESTEROL, LOWERS
INFECTIOUS DISEASES
• VIRAL, ANTI-: Columbia Sk

**STOMACH/DIGESTIVE
DISORDERS**
• DIGESTION, INHIBITS: Inhibits
Trypsin, Amylase

Dose

9 - 18 gm

Common Name

Hyacinth Bean

Contraindications

Not: Intermittent Fever/Chills

Not: Cold Disorders

Notes

Raw: Used For Summer Heat
Fried: To Strengthen SP, Stopping Diarrhea

DA DOU HUANG JUAN
(DOU JUAN)

大豆黄卷
（大豆黄卷）

SEMEN
GLYCINES GERMINATUM

Traditional Functions:

1. Clears Summer Heat and Dampness
2. Relieves the surface

Traditional Properties:

Enters: SP, ST,

Properties: SW, N

Indications:

BOWEL RELATED DISORDERS
• DIARRHEA
CHEST
• CHEST, FULLNESS
EXTREMITIES
• EXTREMITIES, PARALYSIS OF
FEVERS
• FEVER, DAMPNESS, JOINT PAIN
FLUID DISORDERS
• EDEMA
HEAT
• SUMMER HEAT DAMPNESS:

Early With Jont Pain, Heaviness
Sensation, Little Sweating, Greasy
Tongue
INFECTIOUS DISEASES
• FEBRILE DISEASES, EARLY:
With Jont Pain, Heaviness Sensation,
Little Sweating, Greasy Tongue
• INFLUENZA, INITIAL STAGE:
With Jont Pain, Heaviness Sensation,
Little Sweating, Greasy Tongue
MENTAL STATE/
NEUROLOGICAL DISORDERS

• PARALYSIS, EXTREMITIES
MUSCULOSKELETAL/
CONNECTIVE TISSUE
• ARTHRITIS, PAIN
• TENDONS, SPASMS
SKIN
• HYPERHIDROSIS
URINARY BLADDER
• DYSURIA
• URINATION, LACK OF:
(Uropenia)

Clinical/Pharmaceutical Studies:

ENDOCRINE RELATED
DISORDERS
• ESTROGEN-LIKE: Oral/Injection

MUSCULOSKELETAL/
CONNECTIVE TISSUE

• ANTISPASMODIC IN SMOOTH
MUSCLE

Dose
9 - 15 gm

Common Name
Young Soybean Sprout
Notes
Not With Long Dan Cao (Traditional)

HE YE
(HAN LIAN YE)

荷葉
（荷叶）

FOLIUM
NELUMBINIS NUCIFERAE

Traditional Functions:

1. Treats Summer Heat-Dampness patterns
2. Improves the digestion
3. Raises and clears the Yang of the Spleen after attack by Summer Heat
4. Arrests bleeding
5. Dissipates Blood Stasis-Ecchymosis

Traditional Properties:

Enters: ST, SP, LV,

Properties: BIT, <SW, N

Indications:

BOWEL RELATED DISORDERS
• DIARRHEA: Spleen Deficient,
Especially Post Summer Heat
FLUID DISORDERS
• DAMPNESS
• EDEMA
• SUMMER DAMPNESS
HEAT
• SUMMER HEAT COMPLEX:
Fever, Irritability, Excess Sweating,
Scanty Urine, Diarrhea

HEMORRHAGIC DISORDERS
• BLEEDING, IN LOWER JIAO:
Heat/Stagnation
• EPISTAXIS
• HEMAFECIA
• HEMATEMESIS
• HEMATURIA
• HEMORRHAGE: Raise The Yang
To Stop
INFECTIOUS DISEASES
• COMMON COLD, IN SUMMER

W/DAMPNESS
SEXUALITY, FEMALE:
GYNECOLOGICAL
• MENORRHAGIA
STOMACH/DIGESTIVE
DISORDERS
• DIGESTION, ENHANCES
• INDIGESTION
URINARY BLADDER
• DYSURIA W/HEMATURIA

Clinical/Pharmaceutical Studies:

BLOOD RELATED DISORDERS/
TOPICS
• BLOOD PRESSURE, LOWERS:

Vasodilation
INFECTIOUS DISEASES

• BACTERIAL, ANTI-: Shigella,
Eberthella Typhosa

Dose
3 - 30 gm
Common Name
Lotus Leaf

Contraindications
Not: Def/Cold Bleeding
Notes
Used More In Cooking
Fresh Leaves Stronger

LU DOU

綠 豆
(绿 豆)

SEMEN PHASEOLI RADIATI

Traditional Functions:

1. Clears and dissipates Summer Heat and Dampness
2. Relieves toxins:used as antidote to Fu Zi and fava beans

Traditional Properties:

Enters: ST, HT,

Properties: SW, <C

Indications:

FLUID DISORDERS
• THIRST: Summer Heat
HEAT
• SUMMER HEAT: Agitation, Frustration, Irritability, Fever, Helps Prevent Occurance Of
INFECTIOUS DISEASES

• COMMON COLD, IN SUMMER W/DAMPNESS
KIDNEYS
• DIURETIC, MILD
MENTAL STATE/ NEUROLOGICAL DISORDERS
• AGITATION/FRUSTRATION:

Summer Heat
• RESTLESSNESS: Heat
ORAL CAVITY
• ORAL ULCERS
SKIN
• CARBUNCLES
• ULCERS, TOXIC

Clinical/Pharmaceutical Studies:

SKIN
• BURNS: 1ST-2nd Degree w/

Alcohol & Borneol As Paste
TRAUMA, BITES, POISONINGS

• POISONING, PESTICIDES: Good

Dose

Cooking

Common Name

Mung Bean

Contraindications

Not: Pregnancy

Not: Diarrhea From Def Cold SP/ST

Notes

120 gm w/60gm Gan Cao For Fu Zi Toxicity

QING HAO

青蒿

HERBA ARTEMISIAE APIACEAE

Traditional Functions:

1. Clears Summer Heat
2. Clears deficiency Heat and fevers
3. Cools the Blood and arrests bleeding

Traditional Properties:

Enters: LV, GB,

Properties: BIT, C

Indications:

FEVERS
• CHILLS, FEVER, ALTERNATING
• FEVER: Blood Deficient/ Post Febrile Diseases
• FEVER, TIDAL
• FEVER, UNRELENTING
• STEAMING BONE FEVER: Yin Deficient Heat
HEAT

• HEAT STROKE, SUMMER
• HEAT, EXHAUSTION W/ SURFACE COMPLEX
• SUMMER HEAT: Low Fever, No Sweating, Vertigo, Chest Constriction
• YING STAGE HEAT
HEMORRHAGIC DISORDERS
• EPISTAXIS: Blood Heat

INFECTIOUS DISEASES
• COMMON COLD, IN SUMMER W/ DAMPNESS
• FEBRILE DISEASES
• MALARIA: 20-40 gm
• MALARIA, CHILLS, FEVER OF
LIVER
• JAUNDICE

SIX STAGES/ CHANNELS
• SHAO YANG STAGE DISEASE
SKIN
• DIAPHORETIC, WEAK
• PRURITUS
• PURPURA
• SCABIES
• SORES, INTRACTABLE

Clinical/Pharmaceutical Studies:

HEAT
• HEAT STROKE: 15-20 g Added To Boiling Water, Take As Tea
IMMUNE SYSTEM RELATED DISORDERS/ TOPICS

Subside, 2-3 Months To Disappear
INFECTIOUS DISEASES
• ANTIBIOTIC: Dematomycoses, Leptospirosis
• MALARIA: Oral Dose

Not Aqua ext-Inhibits Maturation Of Parasite
LUNGS
• ASTHMA, BRONCHIAL: Volatile Oil, Needs At Least About 1 Month Treatment

Borneol Predissolved In Alcohol, Apply With Cotton Swabs, 3-4x/Day
• SKIN, SEBORRHEIC DERMATITIS: 10 Catties Of Fresh Herb Decocted To 6-7, Add 30-35 g

---

Clinical/Pharmaceutical Studies:

- LUPUS ERYTHEMATOSUS: Active Ingredient, Arteannuin, Given Orally, 0.1 g, 2x/Day, 1ST Month, 0.1 g, 3x/Day, 2nd Month, 0.1 g, 4x/Day, 3rd Month, Achieve Some Remission In All Patients, But First Few Days Worsened With Tingling Sensation, Ok After 2 Weeks, Takes 50 Days To See Improvement, *May Use 36-54 g Honeyed Herb Powder, Took 1 Month For Rash To Must Be High To Avoid High Relapse Rate, Give IM Or 800 mg/kg/Day Of Active Ingredient, Arteannuin, Also Use Huang Qi, Dang Shen With Herbs Or Extract To Reduce Relapse, *100% Cure For Tertian Stage With Tablet Of Dilute Alcohol Extract, For 72-86 g Crude Drug Equivalent Taken In Divided Doses Over 3 Days
- MALARIA, ANTI-: Ether/ Dilute Alcohol Extracts,

- BRONCHITIS, CHRONIC: Volatile Oil
PARASITES
- LIVER FLUKES: (Chlonorchiasis), Small Positive Trial
- SCHISTOSOMA, ANTI-: IM Injection/Oral Of Oil Preparation
SKIN
- FUNGAL, ANTI-: Aqueous Extract
- PRURITUS: 10 Catties Of Fresh Herb Decocted To 6-7, Add 30-35 g

Borneol Predissolved In Alcohol, Apply With Cotton Swabs, 3-4x/Day
- URTICARIA: 10 Catties Of Fresh Herb Decocted To 6-7, Add 30-35 g Borneol Predissolved In Alcohol, Apply With Cotton Swabs, 3-4x/Day
TRAUMA, BITES, POISONINGS
- MOSQUITO REPELLANT: Acetone Extract, Lasted More Than 2 Hrs

Dose

4.5 - 9.0 gm

Common Name

Wormwood

Contraindications

Not: Postpartum Women w/Def Blood/Cold Def SP/ST

Not: w/Diarrea

Notes

Do Not Boil A Long Time

To Dispel Fever: 15-24gm

Few Malaria Patients Developed GI Symptoms, Low Toxicity

XI GUA

西瓜
（西瓜）

FRUCTUS CITRULLUS VULGARIS

Traditional Functions:

1. Clears Summer Heat and controls thirst
2. Purges Fire and removes restlessness

Traditional Properties:

Enters: ST, HT, UB,

Properties: SW, C

Indications:

FLUID DISORDERS
- EDEMA
- THIRST: Fluid Injury
HEAT
- SUMMER HEAT W/O DAMPNESS:

Significant Thirst, Dry Heaves, Scanty Urine
INFECTIOUS DISEASES
- COMMON COLD, IN SUMMER W/DAMPNESS

ORAL CAVITY
- ORAL ULCERS
URINARY BLADDER
- URINATION, SCANTY, DIFFICULT: Summer Heat

Clinical/Pharmaceutical Studies:

KIDNEYS

- DIURETIC: Increases Urea

Formation In Liver

Dose

Eaten

Common Name

Watermelon Fruit

Contraindications

Not: Excess Cold Dampness/Cold Def In Middle Jiao

Clear Heat And Toxins

BA JIAO GEN

芭蕉根

MUSAE CAUDEX

Traditional Functions:

1. Purges fire
2. Helps soothe Wasting and Thirsting syndrome

Traditional Properties:

Enters: SP, LV,

Properties: SW, >C

Indications:

BOWEL RELATED DISORDERS
• FLATULENCE: Evil Heat
ENDOCRINE RELATED
  DISORDERS
• DIABETES
HEAD/NECK
• HEADACHE
HEAT

• HEAT, ACCUMULATED
LIVER
• JAUNDICE
MENTAL STATE/
  NEUROLOGICAL DISORDERS
• RESTLESSNESS
ORAL CAVITY
• MOUTH, DRY

• TOOTHACHE: Wind
SKIN
• BACK, BOILS ON
• BOILS
• URTICARIA
URINARY BLADDER
• DYSURIA W/HEMATURIA

Clinical/Pharmaceutical Studies:

FEVERS

• ANTIPYRETIC: Aqueous Extract,   Strong

Dose

15 - 30 gm

BA JIAO LIAN

八角連
（八角连）

RHIZOMA PODOPHYLLI

Traditional Functions:

1. Clears toxic Heat
2. Dissolves Phlegm, disperses nodules, removes swelling and stagnation

Traditional Properties:

Enters: LU,

Properties: BIT, SP, N

Indications:

INFECTIOUS DISEASES
• SCROFULA
ORAL CAVITY

• TONSILLITIS, ACUTE
SKIN
• BOILS

TRAUMA, BITES, POISONINGS
• TRAUMA, INTERNAL/
  EXTERNAL

Clinical/Pharmaceutical Studies:

CANCER/TUMORS/SWELLINGS/
  LUMPS
• CANCER, ANTI-: Similar To

Convolvulin
SEXUALITY, FEMALE:

GYNECOLOGICAL
• UTERUS, STIMULATES

Dose

6 - 12 gm

Common Name

Podophyllum

BAI HUA LIAN

白花連
(白花连)

RADIX RAUWOLFIAE VERTICILLATAE

Traditional Functions:

1. Clears Wind Heat and disperses toxic swellings
2. Subdues Liver fire

Traditional Properties:

Enters:

Properties: BIT, C

Indications:

ABDOMEN/
  GASTROINTESTINAL TOPICS
• ABDOMEN, PAIN OF
BOWEL RELATED DISORDERS
• DIARRHEA
EARS/HEARING DISORDERS
• DIZZINESS

HEAD/NECK
• HEADACHE
HEAT
• SUMMER HEAT W/SEVERE
  DIGESTIVE PROBLEMS
INFECTIOUS DISEASES
• COMMON COLD, FEVER OF

• MEASLES, GERMAN
ORAL CAVITY
• THROAT, SORE, SWOLLEN
STOMACH/DIGESTIVE
  DISORDERS
• VOMITING

Clinical/Pharmaceutical Studies:

CIRCULATION DISORDERS
• HYPOTENSION: From Reserpine

MENTAL STATE/
NEUROLOGICAL DISORDERS

• HYPNOTIC: Reserpine
• SEDATIVE: Reserpine

Dose

9 - 15 gm

BAI HUA SHE SHE CAO

白花蛇舌
草

HERBA OLDENLANDIAE DIFFUSAE
(HEDYOTIS DIFFUSAE)

Traditional Functions:

1. Clears Heat, resolves toxic Heat and reduces abscesses
2. Clears Damp Heat jaundice and promotes urination
•

Traditional Properties:

Enters: LI, ST, LV,

Properties: BIT, SW, C

Indications:

ABDOMEN/
  GASTROINTESTINAL TOPICS
• INTESTINES, ABSCESS
CANCER/TUMORS/SWELLINGS/
  LUMPS
• GASTROINTESTINAL CANCER
• TUMORS, MALIGNANT

LIVER
• JAUNDICE: Damp Heat
LUNGS
• COUGH: Lung Heat
ORAL CAVITY
• LARYNGITIS
• TONSILLITIS

SKIN
• BOILS
• SORES, TOXIC
TRAUMA, BITES, POISONINGS
• SNAKE BITES
URINARY BLADDER
• URINARY TRACT INFECTIONS

Clinical/Pharmaceutical Studies:

ABDOMEN/ •
GASTROINTESTINAL
TOPICS
• APPENDICITIS: 15 gm +
  Ye Ju Hua, Hai Jin Sha
• APPENDICITIS, ACUTE,
  SIMPLE: 60 g, 2-3 Doses/
  Day, Cure 6-8 Days,
  Severe Cases Add Ye Ju
  Hua, Hai Jin Sha Or Da
  Huang, Chi Shao/Liver
  Heat Purgative Decoction
  Of Long Dan Cao, Life-

Chief Herb
• FIBROSARCOMA: Chief
  Herb
• RECTAL CANCER:
  Chief Herb
• TUMOR, ANTI-: High
  Dose-Various Leukemias
FEVERS
• FEVER, HIGH
GALL BLADDER
• BILIARY TRACT
  INFECTION: Used With
  Other Herbs

Results Better Than
Western Medicine
• LIVER, REDUCED
  DAMAGE TO: Three
  Herb Decoction (Bai Hua
  She She Cao, 2 Parts, Xia
  Ku Cao, 2, Gan Cao, 1),
  Reduced SGPT, Cell
  Damage
LUNGS
• BRONCHITIS,
  CHRONIC: Mild/Simple
  Cases Cured Easier, With

• CERVIX, CANCINOMA:
  Chief Herb
• PELVIC
  INFLAMMATORY
  DISEASE, CHRONIC:
  Pelvic Inflammatory
  Disease Decoction (Bai
  Hua She She Cao, Liang
  Mian Zhen, Radix
  Cudraniae) For Deficient
  Patients, Add Dang Gui,
  Radix Fici
  Simplicissimatis)

Clinical/Pharmaceutical Studies:

Saving Immortal Decoction
- ENTERITIS: Yan Ning Infusion (Bai Hua She She Cao, Herba Monochasmae Savatieri, Ya Zhi Cao)
- GASTROENTERITIS, ACUTE
- GASTROINTESTINAL TRACT: Regulatory Effect With Abnormal Function
- PERITONITIS, MILD LOCAL: 60 g, 2-3 Doses/Day, Cure 6-8 Days, Severe Cases Add Ye Ju Hua, Hai Jin Sha Or Da Huang, Chi Shao/Liver Heat Purgative Decoction Of Long Dan Cao, Life-Saving Immortal Decoction

BOWEL RELATED DISORDERS
- DYSENTERY, BACILLARY, ACUTE: Yan Ning Infusion (Bai Hua She She Cao, Herba Monochasmae Savatieri, Ya Zhi Cao)

CANCER/TUMORS/SWELLINGS/LUMPS
- ANTINEOPLASTIC: High Dose-Leukemia
- BREAST CANCER: Chief Herb
- CANCER: Added To Conventional Chemo, 30-60 g, Sometimes Alcohol Extract, With Tian Men Dong, Synergistic With Other Antineoplastic Herbs
- CERVICAL CANCER:

HEART
- CARDIOTONIC

IMMUNE SYSTEM RELATED DISORDERS/TOPICS
- IMMUNE SYSTEM ENHANCEMENT: Increases Phagocytic Activity Of Leukocytes, Antiinfective
- LYMPHATITIS

INFECTIOUS DISEASES
- BACTERIAL, ANTI-: Weak--Staph Aureus, Shigella
- MUMPS: 120 g Decoction Fresh Herb, 2-3 Days To Cure
- TYPHOID FEVER, CHILDHOOD: With Di Yu

KIDNEYS
- NEPHRITIS, ACUTE: Add Bai Mao Gen, etc, e.g.--Imperata-Plantago Decoction (Bai Hua She Cao, Bai Mao Gen, Che Qian Cao, Shan Zhi Zi, Zi Su Ye)
- PYELONEPHRITIS: Add Phyllanthus Urinaria, Glechoma Longituba

LIVER
- HEPATITIS, ACUTE, VIRAL: Lowers SGPT
- HEPATITIS, CHRONIC ACTIVE: With Shan Dou Gen, etc/Three Herb Decoction Syrup (Bai Hua She Cao, Xia Ku Cao, Gan Cao) , 28 Days,

Crude Extract, Pig Bile/Deoxycholic Acid
- PNEUMONIA, LOBAR: Herb Decoction Cured
- RESPIRATORY TRACT INFECTION, UPPER: Yan Ning Infusion (Bai Hua She She Cao, Herba Monochasmae Savatieri, Ya Zhi Cao)

MENTAL STATE/NEUROLOGICAL DISORDERS
- HYPNOTIC
- SEDATIVE

ORAL CAVITY
- GINGIVITIS
- LARYNGITIS
- PHARYNGITIS, ACUTE/CHRONIC
- STOMATITIS
- TONSILLITIS: Yan Ning Infusion (Bai Hua She She Cao, Herba Monochasmae Savatieri, Ya Zhi Cao)
- TOOTHACHE: Crushed Fresh Herb Acted As Analgesic

PAIN/NUMBNESS/GENERAL DISCOMFORT
- ANALGESIC

SEXUALITY, FEMALE: GYNECOLOGICAL
- ADNEXITIS
- BREASTS, CANCER: Chief Herb
- CERVICITIS: 1:1 Decoction With Pu Yin Gen, Apply Locally To Cervix

SEXUALITY, MALE: UROLOGICAL TOPICS
- EPIDIDYMAL STASIS: 30 g, 3-4 Weeks, Can Help When Complicated With Corditis/Epididymitis
- SPERMATOGENIC, ANTI-: Arrested Developement Of Spermatogonia After 3 Weeks Oral Administration

SKIN
- ACNE VULGARIS: Good Short Term Effects
- BOILS
- BURNS, SEPTICEMIA
- TINEA VERSICOLOR: Fresh Herb
- VERRUCA VULGARIS: Fresh Herb

STOMACH/DIGESTIVE DISORDERS
- STOMACH, CANCER: With Bai Mao Gen, Yi Yi Ren, Brown Sugar

TRAUMA, BITES, POISONINGS
- INFLAMMATORY, ANTI-
- INSECT BITES: Reduced Effect Of Scorpion Bite
- SNAKE BITES: With White Wine Or Decoction With Han Lian Cao
- WOUNDS: With Han Lian Cao In Decoction, * Crushed Fresh Acted As Analgesic

URINARY BLADDER
- URINARY TRACT INFECTIONS

Dose

15 - 60 gm

Contraindications

Not: Pregnancy

Notes

High Doses For Cancer: Up To 150 gm

BAI JIANG CAO

败醬草
(败酱草)

HERBA PATRINIA
(THLASPI)

Traditional Functions:

1. Vitalizes Blood congealed by Heat
2. Clears Heat, toxic Heat and dissipates pus

Traditional Properties:

Enters: LI, ST, LV,

Properties: SP, BIT, <C

Indications:

ABDOMEN/
GASTROINTESTINAL TOPICS
- APPENDICITIS W/PAIN
- INTESTINES, ABSCESS

BLOOD RELATED DISORDERS/
TOPICS
- BLOOD STASIS

CANCER/TUMORS/SWELLINGS/
LUMPS
- SWELLINGS: Topical, Too

CHEST
- CHEST, PAIN, OBSTRUCTION: Heat Induced Stagnant Blood

EYES
- CONJUNCTIVITIS, ACUTE

FLUID DISORDERS

- EDEMA

LIVER
- HEPATITIS, ACUTE, ICTERIC

LUNGS
- LUNGS, ABSCESS
- LUNGS, ABSCESS W/PURULENT VOMIT

PAIN/NUMBNESS/GENERAL
DISCOMFORT
- PAIN, OBSTRUCTION: Chest, Abdomen

SEXUALITY, FEMALE:
GYNECOLOGICAL
- BREASTS, SWOLLEN, PAINFUL, ABSCESS
- DYSMENORRHEA, PAIN

- ENDOMETRITIS, PAIN
- LEUKORRHEA, PINKISH W/ WHITE MATTER
- POSTPARTUM, BLOOD STASIS, HEAT
- POSTPARTUM, PAIN

SKIN
- BOILS, TOXIC: Heat, Toxins, Swellings
- ERYSIPELAS
- HYPEREMIA
- LESIONS, SWOLLEN
- SORES: Topical, Too

TRAUMA, BITES, POISONINGS
- INFLAMMATION
- POST OPERATIVE PAIN

Clinical/Pharmaceutical Studies:

ABDOMEN/
GASTROINTESTINAL
TOPICS
- APPENDICEAL ABSCESS: Herb With Yi Yi Ren, Hong Teng
- APPENDICITIS, ACUTE: Distillate, 2 Gr/ml, 2-4 ml, 2-4x/Day, IM Injection, 2-15 Days
- PANCREATITIS, ACUTE: Distillate, 2 Gr/ml, 2-4 ml, 2-4x/Day, IM Injection, 2-15 Days

BLOOD RELATED
DISORDERS/TOPICS
- BLOOD CELLS, WHITE: May Decrease w/Large Doses
- BLOOD, VITALIZES IN VENA PORTAE

BOWEL RELATED
DISORDERS
- COLITIS, CHRONIC, NONSPECIFIC: Retention Enema Of Yi Yi Ren, Fu Zi, Herb

GALL BLADDER
- BILE DUCT INFLAMMATION/ INFECTION

INFECTIOUS DISEASES
- BACTERIAL, ANTI-: Weak, Staph, Strep
- INFLUENZA: Antipyretic In Granule Infusion Form
- MUMPS: Very Effective 24 Hrs, Decoc + Extl Appl Fresh Herb, Shi Gao, Egg White With Herb Decoction, 10-15 g, 3-4x/

Day, 90% Symptom-Free In 24 Hrs, May Need 2nd Application

LIVER
- LIVER, CELL REGENERATION: Fruit Stem
- LIVER, CELLS, PREVENTS DEGENERATION

LUNGS
- PNEUMONIA: Distillate, 2 Gr/ml, 2-4 ml, 2-4x/Day, IM Injection, 2-15 Days
- TUBERCULOSIS, PULMONARY INFILTRATIVE: Orally, Syrup Similar To Isoniazid, Streptomycin

MENTAL STATE/

NEUROLOGICAL
DISORDERS
- INSOMNIA: 20% Tincture, 10 ml/Dose, 2-3x/ Day, Slow Onset, 3-6 Days After Start Of Treatment, No Morning After Effects
- PSYCHOSIS, SEVERE: 20% Tincture, 10 ml/Dose, 2-3x/Day, Slow Onset, 3-6 Days After Start Of Treatment, No Morning After Effects
- SEDATIVE: Volatile Oil/ ETOH Extract, Orally, 2x As Strong As Valerian

ORAL CAVITY
- TONSILLITIS: Distillate, 2 Gr/ml, 2-4 ml, 2-4x/Day, IM Injection, 2-15 Days

Dose

3 - 30 gm

Contraindications

Not: Def SP/ST

Notes

May Cause Nausea, Dizziness

BAI LIAN

白蘞
(白蘞)

RADIX AMPELOPSIS

Traditional Functions:

1. Closes lesions and toxic swellings
2. Clears Heat and removes toxins
3. Disperses tumors and controls pain
4. Promotes tissue regeneration and healing of wounds

Traditional Properties:

Enters: ST, SP, LV, HT,

Properties: SP, BIT, <C

Indications:

BOWEL RELATED DISORDERS
• HEMORRHOIDS, BLOODY
STOOL
INFECTIOUS DISEASES
• SCROFULA
SEXUALITY, FEMALE:

GYNECOLOGICAL
• LEUKORRHEA, PINK/WHITE
DISCHARGE
SKIN
• BOILS, TOXIC: Heat, Toxins,
Swellings

• BURNS: Scalds
• SKIN, SORES, SWOLLEN: Heat,
Toxins, Swelling
• SORES, WEEPING
• SUPPURATION

Clinical/Pharmaceutical Studies:

INFECTIOUS DISEASES
• BACTERIAL, ANTI-

SKIN

• FUNGAL, ANTI-: Many

Dose

3 - 9 gm

Common Name

Ampelopsis

Contraindications

Not: SP/ST Def w/Cold

BAI TOU WENG

白頭翁
（白头翁）

RADIX
PULSATILLAE CHINENSIS

Traditional Functions:

1. Clears toxic Heat: for dysentery-like disorders
2. Clears Heat and cools Blood

Traditional Properties:

Enters: LI, ST,

Properties: BIT, C

Indications:

BOWEL RELATED DISORDERS
• DIARRHEA: Damp Heat
• DYSENTERY: Blood Heat
• DYSENTERY, BLOODY STOOL:
Toxic Heat
• HEMORRHOIDS, BLOODY

STOOL
• HEMORRHOIDS, INTERNAL
HEMORRHAGIC DISORDERS
• EPISTAXIS
• HEMAFECIA: Heat, Intense
• HEMORRHAGE: Cool Blood To

Stop
INFECTIOUS DISEASES
• MALARIA
• SCROFULA, ULCERATED
PARASITES
• AMOEBIC DYSENTERY

Clinical/Pharmaceutical Studies:

ABDOMEN/
GASTROINTESTINAL TOPICS
• ENTERITIS
BOWEL RELATED DISORDERS
• DIARRHEA: Giardia, Trichomonas
• DIARRHEA, INFANTILE
• DYSENTERY, ACUTE/CHRONIC
W/BLEEDING: Bai Tou Weng Tang
(Bai Tou Weng, Huang Lian, Hang
Bai, Qin Pi) –Give As Fresh
Decoction, Storage Reduces Effect
Against, "60-100 g Of Dried Herb In
3-4 Doses, Cured In 2 Days,
"Superior To Chloramphenicol"
• DYSENTERY, AMOEBIC: Needs
High Dose To Cure, Otherwise
Inhibits, "Superior To Emetine,
Chiniofon, Carbasone", Dose–
Decoction 9-30 g/Day, 3x/Day After
Meals Or As Enema, Powder–2 g, 3-
4x/Day, Improved In 3 Days, Cure In
Average 8 Days
CANCER/TUMORS/SWELLINGS/
LUMPS

BLOOD VESSELS
ENDOCRINE RELATED
DISORDERS
• GOITER, ENDEMIC
EYES
• OPTHALMOPATHY: Wind Heat,
Use As Main Herb
HEART
• CARDIOTONIC: Similar To
Digitalis, Whole Herb w/o Root
INFECTIOUS DISEASES
• BACTERIAL, ANTI-: Fresh/
Decoction/Alcohol Extract--Shigella
Dys., Staph Aureus, Pseudomonas,
B.Subtilis, Amoebic Trophozoites,
Synergizes With Streptomycin
• CANDIDA ALBICANS: Bai Tou
Weng Decoction
• INFLUENZA: Weak Inhibitory
Effect, Aqueous Extract
• MUMPS: Excellent, Dose--Fry
Powder Herb With Egg, Eat As Food,
Marked Results In 7-8 Hours, 24
Hrs For More Serious Cases

Decoction
• YEAST: Bai Tou Weng Decoction
MENTAL STATE/
NEUROLOGICAL DISORDERS
• SEDATIVE: Alcohol Extract
PAIN/NUMBNESS/GENERAL
DISCOMFORT
• ANALGESIC: Alcohol Extract
PARASITES
• ANTIPARASITIC: Endamoiba
Histol. (High Doses) , Trichomonas
Vaginitis (5% Oral) .
• WORMS
SEXUALITY, FEMALE:
GYNECOLOGICAL
• UTERINE BLEEDING,
FUNCTIONAL: With Browned Di
Yu
SKIN
• FUNGAL INFECTIONS: Bai Tou
Weng Decoction
• NEURODERMATITIS
TRAUMA, BITES, POISONINGS
• FAVISM

Clinical/Pharmaceutical Studies:

- CANCER: IV Injection, Helped Squamous Cell Carcinoma, Lung Melanoma
- **CIRCULATION DISORDERS**
- VASODILATOR, PERIPHERAL
- SCROFULA, ULCERATED, SLOW HEALING: Liquor Of With Xia Ku Cao
- TRYPANOSOMA: Bai Tou Weng
- SURGERY, INFECTIONS FROM/ WOUNDS
- WOUNDS, PSEUDOMONAS INFECTION

Dose
9 - 15 gm

Common Name
Chinese Anemone Root

Contraindications
Not: Chronic Dysentery w/Weak SP/ST

Notes
Low Toxicity
Strongly Irritates Skin, Mucosa, Long Storage Reduces Low Toxicity For Decoction

---

BAI XIAN PI

白鲜皮

CORTEX DICTAMNI DASYCARPI RADICIS

Traditional Functions:
1. Clears Heat and relieves toxins while drying Dampness
2. Expels Wind Damp Bi
3. Removes Damp and stops itching

Traditional Properties:
Enters: SP, ST,

Properties: BIT, C

Indications:

HEAT
- DAMP HEAT
INFECTIOUS DISEASES
- LEPROSY
- RUBELLA
- SYPHILIS
LIVER
- JAUNDICE: Damp Heat
MUSCULOSKELETAL/ CONNECTIVE TISSUE
- JOINTS, PAIN, SWELLING, RED:

Hot Bi
PAIN/NUMBNESS/GENERAL DISCOMFORT
- BI, JOINT PAIN: Damp
SEXUALITY, FEMALE: GYNECOLOGICAL
- LEUKORRHEA: Damp Heat
- METRORRHAGIA
SKIN
- CARBUNCLES: Wind Heat/Damp

Heat
- ECZEMA: Damp Heat
- FUNGAL INFECTIONS
- RASHES: Wind Heat/Damp Heat
- RASHES, PRURITIC: Wind Damp
- SCABIES
- SKIN, DISORDERS: Wind Heat/ Damp Heat
- SORES, INTRACTABLE
- ULCERS, WIND

Clinical/Pharmaceutical Studies:

FEVERS
- ANTIPYRETIC: Oral
HEART
- CARDIAC STIMULANT

INFECTIOUS DISEASES
- BACTERIAL, ANTI-
SEXUALITY, FEMALE: GYNECOLOGICAL

- UTERUS, STIMULATES
SKIN
- FUNGAL, ANTI-: Many

Dose
4.5 - 9.0 gm

Common Name
Chinese Dittany Root Cort

Contraindications
Not: Def Cold Conditions

BAN LAN GEN

板籃根
（板籃根）

RADIX ISATIDIS SEU BAPHICACANTHI

Traditional Functions:
1. Clears Heat, relieves toxic Heat and soothes the throat
2. Cools Blood Heat
3. Clears Damp Heat jaundice

Traditional Properties:
Enters: LU, ST, LV,

Properties: BIT, C

Indications:

FEVERS
- FEVER

HEMORRHAGIC DISORDERS
- EPISTAXIS
- HEMATEMESIS

INFECTIOUS DISEASES
- INFECTIONS
- INFLUENZA W/FEVER

- MENINGITIS
- MUMPS
- VIRAL INFECTIONS

LIVER
- JAUNDICE: Damp Heat

ORAL CAVITY
- THROAT INFECTIONS

SKIN

- BOILS
- ERYSIPELAS
- MACULA, FROM ACUTE
  INFECTIOUS DISEASES
- RASHES, INCOMPLETE
  EXPRESSION OF: Blood Heat,
  Wind

Clinical/Pharmaceutical Studies:

**CANCER/TUMORS/
SWELLINGS/LUMPS**
- CANCER, ANTI-
- LEUKEMIA, CHRONIC
  MYELOGENOUS: w/Ma
  Li Lan, Ok Long Term

EYES
- CONJUNCTIVITIS,
  FULMINANT: 10% Eye
  Drops, Better Than 0.5%
  Chloramphenicol, 4 Days
  For Cure

INFECTIOUS DISEASES
- ANTIBIOTIC: Alcohol
  Differs From Water Extract,
  Very Broad Spectrum–
  Shigella, Salmonella
- CHICKEN POX: IM
  Injection Of 50% Solution,
  2 ml/Day, Lowered

Temperature In 1-3 Days
- DIPHTHERIA: Herb
  Decoction, 1 g/ml, 3-4
  Days, 20 ml For 3 Yrs, 25
  ml, 3-5 Yrs, 35 ml 10+Yrs,
  3x/Day, Stop Dose 3 Days
  After Sloughing Of
  Pseudomembrane, Lack Of
  Symptoms
- ENCEPHALITIS B:
  Good, 90% With Other
  Treatment, Too, Early
  Treatment Important, 30-
  60 gm Daily, 7-10 Days,
  Up To 14 Days For Serious
  Cases
- HERPES SIMPLEX: 50%
  Herb Injection 2 ml IM, 1-
  2x/Day

- HERPES ZOSTER: 50%
  Herb Injection 2 ml IM, 1-
  2x/Day
- INFLUENZA: Injection
  Can Prevent
- LEPTOSPIROSIS: At
  High Doses (1:100)
- MENINGITIS,
  EPIDEMIC
  CEREBROSPINAL: Oral
  Decoction, All Symptoms
  Improved By 9th Day
- MONONUCLEOSIS,
  INFECTIOUS: IM
  Injection Plus Decoction,
  Cure In 3-5 Days, Worked
  Best In Young Children, 1-
  7 Yrs, 1-2 ml, Greater
  Than 8 Yrs, 2 ml, 2x/Day

- MUMPS: Treat With 100%
  Injection, 1-6 ml, 2-4 X/
  Day, Best If Taken
  Prophylactically
- VIRAL INFECTIONS

LIVER
- HEPATITIS, ACUTE
- HEPATITIS, CHRONIC/
  ACUTE: Injection/
  Decoction

SKIN
- SKIN, PITYRIASIS
  ROSEA: 50% Herb
  Injection 2 ml IM, 1-2x/
  Day
- WARTS, VIRAL: Slow, 3-
  4 Week Course, 50% Herb
  Injection 2 ml IM, 1-2x/
  Day

Dose

9 - 30 gm

Common Name

Woad Root

Contraindications

Not: Weak People

Not: w/o Fire Poison

Notes

Give Every 4 Hrs For Highest Blood Level

Low Toxicity, No Side Effects Orally/Topical

May Give Up To 60 gm

BAN ZHI LIAN

半枝蓮
（半枝莲）

HERBA
SCUTELLARIAE BARBATAE

Traditional Functions:

1. Clears Heat and toxins
2. Clears Blood Heat, Blood stasis and stops bleeding

Traditional Properties:

Enters: LU, ST, LV,

Properties: BIT, C

Indications:

BOWEL RELATED DISORDERS
- DYSENTERY, RED

**CANCER/TUMORS/SWELLINGS/
LUMPS**
- CANCER, SWELLINGS

HEMORRHAGIC DISORDERS
- EPISTAXIS
- HEMOPTYSIS

INFECTIOUS DISEASES

- SCROFULA

LIVER
- HEPATITIS
- JAUNDICE
- LIVER, CIRRHOSIS W/ASCITES

LUNGS
- LUNGS, ABSCESS

ORAL CAVITY
- THROAT, PAIN, SWELLING

SKIN
- BOILS
- BURNS

TRAUMA, BITES, POISONINGS
- BITES, SNAKE, INSECT
- TRAUMA
- WOUNDS, INFECTED

URINARY BLADDER
- URINATION, BLOODY

Clinical/Pharmaceutical Studies:

INFECTIOUS DISEASES   • BACTERIAL, ANTI-: Acute   Leukemic Granulocytes

Dose
Fresh Juice

Common Name
Barbat Skullcap

Contraindications
Not: Pregnancy

Notes
Usually Fresh Juice Used

CAO HE CHE
(ZHONG LOU /QUAN SHEN)

草河車
（草河车）

RHIZOMA
POLYGONI BISTORTAE

Traditional Functions:

1. Clears Heat and resolves toxic Heat
2. Decreases swelling and masses--resolves Phelgm
3. Relieves spasms

Traditional Properties:

Enters: LV,

Properties: BIT, C, TX

Indications:

**CANCER/TUMORS/SWELLINGS/
LUMPS**
• CANCER, EARLY STAGE
INFECTIOUS DISEASES
• FOCAL INFECTIONS
• INFECTIONS, SEVERE
• SCROFULA

• TETANUS
**MENTAL STATE/
NEUROLOGICAL DISORDERS**
• CONVULSIONS: Hand, Feet
• EPILEPSY
ORAL CAVITY

• THROAT, SORE
SKIN
• BOILS
TRAUMA, BITES, POISONINGS
• MOSQUITO BITES
• SNAKE BITES

Clinical/Pharmaceutical Studies:

**CANCER/TUMORS/SWELLINGS/
LUMPS**
• CANCER, ANTI-: Cervical Cancer,
  Water Extract
INFECTIOUS DISEASES

• BACTERIAL, ANTI-: Shigella,
Bacillus Enteritidis, B.Typhi, Staph
Aureus, Streptococcus,
Meningococcus

LUNGS
• ANTITUSSIVE: Histamine Induced
  Bronchial Spasms (Another Species,
  Paris Polyphylla-As Zao Xiu)

Dose
6 - 15 gm

Common Name
Alpine Knotweed

Notes
(See Zao Xiu, Also)
Only For Severe Infections
5-10 Qian For Cancers

CHA CHI HUANG

茶匙潢
（茶匙潢）

HERBA
MALACHII

Traditional Functions:

1. Clears Heat and toxins
2. Vitalizes the Blood and disperses swelling

Traditional Properties:

Enters: LU,

Properties: SO, N

Indications:

BOWEL RELATED DISORDERS
• DYSENTERY
• HEMORRHOIDS
CIRCULATION DISORDERS

• HYPERTENSION
LUNGS
• PNEUMONIA
SEXUALITY, FEMALE:

GYNECOLOGICAL
• UTERINE BLEEDING
SKIN
• BOILS

Dose
15 - 30 gm

Common Name
Malachium

CHANG SHAN

常 山

RADIX DICHORAE FEBRIFUGAE

Traditional Functions:

1. Clears Heat and resolves Phlegm
2. Induces vomiting
3. Treats malaria

Traditional Properties:

Enters: LU, HT, LV,

Properties: BIT, SP, C, TX

Indications:

CHEST
• CHEST/RIB DISTENSTION, FULLNESS
INFECTIOUS DISEASES

• MALARIA, CHILLS, FEVER OF
• MALARIA, SPECIFIC FOR
PHLEGM
• PHLEGM, FLUID, LINGERING

STOMACH/DIGESTIVE DISORDERS
• VOMITING

Clinical/Pharmaceutical Studies:

ABDOMEN/ GASTROINTESTINAL TOPICS
• INTESTINES, INHIBITS
BLOOD RELATED DISORDERS/TOPICS
• BLOOD PRESSURE, LOWERS
CANCER/TUMORS/ SWELLINGS/LUMPS
• TUMORS, EHRLICH ASCITES CELLS: Eliminates
FEVERS

• FEVER, REDUCES: Greater Than Aspirin
HEART
• ARRHYTHMIAS: Oral, Stir Fried Chang Shan, LU Ti Cao (Herba Pyrolae) , Roasted Huang Qi, Xuan Shen, Dang Shen)
INFECTIOUS DISEASES
• MALARIA: Kills Parasites, Symptoms, Fevers, 26x Quinine, Many Variations, With Huo

Xiang As Tablet Before Meals, Tertian Malaria Responded Best, Better Than Chloroguanide, Quinacrine, *May Compound With Ban Xia, Chai Hu, Huo Xiang, Chen Pi To Control Symptoms, Prevent Relapse
• VIRAL, ANTI-: Flu
PARASITES
• AMOEBIC, ANTI-: Stronger Than Emetine

• GIARDIA: Decoction, 3-9 g/Day In 2-3 Doses For 7 Days
SEXUALITY, FEMALE: GYNECOLOGICAL
• UTERUS, CONTRACTIONS
STOMACH/DIGESTIVE DISORDERS
• EMETIC: Very Strong
TRAUMA, BITES, POISONINGS
• TOXIC: Causes Vomiting

Dose

3 - 9 gm

Precautions

Watch: Chronic Patient

Notes

Strong Side Effects: Vomiting, Nausea-Use Bing Lang

To Counter, Although Increases Toxicity, Stir Fry With Ginger Juice/Yellow Wine Or Use Ban Xia, Huo Xiang, Chen Pi To Reduce Effect, Initially About 40% Of Patients May Vomit With Use

See Shu Qi (Leaf Of This Plant 5x Strength Of Root)

CHUAN XIN LIAN

穿心蓮
(穿心蓮)

HERBA ANDROGRAPHIS PANICULATAE

Traditional Functions:

1. Clears Heat and resolves toxic Heat

Traditional Properties:

Enters: LU, UB, ST, LI,

Properties: >BIT, C

Indications:

ABDOMEN/ GASTROINTESTINAL TOPICS
• APPENDICITIS W/PAIN
• ENTERITIS, ACUTE
• GASTROINTESTINAL TRACT INFECTION, ACUTE
BOWEL RELATED DISORDERS
• DIARRHEA

KIDNEYS
• NEPHRITIS
LUNGS
• ASTHMA
• BRONCHITIS
• COUGH: Lung Heat
• LUNGS, ABSCESS
• LUNGS, ABSCESS W/PURULENT

ORAL CAVITY
• THROAT PAIN
• TONSILLITIS
SKIN
• BOILS, TOXIC: Heat, Toxins, Swellings
• DERMATITIS, PUSTULAR
URINARY BLADDER

Indications:

- DYSENTERY, RED
  EARS/HEARING DISORDERS
- OTITIS MEDIA, PURULENT

- VOMIT
- LUNGS, DYSPNEA: Lung Heat
- PNEUMONIA

- URETHRITIS
- URINARY TRACT INFECTIONS:
  Acute

Clinical/Pharmaceutical Studies:

ABDOMEN/
GASTROINTESTINAL
TOPICS
- ENTERITIS
- INTESTINES,
  TRICHOMONIASIS: Use
  As An Enema
BOWEL RELATED
DISORDERS
- DYSENTERY,
  BACILLARY
CANCER/TUMORS/
SWELLINGS/LUMPS
- CANCER: Malignant
  Hydatidiform Mole
  (Choriocarcinoma)
CIRCULATION
DISORDERS
- BLOOD VESSELS,
  DILATES
- THROMBOANGIITIS
  OBLITERANS: Best For
  Heat, Toxin Type, IV
  Injection
EARS/HEARING
DISORDERS
- EARS, OTITIS MEDIA,
  SUPPURATIVE
ENDOCRINE RELATED
DISORDERS
- HORMONES: Intensifies
  Adrenocortical Function
FEVERS
- ANTIPYRETIC
GALL BLADDER

- GALL BLADDER,
  BILIARY TRACT
  INFECTION: Compound
  Formula Effective
IMMUNE SYSTEM
RELATED DISORDERS/
TOPICS
- IMMUNE SYSTEM:
  Increase WBC Activity
INFECTIOUS DISEASES
- BACTERIAL, ANTI-:
  Equivocal-Staph, Strep,
  Aqueous Extract Was
  Strongly Inhibitory Against
  Shigella, Pneumococci,
  Spirochettes
- CHICKEN POX
- COMMON COLD
- ENCEPHALITIS B,
  EPIDEMIC
- HERPES ZOSTER
- INFECTIOUS DISEASES:
  Many (Listed
  Individually), ETOH
  Extract
- INFLUENZA: Powder/
  Aqueous Extract, Powder
  More Effective
- LEPROSY: Effective
- LEPTOSPIROSIS: The
  Tablet Of The Total
  Lactones, 87% Cure Rate
- PAROTITIS
- TYPHOID FEVER: Can

Be Used With Other Herbs
- VIRAL, ANTI-
KIDNEYS
- PYELONEPHRITIS,
  ACUTE: Tablet, Similar
  To But Less Side Effects
  Than Nitrofurantoin
LIVER
- HEPATITIS,
  FULMINANT: With
  Western Drugs
LUNGS
- BRONCHITIS: Powder/
  Aqueous Extract, Powder
  More Effective
- BRONCHITIS,
  ASTHMATIC
- PNEUMONIA,
  EPIDEMIC ASTHMATIC
- PNEUMONIA, LOBAR:
  Powder/Aqueous Extract,
  Powder More Effective
- PNEUMONIA, VIRAL:
  Powder/Aqueous Extract,
  Powder More Effective
- RESPIRATORY TRACT
  INFECTION: Good For
  Viral Infections, Too
- TUBERCULOSIS:
  Especially Exudative Type,
  Synergizes With Isoniazid
ORAL CAVITY
- PHARYNGOLARYNGITIS
- TONSILLITIS, ACUTE:

Powder/Aqueous Extract,
Powder More Effective, *
May Add Sodium Bisulfite
As Adduct, 92% Effective
PARASITES
- TRICHOMONIASIS,
  INTESTINAL: Use As An
  Enema
SEXUALITY, EITHER
SEX
- CONTRACEPTIVE
SEXUALITY, FEMALE:
GYNECOLOGICAL
- ABORTIFACIENT: Oral
  Ok, But Intrauterine Or IV,
  IP Routes Better
- CERVIX, EROSION OF
- PELVIC
  INFLAMMATION
- VAGINITIS
SKIN
- BURNS
- ECZEMA
- NEURODERMATITIS
- SKIN, INFECTIONS
TRAUMA, BITES,
POISONINGS
- INFLAMMATORY, ANTI-
- SNAKE BITES: ETOH
  Extract Is Muscarinic vs
  Cobra Venom, Other
  Snakes, Too, Used
  Compound Formula, Takes
  3-5 Days For Cure

Dose

9 - 15 gm

Precautions

Watch: Prolonged Overdosing-May Impair ST Qi

Notes

Very Bitter: Pack In Capsules

Cheap Substitute For Huang Lian

Few Toxic Side Effects
Large Doses May Upset The Stomach, Possible
Vomiting

DA QING YE

大青葉
(大青叶)

FOLIUM
DAQINGYE

Traditional Functions:

1. Clears Heat and resolves toxic Heat, reduces swelling
2. Cools Blood: reduces skin problems from Blood Heat

Traditional Properties:

Enters: LU, ST, HT,

Properties: BIT, C

Indications:

FEVERS
- FEVER, HIGH

HEAT
- BLOOD HEAT BLOTCHES/ERUPTIONS IN THROAT, MOUTH, SKIN
- FIRE POISON
- HEAT DISEASES W/ ACUTE ONSET

- QI LEVEL HEAT DISORDERS
- XUE LEVEL HEAT

INFECTIOUS DISEASES
- COMMON COLD
- EPIDEMIC INFECTIOUS DISEASES
- INFLUENZA
- INFLUENZA, BACTERIAL

- MENINGITIS
- MUMPS

LUNGS
- LUNGS, TOXIC HEAT
- PNEUMONIA

MENTAL STATE/ NEUROLOGICAL DISORDERS
- MENTAL DULLNESS

ORAL CAVITY

- PHARYNGITIS
- THROAT, PAIN, SWOLLEN

SKIN
- BOILS
- ERYTHEMA
- FURUNCLES, TOXIC
- RASHES, INCOMPLETE EXPRESSION OF: Blood Heat, Wind

Clinical/Pharmaceutical Studies:

ABDOMEN/ GASTROINTESTINAL TOPICS
- GASTROENTERITIS

BLOOD RELATED DISORDERS/ TOPICS
- LYMPHOCYTOSIS, ACUTE INFECTIOUS: Decoction Cured

BOWEL RELATED DISORDERS
- DIARRHEA, INFANTILE: Good Effects
- DYSENTERY, AMOEBIC
- DYSENTERY, BACILLARY, ACUTE: Fever Down 1 Day After Decoction, Normal 5 Days

EYES
- KERATITIS, HERPES SIMPLEX: Eye Wash, Soak Cornea 15-20

Minutes, Then Add Tetracycline Ointment, 1x/Day

FEVERS
- ANTIPYRETIC: Reduces Fever From Infections

INFECTIOUS DISEASES
- BACTERIAL, ANTI-: Salmonella, Staph Aureus, B. Diphtheria, Leptospirosis, N.Meningitidis
- ENCEPHALITIS B: Mild To Moderate Cases
- INFLUENZA, PROPHYLAXIS, TREAT: 2x/Day Decoction, 2-3 Days For Cure
- MEASLES: w/Pu Gong Ying, Shortens Illness, Reduces Symptoms, Greater Than Sulfonamides

- MUMPS: Symptomatic Relief After 2 Doses Of Decoction, Cure In 3-4 Days
- RHEUMATIC FEVER
- VIRAL PROPHYLAXIS

LIVER
- HEPATITIS, ANICTERIC, INFECTIOUS: Good, Cure Rate 86% With Decoction

ORAL CAVITY
- PERIODONTITIS
- TONSILLITIS: Use Decoction To Cure, 75% Rate

SEXUALITY, FEMALE: GYNECOLOGICAL
- CERVICITIS

Dose
9 - 15 gm

Common Name
Woad Leaf

Contraindications
Not: Cold Def SP/ST

Notes
Take Every 6 Hrs For Best Effect
May Take Up To 30-60 gm
May Give GI Disturbances To Some

DI DAN TOU

地膽頭
（地胆头）

HERBA ELEPHANTOPI

Traditional Functions:

1. Clears Heat and purges Fire
2. Benefits water metabolism and promotes urination

Traditional Properties:

Enters: LU,

Properties: BIT, SP, BL, C

Indications:

FEVERS
- FEVER: Pneumonia

FLUID DISORDERS
- DAMPNESS
- EDEMA

LIVER
- HEPATITIS

LUNGS
- BRONCHITIS

- PNEUMONIA: Fever, Cough Of

MUSCULOSKELETAL/ CONNECTIVE TISSUE
- ARTHRITIS, PAIN: Wind, Bi

Clinical/Pharmaceutical Studies:

INFECTIOUS DISEASES
- BACTERIAL, ANTI-: Inhibits Staph, Strep, Shigella, Bacillus Typhi

KIDNEYS
- DIURETIC

TRAUMA, BITES, POISONINGS

- INFLAMMATORY, ANTI-: Arthritis

Dose

15 - 30 gm

Common Name

Elephantopus

Notes

This Herb Is Used As A Substitute For Pu Gong Ying

GE HUA   葛花   FLOS PUERARIAE

Traditional Functions:

1. Clears Heat in the Stomach and relieves alcoholic intoxication

Traditional Properties:

Enters: ST,

Properties: SW, N

Indications:

ABDOMEN/
  GASTROINTESTINAL TOPICS
• ABDOMEN, DISTENTION OF
• INTESTINES, HEMORRHAGE
FEVERS
• FEVER, HIGH
FLUID DISORDERS
• THIRST

HEAD/NECK
• HEADACHE: Stomach Heat
HEMORRHAGIC DISORDERS
• HEMAFECIA
• INTESTINAL HEMORRHAGE
MENTAL STATE/
  NEUROLOGICAL DISORDERS
• INTOXICATION, ALCOHOLIC:

Fidgets, Thirst
STOMACH/DIGESTIVE
  DISORDERS
• VOMITING: Stomach Heat
TRAUMA, BITES, POISONINGS
• HANGOVER: Headache, Thirst,
  Distension

Dose

3 - 12 gm

Common Name

Pueraria Flower

GUAN ZHONG   貫眾   RHIZOMA GUANZHONG
(GUAN CHONG)   （贯众）   (BLECHNI/ET. AL.)

Traditional Functions:

1. Clears Heat and resolves toxic Heat
2. Stops bleeding caused by Heat
3. Kills parasites
4. Topical use for head sores and baldness

Traditional Properties:

Enters: SP, LV,

Properties: BIT, C, <TX

Indications:

HEAD/NECK
• BALDNESS
HEMORRHAGIC
  DISORDERS
• EPISTAXIS
• HEMAFECIA
• HEMOPTYSIS
• HEMORRHAGE:
  Astringe To Stop
INFECTIOUS DISEASES

• EPIDEMIC DISEASES
• INFLUENZA
• MEASLES
• MENINGITIS
• MUMPS
LUNGS
• PNEUMONIA
PARASITES
• HOOKWORMS
• PINWORMS

• ROUNDWORMS
• TAPEWORMS
SEXUALITY, FEMALE:
  GYNECOLOGICAL
• MENORRHAGIA:
  Avalanche & Leakage
  (Charred, Use w/Other
  Herbs)
• MENSTRUATION,

DISORDERS OF:
Constrict Uterus, Stimulate
Chong
• UTERINE BLEEDING:
  Hot
SKIN
• BOILS
• SORES: Damp Heat
• SORES, HEAD

Clinical/Pharmaceutical Studies:

• WATER PURIFIER:
  Works Quickly
BLOOD RELATED
  DISORDERS/TOPICS
• EOSINOPHILIA,
  TROPICAL: With Di
  Long, Gan Cao

(Guan Zhong, Da Qing Ye,
Gan Cao) To Prevent Flu,
Low Incidence Compared
To Controls, Pill May Be
Curative, Too, *Best To
Use As Fumigant, Too (See
Flu)

• TUBERCULOSIS,
  PULMONARY,
  HEMORRHAGE OF: 60
  g Decoction, Divided In 3-
  4 Doses/Fluid Extract, 4x/
  Day, Bleeding Stopped 1-5
  Days

To Expel Fetus, Mother
Remained Healthy, Action
May Be Species
Dependent
• ABORTION, BLEEDING
  AFTER: Injection Of
  Extract

Clinical/Pharmaceutical Studies:

ENDOCRINE RELATED DISORDERS
- HORMONE-LIKE: Estrogen

HEMORRHAGIC DISORDERS
- GASTROINTESTINAL BLEEDING, UPPER: 60 g Decoction, Divided In 3-4 Doses/Fluid Extract, 4x/Day, Bleeding Stopped 1-5 Days
- HEMOSTATIC

INFECTIOUS DISEASES
- BACTERIAL, ANTI-: Bacteriostatic, Many, Mild, Shigella, Salmonella, E. Coli, Pseudomonas, Proteus, Staph.Aureus
- COMMON COLD: Treat Drinking Water, Folk Medicine, "Herb Granules As Prophylaxis, 2x/Week, " Fu Fang Guan Zhong Pian

- INFLUENZA: Gui Guan Xiang--Incense Made Of Gui Zhi/Guan Zhong With Or Without Moxa, Used As Fumigant When Flu Present
- MEASLES
- MENINGITIS, EPIDEMIC
- VIRAL, ANTI-: Asian Flu, Strongly Inhibits Multiple Strains, Other Viruses

LUNGS
- BRONCHIECTASIS: 60 g Decoction, Divided In 3-4 Doses/Fluid Extract, 4x/Day, Bleeding Stopped 1-5 Days
- BRONCHITIS, CHRONIC
- PNEUMONIA, CHILDHOOD: By Adenovirus

MENTAL STATE/ NEUROLOGICAL DISORDERS
- HYPNOTIC
- SEDATIVE

PAIN/NUMBNESS/ GENERAL DISCOMFORT
- ANALGESIC

PARASITES
- ASCARIASIS
- SCHISTOSOMIASIS
- TAPEWORMS: Paralyzises, Needs Purgative

SEXUALITY, FEMALE: GYNECOLOGICAL
- ABORTIFACIENT: Extract Can Terminate Early Pregnancy, 10-15 ml Of Extract (In Mice) , Injection Also, 500 mg/kg PO Of Extract, 24-41 Hrs

- MENORRHAGIA: With Wu Ling Zhi
- POSTPARTUM, HEMORRHAGE
- UTERUS, STIMULATES: Water Extract

SKIN
- FUNGAL INFECTIONS: Some

TRAUMA, BITES, POISONINGS
- INFLAMMATORY, ANTI-
- LEAD POISONING: Decoction Of Guan Zhong, Dioscorea Hypogauca)
- WOUNDS: Zhi Xue Jing (Guan Zhong, Quan Shen, etc) For Topical Application, Stops Bleeding, Pain, Inflammation

URINARY BLADDER
- CHYLURIA: Carbonized

Dose
3 - 15 gm

Contraindications
Not: Pregnant/Children/GI Ulcer

Notes
See: Dong Bei Guan Zhong

Can Be Several Ferns, Dryopteris Most Toxic

Carbonized Herb Used To Stop Bleeding

HAI JIN SHA

SPORA LYGODII

Traditional Functions:
1. Clears Heat, stones and regulates and promotes urination

Traditional Properties:
Enters: SI, UB

Properties: SW, C

Indications:

URINARY BLADDER
- DYSURIA
- URETHRITIS, ACUTE

- URINARY STONES
- URINATION, DYSFUNCTION: Damp Heat

- URINATION, LACK OF
- URINATION, PAINFUL

Clinical/Pharmaceutical Studies:

KIDNEYS

- DIURETIC

Dose
6 - 12 gm

Common Name
Japanese Fern Spores

HAI JIN SHA CAO
(JIN SHA TENG)

海金砂草

HERBA LYGODII JAPONICI

Traditional Functions:
1. Clears Heat, stones and regulates and promotes urination
2. Clears Heat and resolves toxic Heat

Traditional Properties:
Enters: SI, UB,

Properties: SW, C

Indications:

GALL BLADDER
- GALL BLADDER, STONES

HEMORRHAGIC DISORDERS
- HEMATURIA: Damp Heat
- HEMOPTYSIS

INFECTIOUS DISEASES
- MUMPS

LIVER
- HEPATITIS

LUNGS
- PNEUMONIA

MUSCULOSKELETAL/ CONNECTIVE TISSUE
- BACK, LOWER SPRAIN

ORAL CAVITY
- THROAT, PAIN, SWOLLEN
- TOOTHACHE

URINARY BLADDER

- URETHRITIS, ACUTE
- URINARY STONES: Damp Heat
- URINARY TRACT INFECTIONS: Damp Heat
- URINARY TRACT STONES
- URINATION, PAINFUL, DRIBBLING, CONCENTRATED, RED/YELLOW/TURBID

Clinical/Pharmaceutical Studies:

INFECTIOUS DISEASES
- BACTERIAL, ANTI-: Staph.

Aureus, Strep, Salmonella, B.Typhi, Pseudomonas

KIDNEYS
- DIURETIC

Dose

9 - 60 gm

Common Name

Climbing/Japanese Fern

Notes

Wrap Or Strain For Decoction

JIN DI LUO

錦地羅
(锦地罗)

HERBA DROSERAE

Traditional Functions:

1. Clears Heat and removes toxins

Traditional Properties:

Enters: LU

Properties: SW, BL, CL

Indications:

BOWEL RELATED DISORDERS
- DYSENTERY

CHILDHOOD DISORDERS
- MALNUTRITION, CHILDHOOD

EARS/HEARING DISORDERS
- OTITIS MEDIA, PURULENT

LUNGS

- COUGH: Lung Heat

ORAL CAVITY
- THROAT, SORE

Dose

6 - 15 gm

Common Name

Drosera

JIN GUO LAN

金果攬
(金果揽)

RADIX TINOSPORAE

Traditional Functions:

1. Clears Heat and relieves toxins
2. Soothes the throat and reduces pain

Traditional Properties:

Enters: LU, ST,

Properties: BIT, C

Indications:

- VETERINARY MEDICINE

CANCER/TUMORS/SWELLINGS/ LUMPS
- TOXIC SWELLINGS

EYES
- EYES, CONGESTED

HEMORRHAGIC DISORDERS

- EPISTAXIS
- HEMATEMESIS

LUNGS
- COUGH: Heat

ORAL CAVITY
- THROAT, SORE

SKIN

- CARBUNCLES: External Application
- FURUNCLES
- HYPEREMIA

TRAUMA, BITES, POISONINGS
- INFECTED WOUNDS
- INSECT BITES: Topical

Dose

2.4 - 9.0 gm

JIN YIN HUA

金銀花
（金银花）

FLOS LONICERAE JAPONICAE

Traditional Functions:

1. Clears Heat and resolves toxic Heat
2. Clears Damp Heat in the Lower Burner
3. Dispels Wind Heat
4. Dispels Summer Heat

Traditional Properties:

Enters: LU, ST,

Properties: SW, C

Indications:

ABDOMEN/ GASTROINTESTINAL TOPICS
• APPENDICITIS W/PAIN
• ENTERITIS
• INTESTINES, ABSCESS
BOWEL RELATED DISORDERS
• DYSENTERY, RED: Damp Heat
• STOOLS, BLOODY
EYES
• EYES, SORES/SWELLINGS
FEVERS
• FEVER: Wind Heat
HEAD/NECK
• HEADACHE: Wind Heat
HEAT
• HEAT: In Yang Ming, Qi Level
• SUMMER HEAT, EXPELS
• TOXIC HEAT
• WEI STAGE HEAT
INFECTIOUS DISEASES

• COMMON COLD: Wind Heat
• FEBRILE DISEASES: With High Fever, Thirst
LUNGS
• LUNG HEAT
• LUNGS, ABSCESS W/PURULENT VOMIT
MUSCULOSKELETAL/ CONNECTIVE TISSUE
• JOINTS, PAIN, SWELLING, RED: Hot Bi, Toxic Heat With Stasis
NOSE
• SINUSITIS: Heat, Needs Sinusitis Herbs Plus
ORAL CAVITY
• THROAT INFECTIONS/ SWELLINGS, PAINFUL
• THROAT, SORE: Wind Heat
SEXUALITY, FEMALE: GYNECOLOGICAL

• BREASTS, SORES/SWELLINGS
• BREASTS, SWOLLEN, PAINFUL, ABSCESS
SKIN
• ABSCESS
• FUNGAL INFECTIONS
• RASHES, INCOMPLETE EXPRESSION OF: Early Stage/ Blood Heat, Wind
• RASHES, W/PRURITUS: Clears Wind
• SCABIES
• SKIN, SORES, SWOLLEN, TOXIC: Relieves Surface Complex/Heat, Toxins, Swelling
• ULCERS, INTRACTABLE/ MALIGNANT
URINARY BLADDER
• URINATION, PAINFUL

Clinical/Pharmaceutical Studies:

ABDOMEN/ GASTROINTESTINAL TOPICS
• APPENDICITIS W/ PERFORATION
BLOOD RELATED DISORDERS/TOPICS
• BLOOD PRESSURE, LOWERS: w/Ju Hua
• CHOLESTEROL, LOWERS: Slightly
• CHOLESTEROL, LOWERS ABSORPTION
BOWEL RELATED DISORDERS
• DIARRHEA, INFANTILE: Retention Enema Of Finely Powdered Herb In Water, Less Than 6 Months, 1 g/10 ml Water, 6-12 Months, 1.5 g/15 ml, 1-2 Yrs, 2-3 g/20-30 ml, 2x/ Day
• DYSENTERY, BACILLARY: 6-15 g (15-

Of Vine, Ren Dong Teng) As Oral Dose/Day Or As Wash
• CONJUNCTIVITIS, CHRONIC
• KERATITIS
• ULCERS, CORNEAL
FEVERS
• ANTIPYRETIC
IMMUNE SYSTEM RELATED DISORDERS/ TOPICS
• IMMUNE SYSTEM ENHANCEMENT: Increased Phagocytosis
INFECTIOUS DISEASES
• BACTERIAL, ANTI-: (Broad Spectrum) , Strep, Staph, Salmonella, TB, B. Dysenteriae, B.Typhi, Meningococcus, Leptospirae, Pneumonococcus, Synergistic With Lian Qiao, Can Be Used With

• TYPHOID FEVER: With Lian Qiao, Pu Gong Ying, Zi Hua Di Ding
• VIRAL, ANTI-: Strong: Flu (Pr8)
KIDNEYS
• DIURETIC
LUNGS
• LUNGS, ABSCESS: 6-15 g (15-100 g Of Vine, Ren Dong Teng) As Oral Dose/ Day Or As Wash
• PNEUMONIA, LOBAR: 6-15 g (15-100 g Of Vine, Ren Dong Teng) As Oral Dose/Day Or As Wash
• RESPIRATORY TRACT INFECTION, UPPER: 6-15 g (15-100 g Of Vine, Ren Dong Teng) As Oral Dose/Day Or As Wash
• TUBERCULOSIS, PULMONARY: IM Injection, Improved Symptoms

• TONSILLITIS, ACUTE: IM Injection
SEXUALITY, FEMALE: GYNECOLOGICAL
• CERVIX, EROSION OF: Fluid Extract Or Powder Or Herb With Gan Cao, Applied Vaginally With Cotton Balls
• MASTITIS, ACUTE: 6-15 g (15-100 g Of Vine, Ren Dong Teng) As Oral Dose/Day Or As Wash
• UTERUS, STIMULATES
SKIN
• CARBUNCLES: 6-15 g (15-100 g Of Vine, Ren Dong Teng) As Oral Dose/ Day Or As Wash
• DERMATITIS
• ERYSIPELAS: 6-15 g (15-100 g Of Vine, Ren Dong Teng) As Oral Dose/Day Or As Wash
• URTICARIA: Decoction

Clinical/Pharmaceutical Studies:

100 g Of Vine, Ren Dong Teng) As Oral Dose/Day Or As Wash

CANCER/TUMORS/ SWELLINGS/LUMPS
• ANTINEOPLASTIC: Sarcoma 180, Ehrlich Carcinoma

EYES
• CONJUNCTIVITIS, ACUTE: 6-15 g (15-100 g

Penicillin Against Drug Resistant Bacteria
• COMMON COLD: Yin Qiao San, If Taken In Early Stage
• LEPTOSPIROSIS: With Qian LI Guang (Seneciao Scandens) , Ren Dong Teng, Helped Treat And Prevent, Injection, 2-4 Days To Improve

MENTAL STATE/ NEUROLOGICAL DISORDERS
• CNS, STIMULANT: 1/ 6th Of Caffeine

MUSCULOSKELETAL/ CONNECTIVE TISSUE
• ANTISPASMODIC: Small Intestines

ORAL CAVITY

Of Fresh Herb

STOMACH/DIGESTIVE DISORDERS
• ULCERS, GASTRIC: Mildly Preventative, Extract Slightly Inhibits Occurrence Of

TRAUMA, BITES, POISONINGS
• INFLAMMATORY, ANTI-

Dose

6 - 30 gm

Common Name

Honeysuckle Flower

Contraindications

Not: Cold, Def SP/ST Diarrhea

Not: Yin Or Def Qi Sores/Ulcers

Notes

May Apply Topically
Possible To Increase Up To 120 gm For Serious Cases

LIAN QIAO
(LIAN JIAO)

連翹
(连翘)

FRUCTUS FORSYTHIAE SUSPENSAE

Traditional Functions:

1. Dispels Wind Heat
2. Clears Heat and resolves toxic Heat
3. Disperses accumulations and swellings and drains pus

Traditional Properties:

Enters: LU, HT, LV, GB,

Properties: BIT, CL

Indications:

ABDOMEN/ GASTROINTESTINAL TOPICS
• APPENDICITIS W/PAIN

ENDOCRINE RELATED DISORDERS
• THYROID, ENLARGEMENT

FEVERS
• FEVER, HIGH W/THIRST, DELIRIUM
• FEVER, SIGNIFICANT: Wind Heat

HEAD/NECK
• HEADACHE: Wind Heat

HEAT
• HEAT: In Yang Ming, Qi Level/Wei Level
• WEI & QI STAGE HEAT

IMMUNE SYSTEM RELATED DISORDERS/TOPICS
• LYMPH GLANDS, ENLARGEMENT, CHRONIC: Phlegm Nodules

• LYMPH NODES, INFLAMED
• PURPURA, ALLERGENIC

INFECTIOUS DISEASES
• COMMON COLD: Wind Heat
• FEBRILE DISEASES
• FOCAL INFECTIONS: Boils, Abscesses
• GONORRHEA
• SCROFULA

LUNGS
• LUNGS, ABSCESS W/PURULENT VOMIT

MUSCULOSKELETAL/ CONNECTIVE TISSUE
• JOINTS, PAIN, SWELLING, RED: Hot Bi, Toxic Heat With Stasis

NOSE
• SINUSITIS: Heat, Needs Sinusitis Herbs Plus

ORAL CAVITY
• THROAT, PAIN, SWOLLEN

SEXUALITY, FEMALE:

GYNECOLOGICAL
• BREASTS, SWOLLEN, PAINFUL, ABSCESS

SKIN
• BOILS, TOXIC: Heat, Toxins, Swellings
• ERYSIPELAS
• ERYTHEMA
• PURPURA, ALLERGENIC
• RASHES, INCOMPLETE EXPRESSION OF: Early Stage/ Blood Heat, Wind
• RASHES, W/PRURITUS: Clears Wind
• SKIN, SORES, SWOLLEN, TOXIC: Relieves Surface Complex/Heat, Toxins, Swelling

URINARY BLADDER
• URINATION, PAINFUL, DRIBBLING, CONCENTRATED, RED/YELLOW/TURBID

Clinical/Pharmaceutical Studies:

BLOOD RELATED DISORDERS/TOPICS
• THROMBOCYTOPENIC PURPURA: 30 g, Decoction For 2-7 Days

• PURPURA, ANAPHYLACTOID: 30 g, Decoction For 2-7 Days

INFECTIOUS DISEASES
• BACTERIAL, ANTI-:

Before Meals, 5-10 Days

LIVER
• HEPATITIS, ACUTE, VIRAL: 1:1 Syrup, 10 ml, 3x/Day Orally For 1

SKIN

Qiao, Xia Ku Cao, Xuan Dong, Mu LI, May Be Also Ground With Sesame Seeds, Take 5 g, 3x/Day

---

Clinical/Pharmaceutical Studies:

EYES
- RETINAL HEMORRHAGE: 30-35 g Decoct Over Low Heat, 3 Doses Before Meals, 20-27 Days For Marked Improvement

FEVERS
- ANTIPYRETIC: Injected

HEART
- CARDIOTONIC

IMMUNE SYSTEM RELATED DISORDERS/ TOPICS
- IMMUNE SYSTEM ENHANCEMENT: Antiinflammatory, Increased Antibody Formation, Qing Dan Injection (Lian Qiao, Jin Yin Hua, Pu Gong Ying, Chai Hu, Huang Qin, Qing Pi, Da Huang, Long Dan Cao, Dan Shen, Ban Xia (Treated) , Dan Zhu Ye)

Broad Spectrum Both Gram +/-, Shigella, Staph, TB, Diplococcus Pneumoniae, Pertussis, etc
- COMMON COLD, EARLY STAGE: Jin Yin Hua, Lian Qiao Powder, * Sang Ju Yin
- FEBRILE DISEASES: Jin Yin Hua, Lian Qiao Powder, *Sang Ju Yin
- LEPTOSPIROSIS: Weak
- PULMONARY TUBERCULOSIS: Lian Qiao, Xia Ku Cao, Xuan Dong, Mu LI, May Be Also Ground With Sesame Seeds, Take 5 g, 3x/Day, May Take Herb Alone
- VIRAL, ANTI-: Flu

KIDNEYS
- DIURETIC
- NEPHRITIS, ACUTE: 30 g Decocted Low Heat To 150 ml, Take 3x/Day

Month, Rapidly Lowers SGPT
- LIVER, DAMAGE: Lowers SGPT Enzymes, Reduced Degeneration, 100% Decoction

LUNGS
- LUNGS, ABSCESS: Endobronchial Instillation With IM Injection, 1 g/ml, Took Up To 50 Treatments
- RESPIRATORY TRACT INFECTION, UPPER: Jin Yin Hua, Lian Qiao Powder, *Sang Ju Yin

MENTAL STATE/ NEUROLOGICAL DISORDERS
- STIMULANT: CNS

PARASITES
- ANTIPARASITIC: Weak

SEXUALITY, FEMALE: GYNECOLOGICAL
- CERVIX, LYMPH NODE TUBERCULOSIS: Lian

Not: Def Qi w/Fevers

Not: Ulcerated Abscesses

Not: Yin Def Blood Heat

Not: Ulcers

Not: Yin Def

Not: Purulent Abscess

- PURPURA, ANAPHYLACTOID: 30 g, Decoction For 2-7 Days
- SKIN, INFECTIONS, DECUBITUS ULCER: Pu Gong Ying, Jin Yin Hua, Chai Hu, Da Huang, Quan Shen, Tao Ren, Chi Shao, Mu Dan Pi, Externally 1-2x/Day, 8-46 Days

STOMACH/DIGESTIVE DISORDERS
- ANTIEMETIC: Inhibits Vomiting Center In Medulla, Can Suppress Vomiting From Digitalis

TRAUMA, BITES, POISONINGS
- INFLAMMATORY, ANTI-: Herb Or Injection Of Preparation (Jin Yin Hua, Ban Lan Gen, Huang Lian, Lian Qiao, Gou Teng, Gan Cao, Long Dan Cao, Guan Zhong, Zhi Mu, Shi Gao)

Dose
6 - 15 gm

Common Name
Forsythia Fruit

Contraindications
Not: Def SP/ST w/Diarrhea

LONG KUI

龍葵
（龙葵）

HERBA SOLANI

Traditional Functions:
1. Clears Heat and relieves toxins
2. Promotes Blood circulation and disperses swelling

Traditional Properties:
Enters: LU, LV

Properties: BIT, BL, SW, C

Indications:

LIVER
- HEPATITIS, ACUTE

LUNGS
- BRONCHITIS, CHRONIC

SKIN
- ABSCESS
- CARBUNCLES
- ERYSIPELAS

- FURUNCLES

TRAUMA, BITES, POISONINGS
- SPRAINS
- TRAUMA, EXTERNAL

Clinical/Pharmaceutical Studies:
- SHOCK, HISTAMINE
- SHOCK, INSULIN

BLOOD RELATED DISORDERS/TOPICS
- BLOOD GLUCOSE, INCREASES: Injected
- BLOOD PRESSURE, LOWERS: Injection
- BLOOD, COAGULATON

- VERTIGO: Blood Deficiency, Used Syrup

ENDOCRINE RELATED DISORDERS
- SHOCK, INSULIN

FEVERS
- ANTIPYRETIC

IMMUNE SYSTEM RELATED DISORDERS/

Divide, Take 3x/Day, For 10 Days, Best Results In Simple Type, Fruit May Be Better
- EXPECTORANT

MENTAL STATE/ NEUROLOGICAL DISORDERS
- CNS, STIMULANT

Of 30 gm Orally, 2 Doses/ Day, 7-25 Days, Marked Antipruritic
- ECZEMA: Decoction Of 30 gm Orally, 2 Doses/Day, 7-25 Days, Marked Antipruritic
- FUNGAL, ANTI-: Strong
- URTICARIA: Press

Clinical/Pharmaceutical Studies:

REDUCES
- **LEUKOPENIA:**
Decoction Of Chuan Xiong,
Long Kui

**CANCER/TUMORS/
SWELLINGS/LUMPS**
- **CANCER:** Cervical,
Esophagus, Breast, Lung,
Liver–Decoction/Injection,
Helped Symptoms In Most,
Some Had Remission

**CIRCULATION
DISORDERS**
- **HYPERTENSION:**
Decocted Then
Concentrated To Paste,
Then Pills, 0.2 g, 10-20
Pills In 1-2 Doses/Day, For
10 Days, Hypotension
Began In 2-7 Days

**EARS/HEARING
DISORDERS**

TOPICS
- **ALLERGIES,**
PROTECTS AGAINST
- **IMMUNE RESPONSE:**
Stimulates Antibody
Formation

INFECTIOUS DISEASES
- **BACTERIAL, ANTI-:**
Staph.Aureus, Shigella, S.
Typhi, Roteus, E.Coli,
Pseudomonas Aeruginosa,
Virio Cholerae

LUNGS
- **ANTIASTHMATIC**
- **ANTITUSSIVE:** 60%
ETOH Extract Of Fruit
Showed Marked Effect
- **BRONCHITIS,**
CHRONIC: Compound
Long Kui Tablet (Long Kui
30 g, Jie Geng 10 g, Gan
Cao 3 g Daily Dose)

**PAIN/NUMBNESS/
GENERAL
DISCOMFORT**
- **ANALGESIC**

**SEXUALITY, FEMALE:
GYNECOLOGICAL**
- **CERVIX, EROSION OF:**
Decoction Then
Concentrated, Applied
With Stringed Cotton Ball,
Remove After 24 Hrs,
Treat 1-2 X/Week For
Minimum 8 Applications
- **LEUKORRHEA:** 30 Gr
Long Kui, 30 gm Ji Guan
Hua (Flos Celosiae
Cristatae) Decocted
Together, Orally 2 Doses/
Day

SKIN
- **BURNS**
- **DERMATITIS:** Decoction

Whole Plant, Less Roots,
Into Balls Then Rub
Locally Until Green Stain
Forms, 2-3x/Day, Cured 4-
5 Days

**TRAUMA, BITES,
POISONINGS**
- **INFLAMMATORY, ANTI-
:** Cortisone-Like
- **SNAKE BITES:** 300%
Decoction Gave 10%
Protection Against Cobra
Venom In Mice, Increased
To 50% If Mu Gua,
Japanese Form Of Kuan
Dong Hua (Petasites
Japonicus Fruit) Added (1:
1:1) , *1:1 Long Kui, He
Ye Made Into Paste For
Topical Application Plus
Oral Chinese Medications,
100%

Dose

15 - 30 gm

Common Name

Nightshade

Contraindications

Not: Pregnancy

Notes

Has Possible Mild Atropine-Like Actions

LOU LU

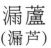

漏蘆
(漏芦)

RADIX
RHAPONTICI SEU
ECHINOPS

Traditional Functions:

1. Subdues Heat and relieves toxic Heat
2. Promotes lactation

Traditional Properties:

Enters: LI, ST,

Properties: BIT, SA, C

Indications:

BOWEL RELATED DISORDERS
- **HEMORRHOIDS**

INFECTIOUS DISEASES
- **SCROFULA**

SEXUALITY, FEMALE:

GYNECOLOGICAL
- **LACTATION, INSUFFICIENT**
- **MASTITIS, ACUTE**

SKIN
- **BOILS, ON BACK**

- **SKIN, SUPPURATIVE**
INFECTIONS W/PAIN
- **SORES/ULCERS, INITIAL STAGE**

TRAUMA, BITES, POISONINGS
- **INFLAMMATION**

Clinical/Pharmaceutical Studies:

**BLOOD RELATED DISORDERS/
TOPICS**
- **BLOOD PRESSURE, LOWERS**

**MENTAL STATE/
NEUROLOGICAL DISORDERS**
- **STRYCHNINE-LIKE TO CNS**

SKIN
- **FUNGAL, ANTI-:** Aqueous
Extract, Skin, Restrains Growth

Dose

3 - 12 gm

Contraindications

Not: Pregnancy
Not: Def Qi

MA BO

馬勃
（马勃）

FRUCIFICATIO LASIOSPHAERAE

Traditional Functions:

1. Clears Heat, relieves toxic Heat and soothes the throat
2. Stops bleeding: topical application for oral cavity and lips

Traditional Properties:

Enters: LU,

Properties: SP, N

Indications:

HEMORRHAGIC DISORDERS
* BLEEDING, LIPS/ORAL CAVITY: Topical
* HEMATEMESIS
* HEMORRHAGE: Topical

LUNGS
* COUGH: Wind Heat/Lung Heat
* LUNG HEAT: Cough
ORAL CAVITY
* LARYNGITIS

* THROAT, PAIN, SWOLLEN
SKIN
* ULCERS, SKIN: External
TRAUMA, BITES, POISONINGS
* FROSTBITE BLEEDING: Topical

Clinical/Pharmaceutical Studies:

* ASTRINGENT
FEVERS
* ANTIPYRETIC
HEMORRHAGIC DISORDERS
* HEMOSTATIC

INFECTIOUS DISEASES
* BACTERIAL, ANTI-: Staph A., Pseudomonas, Proteus, Strep Pneum., etc
ORAL CAVITY

* MOUTH, BLEEDING: Topical
SKIN
* FUNGAL, ANTI-: Aqueous Extract

TRAUMA, BITES, POISONINGS
* INFLAMMATORY, ANTI-
* TRAUMA, BLEEDING: Especially Nose

Dose

1.5 - 9.0 gm

Common Name

Puffball

Contraindications

Not: Chronic Cough

Notes

Use Mask, Very Dusty
Separate In Decoction w/Filter Paper--Upsets Stomach
Throat Only

MA CHI XIAN

馬齒莧
（马齿苋）

HERBA PORTULACAE OLERACEAE

Traditional Functions:

1. Clears Heat, relieves toxins, cools the Blood and controls diarrhea
2. Clears Damp Heat and toxins in the skin
3. Expels intestinal parasites
4. Relieves pain and swelling of wasp or snake bites
5. Controls postpartum bleeding

Traditional Properties:

Enters: LI, SP, LV,

Properties: SO, C

Indications:

BLOOD RELATED DISORDERS/ TOPICS
* ACCUMULATION OF BLOOD
BOWEL RELATED DISORDERS
* DIARRHEA: Damp Heat
* DYSENTERY, BLOODY STOOL, PUS: Toxic Heat/Damp Heat
HEMORRHAGIC DISORDERS
* HEMAFECIA: Heat
* HEMATURIA: Heat
* HEMORRHAGE: Cool Blood To

Stop
SEXUALITY, FEMALE: GYNECOLOGICAL
* LEUKORRHEA, BLOOD TINGED
* MENSTRUATION, DISORDERS OF: Clear Chong, Ren/Constrict Uterus, Stimulate Chong
* POSTPARTUM, UTERINE BLEEDING
SKIN
* CARBUNCLES

* ERYSIPELAS
* FURUNCLES
* SKIN, SORES, SWOLLEN, TOXIC: Topical
* SORES: Damp Heat
TRAUMA, BITES, POISONINGS
* SNAKE BITES
* WASP STINGS
URINARY BLADDER
* URINATION, DRIBBLING: Heat

Clinical/Pharmaceutical Studies:

ABDOMEN/ GASTROINTESTINAL TOPICS
• APPENDICITIS: w/Pu Gong Ying
BOWEL RELATED DISORDERS
• DYSENTERY: Decoction,

Fresh 90% Acute, 60% Chronic, Sulfa-Like Effectiveness
CIRCULATION DISORDERS
• VASOCONSTRICTOR
INFECTIOUS DISEASES
• BACTERIAL, ANTI-:

ETOH Extract–Shigella, Salmonella, Staph, B.Typhi, E.Coli
KIDNEYS
• DIURETIC
PARASITES
• HOOKWORMS: Decoction

SEXUALITY, FEMALE: GYNECOLOGICAL
• UTERUS, STIMULATES: Causes Contractions, Similar To Ergometrine
SKIN
• FUNGAL, ANTI-: Varies

Dose

6 - 60 gm

Common Name

Purslane

Contraindications

Not: Pregnancy

Not: Cold Def SP/ST

MU MIAN HUA

木棉花

FLOS GOSSAMPINI

Traditional Functions:

1. Clears Heat and removes toxins
2. Promotes diuresis
3. Controls bleeding

Traditional Properties:

Enters: UB

Properties: SW, CL

Indications:

BOWEL RELATED DISORDERS
• DIARRHEA
• DYSENTERY, RED

SEXUALITY, FEMALE: GYNECOLOGICAL
• UTERINE BLEEDING

SKIN
• SUPPURATION

Clinical/Pharmaceutical Studies:

• HISTAMINE: Contains 6mg/gm In   Bud

Dose

6 - 9 gm

Common Name

Cotton Flower

PU GONG YING

蒲公英

HERBA TARAXACI MONGOLICI CUM RADICE

Traditional Functions:

1. Clears Heat and relieves toxins--particularly Liver Heat
2. Reduces abscesses and dissipates nodules, particularly if firm and hard
3. Promotes lactation in cases where it is insufficient or absent from Heat
4. Promotes urination and clears Heat

Traditional Properties:

Enters: ST, LV,

Properties: BIT, SW, C

Indications:

ABDOMEN/ GASTROINTESTINAL TOPICS
• APPENDICITIS W/PAIN
• INTESTINES, ABSCESS
IMMUNE SYSTEM RELATED DISORDERS/TOPICS
• LYMPH NODES, SWELLING
INFECTIOUS DISEASES
• SCROFULA

CONNECTIVE TISSUE
• JOINTS, PAIN, SWELLING, RED: Hot Bi, Toxic Heat With Stasis
SEXUALITY, FEMALE: GYNECOLOGICAL
• BREASTS, SWOLLEN, PAINFUL, ABSCESS
• LACTATION, INSUFFICIENT: Heat

Swellings
• FURUNCLES: Toxic
• SKIN, SORES, SWOLLEN: Heat, Toxins, Swelling
• SORES, FIRM, HARD: Topical, Too
STOMACH/DIGESTIVE DISORDERS
• STOMACH FIRE

Indications:

LIVER
- HEPATITIS
- JAUNDICE: Damp Heat
- LIVER HEAT: Red, Swollen Eyes

MUSCULOSKELETAL/
- MASTITIS, ACUTE

SKIN
- ABSCESS
- BOILS, TOXIC: Heat, Toxins,

URINARY BLADDER
- URINATION, PAINFUL, DRIBBLING, CONCENTRATED, RED/YELLOW/TURBID

Clinical/Pharmaceutical Studies:

ABDOMEN/ GASTROINTESTINAL TOPICS
- APPENDICITIS, ACUTE: With Ma Chi Xian, *Bai Jiang Cao, Pu Gong Ying Tang, Lan Wei Qing Hua Decoction (Appendicitis Resolving Decoction) (Pu Gong Ying, Jin Yin Hua, Da Huang, Chi Shao, Chuan Lian Zi, Tao Ren, Gan Cao, Mu Dan Pi) – Not Effective For Chronic/ Recurrent Appendicitis

BOWEL RELATED DISORDERS
- LAXATIVE, MILD

CANCER/TUMORS/ SWELLINGS/LUMPS
- LUNG CANCER: Active Against

EARS/HEARING DISORDERS
- EARS, OTITIS MEDIA: Milky Juice Of Fresh Plant Into Ear

EYES
- CONJUNCTIVITIS: Herb, Ju Hua/Ye Ju Hua Decoction Oral, Second Cooking, Luke Warm Use As An Eye Wash

GALL BLADDER
- BILE SECRETION: Increases 40%, Through Action On Liver, Greater Than Yin Chen, Major Component Is Resin
- CHOLECYSTITIS, ACUTE: Hai Jin Sha, Lian Qian Cao, Jiang Huang, Chuan Lian Zi, Nian Shen Cao With Acupuncture/ Small Doses Of Antispasmodics
- CHOLECYSTITIS, CHRONIC: Herb, Xia Ku Cao, Che Qian Cao, Yin Chen
- GALL BLADDER, SPASMS: Extract
- GALL BLADDER, STONES: Extract

HEAD/NECK
- NECK, CELLULITIS OF: Topical Paste Of Fresh Herb/Ointment Of Herb Root

HEART
- ANGIOMA, CONGENITAL: (Usually Benign Tumor, Consisting Of Blood Vessels) Use Milky Juice Of

IMMUNE SYSTEM RELATED DISORDERS/ TOPICS
- IMMUNE SYSTEM ENHANCEMENT

INFECTIOUS DISEASES
- BACTERIAL, ANTI-: Aqueous Extract, Synergized With Trimethoprim--Staph A., Echo, Leptospira, TB, Pseudo, Strep, Neisseria, Diplococcus Pneumoniae, Diphteriae, Proteus Vulgaris, Shigella Dysenteriae
- INFECTIONS: Especially Effective Against Those Caused By Gram+ Bacteria Or Drug Resistant Strains Of Staph, Strep
- PAROTITIS: Fresh Herb/ With Zi Hua Di Ding Crushed Together, Mix With Egg White Into Paste, Use To Treat Topically
- VIRAL, ANTI-: Echo

KIDNEYS
- DIURETIC
- PYELONEPHRITIS: With Jin Yin Hua, Di Gu Pi, Mu Dan Pi, Zhi Mu

LIVER
- HEPATITIS, ACUTE, ICTERIC: Decoction Accelerated Recovery Of Liver Function
- LIVER, TOXINS DAMAGED: Helped

Reduce Effects Of As 200% Decoction

LUNGS
- BRONCHITIS, ACUTE: See: Lung Topic, Respiratory Tract Infections (Pu Gong Ying)
- RESPIRATORY TRACT, UPPER INFECTION: 30-60 g Decoction, Decoct With White Wine To Speed Effect, Use With Zi Hua Di Ding, Zi Su Ye, Gan Jiang, Ye Ju Hua, Da Qing Ye Or Ban Lan Gen

MUSCULOSKELETAL/ CONNECTIVE TISSUE
- OSTEOMYELITIS

ORAL CAVITY
- MOUTH, SUBMAXILLARITIS: Topical Paste Of Fresh Herb/Ointment Of Herb Root
- PHARYNGO-LARYNGITIS: See: Lung Topic, Respiratory Tract Infections (Pu Gong Ying)
- THROAT, SORE, ACUTE: See Respiratory Tract Infections (Pu Gong Ying)
- TONSILLITIS, ACUTE: See: Lung Topic, Respiratory Tract Infections (Pu Gong Ying) , *Ju Hua Tang (Pu Gong Ying, Ju Hua, Ban Lan Gen, Mai Dong, Jie Geng, Gan Cao

SEXUALITY, FEMALE: GYNECOLOGICAL
- CERVIX, EROSION OF: Solution Of Herb, Ya Zhi Cao/Herb Powder, Zi He Che
- LACTATION, INCREASES
- MASTITIS, ACUTE: Best In Early, Non-Suppurative Forms, *30 g As Decoction, 1-2x/Day

Warmed Over Low Heat, Take With Some Wine, * May Take Herb With Ye Ju Hua/Jin Yin Hua, Lian Qiao, Tian Hua Fen, Qing Pi, Chuan Shan Jia, Chai Hu Plus Treat Infection Area With Herb With Alum, Rapid Results, *Soak In A Dry Wine, 1:5 For 5-7 Days, Take Orally, 15ml 3x/ Day, Best In Early Treated Cases (Less Than 4 Days Old) , *36 g Decoction With LU Jiao Shuang, Some Weak Rice Wine With Topical Application, 80% Marked Improvement

SKIN
- BACK, CELLULITIS OF: Topical Paste Of Fresh Herb/Ointment Of Herb Root
- BOILS: Decoction Singly Or Complex Herbal Formula/Topical Application Or Fresh, Crushed Herb
- BURNS, MILD: Fresh Root Juice
- FUNGAL, ANTI-: Skin

STOMACH/DIGESTIVE DISORDERS
- GASTRITIS, CHRONIC: 15 g Decocted 2x With Tablespoon Rice Wine, Combined Decoction , 3 Doses, After Meals
- STOMACHIC
- ULCERS, GASTRIC/ DUODENAL: Root Powder, 1.5g, 3x/Day After Eating

TRAUMA, BITES, POISONINGS
- SNAKE BITES: (Pit Viper) With Radix/Herba Cirsium Japonicum, Ma Chi Xian, Wu Ling Zhi, Shang LU? (Phytolacca Acinosa)

Dose
6 - 30 gm

Common Name
Dandelion

Contraindications
Not: Def, Cold Syndrome

Notes
Internal Or External Application

Overdose: May Cause Diarrhea

May Increase To 60 gm

Few Side Effects, Sometimes Nausea, Vomiting,
Stomache, Diarrhea

QING DAI   青黛   INDIGO PULVERATA LEVIS

Traditional Functions:

1. Clears Heat and resolves toxic Heat
2. Cools Blood: reduces skin problems from Blood Heat

Traditional Properties:

Enters: LU, LV, ST,

Properties: BIT, C

Indications:

CHILDHOOD DISORDERS
• CONVULSIONS, CHILDHOOD
FEVERS
• FEVER, HIGH: Children
HEMORRHAGIC DISORDERS
• EPISTAXIS
• HEMOPTYSIS
INFECTIOUS DISEASES
• MUMPS
• PESTILENT DISEASES
LUNGS
• LUNG HEAT: Cough

MENTAL STATE/
  NEUROLOGICAL DISORDERS
• CONVULSIONS, FEVER, ACUTE
MUSCULOSKELETAL/
  CONNECTIVE TISSUE
• SPASMS, W/FEVER, ACUTE
ORAL CAVITY
• MOUTH, INFLAMMATION:
  Topical
• ORAL INFLAMMATION: Topical
• THROAT, SORE: Topical
• THRUSH

SKIN
• BOILS
• DERMATITIS
• ECZEMA, CHRONIC
• ERYSIPELAS
• MACULA
• PAPULES
• SKIN, SORES, SWOLLEN, TOXIC:
  Topical
TRAUMA, BITES, POISONINGS
• WOUNDS, INFECTED

Clinical/Pharmaceutical Studies:

CANCER/TUMORS/
  SWELLINGS/LUMPS
• ANTINEOPLASTIC:
  Indirubin, Moderate
  Activity, Injections
  Stronger, Lung, Breast
  Cancer

• LEUKEMIA, CHRONIC
  GRANULOCYTIC: Dang
  Gui LU Hui Pian, Qing
  Dai More Effective Alone,
  But Indirubin Better
  Therapeutic Effects, Faster,
  Lower Dose, Milder Side

Effects
INFECTIOUS DISEASES
• BACTERIAL, ANTI-:
  ETOH Extract-Staph
  Aureus, Cholera, Bacillus
  Anthracis, Shegella
• MUMPS: Topical With

Vinegar
LIVER
• HEPATITIS, VIRAL
• LIVER, PROTECTANT
SKIN
• ECZEMA: Topical
  Ointment

Dose
0.9 - 3.9 gm

Common Name
Natural Indigo

Contraindications
Not: Cold Stomach

Notes
Made From Da Qing Ye
Some Abdominal Pain, Diarrhea, Nausea From Oral Use

REN DONG TENG   忍冬藤   CAULIS/FOLIUM
(JIN YIN HUA TENG)   LONICERAE

Traditional Functions:

1. Clears Heat and resolves toxic Heat
2. Clears Damp Heat in the Lower Burner
3. Dispels Wind Heat
4. Dispels Summer Heat
5. Opens the channels and reduces Wind Damp Heat pain

Traditional Properties:

Enters: LU, HT,

Properties: SW, C

Indications:

BOWEL RELATED DISORDERS
• DYSENTERY
INFECTIOUS DISEASES
• COMMON COLD W/FEVER

LIVER
• HEPATITIS, INFECTIOUS
**MUSCULOSKELETAL/
CONNECTIVE TISSUE**

• ARTHRITIS, RHEUMATIC: Wind
Damp Bi
• JOINTS, PAIN, SWELLING, RED:
Hot Bi

Clinical/Pharmaceutical Studies:

**BLOOD RELATED DISORDERS/
TOPICS**
• BLOOD GLUCOSE, INCREASES:
Oral Decoction
INFECTIOUS DISEASES
• BACTERIAL, ANTI-: Stap Aureus,
B.Subtilis

KIDNEYS
• DIURETIC: Mild
LIVER
• HEPATITIS, INFECTIOUS: 60 g
Decoction, 2x/Day, 15 Days, Helps
Symptoms, Recovered Liver

Functions
**MUSCULOSKELETAL/
CONNECTIVE TISSUE**
• ANTISPASMODIC
TRAUMA, BITES, POISONINGS
• INFLAMMATORY, ANTI-

Dose

9 - 30 gm

Common Name

Honeysuckle Stem

Contraindications

Not: Cold, Deficient Patient

SHAN DOU GEN   山豆根   RADIX
                                        SOPHORAE
                                        SUBPROSTRATAE

Traditional Functions:

1. Relieves Lung Heat cough
2. Removes toxic Heat, soothes throat, disperses swelling and controls pain

Traditional Properties:

Enters: LU, LI, HT,

Properties: BIT, C

Indications:

**ABDOMEN/
GASTROINTESTINAL TOPICS**
• ABDOMEN, PAIN OF
BOWEL RELATED DISORDERS
• CONSTIPATION
• DYSENTERY
• HEMORRHOIDS: With Powder
**CANCER/TUMORS/SWELLINGS/
LUMPS**
• SWELLINGS, HEAT: Topical
• SWELLINGS, PAIN: Topical
Powder
• THROAT CANCER
• URINARY BLADDER CANCER
HEAD/NECK

• HEAD, ULCERS: Topical
HEAT
• HEAT, ACCUMULATED
LIVER
• JAUNDICE, ACUTE
LUNGS
• COUGH: Lung Heat
• DYSPNEA
• LUNG CANCER
**MENTAL STATE/
NEUROLOGICAL DISORDERS**
• RESTLESSNESS W/THIRST
ORAL CAVITY
• ABSCESS, THROAT

• GUMS, PAIN, SWELLING
• MOUTH, SORE
• THROAT ABSCESS
• THROAT CANCER
• THROAT, PAIN, SWOLLEN
SKIN
• SCABIES: Topical
TRAUMA, BITES, POISONINGS
• DOG BITES: Topical
• INSECT BITES: Topical Powder
• SNAKE BITES: Topical Powder
• SPIDER BITE: Topical Powder
URINARY BLADDER
• URINARY BLADDER CANCER

Clinical/Pharmaceutical Studies:

**ABDOMEN/
GASTROINTESTINAL
TOPICS**
• ENTERITIS
**BLOOD RELATED
DISORDERS/TOPICS**
• BLOOD, WBC: Increases,
Can Be Used With
Radiation/Chemo Therapy
To Reduce WBC Loss,
Purified Alkaloid Injected,
200-400 mg 1-2x/Day, 4-

SWELLINGS/LUMPS
• ANTINEOPLASTIC:
Cervical Cancer, et al
FEVERS
• ANTIPYRETIC
HEART
• ARRHYTHMIAS:
Purified Alkaloids, 0.25 g/
Tab, 2-4 Tabs 3x/Day For 1
Week, 4-6 Tabs 3x/Day
2nd Week, Good Results,
Better For Premature Beats,

(Strong) , TB, Cholera
LUNGS
• ASTHMA: Histamine
Induced, Or Ku Shen
• BRONCHITIS,
CHRONIC ASTHMATIC:
Pure Alkaloid In 100 mg
Caps, 3x/Day For 10 Days,
88-100% Effective, Some
Short Term Dizziness,
Stomach Discomfort
ORAL CAVITY

Course, Good Effect
• ENDOMETRITIS: :
Injection Of Purified
Alkaloids, 50-100 mg, 2-3x/
Day For 10 Days, 1-3
Courses
• PELVIC
INFLAMMATORY
DISEASE, CHRONIC:
Injection Of Purified
Alkaloids, 50-100 mg, 2-3x/
Day For 10 Days, 1-3

Clinical/Pharmaceutical Studies:

37 Days, Radiation Group
Better Response, Results
In 1 Week
**BOWEL RELATED
DISORDERS**
• DYSENTERY,
BACILLARY: Purified,
0.3 g/Tab, 2-3 Tabs, 3x/
Day, Same As Antibiotics
CANCER/TUMORS/

Results After 1 Week
**IMMUNE SYSTEM
RELATED DISORDERS/
TOPICS**
• ALLERGIES: Markedly
Suppressed With Injection
INFECTIOUS DISEASES
• BACTERIAL, ANTI-:
Beta Strep, Shigella,
Proteus, E.Coli, Staph

• LARYNGITIS
• TONSILLITIS
**SEXUALITY, FEMALE:
GYNECOLOGICAL**
• CERVIX, EROSION OF:
Apply Sterilized, 1-3 Days,
10 Applications, 78%
Effective, Foam Spray Of
Purified Alkaloids Used,
Too, 2x/Week 5 Sprays =

Courses
SKIN
• ALLERGIES: Markedly
Suppressed With Injection
• FUNGAL, ANTI-:
Dermatophytes, Fungi
**STOMACH/DIGESTIVE
DISORDERS**
• ULCERS, GASTRIC:
Prevented By Injection

Dose

4.5 - 12.0 gm

Contraindications

Not: Diarrhea From Cold Def SP

Precautions

Watch: Nausea

Notes

Safe Anticancer, No Reduction Of WBC
pwdr: 2-6 gm
Active Components Similar To Ku Shen

SHE GAN

射干

RHIZOMA BELAMCANDAE CHINENSIS

Traditional Functions:

1. Removes toxic Heat, soothes throat, controls pain
2. Descends Qi and resolves Phlegm
3. Disperses Blood stagnation and removes swellings

Traditional Properties:

Enters: LU, LV,

Properties: BIT, C

Indications:

**ABDOMEN/
GASTROINTESTINAL TOPICS**
• ABDOMEN, MASS
**CANCER/TUMORS/SWELLINGS/
LUMPS**
• SWELLINGS, PAIN: Topical
CHEST
• CHEST, DISTRESS, FULLNESS
INFECTIOUS DISEASES
• MALARIA W/LUMP
LUNGS
• COUGH: Lung Heat/Qi Reflux

• COUGH IN CHILDREN
• COUGH, PROFUSE SPUTUM:
Lung Heat
• COUGH, WHEEZING W/SPUTUM
OBSTRUCTION
• HYPERPNEA
• LUNGS, DYSPNEA: Lung Heat
• TUBERCULOSIS
ORAL CAVITY
• GLOTTIS, EDEMA
• LARYNGITIS, ACUTE

• THROAT OBSTRUCTION,
PHLEGM, SALIVA
• THROAT, PAIN, SWOLLEN
• THROAT, SORE, BI NUMBNESS
PHLEGM
• PHLEGM OBSTRUCTION
**SEXUALITY, FEMALE:
GYNECOLOGICAL**
• AMENORRHEA
SKIN
• ULCERS, TOXIC: External

Clinical/Pharmaceutical Studies:

**BLOOD RELATED DISORDERS/
TOPICS**
• BLOOD PRESSURE, LOWERS,
ETHANOL
FEVERS
• ANTIPYRETIC
INFECTIOUS DISEASES
• BACTERIAL, ANTI-

• VIRAL, ANTI-: Pharyngitis
Causing
ORAL CAVITY
• PHARYNGITIS: Antiviral, High
Doses
• SALIVATION, INCREASES
**PAIN/NUMBNESS/GENERAL
DISCOMFORT**

• ANALGESIC
SKIN
• DERMATITIS, FIELD: Topical w/
Salt
• FUNGAL, ANTI-: As Decoction,
Many Skin
TRAUMA, BITES, POISONINGS
• INFLAMMATORY, ANTI-

Dose

3 - 9 gm

Contraindications

Not: Pregnancy
Not: Def SP Diarrhea

SHI SHANG BAI

石上柏

HERBA SELAGINELLAE DOEDERLEINII

Traditional Functions:

1. Clears Heat and eliminates toxic Heat
2. Clears Damp Heat
3. Disperses Blood stagnation, accumulations and swellings
4. Shrinks masses and disperses accumulation

Traditional Properties:

Enters: LV, LU

Properties: SW, SP, N,

Indications:

CANCER/TUMORS/SWELLINGS/ LUMPS
• CANCER: Lung, Skin, Throat, Nasal, Liver
FEVERS
• FEVER: Lung Heat
FLUID DISORDERS
• ASCITES, FROM LIVER CIRRHOSIS: Damp Heat
IMMUNE SYSTEM RELATED DISORDERS/TOPICS

• ADENITIS: (Inflammation Of Lymph Gland)
LIVER
• ASCITES, LIVER CIRRHOSIS: Damp Heat
• HEPATITIS, CHRONIC
• JAUNDICE: From Liver Cirrhosis: Damp Heat
• LIVER, CIRRHOSIS
LUNGS
• COUGH: Lung Heat

• LUNG INFLAMMATION, UPPER AREA
• PNEUMONIA
ORAL CAVITY
• THROAT, SORE: Lung Heat
SKIN
• ULCERS, SKIN: Lung Heat
URINARY BLADDER
• URINARY BLADDER DAMP HEAT

Clinical/Pharmaceutical Studies:

CANCER/TUMORS/SWELLINGS/ LUMPS
• TUMORS, LIVER, LUNG,

THROAT, NOSE W/CHEMO/ RADIATION THERAPY
SEXUALITY, FEMALE:

GYNECOLOGICAL
• MOLE, MALIGNANT HYDATIDIFORM

Dose

15 - 60 gm

Common Name

Greater Selaginella

Notes

Use Up To 60 g For Cancers
Fresh Material Used Generally: 60-240 g

SHU QI

蜀漆

FOLIUM /PLANTULA DICHORAE FEBRIFUGAE

Traditional Functions:

1. Relieves malaria

do radix Dichrose

Traditional Properties:

Enters: LU, HT, LV

Properties: BIT, SP, C, TX

Indications:

INFECTIOUS DISEASES

• MALARIA

• MALARIA, CHILLS, FEVER OF

Clinical/Pharmaceutical Studies:

INFECTIOUS DISEASES

• MALARIA, ANTI-: Greater Than

Chan Shan

Dose

3 - 18 gm

Notes

5x As Effective As Chang Shan (Root) Against Malaria

SHU YANG QUAN
(BAI MAO TENG)

蜀羊泉/
白毛藤

HERBA SOLANI LYRATI

Traditional Functions:

1. Clears Heat and removes toxins
2. Promotes diuresis
3. Removes Wind

Traditional Properties:

Enters:

Properties: SW, C

Indications:

FLUID DISORDERS
• ASCITES
• EDEMA
INFECTIOUS DISEASES
• MALARIA
LIVER

• JAUNDICE
MUSCULOSKELETAL/
  CONNECTIVE TISSUE
• ARTHRITIS, PAIN
SKIN

• ERYSIPELAS
• FURUNCLES
URINARY BLADDER
• LIN DISEASE, PAINFUL
  URINATION SYNDROME

Clinical/Pharmaceutical Studies:

CANCER/TUMORS/SWELLINGS/
LUMPS
• CANCER, ANTI-: With Da Zao (1:
  1) :Inhibits Ascitic Carcinoma

IMMUNE SYSTEM RELATED
DISORDERS/TOPICS
• IMMUNE SYSTEM
  ENHANCEMENT: With (1:1) Da

Jao, Increase Antibody Formation
And Non-Specific Immune Response
SKIN
• FUNGAL, ANTI-: Some

Dose

15 - 24 gm

Common Name

Climbing Nightshade

SHUI XIAN GEN

水仙根

BULBUS NARCISSI

Traditional Functions:

1. Dispels Heat and Wind
2. Reduces swelings, drains pus

Traditional Properties:

Enters: HT, LU

Properties: BIT, MILD, SP

Indications:

SKIN
• BOILS

TRAUMA, BITES, POISONINGS

• INSECT BITES

Clinical/Pharmaceutical Studies:

CANCER/TUMORS/SWELLINGS/
LUMPS
• CANCER, ANTI-: Myoma, Ehrlich
  Ascitic Cancer

INFECTIOUS DISEASES
• VIRAL, ANTI-: Lymphocytic
  Choriomeningitis
SEXUALITY, FEMALE:

GYNECOLOGICAL
• UTERUS, CONTRACTION
  EFFECT

Dose

Topical

Common Name

Chinese Sacred Lilly

Notes

Topical Application Of Pounded Material

TIAN JI HUANG

田基黄
（田基黄）

HERBA HYPERICI

Traditional Functions:

1. Clears Heat and removes toxins
2. Clears Damp Heat

Traditional Properties:

Enters: LU

Properties: BIT, SW, BL, C

Indications:

ORAL CAVITY
• TONSILLITIS
SKIN

• DERMATOSIS: (Non-Inflammatory Skin Disorder) As Lotion

TRAUMA, BITES, POISONINGS
• TRAUMA, INTERNAL/EXTERNAL

Clinical/Pharmaceutical Studies:

BLOOD RELATED DISORDERS/TOPICS
• BLOOD PRESSURE, LOWERS:

Slight
INFECTIOUS DISEASES
• BACTERIAL, ANTI-: Oxidized

Extract–Mycobacterium, Pneumoccus, Staph, Cholerae, Shigella

Dose

15 - 60 gm

Common Name

ST John's Wort (Related To)

Notes

Hypericin May Cause Photosensitive Dermatitis & Hair Loss

TU FU LING

土茯苓
（土茯苓）

RHIZOMA SMILACIS GLABRAE

Traditional Functions:

1. Clears Damp Heat toxins
2. Clears Damp Heat from the skin
3. Dispels Dampness and opens the channels

Traditional Properties:

Enters: ST, LV,

Properties: SW, BL, N

Indications:

BOWEL RELATED DISORDERS
• DIARRHEA: Spleen Weak
EXTREMITIES
• LIMBS, PAINFUL CONTRACTURE OF LIGAMENTS, BONES
IMMUNE SYSTEM RELATED DISORDERS/TOPICS
• LYMPH NODES, PAIN
INFECTIOUS DISEASES
• LEPTOSPIROSIS
• SYPHILIS
KIDNEYS

• DIURETIC, MILD
LIVER
• JAUNDICE: Damp Heat
MUSCULOSKELETAL/CONNECTIVE TISSUE
• ARTHRITIS, RHEUMATOID
• JOINTS, PAIN: Damp Heat
• SPASMS, MUSCLES-TENDONS
SEXUALITY, FEMALE: GYNECOLOGICAL
• LEUKORRHEA: Damp Heat
SKIN

• ABSCESS
• CARBUNCLES
• ECZEMA: Damp Heat
• FURUNCLES
• SKIN, SORES: Damp Heat
• SKIN, ULCERS, RED BAYBERRY, TOXIC
• ULCERS, MALIGNANT
URINARY BLADDER
• URINATION, PAINFUL, DRIBBLING, CONCENTRATED, RED/YELLOW/TURBID

Clinical/Pharmaceutical Studies:

CANCER/TUMORS/SWELLINGS/LUMPS
• CANCER, ANTI-: (Need 500-750g)
• TUMOR, ANTI-: (Need 30-60 g)
INFECTIOUS DISEASES

• LEPTOSPIROSIS: Prevents/Active Stage, Too
• SYPHILIS: w/Jin Yin Hua, Gan Cao, Bai Xian Pi, Ma Chi Xian, Pu

Gong Ying (Very Good For 2/3 Stage)
TRAUMA, BITES, POISONINGS
• MERCURY POISONING, NEUTRALIZES

Dose

9 - 30 gm

Common Name

Glabrous Breenbrier Rz

Contraindications

Not: w/Black Tea (Tannin)

Precautions

Watch: Def LV/KI Yin

TU NIU XI

土牛膝

RADIX ACHYRANTHIS

Traditional Functions:

1. Subdues and eliminates the toxic Heat

Traditional Properties:

Enters: KI, LV,

Properties: BIT, SO, N

Indications:

INFECTIOUS DISEASES
• DIPHTHERIA, SORE THROAT
ORAL CAVITY

• THROAT, SORE, SWOLLEN
SKIN
• ABSCESS

TRAUMA, BITES, POISONINGS
• SNAKE BITES: Antidote

Clinical/Pharmaceutical Studies:

INFECTIOUS DISEASES
• DIPHTHERIA: Decoction/Powder,

Treatment/Toxin Antidote
LUNGS

• PNEUMONIA, CHILDHOOD: By Adenovirus

Dose

15 - 30 gm

Contraindications

Not: Pregnancy

WO NIU

蜗牛
(蜗牛)

EULOTAE

Traditional Functions:

1. Clears Heat, removes toxins and disperses swelling

Traditional Properties:

Enters: GB, LV

Properties: SA, C

Indications:

BOWEL RELATED DISORDERS
• HEMORRHOIDS
• RECTAL PROLAPSE
ENDOCRINE RELATED
 DISORDERS
• DIABETES

FEVERS
• FEVER, SPASMS OF
INFECTIOUS DISEASES
• SCROFULA
ORAL CAVITY

• PHARYNGOLARYNGITIS
SKIN
• SORES, PUSTULAR
TRAUMA, BITES, POISONINGS
• INSECT BITES

Dose

30 - 60 gm

Common Name

Snail

Notes

Burnt To Ashes Or Shell

WU HUAN ZI

無患子
(无患子)

SEMEN SAPINDI

Traditional Functions:

1. Clear Heat and dispels Phlegm
2, Disperses accumulation
3. Kills intestinal parasites

Traditional Properties:

Enters: LU, LI

Properties: BIT, N

Indications:

CANCER/TUMORS/SWELLINGS/
  LUMPS
• SWELLINGS, TOXIC
CHILDHOOD DISORDERS
• MALNUTRITION, CHILDHOOD
LUNGS

• COUGH, WHEEZING
ORAL CAVITY
• THROAT, SORE, SWOLLEN
SEXUALITY, FEMALE:
  GYNECOLOGICAL
• LEUKORRHEA

SKIN
• SCABIES
STOMACH/DIGESTIVE
  DISORDERS
• INDIGESTION

Dose

9 - 30 gm

Common Name

Soapberry

YA DAN ZI

鴉膽子
(鸦胆子)

FRUCTUS BRUCAE JAVANICAE

Traditional Functions:

1. Clears Heat and dries Dampness
2. Eliminates worms
3. Removes warts and corns when used topically
4. Clears dysentery-like disorders, particularly chronic or intermittent
5. Treats intermittent fever and chills which are malaria-like

Traditional Properties:

Enters: LI,

Properties: BIT, C, TX

Indications:

BOWEL RELATED DISORDERS
• DIARRHEA, CHRONIC,
  INTERMITTENT W/HARD/SOFT
  STOOL: Cold Stagnation
• DYSENTERY, AMOEBIC
• HEMORRHOIDS
EXTREMITIES

• CORNS: Topical
• PLANTAR WARTS: Topical
INFECTIOUS DISEASES
• MALARIA, CHILLS, FEVER OF
• MALARIA-LIKE SYNDROMES
PARASITES
• HOOKWORMS

• PINWORMS
SEXUALITY, FEMALE:
  GYNECOLOGICAL
• TRICHOMONAS, VAGINAL:
  Topical
SKIN
• WARTS: Topical

Clinical/Pharmaceutical Studies:

BOWEL RELATED DISORDERS
• DYSENTERY: No Effect-Shigella,
  Salmonella But Endamoiba, Malaria,
  et al
• DYSENTERY, AMOEBIC: Oral
  Ingestion, Better If Given
  Concurrently With Enema, Too
CANCER/TUMORS/SWELLINGS/
  LUMPS
• BREASTS, NIPPLE TUMORS:
  Use Oil As A Cytotoxin
• CERVICAL CANCER: Squamous,
  Oil Injection With IM Dose
• ESOPHAGEAL CANCER
• SKIN, CANCER: Paste, Aqueous
  Extract Will Kill Cells, But Also
  Normal Cells

MENTAL STATE/
  NEUROLOGICAL DISORDERS
• CNS, INHIBITOR
PARASITES
• AMOEBIC, ANTI-: Aqueous
  Extract, Killed On Contact, 1/5 To 1/
  10 Of Emetine
• ANTIPARASITIC: Inhibits Amoeba,
  Malaria, Tapeworm, Pinworm,
  Round Worms
• MOSQUITOES: Larva, Eggs Killed
  On Contact By 5-10% Extract, 18-48
  Hrs
• PINWORMS
• ROUNDWORMS
• SCHISTOSOMIASIS: By Itself Or
  With Hua Jiao Pi, Long Treatment,

SEXUALITY, FEMALE:
  GYNECOLOGICAL
• BREASTS, NIPPLE TUMORS:
  Use Oil As A Cytotoxin
• CERVIX, CANCINOMA:
  Squamous, Oil Injection With IM
  Dose
• VAGINITIS, TRICHOMONAS: 88%
  Negative, Local Perfusion Of
  Decoction
SKIN
• KELOIDS
• PAPILLOMAS: Throat, Ear, Causes
  Necrosis Of Cells, Topical
  Application Of Oil
• SKIN, CANCER: Paste, Aqueous
  Extract Will Kill Cells, But Also

Clinical/Pharmaceutical Studies:

- TUMOR, ANTI-, NIPPLES
  ESPECIALLY: Oil
  EXTREMITIES
- CORNS

20-40 Days, 100% Stool Negative
- TAPEWORMS
- TRICHOMONAS
- WHIPWORMS

Normal Cells
- WARTS: Body, Hands, Genital,
  Causes Necrosis Of Cells, Topical
  Application Of Oil

Dose

15 - 90 gm

Contraindications

Not: Def SP/ST

Precautions

Watch: Children & Pregnancy

Notes

May Cause Nausea/Vomit

Used Singly Or With Long Yan Rou
Or 10-15 Seeds, 3x/Day
Topical Application Causes Strong Irritation, Orally
May Cause Abdominal Discomfort, Nausea, Pain,
Diarrhea, Dizziness, Lassitude
Usual Mild Side Effects, But 78% Of Patients Had
Reactions
Possible Allergic Reaction To Topical Application

YU XING CAO

魚腥草
(鱼腥草)

HERBA
HOUTTUYNIAE CORDATAE

Traditional Functions:

1. Clears Heat and toxins, reduces swellings and abscesses in Lungs
2. Clears Heat and drains Dampness

Traditional Properties:

Enters: LU,

Properties: SP, <C

Indications:

BOWEL RELATED DISORDERS
- COLITIS
- DIARRHEA: Damp Heat In Large
  Intestine
- HEMORRHOIDS
- RECTAL PROLAPSE
HEMORRHAGIC DISORDERS
- HEMOPTYSIS W/PUS
INFECTIOUS DISEASES
- MALARIA

LUNGS
- COUGH: Lung Heat
- LUNG INFECTION
- LUNGS, ABSCESS W/
  HEMOPTYSIS, PUS
- LUNGS, ABSCESS W/PURULENT
  VOMIT
- LUNGS, DYSPNEA: Lung Heat
PARASITES

- WORM POISONING
SKIN
- CARBUNCLES
TRAUMA, BITES, POISONINGS
- INSECT BITES
URINARY BLADDER
- URINATION, PAINFUL,
  DRIBBLING, CONCENTRATED,
  RED/YELLOW/TURBID

Clinical/Pharmaceutical Studies:

BLOOD RELATED DISORDERS/
  TOPICS
- BLOOD PRESSURE, LOWERS
CANCER/TUMORS/SWELLINGS/
  LUMPS
- ANTINEOPLASTIC
- CANCER
CIRCULATION DISORDERS
- CAPILLARY WALLS,
  STRENGTHENS
- VASODILATOR IN KIDNEY
EARS/HEARING DISORDERS
- EARS, CHRONIC SUPPURATIVE
  OTITIS MEDIA: Ear Drops Of
  Distillate Of Herb, 95% Cure
EXTREMITIES
- HANDS, FUNGAL INFECTIONS
  OF
HEMORRHAGIC DISORDERS
- HEMOSTATIC
IMMUNE SYSTEM RELATED
  DISORDERS/TOPICS

Tablet When Known Contaminated
Water, Will Protect Against, *May
Add Qing Hao
- SURGICAL INFECTIONS: Helps
  Prevent Or Cure
- TUBERCULOSIS, ANTI-
- VIRAL, ANTI-: Decoction, Flu,
  Echo
KIDNEYS
- DIURETIC
- NEPHRITIS, CHRONIC
- VASODILATOR IN KIDNEY
LUNGS
- ANTITUSSIVE
- BRONCHITIS, CHRONIC:
  Injection Form/Concentrated Form
  Orally With Aster Agerotoides
  (Echinacea-Like Species?)
- BRONCHITIS, CHRONIC,
  GERIATRIC: With Gnaphalium
  Affine
- LUNGS, ABSCESS

- TUBERCULOSIS: Injection Form
- TUBERCULOSIS, PULMONARY
MENTAL STATE/
  NEUROLOGICAL DISORDERS
- CONVULSIVE, ANTI-
- SEDATIVE: Mild
NOSE
- RHINITIS, ATROPHIC: Nose Drop
  Preparation
- SINUSITIS, MAXILLARY,
  CHRONIC: Perfusion With Extract
PAIN/NUMBNESS/GENERAL
  DISCOMFORT
- ANALGESIC
SEXUALITY, FEMALE:
  GYNECOLOGICAL
- ADNEXITIS: Injection Form
- CERVICITIS, CHRONIC: Cotton
  Impregnated With/Injection Form
- PELVIC INFLAMMATION
SKIN
- BOILS: Local Application

Clinical/Pharmaceutical Studies:

- IMMUNE SYSTEM: Very Good, Increases WBC Phagocytosis, Other Activity

INFECTIOUS DISEASES
- ANTIBIOTIC: Strep Pneum, Staph A., TB, Gonococci, Acid-Resistant Bacteria
- FUNGAL INFECTIONS, HANDS
- HERPES SIMPLEX: Very Effective, Use Distilled Topical
- INFLUENZA
- LEPTOSPIROSIS: 15-30 g In

- LUNGS, CHRONIC OBSTRUCTIVE DISEASE: Best Injected In Acu-Pts
- PNEUMONIA: Injection Form, Bacterial/Bronchial/Childhood
- PNEUMONIA, LOBAR: With Jie Geng
- PULMONARY ABSCESSES: High Dose-30-60 gm
- RESPIRATORY TRACT INFECTION, UPPER

- PSORIASIS
- SKIN, DISORDERS: Use Distilled Topical

STOMACH/DIGESTIVE DISORDERS
- APPETITE, INCREASES: Eating Raw Herb

TRAUMA, BITES, POISONINGS
- INFLAMMATORY, ANTI-
- SURGERY, INFECTIONS FROM: Helps Prevent Or Cure

Dose

9 - 30 gm

Contraindications

Not: Def Cold Cases

Not: Yin Furuncles

Notes

Mild Side Effects: Fishy Breath

Note: Heating Eliminates Antibacterial Effect

ZAO XIU
(CHONG LOU/QI YE YI ZHI HUA)

蚤休

RHIZOMA PARIS

Traditional Functions:

!. Clears Heat and toxins
2. Resolves Phlegm
3. Disperses accumulated masses
4. Subdues Wind and stops spasms

Traditional Properties:

Enters: HT, LV

Properties: BIT, <C, <TX, N

Indications:

ABDOMEN/ GASTROINTESTINAL TOPICS
- APPENDICITIS W/PAIN

BLOOD RELATED DISORDERS/ TOPICS
- SEPTICOPYEMEIA: (Septicemia, Pyemia Together)

CANCER/TUMORS/SWELLINGS/ LUMPS
- CANCER: 15-30 gm

EXTREMITIES
- FEET, CONVULSIONS
- HANDS, CONVULSIONS

INFECTIOUS DISEASES
- SCROFULA
- TETANUS

MENTAL STATE/ NEUROLOGICAL DISORDERS
- CONVULSIONS, CHILDHOOD FROM FEVERS

- EPILEPSY

ORAL CAVITY
- THROAT, SORE

SKIN
- CARBUNCLES

TRAUMA, BITES, POISONINGS
- INFLAMMATION, ACUTE, PYOGENIC
- MOSQUITO BITES
- SNAKE BITES

Clinical/Pharmaceutical Studies:

CANCER/TUMORS/SWELLINGS/ LUMPS
- CERVICAL CANCER

INFECTIOUS DISEASES
- BACTERIAL, ANTI-: B. Dysenteriae, B.Typhi, B.Paratyphi,

Streptococci, Meningococci, etc, (May Be Stonger Than Huang Lian)

LUNGS
- ANTIASTHMATIC
- ANTITUSSIVE: Protects From Bronchial Histamine Spasms

- ASTHMA: Reduces Histamine Induced Bronchial Spasms

SEXUALITY, FEMALE: GYNECOLOGICAL
- CERVIX, CANCINOMA

Dose

6 - 9 gm

Common Name

Paris Rhizome

Contraindications

Not: Pregnancy

Not: Weak Persons

Notes

15-30 gm For Cancers

Related To Similar Herb, Quan Shen, Rz Polygoni Bistortae (Hsu P 220) Which Has Similar Uses And Properties

---

ZI HUA DI DING   紫花地丁   HERBA VIOLAE CUM RADICE

Traditional Functions:

1. Clears Heat and and resolves toxic Heat
2. Clears Hot sores: used both internally and externally

Traditional Properties:

Enters: HT, LV,

Properties: SP, BIT, C

Indications:

ABDOMEN/ GASTROINTESTINAL TOPICS
• APPENDICITIS W/PAIN
• INTESTINES, ABSCESS

EARS/HEARING DISORDERS
• EARS, SWOLLEN, PAINFUL: Toxic Heat

EYES
• EYES, PAIN, SWOLLEN, RED

INFECTIOUS DISEASES
• MUMPS
• SCROFULA

ORAL CAVITY
• THROAT, SORE, SWOLLEN: Toxic Heat

SEXUALITY, FEMALE: GYNECOLOGICAL
• BREASTS, ABSCESS OF

SKIN
• ABSCESS, HEAD, BACK: Hot, Topical, Too
• ERYSIPELAS
• FURUNCLES, DEEP ROOTED

• SKIN, DISORDERS: From Heat & Dampness
• SKIN, INFECTIONS, PYROGENIC, ACUTE
• SKIN, SORES, SWOLLEN: Heat, Toxins, Swelling
• SORES, HEAD, BACK: Hot, Topical, Too
• ULCERS, TOXIC

TRAUMA, BITES, POISONINGS
• SNAKE BITES

Clinical/Pharmaceutical Studies:

FEVERS
• ANTIPYROGENIC

INFECTIOUS DISEASES

• ANTIBIOTIC: TB, B.Dysenteriae, B.Pneumoniae, Spirochettes, et al

TRAUMA, BITES, POISONINGS
• INFLAMMATORY, ANTI-

Dose

9 - 15 gm

Common Name

Yedeon's Violet

Contraindications

Not: Def Cold

Notes

Single Herb: 30-60 gm

Purgatives

DA HUANG

大黃
（大黃）

RHIZOMA RHEI

Traditional Functions:

1. Purges excess Heat by moving the stool
2. Breaks up stagnant accumulations
3. Vitalizes and cracks congealed Blood
4. Drains Damp Heat via the stool
5. Clears Blood Heat and reckless Blood Heat
6. Clears Heat and Fire toxins--topically or internally
7. Regulates menstruation

Traditional Properties:

Enters: LI, ST, PC, LV,

Properties: BIT, C

Indications:

ABDOMEN/ GASTROINTESTINAL TOPICS
• ABDOMEN, MASS, IMMOBILE: Blood Stagnation
• ABDOMEN, PAIN OF: Food Stagnation
• ABDOMEN, PAIN OF, TENESMUS
• INTESTINES, ABSCESS W/ BLOOD STAGNATION
• INTESTINES, EXCESS HEAT: High Fever, Profuse Sweat, Thirst, Constipation, Abdominal Distension, Pain, Delirium
• INTESTINES, OBSTRUCTION, INCOMPLETE

BOWEL RELATED DISORDERS
• CONSTIPATION: Cold Accumulation/Excess/Heat/Heat Entanglement With Side Flow/Yang Ming Stage/Excess Heat In Intestine
• DIARRHEA: Food Stagnation, Most Herbs, Cooked, Charred
• DIARRHEA, EARLY STAGE
• DYSENTERY, EARLY: Acute, Hot
• HEMORRHOIDS, PAIN, SWELLING
• TENESMUS

CANCER/TUMORS/SWELLINGS/ LUMPS
• TUMORS: Blood Stasis, Herbs Used Other Than Vitalize Blood
• TUMORS, GYNECOLOGICAL

CHEST

• CHEST, STUFFINESS/FULLNESS

EYES
• EYES, HOT, SWOLLEN, PAINFUL: Blood Level Heat

FEVERS
• FEVER: Blood Level

FLUID DISORDERS
• EDEMA
• EDEMA, SEVERE: Excess Constitution

HEMORRHAGIC DISORDERS
• EPISTAXIS W/CONSTIPATION: Blood Heat
• HEMAFECIA: From Hemorroids/ Heat Stagnation
• HEMATEMESIS, W/ CONSTIPATION: Blood Heat
• HEMORRHAGE: Blood Stasis Caused, Charred/Fried Herbs/Cool Blood To Stop

INFECTIOUS DISEASES
• INFECTIONS: Topical, Too

LIVER
• JAUNDICE: Damp Heat

MENTAL STATE/ NEUROLOGICAL DISORDERS
• DELIRIUM: Yang Ming Stage/ Excess Heat In Intestine
• MANIC AGITATION

MUSCULOSKELETAL/ CONNECTIVE TISSUE
• JOINTS, PAIN, SWELLING, RED: Hot Bi, Toxic Heat With Stasis

PAIN/NUMBNESS/GENERAL

DISCOMFORT
• PAIN, FIXED: Blood Stagnation

SEXUALITY, FEMALE: GYNECOLOGICAL
• AMENORRHEA: Blood Stasis, In Addition To Vitalize Blood Herbs
• DYSMENORRHEA
• POSTPARTUM, ABDOMINAL PAIN: Blood Stasis

SIX STAGES/CHANNELS
• YANG MING ORGAN SYNDROME: High Fever, Profuse Sweat, Thirst, Constipation, Abdominal Distension, Pain, Delirium

SKIN
• BOILS, TOXIC: Heat, Toxins, Swellings, Topical
• BURNS: Topical, Too
• SKIN, SORES, SWOLLEN: Heat, Toxins, Swelling
• SKIN, SORES, SWOLLEN, TOXIC: Topical
• SKIN, SUPPURATIVE DISEASES: Topical
• SORES: Toxic Heat In Blood Level

STOMACH/DIGESTIVE DISORDERS
• FOOD ACCUMULATION W/ PALPABLE MASS

TRAUMA, BITES, POISONINGS
• TRAUMA, INJURIES: Blood Stagnation/Die Da

Clinical/Pharmaceutical Studies:

- ASTRINGENT: Tannic Acid Content, As After Effect

ABDOMEN/ GASTROINTESTINAL TOPICS
- ABDOMEN, DISTENTION OF, SEVERE: External Plaster With Vinegar On K1, Every 2 Hours
- APPENDICITIS, ACUTE: Da Cheng Qi Tang, Da Chai Hu Tang, San Huang Tang
- INTESTINES, SPASMS: Stronger Than Papaverine In Reducing
- PANCREAS, INCREASES SECRETIONS
- PANCREATITIS, ACUTE: Da Cheng Qi Tang, Da Chai Hu Tang, San Huang Tang

BLOOD RELATED DISORDERS/ TOPICS
- BLOOD CLOTTING TIME, SHORTENS
- BLOOD PRESSURE, LOWERS
- CHOLESTEROL, LOWERS
- THROMBOCYTOPENIA

BOWEL RELATED DISORDERS
- PURGATIVE: Bacteria In Intestine Increases Effect, 6-8 Hrs After Oral Intake, May Produce Secondary Constipation--Tannin

CANCER/TUMORS/SWELLINGS/ LUMPS
- ANTINEOPLASTIC: Melanoma, Breast Tumors, Liver Cancer
- LIVER CANCER: Inhibits
- MELANOMA, INHIBITS
- TUMOR, ANTI-: Liver, Melanoma, Lyphosarcoma, Breast
- TUMORS: May Cause Remission Of

CIRCULATION DISORDERS
- HYPERTENSION

EARS/HEARING DISORDERS
- EARS, SUPPURATIVE OTITIS MEDIA

EXTREMITIES
- LEGS, ULCERS

EYES
- CONJUNCTIVITIS, ACUTE

GALL BLADDER
- BILE SECRETION, INCREASES
- CHOLAGOGUE
- CHOLECYSTITIS: Da Cheng Qi Tang, Da Chai Hu Tang, San Huang Tang

HEAD/NECK
- FOLLICULITIS: Especially Staph A. Caused

HEMORRHAGIC DISORDERS
- EPISTAXIS
- HEMOPTYSIS: 1-2 Doses Of 2 g Will Stop
- HEMORRHAGE: w/Ming Fan As Powder
- HEMOSTATIC

IMMUNE SYSTEM RELATED DISORDERS/TOPICS
- ALLERGIC, ANTI-

INFECTIOUS DISEASES
- ANTIBIOTIC: Bacteriostatic To Gram+/-, Staph Aureus, Strep.
- BACTERIAL, ANTI-: Staph. Aureus, Streptococci, Pneumococci, B.Dysenteriae, Diphteriae, B.Typhi, Pseudomonas, Et.Al.
- CELLULITIS
- FEBRILE DISEASES, ACUTE: Da Cheng Qi Tang, Da Chai Hu Tang, San Huang Tang
- GONORRHEA: Used Rhein From Da Huang
- HERPES ZOSTER
- TYPHOID FEVER: Hu Jun Tang (Da Huang, Shi Gao, et al) , SI Huang Mixture (Huang Lian, Da Huang, Huang Qin, Huang Bai)
- VIRAL, ANTI-: Flu, Strongly Inhibits

KIDNEYS

- DIURETIC

LIVER
- HEPATITIS: Yin Chen Tang w/Da Huang
- LIVER, CANCER: Inhibits

ORAL CAVITY
- GUMS, ABSCESS
- LIPS, ULCERS
- PHARYNGOLARYNGITIS
- ULCERS, MOUTH: Topical

PARASITES
- ANTIPARASITIC
- SCHISTOSOMIASIS, COMPLICATIONS OF, BLEEDING ESOPHAGUS: Powder With Bai Shao, Glucose, Taken Orally, 1 Week

SEXUALITY, FEMALE: GYNECOLOGICAL
- ABORTION, BLEEDING AFTER
- BREASTS, TUMORS, INHIBITS
- LACTATION: Active Ingredients Excreted In Milk
- MENORRHAGIA
- UTERINE BLEEDING

SKIN
- BOILS
- BURNS
- ECZEMA
- FUNGAL, ANTI-: Aqueous/Ether/ Alcohol Extracts
- IMPETIGO CONTAGIOSA
- PRURITUS
- SKIN, DISORDERS
- SKIN, INFLAMMATIONS: Topical

STOMACH/DIGESTIVE DISORDERS
- STOMACHIC: Bitter Taste In Low Dose Stimulate Gastric Secretion And Appetite

TRAUMA, BITES, POISONINGS
- INFLAMMATORY, ANTI-
- TRAUMA, BLEEDING: With Ming Fan As Powder

Dose

3 - 12 gm

Common Name

Rhubarb Rhizome

Contraindications

Not: Pregnancy/Menstruation
Not: Nursing Mothers

Notes

Excess Conditions Only
Fried With Wine: Vitalizes Blood
Overboiling Weakens Purgation

Small Doses Can Constipate

To Empy Bowels Needs 9-12 g

Fever/Inflammation: 6g

Purgative Effect Mediated By Intestinal Bacterial Flora, Individual Variations Can Change Degree Of Purgation, May Actually Constipate In Some, More Often In Deficiency Patterns

Antidote To Intestinal Spasms: Either--E Jiao, Belladona, Menthol, Clove Oil, They Do Not Stop Purgation, Though

Long Term Use May Cause Liver Cirrhosis And Electrolyte Disturbances

FAN XIE YE
番瀉葉
（番泻叶）
FOLIUM SENNAE

Traditional Functions:

1. Purges excess Heat by moving the stool

Traditional Properties:

Enters: LI,

Properties: SW, BIT, C

Indications:

ABDOMEN/
GASTROINTESTINAL TOPICS
• ABDOMEN, FULLNESS OF
• ACCUMULATION
BOWEL RELATED DISORDERS

• CONSTIPATION: Habitual
Constipation/Heat
CHEST
• CHEST, DISTENTION
FLUID DISORDERS

• EDEMA, SEVERE: Excess
Constitution
STOMACH/DIGESTIVE
DISORDERS
• FOOD STAGNATION

Clinical/Pharmaceutical Studies:

BOWEL RELATED DISORDERS
• CONSTIPATION, ACUTE
• LAXATIVE, STRONG: Contracts
Colon, Similar To Da Huang
INFECTIOUS DISEASES

• BACTERIAL, ANTI-
MENTAL STATE/
NEUROLOGICAL DISORDERS
• CURARE, ANTI-

SEXUALITY, FEMALE:
GYNECOLOGICAL
• POSTPARTUM, CONSTIPATION:
Very Effective

Dose
1.5 - 9.0 gm
Common Name
Senna Leaf

Contraindications
Not: Pregnancy

Not: Menstruation Or Lactating Mothers
Notes
Overdose: Abdominal Pain, Nausea

LU HUI
蘆薈
（芦荟）
HERBA ALOES

Traditional Functions:

1. Clears Heat and moves the stool
2. Clears Heat and cools the Liver
3. Kills parasites
4. Improves digestion in cases of childhood nutritional impairment

Traditional Properties:

Enters: LI, ST, LV,

Properties: BIT, C

Indications:

BLOOD RELATED DISORDERS/
TOPICS
• ANEMIA
BOWEL RELATED DISORDERS
• CONSTIPATION: Heat
Entanglement
• CONSTIPATION, CHRONIC
CHILDHOOD DISORDERS
• NUTRITIONAL IMPAIRMENT,
CHILDHOOD
EARS/HEARING DISORDERS
• DIZZINESS: Excess Liver Channel
Heat/Heat Accumulation
• TINNITUS: Excess Liver Channel
Heat

• FEVER: Excess Liver Channel Heat
HEAD/NECK
• HEADACHE: Excess Liver
Channel Heat
INFECTIOUS DISEASES
• FUNGAL INFECTIONS: Damp,
Use Topical
LIVER
• LIVER CHANNEL HEAT W/
CONSTIPATION
MENTAL STATE/
NEUROLOGICAL DISORDERS
• CONVULSIONS
• EPILEPSY, INFANTILE
• INSOMNIA

DISORDERS/TOPICS
• MALNUTRITION: From Heat
• MALNUTRITION FEVER
ORAL CAVITY
• CARIES: External Application
PARASITES
• ASCARIASIS
SEXUALITY, FEMALE:
GYNECOLOGICAL
• AMENORRHEA
SKIN
• BURNS
STOMACH/DIGESTIVE
DISORDERS
• EPIGASTRIC DISCOMFORT:

Indications:

- VERTIGO: Liver Yang/Fire Rising
EYES
- EYES, RED: Heat Accumulation
FEVERS

- IRRITABILITY: Excess Liver
  Channel Heat/Heat Accumulation
- RESTLESSNESS
NUTRITIONAL/METABOLIC

Excess Liver Channel Heat
TRAUMA, BITES, POISONINGS
- INSECT BITES

Clinical/Pharmaceutical Studies:

BOWEL RELATED DISORDERS
- COLON CONTRACTIONS,
  STRONG: Oral/Enema Form
- PURGATIVE, STRONG
**CANCER/TUMORS/SWELLINGS/
LUMPS**
- ANTINEOPLASTIC: Tumors,
  Liver Cancer, ETOH Extract
EYES

- EYES, LACERATIONS, ETC: 10%
  Solution Of Speeds Healing
HEART
- CARDIAC INHIBITOR
SKIN
- BURNS: 10% Solution Speeds
  Healing
- FUNGAL, ANTI-: Many, Aqueous

Extract
- SKIN, ULCERS, INHIBITS:
  Inhibits Histamine Synthesis
- SORES: 10% Solution Shortens
  Healing Time
**STOMACH/DIGESTIVE
DISORDERS**
- STOMACHIC

Dose

1.5 - 4.5 gm

Common Name

Dried Aloe Leaf Juice

Contraindications

Not: Pregnancy

Not: Def SP/ST w/Anorexia/Diarrhea

Notes

Pills Usually With Other Herbs, Not Decoction
Use 0.3-0.6 gm As Laxative

MANG XIAO

芒硝
(芒硝)

MIRABILITUM

Traditional Functions:

1. Purges excess Heat by moving the stool
2. Clears Heat and reduces swelling
3. Moistens dryness of intestines
4. Softens firm masses

Traditional Properties:

Enters: LI, ST,

Properties: SA, BIT, >C

Indications:

**ABDOMEN/
GASTROINTESTINAL TOPICS**
- APPENDICITIS W/PAIN
- INTESTINES: Cold/Heat
BOWEL RELATED DISORDERS
- CONSTIPATION: Excess Heat/
  Heat Entanglement With Side Flow
- HEMORRHOIDS, PAIN,
  SWELLING
**CANCER/TUMORS/SWELLINGS/
LUMPS**
- SWELLINGS, PAIN

EYES
- EYES, PAIN, RED, SWOLLEN
FLUID DISORDERS
- FLUID RETENTION, CHRONIC
ORAL CAVITY
- MOUTH, ULCERS, SWOLLEN
- THROAT, SWOLLEN,
  ULCERATED
PHLEGM
- PHLEGM STAGNATION,
  ACCUMULATION IN CHEST

**SEXUALITY, FEMALE:
GYNECOLOGICAL**
- MASTITIS
SKIN
- SKIN, LESIONS, RED
- SKIN, SORES, SWOLLEN, TOXIC:
  Topical
**STOMACH/DIGESTIVE
DISORDERS**
- FOOD STAGNATION
- STOMACH COLD/HEAT

Clinical/Pharmaceutical Studies:

**ABDOMEN/
GASTROINTESTINAL
TOPICS**
- APPENDICITIS: Topical
  With Da Huang, Vinegar,
  Garlic On Abdominal Wall,
  Especially Lower Right

Quad, Increased
Lymphocytic Action,
Reduces Inflammation,
Increases Peristalsis In
Smalll Intestine
BOWEL RELATED

DISORDERS
- PURGATIVE: Increases
  Water Thru Osmosis-Drink
  Large Amts Water
**IMMUNE SYSTEM
RELATED DISORDERS/**

TOPICS
- IMMUNE SYSTEM:
  Increases Phagocytosis
KIDNEYS
- DIURETIC: When
  Injected

Dose
3 - 12 gm
Common Name
Mirabilite

Contraindications
Not: Pregnancy
Not: w/Sulfur Or San Leng
Notes
Drink Large Amounts Of Water

SONG ZI
松子仁
FRUCTUS PINI TABULAEFORMIS

Traditional Functions:
1. Moistens the intestines and facilitates passage of stool
2. Benefits the Qi
3. Dispels Wind

Traditional Properties:
Enters: LU, LI, SP,

Properties: BIT, W

Indications:

BOWEL RELATED DISORDERS
• CONSTIPATION: Intestinal Dryness
• HEMORRHOIDS: Deficient

ENERGETIC STATE
• DEBILITY: Qi Deficient
MUSCULOSKELETAL/

CONNECTIVE TISSUE
• ARTHRITIS, RHEUMATOID: Cold, Wind

Dose
4.5 - 9.0 gm
Common Name
Pine Seeds

Purgatives: Moist Laxatives

BI MA ZI   蓖麻子   *SEMEN*
                         （蓖麻子）   *RICINI*

Traditional Functions:

1. Decreases swelling and removes toxins
2. Drains out pus and extracts toxins: External application
3. Moistens intestines and promotes bowel movement

Traditional Properties:

Enters: SP, LV, KI,

Properties: SP, SW, N, TX

Indications:

BOWEL RELATED DISORDERS
• CONSTIPATION, DRY STOOL
**CANCER/TUMORS/SWELLINGS/
LUMPS**
• SWELLINGS
• TOXIC SWELLINGS: Topical
CIRCULATION DISORDERS
• STROKE, FACIAL DEVIATIONS
FROM
HEAD/NECK

• FACE, DEVIATIONS FROM
STROKE
• FACE, PARALYSIS
**IMMUNE SYSTEM RELATED
DISORDERS/TOPICS**
• LYMPH NODES, SWELLING:
Topical
INFECTIOUS DISEASES
• SCROFULA
ORAL CAVITY

• THROAT, SORE
SKIN
• BOILS
• FURUNCLES
• SKIN, INFECTIONS W/PUS
• SKIN, ULCERS
• SORES, SUPPURATIVE: Topical
TRAUMA, BITES, POISONINGS
• SPLINTERS: External Paste To
Remove

Clinical/Pharmaceutical Studies:

**BLOOD RELATED
DISORDERS/TOPICS**
• HEMOLYTIC
**BOWEL RELATED
DISORDERS**
• CONSTIPATION: Ricinic
Oil Is Safe, But Not In
Pregnant/Menstruating
Women, Causes Mild
Congestion Of Pelvic
Organs, 5-20 ml Or
Emulsion, 30 ml, Give In
Morning On Empty
Stomach
• PURGATIVE: Cathartic,
Irritates Small Intestine, 1-
2 Bowel Movements, 2-6
Hrs After, No Colic,
Greater Dose Does Not
Increase Effect
CANCER/TUMORS/

SWELLINGS/LUMPS
• ANTINEOPLASTIC:
Cancer Cells Are Very
Sensitive To Ricin
• CRANIOCERVICAL
AREA CANCER: Ricin
As Cream/Ointment, 3-5%
And 3% DMSO, Topical
Application, 1x/Day, 5-6x/
Week For 1-2 Months
• SKIN, CANCER: 3-5%
Ricin Ointment, 1x/Day,
66% Marked Effect Or
Cure
FEVERS
• PYROGENIC: Very
Potent, Injected
HEAD/NECK
• FACE, NERVE
PARALYSIS: 10 Days To
Cure, Crushed Kernal To

Mandibular Joint, Corner
Of Mouth, 1x/Day
**IMMUNE SYSTEM
RELATED DISORDERS/
TOPICS**
• IMMUNE REACTION:
Strongly Antigenic,
Increases Antibody
Production, Allergic
Reaction
INFECTIOUS DISEASES
• TETANUS: Root Of Herb
Used
LUNGS
• BRONCHITIS,
CHILDHOOD: Root Of
Herb Used
**MENTAL STATE/
NEUROLOGICAL
DISORDERS**

• EPILEPSY: Root Of Herb
Used
SKIN
• SKIN, CANCER: 3-5%
Ricin Ointment, 1x/Day,
66% Marked Effect Or
Cure
**STOMACH/DIGESTIVE
DISORDERS**
• GASTROPTOSIS: Bi Ma
Zi Wu Be Zi Plaster (50:1
Of Herbs) Topical
Application To Du20 (Bai
Hui) Acupoint, 5 Days,
Symptoms Improved,
Some Cured
**TRAUMA, BITES,
POISONINGS**
• CYTOTOXIC:
Agglutinates Cells

Dose

ext.Use

Common Name

Castor Bean

Notes

External Use Only

20 Pieces Can Cause Death, Ricin Is 22x > Hydrogen
Cyanide
Toxic Symptoms: Has Latent Period, Headache, GI
Distress, Fever, Anuria, Cold Sweats, Spasms,
Prostration
Ricin Is A Large Protein

FENG MI   蜂蜜   *MEL*

Traditional Functions: **Traditional Properties:**

1. Strengthens the Middle Burner and moistens dryness   Enters: LU, LI, SP,
2. Controls pain, removes toxins
3. Nourishes and moistens the Lung   Properties: SW, N

Indications:

BOWEL RELATED DISORDERS
• CONSTIPATION: Intestinal
  Dryness
HERBAL FUNCTIONS
• HERBAL PREPARATION
LIVER
• HEPATITIS, CHRONIC
LUNGS

• COUGH: Lung Dry
• COUGH, CHRONIC
NOSE
• SINUSITIS
ORAL CAVITY
• THROAT, SORE
• ULCERS, ORAL

SKIN
• SCALDS
STOMACH/DIGESTIVE
  DISORDERS
• STOMACH, ACHE
TRAUMA, BITES, POISONINGS
• POISONING, ACONITINE

Clinical/Pharmaceutical Studies:

BOWEL RELATED DISORDERS
• APERIENT
• LAXATIVE, EMOLLIENT
INFECTIOUS DISEASES

• BACTERIAL, ANTI-
LUNGS
• ANTITUSSIVE
• EXPECTORANT

NUTRITIONAL/METABOLIC
  DISORDERS/TOPICS
• NUTRITIONAL

Dose   **Common Name**

3 - 30 gm   Honey

HUO MA REN   火麻仁   *SEMEN*
(MA ZI REN)   （火麻仁）   *CANNABIS SATIVAE*

Traditional Functions: **Traditional Properties:**

1. Moistens, lubricates and nourishes the intestines   Enters: LI, SP, ST,
2. Nourishes the Yin
3. Clears Heat and promotes healing of sores   Properties: SW, N

Indications:

BOWEL RELATED DISORDERS
• CONSTIPATION: Intestinal
  Dryness
• CONSTIPATION, POST FEBRILE

DISEASE
• CONSTIPATION, POSTPARTUM
SKIN
• SORES, AUXILLARY HERB FOR:

Topical, Too
• ULCERS: Auxillary Herb For,
  Topical, Too

Clinical/Pharmaceutical Studies:

BLOOD RELATED DISORDERS/
  TOPICS
• BLOOD PRESSURE, LOWERS:

Slow Action Over 5-6 Weeks
BOWEL RELATED DISORDERS
• LAXATIVE: Fatty Oil, Plus

Stimulates Mucosa, Increasing
Peristalsis

Dose
9 - 30 gm

Common Name
Marijuana Seeds

Contraindications
Not: With Diarrhea

Notes
Break Up Seeds
Prolonged Ingestion May Result In Sperma/Leukorrhea
Overdose: Toxic, Nausea/Vomiting, Nervous Disorders

YU LI REN

鬱李仁
(郁李仁)

SEMEN PRUNI

Traditional Functions:

1. Moistens and lubricates the intestines
2. Promotes the removal of water and reduces swelling

Traditional Properties:

Enters: LI, SP, SI,

Properties: SP, BIT, SW, N

Indications:

ABDOMEN/
GASTROINTESTINAL TOPICS
• LARGE INTESTINE, QI
  STAGNATION
BOWEL RELATED DISORDERS
• CONSTIPATION: Fire/Intestinal
  Dryness/Stagnat Qi In Intestines
• CONSTIPATION W/EDEMA,

DYSURIA
EXTREMITIES
• LEG QI
FLUID DISORDERS
• ASCITES
• EDEMA, DYSURIA,
  CONSTIPATION
• EDEMA, LIMBS

QI RELATED DISORDERS/
TOPICS
• LARGE INTESTINE QI
  STAGNATION
URINARY BLADDER
• URINATION, NON-SMOOTH
  FLOW

Clinical/Pharmaceutical Studies:

BLOOD RELATED DISORDERS/
TOPICS
• BLOOD PRESSURE, LOWERS

BOWEL RELATED DISORDERS
• CONSTIPATION: Stool, Moistens,
  Greater Than Huo Ma Ren

KIDNEYS
• DIURETIC: For Edema

Dose
3 - 12 gm

Common Name
Bush Cherry Pit

Contraindications
Not: Pregnancy Or Body Fluid Depletion

Purgatives: Cathartics To Transform Water

BA DOU   巴豆   *SEMEN CROTONIS*

Traditional Functions:

1. Purges Cold accumulation
2. Expells Phlegm and benefits throat
3. Circulates fluid and reduces edema
4. Kills parasites

Traditional Properties:

Enters: LI, ST,

Properties: SP, H, >TX

Indications:

ABDOMEN/ GASTROINTESTINAL TOPICS
- ABDOMEN, PAIN OF, DISTENTION

BOWEL RELATED DISORDERS
- CONSTIPATION: Cold Accumulation
- CONSTIPATION W/GI PAIN, DISTENTION
- DIARRHEA

CHEST
- CHEST, PAIN, DISTENTION

COLD
- PURGES COLD ACCUMULATION, STAGNATION

FLUID DISORDERS
- EDEMA

LUNGS
- BREATHING, RAPID: pwdr Blown In Throat To Cause Vomiting
- SUFFOCATION: pwdr Blown In Throat To Cause Vomiting
- TRACHEA, EXCESS SPUTUM BLOCKING: pwdr Blown In Throat

To Cause Vomiting

ORAL CAVITY
- PHARYNGITIS: pwdr Blown In Throat To Cause Vomiting
- THROAT WIND/BI

SKIN
- BOILS: Topical
- DERMATITIS: Topical
- FUNGAL INFECTIONS: Topical
- SCABIES: Topical
- ULCERS, EVIL: Topical
- WARTS: Topical

Clinical/Pharmaceutical Studies:

ABDOMEN/ GASTROINTESTINAL TOPICS
- APPENDICITIS: Ding Yong Pill (Ba Dou, Realgar, Da Huang)
- INTESTINES, OBSTRUCTION/POST SURGERY ADHESION: Use Defatted Seed, Capsule Of 150-300 mg Each, Dose--1-2 Caps, Repeat If Necessary In 3-4 Hrs, If No Response In 48 Hrs, Needs Immediate Surgery
- PANCREAS, INCREASES SECRETIONS

BOWEL RELATED DISORDERS
- DIARRHEA, CHRONIC: Ba Dou Liu Huang Pill, Cold Type
- PURGATIVE: Very Drastic, Can Last 10-15hrs

CANCER/TUMORS/ SWELLINGS/LUMPS
- CARCINOGENIC: (Cofactor) Effect To Mucosa

GALL BLADDER
- BILE SECRETION, INCREASES
- BILIARY COLIC: Increases Secretion Of Bile, *100 mg Caps/3-4 Hrs

Until Purgation, Colic Is Then Reduced, Do Not Exceed 400 mg/24 Hrs

HEAD/NECK
- FACE, PARALYSIS OF

INFECTIOUS DISEASES
- ENCEPHALITIS B: Injections Of 5% Solution
- MALARIA: Daily Dose Of 0.6 gm Oral Or Local Application To Superior External Region Of Ear With Defatted Seed

LIVER
- LIVER, CIRRHOSIS W/ ASCITES: Ba Dou Pill (Ba Dou, Da Zao, LU Dou, Hu Jiao

PARASITES
- ASCARIASIS, IN BILE DUCT: 100 mg Caps/3-4 Hrs Until Purgation, Colic Is Then Reduced, Do Not Exceed 400 mg/24 Hrs

SEXUALITY, FEMALE: GYNECOLOGICAL
- MASTITIS, ACUTE: Ba Dou Sha Ren Pill (Ba Dou, Sha Ren, Da Zao) , Not When Abscess Already Formed

SKIN
- BLISTERS, CAUSE OF
- NEURODERMATITIS: With Realgar, Applied Topically

Dose
0.15 - 0.30 gm

Common Name
Croton

Contraindications
Not: w/Heat S/S (Use Da Huang Instead)
Not: Pregnancy
Not: w/Qian Niu Zi/Qian Niu Hua
Not: With Hot Food/Drinks
Not: Weak Constitution

Notes
Usually Used As Pills

Toxic: 1 gm/20 Drops Of Croton Oil Lethal

Causes Severe Diarrhea

Irritates Skin, May Cause Contact Dermatitis

Possible Hypotension, Shock From Too Much
Emergency Treatment: Induce Vomiting, Egg Whites,
Animal Charcoal, IV Glucose-Saline, Respiratory
Stimulants
Antidote: Cooled Decoction Of Huang Lian, Huang Bai,
Or Luo Dou Soup, Soya Bean Juice, Or Water

GAN SUI   甘遂   RADIX EUPHORBIAE KANSUI

Traditional Functions:

1. Expels fluids accumulated in the chest and abdomen
2. Used topically to clear Heat and reduce swelling and lumps
3. Moves the stool

Traditional Properties:

Enters: LU, SP, KI,

Properties: BIT, C, TX

Indications:

ABDOMEN/
  GASTROINTESTINAL TOPICS
• ABDOMEN, LUMPS
BOWEL RELATED DISORDERS
• CONSTIPATION
CHEST
• HYDROTHORAX
FLUID DISORDERS
• ASCITES, DYSPNEA
• EDEMA, GENERALIZED
• EDEMA, SEVERE: Excess
  Constitution

HEAD/NECK
• FACE, EDEMA
LIVER
• LIVER, CIRRHOSIS
LUNGS
• PLEURISY
MENTAL STATE/
  NEUROLOGICAL DISORDERS
• EPILEPSY, DUE TO PHLEGM
  MASKING ORIFICES
PHLEGM

• PHLEGM FLUID
SKIN
• SKIN, LESIONS, EARLY STAGE,
  SWOLLEN, NODULAR, PAINFUL:
  Topical--Damp Heat
TRAUMA, BITES, POISONINGS
• INFLAMMATION
URINARY BLADDER
• DYSURIA
• URINATION, DECREASED
• URINATION, RETENTION

Clinical/Pharmaceutical Studies:

BOWEL RELATED DISORDERS
• LAXATIVE, EMOLLIENT
• PURGATIVE: Intense Diarrhea

KIDNEYS
• DIURETIC: Effect Not Shown For
  Herb

PAIN/NUMBNESS/GENERAL
  DISCOMFORT
• ANALGESIC

Dose
0.6 - 1.5 gm

Contraindications
Not: Pregnancy
Not: w/Gan Cao, More Toxic

Notes
Best: Pill/Powder

Stir Fry For Internal Use

Violent, May Cause Anal Passsing Of Water
Put In Caps To Avoid Nausea
pwdr: 0.3-0.6 gm

HONG DA JI   紅大薊   RADIX KNOXIAE
(DA JI)   (红大薊)   (EUPHORBIA PEKINESIS)

Traditional Functions:

1. Promotes urination and bowel movements
2. Purges localized fluid to relieve swellings

Traditional Properties:

Enters: LU, SP, KI,

Properties: BIT, C, TX

Indications:

CHEST
- CHEST, CONGESTION/ FULLNESS
- CHEST, LATERAL PAIN: Ascites

FLUID DISORDERS
- ASCITES
- EDEMA

IMMUNE SYSTEM RELATED DISORDERS/TOPICS
- LYMPH GLANDS,

ENLARGEMENT, CHRONIC:
Phlegm Nodules
LUNGS
- BREATHING, LABORED: Ascites

MENTAL STATE/ NEUROLOGICAL DISORDERS
- EPILEPSY

PHLEGM
- PHLEGM FLUID

ACCUMULATION
- PHLEGM, STICKY

SKIN
- CARBUNCLES
- SORES, TOXIC, RED, SWOLLEN, PAINFUL: Topical

STOMACH/DIGESTIVE DISORDERS
- APPETITE, LOSS OF

Clinical/Pharmaceutical Studies:

BLOOD RELATED DISORDERS/ TOPICS
- BLOOD PRESSURE, LOWERS: Dilates Peripheral Blood Vessels

BOWEL RELATED DISORDERS
- PURGATIVE

INFECTIOUS DISEASES
- BACTERIAL, ANTI-: Staph. Aureus, Streptococci, Pneumococci, Pseudomonas, Et.Al.

KIDNEYS

- DIURETIC

MENTAL STATE/ NEUROLOGICAL DISORDERS
- PSYCHOLOGICAL DISORDERS: Mania, Schizophrenia

Dose

1.5 - 3.0 gm

Common Name

Knoxia

Contraindications

Not: Pregnancy

Not: w/Gan Cao, Will Inhibit Diuretic/Purgative Action

JING DA JI
(DA JI)

京大戟

RADIX EUPHORBIAE PEKINENSIS

Traditional Functions:

1. Expels water from the chest and flanks
2. Used topically to disperse lumps and reduce swellings

Traditional Properties:

Enters: LU, SP, KI,

Properties: BIT, SP, C, TX

Indications:

ABDOMEN/ GASTROINTESTINAL TOPICS
- ABDOMEN, DISTENTION OF

CHEST
- CHEST, FULLNESS

FLUID DISORDERS
- ASCITES

- EDEMA, CHEST, FLANKS
- FLUID ACCUMULATION IN CHEST, FLANKS

INFECTIOUS DISEASES
- TUBERCLE

MENTAL STATE/ NEUROLOGICAL DISORDERS

- EPILEPSY
- MENTAL DISORDERS

SKIN
- CARBUNCLES
- SORES, SWOLLEN, TOXIC, PAINFUL: Topical

Clinical/Pharmaceutical Studies:

BLOOD RELATED DISORDERS/ TOPICS
- BLOOD PRESSURE, LOWERS

BOWEL RELATED DISORDERS
- PURGATIVE

CIRCULATION DISORDERS
- BLOOD VESSELS, VASODILATES: Vasodialator Of Peripheral Blood Vessels

FLUID DISORDERS

- ASCITES, FROM SCHISTOSOMIASIS

INFECTIOUS DISEASES
- BACTERIAL, ANTI-: Staph Aureus, Streptococci, Pneumococci, etc

KIDNEYS
- DIURETIC, NOT SHOWN
- NEPHRITIS, ACUTE/CHRONIC:

Reduces Edema In 1 Week, Side Effects Noted

MENTAL STATE/ NEUROLOGICAL DISORDERS
- MANIA
- SCHIZOPHRENIA

PARASITES
- ASCITES, FROM SCHISTOSOMIASIS

Dose

1.5 - 3.0 gm

Common Name

Peking Spurge Root

Contraindications

Not: Pregnancy

Not: Cold Deficient Edema

Precautions

Watch: Weak Patients

Notes

Incompatible With Gan Cao Less Effective/More Toxic

pwdr: 1-1.2 gm

QIAN NIU ZI

牽牛子
(牽牛子)

SEMEN PHARBITIDIS

Traditional Functions:

1. Purges out water and excess Heat from the Stomach or Intestines
2. Promotes the removal of water, reduces swelling and moves the stool
3. Expels intestinal parasites
4. Reduces food stagnation
5. Dispels Phlegm and congested fluids from the Lungs

Traditional Properties:

Enters: LU, LI, KI,

Properties: BIT, SP, C, TX

Indications:

ABDOMEN/ GASTROINTESTINAL TOPICS
• ABDOMEN, DISTENTION OF: Excess Heat In Stomach/Intestines
• ABDOMEN, FULLNESS OF: Lungs Obstructed By Congested Fluids
• ABDOMEN, PAIN OF: Food Stagnation/Ascariasis
BOWEL RELATED DISORDERS
• CONSTIPATION: Heat Entanglement

• CONSTIPATION, SEVERE: Excess Heat In Stomach/Intestines
CHEST
• CHEST, FULLNESS: Lungs Obstructed By Congested Fluids
EXTREMITIES
• LEGS, EDEMA
FLUID DISORDERS
• ASCITES, WORMS
• EDEMA
• EDEMA, SEVERE: Excess Constitution

LUNGS
• COUGH: Lungs Obstructed By Congested Fluids
• DYSPNEA
• WHEEZING: Lungs Obstructed By Congested Fluids
PARASITES
• ASCITES W/WORMS
• HOOKWORMS
• PINWORMS
• ROUNDWORMS
• TAPEWORMS

• WORMS, W/ASCITES, KILLS
PHLEGM
• CONGESTED PHLEGM
• PHLEGM FLUID
• PHLEGM RETENTION
STOMACH/DIGESTIVE DISORDERS
• FOOD STAGNATION
URINARY BLADDER
• URINATION, DIFFICULT: Excess Heat In Stomach/Intestines
• URINATION, SCANTY

Clinical/Pharmaceutical Studies:

BOWEL RELATED DISORDERS
• LAXATIVE, STRONG
KIDNEYS
• DIURETIC

PARASITES
• ANTIPARASITIC: Weak
• FLAT WORMS
• ROUNDWORMS

STOMACH/DIGESTIVE DISORDERS
• NAUSEA/VOMITING, INDUCES

Dose

3 - 30 gm

Common Name

Morning Glory Seeds

Contraindications

Not: Pregnancy

Not: w/Ba Dou

Not: SP/ST Weakness

Notes

Pill Form

Toxic To GI Tract, Kidneys

Overdose: Abdominal Pain, Vomiting

pwdr: 1.5-15gm

SHANG LU

商陸
（商陆）

RADIX PHYTOLACCAE

Traditional Functions:

1. Expels water in excess edema conditions
2. Used topically as the fresh herb to reduces sores and carbuncles

Traditional Properties:

Enters: LU, SP, KI, LI

Properties: BIT, C, TX

Indications:

ABDOMEN/
GASTROINTESTINAL TOPICS
• ABDOMEN, DISTENTION OF
CANCER/TUMORS/SWELLINGS/
LUMPS
• TUMORS
CHEST
• CHEST, DISTENTION, DISTRESS
FLUID DISORDERS
• ASCITES

• EDEMA, CONSTIPATION,
SEVERE, DIFFICULT URINATION:
Excessive
• EDEMA, SEVERE: Excess
Constitution
ORAL CAVITY
• THROAT BI W/OBSTRUCTION:
(Numbness) , Topical
• THROAT, SORE
SKIN

• ABSCESS
• SKIN, SORES, SWOLLEN, TOXIC:
Topical
• ULCERS, EVIL: Topical
TRAUMA, BITES, POISONINGS
• WOUNDS, INCISED: Toxic
URINARY BLADDER
• URINATION, DIFFICULT W/
EDEMA: Excess
• URINATION, SCANTY

Clinical/Pharmaceutical Studies:

BLOOD RELATED DISORDERS/
TOPICS
• THROMBOCYTOPENIC
PURPURA: 100% Decoction, 2-4
Days For Petechiae To Fade, Up To 2
Weeks To Go Away
BOWEL RELATED DISORDERS
• PURGATIVE: Large Dose Of
Extract, Intense
FLUID DISORDERS
• ASCITES: Good Diuretic Effect
• EDEMA, CARDIOGENIC: Good
Diuretic Effect
HEMORRHAGIC DISORDERS
• HEMOPTYSIS
IMMUNE SYSTEM RELATED
DISORDERS/TOPICS
• ANAPHYLACTIC PURPURA
INFECTIOUS DISEASES
• ANTIBIOTIC: Strep., Pneumo.
• VIRAL, ANTI-: Tobacco Mosaic

KIDNEYS
• DIURETIC: Mixed Findings
• NEPHRITIS, CHRONIC/ACUTE:
Good Diuretic Effect
LUNGS
• ANTITUSSIVE: Decoction/
Tincture Weak Action, Alkaloids PO
Pronounced Effect
• ASTHMA
• BRONCHITIS, CHRONIC: Best In
Simple Type, ETOH Extract Tablet,
Honey Pill, ETOH Extract Best At
87-95% Short-Term Control
• EXPECTORANT: Decoction
Strong, IP Stronger, Herb Decoction
Stronger Than Jie Geng, Tincture/
Aqueous Extract Weaker, Enhances
Ciliary Movement
MENTAL STATE/
NEUROLOGICAL DISORDERS

• CONVULSIVE: Phytolaccatoxin,
Stimulates Respiratory Center
SEXUALITY, MALE:
UROLOGICAL TOPICS
• SPERMICIDAL ACTION:
Steroidal Saponin Extract
SKIN
• ANAPHYLACTIC PURPURA
• FUNGAL, ANTI-
• PSORIASIS: Tablet 81% Effective,
Best In Arthritic/Simple Psoriasis, 9
g/Day In 3 Doses PO
STOMACH/DIGESTIVE
DISORDERS
• EMETIC
TRAUMA, BITES, POISONINGS
• INFLAMMATORY, ANTI-: ETOH
Extract, Orally
• RADIATION, ANTI-: 100%
Decoction Helped Platelet Recovery

Dose

2.4 - 9.0 gm

Common Name

Poke Root

Contraindications

Not: Pregnancy
Not: Qi Def Edema

Notes

Toxic-Only Excess Conditions, May Produce

Convulsions, Death In Overdose
Large Oral Dose May Cause: Diarrhea, Heart Disorders,
Paralysis
Herb Treatment To Reduce Toxicity: Prolonged (2 Hrs)
Decoction, Honey Pill/Syrup, ETOH Extract Reduced
All Adverse Effects
Red 2x More Toxic White Herb
Causes Vomiting 1-10 g/kg

TING LI ZI

葶藶子
（葶苈子）

SEMEN LEPIDII

Traditional Functions:

1. Redirects Lung Qi downward and eliminates Phlegm
2. Expels water and drains edema
3. Relieves asthma

Traditional Properties:

Enters: LU, UB,

Properties: SP, BIT, C

Indications:

CHEST
• CHEST, DISTENTION FROM WATER
FLUID DISORDERS
• ASCITES, DIFFICULT URINATION: Excess Lung/Bladder Qi Obstruction
• EDEMA: Dampness, Evil Fluid

• EDEMA, HEAD & FACE, CHRONIC
LUNGS
• ASTHMA, ACUTE FROM WATER RETENTION: Excess
• COUGH: Lung Heat
• COUGH, COPIOUS SPUTUM,

GURGLING SOUND: Lung Heat/Phlegm
• LUNGS, ABSCESS
• LUNGS, DYSPNEA: Lung Heat
URINARY BLADDER
• URINATION, DIFFICULT
• URINATION, SCANTY

Clinical/Pharmaceutical Studies:

HEART
• CARDIOTONIC: Increases Output, Needs Large Dose
• COR PULMONALE, CHRONIC WITH CARDIAC FAILURE

KIDNEYS
• DIURETIC
LUNGS
• EXPECTORANT: Oil Of

ORAL CAVITY
• PHARYNGITIS: Oil Alleviates
• THROAT, PHLEGM IN: Oil Alleviates

Dose

3 - 9 gm

Common Name

Woods Whitlow Grass

Contraindications

Not: In Cough/Wheeze From Def LU Qi

Not: Edema From Def SP

WU JIU GEN PI

烏桕根皮
（乌桕根皮））

CORTEX RADICIS SAPII

Traditional Functions:

1. Purges water, removes fluid
2. Disperses accumulations and removes toxins
3. Kills intestinal parasites

Traditional Properties:

Enters: LU, SP, KI,

Properties: BIT, W, TX

Indications:

ABDOMEN/ GASTROINTESTINAL TOPICS
• ABDOMEN, DISTENTION OF
• ABDOMEN, MASS
BOWEL RELATED DISORDERS

• CONSTIPATION
FLUID DISORDERS
• ASCITES
• EDEMA
SKIN

• FURUNCLES: Damp
• SCABIES
URINARY BLADDER
• URINARY RETENTION

Dose

9 - 12 gm

Common Name

Vegetable Tallow Root Bar

XU SUI ZI

續隨子
(续随子)

SEMEN EUPHORBIA LATHYRIDIS

Traditional Functions:

1. Purges water, removes fluid
2. Dissipates edema
3. Breaks up stagnated Blood and dissipates abdominal tumors

Traditional Properties:

Enters: KI, LV,

Properties: SP, W, TX

Indications:

ABDOMEN/
GASTROINTESTINAL TOPICS
• ABDOMEN, DISTENTION OF
BLOOD RELATED DISORDERS/
TOPICS
• BLOOD STASIS
BOWEL RELATED DISORDERS
• CONSTIPATION
CANCER/TUMORS/SWELLINGS/
LUMPS
• TUMORS, GYNECOLOGICAL
FLUID DISORDERS

• EDEMA
• EDEMA, PULMONARY
PARASITES
• SCHISTOSOMIASIS
PHLEGM
• PHLEGM FLUID RETENTION
SEXUALITY, FEMALE:
GYNECOLOGICAL
• AMENORRHEA
SKIN
• FUNGAL INFECTIONS: Topical

• SCABIES: Topical
• WARTS: Topical
STOMACH/DIGESTIVE
DISORDERS
• FOOD ACCUMULATION,
OVERNIGHT
TRAUMA, BITES, POISONINGS
• SNAKE BITES: Topical
URINARY BLADDER
• DYSURIA
• URINARY RETENTION

Clinical/Pharmaceutical Studies:

BOWEL RELATED DISORDERS
• PURGATIVE: Intense Diarrhea,
Toxic

CANCER/TUMORS/SWELLINGS/
LUMPS

• ANTICARCINOGENIC: Acute
Monocytic Leukemia

Dose

0.9 - 4.5 gm

Common Name

Lathyrol Spurge

Contraindications

Not: Pregnancy

Not: Weak Constitution Or Loose Stool

Notes

Toxic
Usually Pills/Powder

YUAN HUA

芫花

FLOS DAPHNES GENKWA

Traditional Functions:

1. Expels fluid from the chest, abdomen and flanks
2. Relieves cough and Phlegm

Traditional Properties:

Enters: LU, LI, KI,

Properties: BIT, SP, W, TX

Indications:

ABDOMEN/
GASTROINTESTINAL TOPICS
• ABDOMEN, DISTENTION OF
• SUBCOSTAL PAIN
BOWEL RELATED DISORDERS
• CONSTIPATION
CHEST
• CHEST, ACCUMULATION OF
FLUIDS
FLUID DISORDERS

• EDEMA, SEVERE: Excess
Constitution
• EDEMA, SEVERE OF
HYPOTHORAX
• FLUID RETENTION,
LOCALIZED
LUNGS
• ASTHMA, CARDIAC
• BRONCHITIS, CHRONIC
• COUGH

• COUGH IN CHILDREN
• DYSPNEA: Soft Phlegm Mass
PHLEGM
• PHLEGM, SOFT MASS
SKIN
• SCABIES
• SKIN, DISORDERS
STOMACH/DIGESTIVE
DISORDERS
• EPIGASTRIC DISTENTION

Clinical/Pharmaceutical Studies:

BOWEL RELATED DISORDERS
• PURGATIVE: Increase Peristalsis--Diarrhea, Abdominal Pain

FLUID DISORDERS
• ASCITES: Powder, 1.5 -2.5 g/Day For 4-5 Days

INFECTIOUS DISEASES
• BACTERIAL, ANTI-

KIDNEYS
• DIURETIC: Not With Large Doses And With Diarrhea
• KIDNEY FAILURE, CHRONIC

LIVER
• HEPATITIS, ACUTE, CHRONIC: Tablet Of Aqueous Extract, Normalized SGPT, Symptom Improvement

LUNGS
• ANTITUSSIVE: Oral Of Water-Alcohol Extract Or The Vinegar/Benzene-Processed Herb
• BRONCHITIS, CHRONIC: Vinegar/Benzene-Prepared Herb
• EXPECTORANT

PARASITES
• FILARIASIS
• ROUNDWORMS: Inhibits Movement

SEXUALITY, FEMALE:

GYNECOLOGICAL
• ABORTIFACIENT: Sodium Carbonate Extract Of Root Bark, Local Injection Strongest, All Forms Of Extract Work, Labor Induced In 30 Hrs Average
• MASTITIS

SKIN
• FUNGAL, ANTI-: 1:4 Aqueous Extract

TRAUMA, BITES, POISONINGS
• FROSTBITE
• TOXIC, INCREASED W/GAN CAO

Dose

1.5 - 3.0 gm

Common Name

Daphne Flower

Contraindications

Not: Pregnancy

Not: w/Gan Cao (Counteracts) Makes More Toxic
Not: Weak Constitution

Notes

pwdr: 0.6-1.9 gm
May Develop Neurological/Digestive Symptoms

Expel Wind Dampness

BAI HUA SHE

白花蛇

AGKISTRODON SEU BUNGARUS

Traditional Functions:

1. Dispels Wind and Dampness and activates the channels
2. Dispels Wind from the skin
3. Relieves and stabilizes spasms

Traditional Properties:

Enters: SP, LV,

Properties: SW, SA, W, TX

Indications:

CHILDHOOD DISORDERS
- INFANTILE SPASMS/ CONVULSIONS

CIRCULATION DISORDERS
- STROKE SYNDROME

EXTREMITIES
- ARMS, NUMB, WEAK, CHRONIC
- EXTREMITIES, PARALYSIS OF: Wind Damp
- LEGS, NUMB, WEAKNESS, CHRONIC

HEAD/NECK
- FACE, PARALYSIS: Windstroke

INFECTIOUS DISEASES
- LEPROSY
- TETANUS: Spasms Of

MENTAL STATE/ NEUROLOGICAL DISORDERS
- CONVULSIONS, FRIGHT IN YOUNG CHILDREN
- HEMIPLEGIA: Windstroke
- NEUROLOGICAL PROBLEMS
- PARALYSIS, EXTREMITIES: Wind Damp
- SEIZURES: Any Kind
- TREMORS: Any Kind

MUSCULOSKELETAL/ CONNECTIVE TISSUE
- ARTHRITIS: For Expelling Wind Damp
- ARTHRITIS, PAIN
- ARTHRITIS, RHEUMATIC: Pain

- CRAMPS
- SPASMS: Any Kind

PAIN/NUMBNESS/GENERAL DISCOMFORT
- BI, WIND DAMP, CHRONIC: Open Luo, Arrest Pain
- NUMBNESS, EXTREMITIES

SKIN
- FUNGAL INFECTIONS
- RASHES: Any Kind
- SCABIES
- SKIN, NUMBNESS
- SORES, INTRACTABLE
- ULCERS, RED BAYBERRY

WIND DISORDERS
- WIND DAMP, CHRONIC

Clinical/Pharmaceutical Studies:

BLOOD RELATED DISORDERS/ TOPICS
- BLOOD, COAGULATION, INCREASES

CIRCULATION DISORDERS
- HYPERTENSION

- VASODILATOR: Injected

MENTAL STATE/ NEUROLOGICAL DISORDERS
- HYPNOTIC
- SEDATIVE
- TRANQUILIZING

MUSCULOSKELETAL/ CONNECTIVE TISSUE
- ANTISPASMODIC

PAIN/NUMBNESS/GENERAL DISCOMFORT
- ANALGESIC

Dose

3.00 - 6.00 gm

Common Name

Multibanded Krait

Contraindications

Not: Def Yin w/Heat

Precautions

Watch: Def Blood

Notes

No Side Effects From 30-60 gm Decoction

Prolonged Use: Possible Dry Mouth

CAN SHA

蠶砂
(蚕砂)

EXCREMENTUM BOMBYCIS MORI

Traditional Functions:

1. Dispels Wind and Dampness
2. Harmonizes the Stomach and transforms turbid Dampness

Traditional Properties:

Enters: SP, ST, LV,

Properties: SW, SP, W

Indications:

ABDOMEN/
GASTROINTESTINAL
TOPICS
• ABDOMEN, PAIN OF:
  Severe Dampness
• BORBORYGMUS:
  Severe Dampness
BOWEL RELATED
DISORDERS
• DIARRHEA: Severe
  Dampness
EXTREMITIES
• CALF MUSCLE SPASMS:
  Severe Dampness

• LEG QI: Cold Dampness
• LEGS, COLD PAIN OF
• LEGS, SWOLLEN,
  PAINFUL (BERIBERI,
  LEG QI) : Cold Dampness
• LOINS, COLD PAIN OF
EYES
• EYES, IRRITATION:
  External
INFECTIOUS DISEASES
• CHOLERA, CALF
  MUSCLE SPASMS
• MEASLES
MUSCULOSKELETAL/

CONNECTIVE TISSUE
• ARTHRITIS: For
  Expelling Wind Damp
• CRAMPS: Severe
  Dampness
• JOINTS, PAIN OF
  RHEUMATISM
• SPASMS, IN ABDOMEN,
  LEGS
NUTRITIONAL/
METABOLIC
DISORDERS/TOPICS
• BERIBERI: Cold
  Dampness

PAIN/NUMBNESS/
GENERAL
DISCOMFORT
• BI, WIND DAMP
SKIN
• ECZEMA: Cold
  Dampness
• SKIN, SORES: Cold
  Damp
STOMACH/DIGESTIVE
DISORDERS
• VOMITING: Severe
  Dampness

Clinical/Pharmaceutical Studies:

HEMORRHAGIC DISORDERS   • HEMOSTATIC

Dose

3 - 15 gm

Common Name

Silkworm Feces

CANG ER ZI

蒼耳子
(苍耳子)

FRUCTUS
XANTHII

Traditional Functions:

1. Opens up the nasal passages
2. Dispels Wind and expels Dampness
3. Release exterior Wind and reduces pain

Traditional Properties:

Enters: LU, LV,

Properties: SW, <BIT, W, TX

Indications:

EXTREMITIES
• LEG QI: Cold Dampness
• LEGS, SWOLLEN,
  PAINFUL (BERIBERI,
  LEG QI) : Cold Dampness
• LIMBS,
  CONTRACTURES
• LIMBS, CRAMPS/NUMB
FLUID DISORDERS
• DAMPNESS,
  EXTERNAL--SURFACE
  COMPLEX
HEAD/NECK
• HEADACHE: Wind Cold/
  Damp

• HEADACHE,
  SPLITTING RADIATING
  TO BACK OF NECK:
  Exterior
INFECTIOUS DISEASES
• LEPROSY
MUSCULOSKELETAL/
CONNECTIVE TISSUE
• ARTHRITIS: Wind Damp
  Cold Bi
• ARTHRITIS,
  RHEUMATIC
• LUMBAGO, CHRONIC
NOSE
• NOSE, RUNNY

• RHINITIS, ALLERGIC
• RHINITIS, CHRONIC
• SINUSITIS W/
  HEADACHE
• SINUSITIS, W/
  HEADACHE/RUNNY
  NOSE
NUTRITIONAL/
METABOLIC
DISORDERS/TOPICS
• BERIBERI: Cold
  Dampness
PAIN/NUMBNESS/
GENERAL
DISCOMFORT

• BI, WIND DAMP
• BODY, NUMBNESS,
  PAIN
SKIN
• ECZEMA: Cold
  Dampness
• RASHES, PRURITIC:
  Wind Damp
• SCABIES: With Pruritus
• SKIN, ITCHING
• SKIN, SORES: Cold
  Damp
• SKIN, SORES, W/
  PRURITUS
• ULCERS, SKIN

Clinical/Pharmaceutical Studies:

BLOOD RELATED
DISORDERS/TOPICS
• BLOOD GLUCOSE,
  REDUCES: Oral Weaker
  Than Injection
IMMUNE SYSTEM
RELATED DISORDERS/
TOPICS

Chicken Eggs, Then
Boiled, Give 1x/Day For 3
Days, If Relapse Then
Give Additional Doses
• SYPHILITIC
  NEURALGIA
LUNGS
• ANTITUSSIVE: 100%

Days, Takes 3-5 Injections
For Effects, Best For
Sprain, Rheumatic Pain
Not Sciatica,
Osteoarthrosis
NOSE
• ALLERGIC RHINITIS:
  Herb Powder Macerate In

• SINUSITIS,
  PARANASAL, CHRONIC:
  As Honey Pill, 3 g/Pill, 1-
  2 Pills, Or Tab, 1.5 g/Tab,
  2 Tabs, 3x/Day For 2
  Weeks, *Fluidextract Of
  Herb With Xin Yi Hua, Jin
  Yin Hua, Ju Hua, Qian Cao

Clinical/Pharmaceutical Studies:

- ALLERGIC RHINITIS: Herb Powder Macerate In ETOH, 12 Days, Percolate With ETOH, Evaporate, Make Tablets Each Equivalent To 1.5 g Of Crude Herb, Dose--2 Tabs, 3x/Day For 2 Weeks, 72% Effective

INFECTIOUS DISEASES
- ANTIBIOTIC: Slight, Staph.A
- BACTERIAL, ANTI-: Staph
- MALARIA: 100 g, Crushed, Decocted, Filtered, Added To

Decoction
- BRONCHITIS, CHRONIC: With Oral Dose Of Stir Fried Seeds, 83% Even A Year After Treatment

MUSCULOSKELETAL/ CONNECTIVE TISSUE
- ANTIRHEUMATIC
- ANTISPASMODIC
- ARTHRITIS, CHRONIC: Decoction
- BACK, LOWER PAIN: Injection In Pain Points Of Alcohol Precipitated Decoction On Alternate

ETOH, 12 Days, Percolate With ETOH, Evaporate, Make Tablets Each Equivalent To 1.5 g Of Crude Herb, Dose--2 Tabs, 3x/Day For 2 Weeks, 72% Effective
- RHINITIS, CHRONIC: Good 30-40 Seeds Crushed With Ounce Of Sesame Oil, Fry Over Low Heat, Cool, Apply To Nasal Cavities With Cotton Swabs 2-3 X/ Day For 2 Weeks, Almost 100% Cure With No Relapse

Gen, Orally, Greater Than 80% Effective

ORAL CAVITY
- TOOTHACHE, REFRACTORY

PAIN/NUMBNESS/ GENERAL DISCOMFORT
- ANALGESIC

SEXUALITY, FEMALE: GYNECOLOGICAL
- MASTITIS, ACUTE

SKIN
- FUNGAL, ANTI-
- SCABIES
- URTICARIA

Dose

3 - 9 gm

Common Name

Cocklebur Fruit

Contraindications

Not: Headache From Blood Def

Notes

Overdose: Vomiting, Diarrhea, Abdominal Pain

Toxicity Removed By Decocting, Heat, Rinsing With Water

Toxic Dose: >100 g, Symptoms In 12 Hrs, Liver, Kidney, CNS Toxin

Possible Exfoliative Dermatitis From External Wash Of Herb Decoction

---

CHOU WU TONG
(BA JIAO WU TONG)

臭梧桐

FOLIUM CLERONDENDRI, RAMULUS ET

Traditional Functions:

1. Dispels Wind and Dampness
2. Lowers blood pressure

Traditional Properties:

Enters: LV, SP

Properties: SP, BIT, SW, CL

Indications:

BOWEL RELATED DISORDERS
- DYSENTERY
- HEMORRHOIDS

CIRCULATION DISORDERS
- HYPERTENSION: Folk Remedy

HEAD/NECK
- MIGRAINE

INFECTIOUS DISEASES

- MALARIA

MENTAL STATE/ NEUROLOGICAL DISORDERS
- HEMIPLEGIA

MUSCULOSKELETAL/ CONNECTIVE TISSUE
- ARTHRITIS: For Expelling Wind Damp

PAIN/NUMBNESS/GENERAL DISCOMFORT
- BI, WIND DAMP, CHRONIC: Open Luo, Arrest Pain

SKIN
- CARBUNCLES
- ECZEMA
- TINEA MANUUM

Clinical/Pharmaceutical Studies:

CIRCULATION DISORDERS
- HYPERTENSION: Water Soluble Components, Superior To Du Zhong, Less Than Rauwolfia (Reserpine Source) , 16-57% Decrease In 3-10 Days Of Treatment, Prolonged Storage Of Herb Reduced

Rebound BP Increase In 2 Weeks, Use 2-4 g/Day To Maintain, *Better Than Rauwolfia Preparations, Synergistic With Di Long

INFECTIOUS DISEASES
- MALARIA: Tabs 0.25 g/ Tab, 10 Tabs/6 Hrs For 2 Days, 5 Tabs/3x/Day For 7 Days, All Symptoms

Doses/Day, 10=1 Course, 3 Courses Markedly Effective, But Slow, Unstable

MENTAL STATE/ NEUROLOGICAL DISORDERS
- SEDATIVE: Synergistic With Di Long, Greater Than Reserpin, No

Xian Cao/Gui Zhen Cao
- RHEUMATISM

PAIN/NUMBNESS/ GENERAL DISCOMFORT
- ANALGESIC

SKIN
- PRURITUS

TRAUMA, BITES, POISONINGS

Clinical/Pharmaceutical Studies:

Effect, Best To Harvest Before Flowering, *As Tablet, 10-16 g In 3-4 Doses/Day, Marked Results In 5 Weeks, Increased Effects With Longer Therapy, Symptoms Improved, Too,

Controlled In 4 Days, 98% Plasmodium Free In 7 Days, No Relapse In 3 Months

LUNGS
• BRONCHITIS, CHRONIC: Fresh Herb, 200 g As Decoction, 3

Hypnotic Effect
• TRANQUILIZING
MUSCULOSKELETAL/ CONNECTIVE TISSUE
• ARTHRITIS, RHEUMATIC: Excellent When Combined With Xi

• INFLAMMATORY, ANTI- : 20 g/kg Orally 1/Day For 5 Days=300 mg/kg IP Aspirin, Synergistic With Xi Xian Cao/Nian Shen Cao (Herba Bidentis Bipinnatae)

Dose
9 - 30 gm

Common Name
Hairy Clerodendrum/Chinese Par

Contraindications
Not: Hypotensive Patients

Notes
For Hypertension, Add Last
Do Not Boil For A Long Time
No Adverse Effects, High Doses (e.g. Bronchitis)
Nausea, Arrhythmia Possible

DU HUO

獨活
（独活）

RADIX DUHUO

Traditional Functions:

1. Expels Wind Dampness
2. Promotes the circulation of the channels, relieves pain
3. Releases the exterior and disperses Cold

Traditional Properties:

Enters: KI, UB,

Properties: BIT, SP, W

Indications:

EXTREMITIES
• ARMS, PAIN
• FEET, CONVULSIONS PAIN OF
• HANDS, CONVULSIONS, PAIN OF
• LEGS, ACHING, PAINS
FLUID DISORDERS
• DAMPNESS, EXTERNAL: Surface Complex
HEAD/NECK
• HEADACHE: Common Cold/Wind Cold Damp

INFECTIOUS DISEASES
• COMMON COLD: Headache, Fever, Body Aches Of
MUSCULOSKELETAL/ CONNECTIVE TISSUE
• ARTHRITIS: Wind Damp Cold Bi
• ARTHRITIS, PAIN: Wind Damp, Especially Lower Body
• BACK, LOWER PAIN: Aches, Pains
• KNEES, LOINS, PAIN, ACHING

OF
• UPPER BODY, ACHES, PAIN: Used With Qiang Huo
ORAL CAVITY
• TOOTHACHE: Wind, Cold, Damp
PAIN/NUMBNESS/GENERAL DISCOMFORT
• BI, WIND DAMP COLD
• NUMBNESS, EXTREMITIES
SKIN
• PRURITUS

Clinical/Pharmaceutical Studies:

CIRCULATION DISORDERS
• HYPERTENSION: Transient, Alcohol Extract Stronger
EYES
• PHOTOSENSITIZING: May Cause Dermatitis From External Or Internal Use
INFECTIOUS DISEASES
• ANTIBIOTIC: TB, E.Coli, Shigella, Proteus, Salmonella, Pseudomonas, Cholerae
LUNGS
• BRONCHITIS, CHRONIC: Decoction, 74% Showed Some

Response, 7% Marked, Some Cough Suppressing Effects
• TUBERCULOSIS: Night Sweats
MENTAL STATE/ NEUROLOGICAL DISORDERS
• CNS, STIMULANT
• HYPNOTIC: Oral/Injection
• SEDATIVE: Decoction, Fluid Extract
• TRANQUILIZING: Oral/Injection
MUSCULOSKELETAL/ CONNECTIVE TISSUE
• ANTISPASMODIC
• ARTHRITIS: Reduces

Inflammation Of Joints, Volatile Injection
PAIN/NUMBNESS/GENERAL DISCOMFORT
• ANALGESIC: Heat
SKIN
• VITILIGO: Use In Photosensitizing Ability To Increase Pigment, Orally, Topically
STOMACH/DIGESTIVE DISORDERS
• ULCERS, GASTRIC: Some Action
TRAUMA, BITES, POISONINGS
• INFLAMMATORY, ANTI-

Dose
3 - 9 gm

Contraindications
Not: Def Yin/Blood With Heat And Pain

Notes
Toxic: Photosensitivity With Rx Heraclei Form
Possible Numbness Of Tongue, Nausea, Vomiting

HAI FENG TENG

海風藤
（海风藤）

CAULIS PIPERIS

Traditional Functions:
1. Dispels Wind Dampness
2. Circulates all the channels
3. Disperses Cold and reduces pain

Traditional Properties:
Enters: LV,

Properties: SP, BIT, <W

Indications:

ABDOMEN/ GASTROINTESTINAL TOPICS
• ABDOMEN, PAIN OF: Spleen/ Stomach Cold
BOWEL RELATED DISORDERS
• DIARRHEA: Spleen/Stomach Cold
MUSCULOSKELETAL/ CONNECTIVE TISSUE
• ARTHRITIS: Wind Cold Damp Bi, For Opening The Luo Channels

• BACK, LOWER PAIN: Wind Cold Damp Bi
• CRAMPS: Wind Cold Damp Bi
• JOINTS, STIFF: Wind Cold Damp Bi
• KNEES, SORE: Wind Cold Damp Bi
• MUSCLES, SPASMS: Wind Cold Damp Bi
PAIN/NUMBNESS/GENERAL

DISCOMFORT
• BI PAIN, WIND COLD DAMP
SPLEEN
• SPLEEN STOMACH DEFICIENCY, COLD
STOMACH/DIGESTIVE DISORDERS
• EPIGASTRIC PAIN: Spleen/ Stomach Cold

Clinical/Pharmaceutical Studies:

CANCER/TUMORS/SWELLINGS/ LUMPS
• ANTINEOPLASTIC: Some Effect

MUSCULOSKELETAL/ CONNECTIVE TISSUE
• ANTIRHEUMATIC

PAIN/NUMBNESS/GENERAL DISCOMFORT
• ANALGESIC: Arthritic Pain

Dose
9 - 15 gm

Contraindications
Not: Pregnancy

HAI TONG PI

海桐皮

CORTEX ERYTHRINAE VARIEGATAE

Traditional Functions:
1. Dispels Wind Dampness
2. Clears the channels
2. Promotes urination and reduces swelling
3. Kills parasites and treats itching skin lesions

Traditional Properties:
Enters: SP, KI, LV,

Properties: BIT, SP, N

Indications:

BOWEL RELATED DISORDERS
• DIARRHEA
EXTREMITIES
• LEGS, PAIN: Wind Damp Bi
FLUID DISORDERS
• EDEMA, SUPERFICIAL: Dampness
HEAT

• ARTHRITIS: For Opening The Luo Channels
• ARTHRITIS, RHEUMATIC: Wind Damp
• BACK, PAIN: Wind Damp Bi
• BACKACHES, PAIN: Wind Damp Bi
• KNEES, PAIN: Wind Damp Bi

Gargle
PAIN/NUMBNESS/GENERAL DISCOMFORT
• BI, WIND DAMP: Extremities
SKIN
• CARBUNCLES
• RASHES
• SCABIES

Indications:

- DAMP HEAT DISCHARGING TO
  INTERIOR
**MUSCULOSKELETAL/
CONNECTIVE TISSUE**

ORAL CAVITY
- CARIES, TOOTHACHE: Gargle
- TOOTHACHE, FROM CARIES:

- SKIN, DISORDERS: Use
  Externally/Internally
- SKIN, LESIONS, ITCHY

Clinical/Pharmaceutical Studies:

INFECTIOUS DISEASES
- ANTIBIOTIC: Dermatomycoses,
  Staph.Aureus
**MENTAL STATE/
NEUROLOGICAL DISORDERS**

- SEDATIVE
- TRANQUILIZING
SKIN
- FUNGAL, ANTI-: Aqueous Extract,
  Skin Fungi

- PRURITUS
TRAUMA, BITES, POISONINGS
- CURARE-LIKE: Numbs, Relaxes
  Striated Muscle

Dose

3 - 30 gm

Contraindications

Not: Def Blood

Notes

Large Doses May Cause Arrhythmia And Low Blood
Pressure

HU GU

虎骨
(虎骨)

OS
TIGRIS

Traditional Functions:

1. Disperses Wind and Cold
2. Strengthens the tendons and bones
3. Dispels Wind and Dampness, stops pain
3. Subdues fearfulness

Traditional Properties:

Enters: KI, LV,

Properties: SP, SW, W

Indications:

**CANCER/TUMORS/SWELLINGS/
LUMPS**
- NODULAR WIND PAIN
EXTREMITIES
- EXTREMITIES, PARALYSIS OF
- LEGS, WEAK, PAIN
- LIMBS, SPASMS
HEART
- PALPITATIONS
MENTAL STATE/

NEUROLOGICAL DISORDERS
- CONVULSIONS
- EPILEPSY
- FEARFULNESS
- PARALYSIS, EXTREMITIES
**MUSCULOSKELETAL/
CONNECTIVE TISSUE**
- ARTHRITIS
- BACK, LOWER STIFF
- BONES, COLD PAIN IN

- BONES, STRENGTHENS
- JOINTS, PAIN: Damp Bi With
  Liver Kidney Weakness;Endangered
  Species!
- KNEES, WEAK, PAIN
- SPASMS
**PAIN/NUMBNESS/GENERAL
DISCOMFORT**
- BI, WIND COLD: Joints
- PAIN, SEDATES

Clinical/Pharmaceutical Studies:

EXTREMITIES
- LEGS, ATROPHY OF
BONES
- LIMBS, SPASMS
**MENTAL STATE/
NEUROLOGICAL
DISORDERS**
- SEDATIVE
**MUSCULOSKELETAL/
CONNECTIVE TISSUE**
- ANTIRHEUMATIC

- ANTISPASMODIC
- ARTHRITIS: Soak In
  Wine, Tiger Bone Papaye
  Wine (Mu Gua, Chuan
  Xiong, Dang Gui, Niu Xi,
  Hong Hua, Qin Jiao, Feng
  Fang, Tian Ma, Wu Jia Pi,
  Xu Duan, Huang Jing,
  Sang Zhi) , *Tiger Bone
  Myrrh Pill (Hu Gu, Mo

Yao, Quan Xie, Wu Gong)
- BACK, LOWER PAIN,
  SPASMS
- OSTALGIA
**PAIN/NUMBNESS/
GENERAL
DISCOMFORT**
- ANALGESIC: 1 g/kg
**TRAUMA, BITES,
POISONINGS**

- FRACTURES: Promotes
  Healing, Compound Bone
  Healing (Hu Gu, Zi Ran
  Tong, Xue Jie, She Xiang,
  Zhe Chong, et al) , Zi Ran
  Tong With Hu Gu Found
  To Be Most Important, In
  Equal Amounts
- INFLAMMATORY, ANTI-
  : Significant, Arthritis

Dose
9 - 15 gm

Common Name
Tiger Bone

Precautions
Watch: Def Blood w/Fire Rising

Notes
Can Substitute Leopard Bone (Bao Gu) Or Dog (Gou Gu) , But Dog Is Hot

Tigers Are An Endangered Species! This Herb Is For Traditional Reference Only.

JI GU CAO

雞骨草
（鸡骨草）

HERBA ABRI

Traditional Functions:

1. Vitalizes stagnant Blood
2. Helps to mend bones
3. Relieves Wind Damp Bi

Traditional Properties:

Enters: LV,

Properties: SP, W

Indications:

LIVER
• HEPATITIS
• JAUNDICE
MUSCULOSKELETAL/

CONNECTIVE TISSUE
• OSTEOARTHRITIS
• RHEUMATISM
TRAUMA, BITES, POISONINGS

• FRACTURES, USED TO SET
• TRAUMA, INTERNAL/
  EXTERNAL

Clinical/Pharmaceutical Studies:

**BLOOD RELATED DISORDERS/
 TOPICS**
• BLOOD, RED, REDUCES

HEMOLYSIS OF
TRAUMA, BITES, POISONINGS

• INFLAMMATORY, ANTI-:
  Reduces Inflammation Of Joints

Dose
9 - 15 gm

Common Name
Chinese Prayer Beads

Notes
Constituent: Abrine (N-Methyltryptophan)

KUAN JIN TENG

寬筋藤
（宽筋藤）

RAMUS TINOSPORAE SINENSIS

Traditional Functions:

1. Dispels Wind Dampness and relaxes the tendons
2. Relaxes tendons and activates the channels

Traditional Properties:

Enters: LV,

Properties: BIT, <C, SW

Indications:

EXTREMITIES
• LIMBS, SPASMS
**MUSCULOSKELETAL/
CONNECTIVE TISSUE**
• ARTHRITIS

• CRAMPS: Hot Bi
• STIFFNESS: Hot Bi
**PAIN/NUMBNESS/GENERAL
DISCOMFORT**

• BI, HOT: Cramping, Stiffness
TRAUMA, BITES, POISONINGS
• TRAUMA: Redness, Swelling, Heat,
  Pain

Dose
15 - 30 gm

Common Name
Chinese Tinospora

Contraindications
Not: Pregnancy/Postpartum

LAO GUAN CAO

老鸛草
(老鸛草)

HERBA ERODII SEU GERANII

Traditional Functions:

1. Expels Wind and Dampness
2. Vitalizes Blood and promotes the circulation of the channels
3. Stops diarrhea
4. Strengthens tendons and helps move muscles

Traditional Properties:

Enters: LV, LI

Properties: SP, BIT, N

Indications:

ABDOMEN/
  GASTROINTESTINAL TOPICS
• ENTERITIS
• INTESTINES, WEAK
BOWEL RELATED DISORDERS
• DIARRHEA
• DYSENTERY

CIRCULATION DISORDERS
• STROKE SYNDROME
MUSCULOSKELETAL/
  CONNECTIVE TISSUE
• ARTHRITIS: For Opening The Luo
  Channels
• ARTHRITIS, ACUTE/CHRONIC

• JOINTS, PAIN
STOMACH/DIGESTIVE
  DISORDERS
• STOMACH, WEAK
TRAUMA, BITES, POISONINGS
• TRAUMA

Clinical/Pharmaceutical Studies:

ABDOMEN/
  GASTROINTESTINAL TOPICS
• INTESTINES, REGULATES:
  Increases Tone Of Smooth Muscles

BOWEL RELATED DISORDERS
• DIARRHEA: Inhibits Peristalsis
INFECTIOUS DISEASES
• BACTERIAL, ANTI-: Staph

Aureus, Streptococci, Pneumoncocci,
Shigella, E.Coli, Typhoid
• VIRAL, ANTI-

Dose

9 - 30 gm

Common Name

Geranium/Cranebill

LIAO DIAO ZHU
(XU CHANG QING)

了刁竹

HERBA PYCNOSTELMAE

Traditional Functions:

1. Expels Wind Damp and stops pain
2. Removes toxins and disperses swellings

Traditional Properties:

Enters: SP, ST, KI,

Properties: SP, W

Indications:

ABDOMEN/
  GASTROINTESTINAL TOPICS
• ABDOMEN, PAIN OF: Cold,
  Deficiency
• ABDOMEN, PAIN OF, UPPER
• HERNIA, PAIN
FLUID DISORDERS
• EDEMA

LUNGS
• ASTHMA
MUSCULOSKELETAL/
  CONNECTIVE TISSUE
• ARTHRITIS
SEXUALITY, FEMALE:
  GYNECOLOGICAL
• UTERUS, PAIN

SKIN
• SWEATING, EXCESSIVE
TRAUMA, BITES, POISONINGS
• CONTUSIONS
• SNAKE BITES
URINARY BLADDER
• URINATION, EXCESS

Clinical/Pharmaceutical Studies:

CIRCULATION DISORDERS
• HYPOTENSION
INFECTIOUS DISEASES

• BACTERIAL, ANTI-: Staph,
  Typhoid, Dysentery
PAIN/NUMBNESS/GENERAL

DISCOMFORT
• ANALGESIC: Joint Pain,
  Abdominal Pain

Dose

3 - 15 gm

Common Name

Paniculate Swallowwort

Contraindications

Not: Boiled Too Long

LU XIAN CAO
(LU HAN CAO/LU TI CAO)

鹿銜草
（鹿銜草）

HERBA
PYROLAE

Traditional Functions:

1. Removes Wind and eliminates Dampness
2. Strengthens the muscles and tendons
3. Vitalizes the Blood and regulates menstruation
4. Nurtures the Kidney Yin
5. Controls bleeding

Traditional Properties:

Enters: LV, KI

Properties: SW, BIT, W

Indications:

EXTREMITIES
• FEET, NUMB
• FEET, WEAKNESS OF
HEART
• PALPITATIONS
HEMORRHAGIC DISORDERS
• EPISTAXIS
• HEMOPTYSIS: Bloody Sputum
MENTAL STATE/
NEUROLOGICAL DISORDERS
• EMOTIONAL DISTRESS
• MENTAL DISORDERS

• NEURASTHENIA
MUSCULOSKELETAL/
CONNECTIVE TISSUE
• ARTHRITIS
• KNEES, NUMB
• KNEES, WEAK
• LUMBAGO
• RHEUMATISM
NUTRITIONAL/METABOLIC
DISORDERS/TOPICS
• BERIBERI
SEXUALITY, FEMALE:

GYNECOLOGICAL
• LEUKORRHEA
• UTERINE BLEEDING
SKIN
• FURUNCLES, MALIGNANT
TRAUMA, BITES, POISONINGS
• INSECT BITES, TOXIC: Use Raw
Juice
• WOUNDS, INCISED: Use Raw
Juice
URINARY BLADDER
• URINATION, PROMOTES

Clinical/Pharmaceutical Studies:

BLOOD RELATED DISORDERS/
TOPICS
• BLOOD GLUCOSE, INCREASES:
By Inhibiting Insulin
• BLOOD PRESSURE, LOWERS:
Vasodilator
BOWEL RELATED DISORDERS
• DIARRHEA, CHILDHOOD
• DYSENTERY, BACILLARY,
ACUTE IN YOUNG CHILDREN
CIRCULATION DISORDERS
• HYPERTENSION
• THROMBOANGIITIS
OBLITERANS: Severe, Used
Methylhydroquinone, Active
Ingredient

ENDOCRINE RELATED
DISORDERS
• INSULIN, INHIBITS
BREAKDOWN IN BLOOD
HEART
• CARDIOTONIC: Weak Hearts,
Vasodilator
• CORONARY HEART DISEASE
• HEART ATTACK: Improved
Symptoms After Treatment
INFECTIOUS DISEASES
• BACTERIAL, ANTI-: Strong,
Broad Band Inhibition, Staph Aureus,
E.Coli, Shigella, Salmonella Typhi,
Proteus
LIVER

• LIVER, ABSCESS: IV Infusion, 3
Days To Control Temperature, 200
mg, 2x/Day, 3 Months To Cure
LUNGS
• LUNG INFECTION: IV Infusion,
200 mg/Day Of Active Ingredient,
Methylhydroquinone
SEXUALITY, EITHER SEX
• CONTRACEPTIVE: 20%
Decoction, PO, May Cause Atrophy
Of Ovary, Uterus
URINARY BLADDER
• URINARY TRACT INFECTIONS:
Controls Acute Symptoms, Did Not
Eliminate Infection

Dose
9 - 30 gm

Common Name
Pyrola

LUO SHI TENG

絡石藤
（络石藤）

CAULIS
TRACHELOSPERMI
JASMINOIDIS

Traditional Functions:

1. Expels Wind and clears the channels
2. Cools the Blood and reduces abscesses and swelling

Traditional Properties:

Enters: HT, KI, LV,

Properties: BIT, <C

Indications:

MUSCULOSKELETAL/
CONNECTIVE TISSUE
- ARTHRITIS, PAIN: Wind Damp Bi
- JOINTS, PAIN, SWELLING, RED:
  Hot Bi

- MUSCLES, SPASMS
ORAL CAVITY
- PHARYNGITIS
- THROAT, OBSTRUCTION
PAIN/NUMBNESS/GENERAL

DISCOMFORT
- BI PAIN, WIND DAMP
SKIN
- ABSCESS, HOT, PAINFUL, RED
- SORES, TOXIC

Clinical/Pharmaceutical Studies:

CIRCULATION DISORDERS
- VASODILATOR, CUTANEOUS
HEART
- CARDIOTONIC: Small Doses
INFECTIOUS DISEASES
- BACTERIAL, ANTI-: Staph,
  Shigella

MENTAL STATE/
NEUROLOGICAL DISORDERS
- CONVULSIONS/RESPIRATORY
  ARREST: Large Dose Can Cause
MUSCULOSKELETAL/
CONNECTIVE TISSUE

- ANTISPASMODIC
- ARTHRITIS
SEXUALITY, FEMALE:
GYNECOLOGICAL
- UTERUS, INHIBITS
  CONTRACTION

Dose
9 - 15 gm

Common Name
Star Jasmine Stem

Notes
Large Dose Can Cause Convulsions, Respiratory Arrest

MU GUA

木瓜
（木瓜）

FRUCTUS CHAENOMELIS LAGENARIAE

Traditional Functions:

1. Relaxes the muscles and tendons and activates blood circulation in the channels
2. Harmonizes the Stomach and dispels Dampness

Traditional Properties:

Enters: SP, LV,

Properties: SO, W, ARO

Indications:

ABDOMEN/
GASTROINTESTINAL TOPICS
- ABDOMEN, PAIN OF
BOWEL RELATED DISORDERS
- DIARRHEA, VIOLENT W/
  SPASMS
EXTREMITIES
- ARMS, CONTORTION OF
- CRAMPS, SEVERE IN CALVES
- LEG QI, EDEMA
- LEGS, PAIN, SWELLING:
  (Beriberi, Leg Qi) Cold Dampness
- LEGS, WEAK, CRAMPS
FLUID DISORDERS
- DAMPNESS, REMOVES

- THIRST: Fluid Injury
LIVER
- LIVER WIND: Spasms
LUNGS
- COUGH, CHRONIC
MUSCULOSKELETAL/
CONNECTIVE TISSUE
- ARTHRITIS: For Expelling Wind
  Damp
- ARTHRITIS, PAIN: Dampness
- BACK, LOWER WEAK
- JOINTS, PAIN: Damp Bi
NUTRITIONAL/METABOLIC
DISORDERS/TOPICS

- BERIBERI, SWELLING OF
PAIN/NUMBNESS/GENERAL
DISCOMFORT
- BI, DAMP: Pain
- NUMBNESS W/SPASMS,
  CONTRACTURES: Blood
  Deficiency Bi
SKIN
- ECZEMA: Cold Dampness
- SKIN, SORES: Cold Damp
STOMACH/DIGESTIVE
DISORDERS
- DYSPEPSIA
- VOMITING

Clinical/Pharmaceutical Studies:

BLOOD RELATED DISORDERS/
TOPICS
- BLOOD, INCREASES
  PRODUCTION OF: Malic Acid
  Increases Absorption Of Iron
INFECTIOUS DISEASES
- BACTERIAL, ANTI-: Malic Acid

Inhibits Growth
KIDNEYS
- DIURETIC: Dramatic Increase
MUSCULOSKELETAL/
CONNECTIVE TISSUE
- ANTISPASMODIC: Limbs, GI
  Tract

STOMACH/DIGESTIVE
DISORDERS
- ANTIEMETIC
- DIGESTIVE
TRAUMA, BITES, POISONINGS
- INFLAMMATORY, ANTI-:
  Arthritis

Dose
4.5 - 9.0 gm
Common Name
Chinese Quince Fruit

Contraindications
Not: Exterior Conditions

Not: Lumbago From Yin Def
Notes
Excess Can Harm Teeth And Bones

QI YE LIAN

七葉蓮
（七叶莲）

RADIX/CAULIS/FOLIUM SCHEFFLERA

Traditional Functions:

1. Relaxes the muscles and tendons
2. Open the channels, reduces swelling and reduces pain

Traditional Properties:

Enters:

Properties: BIT, W

Indications:

MUSCULOSKELETAL/ CONNECTIVE TISSUE
• ARTHRITIS, RHEUMATIC
• BACK, LOWER PAIN
• JOINTS, PAIN

PAIN/NUMBNESS/GENERAL DISCOMFORT
• PAIN, GENERAL
STOMACH/DIGESTIVE DISORDERS

• STOMACH, ACHE
TRAUMA, BITES, POISONINGS
• FRACTURES
• SPRAINS

Clinical/Pharmaceutical Studies:

HEAD/NECK
• HEADACHE, NEUROGENIC: (See "Pain/Numbness/General Discomfort Topic, Analgesic" Entry For Details)
• HEADACHE, OCCIPTIAL NEURALGIA: (See "Pain/ Numbness/General Discomfort Topic,

Analgesic" Entry For Details)
• MIGRAINE: (See "Pain/ Numbness/General Discomfort Topic, Analgesic" Entry For Details)
LUNGS
• BRONCHITIS: Injected, Fast Onset, 10-15 Min, Lasted 3-6 Hrs-10 gm Of Crude Drug Equivalent

MENTAL STATE/ NEUROLOGICAL DISORDERS
• CONVULSIVE, ANTI-: ETOH Extract
• HYPNOTIC
• SEDATIVE
• TRIGEMINAL NEURALGIA: (See "Analgesic" Entry For Details)

PAIN/NUMBNESS/ GENERAL DISCOMFORT
• ANALGESIC: 80-90%, Induced Sleep, Too, Lasted 8-12 Hours, Less If Infection Involved– Decocted 2x, Then ETOH Extracted/Precipitated-3-5 Tabs Of 0.3 gm Postprandial

Dose
9 - 15 gm
Contraindications
Not: Pregnancy

Notes
Available As Crude Extract In Patent Medicine Of Same Name

Nausea Possible, Take After Meals

Drowsiness Possible

QIAN NIAN JIAN

千年健

RHIZOMA HOMALOMENAE OCCULTAE

Traditional Functions:

1. Dispels Wind and Dampness
2. Strengthens the tendons and bones

Traditional Properties:

Enters: KI, LV,

Properties: SP, BIT, <SW, W

Indications:

GERIATRIC TOPICS
• WIND COLD BI, IN ELDERLY:
Wind Cold Damp Bi, Topical, Too
**MUSCULOSKELETAL/
CONNECTIVE TISSUE**
• ARTHRITIS: Wind, Cold Damp Bi,
Commonly Used With Elderly

• BONES, SOFTNESS: Fortifying
• JOINTS, PAIN: Damp Bi With
Liver Kidney Weakness/Wind Cold
Damp Bi
• MUSCLES, WEAK: Fortifying
PAIN/NUMBNESS/GENERAL

DISCOMFORT
• BI, WIND DAMP COLD:
Superficial Or Deep, Tonifying
Effect
TRAUMA, BITES, POISONINGS
• TRAUMA, PAIN, SWELLING

Dose
4.5 - 9.0 gm

Precautions
Watch: Def Yin Conditions

QIN JIAO

秦艽

RADIX
GENTIANAE
MACROPHYLLAE

Traditional Functions:

1. Dispels Wind and Dampness
2. Removes Yin deficiency Heat
3. Clears Damp Heat jaundice
4. Moistens the intestines and facilitates passage of stool

Traditional Properties:

Enters: ST, LV, GB,

Properties: BIT, SP, N

Indications:

BOWEL RELATED DISORDERS
• CONSTIPATION, FROM
DRYNESS
CHILDHOOD DISORDERS
• MALNUTRITION FEVER,
CHILDHOOD
EXTREMITIES
• ARMS, SPASMS
• CRAMPS, ESPECIALLY
EXTREMITIES
• LEGS, SPASMS
FEVERS
• FEVER, LOW GRADE, CHRONIC
DISEASES
• STEAMING BONE FEVER: Yin
Deficient Heat
• STEAMING BONE FEVER W/

SWEAT
FLUID DISORDERS
• DAMPNESS, EXTERNAL:
Surface Complex
HEAT
• HEAT, EXHAUSTION W/
SURFACE COMPLEX
HEMORRHAGIC DISORDERS
• HEMAFECIA
• HEMATURIA
**IMMUNE SYSTEM RELATED
DISORDERS/TOPICS**
• ALLERGIC INFLAMMATION
LIVER
• HEPATITIS
• JAUNDICE, ACUTE/INFANTS:
Damp Heat

**MUSCULOSKELETAL/
CONNECTIVE TISSUE**
• ARTHRITIS: For Opening The Luo
Channels/Wind Damp Cold Bi
• ARTHRITIS, WHOLE BODY PAIN
• JOINTS, PAIN, SWELLING, RED:
Hot Bi
• LIGAMENTS, RELAXES
• SPASMS, PAINFUL
**PAIN/NUMBNESS/GENERAL
DISCOMFORT**
• ARTHRITIS, WHOLE BODY PAIN
• BI, WIND DAMP COLD: Joints
**YIN RELATED DISORDERS/
TOPICS**
• YIN DEFICIENCY W/FEVER

Clinical/Pharmaceutical Studies:

**BLOOD RELATED
DISORDERS/TOPICS**
• BLOOD PRESSURE,
LOWERS: Aqueous/
Ethanol Extract, Short
Term
• HYPERGLYCEMIC: 30
Min After For 3 Hrs
FEVERS
• ANTIPYRETIC
**IMMUNE SYSTEM
RELATED DISORDERS/
TOPICS**
• ANAPHYLACTIC
SHOCK: IP Injection

INFECTIOUS DISEASES
• ANTIBIOTIC: Inhibits
Staph Areus, Strep. Pneum.,
Shigella, Vibrio Cholerae,
Many Fungi, Leptospirosis
(Need High Doses) ,
Typhoid, Dysentery
• MENINGITIS,
EPIDEMIC
CEREBROSPINAL: Cure
By Injection, IM 0.625 g
(Crude) /ml, 2-5 ml Every 6
Hrs, 3-7 Days, No Side
Effects
LUNGS

• ASTHMA: Abated
**MENTAL STATE/
NEUROLOGICAL
DISORDERS**
• CNS, STIMULANT:
Large Doses
• SEDATIVE: Small Doses,
Synergistic With Other
Sedatives
• TRANQUILIZING
**PAIN/NUMBNESS/
GENERAL
DISCOMFORT**
• ANALGESIC: Synergistic
w/Yan Hu Suo, Tian Xian

Zi, Cao Wu
SKIN
• FUNGAL, ANTI-:
Aqueous Extract, Common
Skin
**TRAUMA, BITES,
POISONINGS**
• ANAPHYLACTIC
SHOCK: IP Injection
• ANTIHISTAMINE
• INFLAMMATORY, ANTI-
: Arthritis (=Aspirin) ,
Through Pituitary,
Increases Adrenal Cortex
Activity, Assists Liver

Dose

3 - 12 gm

Contraindications

Not: Frequent Urination Or Pain w/Emaciation
Not: SP Def w/Diarrhea

Notes

Used With Other Drying Wind Damp Herbs

Up To 15-18 gm, Ok

Possible Severe Nausea, Vomiting, Palpitation,
Bradycardia

RONG SHU XU
(LAO GONG XU)

榕樹鬚
（榕树鬚）

RADIX
FICI AERIUS

Traditional Functions:

1. Dispels Wind Heat and removes toxin
2. Vitalizes Blood

Traditional Properties:

Enters:

Properties: BIT, A, N

Indications:

EYES
• CONJUNCTIVITIS
HEAT
• SUMMER HEAT: Severe Digestive
  Disorders
HEMORRHAGIC DISORDERS
• EPISTAXIS
• HEMATURIA W/URINATION

DISTURBANCE
INFECTIOUS DISEASES
• INFLUENZA
• MEASLES, UNERUPTED
LUNGS
• WHOOPING COUGH
ORAL CAVITY

• TONSILLITIS
PAIN/NUMBNESS/GENERAL
  DISCOMFORT
• BI, WIND DAMP: Bone Pain
TRAUMA, BITES, POISONINGS
• FRACTURES
• TRAUMA

Dose

4.5 - 9.0 gm

Common Name

Ficus

SANG ZHI

桑枝

RAMULUS
MORI ALBAE

Traditional Functions:

1. Dispels Wind and Dampness
2. Clears and activates the channels
3. Promotes urination

Traditional Properties:

Enters: LV,

Properties: BIT, SW, N

Indications:

EXTREMITIES
• EXTREMITIES, CONTRACTURE
  OF
• EXTREMITIES, NUMB
• LEGS, EDEMA
FLUID DISORDERS
• EDEMA: Berberi
MUSCULOSKELETAL/

CONNECTIVE TISSUE
• ARTHRITIS, PAIN: Wind Cold/
  Heat
• ARTHRITIS, PAIN, SPASMS:
  Especially Upper Body
• JOINTS, PAIN: Wind Damp Cold
  Bi
• JOINTS, PAIN, SWELLING, RED:

Hot Bi
• JOINTS, SMOOTHES
  MOVEMENT
PAIN/NUMBNESS/GENERAL
  DISCOMFORT
• BI, WIND DAMP: Especially
  Upper Extremities

Clinical/Pharmaceutical Studies:

CANCER/TUMORS/
  SWELLINGS/LUMPS
• TUMOR, ANTI-
CIRCULATION
  DISORDERS
• HYPERTENSION

Sang Zhi Jin Chu Ye)
IMMUNE SYSTEM
  RELATED DISORDERS/
  TOPICS
• IMMUNE EFFECT:
  Increases Lymphocyte

INFECTIOUS DISEASES
• BACTERIAL, ANTI-:
  Typhoid, Staph
• BRUCELLOSIS,
  CHRONIC: Sang Liu
  Tang/Wan (Sang Zhi, Dang

Geranii Seu Erodii
  (Geranium) , Wu Jia Pi)
  Helped Cases
  Unresponsive To
  Antibiotics
PAIN/NUMBNESS/

Clinical/Pharmaceutical Studies:

HEAD/NECK
• HAIR GROWTH: Increases In Rabbits, Sheep, Extract, (Yang Mao

Production, 30 g/Day As Decoction With Other Herbs

Gui, Mo Yao, Mu Gua, Hong Hua, Fang Feng, Liu Zhi (Willow) , Herba

GENERAL DISCOMFORT
• ANALGESIC

Dose

9 - 60 gm

Common Name

Mulberry Twigs

Precautions

Watch: Def Yin Syndrome

SHE TUI

蛇蛻
（蛇蛻）

PERIOSTRACUM SERPENTIS

Traditional Functions:

1. Removes Wind and stops spasms
2. Clears the eyes and removes superficial visual film

Traditional Properties:

Enters: LV,

Properties: SW, SA, N

Indications:

BOWEL RELATED DISORDERS
• FISTULA
• HEMORRHOIDS
EYES
• CORNEAL DISORDERS
• PTERYGIUM
INFECTIOUS DISEASES

• TUBERCULOSIS, BONES: As Powder
MENTAL STATE/ NEUROLOGICAL DISORDERS
• CONVULSIONS, CHILDHOOD
• SEIZURES
ORAL CAVITY

• MOUTH, ULCERS
• THROAT, SORE
SKIN
• CARBUNCLES
• SCABIES
• SKIN, LESIONS: Wind

Clinical/Pharmaceutical Studies:

EYES
• HORDEOLUM: Pieces Soaked In Vinegar, 3 Days

INFECTIOUS DISEASES
• PAROTITIS: 2 Days With Eggs
PARASITES

• BRAIN, CYSTICERCOSIS: Long Term, Some Symptoms Releaved

Dose

4.5 - 9.0 gm

Common Name

Snake Skin Slough

Contraindications

Not: Pregnancy

SHEN JIN CAO

伸筋草

HERBA LYCOPODII

Traditional Functions:

1. Dispels Wind, Cold and Dampness
2. Relaxes the tendons and muscles and clears the channels
3. Vitalizes the Blood

Traditional Properties:

Enters: LV

Properties: BIT, SP, W

Indications:

CIRCULATION DISORDERS
• STROKE, POST: Bending, Stretching Difficulty
FLUID DISORDERS
• EDEMA
MENTAL STATE/

NEUROLOGICAL DISORDERS
• HEMIPLEGIA, DIFFICULTY IN BENDING AND STRETCHING AFTER
MUSCULOSKELETAL/ CONNECTIVE TISSUE

• ARTHRITIS: For Opening The Luo Channels
• JOINTS, NUMBNESS, PAINFUL
TRAUMA, BITES, POISONINGS
• TRAUMA

Clinical/Pharmaceutical Studies:

ABDOMEN/
GASTROINTESTINAL TOPICS
• PERISTALSIS, INCREASES
   SMALL INTESTINES
ENDOCRINE RELATED

DISORDERS
• ESTROGEN-LIKE
FEVERS
• ANTIPYRETIC
INFECTIOUS DISEASES

• BACTERIAL, ANTI-
SEXUALITY, FEMALE:
GYNECOLOGICAL
• UTERUS, STIMULATES

Dose
6 - 15 gm

Contraindications
Not: Pregnancy

Not: With Excess Bleeding

Common Name
Club Moss

SONG JIE
(YOU SONG JIE)

松節
(松节)

LIGNUM
PINI NODI

Traditional Functions:

1. Dispels Wind and dries Dampness
2. Stops pain

Traditional Properties:

Enters: KI, LV,

Properties: BIT, W

Indications:

CANCER/TUMORS/SWELLINGS/
LUMPS
• NODULAR PAIN: Wind
EXTREMITIES
• ARMS, SPASMS: Sudden
• LEGS, SPASMS: Sudden
MUSCULOSKELETAL/
CONNECTIVE TISSUE

• ARTHRITIS, PAIN: Wind Damp
   Cold Bi
• JOINTS, LUBRICATES
• JOINTS, PAIN: Wind Damp Bi
NUTRITIONAL/METABOLIC
DISORDERS/TOPICS
• BERIBERI
ORAL CAVITY

• TEETH, DENTAL CARIES, PAIN
   OF: Wind Pain, Topical
PAIN/NUMBNESS/GENERAL
DISCOMFORT
• BI, WIND DAMP: Joints Pain, Sore
TRAUMA, BITES, POISONINGS
• TRAUMA, PAIN

Clinical/Pharmaceutical Studies:

MUSCULOSKELETAL/
CONNECTIVE TISSUE

• ARTHRITIS, RHEUMATOID:
   Pieces Soaked In Vinegar, 3 Days

• BACK, LOWER PAIN: Injection,
   With Dang Gui

Dose
9 - 15 gm

Precautions
Watch: Def Yin/Blood

Common Name
Knotty Pine Wood

Notes
More External Use In Oil

WEI LING XIAN

威靈仙
(威灵仙)

RADIX
CLEMETIDIS CHINENSIS

Traditional Functions:

1. Expels Wind and activates all twelve channels
2. Dispels Wind Damp and relieves pain
3. Regulates urination
4. Softens and transforms fish bones

Traditional Properties:

Enters: UB,

Properties: SP, SA, W, TX

Indications:

ABDOMEN/
GASTROINTESTINAL TOPICS
• ABDOMEN, ACCUMULATION,

• DAMPNESS: Removes Thru
   Circulation
• EDEMA

• KNEES, PAIN
PAIN/NUMBNESS/GENERAL
DISCOMFORT

Indications:

MASS
- ABDOMEN, MASS

CHEST
- CHEST, PHLEGM FLUID

CIRCULATION DISORDERS
- STROKE

EXTREMITIES
- ARMS, PAIN
- LEGS, PAIN
- LOINS, PAIN

FLUID DISORDERS

HEAD/NECK
- MIGRAINE

MUSCULOSKELETAL/
CONNECTIVE TISSUE
- ARTHRITIS: For Opening The Luo Channels
- ARTHRITIS, WHOLE BODY PAIN: Wind Bi
- BACKACHE
- GOUT
- JOINTS, PAIN IN WHOLE BODY

- BI, WIND: Entire Body
- BI, WIND DAMP, CHRONIC: Open Luo, Arrest Pain

PHLEGM
- PHLEGM FLUID

STOMACH/DIGESTIVE
DISORDERS
- STOMACH PHLEGM FLUID

TRAUMA, BITES, POISONINGS
- BONES, SMALL FISH LODGED IN THROAT

Clinical/Pharmaceutical Studies:

ABDOMEN/
GASTROINTESTINAL
TOPICS
- INTESTINES, STIMULATES

BLOOD RELATED
DISORDERS/TOPICS
- BLOOD PRESSURE, LOWERS

CANCER/TUMORS/
SWELLINGS/LUMPS
- ESOPHAGEAL CANCER: With Ban Lan Gen, Aerial Part Of Euphorbia Lunulata, Tian Nan Xing, Niu Huang (Artificial) , Sal Ammoniac, 11% Remission, Another 80% Had Some Effect
- TUMORS

CHILDHOOD
DISORDERS
- BALANITIS, CHILDHOOD, YOUNG

FLUID DISORDERS
- ANTIDIURETIC

GALL BLADDER
- CHOLECYSTITIS, CHRONIC

INFECTIOUS DISEASES
- BACTERIAL, ANTI-:

Enteritis, Dysentery, Inhibits Staph Aureus, Shigella, Other Gram +/-, Too
- MALARIA

LIVER
- HEPATITIS, ACUTE, ICTERIC, INFECTIOUS: Roasted, Ground, Pork/ Beef Prohibited

MUSCULOSKELETAL/
CONNECTIVE TISSUE
- ARTHRITIS, ANTIINFLAMMATORY: Tincture
- BACK, LOWER: Hypertrophic Spondylitis, Lumbar Muscle Strain: Injection Of Steam Distillate (Volatile Oil) Into Hua To Jia Ji Points, 1 ml Each Point, 2-4 Points/ Day Or Alternate Days, 83-94% Responsive

ORAL CAVITY
- THROAT, FISH BONES LODGED IN: Good, Best Extracted With Acetic Acid, Relaxes Spasms, But Increases Peristalsis, Thus Allowing Bone To

Dislodge, 30 g, May Add Du Huo, Wu Mei, Gan Cao, Make Concentrated Decoction/Use With Vinegar, Give Slowly By Mouth (30-60 Min) , 1-2 Doses/Day, 88% Effective
- THROAT, INTENSIFIES ESOPHAGEAL PERISTALSIS
- TONSILLITIS, ACUTE: Fresh Leaves, As Tea

PAIN/NUMBNESS/
GENERAL
DISCOMFORT
- ANALGESIC: Injected Decoctions

PARASITES
- FILARIASIS
- WORMS, FILARIASIS: Fresh Herb, 500 g, Decoct For 30 Min, Then Boil Liquid With White Wine, 60 g, Brown Sugar 500 g For Short Time, Divide To Take 2x/Day, 5 Days, 75-100% Worm Free

SEXUALITY, FEMALE:
GYNECOLOGICAL
- ABORTION, INDUCES: Wash Root, Sterilize With

Iodine Tincture, 75% Alcohol, Gradually Introduce Into Uterus Until Resistance Felt, 2 Cm Of Root Left Outside Of Cervix, Fix With Gauze, 95% Had Abortion, 15% Incomplete, 24-48 Hrs After
- MASTITIS, ACUTE

SEXUALITY, MALE:
UROLOGICAL TOPICS
- BALANITIS, IN YOUNG CHILDREN

SKIN
- FUNGAL, ANTI-: Candida Albicans, et al
- PSORIASIS: 90 g, Decocted Take Orally, Morning, Evening Until Skin Clears

TRAUMA, BITES,
POISONINGS
- FISH BONES: Can Soften When Extracted With Acetic Acid
- SPRAINS, HELPS REDUCE EFFECTS OF

URINARY BLADDER
- GLUCOSURIA: Controlled

Dose

3 - 12 gm

Common Name

Chinese Clematis Root

Contraindications

Not: Def Qi & Blood (Weak Constitution)

Notes

Prepare With Wine To Increase Effect Against Bi Syndrome

Contact With Fresh Mucus Of Stem May Cause Irritation

WU JIA PI

五加皮

**CORTEX
ACANTHOPANACIS
RADICIS**

Traditional Functions:

1. Dispels Wind Dampness
2. Strengthens the tendons and bones
3. Benefits urination and reduces swelling

Traditional Properties:

Enters: KI, LV,

Properties: SP, W

Indications:

**BOWEL RELATED
DISORDERS**
• FISTULA
  OBSTRUCTION
**CHILDHOOD
DISORDERS**
• RETARDED
  AMBULATION
  DEVELOPMENT,
  CHILDHOOD
EXTREMITIES
• LEG QI: Cold Damp
• LEGS, LOWER, WEAK,
  SORE
FLUID DISORDERS

• EDEMA: Dampness, Evil
  Fluid
GERIATRIC TOPICS
• STANDING,
  PROLONGED, IN
  ELDERLY: Prolonged
  Standing
**MUSCULOSKELETAL/
CONNECTIVE TISSUE**
• ARTHRITIS
• BACKACHE
• JOINTS, PAIN: Damp Bi
  With Liver Kidney
  Weakness/Wind Damp Bi

• KNEES, SORE
• SPASMS, TENDONS,
  BONES
**PAIN/NUMBNESS/
GENERAL
DISCOMFORT**
• BI, WIND DAMP COLD,
  CHRONIC: Liver Kidney
  Deficiency
• NUMBNESS W/SPASMS,
  CONTRACTURES:
  Blood Deficiency Bi
• NUMBNESS, LOINS,
  LEGS

**SEXUALITY, FEMALE:
GYNECOLOGICAL**
• GENITALS, PRURITUS
  IN WOMEN
**SEXUALITY, MALE:
UROLOGICAL TOPICS**
• IMPOTENCE: Mild,
  From Scrotal Dampness
• SCROTUM, ECZEMA
URINARY BLADDER
• DYSURIA
• URINATION,
  DIFFICULT
• URINATION, SCANTY

Clinical/Pharmaceutical Studies:

**CANCER/TUMORS/SWELLINGS/
LUMPS**
• CANCER, REDUCES
  OCCURRANCE OF
ENERGETIC STATE
• ADAPTOGEN: Good
• ENDURANCE, INCREASES
**IMMUNE SYSTEM RELATED
DISORDERS/TOPICS**
• IMMUNE EFFECT: Reduces Loss
  Of Lymphocytes
INFECTIOUS DISEASES

• SHIGELOSIS, LEUKOPENIA OF
KIDNEYS
• DIURETIC
**MUSCULOSKELETAL/
CONNECTIVE TISSUE**
• ARTHRITIS: Antiinflammatory
• MUSCLES, SMOOTH
  STIMULATES: Uterus Esp
**NUTRITIONAL/METABOLIC
DISORDERS/TOPICS**
• METABOLISM, HARMONIZES

**PAIN/NUMBNESS/GENERAL
DISCOMFORT**
• ANALGESIC: Only When Stressed
**SEXUALITY, FEMALE:
GYNECOLOGICAL**
• UTERUS, STIMULATES
TRAUMA, BITES, POISONINGS
• INFLAMMATORY, ANTI-:
  (Hesperidin)
• TOXIC EXPOSURE: Increase
  Tolerance Of

Dose
4.5 - 15.0 gm
Contraindications
Not: Excess Heat

Precautions
Watch: Def Yin w/Heat
Notes
Soak In Wine For Geriatric Joint/Back Pain, Walking
Difficulty

WU SHAO SHE

烏梢蛇
(乌梢蛇)

ZAOCYS DHUMNADES

Traditional Functions:

1. Dispels Wind and Dampness and activates the channels
2. Dispels Wind from the skin
3. Relieves and stabilizes spasms

Traditional Properties:

Enters: SP, LV,

Properties: SW, SA, N

Indications:

HEAD/NECK
- FACE, PARALYSIS

INFECTIOUS DISEASES
- LEPROSY
- TETANUS

**MUSCULOSKELETAL/
CONNECTIVE TISSUE**
- ARTHRITIS: For Expelling Wind
Damp

- CRAMPS
- JOINTS, PAIN: Wind
- SPASMS

**PAIN/NUMBNESS/GENERAL
DISCOMFORT**
- BI, WIND DAMP, CHRONIC:
Open Luo, Arrest Pain

SKIN
- FUNGAL INFECTIONS

- PRURITUS: Wind
- RASHES
- SCABIES
- SKIN, DISORDERS: Heat &
Dampness
- SKIN, NUMBNESS
- SKIN, SORES, INTRACTABLE
- URTICARIA

Clinical/Pharmaceutical Studies:

**BLOOD RELATED DISORDERS/
TOPICS**
- BLOOD PRESSURE, LOWERS:

Vasodilates
**MENTAL STATE/
NEUROLOGICAL DISORDERS**

- TRANQUILIZING: Less Than Bai
Hua She

Dose

4.5 - 9.0 gm

Common Name

Black-Striped Snake

Notes

(Same As Bai Hua She, But Weaker)

Powder: 3 gm

XI XIAN CAO
(XI JIAN CAO)

稀薟草
（稀莶草）

HERBA
SIEGESBECKIAE
ORIENTALIS

Traditional Functions:

1. Expels Wind and Dampness
2. Clears the channels and strengthens the tendons and bones
3. Clears Heat and relieves toxins
4. Calms the spirit
5. Clears Heat and pacifies the Liver
6. Transforms Damp Heat in the skin

Traditional Properties:

Enters: SP, KI, LV,

Properties: BIT, C,

Indications:

**CANCER/TUMORS/SWELLINGS/
LUMPS**
- TUMORS

CIRCULATION DISORDERS
- HYPERTENSION
- STROKE, POST

EARS/HEARING DISORDERS
- DIZZINESS: Liver Yang Rising

EXTREMITIES
- ARMS, NUMB: Bi
- LEGS, NUMB, WEAK
- LEGS, UPPER, WEAK
- LIMBS, ACHING

HEAD/NECK
- FACE, PARALYSIS
- HEADACHE: Liver Yang Rising

INFECTIOUS DISEASES

- MEASLES

LIVER
- LIVER YANG RISING

**MENTAL STATE/
NEUROLOGICAL DISORDERS**
- FORGETFULNESS
- HEMIPLEGIA
- INSOMNIA
- IRRITABILITY

**MUSCULOSKELETAL/
CONNECTIVE TISSUE**
- ARTHRITIS: For Expelling Wind
Damp
- ARTHRITIS, RHEUMATOID:
Wind Damp Bi
- BACK, NUMB, WEAK

- JOINTS, PAIN
- JOINTS, PAIN, SWELLING, RED:
Hot Bi
- KNEES, WEAK

**PAIN/NUMBNESS/GENERAL
DISCOMFORT**
- BI, WIND DAMP HEAT

SEXUALITY, EITHER SEX
- PRURITUS, EXTERNAL
GENITALIA: Use Internal

SKIN
- ECZEMA: Wind Damp
- RASHES: Damp Wind
- SKIN, SUPPURATIVE
INFECTIONS: Wind Damp
- SORES: Damp Heat

Clinical/Pharmaceutical Studies:

**BLOOD RELATED
DISORDERS/TOPICS**
- BLOOD PRESSURE,
LOWERS: Decoctions/

Of Neurotic Symptoms,
Too
INFECTIOUS DISEASES
- MALARIA, ACUTE

CONNECTIVE TISSUE
- ARTHRITIS,
RHEUMATIC: Xi Xian
Chou Wu Wan (Xi Xian

Days, Herb Effective With
Stem Of Piper Futokadsura,
etc
SKIN

Clinical/Pharmaceutical Studies:

Alcohol Extracts, Concentrated Decoction, 3 g, Di Gu Pi 10 g Divided In 2-3 Doses/As Tablet 1.5 g, 2-3x/Day, 85% Some Effect, Some Improvement

EPISODES: 15 Q/Day Decoction Controls, (Report May Not Be Reliable)
MUSCULOSKELETAL/

Cao, Chou Wu Tong) , Used Sucessfully Often, Initial Dose, 6-8 g Gradually Increase Dose To 12-15 g, 2x/Day For 18

• PRURITIC, ANTI-
TRAUMA, BITES, POISONINGS
• INFLAMMATORY, ANTI-
: Arthritis

Dose

9 - 30 gm

Common Name

Siegesbeckia

Contraindications

Not: Def Yin/Blood

Notes

No Known Adverse Effects, Even With Prolonged Oral Use

XUN GU FENG

尋骨風
（寻骨风）

HERBA ARISTOLOCHIAE

Traditional Functions:

1. Dispels Wind and opens and promotes the flow of the channels

Traditional Properties:

Enters:

Properties: BIT, N

Indications:

ABDOMEN/
GASTROINTESTINAL TOPICS
• ABDOMEN, PAIN OF
INFECTIOUS DISEASES

• MALARIA
MUSCULOSKELETAL/
CONNECTIVE TISSUE

• ARTHRITIS, PAIN
SKIN
• ABSCESS, SWELLING

Clinical/Pharmaceutical Studies:

CANCER/TUMORS/SWELLINGS/
LUMPS
• CANCER, ANTI-: Ascitic Tumor,

Subcutaneous Cancers
MUSCULOSKELETAL/
CONNECTIVE TISSUE

• ARTHRITIS: Volitile Oil And
Alkaloids

Dose

9 - 15 gm

Common Name

Hairy Birthwort

Fragrant Herbs That Transform Dampness

BAI DOU KOU
(DOU KOU)

白豆蔻

FRUCTUS
AMOMI CARDAMOMI

Traditional Functions:

1. Dries Dampness
2. Harmonizes and warms the Center and causes rebellious Qi to descend
3. Moves the Qi and relieves and strengthens the Stomach

Traditional Properties:

Enters: LU, SP, ST,

Properties: SP, W, ARO

Indications:

**ABDOMEN/
GASTROINTESTINAL TOPICS**
• ABDOMEN, DISTENTION OF:
Damp Heat
• ABDOMEN, PAIN OF, UPPER:
Cold
• GASTROINTESTINAL
FULLNESS
BOWEL RELATED DISORDERS
• DIARRHEA: Cold Dampness (Add
Warm Interior Herbs, Too) /Spleen
Defienct With Qi Stagnation
CHEST
• CHEST, CONSTRICTION: Damp
Warm Febrile Diseases

• CHEST, FULLNESS
INFECTIOUS DISEASES
• FEBRILE DISEASES: Damp Warm
SPLEEN
• SPLEEN STOMACH
DEFICIENCY, COLD
• SPLEEN STOMACH, DAMPNESS
• SPLEEN STOMACH, QI
STAGNATION
**STOMACH/DIGESTIVE
DISORDERS**
• ANOREXIA: Damp Heat, Febrile
Diseases/Spleen/Stomach Qi
Stagnation
• BELCHING

• DYSPEPSIA, IN PULMONARY
DISEASES/GENERAL DEBILITY
• EPIGASTRIC DISTENTION:
Spleen/Stomach Qi Stagnation
• FOOD STAGNATION: Overnight
• FOOD, AID TO DIGESTION
• HICCUPS: Qi Deficiency-Cold/
Dampness
• INDIGESTION
• VOMITING: Spleen Stomach Cold,
Deficient/Stomach Cold/Qi
Deficiency–Dampness/Cold
TRAUMA, BITES, POISONINGS
• ALCOHOLIC INTOXICATION

Clinical/Pharmaceutical Studies:

**ABDOMEN/
GASTROINTESTINAL TOPICS**
• PERISTALSIS, INCREASES
BOWEL RELATED DISORDERS
• FLATULENCE: Inhibits
Fermentation

INFECTIOUS DISEASES
• BACTERIAL, ANTI-: Shigella
LUNGS
• TUBERCULOSIS: Antitubercular-
Synergizes Streptomycin

**STOMACH/DIGESTIVE
DISORDERS**
• ANTIEMETIC
• STOMACHIC: Increases Secretion
Of Gastric Juice

Dose
1.5 - 6.0 gm
Common Name
Cardamon Fruit (White)

Contraindications
Not: Def Yin & Blood
Precautions
Watch: w/o Cold Damp
Notes
If Powder Used: 1.5-3 gm

CANG ZHU

蒼朮
(苍术)

RHIZOMA
ATRACTYLODIS

Traditional Functions:

1. Dries Dampness, promotes urination and strengthens the Spleen
2. Removes Wind Damp bi
3. Clears Damp Heat pouring downwards
4. Benefits night blindness
5. Releases the exterior and causes sweating

Traditional Properties:

Enters: SP, ST,

Properties: SP, BIT, W, ARO

Indications:

ABDOMEN/
GASTROINTESTINAL
TOPICS
• ABDOMEN,
DISTENTION OF: Damp
Heat
• ABDOMEN,
DISTENTION OF, PAIN
• GASTROINTESTINAL
DISTURBANCES
BOWEL RELATED
DISORDERS
• DIARRHEA: Cold
Dampness (Add Warm
Interior Herbs, Too) /
Spleen Dampness/Spleen
Deficiency
EXTREMITIES
• LEG QI: Damp Heat
• LEGS, SWOLLEN,
PAINFUL (BERIBERI,
LEG QI) : Cold Dampness
EYES
• NIGHT BLINDNESS

FLUID DISORDERS
• DAMPNESS,
EXTERNAL: Surface
Complex
• EDEMA
• EDEMA, DISTENTION,
FULLNESS
HEAD/NECK
• HEADACHE: Wind Cold
Damp Evil
MUSCULOSKELETAL/
CONNECTIVE TISSUE
• ARTHRITIS: Wind Damp
Cold Bi
• JOINTS, PAIN: Wind
Cold Damp Bi
• JOINTS, PAIN,
SWELLING, RED: Hot
Bi
• JOINTS, SORE,
SWELLING: Damp Heat
• RHEUMATIC
ARTHRITIS

NUTRITIONAL/
METABOLIC
DISORDERS/TOPICS
• BERIBERI: Cold
Dampness
PAIN/NUMBNESS/
GENERAL
DISCOMFORT
• BI, WIND DAMP: w/
Fang Feng
• BODY SORENESS:
Wind Cold Damp Evil
PHLEGM
• DAMP PHLEGM
SEXUALITY, FEMALE:
GYNECOLOGICAL
• LEUKORRHEA: Cold,
Damp/Damp Heat
SKIN
• ECZEMA: Cold
Dampness/Damp Heat
• SKIN, SORES: Cold
Damp/Damp Heat

• SORES, OOZING YIN
SORES: Wind Cold Damp
Evil
SPLEEN
• SPLEEN STOMACH,
DAMPNESS
STOMACH/DIGESTIVE
DISORDERS
• ANOREXIA: Spleen
Dampness
• EPIGASTRIC
DISTENTION: Spleen
Dampness
• HICCUPS: Qi Deficiency-
-Dampness
• INDIGESTION
• NAUSEA/VOMITING:
Spleen Dampness
• VOMITING: Qi
Deficiency–Dampness
URINARY BLADDER
• UROPENIA: Kidney
Weakness

Clinical/Pharmaceutical Studies:

ABDOMEN/
GASTROINTESTINAL
TOPICS
• ABDOMEN,
DISTENTION OF, UPPER:
Ping Wei San (Cang Zhu,
Hou PO, Chen Pi, Gan Cao) ,
With Ginger Soup Or
Boiled Water
• ABDOMEN, PAIN OF:
Ping Wei San (Cang Zhu,
Hou PO, Chen Pi, Gan Cao) ,
With Ginger Soup Or
Boiled Water
• INTESTINES,
GURGLING: Ping Wei
San (Cang Zhu, Hou PO,
Chen Pi, Gan Cao) , With
Ginger Soup Or Boiled
Water
BLOOD RELATED

DISORDERS/TOPICS

ENERGETIC STATE
• TONIFIES
EYES
• NIGHT BLINDNESS:
Not So, Very Little Vit A
As Previously Thought
HEART

• TACHYCARDIA, SINUS:
IM Injection Of Herb
Preparation (Not
Mentioned) , 3-5 Days

Treatment
INFECTIOUS DISEASES
• BACTERIAL, ANTI-:
With Ai Ye, As Incense
Fumigant, Lasts 6-8 Hrs,
Almost Equal To
Formaldhyde, Used
Successfully In Nurseries

To Stop Spread Of

Ye, Against Bacterial/Viral
Form
• BRONCHITIS,
CHRONIC: Use Of
Incense Of Cang Zhu, Ai
Ye, 7-14 Days Improved
Cough, Dyspnea,

Expectoration
MENTAL STATE/
NEUROLOGICAL
DISORDERS

• TRANQUILIZING:
Volatile Oil, Low Dose
SEXUALITY, FEMALE:
GYNECOLOGICAL
• ABORTIFACIENT: Up
To 8 Weeks Pregnant, :
Ping Wei San (Cang Zhu,
Hou PO, Chen Pi, Gan Cao) ,
With Mang Xiao, Up To
2 Doses Needed

Day 15-30 Minutes,
Powder Of Cang Zhu, Da
Feng Zi, Ku Shen, Fang
Feng, Bai Xian Pi, Gall Of
Melaphis Chinensis, Song
Xiang, Huang Bai, (Nan)
He Shi, Cure In 20-40

Days
• SKIN, DISORDERS:
Pruritus, Erythema
Multiforme Exudation,

Chronic, Acute Urticaria,
Allergic Dermatitis,
Pediatric Pruritus, IM
Injection Of Herb Oil For 1-
5 Weeks
STOMACH/DIGESTIVE
DISORDERS
• GASTRITIS, ACUTE,

CHRONIC: Ping Wei San,

Clinical/Pharmaceutical Studies:

- BLOOD PRESSURE, RAISES
BOWEL RELATED DISORDERS
- DIARRHEA: Ping Wei San, With Ginger Soup Or Boiled Water
- FLATULENCE: Stimulates Peristalsis
CANCER/TUMORS/ SWELLINGS/LUMPS
- ESOPHAGEAL CANCER: Volitile Oil Inhibited In Vitro At High Doses
ENDOCRINE RELATED DISORDERS
- DIABETES MELLITUS: Reduces Blood Glu, Significant After 10 Days, Then Continues Lower

Diseases
- MALARIA: Powder Of Cang Zhu, Du Huo, Chuan Xiong, Gui Zhi Wrapped In Gauze, Inserted In Nostrils May Control Malaria Symptoms, Preventing Relapse, Old Study, No Reconfirmation Recently
- VIRAL, ANTI-: Influenza, et al With Ai Ye, As Incense Fumigant, Lasts 6-8 Hrs, Almost Equal To Formaldhyde, Used Successfully In Nurseries To Stop Spread Of Diseases
LUNGS
- BRONCHITIS: With Ai

- LABOR, INDUCES, W/ INTRAUTERINE FETAL DEATH: Ping Wei San (Cang Zhu, Hou PO, Chen Pi, Gan Cao) , With Mang Xiao, Up To 2 Doses Needed
- LEUKORRHEA, PROFUSE YELLOW: Er Miao San (Cang Zhu, Huang Bai)
SKIN
- DIAPHORETIC
- ECZEMA: Er Miao San (Cang Zhu, Huang Bai) , Oral And External Application
- NEURODERMATITIS: Fumigate Skin Lesions 2x/

With Ginger Soup Or Boiled Water
- STOMACHIC
- VOMITING: Ping Wei San, With Ginger Soup Or Boiled Water
TRAUMA, BITES, POISONINGS
- STREPTOMYCIN TOXICITY: Prevents, Treats Ototoxicity, Circumoral Numbness, Oral Tablet
URINARY BLADDER
- EXCRETION: Increases Salts Excretion, Not Diuretic:Increase Ion Output, Not So Much Fluids

Dose

3 - 9 gm

Contraindications

Not: With Excess Sweating w/Def Qi

Not: Def Yin w/Internal Heat

Precautions

Watch: Loose Stool

Watch: Drying

CAO DOU KOU
(DOU KOU)

草豆蔻

SEMEN ALPINIAE KATSUMADAI

Traditional Functions:

1. Dissipates Cold by warming and dries Dampness
2. Warms the Stomach, strengthens Spleen Yang
3. Promotes Qi circulation, reduces vomiting

Traditional Properties:

Enters: SP, ST,

Properties: SP, W, ARO

Indications:

ABDOMEN/ GASTROINTESTINAL TOPICS
- ABDOMEN, DISTENTION OF: Damp Heat
- ABDOMEN, FULLNESS OF
- ABDOMEN, PAIN OF: Cold
BOWEL RELATED DISORDERS
- DIARRHEA, CHRONIC: Spleen Cold, Deficient
CHEST

- CHEST, CHILLS, PAIN
SPLEEN
- SPLEEN DEFICIENCY, COLD
- SPLEEN STOMACH, DAMPNESS, COLD
STOMACH/DIGESTIVE DISORDERS
- ACID REGURGITATION
- ANOREXIA: Spleen Cold,

Deficient
- BELCHING: Stomach Reflux
- DYSPHAGIA
- EPIGASTRIC PAIN: Cold
- HICCUPS: Qi Deficiency-Cold
- STOMACH, PAIN: Spleen Stomach Cold, Damp
- VOMITING: Qi Deficiency-Cold/ Spleen Stomach Cold, Damp

Clinical/Pharmaceutical Studies:

ABDOMEN/ GASTROINTESTINAL TOPICS

- INTESTINES, STIMULATES:

Aqueous Extract, Low Doses

Dose

2.4 - 6.0 gm

Common Name

Katsumada's Galangal Seed

Contraindications

Not: Def Yin

Not: w/o Cold Dampness

CAO GUO

草果

FRUCTUS AMOMI TSAO-KO

Traditional Functions:

1. Dissipates Cold by warming and dries Dampness
2. Relieves malaria
3. Removes fullness and Phlegm

Traditional Properties:

Enters: SP, ST,

Properties: SP, W

Indications:

ABDOMEN/ GASTROINTESTINAL TOPICS
• ABDOMEN, PAIN OF: Cold
BOWEL RELATED DISORDERS
• DIARRHEA
CHEST
• CHEST, PAIN: Cold
• CHEST, STUFFINESS/FULLNESS
FEVERS
• FEVER, CHILLS INTERMITTENT
• FEVER, DAMPNESS

INFECTIOUS DISEASES
• MALARIA, CHILLS, FEVER OF
• MALARIA-LIKE SYNDROMES
PHLEGM
• PHLEGM FLUID W/MASS SENSATION
SKIN
• DIAPHORETIC, WEAK
SPLEEN
• SPLEEN STOMACH

DEFICIENCY, COLD
STOMACH/DIGESTIVE DISORDERS
• ACID REGURGITATION
• EPIGASTRIC PAIN
• FOOD STAGNATION: Excess Meat Eating
• NAUSEA/VOMITING: Spleen Stomach Cold, Deficient
• STOMACH REFLUX

Dose

2.4 - 9.0 gm

Contraindications

Not: Def Qi/Blood
Not: w/o Cold/Damp

GAN SONG XIANG
(GAN SUNG)

甘松香

RHIZOMA NARDOSTACHYTIS

Traditional Functions:

1. Regulates the Qi
2. Disperses Cold and controls pain

Traditional Properties:

Enters: SP, ST

Properties: SW, W

Indications:

ABDOMEN/ GASTROINTESTINAL TOPICS
• ABDOMEN, DISTENTION OF/

PAIN
CHEST
• CHEST, DISTENTION/PAIN

ORAL CAVITY
• TOOTHACHE

Clinical/Pharmaceutical Studies:

MENTAL STATE/ NEUROLOGICAL
DISORDERS
• TRANQUILIZING:

Similar To Valerian, Lower

Toxicity (Essential Oil)

Dose

3.0 - 4.5 gm

Common Name

Chinese Spikenard

HOU PO HUA
(CHUAN PO HUA)

厚樸花
(厚朴花)

FLOS MAGNOLIA OFFICIANLIS

Traditional Functions:

1. Dries Dampness by aromatic stimulation
2. Promotes Qi circulation in Spleen and Stomach

Traditional Properties:

Enters: SP, ST

Properties: SP, BIT, W

Indications:

**ABDOMEN/
GASTROINTESTINAL
TOPICS**
• ABDOMEN,
DISTENTION OF: Food
Stagnation/Stagnant Qi/
Turbid Dampness
• ABDOMEN, PAIN OF:
Food Stagnation
**BOWEL RELATED
DISORDERS**
• DIARRHEA: Food
Stagnation, With Most

Herbs, Cooked, Charred
CHEST
• CHEST, DISTENTION:
Food Stagnation
• CHEST, FULLNESS:
Stagnant Qi/Turbid
Dampness
LUNGS
• ASTHMA
• COUGH
• WHEEZING, COUGH,
CHEST CONSTRICTION:
Phlegm Obstruction

SPLEEN
• SPLEEN STOMACH
DISHARMONY
• SPLEEN STOMACH,
DAMPNESS
**STOMACH/DIGESTIVE
DISORDERS**
• ACID REGURGITATION
• ANOREXIA: Food
Stagnation
• EPIGASTRIC
DISTENTION,

FULLNESS
• FOOD STAGNATION
• FOOD STAGNATION,
DAMPNESS
• HICCUPS: Qi Deficiency-
-Dampness
• STOMACH, ACHE:
Stagnant Qi/Turbid
Dampness
• VOMITING: Food
Stagnation/Qi Deficiency–
Dampness

Clinical/Pharmaceutical Studies:

**BLOOD RELATED DISORDERS/
TOPICS**
• BLOOD PRESSURE, LOWERS:
Tinture IV/IP Injection
CIRCULATION DISORDERS
• VASOCONSTRICTOR: Perpheral
Blood Vessels

INFECTIOUS DISEASES
• BACTERIAL, ANTI-: Typhoid,
Dysentery, E.Coli, Staph.Aureus
**MUSCULOSKELETAL/
CONNECTIVE TISSUE**
• ANTISPASMODIC: Decoction, Of
Smooth, Striated Muscle

PARASITES
• ROUNDWORMS: Eliminates
**STOMACH/DIGESTIVE
DISORDERS**
• INDIGESTION, MILD
• STOMACHIC

Dose

3 - 9 gm

Common Name

Magnolia Flower

Contraindications

Not: Yin Or Fluid Deficiency

HOU PO
(CHUAN PO)

厚樸
(厚朴)

CORTEX
MAGNOLIAE OFFICINALIS

Traditional Functions:

1. Dries Dampness
2. Promotes Qi circulation
3. Descends Qi and relieves cough and wheezing
4. Disperses food stagnation
5. Descends reflux and warms and transforms Phlegm

Traditional Properties:

Enters: LU, LI, SP, ST,

Properties: BIT, SP, W, ARO

Indications:

**ABDOMEN/
GASTROINTESTINAL TOPICS**
• ABDOMEN, DISTENTION OF:
Damp Heat/Dampness
• ABDOMEN, PAIN OF
BOWEL RELATED DISORDERS
• CONSTIPATION, MOIST
• DIARRHEA: Cold Dampness (Add
Warm Interior Herbs, Too)
• DYSENTERY

CHEST
• CHEST, CONSTRICTION
LUNGS
• COUGH: Cold Phlegm/Surging
Phlegm
• COUGH, PROFUSE SPUTUM
• DYSPNEA: Surging Phlegm
• LUNG QI CONGESTION W/
SPUTUM

• WHEEZING, PHLEGM
**STOMACH/DIGESTIVE
DISORDERS**
• ANOREXIA
• BELCHING
• FOOD CONGESTION
• GASTRALGIA
• HICCUPS
• NAUSEA/VOMITING

Clinical/Pharmaceutical Studies:

**ABDOMEN/
GASTROINTESTINAL
TOPICS**
• ABDOMEN,
DISTENTION OF: With

Greater Than 50 kg
• INTESTINES,
PERISTALSIS,
INCREASES
• INTESTINES,

• DYSENTERY,
BACILLARY: Powdered,
3 g/Dose, 2-3x/Day
• FLATULENCE: Reduces
HEART

DISORDERS
• CNS, DEPRESSES: Ether
Extract IP Injection,
Lessened Stimulation Of
Methamphetamine

Clinical/Pharmaceutical Studies:

Qing Pi, 9 g Each, Da Huang, 6 g, Oral Decoction
- ABDOMEN, DISTENTION OF, GAS DURING PANHYSTERECTOMY: 5-7.5 g Powdered If Less Than 50 kg/7.5-10, If Greater Than 50 kg
- ENTERITIS, ACUTE
- GASTROINTESTINAL STIMULATION
- INTESTINES, GAS, FROM PANHYSTERECTO MY: 5-7.5 g Powdered If Less Than 50 kg/7.5-10 If

VOLVULUS: 5-7.5 g Powdered If Less Than 50 kg/7.5-10 g If Greater Than 50 kg

BLOOD RELATED DISORDERS/TOPICS
- BLOOD PRESSURE, LOWERS

BOWEL RELATED DISORDERS
- CONSTIPATION: With Qing Pi, 9 g Each, Da Huang, 6 g, Oral Decoction
- DYSENTERY, AMOEBIC: 10 ml (6 g Of Herb) Decoction Orally, 2x/Day, 3-9 Days

- HEART RATE, INCREASES

INFECTIOUS DISEASES
- ANTIBIOTIC: Broad Specturm, Heat Stable-- Strep Pneum, Strep, Shigella, Staph A. (Greater Than Huang Lian For Staph, 5-10x, Less Than For Other Bacteria)
- VIRAL, ANTI-: Hepatitis

LUNGS
- PNEUMONIA, ANTI-STREP
- RESPIRATION RATE, INCREASES

MENTAL STATE/ NEUROLOGICAL

MUSCULOSKELETAL/ CONNECTIVE TISSUE
- MUSCLES, RELAXANT: Lasts 3 Hrs, Injection

PARASITES
- ANTIHELMINTIC: Ascaris

SKIN
- FUNGAL, ANTI-: Skin
- FURUNCLES: 25% Ointment Of Powder w/ Vaseline, Topical

STOMACH/DIGESTIVE DISORDERS
- STOMACHIC
- ULCERS, GASTRIC: Inhibits

Dose
3 - 9 gm

Common Name
Magnolia Bark

Contraindications
Not: Spleen, Stomach Deficiency

Precautions
Watch: Pregnancy

Notes
Add Slices Later To Decoction

Slices Stronger Than Strips

Very Safe Orally

HUO XIANG

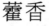 藿香

HERBA AGASTACHES SEU POGOSTEMI

Traditional Functions:

1. Aromatically dries Dampness
2. Harmonizes the Center, moves Qi and stops vomiting
3. Releases the Exterior and expels Cold and Dampness
4. Dispels Summer Heat and dries Dampness in Spleen and Stomach

Traditional Properties:

Enters: LU, SP, ST,

Properties: SP, <W

Indications:

ABDOMEN/ GASTROINTESTINAL TOPICS
- ABDOMEN, DISTENTION OF: Dampness From Spleen Transportation Function Loss/Damp Heat
- ABDOMEN, PAIN OF/ CRAMP

BOWEL RELATED DISORDERS
- DIARRHEA: Cold Dampness (Add Warm Interior Herbs, Too) / Dampness From Spleen Transportation Function Loss

CHEST
- CHEST, FULLNESS,

Transportation Function Loss

EXTERIOR CONDITIONS
- EXTERIOR PATHOGEN W/SPLEEN DISORDERS

FLUID DISORDERS
- DAMPNESS, CONGESTED IN SPLEEN
- DAMPNESS, EXTERNAL--SURFACE COMPLEX

HEAD/NECK
- HEADACHE

HEAT
- SUMMER HEAT: With Stomach Ache, Nausea, Abdominal Distension

INFECTIOUS DISEASES

- COMMON COLD, IN SUMMER W/ DAMPNESS

SEXUALITY, FEMALE: GYNECOLOGICAL
- MORNING SICKNESS: Gestational Foul Obstruction--Cold

SIX STAGES/ CHANNELS
- TAI YANG STAGE W/ STOMACH ACHE, NAUSEA, ABDOMINAL DISTENTION

SPLEEN
- EXTERNAL PATHOGEN W/SPLEEN DISORDERS
- SPLEEN DAMPNESS CONGESTED
- SPLEEN STOMACH,

- ANOREXIA: Dampness From Spleen Transportation Function Loss
- EPIGASTRIC DISTENTION: Dampness From Spleen Transportation Function Loss
- HICCUPS: Qi Deficiency--Dampness
- NAUSEA, EXTERIOR CONDITION
- NAUSEA/VOMITING: Dampness From Spleen Transportation Function Loss
- STOMACH, ACHE, EXTERIOR CONDITION
- VOMITING: Dampness

Indications:

OPPRESSION
ENERGETIC STATE
• FATIGUE: Dampness
From Spleen

• COMMON COLD W/
DAMPNESS: Stomach
Ache, Nausea, Abdominal
Distension

DAMPNESS
**STOMACH/DIGESTIVE
DISORDERS**

From Spleen
Transportation Function
Loss

Clinical/Pharmaceutical Studies:

BOWEL RELATED DISORDERS
• DIARRHEA: Tranquilizes GI
Nerves
FEVERS
• ANTIPYRETIC: Relaxes Blood
Capillaries
INFECTIOUS DISEASES
• ANTIBIOTIC: Many Fungi,

Leptospirosis (Need High Doses) ,
Staph.Aureus, Strep, Pneumococci,
E.Coli, B.Dysenteriae, Spirochete
• LEPTOSPIROSIS: At High Doses
(31mg/ml)
SKIN
• DIAPHORETIC

• FUNGAL, ANTI-: Strongly Inhibits
Common Ones
**STOMACH/DIGESTIVE
DISORDERS**
• ANTIEMETIC: Tranquilizes GI
Nerves
• STOMACHIC

Dose

4.5 - 15.0 gm

Common Name

Patchouli

Contraindications

Not: Def Yin w/Heat

Not: ST Fire

LUO LE

罗 勒
（罗勒）

**HERBA
OCIMI**

Traditional Functions:

1. Harmonizes the Spleen and Stomach
2. Disperses food stagnation and expels the Evil

Traditional Properties:

Enters: LU, SP, ST, LI

Properties: SP, W

Indications:

KIDNEYS
• KIDNEY DISEASES
ORAL CAVITY
• GINGIVA, ULCERS OF
SEXUALITY, FEMALE:

GYNECOLOGICAL
• POSTPARTUM, PAIN: Blood
Stagnation
• PREGNANCY, PAIN DURING:

Blood Stagnation
**STOMACH/DIGESTIVE
DISORDERS**
• STOMACH, SPASMS

Dose

6 - 9 gm

Common Name

Sweet Basil

PEI LAN
(JA LANG)

佩 蘭
（佩兰）

**HERBA
EUPATORII FORTUNEI**

Traditional Functions:

1. Aromatically dries Dampness and harmonizes the Center
2. Removes Summer Heat, Dampness

Traditional Properties:

Enters: SP, ST,

Properties: SP, N

Indications:

**ABDOMEN/
GASTROINTESTINAL TOPICS**
• ABDOMEN, DISTENTION OF:
Damp Heat

Confinement
HEAD/NECK
• HEADACHE
HEAT

• HALITOSIS
SPLEEN
• EXTERNAL PATHOGEN W/
SPLEEN WEAKNESS

Indications:

- ABDOMEN, MASS: w/o Hunger
CHEST
- CHEST, CONSTRICTION:
Dampness
EXTERIOR CONDITIONS
- EXTERIOR PATHOGEN W/
SPLEEN WEAKNESS
EYES
- EYES, IRRITATION
FEVERS
- FEVER
FLUID DISORDERS
- DAMPNESS, TURBID: Internal

- SUMMER HEAT DAMPNESS:
Nausea
INFECTIOUS DISEASES
- COMMON COLD, IN SUMMER
W/DAMPNESS
LIVER
- JAUNDICE: Spleen Deficiency
With Sweet Taste In Mouth
**MUSCULOSKELETAL/
CONNECTIVE TISSUE**
- ARTHRITIS, WHOLE BODY
ORAL CAVITY

- SPLEEN STOMACH, DAMPNESS
**STOMACH/DIGESTIVE
DISORDERS**
- ANOREXIA: Dampness
- HICCUPS: Qi Deficiency–
Dampness
- INDIGESTION
- NAUSEA/VOMITING: Dampness/
Summer Heat
- STOMACH, FULLNESS
- VOMITING: Qi Deficiency–
Dampness

Clinical/Pharmaceutical Studies:

FEVERS
- ANTIPYRETIC
INFECTIOUS DISEASES

- VIRAL, ANTI-: Hepatitis, Flu
KIDNEYS
- DIURETIC

**STOMACH/DIGESTIVE
DISORDERS**
- STOMACHIC

Dose

4.5 - 9.0 gm

Contraindications

Not: Def Yin, Qi

Notes

Ethanol Extract Can Cause Anesthetic Action, But Toxic

SHA REN
(SUO SHA)

砂仁

FRUCTUS/SEMEN
AMOMI

Traditional Functions:

1. Warms the Spleen, moves the Qi and stops diarrhea
2. Dries Dampness and stops vomiting
3. Calms the fetus, stops miscarriage
4. Used in preparing tonifying herbs to reduce their stagnation-causing action

Traditional Properties:

Enters: SP, ST, KI,

Properties: SP, W, ARO

Indications:

**ABDOMEN/
GASTROINTESTINAL TOPICS**
- ABDOMEN, DISTENTION OF:
Damp Heat
- ABDOMEN, DISTENTION OF/
PAIN: Spleen Stomach Stagnant Qi
- ABDOMEN, PAIN OF: Cold
- GAS, GASTROINTESTINAL
BOWEL RELATED DISORDERS
- DIARRHEA: Food Stagnation,
Most Herbs, Cooked, Charred/
Spleen Deficient With Qi Stagnation
- DIARRHEA, CHRONIC: Cold
- DYSENTERY: Cold

ENERGETIC STATE
- HERBS, TONIFYING: Add To
Prevent Stagnation
**SEXUALITY, FEMALE:
GYNECOLOGICAL**
- FETUS, RESTLESS: Qi Stagnation
- MISCARRIAGE, THREATENED
- MORNING SICKNESS:
Gestational Foul Obstruction–Cold
SPLEEN
- SPLEEN STOMACH, DAMPNESS
**STOMACH/DIGESTIVE
DISORDERS**
- ANOREXIA: Spleen Stomach

Stagnant Qi
- BELCHING
- EPIGASTRIC DISTENTION/PAIN:
Spleen Stomach Stagnant Qi:Spleen
Stomach
- FOOD ACCUMULATION,
OVERNIGHT
- FOOD STAGNATION
- HICCUPS: Qi Deficiency–
Dampness/Cold
- INDIGESTION
- NAUSEA/VOMITING
- VOMITING: Qi Deficiency–
Dampness/Cold

Clinical/Pharmaceutical Studies:

**ABDOMEN/
GASTROINTESTINAL TOPICS**
- INTESTINES, SPASMS,

**RELAXES
STOMACH/DIGESTIVE
DISORDERS**

- ANTIEMETIC
- STOMACHIC

Dose
1.5 - 6.0 gm

Common Name
Grains-Of-Paradise Fruit

Contraindications
Not: Def Yin w/Heat

Notes
Used To Process Di Huang

Drains Dampness

BAN BIAN LIAN

半邊蓮
（半边莲）

HERBA LOBELIAE CHINENSIS CUM RADICE

Traditional Functions:

1. Promotes urination, reduces swelling and clears Heat
2. Cools the Blood and removes toxins

Traditional Properties:

Enters: LU, HT, SI,

Properties: SW, N, SP

Indications:

ABDOMEN/ GASTROINTESTINAL TOPICS
• INTESTINES, INFLAMMATION OF

BOWEL RELATED DISORDERS
• DYSENTERY

CANCER/TUMORS/SWELLINGS/ LUMPS
• CANCER: Stomach, Rectal, Liver
• SWELLINGS, TOXIC: Topical

FLUID DISORDERS
• ASCITES

• EDEMA: Dampness, Evil Fluid
• EDEMA, NEPHRITIC

KIDNEYS
• DIURETIC, MILD

LIVER
• LIVER, CIRRHOSIS

LUNGS
• DYSPNEA

ORAL CAVITY
• TONSILLITIS

PARASITES
• SCHISTOSOMIASIS, END STAGE:

Uropenia Of

SKIN
• ECZEMA
• FURUNCLES: Topical

TRAUMA, BITES, POISONINGS
• INSECT BITES
• SNAKE BITES: Topical, Too
• WASP STINGS: Topical, Too

URINARY BLADDER
• URINATION, PAINFUL, DRIBBLING: Concentrated, Red/ Yellow/Turbid

Clinical/Pharmaceutical Studies:

BLOOD RELATED DISORDERS/TOPICS
• BLOOD PRESSURE, LOWERS: Not Well Absorbed By GI Tract, Injection Of Aqueous Extract Better

BOWEL RELATED DISORDERS
• LAXATIVE, MILD

GALL BLADDER
• GALL BLADDER, BILE SECRETION, INCREASES: IV Injection Of Alcohol Precipitated Decoction, 2x Increase

HEMORRHAGIC DISORDERS
• HEMOSTATIC: Lowers Bleeding Time

INFECTIOUS DISEASES
• HERPES ZOSTER:

Apply Crushed Herb And She Mei (Herba Duchesneae) To Skin

KIDNEYS
• DIURETIC: Prolonged, Strong
• NEPHRITIS, ACUTE W/ EDEMA: Injection, With 4-8 g Crude Herb/Dose, IM, 2-3x/Day, 7-14 Days

LUNGS
• RESPIRATION, STIMULATES
• WHOOPING COUGH: With Shi Hu Shui

MENTAL STATE/ NEUROLOGICAL DISORDERS
• CNS: Lobeline Similar To Nicotine, But Only 5-20% As Strong

PARASITES
• SCHISTOSOMIASIS,

MID-STAGE: 30 g Or With Dang Gui, Dan Shen, Fu Ling, Da Fu Pi As Decoction, 30 Day Course, 64% Effective

SKIN
• CARBUNCLES, INITIAL STAGE: With Tian Nan Xiang Crushed Then Add Small Amount Xiong Huang For Topical Application, Change Dressing 2-3x/Day
• ECZEMA, SUBACUTE: Wet Compress Or Topical Application Of Decoction, Prompt
• FUNGAL INFECTIONS: Tinea Mannum, Capitis: Wet Compress Or Topical Application Of Decoction, Prompt
• FUNGAL, ANTI-: Many

STOMACH/DIGESTIVE DISORDERS
• APPETITE SUPPRESSENT: Oral Administration--Acted On Satiety Center, Adrenal Medulla To Cause Hyperglycemia, GI Tract, Inhibition Of Intestinal Motility
• VOMITING, CAUSES: Lobeline

TRAUMA, BITES, POISONINGS
• SNAKE BITES: Need To Take Within 30 Min Before Or After Bite To Help, 30-120 g, Fresh Herb In 3 Doses, Apply To Wound, Too, Need 5-6 Days Treatment, Better Than Procaine Block

Dose

9 - 36 gm

Common Name

Chinese Lobelia w/Root

Contraindications

Not: Def Patterns

Notes

For Snakebite: 30-60 gm

Non Toxic, Even After Long Use

BEI XIE
(BI XIE)

萆 解

RHIZOMA
DIOSCOREAE SATIVAE

Traditional Functions:

1. Resolves turbid urine, separating the pure from the turbid
2. Expels Wind Cold Damp Bi
3. Clears Damp Heat from the skin

Traditional Properties:

Enters: ST, UB, LV,

Properties: BIT, N

Indications:

EXTREMITIES
- **LEGS, STIFF/NUMB:**
  Wind Damp/Damp Heat Bi-
  Mild
FLUID DISORDERS
- **EDEMA:** Dampness, Evil
  Fluid
INFECTIOUS DISEASES
- SYPHILIS
**MUSCULOSKELETAL/
CONNECTIVE TISSUE**
- ARTHRITIS, FROM
  URIC ACID
- ARTHRITIS,

RHEUMATIC
- **JOINTS, PAIN,**
  SWELLING, RED: Hot
  Bi
- **KNEES, PAIN**
- **MUSCLES, ACHES:**
  Wind Damp/Damp Heat Bi-
  Mild
**PAIN/NUMBNESS/
GENERAL
DISCOMFORT**
- BI, DAMP HEAT: Mild
- BI, WIND DAMP HEAT:
  Lower Back Pain, Leg

Stiffness, Numbness,
Muscle Aches-Mild
**SEXUALITY, FEMALE:
GYNECOLOGICAL**
- **LEUKORRHEA:**
  Dampness In Lower Jiao/
  Damp Heat
**SEXUALITY, MALE:
UROLOGICAL TOPICS**
- PENILE PAIN
SKIN
- **ECZEMA:** Damp Heat
- FURUNCLES, TOXIC
- LESIONS: Damp Heat

- **SORES, PUSTULAR:**
  Damp Heat
URINARY BLADDER
- DRIBBLING W/PAIN
- **URINATION,
  DRIBBLING**
- **URINATION,
  FREQUENT**
- **URINATION, PAINFUL:**
  Dribbling, Concentrated,
  Red/Yellow/Turbid
- **URINATION, TURBID:**
  Dampness In Lower Jiao

Clinical/Pharmaceutical Studies:

INFECTIOUS DISEASES
- BACTERIAL, ANTI-
LUNGS
- ANTITUSSIVE
- BRONCHITIS
- EXPECTORANT

**MUSCULOSKELETAL/
CONNECTIVE TISSUE**
- **ARTHRITIS:** Rheumatism
PARASITES
- ANTIPARASITIC: Intestinal

SEXUALITY, EITHER SEX
- **CONTRACEPTIVE:** Used In
  Manufacture Of
SKIN
- FUNGAL, ANTI-: Many

Dose

9 - 15 gm

Common Name

Fish-Poison Yam

Contraindications

Not: Def KI Yin

BI ZI CAO

筆仔草
(笔仔草)

HERBA
POGONATHERI

Traditional Functions:

1. Clears Heat and promotes urination

Traditional Properties:

Enters: SP, KI, UB,

Properties: SW, CL

Indications:

BOWEL RELATED DISORDERS
• DIARRHEA
ENDOCRINE RELATED DISORDERS
• DIABETES
FLUID DISORDERS

• THIRST: Febrile Diseases
HEMORRHAGIC DISORDERS
• HEMATURIA
LIVER
• JAUNDICE: Hepatic
MENTAL STATE/

NEUROLOGICAL DISORDERS
• RESTLESSNESS: Febrile Diseases
URINARY BLADDER
• DYSURIA
• URINATION, TURBID

Dose
9 - 15 gm

Common Name
Golden Hair Grass

BIAN XU

編蓄
(編蓄)

HERBA
POLYGONI AVICULARIS

Traditional Functions:

1. Promotes urination and clears Damp Heat from the bladder
2. Clears Heat and kills worms
3. Clears damp skin lesions and stops itching

Traditional Properties:

Enters: UB,

Properties: BIT, <C

Indications:

BOWEL RELATED DISORDERS
• DYSENTERY, RED
CHILDHOOD DISORDERS
• ASCARIASIS, CHILDHOOD
FLUID DISORDERS
• EDEMA: Dampness, Evil Fluid
INFECTIOUS DISEASES
• GONORRHEA
LIVER
• JAUNDICE
PARASITES
• HOOKWORMS

• PARASITES, INTESTINAL
• PINWORMS
• TAPEWORMS
SEXUALITY, EITHER SEX
• ULCERS/PRURITUS OF
  EXTERNAL GENITALS
SEXUALITY, FEMALE:
GYNECOLOGICAL
• TRICHOMONAS, VAGINAL:
  External Application
SKIN
• ECZEMA: External Application

• SCABIES
• SKIN, LESIONS, ITCHY: Damp
• TINEA FUNGUS: Itching
URINARY BLADDER
• URETHRITIS
• URINATION, DRIBBLING: Heat
• URINATION, PAINFUL: Damp
  Heat
• URINATION, PAINFUL,
  DRIBBLING: Concentrated, Red/
  Yellow/Turbid

Clinical/Pharmaceutical Studies:

**BLOOD RELATED DISORDERS/
TOPICS**
• BLOOD PRESSURE, LOWERS:
  Aqueous/ETOH Extract, Injected
BOWEL RELATED DISORDERS
• DYSENTERY, BACILLARY: Paste
  From Sugar
GALL BLADDER
• CHOLAGOGUE: Increases Bile

Secretion
INFECTIOUS DISEASES
• BACTERIAL, ANTI-: B.
  Dysenteriae, Microsporon Lanosum
KIDNEYS
• DIURETIC
PARASITES
• ANTIHELMINTIC
SEXUALITY, FEMALE:

GYNECOLOGICAL
• UTERINE BLEEDING,
  POSTPARTUM
• UTERUS, INCREASES TONICITY
SKIN
• FUNGAL, ANTI-: Many
TRAUMA, BITES, POISONINGS
• WOUNDS: Astringent

Dose
4.5 - 18.0 gm

Common Name
Knotweed

Contraindications
Not: With Difficult Urination From Weak Abdomen

Notes
Too Much Will Damage Essential Qi
May Cause Dermatitis/GI Disturbance
Single Herb: Up To 30 gm

CHA YE

茶葉
(茶叶)

FOLIUM CAMELLIAE

Traditional Functions:

1. Clears the eyes and head
2. Quenches thirst and calms restlessness
3. Resolves Phlegm
4. Clears food stagnation
5. Promotes urination and relieves toxins

Traditional Properties:

Enters: LU, ST, HT,

Properties: BIT, SW, CL

Indications:

BOWEL RELATED DISORDERS
• DYSENTERY, MALARIAL
EARS/HEARING DISORDERS
• DIZZINESS
FLUID DISORDERS
• THIRST

HEAD/NECK
• HEADACHE
MENTAL STATE/
NEUROLOGICAL DISORDERS
• FIDGETS
• SLEEPINESS

PHLEGM
• PHLEGM, STAGNANT
STOMACH/DIGESTIVE
DISORDERS
• INDIGESTION

Clinical/Pharmaceutical Studies:

CIRCULATION DISORDERS
• BLOOD VESSELS, DILATES,
PERIPHERAL
FLUID DISORDERS
• DIURETIC, STONGER THAN
CAFFEINE
HEART
• CORONARY ARTERIES,

DILATES
• HEART, STIMULATES: Directly
Stimulates
INFECTIOUS DISEASES
• BACTERIAL, ANTI-:
Bacteriostatic To Bacillus
Dysenteriae
LUNGS

• ASTHMA, BRONCHIAL: Relaxes
Smooth Muscles
• BRONCHIAL SMOOTH
MUSCLES RELAXANT: Bronchial
MENTAL STATE/
NEUROLOGICAL DISORDERS
• CNS, STIMULANT

Dose

3 - 9 gm

Common Name

Tea

CHE QIAN CAO

車前草
(车前草)

HERBA PLANTAGINIS

Traditional Functions:

1. Promotes urination, clears Heat and stops diarrhea
2. Stops bleeding
3. Clears Heat and toxins

Traditional Properties:

Enters: LI, SI,

Properties: SW, C

Indications:

BOWEL RELATED DISORDERS
• DIARRHEA
• DYSENTERY, ACUTE
HEART
• CARDITIS
HEMORRHAGIC DISORDERS
• BLEEDING
• HEMATURIA
• HEMOSTATIC
INFECTIOUS DISEASES

• GONORRHEA
KIDNEYS
• NEPHRITIS
LIVER
• JAUNDICE
LUNGS
• COUGH, PHLEGM
• LUNGS, ACUTE INFECTION OF
SEXUALITY, FEMALE:
GYNECOLOGICAL

• LEUKORRHEA
SKIN
• CARBUNCLES
• FURUNCLES
URINARY BLADDER
• URINARY SYSTEM, ACUTE
INFECTION
• URINATION, PROMOTES
• URINATION, SCANTY

Clinical/Pharmaceutical Studies:

ABDOMEN/
 GASTROINTESTINAL TOPICS
• INTESTINES, REDUCES SPASMS
• INTESTINES, STIMULATES
BOWEL RELATED DISORDERS
• DYSENTERY, BACILLARY,
 CHRONIC: 60-120 ml Decoction/
 Day, Fever Down In 2 Days,
 Symptoms Gone In 10 Days, In
 Children, Too
CANCER/TUMORS/SWELLINGS/
 LUMPS
• TUMOR, ANTI-
EYES
• EYES, DISEASES OF
HEART
• HEART, AFFECTS RATE: Small
 Doses Decrease Heart Rate, Increase
 Amplitude
INFECTIOUS DISEASES
• BACTERIAL, ANTI-: General,
 Spirochettes
KIDNEYS
• DIURETIC
• KIDNEY STONES: 15-30 g
• NEPHRITIS W/EDEMA: 15-30 g
• PYELONEPHRITIS: 15-30 g
LIVER
• HEPATITIS, ACUTE, ICTERIC: 60
 g/Day, 5-7 Days To Restore Appetite,
 14 Days To Subside Jaundice, Liver
 Functions Returned
LUNGS
• BRONCHITIS: Antitussiuve,
 Expectorant, 30 gm/Day, 1-2 Weeks
• COUGH: Controls
• EXPECTORANT
• RESPIRATORY TRACT
 INFECTION, UPPER: Antitussiuve,
 Expectorant, 30 gm/Day
• TUBERCULOSIS, LARYNGEAL/
 ULCERS: Injection
• WHOOPING COUGH:
 Antitussiuve, Expectorant, 30 gm/
 Day
SEXUALITY, FEMALE:
 GYNECOLOGICAL
• UTERUS, STIMULATES
SKIN
• FUNGAL, ANTI-
• ULCERS, STOMACH/SKIN:
 Reduces-Especialy Gastric
STOMACH/DIGESTIVE
 DISORDERS
• STOMACH, PROLONGS TIME
 FOOD IN
• ULCERS, GASTRIC/SKIN:
 Reduces-Especialy Gastric
TRAUMA, BITES, POISONINGS
• INFLAMMATORY, ANTI-
URINARY BLADDER
• DYSURIA: 15-30 g

Dose
9 - 30 gm

Common Name
Plantain

Contraindications
Not: Kidney Def Spermatorrhea

Notes
Juice Used Often

CHE QIAN ZI

車前子
（车前子）

SEMEN PLANTAGINIS

Traditional Functions:

1. Promotes urination, clears Heat and stops diarrhea
2. Clears Heat in the Liver and brightens the eyes
3. Disperses Phlegm, controls coughs

Traditional Properties:

Enters: LU, SI, KI, UB, LV,

Properties: SW, BL, C

Indications:

BOWEL RELATED DISORDERS
• DIARRHEA: Evil Fluid Dampness/
 Damp Heat
EARS/HEARING DISORDERS
• VERTIGO
EYES
• CATARACTS: Liver Kidney
 Deficient
• EYES, DRY: Liver Kidney
 Deficient
• EYES, PAIN, SWOLLEN, RED:
 Liver Heat
• EYES, PROBLEMS: Liver Heat/
 Liver Kidney Deficient
• EYES, RED, CONGESTED: Liver
 Heat
• PHOTOPHOBIA
FLUID DISORDERS
• EDEMA: Dampness, Evil Fluid
• EDEMA, ANY TYPE
INFECTIOUS DISEASES
• GONORRHEA
LUNGS
• COUGH: Lung Heat
• COUGH, COPIOUS SPUTUM:
 Lung Heat
• LUNGS, DYSPNEA: Lung Heat
SEXUALITY, FEMALE:
 GYNECOLOGICAL
• LEUKORRHEA: Damp Heat
SKIN
• ECZEMA: Damp Heat
• SKIN, SORES: Damp Heat
URINARY BLADDER
• DYSURIA
• URINARY TRACT INFECTIONS
• URINATION, PAINFUL,
 DRIBBLING, CONCENTRATED,
 RED/YELLOW/TURBID
• URINATION, SCANTY

Clinical/Pharmaceutical Studies:

BLOOD RELATED DISORDERS/
 TOPICS
• BLOOD PRESSURE, LOWERS
BOWEL RELATED DISORDERS
• DIARRHEA W/INDIGESTION
KIDNEYS
• DIURETIC: Unknown Ingredient,
 Recently No Evidence Seen
• KIDNEY STONES: 3-10 g
• NEPHRITIS W/EDEMA: 3-10 g
DISLOCATION: 5% Solution
 Injected
SEXUALITY, FEMALE:
 GYNECOLOGICAL
• MALPOSITION OF FETUS (8 MO)

Clinical/Pharmaceutical Studies:

CHILDHOOD DISORDERS
- INDIGESTION, DIARRHEA, CHILDHOOD
- INFANTILE DYSPEPSIA: 2-3 Days, Stir-Fried, Crushed Oral--4-12 Months, 0.5g/Dose, 1-2 Yrs, 1 g/Dose, 3-4x/Day

HEAD/NECK
- TMJ DISLOCATION

- PYELONEPHRITIS: 3-10 g

LUNGS
- ANTITUSSIVE: Definite
- EXPECTORANT

MUSCULOSKELETAL/ CONNECTIVE TISSUE
- JOINT CAPSULES, TIGHTENS IF LOOSE W/RECURRENT

SKIN
- ABSCESS, INHIBITS PUS FORMATION: Powdered Seed Ointment
- SKIN, INFLAMMATIONS: Reduced, Powdered Seed Ointment

URINARY BLADDER
- DYSURIA: 3-10 g

Dose

4.5 - 15.0 gm

Common Name

Plantago Seeds

Contraindications

Not: Pregnancy

Precautions

Watch: Exhausted Yang Qi/Def KI Spermatorrhea/Overwork

Notes

Wrap For Herbal Decoctions

CHI XIAO DOU

赤小豆

SEMEN PHASEOLI CALCARATI

Traditional Functions:

1. Promotes urination and clears Heat
2. Disperses congealed Blood, removes swelling, and detoxifies toxic Heat
3. Clears Damp Heat, relieving jaundice

Traditional Properties:

Enters: HT, SI,

Properties: SW, SO, N

Indications:

BOWEL RELATED DISORDERS
- DIARRHEA: Damp Heat
- DYSENTERY: Damp Heat

CANCER/TUMORS/SWELLINGS/ LUMPS
- SWELLINGS

EXTREMITIES
- LEG QI, EDEMA

FLUID DISORDERS

- EDEMA: Abdominal Swelling, Fullness

HEAT
- SUMMER HEAT DAMPNESS

LIVER
- JAUNDICE: Damp Heat, Mild

NUTRITIONAL/METABOLIC DISORDERS/TOPICS
- BERIBERI: Leg Qi

SKIN
- CARBUNCLES, TOXIC
- FURUNCLES
- SKIN, SUPPURATIVE INFECTIONS
- SORES, SWOLLEN, TOXIC

URINARY BLADDER
- DYSURIA
- URINATION, SCANTY

Clinical/Pharmaceutical Studies:

INFECTIOUS DISEASES
- BACTERIAL, ANTI-: Staph. Aureus, B.Dysenteriae, B.Typhi, Et.

Al.
- MUMPS

KIDNEYS

- DIURETIC

LIVER
- LIVER, CIRRHOSIS W/ASCITES

Dose

9 - 15 gm

Common Name

Aduki Bean

Precautions

Watch: Pregnancy

Notes

Can Lead To Dryness
Used Mainly As Food: 30-120 gm

DENG XIN CAO

燈心草
（灯心草）

MEDULLA JUNCI EFFUSI

Traditional Functions:

1. Promotes urination and filters out Dampness and Heat
2. Lowers Heart Fire

Traditional Properties:

Enters: LU, HT, SI,

Properties: SW, BL, <C

Indications:

BOWEL RELATED DISORDERS
• DIARRHEA, POSTPARTUM
CHILDHOOD DISORDERS
• SLEEP DISORDERS WITH
  SCANTY URINE, IRRITABILITY,
  CHILDHOOD
FLUID DISORDERS
• EDEMA
• WATER RETENTION
HEART
• HEART KIDNEY DISHARMONY
• RESTLESS HEART
HEMORRHAGIC DISORDERS
• HEMATURIA

INFECTIOUS DISEASES
• GONORRHEA
KIDNEYS
• DIURETIC, MILD
LIVER
• JAUNDICE
MENTAL STATE/
  NEUROLOGICAL DISORDERS
• INSOMNIA: Heart Kidney
  Discommunication
• NOCTURNAL CRYING
• RESTLESSNESS
• SLEEP, RESTLESS: Kidney Heart
  Discommunication

ORAL CAVITY
• THROAT, NUMB: External
• THROAT, SORE
SEXUALITY, FEMALE:
  GYNECOLOGICAL
• LACTATION, INSUFFICIENT
URINARY BLADDER
• DRIBBLING
• DYSURIA
• URINARY RETENTION
• URINARY TRACT INFECTIONS
• URINATION, DRIBBLING: Heat
• URINATION, SCANTY W/HEAT
  DISORDERS

Dose

1.5 - 3.0 gm

Common Name

Rush Pith

Contraindications

Not: Pregnancy

Precautions

Watch: Def Cold SP/ST

DI FU ZI

地膚子
（地肤子）

FRUCTUS KOCHIAE SCOPARIAE

Traditional Functions:

1. Promotes urination and clears Heat
2. Expels Damp Heat from the skin and stops itching

Traditional Properties:

Enters: UB,

Properties: SW, BIT, C

Indications:

FLUID DISORDERS
• EDEMA: Dampness, Evil Fluid
KIDNEYS
• DIURETIC: Mild
• NEPHRITIS
SEXUALITY, EITHER SEX
• GENITALS, PRURITUS, SORES:
  Damp Heat, Topical, Too
SEXUALITY, FEMALE:
  GYNECOLOGICAL

• LEUKORRHEA: Damp Heat
SKIN
• BOILS, MALIGNANT
• ECZEMA: Damp Heat, Topical,
  Too
• PRURITUS: Wind Heat, Topical,
  Too
• RASHES, PRURITIC: Wind Damp
• SCABIES: Topical, Too
• SKIN, RASHES: Topical, Too

• SKIN, SORES: Damp Heat
• ULCERS, EVIL: Topical, Too
• URTICARIA
URINARY BLADDER
• URINARY TRACT INFECTIONS,
  ACUTE
• URINATION, DRIBBLING: Heat
• URINATION, PAINFUL: Damp
  Heat In UB
• URINATION, SCANTY

Clinical/Pharmaceutical Studies:

INFECTIOUS DISEASES
• BACTERIAL, ANTI-
KIDNEYS

• DIURETIC
SKIN

• FUNGAL, ANTI-: Aqueous Extract,
  Many

Dose
3 - 15 gm

Common Name
Broom Cypress/Kochia Seed

Contraindications
Not: With Hai Piao Xiao

Not: w/o Damp Heat

DONG GUA PI   冬瓜皮   EXOCARPIUM BENINCASAE

Traditional Functions:

1. Promotes urination and reduces edema
2. Clears Summer Heat and relieves thirst

Traditional Properties:

Enters: LU, SP,

Properties: SW, <C

Indications:

FLUID DISORDERS
• EDEMA: Dampness, Evil Fluid
• THIRST, ESPECIALLY IN

SUMMER
HEAT
• SUMMER HEAT

URINARY BLADDER
• URINATION, SCANTY

Clinical/Pharmaceutical Studies:

KIDNEYS   • DIURETIC

Dose
15 - 30 gm

Common Name
Chinese Wax-Gourd Peel

Contraindications
Not: Edema From Malnutrition

DONG GUA REN   冬瓜仁   SEMEN BENINCASAE HISPIDAE
(DONG GUA ZI)

Traditional Functions:

1. Clears Heat, eliminates sputum
2. Clears Heat and promotes discharge of pus
3. Clears Heat and drains Dampness in the Lower Burner

Traditional Properties:

Enters: LU, LI, ST, SI,

Properties: SW, C

Indications:

ABDOMEN/
GASTROINTESTINAL TOPICS
• ABDOMEN, DISTENTION OF,
  RESTLESS
• APPENDICITIS W/PAIN
• INTESTINES, ABSCESS
• INTESTINES, DAMP HEAT
EXTREMITIES
• LEGS, SWELLING
FLUID DISORDERS

• ASCITES
• THIRST, CONSUMPTIVE
• WATER RETENTION
HEAT
• DAMP HEAT IN LUNG/
  INTESTINES
LUNGS
• COUGH, THICK SPUTUM: Heat
  Phlegm
• LUNG DAMP HEAT

• LUNGS, ABSCESS
• LUNGS, ABSCESS W/PURULENT
  VOMIT
MENTAL STATE/
NEUROLOGICAL DISORDERS
• IRRITABILITY
• RESTLESSNESS
SEXUALITY, FEMALE:
GYNECOLOGICAL
• LEUKORRHEA: Damp Heat

Dose
15 - 30 gm

Common Name
Winter Melon

Precautions
Watch: Damp-Cold Cases Or Loose BM

DONG KUI ZI

冬葵子

SEMEN ABUTILONI SEU MALVAE

Traditional Functions:

1. Promotes urination and the circulation of fluids
2. Promotes lactation and benefits the breasts
3. Moistens the intestines and facilitates passage of stool

Traditional Properties:

Enters: LI, SI,

Properties: SW, C

Indications:

BOWEL RELATED DISORDERS
• CONSTIPATION: Intestinal Dryness, As Adjunct
• PURGATIVE: Mild
FLUID DISORDERS
• EDEMA: Auxillary Herb
• EDEMA, CONSTIPATION
INFECTIOUS DISEASES

• GONORRHEA
SEXUALITY, FEMALE: GYNECOLOGICAL
• BREASTS, ABSCESS OF: Early Stage
• BREASTS, DISTENTION, PAIN
• ECLAMPSIA: Edema Of

• LACTATION, INSUFFICIENT
URINARY BLADDER
• DYSURIA
• URINARY TRACT INFECTIONS, ACUTE
• URINATION, SANDY
• URINATION, SCANTY

Dose

3 - 15 gm

Common Name

Musk Mallow Seeds

Contraindications

Not: Diarrhea w/Def SP

Precautions

Watch: Pregnancy

FU LING
(BAI FU LING)

茯苓
(茯苓)

SCLEROTIUM PORIAE COCOS

Traditional Functions:

1. Promotes urination and filters out Dampness
2. Reinforces the Spleen and harmonizes the Middle Burner
3. Helps the Spleen to transform Phlegm
4. Calms the Heart and pacifies the Spirit

Traditional Properties:

Enters: LU, SP, HT, UB,

Properties: SW, BL, N

Indications:

ABDOMEN/ GASTROINTESTINAL TOPICS
• ABDOMEN, DISTENTION OF
BOWEL RELATED DISORDERS
• DIARRHEA: Cold Dampness (Add Warm Interior Herbs, Too) / Dampness/Fluid Stagnation/Spleen Deficient
CANCER/TUMORS/ SWELLINGS/LUMPS
• SWELLINGS, INFLAMMED
EARS/HEARING DISORDERS
• DIZZINESS: Spleen Deficient, Congested

Fluids With Phlegm Rising
ENERGETIC STATE
• WEAKNESS: Qi Deficiency
FLUID DISORDERS
• EDEMA: Dampness, Evil Fluid/Spleen Deficiency
• EDEMA, ASCITES
• EDEMA, GENERALIZED
• EDEMA, SCANTY URINE
HEAD/NECK
• HEADACHE: Spleen Deficient, Congested Fluids With Phlegm Rising
HEART
• PALPITATIONS: Spleen Deficient, Congested Fluids With Phlegm Rising
LIVER

• JAUNDICE, YIN
LUNGS
• COUGH: Cold Phlegm/ Phlegm Fluid
• LUNGS, DYSPNEA: Cold Phlegm
MENTAL STATE/ NEUROLOGICAL DISORDERS
• FORGETFULNESS
• INSOMNIA
ORAL CAVITY
• TONGUE, THICK, GREASY
PHLEGM
• SPUTUM: Lungs
SPLEEN
• SPLEEN DEFICIENCY W/DAMPNESS
• SPLEEN STOMACH,

DAMPNESS
STOMACH/DIGESTIVE DISORDERS
• ANOREXIA: Spleen Deficient, Dampness
• DIGESTIVE DISORDERS-DAMP
• EPIGASTRIC DISTENTION: Spleen Deficient, Dampness
• VOMITING
URINARY BLADDER
• URINATION, DIFFICULT: Dampness/ Fluid Stagnation
• URINATION, PAINFUL, DRIBBLING: With Deficiency Cold
• URINATION, SCANTY: Damp Heat

Clinical/Pharmaceutical Studies:

BLOOD RELATED DISORDERS/TOPICS
• BLOOD GLUCOSE, REDUCES

BOWEL RELATED DISORDERS
• DIARRHEA: Spleen Stomach Deficiency:Wei Ling Tang

CANCER/TUMORS/ SWELLINGS/LUMPS
• ANTINEOPLASTIC: High Inhibition Against Sarcoma

FLUID DISORDERS
• EDEMA, NEPHRITIC/ CARDIAC: Wu Ling San/ Fu Ling Dao Shui Tang (Fu Ling, Ze Xie, Sang Bai Pi, Chen Pi, Mu Xiang, Mu Gua, Sha Ren, Bai Zhu, Zi Su Ye, Zi Su Zi, Bing Lang, Mai Dong, Tong Cao, Da Fu Pi)

IMMUNE SYSTEM RELATED DISORDERS/ TOPICS
• IMMUNE SYSTEM ENHANCEMENT: Oral With Dang Shen, Bai Zhu Significantly Increased

INFECTIOUS DISEASES
• BACTERIAL, ANTI-: Inhibits, Staph Aureus, TB, Proteus, Leptospirae (ETOH Extract Only)

KIDNEYS
• DIURETIC: Slow, Prolonged, But Not Shown In Normal Doses (Slight At 15+g), More ETOH Extract

LIVER
• LIVER, PROTECTANT

MENTAL STATE/ NEUROLOGICAL DISORDERS
• INSOMNIA: With Suan Zao Ren (9-18 g) , Decocted
• SEDATIVE: Antagonizes Caffeine Excitation
• TRANQUILIZING

MUSCULOSKELETAL/ CONNECTIVE TISSUE
• MUSCLES, SMOOTH RELAXES

NUTRITIONAL/ METABOLIC DISORDERS/TOPICS
• NUTRITIVE

SEXUALITY, FEMALE/ GYNECOLOGICAL
• POSTPARTUM, JAUNDICE: Wu Ling San/ Fu Ling Dao Shui Tang

(Fu Ling, Ze Xie, Sang Bai Pi, Chen Pi, Mu Xiang, Mu Gua, Sha Ren, Bai Zhu, Zi Su Ye, Zi Su Zi, Bing Lang, Mai Dong, Tong Cao, Da Fu Pi)
• PREGNANCY, HYDRAMINON: (Excess Fluid In Amnionic Sac) Best For Chonic, Single-Fetus Pregnacy

STOMACH/DIGESTIVE DISORDERS
• INDIGESTION: Spleen Stomach Deficiency:Wei Ling Tang
• ULCERS, GASTRIC: Slightly Lessens Formation Of

URINARY BLADDER
• URINATION, SCANTY

Dose
9 - 18 gm

Common Name
Tuckahoe/China-Root/Hoelen

Contraindications
Not: Def Cold Frequent Copious Urine

Not: Spermatorrhea/Prolapse Of Urogenital Organs

Notes
For Edema: 30-45 gm

FU LING PI

茯苓皮
（茯苓皮）

CORTEX PORIAE COCOS

Traditional Functions:
1. Promotes urination and filters out Dampness

Traditional Properties:
Enters: UB,

Properties: SW, BL, N

Indications:

ABDOMEN/ GASTROINTESTINAL TOPICS
• ABDOMEN, DISTENTION OF

FLUID DISORDERS
• EDEMA: Dampness, Evil Fluid

KIDNEYS

• DIURETIC, MILD
URINARY BLADDER
• URINATION, SCANTY

Dose
6 gm

Common Name
Tuckahoe Skin

GUANG FANG JI

廣防己
（广防己）

RADIX ARISTOLOCHIAE SEU COCCULI

Traditional Functions:
1. Expels Wind Damp Hot Bi
2. Promotes urination and reduces swelling

Traditional Properties:
Enters: SP, KI, UB,

Properties: >BIT, SP, C

Indications:

EXTREMITIES
• LEG QI
FLUID DISORDERS
• EDEMA, UPPER BODY
• EDEMA, WHEEZING: Facial/
Systemic:Wind

**MUSCULOSKELETAL/
CONNECTIVE TISSUE**
• ARTHRITIS, RHEUMATIC
• JOINT BI W/HEAT
• JOINTS, PAIN, SWELLING
PAIN/NUMBNESS/GENERAL

DISCOMFORT
• ACHES, PAINS, DIFFUSE W/
HEAT
• BODY ACHES, PAINS, DIFFUSE
W/HEAT

Clinical/Pharmaceutical Studies:

**CANCER/TUMORS/SWELLINGS/
LUMPS**
• TUMORS: Inhibits
FEVERS
• ANTIPYRETIC
INFECTIOUS DISEASES

• BACTERIAL, ANTI-
**MUSCULOSKELETAL/
CONNECTIVE TISSUE**
• MUSCLES, SMOOTH: Stimulates,
Large Doses Paralyze

**PAIN/NUMBNESS/GENERAL
DISCOMFORT**
• ANALGESIC: Less Than Morphine
PARASITES
• AMOEBIC, ANTI-

Dose

4.5 - 9.0 gm

Precautions

Watch: Def Yin

HAN FANG JI
(FANG JI)

漢防己
（汉防己）

RADIX
STEPHANIAE
TETRANDRAE

Traditional Functions:

1. Promotes urination and disperses edema and swelling
2. Expels Wind Dampness and controls pain

Traditional Properties:

Enters: LU, SP, KI, UB,

Properties: BIT, SP, C

Indications:

**ABDOMEN/
GASTROINTESTINAL
TOPICS**
• ABDOMEN,
DISTENTION OF
• BORBORYGMUS
**CANCER/TUMORS/
SWELLINGS/LUMPS**
• SWELLINGS: Dampness/
Wind
EXTREMITIES
• ARMS, CONVULSIONS,
PAIN
• FEET, SPASMS, PAIN
• HANDS, SPASMS, PAIN

• LEG QI, DAMP
• LEGS, CONVULSIONS,
PAIN
FLUID DISORDERS
• ASCITES: Dampness In
Lower Jiao
• EDEMA: Dampness, Evil
Fluid
• EDEMA, LEGS/LOWER
BODY
HEART
• CARDIAC FUNCTION
DEFICIENCY
INFECTIOUS DISEASES
• GONORRHEA

**MUSCULOSKELETAL/
CONNECTIVE TISSUE**
• JOINTS, PAIN,
SWELLING, RED: Hot
Bi
• JOINTS, PAIN,
SWELLING, RED, HOT
W/FEVER: Wind Damp
Heat
**NUTRITIONAL/
METABOLIC
DISORDERS/TOPICS**
• BERIBERI: Damp Heat
**SEXUALITY, FEMALE:
GYNECOLOGICAL**

• LEUKORRHEA: Damp
Heat
SKIN
• ECZEMA: Damp Heat
• SKIN, SORES: Damp
Heat
URINARY BLADDER
• DYSURIA
• URINATION, PAINFUL,
DRIBBLING,
CONCENTRATED, RED/
YELLOW/TURBID
• URINATION, SCANTY
WIND DISORDERS
• WIND EDEMA

Clinical/Pharmaceutical Studies:

**BLOOD RELATED
DISORDERS/TOPICS**
• BLOOD PRESSURE,
LOWERS
**BOWEL RELATED
DISORDERS**
• DYSENTERY, AMOEBIC:
40 mg, 3x/Day
Tetrandrine, Orally, Kills
Entamoeba Histolytica,
Greater Than Berberine,
Less Than Emetine

• VASODILATOR IN
KIDNEY
FEVERS
• ANTIPYRETIC
HEART
• ANGINA PECTORIS: IV
Injection Of Tetrandrine
• HEART, INCREASES
CORONARY BLOOD
FLOW
**IMMUNE SYSTEM
RELATED DISORDERS/**

• LUNG CANCER: Short
Term Effect On Advanced,
Tetrandrine With
Radiotherapy
• SILICOSIS
**MENTAL STATE/
NEUROLOGICAL
DISORDERS**
• TRIGEMINAL
NEURALGIA: 400 mg
Tetrandrine 3x/Day
MUSCULOSKELETAL/

400 mg Tetrandrine 3x/
Day
• MUSCLES, RELAXANT,
STRIATED MUSCLES:
High Dose
**PAIN/NUMBNESS/
GENERAL
DISCOMFORT**
• ANALGESIC: Reduced
At High Doses Or w/Yan
Hu Suo, Less Potent Than
Yan Hu Suo

Clinical/Pharmaceutical Studies:

CANCER/TUMORS/
SWELLINGS/LUMPS
• LEUKEMIA: Short Term
WBC Reduction In, With
Tetrandrine
• TUMOR, ANTI-
CIRCULATION
DISORDERS
• HYPERTENSION: Good,
As Tetrandrine Orally,
Effective In All Stages

TOPICS
• ALLERGIC, ANTI-:
Inhibits Allergic Reactions,
Wheezing
INFECTIOUS DISEASES
• BACTERIAL, ANTI-
KIDNEYS
• DIURETIC
• VASODILATOR IN
KIDNEY
LUNGS

CONNECTIVE TISSUE
• ANKYLOSING
SPONDYLITIS WITH
RADICULITIS: 400 mg
Tetrandrine 3x/Day
• BACK, DISK
PROBLEMS: 400 mg
Tetrandrine 3x/Day
• BACK, LOWER PAIN:
Acute, Subacute
Lumbosacral Radiculitis:

• ANESTHETIC: Injection
PARASITES
• AMOEBIC, ANTI-:
Stronger Than Berberine
• ANTIPARASITIC: Weak
TRAUMA, BITES,
POISONINGS
• ANTIHISTAMINE
• INFLAMMATORY, ANTI-
: Adrenals

Dose
4.5 - 15.0 gm

Contraindications
Not: w/Interior Dampness

Precautions
Watch: Def Yin

Notes
Better For Edema, Guan Fang Ji, Better For Arthritis

HUA SHI   滑石   TALCUM

Traditional Functions:

1. Promotes urination and drains Heat from the bladder
2. Clears Heat and releases Summer Heat
3. Absorbs Dampness, as in damp skin lesions
4. Expels Damp Heat through the urine

Traditional Properties:

Enters: ST, UB,

Properties: SW, BL, C

Indications:

ABDOMEN/
GASTROINTESTINAL TOPICS
• ABDOMEN, DISTENTION OF:
Damp Heat
BOWEL RELATED DISORDERS
• DIARRHEA: Damp Heat/Summer
Heat/Evil Fluid Dampness
• DYSENTERY: Heat
FEVERS
• FEVER: Summer Heat
• FEVER, UNRELENTING: Qi
Level Heat With Dampness
FLUID DISORDERS
• EDEMA: Dampness, Evil Fluid
• THIRST: Qi Level Heat With
Dampness
HEAT
• QI LEVEL HEAT W/DAMP

• SUMMER HEAT: Fever, Urination
Difficult, Irritabilty, Thirst
HEMORRHAGIC DISORDERS
• EPISTAXIS
• HEMATEMESIS
• HEMOPTYSIS
INFECTIOUS DISEASES
• COMMON COLD, IN SUMMER
W/DAMPNESS
KIDNEYS
• DIURETIC: Good
• KIDNEY STONES
MENTAL STATE/
NEUROLOGICAL DISORDERS
• IRRITABILITY: Summer Heat
ORAL CAVITY
• MOUTH, DRY
PAIN/NUMBNESS/GENERAL

DISCOMFORT
• BODY, HEAVY FEELING: Qi
Level Heat With Dampness
SKIN
• ECZEMA: Damp Heat
• SKIN, LESIONS: Damp--Topical
TRAUMA, BITES, POISONINGS
• WOUNDS, TRAUMATIC: Topical
URINARY BLADDER
• DYSURIA: Hot
• URINARY STONES
• URINATION, DIFFICULT:
Summer Heat
• URINATION, DRIBBLING: Hot
• URINATION, PAINFUL
• URINATION, RETENTION
• URINATION, SCANTY: Hot

Clinical/Pharmaceutical Studies:

ABDOMEN/
GASTROINTESTINAL TOPICS
• GASTROINTESTINAL, INHIBITS
ABSORPTION OF POISON
BOWEL RELATED DISORDERS
• DIARRHEA: Protects Intestines
From
INFECTIOUS DISEASES

• BACTERIAL, ANTI-: B.Typhi, B.
Paratyphi, Meningococci
SKIN
• SKIN & MUCOUS MEMBRANES,
PROTECTOR FROM TOXINS
STOMACH/DIGESTIVE
DISORDERS

• STOMACH, PROTECTS LINING
OF: In Gastritis, Stops Nausea/
Vomiting
TRAUMA, BITES, POISONINGS
• WOUNDS: Protects Surface,
Absorption Of Secretions, Promotes
Scar Formation

Dose
9 - 12 gm

Common Name
Talcum

Precautions
Watch: Pregnancy

Notes
Prolonged Contact May Stimulate Granuloma Growth In Colon, Vagina

Wrap For Decoction

JIN QIAN CAO

金錢草
(金钱草)

HERBA DESMODII STYRACIFOLII

Traditional Functions:

1. Promotes urination and clears Heat
2. Expels stones from the gall bladder and the urinary bladder
3. Clears Liver channel Heat and Dampness
4. Eliminates toxins and reduces swelling

Traditional Properties:

Enters: LU, KI, LV, GB,

Properties: SW, N

Indications:

EYES
• EYES, RED, SWOLLEN: Liver Heat
FLUID DISORDERS
• EDEMA: Dampness, Evil Fluid
GALL BLADDER
• BILIARY STONES
• GALL BLADDER, STONES
KIDNEYS

• DIURETIC, MILD
• KIDNEY STONES
LIVER
• HEPATITIS
• JAUNDICE: Hepatitis:Liver Heat
SKIN
• ABSCESS
TRAUMA, BITES, POISONINGS
• SNAKE BITES

• TRAUMA, INJURIES, SWELLING
URINARY BLADDER
• DYSURIA
• URINARY BLADDER STONES
• URINARY TRACT STONES
• URINATION, DRIBBLING: Damp Heat
• URINATION, PAINFUL: Damp Heat

Clinical/Pharmaceutical Studies:

BLOOD RELATED DISORDERS/ TOPICS
• CHOLESTEROL: Promotes Accelerated Excretion Of
CIRCULATION DISORDERS
• CEREBRAL ARTERIOSCLEROSIS: Can Help Reduce Cholesterol Plague
GALL BLADDER
• BILE SECRETION, INCREASES ACUTELY
• CHOLECYSTITIS: 30-60 g Decoction With Hu Zhang, 15 g, Yu Jin, 15 g May Be Added For Pain
• GALL BLADDER, STONES
• GALL BLADDER, STONES/ INFECTION: Especially Sandy Stones, Fresh Superior To Dry
HEART
• CARDIOVASCULAR: Increase Coronary Circulation, Lowered Arterial Pressure, Slowed Heart, Decreased Oxygen Consumption
• HEART DISEASE: Can Help Reduce Cholesterol Plague In

Arteriosclerosis
• HEART, DECREASES OXYGEN USE
• HEART, INCREASES CORONARY BLOOD FLOW
INFECTIOUS DISEASES
• BACTERIAL, ANTI-: Tincture Strongly Inhibits Diphteriae, Active Against Staph. Aureus, B.Subtilis, E. Coli, ETOH Extract Inhibited Candida Albicans
• HERPES ZOSTER: Fresh Herb, 250 g Macerated In 100 ml 75% ETOH, 1 Week, Mix Filtrate With Realgar, Apply Topically, 2-3x/Day, Not If Broken Skin
• PAROTITIS: Local Application– Good
• PERTUSSIS
KIDNEYS
• DIURETIC: Calcium/Potassium Salts
LIVER
• HEPATITIS, ICTERIC

• LIVER, DISEASES, CHRONIC: Aid
PARASITES
• SCHISTOSOMIASIS, ADVANCED W/ASCITES: 60 g In 2 Daily Doses As Decoction, Rapid Disappearance Of Symptoms, Ascites
SEXUALITY, FEMALE: GYNECOLOGICAL
• MASTITIS, ACUTE
SKIN
• BURNS: Local Treatment
• ERYSIPELAS: Fresh Herb, 250 g Macerated In 100 ml 75% ETOH, 1 Week, Mix Filtrate With Realgar, Apply Topically, 2-3x/Day, Not If Broken Skin
TRAUMA, BITES, POISONINGS
• ANTIDOTE, TRIPTERGIUM WILFORDII POISONING
URINARY BLADDER
• URINARY BLADDER STONES: Urine Becomes Acidic Which Dissolves Alkaline Induced Stones

Dose
9 - 60 gm

Notes
Low Toxicity: Long Term (>6 Months) , Lrg Dose (>250

g/Day) Use Leads To K+ (Potassium) Depletion: Dizziness, Possible Palpitations, Which Disappears Spontaneously

As Single Herb: 120-150gm

MU TONG

木通

CAULIS AKEBIAE
(MUTONG)

Traditional Functions:

1. Promotes urination and drains Heat from the Heart via the Small Intestine
2. Facilitates lactation and promotes blood circulation

Traditional Properties:

Enters: LU, HT, SI, UB,

Properties: BIT, C

Indications:

BLOOD RELATED DISORDERS/ TOPICS
• ANEMIA
CANCER/TUMORS/SWELLINGS/ LUMPS
• TUMORS: Blood Stasis, Herbs Used Other Than Vitalize Blood
EXTREMITIES
• LEG QI
FLUID DISORDERS
• EDEMA: Dampness, Evil Fluid
HEMORRHAGIC DISORDERS
• HEMATURIA
KIDNEYS
• DIURETIC, MILD
MENTAL STATE/ NEUROLOGICAL DISORDERS
• IRRITABILITY WITH MOUTH SORES/TONGUE
• IRRITABILITY, HEAT SENSATION IN CHEST
• MANIC AGITATION

• RESTLESSNESS
MUSCULOSKELETAL/ CONNECTIVE TISSUE
• ARTHRITIS, RHEUMATIC
• CRAMPS
• JOINTS, PAIN, SWELLING, RED: Hot Bi
• JOINTS, STIFF, PAIN
ORAL CAVITY
• LARYNGITIS
• SORES, MOUTH/TONGUE
• THROAT, SORE
PAIN/NUMBNESS/GENERAL DISCOMFORT
• BODY, PAIN ALL OVER
SEXUALITY, FEMALE: GYNECOLOGICAL
• AMENORRHEA: Blood Stasis, In Addition To Vitalize Blood Herbs
• BREASTS, SWOLLEN, PAINFUL, ABSCESS

• LACTATION, INSUFFICIENT: Heat
• POSTPARTUM, ABDOMINAL PAIN: Blood Stasis
SKIN
• ECZEMA: Damp Heat
• SKIN, SORES: Damp Heat
URINARY BLADDER
• CHYLURIA
• DYSURIA: Damp Heat, With Concentrated Urine
• URINARY BLADDER DYSFUNCTION
• URINARY STONES
• URINARY TRACT INFECTIONS, ACUTE
• URINATION, DRIBBLING
• URINATION, PAINFUL, DRIBBLING, CONCENTRATED, RED/YELLOW/TURBID
• URINATION, SCANTY

Clinical/Pharmaceutical Studies:

ABDOMEN/ GASTROINTESTINAL TOPICS
• INTESTINES, STIMULATES
CANCER/TUMORS/ SWELLINGS/LUMPS
• TUMOR, ANTI-: Aristolochine Active Ingredient, Used With Chemo/Radiotherapy
FLUID DISORDERS
• EDEMA, LIVER CIRRHOSIS, CARDIAC, RENAL: Injection Of Mix Of Mu Tong, Ze Xie, Xia Ku Cao
HEART

• CARDIOTONIC: Similar To Digitalis In Action
HEMORRHAGIC DISORDERS
• HEMATURIA W/ OLIGURIA: 3-9 gm Decoction
IMMUNE SYSTEM RELATED DISORDERS/ TOPICS
• IMMUNE RESPONSE: Increases Ability Of Phagocytosis
INFECTIOUS DISEASES
• BACTERIAL, ANTI-: Gram Positive Bacilli
KIDNEYS
• DIURETIC, STRONG:

Less Than Zhu Ling, Greater Than Dan Zhu Ye
LIVER
• HEPATITIS
LUNGS
• PNEUMONIA, CHILDHOOD
• TUBERCULOSIS
ORAL CAVITY
• MOUTH, ULCERS: 3-9 gm Decoction
• THROAT, SORE
• TONGUE, ULCERS: 3-9 gm Decoction
PAIN/NUMBNESS/ GENERAL DISCOMFORT

• ANALGESIC
SEXUALITY, FEMALE: GYNECOLOGICAL
• LACTATION, INSUFFICIENT/ STOPPED: 3-9 gm Decoction
• UTERUS, INHIBITS
SKIN
• FUNGAL, ANTI-
TRAUMA, BITES, POISONINGS
• INFLAMMATORY, ANTI-
URINARY BLADDER
• URINARY TRACT INFECTIONS, ACUTE: 3-9 gm Decoction

Dose

3 - 9 gm

Contraindications

Not: Pregnancy

Not: w/o Internal Damp Heat

Not: Those With Deficient Essence

Precautions

Watch: Deficient Yin, Easily Injures Fluids

Notes

>60 gm Dose May Cause Acute Renal Failure

QU MAI

瞿麥
（瞿麦）

HERBA DIANTHI

Traditional Functions:

1. Promotes urination and clears Heat
2. Cracks the Blood and opens menstruation
3. Promotes movement of stool

Traditional Properties:

Enters: HT, SI, UB,

Properties: BIT, C

Indications:

BOWEL RELATED DISORDERS
• CONSTIPATION
CANCER/TUMORS/SWELLINGS/LUMPS
• TUMORS: Blood Stasis, Herbs Used Other Than Vitalize Blood
FLUID DISORDERS
• EDEMA: Dampness, Evil Fluid
HEMORRHAGIC DISORDERS
• HEMATURIA
KIDNEYS
• DIURETIC, MILD

SEXUALITY, FEMALE: GYNECOLOGICAL
• ABORTION OF DEAD FETUS
• AMENORRHEA: Blood Stasis, In Addition To Vitalize Blood Herbs
• BIRTH, PROMOTES
• POSTPARTUM, ABDOMINAL PAIN: Blood Stasis
SKIN
• CARBUNCLES
• SKIN, ULCERS, TOXIC EROSIVE
URINARY BLADDER

• DYSURIA
• URINARY OBSTRUCTION
• URINARY TRACT INFECTIONS, ACUTE
• URINATION, DRIBBLING
• URINATION, HOT
• URINATION, PAINFUL, DRIBBLING, CONCENTRATED, RED/YELLOW/TURBID
• URINATION, RETENTION
• URINATION, SANDY

Clinical/Pharmaceutical Studies:

ABDOMEN/GASTROINTESTINAL TOPICS
• PERISTALSIS, INCREASES
BLOOD RELATED DISORDERS/TOPICS
• BLOOD PRESSURE, LOWERS
CANCER/TUMORS/SWELLINGS/LUMPS
• ESOPHAGEAL CANCER: Decoction Fresh Root, 30-

40 g (24-30 g Dried) Alone Or With Ren Shen, Fu Ling, Bai Zhu, Gan Cao
• RECTAL CANCER: Decoction Fresh Root, 30-40 g (24-30 g Dried) Alone Or With Ren Shen, Fu Ling, Bai Zhu, Gan Cao
HEART
• CARDIAC INHIBITOR
INFECTIOUS DISEASES
• BACTERIAL, ANTI-: Pseudomonas, E.Coli, B.

Typhi, Shigella, Staph. Aureus
KIDNEYS
• DIURETIC, STRONG: Flowers Better, Increased Urine Output 5-8 X In Dogs
PARASITES
• ANTIPARASITIC: Inhibits Schistosomiasis
• SCHISTOSOMIASIS: 10% Decoction Kills In 8-12

Minutes
SEXUALITY, FEMALE: GYNECOLOGICAL
• AMENORRHEA: Blood Stasis, With Dan Shen, Chi Shao, Yi Mu Cao
URINARY BLADDER
• CYSTITIS: With Bian Xu, Hai Jin Sha
• URINARY TRACT INFECTIONS, ACUTE: With Bian Xu, Hai Jin Sha

Dose
4.5 - 12.0 gm

Common Name

Fringed Pink Flower

Contraindications

Not: Pregnancy
Not: Def SP/KI

Notes
May Be Increased 18-24 gm

SHENG JIANG PI

生姜皮

CORTEX ZINGIBERIS OFFICINALIS RECENS

Traditional Functions:

1. Promotes urination
2. Reduces superficial edema
3. Harmonizes the Spleen

Traditional Properties:

Enters: SP, UB

Properties: SP, CL

Indications:

FLUID DISORDERS

• ASCITES

• EDEMA, SUPERFICIAL

Dose
3 - 9 gm

Common Name
Ginger Peel

SHI WEI

石葦
(石苇)

FOLIUM PYRROSIAE

Traditional Functions:

1. Clears Damp Heat and stones from the bladder
2. Clears Heat and stops bleeding
3. Transforms Phlegm and reduces coughs

Traditional Properties:

Enters: LU, UB,

Properties: BIT, SW, CL

Indications:

GALL BLADDER
- GALL BLADDER, STONES
HEMORRHAGIC DISORDERS
- HEMATEMESIS: Blood Heat
- HEMATURIA: Blood Heat
INFECTIOUS DISEASES
- GONORRHEA
KIDNEYS
- KIDNEY STONES

LUNGS
- BRONCHITIS, W/COUGH, PROFUSE SPUTUM: Lung Heat
- COUGH: Lung Heat
- LUNGS, DYSPNEA: Lung Heat
SEXUALITY, FEMALE: GYNECOLOGICAL
- MENORRHAGIA
- UTERINE BLEEDING: Blood Heat

URINARY BLADDER
- DRIBBLING
- URINARY INFECTIONS, ACUTE
- URINARY TRACT STONES
- URINATION, PAINFUL: Heat
- URINATION, PAINFUL, DRIBBLING, CONCENTRATED, RED/YELLOW/TURBID

Clinical/Pharmaceutical Studies:

INFECTIOUS DISEASES
- BACTERIAL, ANTI-: Staph.Aureus, E.Coli, Proteus, Amoeba, P.Lingua
KIDNEYS

- GLOMERULO-NEPHRITIS
- NEPHRITIS, GLOMERULE-/PYELO-
- PYELONEPHRITIS

LUNGS
- ANTITUSSIVE: Short Duration, Strong
- ASTHMA: Very Strong
- BRONCHITIS,

CHRONIC: Helps Symptoms, Cell Changes
- EXPECTORANT: Very Strong

Dose
4.5 - 30.0 gm

TONG CAO

通草

MEDULLA TETRAPANACIS PAPYRIFERI

Traditional Functions:

1. Promotes urination and drains Heat
2. Promotes lactation

Traditional Properties:

Enters: LU, ST,

Properties: SW, BL, <C

Indications:

FLUID DISORDERS
- EDEMA
INFECTIOUS DISEASES
- FEBRILE DISEASES: Damp Heat
KIDNEYS
- DIURETIC, MILD
LUNGS

- LUNG HEAT: Cough
SEXUALITY, FEMALE: GYNECOLOGICAL
- BIRTH, INDUCES
- LACTATION, INSUFFICIENT
- LACTATION, PROMOTES
URINARY BLADDER

- DYSURIA: Damp Heat
- URINATION, DRIBBLING
- URINATION, PAINFUL, DRIBBLING, CONCENTRATED, RED/YELLOW/TURBID
- URINATION, RETENTION

Clinical/Pharmaceutical Studies:

KIDNEYS
- DIURETIC

SEXUALITY, FEMALE: GYNECOLOGICAL

- LACTATION, PROMOTES

Dose

2.4 - 6.0 gm

Common Name

Rice Paper Pith

Precautions

Watch: Pregnancy

Watch: Def Qi/Yin

TU YIN CHEN
(BEI YIN CHEN/TU XIANG JU)

土茵陳
（土茵陈）

HERBA ORIGANI
(ARTEMISIA)

Traditional Functions:

1. Releases the Exterior by promoting sweating
2. Regulates the Qi
3. Eliminates Dampness

Traditional Properties:

Enters:

Properties: SP, CL

Indications:

BOWEL RELATED DISORDERS
• DYSENTERY
CHEST
• CHEST, FULLNESS, DISTENTION
CHILDHOOD DISORDERS

• MALNUTRITION, CHILDHOOD
FEVERS
• FEVER
INFECTIOUS DISEASES
• COMMON COLD

LIVER
• JAUNDICE
STOMACH/DIGESTIVE DISORDERS
• VOMITING

Clinical/Pharmaceutical Studies:

GALL BLADDER
• GALL BLADDER, BILE SECRETION, INCREASES
INFECTIOUS DISEASES
• VIRAL, ANTI-: 1:10 Decoction Inhibits Echo Virus, Not Any Others
KIDNEYS

• DIURETIC
LIVER
• HEPATITIS, ICTERIC
LUNGS
• EXPECTORANT
SKIN

• FUNGAL, ANTI-
STOMACH/DIGESTIVE DISORDERS
• DIGESTION, ENHANCES: Promotes Appetite, Improves Digestion

Dose

9 - 15 gm

Common Name

Oregano

Notes

Irritates Stomach In Large Doses, Vomiting

Commonly Used As A Substitute For Yin Chen

YI YI REN

薏苡仁

SEMEN COICIS LACHRYMA-JOBI

Traditional Functions:

1. Promotes urination and filters out Dampness
2. Benefits the Spleen and controls diarrhea
3. Clears Heat and toxins and dissipates pus
4. Expels Wind Damp Bi and spasms
5. Clears Damp Heat

Traditional Properties:

Enters: LU, SP, ST, KI,

Properties: SW, BL, CL

Indications:

ABDOMEN/ GASTROINTESTINAL TOPICS
• ABDOMEN, DISTENTION OF: Damp Heat
• ABSCESS, LARGE

• ASCITES
• EDEMA: Spleen Deficiency
• THIRST
HEAT
• DAMP HEAT, ANY
INFECTIOUS DISEASES

• TENDONS, CONTRACTIONS
PAIN/NUMBNESS/ GENERAL DISCOMFORT
• BI, WIND DAMP: Joint Pain, Chronic Conditions:

• FUNGAL INFECTIONS, FOOT TINEA
• SKIN, SORES: Damp Heat
• WARTS, PLANTERS
SPLEEN
• SPLEEN DEFICIENCY

Indications:

INTESTINE/LUNG
BOWEL RELATED
DISORDERS
• DIARRHEA: Evil Fluid
Dampness/Mild For Spleen
Deficient w/Dampness
EXTREMITIES
• FEET, TINEA
INFECTION
• LEG QI: Damp
• LEGS, SWELLING
FLUID DISORDERS

• TINEA INFECTION,
FEET
LUNGS
• ABSCESS, LUNG/
LARGE INTESTINE
• COUGH
• LUNG ATROPHY
• LUNG FISTULA
• LUNGS, ABSCESS W/
PURULENT VOMIT
MUSCULOSKELETAL/
CONNECTIVE TISSUE

Aches, Stiff, Spasms
SEXUALITY, FEMALE:
GYNECOLOGICAL
• LEUKORRHEA
• MENSTRUATION,
DISORDERS OF:
Constrict Uterus, Stimulate
Chong
SKIN
• CARBUNCLES, SOFT
PUS-FILLED
• ECZEMA: Damp Heat

W/DAMPNESS,
DIARRHEA: Mild
STOMACH/DIGESTIVE
DISORDERS
• DIGESTIVE
DISORDERS: Damp Heat
URINARY BLADDER
• URINATION,
DIFFICULT
• URINATION, SCANTY
• URINATION, TURBID
DRIBBLING

Clinical/Pharmaceutical Studies:

ABDOMEN/
GASTROINTESTINAL
TOPICS
• APPENDICITIS: Yi Yi
Wu Tou Bai Jiang Cao
Tang (Yi Yi Ren, Wu Tou,
Bai Jiang Cao) , Effective
Standard Formula
BLOOD RELATED
DISORDERS/TOPICS
• BLOOD GLUCOSE,
REDUCES: Injection, Oil
Of, Weak Effect
CANCER/TUMORS/
SWELLINGS/LUMPS
• ANTINEOPLASTIC:
Granuloma, Hepatic
Cancer, Believed To Be
Coixenolide
• CANCER, ANTI-:
Acetone Extract Of Oils
• CERVICAL CANCER:
Markedly Inhibited
• STOMACH CANCER:
Digestive Tract, Use Herb,
Teng Liu (?) , He Zi, Ling
Jiao (Trapa Bispinosa) ,
Includes Postoperative,

Advanced Inoperable
Cases, 3 Doses/Day,
Improved Symptoms For
Most, Take More Than 3
Months, No Side Effects
• TUMOR, ANTI-: Acetone
Extract Of Oils, ETOH
Extract
CIRCULATION
DISORDERS
• VASODILATOR,
PERIPHERAL BLOOD
VESSELS, ESPECIALLY:
Oil Of
FEVERS
• ANTIPYRETIC
INFECTIOUS DISEASES
• BACTERIAL, ANTI-:
Decoction Of Root, Staph
Aureus, Strep, B.Anthracis,
Corynebacterium
Diphtheriae
LUNGS
• BRONCHODILATORY
• LUNGS, ABSCESS: Yi
Yi Gen Or Qian Jin Wei
Jing Tang (Has Yi Yi Ren)
• RESPIRATION, OIL OF:

Low Doses Stimulate,
High Doses Inhibits
MENTAL STATE/
NEUROLOGICAL
DISORDERS
• CNS, SEDATIVE:
Counteracts Caffeine
MUSCULOSKELETAL/
CONNECTIVE TISSUE
• MUSCLES, SPASMS,
STRIATED: Relaxes
NUTRITIONAL/
METABOLIC
DISORDERS/TOPICS
• HYPOTHERMIA
PAIN/NUMBNESS/
GENERAL
DISCOMFORT
• ANALGESIC: Aqueous
Extract
PARASITES
• ASCARIASIS: 1:1 Fluid
Extract, 50 ml In 1 Or 3
Doses Preprandial
SEXUALITY, FEMALE:
GYNECOLOGICAL
• ABORTIFACIENT:

Induces Labor, Mid Term
By Chewing, Eating Root
• CERVIX, CANCINOMA:
Markedly Inhibited
SKIN
• WARTS: 30% Cured, 10-
30 g Decoction/Day, 1
Dose, 2-4 Weeks, *60 g
Cooked With Husked Rice
Given As Meal 1x/Day,
Almost 50% Cured In 7-16
Days, Often Warts Will
Become Enlarged, Red,
Inflammed Before
Disappearing
STOMACH/DIGESTIVE
DISORDERS
• STOMACH, CANCER:
Digestive Tract, Use Herb,
Teng Liu (?) , He Zi, Ling
Jiao (Trapa Bispinosa) ,
Includes Postoperative,
Advanced Inoperable
Cases, 3 Doses/Day,
Improved Symptoms For
Most, Take More Than 3
Months, No Side Effects

Dose

9 - 30 gm

Common Name

Job's Tears Seeds

Precautions

Watch: Pregnancy

Notes

Dry Fry For SP Tonification
May Increase: 60-90 gm
No Adverse Reactions From Ingestion

YIN CHEN
(MIAN YIN CHEN/YIN CHEN HAO)

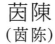
茵 陳
（茵 陈）

HERBA
ARTEMESIAE CAPILLARIS

Traditional Functions:

1. Clears Damp Heat and relieves jaundice from the Liver and Gall Bladder channels
2. Clears Heat and releases Shao Yang Exterior conditions

Traditional Properties:

Enters: SP, ST, LV, GB,

Properties: BIT, C

Indications:

CHEST
- CHEST, CONSTRICTION: Shao Yang

EARS/HEARING DISORDERS
- DIZZINESS: Shao Yang

FEVERS
- CHILLS/FEVER: Shao Yang
- FEVER

GALL BLADDER
- CHOLECYSTITIS

KIDNEYS
- DIURETIC, MILD

LIVER
- HEPATITIS
- JAUNDICE: Damp Heat/Damp Cold
- JAUNDICE, YIN

ORAL CAVITY
- TASTE, BITTER: Shao Yang

SIX STAGES/CHANNELS
- SHAO YANG STAGE DISEASE

SKIN
- RASHES, PRURITIC: Wind Damp

STOMACH/DIGESTIVE DISORDERS
- ANOREXIA: Shao Yang
- NAUSEA: Shao Yang

URINARY BLADDER
- DYSURIA

Clinical/Pharmaceutical Studies:

BLOOD RELATED DISORDERS/TOPICS
- ANTICOAGULANT
- BLOOD PRESSURE, LOWERS: ETOH/ Aqueous Extract
- BLOOD, BILIRUBIN LEVELS LOWERED: w/ Da Huang, Zhi Zi
- CHOLESTEROL, LOWERS: (Mean 96mg%) Also, Blood Lipids (Mean 64mg%) , Oral Use For 3 Weeks, Yin Chen, 24 g As 7 Tabs, 3x/Day For 30 Days, *Ze Xie, Yin Chen, Gan Cao For 1 Month, Lowered Cholesterol Mean 37mg%, *Yin Chen, Ze Xie, Ge Gen

CANCER/TUMORS/ SWELLINGS/LUMPS
- CANCER: Orally, Lethal To Erhlich Ascites

ENDOCRINE RELATED DISORDERS
- DIABETES: Extract Lowers Blood Glucose Level Dose-Dependent

FEVERS
- ANTIPYRETIC: Aqueous Extract, Strong, Decoction Weaker, ETOH Extract, Too

GALL BLADDER
- CHOLAGOGUE
- GALL BLADDER, BILE SECRETION,

STIMULATES: Decoction/ Aqueous Extract/Volatile Oil-Free Extract/ETOH Extract, All Help, Shan Zhi Zi Synergizes
- GALL BLADDER, STONES: Damp Heat Type, 90% Passed Stones, 35% Still Needed Surgery, Lithogogue Decoction No.2 (Yin Chen, Ling Ling Xiang (Sweet Basil) , Yu Jin, Jin Yin Hua, Lian Qiao, Da Huang, Mu Xiang, Zhi Shi, Mang Xiao)

HEART
- CORONARY HEART DISEASE W/ANGINA: Yin Chen, Cang Zhu, Vine Spatholobus Suberectus, E Zhu, For Yang Def Add Fu Zi, With Yin Def Add Xuan Shen

INFECTIOUS DISEASES
- BACTERIAL, ANTI-: Staph Aureus, Strep., B. Dysenteriae, Pneumococci, C.Diphteriae, B.Typhi, B. Subtilis, Mycobacteria, et al
- COMMON COLD: Helps To Treat
- INFLUENZA: Decoction, ETOH Extract Used As Prophylaxis During Time Of Flu Epidemic, No One Caught Flu, May Be Used

To Treat Symptoms, Too
- LEPTOSPIROSIS: Various Strains, 5% Decoction Over Several Days, In Vitro, *Use Yin Chen, Hua Shi, Huang Qin, Bo He, Huo Xiang, Lian Qiao, Mu Tong, Bai Dou Kou
- VIRAL, ANTI-: ETOH Extract Strongly Inhibits Flu

KIDNEYS
- DIURETIC

LIVER
- HEPATITIS, ICTERIC: 1- 1.5 Liang, 3x/Day, 7 Days/ Wih Gan Cao, Da Zao, Sugar 10 Days, For Young Children, *30-45 g, 7 Days PO, Gives Rapid Reduction Of Jaundice, Fever, Size Of Liver, *Yin Chen, Huang Bai, Xhan Zhi Zi, Ban Lan Gen,* Prophylaxis Use Against Viral--Yin Chen, Dan Shen, Ba Qing Ye, Da Zao/With Serissa Serissoides, Tian Ji Huang, Bai Jian Cao, Gan Cao
- LIVER, CELL REGENERATION: w/ Dahuang, Zhizi
- LIVER, PROTECTANT

LUNGS

- ANTIASTHMATIC

MENTAL STATE/ NEUROLOGICAL DISORDERS
- SEDATIVE: Essential Oil

PARASITES
- ASCARIASIS, BILIARY: Oral Decoction, Plus Acupuncture Analgesia Of PC6, Neiguan, "Other Measures", Cure In 4 Days, Pain Gone In 1.5 Days, Much Shorter Than Western Drugs
- ROUNDWORMS: Essential Oil Paralyzes, Decoction In Vitro For Some Varieties

SEXUALITY, FEMALE: GYNECOLOGICAL
- UTERUS, STIMULATES

SKIN
- FUNGAL INFECTIONS: Tinea Corporis, Pedis Treated With 5% Volatile Oil In ETOH (High Boiling Point Fraction) , 2x/ Day, 4 Weeks, 71% Cured, * Fluid Extract Of 25 g/Day Helped Various Tinea
- FUNGAL, ANTI-: High Boiling Point Volatile Oil Of, Heat Stable To Over 100 Degrees C, Apply Topically, Very Strong, Many

Dose

6 - 30 gm

Contraindications

Not: Yin Yellow w/SP Qi Def

Notes

Up To 30 g For Jaundice

Side Effects: If 24 g/Day, 33% Developed Dizziness, Nausea, Distention, Heartburn, All Gradually Disappear

YU MI XU

玉米須
（玉米须）

STYLUS ZEAE MAYS

Traditional Functions:

1. Promotes urination and reduces swelling
2. Clears jaundice
3. Benefits wasting and thirsting syndrome(diabetes)
4. Stops bleeding

Traditional Properties:

Enters: UB, LV, GB

Properties: SW, N

Indications:

CIRCULATION DISORDERS
• HYPERTENSION
ENDOCRINE RELATED DISORDERS
• WASTING & THIRSTING SYNDROME: Diabetes
FLUID DISORDERS
• EDEMA, NEPHRITIC, ACUTE/ CHRONIC
GALL BLADDER

• CHOLECYSTITIS
• GALL BLADDER, STONES
HEMORRHAGIC DISORDERS
• EPISTAXIS
KIDNEYS
• KIDNEY DISEASES
LIVER
• HEPATITIS, ICTERIC
• JAUNDICE: Yin Or Yang
• LIVER, CIRRHOSIS, HEPATIC-

EDEMA
NUTRITIONAL/METABOLIC DISORDERS/TOPICS
• BERIBERI, SWELLING OF
ORAL CAVITY
• GUMS, BLEEDING
URINARY BLADDER
• URINARY TRACT STONES
• URINATION, PAINFUL: Hot LI

Clinical/Pharmaceutical Studies:

BLOOD RELATED DISORDERS/TOPICS
• BLOOD GLUCOSE, REDUCES, DRAMATICALLY
• BLOOD PRESSURE, LOWERS: By Dilation Of Peripheral Capillaries, Over Long Term, IV Only
• PROTHROMBIN, INCREASES, DECREASES CLOT TIME
CIRCULATION DISORDERS

• HYPERTENSION: 15 g As Hot Tea/Day For 2 Months, Reduced BP 170/ 90 To 130/70, Stability Reached After 7 Months
FLUID DISORDERS
• EDEMA: Renal, Liver Cirrhosis, Schistosomiasis, Nutritional, 50 g As Tea, Do Not Exceed Urine Output
GALL BLADDER
• CHOLAGOGUE
• CHOLANGITIS: Increases Bile Secretion,

Decreases Viscosity
• CHOLECYSTITIS: Increases Bile Secretion, Decreases Viscosity
• CHOLELITHIASIS: Fluid Extract, 30-40 Drops/ Tablet 0.8 g, 3-4x/Day
HEMORRHAGIC DISORDERS
• HEMATURIA
KIDNEYS
• DIURETIC, WEAK
• NEPHRITIS, CHRONIC W/EDEMA: Improves

Renal Function
• PROTEIN, INHIBITS EXCRETION
LIVER
• HEPATITIS, NONICTERIC: Fluid Extract, 30-40 Drops/ Tablet 0.8 g, 3-4x/Day
URINARY BLADDER
• CHYLURIA
• DYSURIA
• URINARY STONES
• URINATION, FREQUENT/URGENT

Dose

15 - 60 gm

Common Name

Cornsilk

Notes

Non-Toxic

ZE XIE

澤瀉
（泽泻）

RHIZOMA ALISMATIS

Traditional Functions:

1. Promotes urination and filters out Dampness
2. Drains deficient Kidney fire

Traditional Properties:

Enters: KI, UB,

Properties: SW, BL, C

Indications:

ABDOMEN/ GASTROINTESTINAL TOPICS
• ABDOMEN, DISTENTION OF

• EDEMA, FULLNESS, DISTENTION: Dampness
• THIRST

• PHLEGM, RETENTION
SEXUALITY, FEMALE: GYNECOLOGICAL

Indications:

**BLOOD RELATED DISORDERS/
TOPICS**
• CHOLESTEROLEMIA
BOWEL RELATED DISORDERS
• DIARRHEA: Evil Fluid Dampness
• DIARRHEA, ACUTE: Dampness
• DYSENTERY
EARS/HEARING DISORDERS
• DIZZINESS: Kidney Yin Deficient
With Heat
• TINNITUS: Kidney Yin Deficient
With Heat
EXTREMITIES
• LEGS, EDEMA
FLUID DISORDERS
• EDEMA: Dampness, Evil Fluid

HEAT
• DAMP HEAT
HEMORRHAGIC DISORDERS
• HEMATURIA
KIDNEYS
• DIURETIC, MILD
• KIDNEY YIN DEFICIENCY WITH
HEAT: Tinnitus, Dizziness
• NEPHRITIS
LIVER
• JAUNDICE, YIN
**NUTRITIONAL/METABOLIC
DISORDERS/TOPICS**
• BERIBERI
PHLEGM
• PHLEGM FLUID

• LEUKORRHEA: Damp Heat
**STOMACH/DIGESTIVE
DISORDERS**
• STOMACH, STAGNANT WATER
IN
• VOMITING
URINARY BLADDER
• URINARY TRACT INFECTIONS
• URINATION, DIFFICULT:
Dampness
• URINATION, DRIBBLING
• URINATION, PAINFUL,
DRIBBLING, CONCENTRATED,
RED/YELLOW/TURBID
• URINATION, SCANTY: Damp
Heat

Clinical/Pharmaceutical Studies:

**BLOOD RELATED
DISORDERS/TOPICS**
• BLOOD GLUCOSE,
REDUCES: Similar To
Choline, Lecithin
• BLOOD PRESSURE,
LOWERS: Prolonged
• CHOLESTEROL,
LOWERS: Similar To
Choline, Lecithin, *Tab Of

ETOH Extract 0.15 g, Fine
Powder 0.15 g=2.5 g Herb,
3-4 Tabs, 3-4x/Day PO, 1-
3 Months, Marked
Lowering, Similar To
Clofibrate
FLUID DISORDERS
• EDEMA: With Fu Ling,
Che Qian Zi

INFECTIOUS DISEASES
• BACTERIAL, ANTI-:
Staph, Pneumococci,
Mycobacteria, etc
KIDNEYS
• DIURETIC: Varies With
Season Harvested, Can Be
Marked, Winter Collection
Stronger, Salt Treated Herb

Not Diuretic
• NEPHRITIS, ACUTE:
With Fu Ling, Che Qian Zi
LIVER
• LIVER, ANTI FATTY:
Helps To Recover
URINARY BLADDER
• URINATION, SCANTY:
With Fu Ling, Che Qian Zi

Dose
6 - 45 gm

Common Name
Water Plantain Rhizome

Contraindications
Not: Spermatorrhea/Leukorrhea From Def KI Yang/
Damp Cold

Notes
Mild Digestive Reactions, Soft Stool, Possible Skin
Rash

ZHU LING

豬苓
（猪苓）

SCLEROTIUM
POLYPORI UMBELLATI
(GRIFOLA)

Traditional Functions:

1. Promotes urination, filters out Dampness and dispels Heat

Traditional Properties:

Enters: KI, UB,

Properties: SW, BL, N

Indications:

BOWEL RELATED DISORDERS
• DIARRHEA: Dampness/Evil Fluid
Dampness
FLUID DISORDERS
• ASCITES
• EDEMA: Dampness, Evil Fluid
• EDEMA, DISTENTION/
FULLNESS OF: Dampness

KIDNEYS
• DIURETIC, MILD
LIVER
• JAUNDICE: Dampness
• JAUNDICE, YIN
**SEXUALITY, FEMALE:
GYNECOLOGICAL**
• LEUKORRHEA: Dampness

URINARY BLADDER
• DYSURIA: Dampness
• URINATION, PAINFUL,
DRIBBLING: With Deficiency Cold
• URINATION, PAINFUL, TURBID:
Dampness
• URINATION, SCANTY: Dampness

Clinical/Pharmaceutical Studies:

BLOOD RELATED DISORDERS/ TOPICS
• BLOOD GLUCOSE, REDUCES
CANCER/TUMORS/SWELLINGS/ LUMPS
• ESOPHAGEAL CANCER: Synergistic With Chemotherapy, Protects Bone Marrow, Immune System Enhanced
• TUMOR, ANTI-
HEMORRHAGIC DISORDERS
• HEMATURIA: 6-12 g/Day
IMMUNE SYSTEM RELATED

DISORDERS/TOPICS

• IMMUNE SYSTEM ENHANCEMENT: Extract, ETOH Extract Helps Phagocytosis, T-Cell Transformation
INFECTIOUS DISEASES
• ANTIBIOTIC: ETOH Extract, Staph A., E.Coli
• BACTERIAL, ANTI-: Staph, E. Coli
KIDNEYS
• DIURETIC: Stronger Than Caffeine, Mu Tong, Fu Ling As A Decoction, No Diuresis If As ETOH Extract

LIVER
• LIVER, CIRRHOSIS: Wu Ling San/ Wu Pi Yin
LUNGS
• LUNG CANCER: With Chemotherapy, Improves Symptoms, Reduces Side Effects Of Chemo, Supports Immune System
URINARY BLADDER
• DYSURIA: 6-12 g/Day
• URINARY TRACT INFECTIONS: 6-12 g/Day
• URINATION, CLOUDY: (Dhyluria) Zhu Ling Tang

Dose

6 - 18 gm

Common Name

Grifola

Contraindications

Not: w/o Dampness

Precautions

Watch: Prolonged Use Damages Yin/SP

Notes

No Toxicity Even In Large Doses

ZHU MA GEN
(NING MA GEN)

苧 麻 根
(苧 麻 根)

RADIX BOEHMERIAE

Traditional Functions:

1. Clears Heat and relieves toxins
2. Vitalizes and moves Blood, calming restless fetus
3. Promotes urination

Traditional Properties:

Enters: HT, LV

Properties: SW, C

Indications:

HEMORRHAGIC DISORDERS
• HEMATURIA
INFECTIOUS DISEASES
• GONORRHEA
MENTAL STATE/ NEUROLOGICAL DISORDERS

• RESTLESSNESS W/THIRST: Heat
SEXUALITY, FEMALE: GYNECOLOGICAL
• FETUS, RESTLESS: Threatened Abortion, Blood Deficiency
SKIN

• CARBUNCLES
• ERYSIPELAS
• PIMPLES ON BACK/SHOULDER
• SKIN, TOXIC SWELLINGS
URINARY BLADDER
• DYSURIA

Dose

4.5 - 15.0 gm

Common Name

Boehmeria

Warm The Interior And Expel Cold

BA JIAO HUI XIANG   八角茴香   *FRUCTUS ILLICIUS*

Traditional Functions:

1. Dispels Cold from the Lower Jiao
2. Circulates and moves the Qi

Traditional Properties:

Enters: SP, KI

Properties: SP, SW, W

Indications:

ABDOMEN/
GASTROINTESTINAL TOPICS
• ABDOMEN, PAIN OF: Cold
• HERNIA

MUSCULOSKELETAL/
CONNECTIVE TISSUE
• BACK, LOWER PAIN

NUTRITIONAL/METABOLIC
DISORDERS/TOPICS
• BERIBERI

Clinical/Pharmaceutical Studies:

INFECTIOUS DISEASES
• BACTERIAL, ANTI-: Similar To
Penicillin, Streptomycin, Many

Gram Positive
SKIN

• FUNGAL, ANTI-: Stronger Than 1%
Benzoic Acid, Salicylic Acid

Dose

3 - 6 gm

Common Name

Star Anise

Precautions

Watch: Yin Def With Excess Fire

BI BA   華茇   *FRUCTUS PIPERIS LONGI*
(BI BO)   (荜茇)

Traditional Functions:

1. Warms the Middle and disperses Cold
2. Descends rebellious Qi
3. Reduces toothache pain with topical application

Traditional Properties:

Enters: LI, ST,

Properties: SP, H

Indications:

ABDOMEN/
GASTROINTESTINAL TOPICS
• ABDOMEN, PAIN OF: Cold/
Stomach Cold
• ABDOMEN, PAIN OF, HERNIA-
LIKE: Cold
• BORBORYGMUS
BOWEL RELATED DISORDERS
• DIARRHEA
CHEST

• CHEST, PAIN, COLD
HEAD/NECK
• HEADACHE
HEART
• ANGINA PECTORIS: Chest Bi
Strangulating Pain
NOSE
• RHINITIS
ORAL CAVITY
• TOOTHACHE: Topical

STOMACH/DIGESTIVE
DISORDERS
• ACID REGURGITATION
• HICCUPS: Qi Deficiency-Cold
• NAUSEA/VOMITING: Stomach
Cold
• STOMACH COLD: Nausea,
Vomiting, Abdominal Pain
• VOMITING: Qi Deficiency-Cold

Clinical/Pharmaceutical Studies:

INFECTIOUS DISEASES
• ANTIBIOTIC: Staph A., Bac.Subtl./ Cereus, E.Coli
NUTRITIONAL/METABOLIC DISORDERS/TOPICS
• TEMPERATURE, LOWERS: Vasodilator, Cutaneous, Develops
Tolerance
PAIN/NUMBNESS/GENERAL DISCOMFORT
• ANALGESIC: Helps With Deficient Blood Pain By Stimulating Blood Flow
STOMACH/DIGESTIVE DISORDERS
• STOMACHIC
TRAUMA, BITES, POISONINGS
• INSECTICIDE: Destroys Nervous, Muscular Tissue Of Flies

Dose
1.5 - 4.5 gm
Common Name
Long Pepper Fruit

Contraindications
Not: Any Kind Of Fire--True Heat Or Def Yin Heat
Notes
Harsh On Stomach

BI CHENG QIE

蓽澄茄
（荜澄茄）

FRUCTUS LITSEAE

Traditional Functions:
1. Warms the Middle Jiao and descends rebellious Qi
2. Disperses the Cold and controls pain

Traditional Properties:
Enters: SP, ST, KI, UB,

Properties: SP, W

Indications:

ABDOMEN/ GASTROINTESTINAL TOPICS
• ABDOMEN, PAIN OF: Cold
• ABDOMEN, PAIN OF, COLD, AT UMBILICUS: Spleen Deficient
• BORBORYGMUS: Stomach Cold
• HERNIA: Cold
BOWEL RELATED DISORDERS
• DIARRHEA: Stomach Cold
STOMACH/DIGESTIVE DISORDERS
• ANOREXIA
• BELCHING: Stomach Cold
• HICCUPS: Qi Deficiency-Cold/ Stomach Cold
• STOMACH REFLUX
• STOMACH, PAIN: Cold
• VOMITING: Qi Deficiency-Cold/ Stomach Cold
URINARY BLADDER
• URINATION, PAINFUL, DRIBBLING: With Deficiency Cold
• URINATION, TURBID, CHILDHOOD

Clinical/Pharmaceutical Studies:
• MUCOSA, STIMULATION: Topical Or Absorbtion
INFECTIOUS DISEASES
• BACTERIAL, ANTI-: Schistosoma Japonicum
URINARY BLADDER
• URINARY TRACT INFECTIONS: Volatile Oil Prevents

Dose
1.5 - 3.0 gm
Common Name
Cubebs

CAO WU
(TSAO WU)

草烏
（草乌）

RADIX ACONITI KUSNEZOFFII

Traditional Functions:
1. Restores devastated Yang
2. Warms the Kidney Fire and strengthens the Yang
3. Warms the Kidneys and Spleen
4. Expels Cold, warms the channels and relieves pain: less moving than Fu Zi

Traditional Properties:
Enters: SP, HT, KI,

Properties: >SP, H, >TOX

Indications:
ABDOMEN/ GASTROINTESTINAL TOPICS
• ABDOMEN, PAIN OF, HERNIA-
• PARALYSIS, APOPLEXY
MUSCULOSKELETAL/ CONNECTIVE TISSUE
PAIN/NUMBNESS/GENERAL DISCOMFORT
• BI, COLD

Indications:

LIKE: Cold
MENTAL STATE/
NEUROLOGICAL DISORDERS

• ARTHRITIS: For Expelling Cold,
Dampness
• RHEUMATISM

SKIN
• BOILS
• ULCERS, DEEP, EARLY

Clinical/Pharmaceutical Studies:

CANCER/TUMORS/
SWELLINGS/LUMPS
• SWELLINGS: Promotes
Reduction Of
EXTREMITIES
• LEGS, PAIN: Injection
FEVERS
• ANTIPYRETIC
HEAD/NECK
• FACE, PARALYSIS: San
Wu Syrup (He Shou Wu,
Fu Zi, Cao Wu) , 90%
Cure Rate
HEART
• CARDIOTONIC

INFECTIOUS DISEASES
• COMMON COLD:
Injection, But Toxic
MUSCULOSKELETAL/
CONNECTIVE TISSUE
• ARTHRITIS, PAIN:
Injection
• ARTHRITIS,
RHEUMATIC: Injection
• BACK, LOWER PAIN:
Injection
PAIN/NUMBNESS/
GENERAL
DISCOMFORT

• ANALGESIC: 1/5 Of
Morphine, Processed Herb
Did Not Lose Effect
• ANESTHETIC: Herb
With Yang Jin Hua, Dang
Gui, Chuan Xiong As
Decoction, Granule
Infusion Or Injection, 93%
Effective, Cao Wu, Yang
Jin Hua Are Synergistic
With Mutually Cancelling
Side Effects
• ANESTHETIC, LOCAL:
Active Ingredient 2x That

Of Cocaine, Lasts 40-60
Minutes, Tongue Numbing
May Last 4-5 Hours
• ANESTHETIC,
SURFACE: With Tian
Nan Xiang, Ban Xia, Xi
Xin As Tincture
• NEURALGIA: Injection
TRAUMA, BITES,
POISONINGS
• ANTIHISTAMINE
• INFLAMMATORY, ANTI-
: Active Ingredient,
Hesperidin

Dose

6 - 9 gm

Common Name

Wild Aconite

Contraindications

Not: Pregnancy
Not: Def Yin w/False Cold, True Heat

Notes

Extremely Toxic-Prolonged Cooking Necessary With

Gan Cao, Black Beans
Toxic Components Very Soluble In ETOH
Toxic Symptoms: Salivation, Nausea, Vomiting,
Diarrhea, Dizziness, Blurred Vision, Mouth, Tongue,
Extremities Or Whole Body Numbness, Dyspnea,
Spasms Of Extremities, Unconsciousness, Incontinence,
Arrhythmia, Hypotension, Hypothermia
Antidotes: Atropine, Lidocaine, Procainamide,
Propranol, Honey, LU Dou, Xi Jiao

CHUAN JIAO
(HUA SHAN JIAO)

川椒

FRUCTUS
ZANTHOXYLI BUNGEANI

Traditional Functions:

1. Warms the Spleen and Stomach, controls pain, and disperses Cold
2. Expels round worms and relievs their pain

Traditional Properties:

Enters: SP, ST, KI,

Properties: SP, H, TX

Indications:

ABDOMEN/
GASTROINTESTINAL TOPICS
• ABDOMEN, PAIN OF: Ascariasis
(Aux.Herb) /Cold/Spleen Stomach
Cold, Deficient
BOWEL RELATED DISORDERS
• DIARRHEA: Cold Dampness (Add
Warm Interior Herbs, Too) /Spleen
Stomach Cold, Deficient
• DIARRHEA FROM PARASITES
EXTREMITIES
• LEG QI: Cold Dampness
• LEGS, PAIN, SWELLING: Cold

Dampness, Beriberi, Leg Qi
LUNGS
• COUGH, CHRONIC W/DYSPNEA:
To Store Qi, Stop Cough
NUTRITIONAL/METABOLIC
DISORDERS/TOPICS
• BERIBERI: Cold Dampness
SEXUALITY, FEMALE:
GYNECOLOGICAL
• MENSTRUATION, DISORDERS
OF: Warm Chong, Ren
SKIN
• ECZEMA: Cold Dampness

• SKIN, DISORDERS
• SKIN, SORES: Cold Damp
• ULCERS, DAMP, SKIN
SPLEEN
• SPLEEN STOMACH
DEFICIENCY, COLD: Abdominal
Pain, Vomiting, Diarrhea
STOMACH/DIGESTIVE
DISORDERS
• HICCUPS: Qi Deficiency-Cold
• STOMACH, ACHE: Cold Stomach
• VOMITING: Qi Deficiency-Cold

Clinical/Pharmaceutical Studies:

ABDOMEN/ GASTROINTESTINAL TOPICS
- ABDOMEN, PAIN OF: Acu-Pt Inject
- INTESTINES, SPASMS: Reduces Pain Of With Acu-Point/Intramuscular Injection
- PERISTALSIS: Small Doses Increase, Large Doses Inhibits In SI/ST

BLOOD RELATED

DISORDERS/TOPICS
- BLOOD PRESSURE, LOWERS

GALL BLADDER
- GALL BLADDER DISEASES: Reduces Pain Of With Acu-Point/Intramuscular Injection

INFECTIOUS DISEASES
- BACTERIAL, ANTI-: B. Dysenteriae, Staph.Aureus

KIDNEYS
- DIURETIC, MILD: Small Doses

PAIN/NUMBNESS/ GENERAL DISCOMFORT
- ANESTHETIC: Local Action

PARASITES
- PINWORMS: Enemas With
- ROUNDWORMS: 1 Dose With Sesame Oil Stopped Pain In 30 Minutes
- SCHISTOSOMIASIS, COMPLICATIONS OF: Take Powder
- TAPEWORMS, PORK

SEXUALITY, FEMALE; GYNECOLOGICAL
- LACTATION, INHIBITS: w/Brown Sugar, Stopping In 1-2 Days, Postpartum

SKIN
- FUNGAL, ANTI-

Dose
1.5 - 6.0 gm

Common Name
Szechuan Pepper Fruit

Contraindications
Not: Def Yin w/Heat

Precautions
Watch: Pregnancy

CHUAN WU
(WU TOU)

川烏
(川乌)

RADIX ACONITII

Traditional Functions:

1. Retrieves devastated Yang
2. Warms the Kidney fire and strengthens the Yang of the Kidneys and Heart
3. Warms the Kidneys and Spleen
4. Expels Cold, warms and moves the channels, and relieves pain
5. Eliminates Wind Damp, relieves pain

Traditional Properties:

Enters: SP, HT, KI, LV,

Properties: >SP, H, TOX, BIT

Indications:

ABDOMEN/ GASTROINTESTINAL TOPICS
- ABDOMEN, PAIN OF, HERNIA-LIKE: Cold
- ABDOMEN, PAIN OF, SEVERE: Cold
- HERNIA-LIKE CONDITION

CHEST
- CHEST, PAIN, SEVERE: Heart Pain

EXTREMITIES

- LIMBS, NUMB

HEAD/NECK
- HEADACHE
- HEADACHE, MIGRAINE

HEART
- ANGINA PECTORIS: Chest Bi Strangulating Pain

MUSCULOSKELETAL/ CONNECTIVE TISSUE
- ARTHRITIS: For Expelling Cold, Dampness
- ARTHRITIS, RHEUMATIC
- BACK, LOWER PAIN

PAIN/NUMBNESS/GENERAL DISCOMFORT
- ANESTHETIC, LOCAL: Topical, Tincture
- BI, WIND DAMP COLD
- BI, WIND DAMP, CHRONIC: Open Luo, Arrest Pain

Dose
1.5 - 6.0 gm

Common Name
Aconite

Contraindications
Not: Pregnancy/Def Yin w/False Cold True Heat

Notes
Toxic: Prolonged Cooking Helps, More Soluble In Alcohol, 15-60 Gms Toxic, Use Lidocaine, Atropine, Add Gan Jiang + Gan Cao
See Fu Zi
Very Toxic

DING XIANG 丁香

FLOS CARYOPHYLLI

Traditional Functions:

1. Warms the Spleen and Stomach and descends rebellious Qi
2. Warms the Kidneys and supports the Yang

Traditional Properties:

Enters: SP, ST, KI,

Properties: SP, W

Indications:

ABDOMEN/ GASTROINTESTINAL TOPICS
• ABDOMEN, PAIN OF: Stomach Cold
• ABDOMEN, PAIN OF, HERNIA-LIKE: Cold
BOWEL RELATED DISORDERS
• DIARRHEA: Spleen Defienct With Qi Stagnation/Spleen Stomach Cold, Deficient
SEXUALITY, FEMALE:

GYNECOLOGICAL
• LEUKORRHEA, CLEAR: Cold Deficient Womb
• UTERUS, COLD, DEFICIENT
SEXUALITY, MALE: UROLOGICAL TOPICS
• IMPOTENCE: Kidney Yang Deficient
SPLEEN
• SPLEEN KIDNEY DEFICIENCY, COLD

• SPLEEN STOMACH DEFICIENCY, COLD
STOMACH/DIGESTIVE DISORDERS
• ANOREXIA: Spleen Stomach Cold, Deficient
• BELCHING: Stomach Cold
• HICCUPS: Qi Deficiency-Cold/ Stomach Cold
• VOMITING: Qi Deficiency-Cold/ Stomach Cold

Clinical/Pharmaceutical Studies:

ENDOCRINE RELATED DISORDERS
• ADRENALIN ANTAGONIZING ACTION
INFECTIOUS DISEASES
• ANTIBIOTIC: Many, Staph.Aureus, Strep, Pseudomonas, Shigella
• VIRAL, ANTI-: Pr8 Virus, Flu (Dramatic)
MENTAL STATE/ NEUROLOGICAL DISORDERS
• TRANQUILIZING: IP Injection

ORAL CAVITY
• TOOTHACHE: Oil
PARASITES
• ANTIPARASITIC: Round Worms (Oil Better)
• TAPEWORMS, PORK
SEXUALITY, FEMALE: GYNECOLOGICAL
• UTERUS, STIMULATES: Aqueous/ ETOH Extract
SKIN

• FUNGAL, ANTI-: Tinea, etc, Very Good
STOMACH/DIGESTIVE DISORDERS
• ANTIEMETIC
• CARMINATIVE
• STOMACH, INCREASES SPUTUM IN
• STOMACHIC
TRAUMA, BITES, POISONINGS
• INFLAMMATORY, ANTI-

Dose
0.9 - 4.5 gm
Common Name
Clove Flower-Bud

Contraindications
Not: w/Yu Jin
Not: Fevers, Def Yin
Notes
More Superficial, Acute Problems

DOU CHI JIANG 豆豉姜

RAMUS/RADIX LITSEAE CUBEBAE

Traditional Functions:

1. Expels Wind and Dampness, moves the Qi and reduces pain
2. Moves Qi and Blood and controls pain
3. Relieves the pain of External pathogens

Traditional Properties:

Enters: LU, LV,

Properties: SP, ARO, W

Indications:

INFECTIOUS DISEASES
• COMMON COLD: Headaches, Muscle Aches, Chills Of

PAIN/NUMBNESS/GENERAL DISCOMFORT
• BI, WIND DAMP

ABDOMEN PAIN: Cold
STOMACH/DIGESTIVE DISORDERS

Indications:

MUSCULOSKELETAL/
CONNECTIVE TISSUE
• BACK, LOWER PAIN: Wind
Damp Bi

SEXUALITY, FEMALE:
GYNECOLOGICAL
• DYSMENORRHEA: Blood Stasis
• DYSMENORRHEA, LOW

• STOMACH, ACHE
TRAUMA, BITES, POISONINGS
• TRAUMA, BLOOD STASIS

Clinical/Pharmaceutical Studies:

TRAUMA, BITES, POISONINGS   • MOTION SICKNESS

Dose

1.5 - 60.0 gm

Common Name

Aromatic Listsea Root/Stem

FU ZI

附子

RADIX
ACONITI CARMICHAELI
PRAEPARATA

Traditional Functions:

1. Retrieves devastated Yang
2. Warms the Kidney fire and strengthens the Yang of the Kidneys and Heart
3. Warms the Kidneys and Spleen
4. Expels Cold, warms and moves the channels, and relieves pain

Traditional Properties:

Enters: SP, HT, KI,

Properties: SP, SW, H, TX

Indications:

• SHOCK: With Collapse, 18-24 gm
ABDOMEN/
GASTROINTESTINAL TOPICS
• ABDOMEN, PAIN OF: Cold
• ABDOMEN, PAIN OF, HERNIA-
LIKE: Cold
BOWEL RELATED DISORDERS
• DIARRHEA: Spleen Kidney Yang
Deficient
• DIARRHEA W/UNDIGESTED
FOOD PARTICLES: Devastated
Yang, From Severe Diarrhea:Spleen
Kidney Yang Deficient
• DIARRHEA, VIOLENT: Yang
Collapse
• FISTULA, CHRONIC
• STOOLS, LOOSE: Spleen Kidney
Yang Deficient
COLD
• CHILLS: Devastated Yang, From
Severe Vomit
• COLD: Chronic Diseases With
EXTREMITIES
• EXTREMITIES, COLD:
Devastated Yang, From Severe
Adominal Pain:Spleen Kidney Yang
Deficient
• LIMBS, COLD
• LIMBS, CONTRACTURES

FLUID DISORDERS
• ASCITES
• EDEMA: Yang Deficiency
• EDEMA, EXCESS/INSUFFICIENT
URINATION: Kidney Not
Controlling Water
HEAD/NECK
• HEADACHE, SEVERE
INTERMITTENT
HEART
• ANGINA PECTORIS: Chest Bi
Strangulating Pain
LIVER
• JAUNDICE, YIN
MENTAL STATE/
NEUROLOGICAL DISORDERS
• CONVULSIONS, INFANTILE
CHRONIC
• HEMIPLEGIA
MUSCULOSKELETAL/
CONNECTIVE TISSUE
• ARTHRITIS: For Expelling Cold,
Dampness
• ARTHRITIS, PAIN: Cold
• JOINTS, PAIN: Wind Cold Damp
• TENDONS, PAIN: Wind
ORAL CAVITY
• COLD SORES
PAIN/NUMBNESS/GENERAL

DISCOMFORT
• BI, COLD IN ORGANS
• BI, WIND DAMP COLD
SEXUALITY, EITHER SEX
• INFERTILITY: Uterine Cold Palace
SEXUALITY, FEMALE:
GYNECOLOGICAL
• LEUKORRHEA: Kidney Spleen
Yang Deficiency
SEXUALITY, MALE:
UROLOGICAL TOPICS
• IMPOTENCE: Weak Kidney Fire
• SPERMATORRHEA: Weak Kidney
Fire
SKIN
• SWEATING
• SWEATING, PROFUSE: With
Yang Fleeing
STOMACH/DIGESTIVE
DISORDERS
• GASTRALGIA: Cold
• VOMITING, CLEAR FLUIDS:
Spleen Kidney Yang Deficient
YANG RELATED DISORDERS/
TOPICS
• YANG DEPLETION
YIN RELATED DISORDERS/
TOPICS
• YIN SEPARATING FROM YANG

Clinical/Pharmaceutical Studies:

BLOOD RELATED
DISORDERS/TOPICS
• BLOOD PRESSURE,
LOWERS: Sharp,

• THROMBOANGIITIS
OBLITERANS: Fu Zi
Wen Jing Tang (Fu Zi, Dan
Shen, Huang Qi, Gan Cao,

• CARDIOTONIC:
Stimulates Central Vagus
Nerve
• CONGESTIVE HEART

Breathing Rate
NUTRITIONAL/
METABOLIC
DISORDERS/TOPICS

Clinical/Pharmaceutical Studies:

Transient, *For Renal Hypertension--Fu Zi, Rou Gui

BOWEL RELATED DISORDERS
• DIARRHEA, CHRONIC INFANTILE: Add To Spleen Qi And Astringent Herbs, e.g. Treated Fu Zi, Rou Dou Kou, Lian Zi, Huang Qin, Fu Long Gan, Flower Bud Of Syzygium Aromaticum

CIRCULATION DISORDERS

Hai Ma, Tao Ren, Xi Xin, Dang Gui, Rou Gui, Chi Shao, Da Huang, Jin Yin Hua) Oral With Bi Ba Ointment Topically, 87% Effective
• VASODILATOR

ENDOCRINE RELATED DISORDERS
• ENDOCRINE: Stimulates Adrenals, Pituitary

HEART
• BRADYCARDIA W/ SLIGHT LOWERING BLOOD PRESSURE

FAILURE
• CORONARY ARTERIES, DILATES: Vasodilator, Both Legs, Coronary Vessels
• HEART FAILURE: Injection/SI Ni San/Ren Shen Fu Zi Tang

HEMORRHAGIC DISORDERS
• HEMORRHAGE, ACUTE: Fu Zi, Rou Gui, Ren Shen, Gan Jiang, Gan Cao

LUNGS
• LUNGS: Lowers

• TEMPERATURE, LOWERS: In Both Febrile/ Normal

PAIN/NUMBNESS/ GENERAL DISCOMFORT
• ANALGESIC: Enhanced By Scopolamine, Stronger But Shorter Than Morphine

TRAUMA, BITES, POISONINGS
• INFLAMMATORY, ANTI- : Arthritis In Decoction

Dose

6 - 9 gm

Common Name

Szechuan Aconite Prep Rt.

Contraindications

Not: Pregnancy/Def Yin w/False Cold True Heat

Notes

Toxic: Prolonged Cooking Helps, More Soluble In Alcohol, 15-60 Gms Toxic, Use Lidocaine, Atropine,

Add Gan Jiang + Gan Cao

To Reinforce Tonics: 1.5-6 g

Overdose/Faulty Processed: Possible Burning Mouth, Salivation, Nausea, Numbness Of Extremities/Whole Body, Dizziness, Blurred Vision, Dyspnea, Pallor, Cold, Clammy Skin, Possible Death

Antidote: 1-2% Tannic Acid, If Necessary, Emetics, Activated Charcoal, IV Glucose-Saline, Use Stimulants, Keep Warm

---

GAN JIANG   干姜   RHIZOMA ZINGIBERIS OFFICINALIS

Traditional Functions:

1. Warms the Spleen and Stomach and dispels Cold
2. Prevents the Yang from collapsing and expels interior Cold
3. Warms the Lungs and resolves Cold phlegm
4. Warms the channels and stops deficiency Cold bleeding

Traditional Properties:

Enters: LU, SP, ST, HT, KI,

Properties: SP, H

Indications:

• SHOCK: Cold Limbs, Abdomen

ABDOMEN/ GASTROINTESTINAL TOPICS
• ABDOMEN, COLD, PAIN: Cold, Deficiency
• ABDOMEN, PAIN OF, HERNIA-LIKE: Cold

BOWEL RELATED DISORDERS
• BOWEL MOVEMENT, LOOSE
• CONSTIPATION: Cold Accumulation
• DIARRHEA: Spleen Kidney Yang Deficient

CHEST
• CHEST, COLD, PAINFUL: Cold, Deficiency

EXTREMITIES
• EXTREMITIES, COLD

FLUID DISORDERS
• EDEMA: Yang Deficiency

HEAD/NECK
• PALLOR

LIVER
• JAUNDICE, YIN

LUNGS
• BRONCHITIS, CHRONIC: Thin, White, Foamy Sputum
• COUGH: Cold Phlegm/Cold
• LUNGS, DYSPNEA: Cold Phlegm

MUSCULOSKELETAL/ CONNECTIVE TISSUE
• ARTHRITIS, PAIN: Cold, Damp
• JOINTS, PAIN: Wind Cold Damp Bi

PHLEGM
• SPUTUM, THIN, WATERY WHITE

SEXUALITY, FEMALE: GYNECOLOGICAL
• UTERINE BLEEDING, CHRONIC: Cold, Deficient, Only

SPLEEN
• SPLEEN STOMACH, COLD: Warming

STOMACH/DIGESTIVE DISORDERS
• APPETITE, POOR
• HICCUPS: Qi Deficiency-Cold
• NAUSEA/VOMITING
• VOMITING: Qi Deficiency-Cold

YANG RELATED DISORDERS/ TOPICS
• YANG DEFICIENCY W/COLD LIMBS, WEAK PULSE

Clinical/Pharmaceutical Studies:

**BLOOD RELATED DISORDERS/
TOPICS**
• BLOOD PRESSURE, RAISES: By

Stimulating Vasomotor Center/
Sympathetic Nervous System
STOMACH/DIGESTIVE

DISORDERS
• STOMACHIC
• VOMITING: Antiemetic

Dose

1.5 - 9.0 gm

Not: w/Hot Blood

Common Name

Dried Ginger Rhizome

Precautions

Watch: Pregnancy

Notes

Drying

Contraindications

Not: Def Yin w/Heat

Large Doses: 12-15 gm

GAO LIANG JIANG   高良姜   RHIZOMA ALPINIAE OFFICINARI

Traditional Functions:

1. Warms the Spleen and Stomach and controls pain

Traditional Properties:

Enters: SP, ST,

Properties: SP, W

Indications:

**ABDOMEN/
GASTROINTESTINAL TOPICS**
• ABDOMEN, MASS: Cold
• ABDOMEN, PAIN OF, UPPER
STOMACH: Cold
• ENTERITIS, CHRONIC
BOWEL RELATED DISORDERS
• DIARRHEA: Spleen Cold/Spleen

Kidney Yang Deficient
HEART
• ANGINA PECTORIS: Chest Bi
Strangulating Pain
INFECTIOUS DISEASES
• MALARIA
**STOMACH/DIGESTIVE
DISORDERS**

• DYSPEPSIA
• EPIGASTRIC PAIN: Cold
• HICCUPS: Qi Deficiency-Cold
• VOMITING: Qi Deficiency-Cold/
Spleen Cold
TRAUMA, BITES, POISONINGS
• HANGOVER W/NAUSEA/
VOMITING

Clinical/Pharmaceutical Studies:

INFECTIOUS DISEASES
• ANTIBIOTIC: Anthrax, Staph,
Strep (Hemolytic) , B.Antracis, C.
Diphtheriae, Pseudodiphthericum
Pneumococcus
MUSCULOSKELETAL/

CONNECTIVE TISSUE
• MUSCLES, SMOOTH
STIMULATES: At Low Doses
**PAIN/NUMBNESS/GENERAL
DISCOMFORT**
• ANALGESIC: Greater Than Dried

Ginger
**STOMACH/DIGESTIVE
DISORDERS**
• STOMACHIC: Greater Than Dried
Ginger

Dose

2.4 - 6.0 gm

Common Name

Lesser Galangal Rhizome

Contraindications

Not: Def Yin w/Heat

HU JIAO   胡椒   FRUCTUS PIPERIS NIGRI

Traditional Functions:

1. Warms the Middle Jiao and disperses Cold
2. Strengthens the Stomach and increases appetite

Traditional Properties:

Enters: LI, ST,

Properties: SP, H

Indications:

ABDOMEN/
GASTROINTESTINAL TOPICS
• ABDOMEN, PAIN OF: Cold/
Stomach Cold, Yin Cold
BOWEL RELATED DISORDERS
• DIARRHEA: Stomach Cold

• DYSENTERY
INFECTIOUS DISEASES
• CHOLERA
PHLEGM
• PHLEGM, COLD
STOMACH/DIGESTIVE

DISORDERS
• FOOD ACCUMULATION
• FOOD POISONING
• STOMACH, PROBLEMS: Cold
• VOMITING: Stomach Cold

Clinical/Pharmaceutical Studies:

BOWEL RELATED DISORDERS
• DIARRHEA, CHRONIC, NON-
INFECTIOUS: With Sugar, Orally/
Plaster Of Herb On Navel/Injection
Into Acu-Points
CANCER/TUMORS/SWELLINGS/
LUMPS
• CANCER, PAIN OF: Give Large
Dose
• MALIGNANCIES, PAIN OF: Give

Large Dose
INFECTIOUS DISEASES
• MALARIA: Weak
KIDNEYS
• NEPHRITIS: Placed In Eggs, Then
Steamed, Given Daily
MENTAL STATE/
NEUROLOGICAL DISORDERS
• CONVULSIONS: Similar To

Dilantin, But Slower
• TRANQUILIZING: Significant,
Synergistic With Thiopental
SKIN
• SKIN, STIMULATES: Topical
STOMACH/DIGESTIVE
DISORDERS
• CARMINATIVE
• STOMACHIC: Small Doses

Dose

0.9 - 4.5 gm

Common Name

Black Pepper Fruit

Contraindications

Not: Def Yin w/Heat

ROU GUI

肉桂

CORTEX
CINNAMOMI CASSIAE

Traditional Functions:

1. Warms the Kidneys and strengthens the Yang
2. Warms the Spleen and disperses Cold
3. Dispels cold from the channels, relieves pain and promotes menstruation
4. Leads the Fire back to the Ming Men:Waning Fire of the gate of vitality
5. Generates Qi and Blood

Traditional Properties:

Enters: SP, KI, UB, LV,

Properties: SP, SW, H

Indications:

ABDOMEN/
GASTROINTESTINAL
TOPICS
• ABDOMEN, PAIN OF:
Spleen Stomach Cold,
With Vomiting, Diarrhea
• ABDOMEN, PAIN OF,
HERNIA-LIKE: Cold
• HERNIA: Cold
• HERNIA,
PROTUBERANCE
BLOOD RELATED
DISORDERS/TOPICS
• BLOOD, QI
DEFICIENCY:
Commonly Added To
Formulas, Stimulates
Blood Circulation, Qi Of
Stomach, e.g.Shi Quan Da
Bu Tang/Bao Yuan Tang
• BLOOD, QI
DEFICIENCY, CHRONIC:
Auxillary Herb

SWELLINGS/LUMPS
• TUMORS: Blood Stasis,
Herbs Used Other Than
Vitalize Blood
EXTREMITIES
• LEGS, COLD W/UPPER
BODY HEAT
• LEGS, COLD, WEAK:
Kidney Yang Deficient
FEVERS
• FEVER, UPPER, COLD
IN LOWER
FLUID DISORDERS
• EDEMA: Yang
Deficiency
HEAT
• HEAT ABOVE, COLD
BELOW
KIDNEYS
• KIDNEY YANG
DEFICIENCY
• LIFE GATE FIRE,
INSUFFICIENCY OF

MUSCULOSKELETAL/
CONNECTIVE TISSUE
• BACK, LOWER PAIN:
Kidney Yang Deficient
• BACK, LOWER PAIN W/
UPPER BODY HEAT
• KNEES, SORE
ORAL CAVITY
• MOUTH, DRY W/
LOWER BODY COLD
• THROAT, SORE,
LOWER BODY COLD
• TOOTHACHE, WORSE
AT NIGHT WITH
LOWER BODY COLD
SEXUALITY, FEMALE:
GYNECOLOGICAL
• AMENORRHEA: Blood
Stasis, In Addition To
Vitalize Blood Herbs/Cold
Blood
• DYSMENORRHEA:
Cold Blood

ABDOMINAL PAIN:
Blood Stasis
SEXUALITY, MALE:
UROLOGICAL TOPICS
• IMPOTENCE: Kidney
Yang Deficient
• SPERMATORRHEA:
Kidney Yang Deficient
SKIN
• ABSCESS, CONCAVE,
CLEAR FLUID: Yin
• ABSCESS, YIN,
INTERNAL SINKING OF
• SKIN, SORES,
SWOLLEN, TOXIC:
Helps Healing, Deficiency
• SWEATING, SEVERE,
OIL-LIKE: Floating Yang
• ULCERS, YIN
STOMACH/DIGESTIVE
DISORDERS
• EPIGASTRIC PAIN:
Spleen Stomach Cold

Indications:

BOWEL RELATED DISORDERS
- DIARRHEA: Spleen Kidney Yang Deficient/ Spleen Stomach Cold
- DIARRHEA W/UPPER BODY HEAT
CANCER/TUMORS/

LUNGS
- ASTHMA: Kidney Unable To Grasp Qi
- COUGH, CHRONIC W/ DYSPNEA: To Store Qi, Stop Cough
- WHEEZING: Floating Yang

- INFERTILITY, FEMALE: Uterine Cold Palace
- LEUKORRHEA: Kidney Spleen Yang Deficiency
- MENSTRUATION, DISORDERS OF: Warm Chong, Ren
- POSTPARTUM,

YANG RELATED DISORDERS/TOPICS
- YANG FLOATING FROM DEFICIENCY
YIN RELATED DISORDERS/TOPICS
- YIN/YANG SEPARATION

Clinical/Pharmaceutical Studies:

ABDOMEN/ GASTROINTESTINAL TOPICS
- ABDOMEN, PAIN OF: With Flower Buds Of Syzygium Aromaticum, Each 30 g Ground, 0.6-1.5 g Dose, Can Be Applied To Umbilicus As Plaster
- GASTROINTESTINAL GAS
- GASTROINTESTINAL SPASMS
BLOOD RELATED DISORDERS/ TOPICS
- BLOOD PRESSURE, LOWERS: With Fu Zi
BOWEL RELATED DISORDERS
- COLIC: Oral, 1.0-4.5 g, Topical, Too
- DIARRHEA: With Flower Buds Of Syzygium Aromaticum, Each 30 g Ground, 0.6-1.5 g Dose, Can Be Applied To Umbilicus As Plaster

- FLATULENCE: Oral, 1.0-4.5 g, Topical, Too
CIRCULATION DISORDERS
- HYPERTENSION, ADRENAL
FEVERS
- ANTIPYRETIC
HEART
- HEART, INCREASES CORONARY BLOOD FLOW
INFECTIOUS DISEASES
- ANTIBIOTIC: Strong:Many Gram+
LUNGS
- ASTHMA: UB13 Injection Of Alcohol Extract, 0.15-0.3 ml With 2% Procaine To Make 2ml
MENTAL STATE/ NEUROLOGICAL DISORDERS
- CONVULSIONS: Able To Delay Onset

- SEDATIVE: Reduces Effect Of Strychnine, Amphetamines
PAIN/NUMBNESS/GENERAL DISCOMFORT
- ANALGESIC
PARASITES
- SCHISTOSOMA: Prevents Infestation, Use With Bing Lang, A Wei To Be Effective
SKIN
- FUNGAL, ANTI-: ETOH/Ether Extract, Many Pathogenic
STOMACH/DIGESTIVE DISORDERS
- STOMACH, ACHE: Oral, 1.0-4.5 g, Topical, Too
TRAUMA, BITES, POISONINGS
- RADIATION, PROTECTION: Helps Increase Leukocytes, Platelets

Dose
0.9 - 4.5 gm

Common Name
Saigon Cinnamon Inner Brk

Contraindications
Not: Pregnancy

Notes
Toxic In Large Overdoses, 36 g, Dizziness, Blurred Vision, Cough, Thirst

---

ROU GUI PI   肉桂皮   CORTEX CINNAMONI

Traditional Functions:

1. Warms the Kidneys and strengthens the Yang
2. Warms the Spleen and disperses Cold
3. Dispels Cold from the channels, relieves pain and promotes menstruation
4. Vitalizes the Bood

Traditional Properties:

Enters: SP, KI, LV,

Properties: SP, SW, H

Indications:

ABDOMEN/ GASTROINTESTINAL TOPICS
- ABDOMEN, PAIN OF
- HERNIA, COLD
- WAIST, PAIN: Cold
BLOOD RELATED DISORDERS/ TOPICS
- ANEMIA
BOWEL RELATED DISORDERS
- DIARRHEA
EXTREMITIES

- LEGS, COLD
FEVERS
- FEVER, UPPER, COLD IN LOWER
KIDNEYS
- KIDNEY YANG DEFICIENCY
MUSCULOSKELETAL/ CONNECTIVE TISSUE
- ARTHRITIS, PAIN
- BACK, LOWER PAIN

- KNEES, SORE: Cold
SEXUALITY, FEMALE: GYNECOLOGICAL
- AMENORRHEA
- LOCHIA
SKIN
- ABSCESS, WANDERING
YIN RELATED DISORDERS/ TOPICS
- YIN/YANG SEPARATION

Clinical/Pharmaceutical Studies:

ABDOMEN/
GASTROINTESTINAL TOPICS
• GASTROINTESTINAL PAIN,
  ELIMINATES
CIRCULATION DISORDERS
• BLOOD VESSELS, DILATES:
  Promotes Circulation, Thus Leading
  Herbs
• HYPERTENSION, ADRENAL
FEVERS

• ANTIPYRETIC: Mild
INFECTIOUS DISEASES
• ANTIBIOTIC: Strong:Gram+
LUNGS
• ASTHMA: UB13 Injection
MENTAL STATE/
NEUROLOGICAL DISORDERS
• SEDATIVE: Reduces Effect Of
  Strychnine, Amphetamines

PAIN/NUMBNESS/GENERAL
DISCOMFORT
• ANALGESIC
SKIN
• FUNGAL, ANTI-
STOMACH/DIGESTIVE
DISORDERS
• DIGESTION, ENHANCES
• GAS, DIGESTIVE, ELIMINATES

Dose
0.9 - 3.0 gm

Common Name
Saigon Cinnamon

WU ZHU YU

吴茱萸
（吳茱萸）

FRUCTUS
EVODIAE RUTAECARPAE

Traditional Functions:

1. Dispels Cold and relieves pain
2. Pacifies the Liver and directs rebellious Qi downward
3. Stops vomiting
4. Warms the Spleen, stops diarrhea and expels Cold Dampness
5. Expels pinworms

Traditional Properties:

Enters: SP, ST, KI, LV,

Properties: SP, BIT, H, TX

Indications:

ABDOMEN/
GASTROINTESTINAL
TOPICS
• ABDOMEN, PAIN OF:
  Cold
• ABDOMEN, PAIN OF,
  HERNIA-LIKE: Cold
• FLANK PAIN: Liver
  Stomach Disharmony
• HERNIA, INGUINAL
  DROPPING TO
  SCROTUM
• HERNIA-LIKE
  CONDITION: Cold, Liver
  Channel, Yin
BOWEL RELATED
DISORDERS
• DIARRHEA: Cold
  Dampness (Add Warm
  Interior Herbs, Too) /
  Spleen Kidney Yang
  Deficient/Stomach Cold
CHEST
• CHEST, PAIN: Cold

EXTREMITIES
• LEG QI: Cold Damp
• LEGS, EDEMA
• LEGS, SWOLLEN,
  PAINFUL (BERIBERI,
  LEG QI) : Cold Dampness
FLUID DISORDERS
• EDEMA
HEAD/NECK
• HEADACHE: Liver
  Stomach Phlegm Disorder,
  Jue Yin Stage
LIVER
• LIVER ATTACKING
  STOMACH
MUSCULOSKELETAL/
CONNECTIVE TISSUE
• ARTHRITIS, PAIN:
  Blood Stasis
NUTRITIONAL/
METABOLIC
DISORDERS/TOPICS
• BERIBERI

ORAL CAVITY
• DROOLING: Liver
  Stomach Phlegm Disorder
• MOUTH, ULCERS:
  Topical
• TASTE, DECREASING:
  Liver Stomach Phlegm
  Disorder
PAIN/NUMBNESS/
GENERAL
DISCOMFORT
• NUMBNESS, PAIN:
  Blood Bi
PARASITES
• HOOKWORMS
• PINWORMS
SEXUALITY, FEMALE:
GYNECOLOGICAL
• MENSTRUATION,
  CRAMPS OF: Cold
  (Delayed)
• MENSTRUATION,
  DISORDERS OF:

Constrict Uterus, Stimulate
Chong/Warm Chong, Ren
SKIN
• ECZEMA: Cold
  Dampness
• SKIN, SORES: Cold
  Damp
SPLEEN
• SPLEEN KIDNEY
  DEFICIENCY, COLD
STOMACH/DIGESTIVE
DISORDERS
• ACID REGURGITATION
• EPIGASTRIC PAIN,
  NAUSEA: Liver Stomach
  Phlegm Disorder
• HICCUPS
• REGURGITATION,
  ACIDIC: Liver Stomach
  Disharmony
• VOMITING: Cold
  Stomach/Qi Deficiency--
  Dampness

Clinical/Pharmaceutical Studies:

BOWEL RELATED
DISORDERS
• DIARRHEA, CHRONIC:
  Cold, Deficient/Morning,
  SI Shen Pill (Wu Zhu Yu,
  Bu Gu Zhi, Wu Wei Zi,

Strongly Inhibits,
Pseudomonas, Staph.
Aureus
• VIRAL, ANTI-
MENTAL STATE/
NEUROLOGICAL

Response In 1 Day
PAIN/NUMBNESS/
GENERAL
DISCOMFORT
• ANALGESIC: Similar To
  Amniopyrine Strength,

Black, Grind To Fine
Powder, Make 1:10
Ointment By Mixing With
Vaseline
• ECZEMA, CHILDHOOD
• ECZEMA, EARLY/

Clinical/Pharmaceutical Studies:

Rou Dou Ko)
- IRRITABLE BOWEL SYNDROME: w/Vinegar, Plaster On Navel

CIRCULATION DISORDERS
- HYPERTENSION: Vinegar Plaster On Soles Of Feet, Lowers In 12-24 Hours, *Alcohol Extract/ Granule Infusion, Equivalent 8 g Of Crude Drug 1x/Day For 1 Month, Orally, 77% Effective, * Apply Powder Mixed With Wax To Soles Of Feet At Bedtime

HEAD/NECK
- MIGRAINE: Wu Zhu Yu Tang (Herb, Ren Shen, Da Zao, Sheng Jiang) , Eye Pain, Headache Disappeared, No Recurrence After 4 Months

INFECTIOUS DISEASES
- ANTIBIOTIC: Cholera,

DISORDERS
- CNS, POSSIBLE HALLUCINATIONS: 5-Methoxy-N-Dimethyl-Tryptamine, Rutamine, At High Dose

NUTRITIONAL/ METABOLIC DISORDERS/TOPICS
- BODY TEMPERATURE, RAISES
- TEMPERATURE, BODY: Raises Slightly

ORAL CAVITY
- CANDIDIASIS, ORAL: Apply Powder Mixed With Wax To Soles Of Feet At Bedtime, Good Results
- MOUTH, ULCERS CHILDREN: Bilateral Powder K1, Good Response In 1 Day
- ULCERS, ORAL, IN CHILDREN: Bilateral Powder K1, Good

Similar To Antipyrine
PARASITES
- ANTIPARASITIC: Ascarisis, Liver Flukes, Tapeworms, Decoction/ Alcohol Extract

SEXUALITY, FEMALE: GYNECOLOGICAL
- UTERINE BLEEDING: Decoction/Powder, 6-12 g, Orally In 3 Doses
- UTERUS, DYSTONIA: Decoction/Powder, 6-12 g, Orally In 3 Doses
- UTERUS, STIMULATES: Strong, From Water Soluble Portion

SKIN
- ECZEMA: Grind Herb With Hai Piao Xiao, Sulfur To Fine Powder, 95% Effective, *Burn Wu Zhu Yu With Equal Amounts Sulfur, Use Alcohol In Mix, Stir Continuously Until

SUBACUTE
- FUNGAL, ANTI-: Some
- NEURODERMATITIS: Apply Paste Of Herb Topically Then Moxabustion For 10 Minutes, 4-6 Treatments, 50% Showed Marked Improvement
- SKIN, PUSTULOSIS: Burn Wu Zhu Yu With Equal Amounts Sulfur, Use Alcohol In Mix, Stir Continuously Until Black, Grind To Fine Powder, Make 1:10 Ointment By Mixing With Vaseline, Apply To Pustules

STOMACH/DIGESTIVE DISORDERS
- ANTIEMETIC: Orally With Ginger, Especially Strong, Probably As A Powder
- STOMACHIC

Dose
1.5 - 9.0 gm

Common Name
Evodia Fruit

Contraindications
Not: Def Yin w/Heat

Notes
Large Doses Leads To Visual Hallucinations

XIAO HUI XIANG
(HUI XIANG)

小茴香

FRUCTUS FOENICULI VULGARIS

Traditional Functions:

1. Moves the Qi and harmonizes the Stomach
2. Warms the Spleen and Stomach and relieves pain

Traditional Properties:

Enters: SP, ST, KI, LV,

Properties: SP, W

Indications:

ABDOMEN/ GASTROINTESTINAL TOPICS
- ABDOMEN, PAIN OF: Cold
- ABDOMEN, PAIN OF, BELOW UMBILICUS.
- ABDOMEN, PAIN OF, HERNIA-LIKE: Cold

BOWEL RELATED DISORDERS

- DIARRHEA

QI RELATED DISORDERS/ TOPICS
- QI DISTENTION

SEXUALITY, FEMALE: GYNECOLOGICAL
- MENSTRUATION, DISORDERS OF: Warm Chong, Ren

SEXUALITY, MALE: UROLOGICAL TOPICS
- TESTICLES, PAIN

STOMACH/DIGESTIVE DISORDERS
- ANOREXIA: Stomach Cold
- INDIGESTION: Stomach Cold
- VOMITING: Stomach Cold

Clinical/Pharmaceutical Studies:

ABDOMEN/ GASTROINTESTINAL TOPICS
- ABDOMEN, PAIN OF
- HERNIA, INCARCERATED: Oral Preparations, Lie With Knees Bent, Symptoms Reduced In 30 Min, If None In 1.5 Hrs–Surgery, Long

- FLATULENCE: w/Mu Xiang

CANCER/TUMORS/SWELLINGS/ LUMPS
- CANCER PATIENTS: Chemotherapy/Radiation Side Effects--Take In Enteric Coated Caps

INFECTIOUS DISEASES

SEXUALITY, MALE: UROLOGICAL TOPICS
- HYDROCELE OF TUNICA VAGINALIS: With Salt, Other Herbs In Wine

SKIN
- STIMULANT, LOCAL OF SKIN

Clinical/Pharmaceutical Studies:

Incarcerations Less Effective
- INTESTINES, SPASMS
- PERISTALSIS, INCREASES: Oil
BOWEL RELATED DISORDERS

- ANTIBIOTIC: TB, Synergistic w/
  Streptomycin
LUNGS
- EXPECTORANT

**STOMACH/DIGESTIVE
DISORDERS**
- STOMACHIC: Increases Secretions,
  Appetite

Dose

2.4 - 9.0 gm

Common Name

Fennel Fruit

Precautions

Watch: Def Yin w/Heat

Notes

Stir Bake For Testicular/Urinary Bladder Pain
With Salt To Descend Qi
With Wine To Ascend Qi

Regulate The Qi

CHEN PI
(JU PI/ZHU PI)

陳皮
（陈皮）

PERICARPIUM
CITRI RETICULATAE

Traditional Functions:

1. Regulates the Qi and strengthens the Spleen
2. Dries Dampness and resolves Phlegm
3. Reverses the upward flow of Qi and stops vomiting
4. Helps prevent stagnation when used with tonifying herbs

Traditional Properties:

Enters: LU, SP, ST,

Properties: SP, BIT, W,

Indications:

**ABDOMEN/
GASTROINTESTINAL TOPICS**
• ABDOMEN, DISTENTION OF:
Damp Heat
• ABDOMEN, DISTENTION OF/
FULLNESS: Spleen Stomach Qi
Stagnation
• ABDOMEN, PAIN OF: Food
Stagnation
• GASTROINTESTINAL
DISTENTION
BOWEL RELATED DISORDERS
• DIARRHEA: Cold Dampness (Add
Warm Interior Herbs, Too) /Food
Stagnation, Most Herbs, Cooked,
Charred For This Purpose/Spleen
Defienct With Qi Stagnation
CHEST
• CHEST, DISTENTION

• CHEST, FULLNESS
ENERGETIC STATE
• HERBS, TONIFYING: Reduces
Stagnation From
LIVER
• LIVER QI CONGESTION W/
SUBCOSTAL PAIN
LUNGS
• COUGH: Cold Phlegm
• COUGH, CHEST/DIAPHRAGM
CONSTRICTION, COPIOUS
SPUTUM: Phlegm Damp
• LUNGS, DYSPNEA: Cold Phlegm
**SEXUALITY, FEMALE:
GYNECOLOGICAL**
• BREASTS, SWOLLEN, PAINFUL,
ABSCESS
• MORNING SICKNESS:

Gestational Foul Obstruction--Cold
SPLEEN
• SPLEEN STOMACH,
CONGESTION
• SPLEEN STOMACH, DAMPNESS
**STOMACH/DIGESTIVE
DISORDERS**
• ANOREXIA: Spleen Stomach Qi
Stagnation
• EPIGASTRIC DISTENTION/
FULLNESS: Spleen Stomach Qi
Stagnation
• HICCUPS: Qi Deficiency--
Dampness
• INDIGESTION
• NAUSEA/VOMITING: Any Type
• VOMITING: Qi Deficiency--
Dampness

Clinical/Pharmaceutical Studies:

**ABDOMEN/
GASTROINTESTINAL
TOPICS**
• ABDOMEN,
DISTENTION OF
• ABDOMEN,
DISTENTION OF,
SEVERE: With Cang Zhu,
Hou PO As In Ping Wei
San
• INTESTINES,
REGULATES
**BLOOD RELATED
DISORDERS/TOPICS**
• BLOOD CLOTTING
TIME, SHORTENS
• BLOOD PRESSURE,
RAISES

Hespiridin Reduces
Capillary Fragility,
Unreliable Though
FLUID DISORDERS
• ANTIDIURETIC
GALL BLADDER
• GALL BLADDER, BILE
SECRETION,
INCREASES: Enhanced
With Vit C, K
HEART
• CORONARY ARTERIES,
DILATES
• HEART DISEASE:
Hespiridin Reduces
Capillary Fragility,
Unreliable Though
• HEART, INCREASES

• ANTIASTHMATIC:
Alcohol Extract
• ANTITUSSIVE: Most
Formulas Have Herb In
Them As Syrup/Tincture
• ASTHMA: May Add
With Snake Bile
• BRONCHITIS: Combine
With Snake Bile
• EXPECTORANT:
Volatile Oil
• WHOOPING COUGH: In
Young Children, With
Snake Bile As Powder, 4-
16 Days
**MUSCULOSKELETAL/
CONNECTIVE TISSUE**
• ARTHRITIS,

**SEXUALITY, MALE:
UROLOGICAL TOPICS**
• SPERMICIDAL ACTION:
Hesperidin
SKIN
• BIRTHMARKS:
Hespiridin Reduces
Capillary Fragility,
Unreliable Though
• SUNLIGHT: Protects
From Uv
• ULCERS: Injection, Add
Vit C, K, To Make Oral
Intake Effective
**STOMACH/DIGESTIVE
DISORDERS**
• ANOREXIA
• ANOREXIA, LOOSE/

Clinical/Pharmaceutical Studies:

- CHOLESTEROL, DECREASES
BOWEL RELATED DISORDERS
- FLATULENCE: May Add With Snake Bile
CHEST
- CHEST, DISCOMFORT W/THICK VISCOUS SPUTUM: Dampness, Use With Ban Xia Or Liu Jun Zi Tang
- CHEST, TIGHTNESS
EYES
- DIABETIC RETINITIS: Hespiridin Reduces Capillary Fragility, Unreliable Though
- RETINAL HEMORRHAGE: From Hypertension, Arteriosclerosis--

OUTPUT: Increases Cardiac Output Not Heart Rate-Small Doses
- HEART, STIMULATES: Decoction, Alcohol Extract, 25-50% Of Theophylline
HEMORRHAGIC DISORDERS
- HEMOPHILIA: Hespiridin Reduces Capillary Fragility, Unreliable Though
- HEMOSTATIC
IMMUNE SYSTEM RELATED DISORDERS/TOPICS
- ALLERGIC, ANTI-
INFECTIOUS DISEASES
- BACTERIAL, ANTI-: Staph
- RHEUMATIC FEVER
LUNGS

RHEUMATOID
- MUSCLES, SMOOTH, INHIBITS
NUTRITIONAL/ METABOLIC DISORDERS/TOPICS
- BERIBERI: Vit B1
ORAL CAVITY
- TEETH, DENTAL CARIES: Decreases Incidence Of
SEXUALITY, FEMALE: GYNECOLOGICAL
- MASTITIS, ACUTE, NON-PURULENT: Decoction With Gan Cao, 2-3 Days, Good
- MENORRHAGIA: Hespiridin Reduces Capillary Fragility, Unreliable Though
- UTERUS, RELAXES

MUSHY STOOL: Jian Pi Wan
- ANTIEMETIC
- CARMINATIVE
- DIGESTION, ENHANCES
- DYSPEPSIA
- HICCUPS: With Zhu Ru, Dang Shen
- NAUSEA
- STOMACHIC: Improves Digestion, Passes Gas
TRAUMA, BITES, POISONINGS
- FROSTBITE: Oral Hesperidin For 7 Days Before Exposure, Reduced Effects
- INFLAMMATORY, ANTI-: (Hesperidin)
- TRAUMA, BY COLD: Reduces

Dose
1.5 - 9.0 gm

Common Name
Tangerine Peel

Precautions
Watch: Heat Signs--Red Tongue, Blood In Sputum, Hot Phlegm, Dry Cough

Notes
Longer Stored, Better

CHEN XIANG

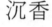
沉香

LIGNUM AQUILARIAE

Traditional Functions:

1. Moves the Qi and relieves pain
2. Descends rebellious Qi: either Lung or Stomach Qi
3. Calms asthma by warming and strengthening the Kidneys in grasping the Qi

Traditional Properties:

Enters: SP, ST, KI,

Properties: SP, BIT, W,

Indications:

ABDOMEN/ GASTROINTESTINAL TOPICS
- ABDOMEN, DISTENTION OF/PAIN: Deficient Cold/Blood Stagnation
- ABDOMEN, PAIN OF, HERNIA-LIKE: Cold
- ABDOMEN, PAIN OF/ PRESSURE/ DISTENTION: Qi Stagnation
- BORBORYGMUS
- WAIST, WEAK: Cold

BLOOD RELATED DISORDERS/TOPICS
- BLOOD, CONGEALED MASSES
BOWEL RELATED DISORDERS
- CONSTIPATION: Deficiency
- DIARRHEA
CHEST
- CHEST, DISTENTION, PAIN
LUNGS
- ASTHMA/WHEEZING: Kidney Deficient

- COUGH, CHRONIC W/ DYSPNEA: To Store Qi, Stop Cough
- EMPHYSEMA, PULMONARY
- WHEEZING: Excess/ Deficient Type
MUSCULOSKELETAL/ CONNECTIVE TISSUE
- BACK, PAIN, COLD: Deficiency Type
- KNEES, WEAK: Cold
SEXUALITY, MALE: UROLOGICAL TOPICS
- SEMINAL FLUID: Cold

STOMACH/DIGESTIVE DISORDERS
- BELCHING
- EPIGASTRIC PAIN
- HICCUPS: Spleen/ Stomach Cold/Qi Deficient
- STOMACH, PAIN/ PRESSURE/ DISTENTION: Qi Stagnation
- VOMITING: Qi Deficiency-Cold
URINARY BLADDER
- URINATION, DRIBBLING

Clinical/Pharmaceutical Studies:

INFECTIOUS DISEASES
- ANTIBIOTIC: Very Strong:Myco. TB, Shigella, Typhoid

MENTAL STATE/ NEUROLOGICAL DISORDERS
- TRANQUILIZING: Essential Oil

PAIN/NUMBNESS/GENERAL DISCOMFORT
- ANALGESIC: Essential Oil

Dose
1.5 - 3.0 gm

Common Name
Aloeswood

Precautions
Watch: Prolapse/Def Qi

Watch: Def Yin w/Heat

Notes
Generally Powder Form Not Decocted

CHUAN LIAN ZI
(ZHUAN LIAN ZI)

川楝子

FRUCTUS MELIAE TOOSENDAN

Traditional Functions:

1. Clears Heat, dries Dampness
2. Regulates Qi and reduces pain
3. Kills intestinal parasites

Traditional Properties:

Enters: ST, SI, LV,

Properties: BIT, C,

Indications:

ABDOMEN/ GASTROINTESTINAL TOPICS
- ABDOMEN, PAIN OF: Damp Heat Qi Stagnation
- ABDOMEN, PAIN OF, HERNIA-LIKE: Cold
- APPENDICITIS W/PAIN
- FLANK PAIN: Damp Heat Qi Stagnation
- HERNIA-LIKE PAIN: Damp Heat Qi Stagnation

CIRCULATION DISORDERS
- SYNCOPE W/HEART PAIN: Heat

GALL BLADDER
- CHOLECYSTITIS, PAIN

HEART
- CARDIAC PAIN
- SYNCOPE W/HEART PAIN: Heat

LIVER
- HEPATITIS: Pain
- LIVER ATTACKING SPLEEN/ STOMACH
- LIVER QI CONGESTION W/ SUBCOSTAL PAIN

PARASITES

- ROUNDWORMS
- TAPEWORMS

SEXUALITY, FEMALE: GYNECOLOGICAL
- BREASTS, SWOLLEN, PAINFUL, ABSCESS

SKIN
- SCALP, TINEA: Topical Powder

STOMACH/DIGESTIVE DISORDERS
- EPIGASTRIC PAIN: Damp Heat Qi Stagnation

Clinical/Pharmaceutical Studies:

INFECTIOUS DISEASES
- ANTIBIOTIC: Staph A.

PAIN/NUMBNESS/GENERAL DISCOMFORT
- ANALGESIC

PARASITES
- ANTIPARASITIC: Pork Tapeworm, Earthworm, Leech

SKIN

- FUNGAL, ANTI-: Candida, Crytococci, Blastomyces, White Ringworm (Monila Albicans)
- SCALDS

Dose
4.5 - 12.0 gm

Common Name
Sichuan Pagoda Tree Fruit

Contraindications
Not: Cold Def SP/ST

Notes
Ripe Fruit Most Toxic
Overdose Symptoms: Nausea, Vomiting, Diarrhea, Dyspnea, Arrhythmias

DA FU PI

大腹皮

PERICARPIUM ARECAE CATECHU

Traditional Functions:

1. Lowers the Qi and relieves stagnation
2. Dispels Dampness in the Stomach and Intestines
3. Circulates fluids and Promotes urination

Traditional Properties:

Enters: LI, SP, ST, SI,

Properties: SP, <W

Indications:

ABDOMEN/ GASTROINTESTINAL TOPICS
- ABDOMEN, DISTENTION OF: Food Stagnation
- ABDOMEN, DISTENTION OF W/ EDEMA

BOWEL RELATED DISORDERS
- CONSTIPATION W/FOOD STAGNATION
- DIARRHEA: Evil Fluid Dampness

EXTREMITIES
- LEGS, PAIN, SWELLING: Cold Dampness (Beriberi, Leg Qi)

FLUID DISORDERS
- EDEMA: Dampness, Evil Fluid
- EDEMA, SUPERFICIAL W/ ABDOMINAL DISTENTION/ FOOD STAGNATION

LIVER
- HEPATITIS, CHRONIC

NUTRITIONAL/METABOLIC DISORDERS/TOPICS
- BERIBERI

QI RELATED DISORDERS/ TOPICS
- QI OBSTRUCTION

SEXUALITY, FEMALE: GYNECOLOGICAL
- MORNING SICKNESS

SKIN
- ECZEMA: Cold Dampness
- SKIN, SORES: Cold Damp

SPLEEN
- SPLEEN STOMACH, DAMPNESS

STOMACH/DIGESTIVE DISORDERS
- BELCHING, SOUR TASTE: Food Stagnation
- EPIGASTRIC DISTENTION: Food Stagnation
- FOOD STAGNATION
- HICCUPS: Qi Deficiency-- Dampness
- INDIGESTION
- REGURGITATION OF FOOD: Food Stagnation
- STOMACH INTESTINES DAMP STAGNATION
- VOMITING: Qi Deficiency-- Dampness

URINARY BLADDER
- URINATION, SCANTY

Clinical/Pharmaceutical Studies:

ABDOMEN/ GASTROINTESTINAL TOPICS
- INTESTINES, STRENGTHENS

CONTRACTIONS & TENSION OF

Dose

4.5 - 9.0 gm

Common Name

Betel Husk

Precautions

Watch: Def Qi

FO SHOU
(FO SHOU GAN)

佛手

FRUCTUS CITRI SARCODACTYLIS

Traditional Functions:

1. Moves the Qi and reduces pain
2. Pacifies the Liver and regulates Qi
3. Harmonizes the Stomach and stregthens the Spleen
4. Regulates the circulation of Lung Qi and disperses Phlegm

Traditional Properties:

Enters: LU, SP, ST, LV,

Properties: SP, SO, BIT, <W

Indications:

ABDOMEN/ GASTROINTESTINAL TOPICS
- ABDOMEN, PAIN OF, DISTENTION
- ABDOMEN, PAIN OF, HERNIA-LIKE: Cold
- FLANK PAIN/DISTENTION: Liver Qi Stagnation

CHEST

SUBCOSTAL PAIN
- LIVER QI CONSTRAINED: Attacking ST

LUNGS
- ASTHMA
- COUGH, PROFUSE SPUTUM
- WHEEZING

PHLEGM
- PHLEGM STAGNATION

STAGNATION
STOMACH/DIGESTIVE DISORDERS
- ANOREXIA: Spleen Stomach Qi Stagnation
- BELCHING: Liver Qi Stagnation
- EPIGASTRIC DISTENTION/PAIN: Spleen Stomach Qi Stagnation
- HICCUPS: Qi Deficiency-Cold

Indications:

- CHEST, FULLNESS
- RIB PAIN: Liver Qi Stagnation
LIVER
- HEPATITIS, INFECTIOUS
- LIVER QI CONGESTION W/

QI RELATED DISORDERS/
TOPICS
- QI STAGNATION
SPLEEN
- SPLEEN STOMACH, QI

- NAUSEA/VOMITING
- STOMACH, FULLNESS
- VOMITING: Qi Deficiency-Cold/
Spleen Stomach Qi Stagnation

Clinical/Pharmaceutical Studies:

ABDOMEN/
GASTROINTESTINAL TOPICS
- ABDOMEN, DISTENTION OF/
PAIN: 6-9 g With Shan Zha, Shen
Qu, Wheat Germ
- GASTROINTESTINAL,
ANTISPASMODIC: Antispamodic
On Duodenum
- INTESTINES, PERISTALSIS,
INHIBITS: Alcohol Extract
GALL BLADDER
- GALL BLADDER DISEASES:
With Subcostal Pain, Abdominal
Distension
- GALL BLADDER, BILIARY
COLIC: Wine Extract Of Single
Herb

HEART
- HEART, INHIBITS: Drops BP
LIVER
- HEPATITIS, INFECTIOUS, IN
CHILDREN: Helpful For
Symptomatic Treatment, Used With
Fruit Of Bai Jiang Cao
LUNGS
- ANTIASTHMATIC: Sichuan Best
For Effect
- BRONCHITIS, CHRONIC: With
Ban Xia, Fu Ling, etc, *30 g With
Honey As Tea, 2 Months
- EMPHYSEMA: 30 g With Honey
As Tea, 2 Months
- EXPECTORANT
MUSCULOSKELETAL/

CONNECTIVE TISSUE
- ANTISPASMODIC
STOMACH/DIGESTIVE
DISORDERS
- ANOREXIA: 6-9 g With Shan Zha,
Shen Qu, Wheat Germ
- BELCHING: 6-9 g With Shan Zha,
Shen Qu, Wheat Germ
- CARMINATIVE
- GASTRITIS, ACUTE: 50 g Boiled
Take In 2 Doses When Cool For 3
Days
- STOMACH, ACHE: 6-9 g With
Shan Zha, Shen Qu, Wheat Germ
TRAUMA, BITES, POISONINGS
- ANTIHISTAMINE

Dose
3.00 - 9.00 gm

Common Name
Finger Citron Fruit

Contraindications
Not: Excess Fire

Precautions
Watch: w/o Stagnant Qi
Watch: Def Yin w/Heat

Notes
Large Doses Up To 30 gm

JIU BI YING

救 必 應
(救必应)

CORTEX
OLOCUS ROTUNDAE

Traditional Functions:

1. Clears Heat, relieves toxins
2. Dispels Dampness
3. Moves the Qi and controls pain

Traditional Properties:

Enters: ST, LV,

Properties: BIT, CL

Indications:

ABDOMEN/
GASTROINTESTINAL TOPICS
- GASTROINTESTINAL
INFLAMMATION, ACUTE
- ULCERS, DUODENAL
INFECTIOUS DISEASES
- COMMON COLD, FEVER OF

LIVER
- HEPATITIS, CHRONIC/ACUTE
MUSCULOSKELETAL/
CONNECTIVE TISSUE
- ARTHRITIS, PAIN
ORAL CAVITY

- THROAT, PAIN, SWOLLEN
- TONSILLITIS
SKIN
- BURNS
TRAUMA, BITES, POISONINGS
- TRAUMA

Dose
9 - 21 gm

Common Name
Iron Holly

JU HE

橘核

SEMEN CITRI RETICULATAE

Traditional Functions:

1. Expedites the free flow of Liver Qi and alleviates pain

Traditional Properties:

Enters: KI, LV,

Properties: BIT, N

Indications:

ABDOMEN/ GASTROINTESTINAL TOPICS
• ABDOMEN, PAIN OF, HERNIA-LIKE: Cold
• HERNIA, PAIN
MUSCULOSKELETAL/

CONNECTIVE TISSUE
• LUMBAGO
PAIN/NUMBNESS/GENERAL DISCOMFORT
• ANALGESIC: Stomach, Muscles, Joints

SEXUALITY, FEMALE: GYNECOLOGICAL
• MASTITIS
SEXUALITY, MALE: UROLOGICAL TOPICS
• TESTICLES, PAIN, SWELLING

Dose

3 - 9 gm

Common Name

Mandarin Orange Seed

Contraindications

Not: Def Qi

JU HONG

橘紅
(橘红)

EXOCARPIUM CITRI GRANDIS

Traditional Functions:

1. Dries Dampness(more than Chen Pi) and expels Phlegm
2. Descends Qi
3. Regulates the Qi and strengthens the Spleen

Traditional Properties:

Enters: LU, SP,

Properties: SP, BIT, W

Indications:

ABDOMEN/ GASTROINTESTINAL TOPICS
• ABDOMEN, DISTENTION OF
LUNGS

• COUGH: Cold Phlegm/Wind Cold
• COUGH, PROFUSE SPUTUM: Phlem Damp/Wind Cold
• LUNGS, DYSPNEA: Cold Phlegm

STOMACH/DIGESTIVE DISORDERS
• DYSPEPSIA
• STOMACH, DISTENTION

Dose

3.0 - 4.5 gm

Common Name

Red Tangerine Peel

Contraindications

Not: Yin Def Dry Cough

Not: Qi Def Chronic Cough

LI ZHI HE

荔枝核

SEMEN LITCHI CHINENSIS

Traditional Functions:

1. Warms the Center and disperses Cold
2. Regulates Qi and relieves pain

Traditional Properties:

Enters: LV, ST

Properties: SW, W

Indications:

ABDOMEN/
GASTROINTESTINAL
TOPICS
• ABDOMEN, PAIN OF
• ABDOMEN, PAIN OF,
HERNIA-LIKE: Cold
• HERNIA-LIKE PAIN,
ESPECIALLY MEN:
Liver Channel Qi

Stagnation
BLOOD RELATED
DISORDERS/TOPICS
• BLOOD DISORDERS
INFECTIOUS DISEASES
• MEASLES,
UNERUPTED
SEXUALITY, FEMALE:

GYNECOLOGICAL
• DYSMENORRHEA
• MENSTRUATION,
DISORDERS OF: Dredge,
Regulate Chong, Ren
SEXUALITY, MALE:
UROLOGICAL TOPICS
• TESTICLES, PAIN

STOMACH/DIGESTIVE
DISORDERS
• EPIGASTRIC PAIN:
Spleen Stomach Qi
Stagnation
• STOMACH, PAIN:
Spleen Stomach Qi
Stagnation (Use High Dose)

Clinical/Pharmaceutical Studies:

BLOOD RELATED DISORDERS/
TOPICS

• BLOOD GLUCOSE, REDUCES: Injected

Dose
4.5 - 30.0 gm

Common Name
Leechee Nut

Notes
Use Only For Cold Damp Qi Stagnation

MEI GUI HUA   玫瑰花   FLOS
                                                    ROSAE RUGOSAE

Traditional Functions:

1. Relieves constrained Liver Qi: especially Liver-Stomach disharmony
2. Removes Blood stagnation and moves the Qi

Traditional Properties:

Enters: SP, LV,

Properties: SW, <BIT, W

Indications:

ABDOMEN/
GASTROINTESTINAL TOPICS
• ABDOMEN, DISTENTION OF
• ABDOMEN, PAIN OF, UPPER
• FLANK PAIN/DISTENTION:
Liver Spleen/Stomach Disharmony
CHEST
• CHEST, CONSTRICTION: Liver
Spleen/Stomach Disharmony
LIVER
• HEPATITIS

• LIVER SPLEEN/STOMACH
DISHARMONY: Chest Constriction,
Flank Pain/Distension, Belching,
Epigastric Pain, Anorexia
SEXUALITY, FEMALE:
GYNECOLOGICAL
• DYSMENORRHEA: Blood Stasis
• MASTITIS, ACUTE
• MENSTRUATION, IRREGULAR:
Blood Stasis
STOMACH/DIGESTIVE

DISORDERS
• ANOREXIA: Liver Spleen/
Stomach Disharmony
• BELCHING: Liver Spleen/Stomach
Disharmony
• EPIGASTRIC PAIN: Liver Spleen/
Stomach Disharmony
• GASTRITIS, CHRONIC
TRAUMA, BITES, POISONINGS
• TRAUMA

Clinical/Pharmaceutical Studies:

GALL BLADDER
• CHOLAGOGUE: Oil

TRAUMA, BITES, POISONINGS
• POISONING, ANTIMONY:

Decoction Antidote To

Dose
1.5 - 9.0 gm

Common Name
Chinese Rose, Young Flower

MU XIANG

木香

**RADIX
SAUSSUREAE SEU
VLADIMIRIAE**

Traditional Functions:

1. Promotes Qi circulation in the Spleen and Stomach
2. Alleviates pain and controls diarrhea
3. Adjusts and regulates stagnant Qi in the intestines
3. Harmonizes the Stomach and prevents stagnation from tonifying herbs

Traditional Properties:

Enters: LI, SP, ST, GB,

Properties: SP, BIT, W

Indications:

**ABDOMEN/
GASTROINTESTINAL
TOPICS**
- ABDOMEN, PAIN OF/
DISTENTION: Spleen
Stomach Qi Stagnation
- APPENDICITIS W/PAIN
- BORBORYGMUS
- ENTERITIS
- FLANK PAIN/
DISTENTION/
SORENESS
**BOWEL RELATED
DISORDERS**
- DIARRHEA: Food
Stagnation, Most Herbs,
Cooked, Charred/Spleen

Defient With Qi
Stagnation
- TENESMUS
CHEST
- CHEST, DISTENTION/
PAIN
ENERGETIC STATE
- HERBS, TONIFYING:
Ameliorates Side Effects
GALL BLADDER
- GALL BLADDER QI
STAGNATION: Flank
Pain/Distension/Soreness
- GALL BLADDER,
STONES
HEART
- ANGINA PECTORIS:

Chest Bi Strangulating
Pain
LIVER
- JAUNDICE
- JAUNDICE, YIN
- LIVER QI STAGNATION
LUMPS
**QI RELATED
DISORDERS/TOPICS**
- QI STAGNATION
**STOMACH/DIGESTIVE
DISORDERS**
- ANOREXIA: Spleen
Stomach Qi Stagnation
- HICCUPS: Qi Deficiency-
Cold
- INDIGESTION

- NAUSEA/VOMITING:
Spleen Stomach Qi
Stagnation
- STOMACH, PAIN: Liver
Qi Stagnation/Disharmony
- STOMACH, PAIN/
DISTENTION: Spleen
Stomach Qi Stagnation
- VOMITING: Qi
Deficiency-Cold
**TRIPLE WARMER (SAN
JIAO)**
- MIDDLE BURNER,
COLD
URINARY BLADDER
- URINARY TRACT
STONES

Clinical/Pharmaceutical Studies:

**ABDOMEN/
GASTROINTESTINAL
TOPICS**
- LARGE INTESTINE,
ANALGESIC
- PERISTALSIS,
INCREASES LARGE
INTESTINES

**BLOOD RELATED
DISORDERS/TOPICS**
- BLOOD PRESSURE,
LOWERS: Similar To
Papaverine
**BOWEL RELATED
DISORDERS**
- FLATULENCE

INFECTIOUS DISEASES
- BACTERIAL, ANTI-:
Typhoid, B.Dysenteriae, E.
Coli, Staph, B.Subtilis
LUNGS
- ANTI-
BRONCHOSPASMA
TIC: (Histamine-Induced) ,

Not: Anemia, Dehydration

Strong
- BRONCHODILATORY
**MUSCULOSKELETAL/
CONNECTIVE TISSUE**
- ANTISPASMODIC IN
SMOOTH MUSCLE
SKIN
- FUNGAL, ANTI-

Dose

1.5 - 9.0 gm

Common Name

Costus Root

Contraindications

Not: Def Yin Or Def Fluids

Notes

Add Later To Decoction
Raw: Qi Stagnation
Baked: Diarrhea

QING MU XIANG
(SHE SHEN)

青木香

**RADIX
ARISTOLOCHIAE**

Traditional Functions:

1. Reduces pain by moving the Qi
2. Clears Heat and relieves toxic Heat

Traditional Properties:

Enters: ST, LV

Properties: BIT, C

Indications:

ABDOMEN/
GASTROINTESTINAL TOPICS
• HERNIA-LIKE CONDITION
BLOOD RELATED DISORDERS/
TOPICS
• BLOOD PRESSURE, LOWERS
BOWEL RELATED DISORDERS

• DIARRHEA: Enteritis
MUSCULOSKELETAL/
CONNECTIVE TISSUE
• ARTHRITIS; RHEUMATOID
SKIN
• CARBUNCLES
• ECZEMA

STOMACH/DIGESTIVE
DISORDERS
• STOMACH, PAIN, DISTENTION
IN PIT
TRAUMA, BITES, POISONINGS
• INSECT BITES
• SNAKE BITES

Clinical/Pharmaceutical Studies:

BLOOD RELATED
DISORDERS/TOPICS
• BLOOD PRESSURE,
LOWERS: Decoction
Stronger
BOWEL RELATED
DISORDERS
• FISTULA
CANCER/TUMORS/
SWELLINGS/LUMPS
• ANTINEOPLASTIC
• CANCER,
RADIOTHERAPY/
CHEMOTHERAPY: Use
As Adjunct To Stabilize
WBC Count
EARS/HEARING
DISORDERS
• EARS,
INFLAMMATORY
DISEASES: Acute Otitis
Media, 5% Ear Drops
From Equal Amounts Herb,
Cheng Xing Shu Powder
With Small Amount
Borneol, Extracted With
Alcohol

EYES
• EYES,
INFLAMMATORY
DISEASES: Local
Application
IMMUNE SYSTEM
RELATED DISORDERS/
TOPICS
• IMMUNE SYSTEM
ENHANCEMENT:
Increases Nonspecific
Antibodies, Phagocytic
Activity
INFECTIOUS DISEASES
• BACTERIAL, ANTI-:
Staph Aureus,
Pseudomonas, E.Coli,
Proteus
LUNGS
• BRONCHIECTASIS
• BRONCHITIS,
CHRONIC: Cleared Up
Purulent Sputum
• PNEUMONIA, POST-
MEASLES: Grind With
Mild/Boiling Water
MENTAL STATE/

NEUROLOGICAL
DISORDERS
• SEDATIVE
MUSCULOSKELETAL/
CONNECTIVE TISSUE
• OSTEOMYELITIS,
CHRONIC
NOSE
• NOSE,
INFLAMMATORY
DISEASES
ORAL CAVITY
• MOUTH,
INFLAMMATORY
DISEASES: Local
Application, Cold Water
Extract
• TEETH, DENTAL
CARIES, ACUTE
PULPITIS: 5%
Suspension Of Herb
Powder In Glycerine
• TONSILLITIS, IN
CHILDREN: Markedly
Reduced Recurrence, With
Antibiotics
SEXUALITY, FEMALE:

GYNECOLOGICAL
• OVARIES, OVIDUCT,
INFLAMMATION OF:
(Adnexitis) Use With
Chemotherapy For Better
Results
SEXUALITY, MALE:
UROLOGICAL TOPICS
• PROSTATITIS: Use With
Chemotherapy For Better
Results
SKIN
• ABSCESS, CHRONIC
• BURNS
• SKIN, ULCERS
STOMACH/DIGESTIVE
DISORDERS
• STOMACH, ACHE:
Tincture/Powder, 95%,
Lasted 6-8 Hrs, From
Various Causes, Ulcers,
Gastritis, etc
TRAUMA, BITES,
POISONINGS
• WOUNDS: Cleared
Surfaces

Dose
6 - 9 gm

Common Name
Birthwort Root

Notes
Oral Extract May Cause Nausea, Anorexia, Dry Mouth,
Constipation

QING PI   青皮   *PERICARPIUM*
CITRI RETICULATAE VIRIDE

Traditional Functions:

1. Dries Dampness and resolves Phlegm
2. Promotes the free flow of Qi in the Liver and reduces pain
3. Relieves food retention and reduces stagnation

Traditional Properties:

Enters: LV, GB,

Properties: BIT, SP, <W

Indications:

ABDOMEN/
GASTROINTESTINAL TOPICS
• ABDOMEN, PAIN OF: Food
Stagnation
• ABDOMEN, PAIN OF, HERNIA-

CHEST
• CHEST, PAIN: Liver Qi Stagnation
INFECTIOUS DISEASES
• MALARIA, CHRONIC W/MASS
FORMATION

• BREASTS, ABSCESS OF: Phlegm
Dampness
• BREASTS, PAIN: Liver Qi
Stagnation
• LACTATION, INSUFFICIENT: w/

Indications:

LIKE: Cold
- GASTROINTESTINAL DISTENTION
- HERNIA-LIKE PAIN: Liver Qi Stagnation
- HYPOCHONDRIAC REGION, PAIN: Liver Qi Stagnation

BLOOD RELATED DISORDERS/ TOPICS
- BLOOD, CONGEALED MASSES: Stagnant Qi

LIVER
- LIVER QI CONGESTION W/ SUBCOSTAL PAIN
- LIVER, CIRRHOSIS
- LIVER, SWELLING OF

PHLEGM
- PHLEGM DAMP: Intermittent Fever, Chills/Breast Abscess

SEXUALITY, FEMALE: GYNECOLOGICAL

Liver Qi Congestion Add
- MENSTRUATION, CRAMPS OF
- UTERUS, FIBROSIS

SPLEEN
- SPLEEN, SWELLING OF

STOMACH/DIGESTIVE DISORDERS
- FOOD CONGESTION PAIN
- INDIGESTION
- STOMACH, PAIN

Clinical/Pharmaceutical Studies:

ABDOMEN/ GASTROINTESTINAL TOPICS
- ABDOMEN, DISTENTION OF, POSTOPERATIVE: Zhi PO Er Qing Tang (Qing Pi, Hou PO, Zhi Shi, Qing Mu Xiang, 1-2 Doses, Helped Patients To Pass Gas In 24 Hrs
- INTESTINES, INHIBITS: Stronger Than Chen Pi

GALL BLADDER
- CHOLECYSTITIS, CHRONIC, PAIN OF: Chai Hu Shu Gan San

LIVER
- HEPATITIS, CHRONIC, PAIN OF: Chai Hu Shu Gan San

LUNGS
- ANTIASTHMATIC: Short Lived
- ASTHMA, BRONCHIAL: Less

Than Isoproterenol, Aminophylline
- EXPECTORANT: Volatile Oil

SKIN
- DIAPHORETIC

STOMACH/DIGESTIVE DISORDERS
- DYSPEPSIA: With Shan Zha, Mai Ya, Shen Qu, etc
- STOMACHIC

Dose

3 - 9 gm

Common Name

Immature Tangerine Peel

Precautions

Watch: Def Qi

Notes

Similar Constituents As Chen Pi

SHI BING

柿 餅
(柿 饼)

FRUCTUS DIOSPYROS

Traditional Functions:

1. Moistens the Lungs and stops bleeding

Traditional Properties:

Enters: LU, ST

Properties: AS, N, BIT

Indications:

BOWEL RELATED DISORDERS
- CONSTIPATION: Raw
- DIARRHEA: Cooked

- DYSENTERY-LIKE DISORDERS: Cooked

- HEMORRHOIDS, BLOODY STOOL: Raw

Common Name

Persimmon

SHI DI

柿 蒂

CALYX DIOSPYROS KAKI

Traditional Functions:

1. Reverses the upward flow of Qi and stops hiccups and belching

Traditional Properties:

Enters: ST,

Properties: BIT, N

Indications:

LUNGS
• COUGH
SKIN
• SKIN, SORES, SWOLLEN, TOXIC:
  Helps Healing, Deficiency

STOMACH/DIGESTIVE
DISORDERS
• BELCHING: Stomach Cold
• HICCUPS: Stomach Cold/Qi

Deficiency-Cold
• VOMITING: Qi Deficiency-Cold
URINARY BLADDER
• NOCTURIA

Clinical/Pharmaceutical Studies:

STOMACH/DIGESTIVE

DISORDERS

• HICCUPS

Dose
4.5 - 9.0 gm

Common Name
Persimmon Calyx

Contraindications
Not: Prolapse Of Urogenital Organs From Qi Def

SU XIN HUA
(MO LI HUA)

素馨花

FLOS
JASMINI OFFICINALIS

Traditional Functions:

1. Dissolves accumulations and regulates the Qi
2. Harmonizes the Middle Jiao
3. Disperses and clears turbidity

Traditional Properties:

Enters: ST, LV,

Properties: SP, W, SW

Indications:

ABDOMEN/
GASTROINTESTINAL TOPICS
• ABDOMEN, PAIN OF

BOWEL RELATED DISORDERS
• DIARRHEA
EYES

• CONJUNCTIVITIS
SKIN
• SKIN, SUPPURATIVE DISEASES

Dose
1.5 - 3.0 gm

Common Name
White Jasmine

SUO LUO ZI

娑羅子
(娑罗子)

FRUCTUS
AESCULI

Traditional Functions:

1. Regulates the Qi and relieves the Middle Jiao
2. Kills intestinal parasites

Traditional Properties:

Enters: SP, LU

Properties: SW, W

Indications:

BOWEL RELATED DISORDERS
• DYSENTERY
CHEST
• CHEST, PAIN FROM SWELLING

CHILDHOOD DISORDERS
• MALNUTRITION, CHILDHOOD
STOMACH/DIGESTIVE

DISORDERS
• STOMACH, PAIN FROM
  SWELLING

Dose
3 - 9 gm

Common Name
Horse Chestnut

TAN XIANG

檀香

LIGNUM
SANTALI ALBI

Traditional Functions:

1. Moves the Qi and relieves pain
2. Dispels Cold
3. Regulates the Qi above the diaphragm

Traditional Properties:

Enters: LU, SP, ST,

Properties: SP, W,

Indications:

ABDOMEN/
GASTROINTESTINAL TOPICS
• ABDOMEN, PAIN OF: Qi
Stagnation
CHEST
• CHEST, PAIN: Qi Stagnation

HEART
• ANGINA PECTORIS: Chest Bi
Strangulating Pain
STOMACH/DIGESTIVE
DISORDERS

• BELCHING
• DYSPEPSIA
• DYSPHAGIA
• EPIGASTRIC PAIN
• VOMITING

Clinical/Pharmaceutical Studies:

ABDOMEN/
GASTROINTESTINAL TOPICS
• INTESTINES, PARALYZES: Oil
Of
IMMUNE SYSTEM RELATED

DISORDERS/TOPICS
• IMMUNE SYSTEM: Increases
White Blood Cells
INFECTIOUS DISEASES
• BACTERIAL, ANTI-: Staph.Albus

KIDNEYS
• DIURETIC
MENTAL STATE/
NEUROLOGICAL DISORDERS
• PARALYTIC EFFECT: Oil

Dose

1.5 - 3.0 gm

Common Name

Sandalwood

Contraindications

Not: Def Yin w/Heat

WU YAO
(TAI WAU)

烏藥
(乌药)

RADIX
LINDERAE
STRYCHNIFOLIAE

Traditional Functions:

1. Moves the Qi and reduces pain
2. Warms the Kidneys and dispels Cold

Traditional Properties:

Enters: LU, SP, ST, KI, UB,

Properties: SP, W

Indications:

ABDOMEN/
GASTROINTESTINAL
TOPICS
• ABDOMEN, PAIN OF:
Cold
• ABDOMEN, PAIN OF,
HERNIA-LIKE: Cold
• ABDOMEN, PAIN OF,
LOWER: Cold/Qi
Stagnation
• ABDOMEN, PAIN OF/
DISTENTION: Spleen
Stomach Qi Stagnation
CHEST
• CHEST, DISTENTION,

PAIN
CIRCULATION
DISORDERS
• STROKE, W/REFLUX
OF QI
KIDNEYS
• KIDNEY DEFICIENCY,
COLD: Frequent
Urination, Urinary
Incontinence
PHLEGM
• PHLEGM
ACCUMULATION
• PHLEGM SURGING
QI RELATED

DISORDERS/TOPICS
• QI FLUSHING UP
• QI STAGNATION
SEXUALITY, FEMALE:
GYNECOLOGICAL
• MENSTRUATION,
CRAMPS OF: Cold/Qi
Stagnation
STOMACH/DIGESTIVE
DISORDERS
• EPIGASTRIC PAIN:
Spleen Stomach Qi
Stagnation
• FOOD STAGNATION

• REGURGITATION
• VOMITING: Stomach
Reflux
URINARY BLADDER
• ENURESIS
• URINARY
INCONTINENCE: Cold
With Kidney Deficient
• URINATION,
FREQUENT: Cold With
Kidney Deficient
• URINATION, PAINFUL,
DRIBBLING: With
Deficiency Cold

Clinical/Pharmaceutical Studies:

ABDOMEN/
GASTROINTESTINAL TOPICS
• GASTROINTESTINAL GAS,
REMOVES: Pai Qi Tang--Wu Yao,
Mu Xiang, Chen Xiang, Hou PO,
Bai Zhu, Chen Pi, Mai Ya
• INTESTINES, RELAXES SMALL
• PERISTALSIS, INCREASES: Pai
Qi Tang--Mu Xiang, Wu Yao--Mild,
Prolonged Action
BLOOD RELATED DISORDERS/
TOPICS
• BLOOD PRESSURE, RAISES
CIRCULATION DISORDERS
• VASODILATOR, LOCAL
INFECTIOUS DISEASES

• ANTIBIOTIC: Staph A., Strep A-
Hemolytic, Pseudomonas
MENTAL STATE/
NEUROLOGICAL DISORDERS
• CNS, STIMULANT: Cerebral
Cortex, Respiration
MUSCULOSKELETAL/
CONNECTIVE TISSUE
• BACK, LOWER PAIN,
RHEUMATIC: Wu Yao, Man Shan
Xiang, Mu Tong--Markedly
Effective
• MUSCLES, RELAXANT, LOCAL
NUTRITIONAL/METABOLIC
DISORDERS/TOPICS
• WEIGHT GAIN AID: Long Term

Use
SKIN
• DIAPHORETIC
STOMACH/DIGESTIVE
DISORDERS
• STOMACHIC
• ULCERS, GASTRIC/DUODENAL:
Wu Yao, Aralia Chinensis (Chung
Ken/Tsung Mu) , Hong Mu Xiang,
Gan Cao, Zhi Shi
URINARY BLADDER
• ENURESIS: Suo Chuan Pill
• URINATION, FREQUENT: Kidney
Qi Weak--Suo Chuan Pill--Wu Yao,
Yi Zhi Ren, etc

Dose
3 - 12 gm

Contraindications
Not: Def Qi Or Internal Heat

Notes
w/Salt To Warm Kidney, Control Urine
w/Wine To Dispel Cold, Pain

XIANG FU
(XIANG FU ZI)

香附

RHIZOMA
CYPERI ROTUNDI

Traditional Functions:

1. Promotes the free flow of Qi in the Liver
2. Regulates menstruation and controls pain

Traditional Properties:

Enters: SJ, LV,

Properties: SP, <BIT, N

Indications:

• STAGNATION
ABDOMEN/
GASTROINTESTINAL TOPICS
• ABDOMEN, FULLNESS OF
• ABDOMEN, PAIN OF: Liver Qi
Stagnation
• HERNIA
• HYPOCHONDRIAC REGION,
PAIN: Liver Qi Stagnation
BOWEL RELATED DISORDERS
• DIARRHEA
CHEST
• CHEST, FULLNESS
• INTERCOSTAL PAIN: Liver Qi
Stagnation
HEAD/NECK
• HEADACHE, ANTE,
POSTPARTUM
HEMORRHAGIC DISORDERS
• HEMAFECIA

• HEMATEMESIS
• HEMATURIA
LIVER
• LIVER QI CONGESTION W/
SUBCOSTAL PAIN
• LIVER QI STAGNATION
• LIVER QI STAGNATION LUMPS
• LIVER SPLEEN/STOMACH
DISHARMONY
MENTAL STATE/
NEUROLOGICAL DISORDERS
• CONVULSIONS
QI RELATED DISORDERS/
TOPICS
• QI/BLOOD CONGESTION
SEXUALITY, FEMALE:
GYNECOLOGICAL
• AMENORRHEA
• BREASTS, DISTENTION: Liver
Qi Stagnation

• DYSMENORRHEA
• ENDOMETRIOSIS
• FETUS, RESTLESS: Qi Stagnation
• LACTATION, INSUFFICIENT: w/
Liver Qi Congestion Add
• LEUKORRHEA
• MENSTRUATION, ABNORMAL
• MENSTRUATION, DISORDERS
OF: Dredge, Regulate Chong, Ren
• MENSTRUATION, IRREGULAR
• MORNING SICKNESS:
Gestational Foul Obstruction--Cold
• UTERINE BLEEDING
STOMACH/DIGESTIVE
DISORDERS
• DYSPEPSIA
• EPIGASTRIC PAIN
• STOMACH, PAIN: Liver Qi
Stagnation

Clinical/Pharmaceutical Studies:

ABDOMEN/
GASTROINTESTINAL
TOPICS
• ABDOMEN, PAIN OF:

INFECTIOUS DISEASES
• BACTERIAL, ANTI-
MENTAL STATE/
NEUROLOGICAL

• DYSMENORRHEA:
Alone 6-9 g Or With Dang
Gui, Ai Ye
• MENSTRUATION,

Grind To Fine pwdr, 3 g
Each Morning, 80%
Effective
• GASTRITIS: Cold Stasis/

Clinical/Pharmaceutical Studies:

With Ai Ye
- **GASTROINTESTINAL DISORDERS**: Oral
- **INTESTINES, DECREASES TENSION**

BOWEL RELATED DISORDERS
- **DIARRHEA**: Oral

ENDOCRINE RELATED DISORDERS
- **HORMONES**: Volatile Oils Contains Estrogen-Like Substance--Weak

FEVERS
- **ANTIPYRETIC**: 6x Aspirin Efficacy
- **FEVER**: Oral

DISORDERS
- **TRANQUILIZING**: ETOH Extract

PAIN/NUMBNESS/ GENERAL DISCOMFORT
- **ANALGESIC**: 20% ETOH Extract, Active Ingredient Equal To Aspirin

PARASITES
- **FILARIASIS**: Fresh Herb 30-60 g In 2 Doses, One In AM, 1 In PM, Symptoms Controlled

SEXUALITY, FEMALE: GYNECOLOGICAL

IRREGULAR: Alone 6-9 g Or With Dang Gui, Ai Ye
- **UTERUS, INHIBITS CONTRACTION, SPASMS**: 5% Fluid Extract, Less Than Dang Gui

SKIN
- **FUNGAL, ANTI-**: Some

STOMACH/DIGESTIVE DISORDERS
- **ANTIEMETIC**
- **EPIGASTRIC PAIN**: With Ai Ye
- **GASTRIC SPASMS**: 120 g Herb, Gan Liang Jiang 90 g (Liang Fu Wan),

Qi Stasis:120 g Herb, Gan Liang Jiang 90 g (Liang Fu Wan), Grind To Fine pwdr, 3 g Each Morning, 80% Effective

TRAUMA, BITES, POISONINGS
- **INFLAMMATORY, ANTI-**: Significant, ETOH Extract, Stronger Than Similar Amount Of Hydrocortisone, 8x Hydrocortisone, With 4x Safety Range, Partial Absorption From Gastrointestinal Tract

Dose

4.5 - 12.0 gm

Common Name

Nut-Grass Rhizome

Contraindications

Not: Def Qi w/o Stagnation

Not: Def Yin Or Heat In Blood

Notes

w/Vinegar For Pain
w/Wine To Penetrate Channels
Rarely Adverse Effects

XIE BAI
(JIU BAI//HAI BAI)

薤白

BULBUS
ALLII

Traditional Functions:

1. Promotes the flow of the Yang and dispels Cold in the chest
2. Moves the Qi and Blood and reduces pain
3. Directs the Qi downward, moistens and reduces stagnation--primarily in the large intestines
4. Disperses accumulations and warms the abdomen

Traditional Properties:

Enters: HT, LU, LI, ST,

Properties: SP, BIT, W

Indications:

ABDOMEN/ GASTROINTESTINAL TOPICS
- **ABDOMEN, PAIN OF**: Cold Qi Stagnation
- **FLANK PAIN**: Turbid Phlegm Causing Cold, Damp Chest Bi

BOWEL RELATED DISORDERS
- **DIARRHEA**: Cold Dampness (Add Warm Interior Herbs, Too)
- **DYSENTERY-LIKE DISORDERS, W/TENESMUS**: Damp Stagnation In Large Intestine
- **TENESMUS**

CHEST
- **CHEST, PAIN**: Blood Obstructing

Heart Channel/Turbid Phlegm Causing Cold, Damp Chest Bi

LUNGS
- **ASTHMA, COUGH**
- **BRONCHITIS**
- **COUGH**: Turbid Phlegm Causing Cold, Damp Chest Bi
- **DYSPNEA**: Turbid Phlegm Causing Cold, Damp Chest Bi
- **PLEURITIS**
- **WHEEZING**: Turbid Phlegm Causing Cold, Damp Chest Bi

MUSCULOSKELETAL/ CONNECTIVE TISSUE
- **BACK, UPPER PAIN**: Turbid

Phlegm Causing Cold, Damp Chest Bi

PAIN/NUMBNESS/GENERAL DISCOMFORT
- **BI, COLD, DAMP CHEST**: Turbid Phlegm

STOMACH/DIGESTIVE DISORDERS
- **DISTENTION**
- **EPIGASTRIC FULLNESS/ DISTENTION**: Cold Qi Stagnation

YANG RELATED DISORDERS/ TOPICS
- **YANG QI STAGNATION**

Clinical/Pharmaceutical Studies:

HEART
- **ANGINA PECTORIS**: Inhibits Smooth Muscles

MUSCULOSKELETAL/ CONNECTIVE TISSUE
- **SMOOTH MUSCLE, INHIBITS**:

Oral Extract First Stimulates Short Term, Then Inhibits

Dose

4.5 - 18.0 gm

Common Name

Chinese Chive Bulb

Precautions

Watch: Def Qi

ZHI KE
(ZHI QIAO)

枳殼
(枳壳)

FRUCTUS AURANTII

Traditional Functions:

1. Disperses stagnant Qi and reduces distension

Traditional Properties:

Enters: SP, ST,

Properties: SO, BIT, <C

Indications:

ABDOMEN/
GASTROINTESTINAL
TOPICS
• ABDOMEN,
DISTENTION OF,
PRESSURE: Food
Stagnation
• GASTROINTESTINAL
GAS
BOWEL RELATED
DISORDERS
• CONSTIPATION: Food

Stagnation
• DIARRHEA: Food
Stagnation, Most Herbs,
Cooked, Charred
• RECTAL PROLAPSE
CHEST
• CHEST, STUFFINESS W/
YELLOW, THICK
SPUTUM
HEART
• ANGINA PECTORIS:
Chest Bi Strangulating

Pain
LIVER
• LIVER QI CONGESTION
W/SUBCOSTAL PAIN
LUNGS
• COUGH: Lung Heat
• LUNGS, DYSPNEA:
Lung Heat
SEXUALITY, FEMALE:
GYNECOLOGICAL
• MENSTRUATION,
DISORDERS OF:

Constrict Uterus, Stimulate
Chong
• UTERUS, PROLAPSE
STOMACH/DIGESTIVE
DISORDERS
• DYSPEPSIA
• EPIGASTRIC QI
FORMATION
• FOOD STAGNATION
• INDIGESTION
• STOMACH, PROLAPSE

Clinical/Pharmaceutical Studies:

ABDOMEN/
GASTROINTESTINAL TOPICS
• INTESTINES, REGULATES,
INCREASES ACTIVITY
BLOOD RELATED DISORDERS/

TOPICS
• BLOOD PRESSURE, RAISES
SEXUALITY, FEMALE:
GYNECOLOGICAL
• UTERUS, INCREASES TONICITY,

CONTRACTION OF
STOMACH/DIGESTIVE
DISORDERS
• STOMACHIC, AROMATIC
BITTER

Dose

3 - 9 gm

Common Name

Bitter Orange

Precautions

Watch: SP/ST Weakness

Notes

Milder Than Zhi Shi, See That Entry, Too
For Uterine Prolapse: 15-30 gm

ZHI SHI

枳實
(枳实)

FRUCTUS AURANTII IMMATURUS

Traditional Functions:

1. Cracks the Qi, purges Phlegm and reduces accumulations
2. Disperses stagnant Qi and relieves food stagnation
3. Moves the Qi downward thus moving the stool

Traditional Properties:

Enters: SP, ST,

Properties: BIT, SO, <C

Indications:

• SHOCK
ABDOMEN/
GASTROINTESTINAL TOPICS
• ABDOMEN, PAIN OF, UPPER

Stagnant Qi, Accumulation
• RECTAL PROLAPSE
CHEST
• CHEST, FULLNESS

GYNECOLOGICAL
• UTERUS, PROLAPSE
SPLEEN
• SPLEEN STOMACH, DAMPNESS

Indications:

- ABDOMEN, PAIN OF/ DISTENTION: Food Stagnation
- GASTROINTESTINAL GAS: Indigestion
- HYPOCHONDRIAC REGION, PHLEGM ACCUMULATION
- SUBCOSTAL REGION, SOFT PHLEGM MASS

BOWEL RELATED DISORDERS
- CONSTIPATION: Food Stagnation/

- CHEST, NUMB ENTANGLEMENT
- CHEST, PHLEGM MASS, SOFT

HEART
- ANGINA PECTORIS: Chest Bi Strangulating Pain

LIVER
- LIVER QI CONGESTION W/ SUBCOSTAL PAIN

SEXUALITY, FEMALE:

STOMACH/DIGESTIVE DISORDERS
- DYSPEPSIA
- EPIGASTRIC DISTENTION/PAIN
- FOOD ACCUMULATION W/ PALPABLE MASS
- INDIGESTION, FOCAL DISTENTION/GAS
- STOMACH, PROLAPSE

Clinical/Pharmaceutical Studies:

- SHOCK, CARDIOGENIC, INFECTIOUS, ANAPHYLACTIC: Injection, Increases Blood Pressure, Does Not Work With Oral Dose

ABDOMEN/ GASTROINTESTINAL TOPICS
- HERNIA
- INTESTINES, PERISTALSIS, INHIBITS, THEN INCREASES

BLOOD RELATED DISORDERS/TOPICS

- BLOOD PRESSURE, RAISES

BOWEL RELATED DISORDERS
- PURGATIVE: Flavonoids In Aqueous Extract
- RECTAL PROLAPSE: Chronic Diarrhea, Decoction, 3x/Day, 5-10 Days

HEAD/NECK
- BRAIN, INCREASES OXYGEN TO

HEART
- HEART FAILURE:

Injection
- HEART, STIMULATES: Small Doses

IMMUNE SYSTEM RELATED DISORDERS/ TOPICS
- ALLERGIC, ANTI-: Inhibits Histamine Release

KIDNEYS
- DIURETIC

LUNGS
- ASTHMA, BRONCHIAL: (Synephrine)

SEXUALITY, FEMALE: GYNECOLOGICAL

- CONTRACEPTIVE, INHIBITS EGG RELEASE
- UTERUS, CONTRACTS: Synergistic With Oxytocin
- UTERUS, PROLAPSE: Decoction, 3x/Day, 5-10 Days

STOMACH/DIGESTIVE DISORDERS
- DIGESTION, INCREASES: Extract Of

TRAUMA, BITES, POISONINGS
- ANTIHISTAMINE

Dose

3 - 9 gm

Common Name

Immature Bitter Orange

Precautions

Watch: Pregnancy

Watch: Cold Def ST

Notes

12-30 g For Prolapse

Low Toxicity, Safe

Relieve Food Stagnation

A WEI
(E WEI)

阿魏

ASAFOETIDA

Traditional Functions:

1. Improves digestion and helps purge undigested meat after overeating
2. Disperses abdominal distension caused by constipation
3. Removes accumulation and kills intestinal parasites
4. Clears toxins

Traditional Properties:

Enters: SP, ST,

Properties: SP, W

Indications:

ABDOMEN/
GASTROINTESTINAL TOPICS
• ABDOMEN, PAIN OF: Cold
• ABDOMEN, SWELLING
BOWEL RELATED DISORDERS
• CONSTIPATION, SWELLING OF
• DYSENTERY
CANCER/TUMORS/SWELLINGS/

LUMPS
• TUMORS
CHEST
• CHEST, DISTENTION, PAIN
• CHEST, PAIN, COLD IN HEART
  REGION
FEVERS
• FEVER, CHILLS

PARASITES
• PARASITES, INTESTINAL
STOMACH/DIGESTIVE
DISORDERS
• EPIGASTRIC COLD, PAIN
• FOOD RETENTION: Meat
  Overeating

Clinical/Pharmaceutical Studies:

BLOOD RELATED DISORDERS/
TOPICS
• BLOOD: Increases Coagulation
  Time
INFECTIOUS DISEASES
• BACTERIAL, ANTI-:
  Mycobacterial
LUNGS

• ASTHMA: Expectorant
• BRONCHITIS: Expectorant
• WHOOPING COUGH: Expectorant
MENTAL STATE/
NEUROLOGICAL DISORDERS
• SEDATIVE EFFECT FROM ODOR
PARASITES

• ANTIPARASITIC
SEXUALITY, FEMALE:
GYNECOLOGICAL
• UTERUS, STIMULATES: Strong
STOMACH/DIGESTIVE
DISORDERS
• CARMINATIVE

Dose
0.9 - 1.5 gm

Common Name
Asafoetida

Contraindications
Not: Pregnancy

Not: Weak SP/ST

GU YA
(DAO YA)

谷芽

FRUCTUS
ORYZAE SATIVAE
GERMINANTUS

Traditional Functions:

1. Eliminates food stagnation and harmonizes and opens the Stomach

Traditional Properties:

Enters: SP, ST,

Properties: SW, N

Indications:

**ABDOMEN/
GASTROINTESTINAL TOPICS**
• ABDOMEN, PAIN OF: Food
Stagnation

**STOMACH/DIGESTIVE
DISORDERS**
• ANOREXIA: Spleen Deficient
• DIGESTION, WEAK: Spleen

Deficient
• INDIGESTION FROM STARCHY
FOODS

Clinical/Pharmaceutical Studies:

**STOMACH/DIGESTIVE
DISORDERS**

• STARCH, DIGESTION: If Not

Toasted Or Decocted

Dose

9 - 15 gm

Common Name

Rice Sprout

Contraindications

Not: By Nursing Mothers

Not: Prolonged Use-Injures KI

Precautions

Watch: Prolonged Cooking Will Reduce Effects

Notes

With Mai Ya, Usually, Tonifies ST Better, 100x Less
Starch Enzymes Than Mai Ya

JI NEI JIN

雞內金
（鸡内金）

ENDOTHELIUM
CORNEUM GIGERAIAE
GALLI

Traditional Functions:

1. Eliminates food stagnaition, promotes digestion
2. Astringes essence and stops leakage
3. Resolves stones

Traditional Properties:

Enters: SP, ST, SI, UB,

Properties: SW, N, A

Indications:

**ABDOMEN/
GASTROINTESTINAL
TOPICS**
• ABDOMEN,
DISTENTION OF
• ABDOMEN, PAIN OF:
Food Stagnation
**BOWEL RELATED
DISORDERS**
• DIARRHEA: Food
Stagnation, Most Herbs,
Need To Be Cooked,
Charred
• DYSENTERY
• STOOLS, UNDIGESTED

FOOD IN: Spleen
Stomach Cold, Deficient
**CHILDHOOD
DISORDERS**
• BED WETTING
• NUTRITIONAL
IMPAIRMENT,
CHILDHOOD
GALL BLADDER
• GALL BLADDER,
STONES
LIVER
• HEPATOMEGALY
ORAL CAVITY
• CANKERS: External

Application
**SEXUALITY, MALE:
UROLOGICAL TOPICS**
• NOCTURNAL
EMISSIONS
• SPERMATORRHEA
SPLEEN
• SPLEEN STOMACH
DEFICIENCY, COLD:
Anorexia, Undigested Food
Particles In BM
• SPLENOMEGALY
**STOMACH/DIGESTIVE
DISORDERS**

• ANOREXIA
• FOOD STAGNATION
• REGURGITATION
• VOMITING
URINARY BLADDER
• URINARY
INCONTINENCE
• URINARY STONES
• URINARY TRACT
STONES
• URINATION,
FREQUENT
• URINATION, NIGHT
FREQUENCY

Clinical/Pharmaceutical Studies:

• ASTRINGENT
**ABDOMEN/
GASTROINTESTINAL
TOPICS**
• ABDOMEN,
DISTENTION OF: Used
With Mai Ya, Shan Zha,
Bai Zhu, Chen Pi
• INTESTINES, GAS,
FROM ABNORMAL
FERMENTATION: Used
With Mai Ya, Shan Zha,

Mai Ya, Shan Zha, Bai Zhu,
Chen Pi
**SEXUALITY, MALE:
UROLOGICAL TOPICS**
• SEMINAL EMISSIONS,
IN LUNG
TUBERCULOSIS
PATIENTS: Baked
Powder, Orally With Water,
3 g, Morning, Evening For
3 Days
STOMACH/DIGESTIVE

Sufficient Enzymes, Used
With Mai Ya, Shan Zha,
Bai Zhu, Chen Pi
• STOMACHIC: Increases
Digestion Function Slowly,
But Lasts, High Heat
Destroys Activity, Use
Raw
**TRAUMA, BITES,
POISONINGS**
• RADIOACTIVE
STRONTIUM

With Water And Drunk
With Sang Piao Xiao, 9 g,
Duan Long Gu, 12 g, Duan
Mu LI, 12 g, Wheat/Barley,
Zhi Gan Cao
• URINATION,
FREQUENT: 9 g Roasted,
Powdered Mixed With
Water And Drunk With
Sang Piao Xiao, 9 g, Duan
Long Gu, 12 g, Duan Mu
LI, 12 g, Wheat/Barley,

Clinical/Pharmaceutical Studies:

Bai Zhu, Chen Pi
BOWEL RELATED
DISORDERS
• STOOLS, MUSHY: Used With Mai Ya, Shan Zha, Bai Zhu, Chen Pi
ENERGETIC STATE
• TONIFIES
ORAL CAVITY
• HALITOSIS: Used With

DISORDERS
• DIGESTION, STIMULATES
• GASTRIC SECRETIONS, INCREASES: 30-37%
• STOMACH: Increase Peristalsis, Evacuation
• STOMACH, DISCOMFORT: Lack Of

EXCRETION, ACCELERATES: Best Effects With Acid Extract, May Be Ammonium Chloride In Herb
URINARY BLADDER
• ENURESIS, CHILDHOOD: 9 g Roasted, Powdered Mixed

Zhi Gan Cao
• URINATION, NOCTURNAL: 9 g Roasted, Powdered Mixed With Water And Drunk With Sang Piao Xiao, 9 g, Duan Long Gu, 12 g, Duan Mu LI, 12 g, Wheat/Barley, Zhi Gan Cao

Dose
3 - 12 gm

Common Name
Chicken Gizzard Lining

Notes
More Effective As Powder Than Decoction (1.5-3 gm Dose)

LAI FU ZI   萊菔子   SEMEN RAPHANI SATIVI

Traditional Functions:

1. Promotes food digestion and dispels distension
2. Redirects Lung Qi downward and eliminates Phlegm

Traditional Properties:

Enters: LU, SP, ST,

Properties: SP, SW, N

Indications:

ABDOMEN/ GASTROINTESTINAL TOPICS
• ABDOMEN, FULLNESS OF
• ABDOMEN, PAIN OF: Food Stagnation
• GASTROINTESTINAL DISTENTION
BOWEL RELATED DISORDERS
• DIARRHEA: Food Stagnation, Most Herbs, Cooked, Charred
• DYSENTERY, TENESMUS OF
• TENESMUS, RECTAL

CHEST
• CHEST, STUFFINESS
LUNGS
• BRONCHITIS, CHRONIC
• COUGH: Cold Phlegm
• COUGH, WHEEZING, CHRONIC W/SPUTUM: Excess
• LUNGS, DYSPNEA: Cold Phlegm
PAIN/NUMBNESS/GENERAL DISCOMFORT
• FOCAL DISTENTION

QI RELATED DISORDERS/ TOPICS
• QI STAGNATION
STOMACH/DIGESTIVE DISORDERS
• ACID REGURGITATION
• BELCHING, SOUR TASTE: Food Stagnation
• FOOD STAGNATION
• INDIGESTION
• NAUSEA/VOMITING

Clinical/Pharmaceutical Studies:

ABDOMEN/ GASTROINTESTINAL TOPICS
• ABDOMEN, DISTENTION OF: Stir Fried Herb With Shan Zha, Mai Ya, Shen Qu
• INTESTINES, OBSTRUCTION: Ascariasis/Adhesions, With Da Huang, Mu Xiang, 3-5 Doses Usually, *With Mang Xiao For Adhesions
BLOOD RELATED DISORDERS/TOPICS
• BLOOD PRESSURE, LOWERS: Aqueous Extract, Significant Slow,

SWELLINGS/LUMPS
• SWELLINGS, PAIN: Powder With Vinegar
CIRCULATION DISORDERS
• HYPERTENSION: 2-5 Weeks Of Using Tablet Lowered BP Significantly, Varying Degrees Of Symptom Improvement, Similar To Reserpine, Each Tab (0.4 g) = 5 g Of Crude Herb, 4-6 Tabs, 2-3x/Day
ENDOCRINE RELATED DISORDERS
• HYPERTHYROIDISM: Disruption Of Thyroxin Synthesis, Also Tan Yin

LUNGS
• BRONCHITIS, CHRONIC: San Zi Yang Qin Tang (Lai Fu Zi, Bai Jie Zi, Zi Su Zi) , *Often With Phlegm Use Tan Yin Wan With Cang Zhu, Bai Zhu, Gan Jiang, Rou Gui Pi, Gan Cao, Fu Zi, Especially For Kidney Spleen Deficient Patterns
• EXPECTORANT
• TUBERCULOSIS, PULMONARY: With Hemoptysis, Use As Radish Juice
MUSCULOSKELETAL/ CONNECTIVE TISSUE

• TRICHOMONAS, VAGINAL: Apply With Cotton Ball Soaked In Radish Juice Or Ground Radish, High Cure Rate
SKIN
• FUNGAL, ANTI-: Inhibited Many
STOMACH/DIGESTIVE DISORDERS
• ACID REGURGITATION: Stir Fried Herb With Shan Zha, Mai Ya, Shen Qu
• BELCHING: Stir Fried Herb With Shan Zha, Mai Ya, Shen Qu
• STOMACHIC: Stir Fried Herb With Shan Zha, Mai

Clinical/Pharmaceutical Studies:

Prolonged
BOWEL RELATED DISORDERS
• COLITIS, ALLERGIC: Retention Enema Of
• CONSTIPATION, CHILDHOOD
• CONSTIPATION, INTRACTABLE
• DIARRHEA FROM INDIGESTION: Retention Enema Of
• DIARRHEA, POST COLON OPERATION: Retention Enema Of
CANCER/TUMORS/

Wan, Markedly Inhibits Thyroid Function, But Herb Not Main Active Ingredient
HEART
• CARDIOTOXIC: Slightly
IMMUNE SYSTEM RELATED DISORDERS/ TOPICS
• COLITIS, ALLERGIC: Retention Enema Of
INFECTIOUS DISEASES
• ANTIBIOTIC: Aqueous Extract, Marked--Staph A., Strep Pneum, E Coli, Can Detoxify Bacterial Toxins

• SPONDYLITIS, HYPERTROPHIC: Osteohyperplasia Pill (See Analgesic Entry)
PAIN/NUMBNESS/ GENERAL DISCOMFORT
• ANALGESIC: As In Osteohyperplasia Pill (Shu Di, Yin Yang Huo, Gu Sui Bu, Rou Cong Rong, LU Ti Cao, Lai Fu Zi, Caulis Spatholobi)
SEXUALITY, FEMALE: GYNECOLOGICAL

Ya, Shen Qu
TRAUMA, BITES, POISONINGS
• INFLAMMATORY, ANTI- : Herb With Rou Cong Rong, Shu Di As In Osteohyperplasia Pill (Shu Di, Yin Yang Huo, Gu Sui Bu, Rou Cong Rong, LU Ti Cao, Lai Fu Zi, Caulis Spatholobi) , *Tan Yin Wan, Too
• TOXINS, DETOXIFIES: Bacterial Toxins, e.g. Tetanus, Diphtheria

Dose
6 - 12 gm

Common Name
Radish Seed

Precautions
Watch: Def Qi

Notes
Raw-Food Stagnation
Toasted-Productive Cough

MAI YA

麥芽
（麦芽）

FRUCTUS HORDEI VULGARIS GEMINANTUS

Traditional Functions:

1. Eliminates food stagnation and harmonizes the Stomach
2. Restrains lactation
3. Promotes the free flow of Liver Qi

Traditional Properties:

Enters: SP, ST,

Properties: SW, N

Indications:

ABDOMEN/ GASTROINTESTINAL TOPICS
• ABDOMEN, DISTENTION OF, PAIN
• ABDOMEN, PAIN OF: Food Stagnation
BOWEL RELATED DISORDERS
• DIARRHEA: Food Stagnation, Most Herbs, Cooked, Charred
CHEST
• INTERCOSTAL DISTENTION: Liver Qi Stagnation
CHILDHOOD DISORDERS

• INFANTS, INDIGESTED MILK IN
LIVER
• LIVER QI CONSTRAINED: Attacking ST
SEXUALITY, FEMALE: GYNECOLOGICAL
• BREASTS, DISTENTION, PAIN
• LACTATION, INHIBITS: When Ceasing Breast Feeding
• LACTATION, INSUFFICIENT
SPLEEN
• SPLEEN DEFICIENCY: Weak Digestion, Anorexia

STOMACH/DIGESTIVE DISORDERS
• ANOREXIA: Spleen Deficient/ Liver Qi Stagnation
• BELCHING: Liver Qi Stagnation
• DIGESTION, WEAK
• DYSPEPSIA, FROM CARBOHYDRATES
• EPIGASTRIC DISTENTION: Liver Qi Stagnation
• FOOD STAGNATION: Starchy Foods

Clinical/Pharmaceutical Studies:

ABDOMEN/ GASTROINTESTINAL TOPICS
• ABDOMEN, PAIN OF, DISTENTION: 9-12 g In Decoction For Mild Cases, * Serious Cases--Mai Ya, Stir Fried, Gu Ya, Stir

10 ml, 3x/Day
LIVER
• HEPATITIS, ACUTE: Powdered With Sugar
MENTAL STATE/ NEUROLOGICAL DISORDERS
• CNS, STIMULANT:

Water
SEXUALITY, FEMALE: GYNECOLOGICAL
• BREASTS, DISTENTION FROM CESSATION OF BREAST FEEDING-- TREATS PAIN, SWELLING

STOMACH/DIGESTIVE DISORDERS
• ANOREXIA: Add Bai Zhu, Dang Shen, *Extract Works Well
• DIGESTION, ENHANCES: Vitamin B & Enzymes

Clinical/Pharmaceutical Studies:

Fried, Shan Zha, Browned, 9 g Each, Lai Fu Zi, Stir Fried, 6g, *Herb Extract, Hordenine, Similar To Epinephrine, Small Amount, Insoluble In

• LACTATION, INSUFFICIENT: 1 Dose Of 120 g In 200 ml Water

• STOMACHIC: Slight Stimulation Of Pepsin, Gastric Acid Secretion

Dose

6 - 120 gm

Common Name

Barley Sprout

Contraindications

Not: Nursing Mothers

Not: Extened Use Hurts KI

Notes

Powder: 6-15 gm

Generally: 12-30 gm

Slightly Toxic Only If Allowed To Mold

Raw: Food Stagnation

Toasted: Used For No Lactation

SHAN ZHA   山楂   *FRUCTUS CRATAEGI*

Traditional Functions:

1. Dissolves food and transforms accumulations
2. Expels Phlegm and eliminates food stagnation
3. Disperses Blood stasis and reduces masses
3. Relieves diarrhea when charred

Traditional Properties:

Enters: SP, ST, LV,

Properties: SO, SW, <W

Indications:

ABDOMEN/ GASTROINTESTINAL TOPICS
• ABDOMEN, DISTENTION OF/PAIN: Food Stagnation, From Meat
• ABDOMEN, MASS
• ABDOMEN, PAIN OF, HERNIA-LIKE: Cold
• HERNIA, PAIN
BLOOD RELATED DISORDERS/TOPICS
• BLOOD, CONGEALED MASSES
BOWEL RELATED DISORDERS
• DIARRHEA: Food Stagnation From Meat,

Most Herbs, Cooked, Charred
• DIARRHEA, CHRONIC: Partially Charred
CANCER/TUMORS/ SWELLINGS/LUMPS
• TUMORS: Blood Stasis, Herbs Used Other Than Vitalize Blood
• TUMORS, GYNECOLOGICAL
CHEST
• CHEST, STUFFINESS, FULLNESS
CHILDHOOD DISORDERS
• INFANTS, INDIGESTION IN FROM IMPROPER NURSING

CIRCULATION DISORDERS
• HYPERTENSION
HEART
• ANGINA PECTORIS: Chest Bi Strangulating Pain
• HEART PAIN
MUSCULOSKELETAL/ CONNECTIVE TISSUE
• BACKACHE
PHLEGM
• PHLEGM FLUID
SEXUALITY, FEMALE: GYNECOLOGICAL
• AMENORRHEA: Blood Stasis, In Addition To Vitalize Blood Herbs
• LACTATION,

STAGNATION OF
• LOCHIA, RETENTION
• MENORRHAGIA
• MENSTRUATION, DISORDERS OF: Constrict Uterus, Stimulate Chong
• POSTPARTUM, ABDOMINAL PAIN: Blood Stasis
• POSTPARTUM, BLEEDING
STOMACH/DIGESTIVE DISORDERS
• ACID REGURGITATION
• DYSPEPSIA
• FOOD STAGNATION: From Meat, Greasy Foods

Clinical/Pharmaceutical Studies:

BLOOD RELATED DISORDERS/TOPICS
• BLOOD PRESSURE, LOWERS: IV, Highly Significant, Lasts 3 Hrs
• CHOLESTEROL, LOWERS
• HYPERLIPIDEMIA: Tabs Of 3.1 g, 5 Ea 3x/Day, 6 Weeks, Quite Marked Reduction Or Use Combination–Shan Zha, Ju Hua, Jin Ying Zi, Yu Zhu, Mao Dong Qing

Chloramphenicol Doesn't Seem To Help
• DYSENTERY, BACILLARY, ACUTE: 20% Solution With Sugar, 1 Week
CIRCULATION DISORDERS
• ATHEROSCLEROSIS
• HYPERTENSION: 2nd Stage, Fruit Syrup, 0.65 g Herb/ml, 20 ml, 3x/Day For 1 Month, Most Improved Sleep, Appetite,

Up To 3-4 Courses
• HEART DISORDERS, KESHAN DISEASES (ENLARGED HEART) : Shan Zha, Wu Wei Zi, Eliminated Most Symptoms With Treatment
• HEART, INCREASES CORONARY BLOOD FLOW
INFECTIOUS DISEASES
• ANTIBIOTIC: Strongly-- Shigella, Pseudo, B. Dysenteriae

Day Oral, 10 Days/Course, 2-4 Courses Required For Cure/Marked Improvement, Lowers SGPT
SEXUALITY, FEMALE: GYNECOLOGICAL
• AMENORRHEA
• MENSTRUATION, DELAYED
• UTERUS, CONTRACTS
SKIN
• PSORIASIS
STOMACH/DIGESTIVE DISORDERS

Clinical/Pharmaceutical Studies:

BOWEL RELATED DISORDERS
• DYSENTERY, BACILLARY: Oral Decoction, 97% Effective, Faster Still Use Ku Shen, Too, One Dose Yields Improvement, Even In Cases Where

BP
• VASODILATOR, SYSTEMIC
HEART
• ANGINA PECTORIS: Tabs Of 1 gm Of ETOH Extract, 5 Ea, 3x/Day For 4 Week Course, May Need

KIDNEYS
• PYELONEPHRITIS: 90 g/ Day Oral In 3 Divided Doses, 7 Days, High Cure Rate
LIVER
• HEPATITIS: Acute Viral/ Chronic, Powder, 3g 3x/

• DIGESTIVE: Increases Gastric Secretion
• DYSPEPSIA: Contains Lipase, Other Enzyme Enhancers To Digest Meat
TRAUMA, BITES, POISONINGS
• FROSTBITE

Dose
6 - 15 gm

Common Name
Hawthorn Fruit

Contraindications
Not: Weak SP/ST

Notes
Charred For Diarrhea/Dysentery
Ripe/Raw: Food Stagnation, Lowers Blood Pressure
Unripe: For Diarrhea

SHEN QU
(LIU QU)

神曲

MASSA FERMENTATA

Traditional Functions:

1. Eliminates food stagnation and harmonizes the Stomach
2. Relieves diarrhea
3. Resolves the surface
4. Aids digestion and absorption when added to pills containing minerals

Traditional Properties:

Enters: SP, ST,

Properties: SW, SP, W

Indications:

ABDOMEN/ GASTROINTESTINAL TOPICS
• ABDOMEN, FULLNESS OF
• ABDOMEN, PAIN OF: Food Stagnation
BOWEL RELATED DISORDERS
• DIARRHEA: Cold Stomach Food Stagnation, Most Herbs, Cooked,

Charred
INFECTIOUS DISEASES
• COMMON COLD W/ INDIGESTION
STOMACH/DIGESTIVE DISORDERS
• ANOREXIA

• DYSPEPSIA
• EPIGASTRIC FULLNESS: Cold Stomach Food Stagnation
• FOOD STAGNATION: Cold Stomach
• STOMACH, FLU
• STOMACH, FULLNESS

Clinical/Pharmaceutical Studies:

STOMACH/DIGESTIVE DISORDERS

• STOMACHIC: From Yeast,

Amylase

Dose
6 - 15 gm

Common Name
Medicated Leaven

Contraindications
Not: w/ST Fire

Precautions
Watch: Pregnancy

Notes
Toast To Enhance Effect On Food Stagnation

Expel Parasites

BING LANG
(BING LANG ZI)

檳榔
（槟榔）

SEMEN
ARECAE CATECHU

Traditional Functions:

1. Kills intestinal parasites and purges them
2. Promotes Qi circulation and reduces food stagnation
3. Promotes urination

Traditional Properties:

Enters: LI, ST,

Properties: SP, BIT, W

Indications:

ABDOMEN/
GASTROINTESTINAL TOPICS
• ABDOMEN, DISTENTION OF:
Damp Heat
• ABDOMEN, PAIN OF: Ascariasis/
Food Stagnation
• ABDOMEN, PAIN OF, HERNIA-
LIKE: Cold
• APPENDICITIS W/PAIN
BOWEL RELATED DISORDERS
• CONSTIPATION
• DIARRHEA: Food Stagnation,
Generally Cooked, Charred
• TENESMUS
EXTREMITIES
• LEGS, PAIN, SWELLING: Cold

Dampness (Beriberi, Leg Qi)
FLUID DISORDERS
• EDEMA: Dampness, Evil Fluid
INFECTIOUS DISEASES
• MALARIA, CHILLS, FEVER OF
NUTRITIONAL/METABOLIC
DISORDERS/TOPICS
• BERIBERI
PARASITES
• FLUKES, BLOOD
• HOOKWORMS
• PINWORMS
• ROUNDWORMS
• TAPEWORMS: Good
• WORMS, FASCIOLOPSIASIS
• WORMS, HELPS TO DRAIN

DEAD ONES OUT
PHLEGM
• PHLEGM, DAMP: Fever/Chills
QI RELATED DISORDERS/
TOPICS
• STAGNANT QI
SKIN
• ECZEMA: Cold Dampness
• SKIN, SORES: Cold Damp
• SWEATING, INCREASES
SPLEEN
• SPLEEN STOMACH, DAMPNESS
STOMACH/DIGESTIVE
DISORDERS
• FOOD STAGNATION

Clinical/Pharmaceutical Studies:

ABDOMEN/
GASTROINTESTINAL
TOPICS
• INTESTINES,
PERISTALSIS,
INCREASES: Sometimes
Diarrhea
EYES
• ANTIMYDRIATIC:
Constricts Pupils
• GLAUCOMA: Prepare
Eye Drops, 200 g To 100
ml, Similar To Pilocarpine
Drops
INFECTIOUS DISEASES
• INFLUENZA: Apply
Extract Into Nose, * Also
Drink Water Mixed With

• VIRAL, ANTI-: Some Flu,
Colds, May Be Tannin
Content
MENTAL STATE/
NEUROLOGICAL
DISORDERS
• ADDICTIVE: Causes
Peridontal Disease,
Discoloration
• CNS, CHOLINERGIC:
Increases Salivation
• MEMORY LOSS:
Inhibits Loss Of Due To
Chlorpromazine
PARASITES
• ASCARIASIS
• HOOKWORMS
• PINWORMS: Paralyzes

• SCHISTOSOMIASIS:
Paralyzes
• TAPEWORMS: 70%
Effective, Paralyzes,
Synergistic With Nan Gua
Zi, *75-100 g PO
Decoction, 94% Effective,
Some Species Require Up
To 200 g On Empty
Stomach, Add Nan Gua Zi,
Lei Wan, Shi Liu Pi To
Increase Effectiveness
• WORMS,
FASCIOLOPSIASIS:
Decotion 40-50 g, 95%
Cured After 3 Treatments,
May Add Chillis,
Bephenium

• WORMS,
TRICHURIASIS
SEXUALITY, FEMALE:
GYNECOLOGICAL
• UTERUS, STIMULATES:
Ethyl Acetate Extract
Causes Spasm In Pregnant
Rats
SKIN
• FUNGAL, ANTI-: Many,
Effectiveness Varies, Use 1:
1 Decoction
STOMACH/DIGESTIVE
DISORDERS
• APPETITE, INCREASES
• DIGESTION,
STIMULATES: Saliva,
Peristalsis

Dose
6 - 90 gm
Common Name
Betel Nut
Contraindications
Not: Weak Spleen With Diarrhea

Notes
Overdose: Vomit, Stupor, Diuresis, Salivation, Spasms
In Stomach
Up To 60 gm Ok
Raw Has More Alkaloids Than Processed (About +50%)
Minimize Vomiting By Taking Cold

DA SUAN   大蒜   *SUBLUS ALLI SATIVI*

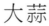

Traditional Functions:

1. Kills parasites
2. Releases the Exterior
3. Promotes urination
4. Strengthens the Stomach and dispels Phlegm
5. Relieves toxins and pus
6. Detoxifies poison

Traditional Properties:

Enters: LU, LI, ST,

Properties: SP, W

Indications:

ABDOMEN/ GASTROINTESTINAL TOPICS
• GASTROENTERIC DISEASES, ACUTE/CHRONIC
BLOOD RELATED DISORDERS/ TOPICS
• CHOLESTEROL, LOWERS
BOWEL RELATED DISORDERS
• DIARRHEA

• DYSENTERY: Good
CIRCULATION DISORDERS
• ARTERIOSCLEROSIS
• HYPERTENSION
INFECTIOUS DISEASES
• FEBRILE DISEASES
LUNGS
• COUGH, SUDDEN

• TUBERCULOSIS, PULMONARY
• WHOOPING COUGH
PARASITES
• HOOKWORMS
• PINWORMS
SKIN
• BOILS, INITIAL STAGE: Topical
• SCALP, RINGWORM

Clinical/Pharmaceutical Studies:

ABDOMEN/ GASTROINTESTINAL TOPICS
• APPENDICITIS: Paste With Mang Xiao, On Lower Right Quad, Increases Peristalsis, Activated Immune Response, Use Gauze Over Mc Burney's Pt, 2 Hrs, Follow With Vinegar, Da Huang Paste--90% Resolution, Used On Uncomplicated Cases With Acupuncture, Oral Herbal Rx
• APPENDICITIS, ACUTE: Bulb Paste Applied Topically
BLOOD RELATED DISORDERS/TOPICS
• HYPERLIPIDEMIA: Pill Made Of Essential Oil Signicant Reduction Of Cholesterol (Least Effect), Triglycerides, Lipoproteins- -0.2 ml/Day For 1 Month
BOWEL RELATED DISORDERS

Stool Or 1-3 Cloves Oral For 5-10 Days Plus Retention Enema With 5% Bulb Solution, Then In Food Afterwards
• DYSENTERY, BACILLARY: Good Effects, 10% Bulb Suspension Orally, 10-40 ml/4 Hrs, Reduce 1/2 When Better, Continue For 2 Weeks, Then, Or Retention Enema, 30-40 ml 1x/Day For 7-10 Days
• DYSENTERY, BACTERIAL: Via Enema, 6-7 Days, Purple, Fresh Bulbs Best
CANCER/TUMORS/ SWELLINGS/LUMPS
• CANCER: Bulb Injection-- Nasopharyngeal, Lymphoepithelioma, Some Lung, Stomach, Least Helpful In Malignant Tumors, Water Extracts-- Liver Cancer With Ascites, MTK Sarcoma III Cells, Diet Of Fresh Garlic

Oil Of, Not Decoction
INFECTIOUS DISEASES
• ANTIBIOTIC: Very Strong, But Variable, Inhibits Many, Inconclusive Clinical Value
• CANDIDA: Oral With Sugar As Paste, Multivitamins
• ENCEPHALITIS B: Via IV Drip
LUNGS
• LUNGS, MYCOSES: Via IV Drip
• TUBERCULOSIS, ENDOBRONCHIAL: Bulb Juice, Short Term Cure, 1-5% Bulb Juice Into Trachea
• WHOOPING COUGH: 95% Effective, 60 g Cut, Macerated For 10 Hrs In 300 ml Boiled Cold Water, Filter, Sweetened With Sugar, 5+Yrs 15 ml/2 Hrs, Less Than 5yrs, 1/2 Dose
PARASITES
• AMOEBIC, ANTI-:

Retention Enema 1/Night For 7 Day Course
• PINWORMS, IN CHILDREN: Via Enema, 1ST, 3rd, 7th Day
SEXUALITY, FEMALE: GYNECOLOGICAL
• TRICHOMONAS, VAGINAL: Eliminates, 50% Pressary Made From Bulb, Gelatin, Glycerin
• UTERUS, STIMULATES: ETOH Extract, Also Increases Tone, Synergized Estradiol Effect On Uterus
SKIN
• FUNGAL INFECTIONS, DEEP: 100% Solution Injection For Candida Albicans, Cryptococcus Meningitis, Lung Fungi, 20-50 ml Addded To Glu- Saline IV
• FUNGAL, ANTI-: Many-- Respiratory Mycoses, Candida
TRAUMA, BITES, POISONINGS
• LEAD POISONING:

Clinical/Pharmaceutical Studies:

- DYSENTERY, AMOEBIC: Oral 1 Piece Purple Garlic Bulb For 7 Days Or

  10% Bulb Liquid, 70-100 ml As Enema 1x/Day, 6 Doses, 2days For Negative

Prevented Breast Cancer In Mice
CIRCULATION

DISORDERS
- ATHEROSCLEROSIS:

Strong (Purple Skin Garlic Best)
- PINWORMS: (Oxyuriasis), 150 g Of Bulb, Crushed, Macerated 24 Hrs In Cold Water, Filter, 20-30 ml In

Treats, Prevents, Bulb Used Alone–4 Cloves, 3x/Day For 1 Month, Helped

Symptoms, Lowered Urine Lead

Dose
6 - 15 gm

Common Name
Garlic Bulb

Notes
High Concentrations-Hemolytic

Cooking Reduces Effect

Long Term Use: May Cause Damp Heat

Local Irritant

DONG BEI GUAN ZHONG   東北貫衆（东北贯众）   *RHIZOMA DRYOPTERIDIS CRASSIRHIZOMAE*

Traditional Functions:

1. Kills intestinal parasites and skin infections
2. Contols bleeding, cools the Blood
3. Clears Heat, removes toxins
4. Vitalizes Blood circulation, disperses stagnant Blood

Traditional Properties:

Enters: ST, LV,

Properties: BIT, CL

Indications:

INFECTIOUS DISEASES
- PAROTITIS, HEAT TOXIN
PARASITES
- HOOKWORMS

- TAPEWORMS
- WORMS, INTESTINAL WITH ABDOMINAL PAIN
SEXUALITY, FEMALE:

GYNECOLOGICAL
- UTERINE BLEEDING: Blood Heat
SKIN
- ABSCESS

Clinical/Pharmaceutical Studies:

PARASITES
- LIVER FLUKES: Filicin Active Ingredient
- ROUNDWORMS, IN BILE DUCT: Concentrated Decoction With Ku Lian Gen Pi, 1-2x/Day, Skip Every

Other Day (Toxic), 4 Days To Expell, 2-6 Doses Needed
- TAPEWORMS: Filicin Active Ingredient
SEXUALITY, FEMALE:

GYNECOLOGICAL
- UTERINE BLEEDING, STOPS WITH INJECTION
- UTERUS, STIMULATES: Strong: Alcohol, Water Extracts

Dose
4.5 - 9.0 gm

Common Name
Dryopteris Rhizome

Contraindications
Not: Weak Patient/Recent Ulcers

Precautions
Watch: Taking With Fatty Foods

Notes
See: Guan Zhong, Can Be Several Ferns

This Species Toxic, Use Others

FEI ZI   榧子   *SEMEN TORREYAE GRANDIS*

Traditional Functions:

1. Kills intestinal parasites
2. Expels accumulations, soothes and lubricates dryness facilitating the passage of stool

Traditional Properties:

Enters: LI, ST,

Properties: SW, A, N

Indications:

ABDOMEN/
GASTROINTESTINAL TOPICS
• ABDOMEN, PAIN OF: Ascariasis
BOWEL RELATED DISORDERS
• CONSTIPATION: Intestinal

Dryness
• HEMORRHOIDS
LUNGS
• COUGH: Lung Dryness
PARASITES

• HOOKWORMS
• PINWORMS
• ROUNDWORMS
• TAPEWORMS
• WORMS, ABDOMINAL PAIN

Clinical/Pharmaceutical Studies:

PARASITES
• HOOKWORMS: 1 Month, 100-150

Gms, Toasted, No Side Effects
• ROUNDWORMS: Not Effective

(In Pigs)
• TAPEWORMS

Dose

9 - 30 gm

Notes

Best Not Decocted, But Toasted Or Made Into Medical
Ball With Honey
Dose: 10-20 Pcs

HE SHI

鶴虱
（鶴虱）

FRUCTUS
CARPESII ABROTANOIDIS
(DAUCI)

Traditional Functions:

1. Expels intestinal parasites and relieves pain of parasites

Traditional Properties:

Enters: SP, ST, LV,

Properties: BIT, SP, N, <TX

Indications:

ABDOMEN/
GASTROINTESTINAL TOPICS
• ABDOMEN, PAIN OF: Worms/
Ascariasis

PARASITES
• HOOKWORMS, ABDOMINAL
PAIN
• PINWORMS, ABDOMINAL PAIN

• ROUNDWORMS, ABDOMINAL
PAIN
• TAPEWORMS, ABDOMINAL
PAIN

Clinical/Pharmaceutical Studies:

CIRCULATION DISORDERS
• VASODILATES
MUSCULOSKELETAL/
CONNECTIVE TISSUE

• ANTISPASMODIC
PARASITES
• HOOKWORMS: 15 Days,
Concentrated Decoctions

• ROUNDWORMS: 15 Days,
Concentrated Decoctions
• TAPEWORMS

Dose

6 - 12 gm

Notes

Other Herbs Usually Used, They Are Stronger In Action
Pills/Powder
Possible Transient Dizziness, Tinnitus, Abdominal Pain

KU LIAN GEN PI

苦楝根皮

CORTEX
MELIAE RADICIS

Traditional Functions:

1. Kills roundworms
2. Used topically to clear Heat and dry Dampness of the skin

Traditional Properties:

Enters: SP, ST, LV,

Properties: BIT, C, TX

Indications:

• LICHEN
ABDOMEN/
GASTROINTESTINAL TOPICS

• LEPROSY
PARASITES
• HOOKWORMS

• VAGINAL TRICHOMONAS
SKIN
• FUNGAL INFECTIONS

Indications:

- ABDOMEN, PAIN OF:
  Roundworm Infestation
  HEAD/NECK
- HEAD, FUNGAL INFECTIONS
  INFECTIOUS DISEASES

- PINWORMS
- ROUNDWORMS
- TAPEWORMS
  SEXUALITY, FEMALE:
  GYNECOLOGICAL

- FURUNCLES, MALIGNANT
- RASHES: Wind
- SCABIES
- SORES

Clinical/Pharmaceutical Studies:

PARASITES
- PINWORMS:
  Concentrated Dose
- ROUNDWORMS: High
  Doses Paralyzes, Low
  Doses Stimulates And
  Exhausts, Detaching Itself
  From Intestinal Wall, *90-
  120 g For Children, 98%

Expelled, *Adults, 35-40
ml Or Syrup (2.5 g Fresh
Herb/ml) , 100% Expelled,
Worms Begin Expulsion 1-
6 Hrs After Herbs, Peaked
24-48 Hrs, Continued For
3-4 Days, Max 8 Days, *
Strong (Sichuan Prov,

Autumn/Winter Harvested
Best)
- TAPEWORMS: Low
  Concentrations-Can Help
  To Release And Expel, 10-
  24 Hrs, High
  Concentrations-Paralyzes
  SKIN

- FUNGAL, ANTI-:
  Various, Cures Head
  Fungal Infections, Tinea, et
  al, Good:Alcohol Extracts
  Best
- SCABIES: Powdered
  With Vinegar, Apply
  Topically

Dose

6 - 15 gm

Common Name

China Tree, Cortex Of Root

Contraindications

Not: For Prolonged Periods
Not: With Liver Disorder/Chronic Diseases

Precautions

Watch: Def SP/ST Or Weakness

Notes

Toxic: May Cause Nausea, Vomiting, Dizziness,
Abdominal Pain, Flushing, Drowsiness, Rarely Blurred
Vision, Pruritus Which Disappear In 2-3 Hrs, Large Oral
Doses May Cause Internal Bleeding, Hypotension,
Circulatory Failure

LEI WAN

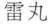

FRUCTIFICATO OMPHALIA
(POLYPORI MYLITTAE)

Traditional Functions:

1. Kills parasites

Traditional Properties:

Enters: LI, ST,

Properties: BIT, C, <TX

Indications:

ABDOMEN/
GASTROINTESTINAL TOPICS
- ABDOMEN, PAIN OF: Ascariasis
- INTESTINES, PARASITES
PARASITES

- ANCYLOSTOMIASIS
- BRAIN, CYSTICERCOSIS
- HOOKWORMS
- INTESTINAL PARASITES

- PINWORMS
- ROUNDWORMS
- TAPEWORMS: Good
- TRICHURIASIS

Clinical/Pharmaceutical Studies:

PARASITES
- ASCARIASIS: ETOH Extract
  Active, Not Aqueous Extract
- HOOKWORMS: Powder In
  Glucose Solution, 40-60 g In 1-3
  Doses, Inconsistent Results, Though
- INTESTINES, TRICHOMONIASIS:
  Decoct Under Low Heat Until
  Boiling, 12 g/Day For 3 Days, 2nd

Course May Be Required, 96% Cure
Rate
- PINWORMS: 2g Powder, Da
  Huang 3 g, Qian Niu Zi 9g With
  Water Early In Morning, Empty
  Stomach
- TAPEWORMS: Destroys Protein
  Of, 20 Gms, 3x/Day For 3 Days As
  Powder Followed By Mang Xiao, 15-

20 g 4th Day, Guan Zhong, Bing
Lang Paralyzes Worms
- WORMS, FILARIASIS: 30 g For 7
  Days
SEXUALITY, FEMALE:
GYNECOLOGICAL
- VAGINITIS, TRICHOMONAS: 5%
  Decoction Will Kill Most In 5
  Minutes

Dose

6 - 9 gm

Common Name

Thunder Ball (Fungus)

Precautions

Watch: Def SP/ST w/Parasites

Notes

Do Not Cook, Destroys Active Enzymes
Possible Transient Nausea With Use

NAN GUA ZI

南瓜子
（南瓜子）

SEMEN CUCURBITAE MOSCHATAE

Traditional Functions:

1. Kills intestinal parasites and relieves their pain
2. Benefits postpartum fluid metabolism, increasing lactation and reducing swelling
3. Harmonizes the Spleen and Stomach
4. Removes Heat and promotes urination

Traditional Properties:

Enters: LI, LV, SP, ST

Properties: SW, W

Indications:

BOWEL RELATED DISORDERS
• CONSTIPATION: Intestinal Dryness
ENDOCRINE RELATED DISORDERS

• DIABETES
PARASITES
• ROUNDWORMS
• TAPEWORMS: Suppository
SEXUALITY, FEMALE:

GYNECOLOGICAL
• LACTATION, INSUFFICIENT
• POSTPARTUM, SWELLING OF HANDS, FEET

Clinical/Pharmaceutical Studies:

LUNGS
• WHOOPING COUGH: Fine Powder Of Browned Seeds With Brown Sugar Solution, 2-3x/Day
PARASITES
• SCHISTOSOMIASIS: Kills Young, Preventative Against Development Of,

Needs High Dose To Kill Adults, *17-64% Short Term Effect, Use Powder, Decotion (10 g/ml), Aqueous Extract (4 g), 30 Day Course, Best Results With Extract
• TAPEWORMS: Paralyzes,

ETOH Extract Can Kill In 45 Minutes-1 Hr, Tapeworms:60-120 gm Powder, +2 Hrs 60-120 gm Bing Lang, +30 Min 15 gm Mang Xiao, Aqueous Extract Of 300 g, 70% Cure Rate, 95% If Single

Dose Of 120 g With Bing Lang
• WORMS
• WORMS, FILARIASIS: 60 g Seeds With 30 g Decoction Of Bing Lang, Mixed In Emulsion, Take On Empty Stomach

Dose

30 - 120 gm

Common Name

Pumpkin Seeds And Husks

Notes

Toxic To Liver In Large Doses
Possible: Dizziness, Nausea, Vomiting, Diarrhea, Easily Controlled Without Stopping Treatment
Synergistic With Bing Lang

SHI JUN ZI

使君子

FRUCTUS QUISQUALIS INDICAE

Traditional Functions:

1. Kills roundworms
2. Strengthens the Spleen and dissipates accumulations

Traditional Properties:

Enters: SP, ST,

Properties: SW, W

Indications:

ABDOMEN/ GASTROINTESTINAL TOPICS
• ABDOMEN, DISTENTION OF/

FEEDING, CHILDHOOD
• NUTRITIONAL IMPAIRMENT, CHILDHOOD

• HOOKWORMS
• PINWORMS
• ROUNDWORMS

Indications:

PAIN: Worms
CHILDHOOD DISORDERS
• INDIGESTION IMPROPER

ENERGETIC STATE
• WEAK CONSTITUTION
PARASITES

**STOMACH/DIGESTIVE
DISORDERS**
• ANOREXIA

Clinical/Pharmaceutical Studies:

PARASITES
• ASCARIASIS: The Best 8 Herbs Are:This Herb, He Shi, Wu Yi, Bing Lang, Guang Zhong, Chuan Lian Zi, Lei Wan, Wu Zhu Yu, *Best Chewed, Not As Effective As Decoction, 1 Large Dose Better Than Several Smaller Doses, Fresh Herb Better, Dose-1 g/Year Of Age With 16 g As

Maximum, Best To Combine With Bing Lang To Increase Effectiveness, Reduce Side Effects
• INTESTINES, TRICHOMONIASIS: Stir Fried To Yellow, Powder Form, Less Than 1 Yr, 3 g/Day In 1-2 Doses, 1-3 Yrs, 4.5 g/Day, Adults 15 g/Day For 3-5 Days, Repeat 1-2 X If Still Some Symptoms, All Cured

• PINWORMS: Water/Alcohol Extract, Age Plus 1 In Grams, 2x/ Day For 3 Days
• ROUNDWORMS: Water/Alcohol Extract
• TAPEWORMS, PORK
SKIN
• FUNGAL, ANTI-: Many With The Aqueous Extract

Dose

4.5 - 12.0 gm

Common Name

Rangoon Creeper Fruit/See

Notes

Overdose: Hiccups, Dizzyness, Nausea/Vomiting, Belching, Diarrhea Side Effects
If Taken With Hot Tea Can Cause Hiccups
If Roasted Less Hiccups

SHI LIU GEN PI

石榴根皮
（石榴根皮）

RADIX GRANATI

Traditional Functions:

1. Kills parasites
2. Astringes the intestines and controls diarrhea

Traditional Properties:

Enters: LI, KI,

Properties: SO, A, W

Indications:

BOWEL RELATED DISORDERS
• DIARRHEA, CHRONIC: Deficient Cold

• DYSENTERY-LIKE DISORDERS
• RECTAL PROLAPSE
PARASITES

• ROUNDWORMS
• TAPEWORMS

Dose

1.5 - 9.0 gm

Common Name

Pomegranate Root

Notes

No Oils/Fats Should Be Taken With Herb, Avoids Toxic Overdose

---

WU YI

蕪夷
（芫夷）

PASTA ULMI MACROCARPI

Traditional Functions:

1. Kills intestinal parasites and expels their accumulation

Traditional Properties:

Enters: SP, ST, LV,

Properties: BIT, SP, W

Indications:

ABDOMEN/
  GASTROINTESTINAL TOPICS
• ABDOMEN, PAIN OF: Ascariasis
CHILDHOOD DISORDERS
• MALNUTRITION, CHILDHOOD

PARASITES
• HOOKWORMS
• PINWORMS
• ROUNDWORMS

• TAPEWORMS
STOMACH/DIGESTIVE
  DISORDERS
• INDIGESTION

Clinical/Pharmaceutical Studies:

PARASITES
• ROUNDWORMS: Alcohol Extracts,

Strong
SKIN

• FUNGAL, ANTI-: Water Extracts
  Significantly Inhibits Many

Dose

3 - 9 gm

Common Name

Stinking Elm Fruit Paste

Contraindications

Not: Def SP/ST

Stop Bleeding

AI YE
(MOXA)

艾葉
（艾叶）

FOLIUM
ARTEMISIAE VULGARIS
(ARGYI)

Traditional Functions:

1. Warms the menses and controls bleeding
2. Warms the womb and pacifies the fetus
3. Disperses Cold and Dampness and relieves pain
4. Expels Phlegm and relieves cough and asthma

Traditional Properties:

Enters: SP, KI, LV,

Properties: BIT, SP, W

Indications:

ABDOMEN/
GASTROINTESTINAL TOPICS
• ABDOMEN, PAIN OF, LOWER:
Cold
BOWEL RELATED DISORDERS
• DYSENTERY, CHRONIC W/
BLOODY STOOL
HEMORRHAGIC DISORDERS
• EPISTAXIS
• HEMATEMESIS
• HEMOPTYSIS
• HEMORRHAGE: Warms Channels
To Stop
LUNGS
• ASTHMA
• COUGH

MUSCULOSKELETAL/
CONNECTIVE TISSUE
• ARTHRITIS: For Expelling Cold,
Dampness
SEXUALITY, EITHER SEX
• INFERTILITY: Cold Womb
SEXUALITY, FEMALE:
GYNECOLOGICAL
• DYSMENORRHEA: Cold
• FETUS, RESTLESS: Threatened
Abortion, Blood Deficiency
• LEUKORRHEA: Kidney Spleen
Yang Deficiency
• MENSTRUATION, DISORDERS
OF: Constricts Uterus, Stimulates

Chong/Warms Chong, Ren
• MENSTRUATION, IRREGULAR
• STERILITY, FEMALE
• UTERINE BLEEDING: Cold/
Prolonged Menstruation
• VAGINAL BLEEDING: Threatened
Miscarriage
• WOMEN'S DISEASES: Bleeding
SKIN
• DERMATITIS: Topical
• DERMATOSIS
• FUNGAL INFECTIONS: Topical
• SCABIES: Topical
TRIPLE WARMER (SAN JIAO)
• LOWER BURNER, WARMS

Clinical/Pharmaceutical Studies:

BLOOD RELATED
DISORDERS/TOPICS
• BLOOD,
COAGULATION:
Reduces Time
BOWEL RELATED
DISORDERS
• DYSENTERY,
BACILLARY: Decoction,
Good Results
FEVERS
• ANTIPYRETIC
IMMUNE SYSTEM
RELATED DISORDERS/
TOPICS
• ALLERGIC, ANTI-: Oral,
Oil, Inhibits Histamines
• ALLERGY, TO DRUGS:
Decoction
• IMMUNE SYSTEM
ENHANCEMENT:

Inhibited
• LEPROSY
• MALARIA: Good, In
Large Doses (15-30 g) ,
Given 2 Hours Before
Symptoms
LIVER
• HEPATITIS, CHRONIC
PERSISTENT/ACTIVE:
Injection Of Distillate
• LIVER, CIRRHOSIS:
Injection Of Distillate
LUNGS
• ANTITUSSIVE: Effect
Peaked 1-2 Hrs, Lasted 4-5
Hrs
• ASTHMA: Leaf Oil, 0.5
ml, Inhibits Spasms,
Sputum, Cough
• ASTHMA, BRONCHIAL:
Decoction

Can Reduce Cough
• TUBERCULOSIS:
Inhibits Bacteria
MENTAL STATE/
NEUROLOGICAL
DISORDERS
• CNS, STIMULANT:
Stimulates, May Cause
Convulsions In Large
Doses
NOSE
• RHINITIS, ALLERGIC:
Decoction
SEXUALITY, EITHER
SEX
• ULCERS, PERINEAL
REGION: Use Moxa
SEXUALITY, FEMALE:
GYNECOLOGICAL
• LEUKORRHEA: Oral
Decotion

Decoction
SKIN
• BURNS: Fumigate
Rooms Or Local Moxa,
Better With Cang Zhu
• DERMATITIS,
ALLERGIC: Decoction
Plus Topical Drugs
• DERMATITIS,
ANCYLOSTOME: Moxa
Helps
• FUNGAL, ANTI-
• PRURITUS: Lotion Of
Herb
• TINEA FUNGUS: Use
Moxa
• ULCERS, PERINEAL
REGION: Use Moxa
• URTICARIA: Decoction
• WARTS: Fresh, Crushed
Leaves, Numerous Times/

Clinical/Pharmaceutical Studies:

Increased Phagocytosis
INFECTIOUS DISEASES
• ANTIBIOTIC: Especially As A Fumigant, Synergistic With Cang Zhu, Mild As Decoction, Many Bacteria

• BRONCHITIS, CHRONIC: Caps Of Oil, 2 Courses Of 10 Days Each/Decoction
• BRONCHODILATORY
• EXPECTORANT: Oral

• UTERINE BLEEDING: Jiao Ai SI Wu Tang (Ai Ye, E Jiao, etc)
• UTERUS, STIMULATES: Strong, From Infusion/

Day, Warts Fell Off 3-10 Days
STOMACH/DIGESTIVE DISORDERS
• STOMACHIC

Dose

3 - 15 gm

Common Name

Mugwort Leaf

Precautions

Watch: Blood Heat
Watch: Def Yin

Notes

Decoction: 30% Had Dry Mouth, Nausea, Vomiting, GI Distress, Diarrhea, The Oil Had Less Side Effects

---

BAI JI

白芨
(白芨)

RHIZOMA BLETILLAE STRIATAE

Traditional Functions:

1. Arrests bleeding in the Lung and Stomach
2. Reduces swelling and promotes tissue regeneration of wounds and sores by topical application

Traditional Properties:

Enters: LU, ST, LV,

Properties: BIT, SW, CL, A

Indications:

EXTREMITIES
• FEET, CRACKED: With Sesame Oil
HEMORRHAGIC DISORDERS
• BLEEDING, TRAUMA, WOUNDS
• EPISTAXIS
• HEMATEMESIS
• HEMOPTYSIS: Lung Deficiency/ Astringe To Stop/Cool Blood To Stop/Deficiency Caused
LUNGS
• COUGH, LUNG EXHAUSTION:

Tuberculosis
• LUNG BLEEDING
• LUNGS, DAMAGE TO
• SILICOSIS
• TUBERCULOSIS, PULMONARY
SKIN
• ABSCESS, INFLAMMATION
• BOILS: External
• BURNS: External
• CHAPPED: With Sesame Oil
• SKIN, LACERATIONS
• SORES: Topical

• SORES, CHRONIC NON-HEALING
• ULCERS, CHRONIC, NONHEALING: Topical
STOMACH/DIGESTIVE DISORDERS
• STOMACH, BLEEDING
• ULCERS, GASTRIC/DUODENAL
TRAUMA, BITES, POISONINGS
• CHILBLAIN
• TRAUMA: Topical

Clinical/Pharmaceutical Studies:

CANCER/TUMORS/SWELLINGS/ LUMPS
• CANCER, ANTI-
HEMORRHAGIC DISORDERS
• HEMOSTATIC: Powder Or w/ Starch, Very Effective Locally
INFECTIOUS DISEASES
• BACTERIAL, ANTI-: Gram Positive Bacteria, Effective Against Endotoxin From Hemophilus

Pertussis
LUNGS
• BRONCHIECTASIS: Long Term Use (3-6 Months) , Lowered Coughing, Hemoptysis, Sputum
• TUBERCULOSIS, PULMONARY: Powder, High Cure Rate
SKIN
• BURNS: Sterile w/Petroleum Jelly For Less Than 11% Body, Change 5-

7 Days
• FUNGAL, ANTI-: "White Scabies"
• ULCERS, BLEEDING
STOMACH/DIGESTIVE DISORDERS
• ULCERS, GASTRIC/SMALL INTESTINE: 9 gm Of Powder Closes Small ST/SI Ulcers In 15-40 Seconds

Dose

3 - 15 gm

Common Name

Bletilla Rhizome

Contraindications

Not: Wind Heat w/Coughing Blood
Not: Early LU Abscess

Not: Excess Heat In LU/ST
Not: Fu Zi/Wu Tou, Counteracts Effects Of Herb

Notes

Ulcers: Can Cause Adhesions In Abdominal Cavity, If Leaks
If Powder Used: 3-9 gm
Decoction: Max: 24-30 gm

BAI MAO GEN

白茅根

RHIZOMA IMPERATAE CYLINDRICAE

Traditional Functions:

1. Cools the Blood and controls bleeding
2. Removes Heat and promotes urination
3. Clears Heat from the Stomach and Lungs

Traditional Properties:

Enters: LU, ST, SI, UB,

Properties: SW, C

Indications:

BLOOD RELATED DISORDERS/ TOPICS
• RECKLESS HOT BLOOD
FLUID DISORDERS
• EDEMA: Dampness, Evil Fluid
• THIRST: Fluid Injury/Stomach Heat
HEMORRHAGIC DISORDERS
• EPISTAXIS: Hot Blood
• HEMATEMESIS: Hot Blood
• HEMATURIA: Hot Blood

• HEMOPTYSIS: Hot Blood
LIVER
• JAUNDICE
LUNGS
• COUGH, ASTHMATIC: Lung Heat
MENTAL STATE/ NEUROLOGICAL DISORDERS
• RESTLESSNESS: Heat
STOMACH/DIGESTIVE DISORDERS
• BELCHING: Stomach Heat

• HICCUPS: Qi Deficiency–Heat
• STOMACH HEAT: Nausea/Thirst, Belching
• VOMITING: Qi Deficiency–Heat
URINARY BLADDER
• DYSURIA W/EDEMA
• URINARY DYSFUNCTION, PAINFUL, HOT
• URINATION, PAINFUL, DRIBBLING, CONCENTRATED, RED/YELLOW/TURBID

Clinical/Pharmaceutical Studies:

HEMORRHAGIC DISORDERS
• EPISTAXIS: Decoction, 250 gm, May Add Ou Jie, He Ye, Xian He Cao
• HEMATURIA: Decoction, 250 gm, May Add Ou Jie, He Ye, Xian He Cao
• HEMOPTYSIS: Decoction, 250 gm, May Add Ou Jie, He Ye, Xian He Cao

• HEMOSTATIC
INFECTIOUS DISEASES
• ANTIBIOTIC: Strong-- Shigella, et al
KIDNEYS
• DIURETIC: Aqueous Extract, Most Prominent After 5-10 Hrs Of Taking
• GLOMERULO- NEPHRITIS, ACUTE/ CHRONIC: 250-500 gm Decoction In 2 Doses/Day

To Cure
• NEPHRITIS, ACUTE: Shortens Duration, Improves Symptoms
LIVER
• HEPATITIS, ACUTE, VIRAL: Decoction, Generally With Che Qian Zi/Cao, Yin Chen Hao, Glechoma Longituba (Lian Qian Cao?)
SEXUALITY, FEMALE:

GYNECOLOGICAL
• MENORRHAGIA: Decoction, 250 gm, May Add Ou Jie, He Ye, Xian He Cao
STOMACH/DIGESTIVE DISORDERS
• STOMACH, BLEEDING: Decoction, 250 gm, May Add Ou Jie, He Ye, Xian He Cao

Dose

9 - 30 gm

Common Name

Woolly Grass Rhizome

Contraindications

Not: Cold Def SP

Notes

Up To 60 gm If Used Alone
Safe In Decoction, May Have Dizziness, Nausea, Slight Diarrhea

---

BAI MAO GEN HUA
(MAO HUA)

白茅根花
（白茅根花）

FLOS IMPERATAE CYLINDRIAE

Traditional Functions:

1. Cools Heat in the Blood and strongly stops bleeding

Traditional Properties:

Enters:

Properties: SW, C

Indications:

HEMORRHAGIC DISORDERS
• EPISTAXIS: Hot Blood

• HEMATEMESIS: Hot Blood
URINARY BLADDER

• URINATION, PAINFUL, LI

Notes   Disorders

Not As Effective As Bai Mao Gen For LI (Urinary Type)

CE BAI YE
(CE BO YE)

侧柏葉
（侧柏叶）

CACUMEN
BIOTAE ORIENTALIS

Traditional Functions:

1. Cools the Blood and controls bleeding
2. Expels Phlegm and alleviates coughs
3. Promotes healing of burns
4. Dispels Wind Damp Bi
5. Clears Damp Heat
6. Promotes hair growth

Traditional Properties:

Enters: LU, LI, LV,

Properties: BIT, A, <C

Indications:

BOWEL RELATED DISORDERS
• DYSENTERY-LIKE DISORDERS
  W/BLEEDING
HEAD/NECK
• ALOPECIA: Blood Heat Complex
• BALDNESS
• HAIR, PREMATURE WHITENING:
  Blood Heat
HEMORRHAGIC DISORDERS
• BLEEDING: Hot Blood
• BLEEDING GUMS
• EPISTAXIS
• HEMAFECIA
• HEMATEMESIS
• HEMATURIA
• HEMOPTYSIS

• HEMORRHAGE: Cool Blood To
  Stop
INFECTIOUS DISEASES
• MUMPS
LUNGS
• BRONCHITIS, CHRONIC
• COUGH: Lung Heat
• COUGH, BLOODY, DIFFICULT
  TO EXPECTORATE SPUTUM
• COUGH, DIFFICULT
  EXPECTORATION
• LUNGS, DYSPNEA: Lung Heat
**MUSCULOSKELETAL/
CONNECTIVE TISSUE**
• ARTHRITIS, PAIN

**SEXUALITY, FEMALE:
GYNECOLOGICAL**
• MENORRHAGIA
• MENSTRUATION, DISORDERS
  OF: Consolidate, Astringe, Clear
  Chong, Ren
• UTERINE BLEEDING
SKIN
• BURNS, EARLY STAGE: Small,
  Moderate Size
• ERYSIPELAS
• PRURITUS, W/OILY SKIN
• SCALDS
TRAUMA, BITES, POISONINGS
• WOUNDS: Topical

Clinical/Pharmaceutical Studies:

**BOWEL RELATED
DISORDERS**
• CONSTIPATION
• DYSENTERY: Dry
  Powder, 7-10 Days
• DYSENTERY,
  BACILLARY, ACUTE:
  18% ETOH Extract, 50 ml,
  3x/Day, 7-10 Days, 88%
  Cured
ENERGETIC STATE
• ASTHENIA
HEAD/NECK
• BALDNESS: Tincture
  (ETOH) Of Fresh Material,
  Hair Growth Proportional
  To Frequency Of
  Application, Rub Onto
  Bald Areas
HEART
• PALPITATIONS
**HEMORRHAGIC
DISORDERS**
• HEMOSTATIC

INFECTIOUS DISEASES
• ANTIBIOTIC: TB, Strep,
  Pneumonia--Alcohol
  Extract
• VIRAL, ANTI-:
  Decoction, 1:40 Inhibited
  Flu, Especially Herpes
LUNGS
• ANTITUSSIVE: Oral
  Ingestion, ETOH Extract
  Of Flavones
• ASTHMA: Dilates
  Bronchial Smooth Muscles,
  Active Principle Extracted
  By Ethyl Acetate
• BRONCHITIS,
  CHRONIC: 70-95%
  Effective Rate, Herb Plus
  e.g. Shan Yao, Yin Yang
  Huo, 15 g Ea, SIGA Levels
  Increased, •60 g/Day In 2
  Doses Of Cone, 15 Days=
  Course, 81% Effective
• EXPECTORANT: ETOH

Extract
• TUBERCULOSIS,
  PULMONARY: Tablet Of
  Extract (= 45 g Crude Herb/
  Day) 6 Months, Helped
  Symptoms, 60%
  Registered Negative TB
  Bacillus
• WHOOPING COUGH:
  Fresh Leaves, Branches, 30
  g Decoct To 100 ml With
  20 ml Honey Added, Less
  Than 2 Yrs, 15-25 ml, 3x/
  Day, Increase With Age
**MENTAL STATE/
NEUROLOGICAL
DISORDERS**
• INSOMNIA
• NEURASTHENIA
• SEDATIVE: Decoction,
  Large Doses
**MUSCULOSKELETAL/
CONNECTIVE TISSUE**
• MUSCLES, SMOOTH,

INHIBITS
SKIN
• BURNS: Ointment For
  Topical Use, Fine pwdr Of
  Carbonized Herb, Boiled
  Sesame/Soy Oil For Small-
  Moderate Sized 1ST
  Degree Burns, Induces
  Antiinflammatory,
  Antiseptic Effects
**STOMACH/DIGESTIVE
DISORDERS**
• ULCERS, GASTRIC/
  DUODENAL: Bleeding,
  Oral Preparations, 3.5
  Days To Stop Bleeding
• ULCERS, PEPTIC
  BLEEDING: 3 Days Of
  Decoction 15 g, Control
  Was 4-5 Days
**TRAUMA, BITES,
POISONINGS**
• INFLAMMATORY, ANTI-

Dose
6 - 18 gm

Common Name
Leafy Twig Of Arborvitae

CHEN ZONG TAN
(ZHONG LU TAN)

陳棕炭
（陈棕炭）

VAGINA TRACHYCARPI CARBONISTA

Traditional Functions:

1. Astringes and arrests bleeding

Traditional Properties:

Enters: LU, LI, LV,

Properties: BIT, N, A

Indications:

ABDOMEN/ GASTROINTESTINAL TOPICS
• INTESTINES, HEMORRHAGE
BOWEL RELATED DISORDERS
• DYSENTERY, RED, WHITE
HEMORRHAGIC DISORDERS
• EPISTAXIS
• HEMAFECIA
• HEMATEMESIS

• HEMORRHAGE: Astringe To Stop
• INTESTINAL HEMORRHAGE
SEXUALITY, FEMALE: GYNECOLOGICAL
• FUNCTIONAL BLEEDING
• LEUKORRHEA
• MENSTRUATION, DISORDERS OF: Consolidate, Astringe Chong, Ren/Constrict Uterus, Stimulate

Chong
SKIN
• FUNGAL INFECTIONS: External
• SCABIES: External
TRAUMA, BITES, POISONINGS
• WOUNDS: External
URINARY BLADDER
• URINATION, DRIBBLING W/ BLOOD

Clinical/Pharmaceutical Studies:

• ASTRINGENT

HEMORRHAGIC DISORDERS

• HEMOSTATIC

Dose
9 - 15 gm

Common Name
Charred Palm Tree Bark

DA JI

大薊
（大薊）

HERBA CIRSII JAPONICI

Traditional Functions:

1. Cools the Blood, stops bleeding and disperses stagnant Blood
2. Reduces swelling and promotes healing of boils and sores by topical application

Traditional Properties:

Enters: SP, LV, HT

Properties: SW, CL

Indications:

CANCER/TUMORS/SWELLINGS/ LUMPS
• SWELLINGS: Topical
FLUID DISORDERS
• EDEMA, SEVERE: Excess Constitution
HEMORRHAGIC DISORDERS
• EPISTAXIS: Blood Heat
• HEMAFECIA: Blood Heat

• HEMATEMESIS: Blood Heat, Very Good
• HEMATURIA: Blood Heat
• HEMOPTYSIS: Blood Heat, Very Good
• HEMORRHAGE: Cool Blood To Stop
SEXUALITY, FEMALE:

GYNECOLOGICAL
• LEUKORRHEA
• MENORRHAGIA
• UTERINE BLEEDING: Blood Heat
SKIN
• ABSCESS: Topical
• FURUNCLES, DEEP ROOTED
• SORES: Topical

Clinical/Pharmaceutical Studies:

BLOOD RELATED DISORDERS/ TOPICS
- BLOOD PRESSURE, LOWERS: Both ETOH/Water Exts

CIRCULATION DISORDERS
- HYPERTENSION: 1-12 Weeks,

Reduce Diastolic Pressuer 10-20mm Hg For Most

HEMORRHAGIC DISORDERS
- HEMOSTATIC: Charred Herb

INFECTIOUS DISEASES

- BACTERIAL, ANTI-

KIDNEYS
- DIURETIC

TRAUMA, BITES, POISONINGS
- INFLAMMATORY, ANTI-

Dose
4.5 - 15.0 gm

Common Name
Japanese Thistle

Contraindications
Not: Cold Def SP/ST

Notes
External For Sores

DI YU   地榆   *RADIX SANGUISORBAE OFFICINALIS*

Traditional Functions:

1. Cools the Blood and controls bleeding
2. Dispels Heat and promotes healing of burns and sores by topical application
3. Stops diarrhea

Traditional Properties:

Enters: LI, ST, LV,

Properties: BIT, SO, <C

Indications:

ABDOMEN/ GASTROINTESTINAL TOPICS
- APPENDICITIS W/PAIN

BOWEL RELATED DISORDERS
- DIARRHEA: Damp Heat
- DYSENTERY: Blood Heat
- DYSENTERY-LIKE DISORDERS W/BLEEDING: Damp Heat
- HEMORRHOIDS, BLOODY STOOL: Damp Heat
- HEMORRHOIDS, PAIN, SWELLING

HEMORRHAGIC DISORDERS
- BLEEDING, ANY TYPE: Hot, Cold, Deficient, *Use w/Huai Hua

Mi For Lower Jiao Bleedng
- EPISTAXIS
- HEMAFECIA: Damp Heat
- HEMATEMESIS
- HEMATURIA
- HEMORRHAGE. Cool Blood To Stop

SEXUALITY, FEMALE: GYNECOLOGICAL
- MENORRHAGIA
- UTERINE BLEEDING: Damp Heat

SKIN
- ABSCESS, EXTERNAL
- BURNS: Good Topical, Decreases Oozing, Promotes Healing, *w/

Huang Lian
- SCALDS: Topical
- SORES: Topical
- ULCERS, SKIN: Topical

STOMACH/DIGESTIVE DISORDERS
- ULCERS, PEPTIC

TRAUMA, BITES, POISONINGS
- INSECT BITES: Topical
- SNAKE BITES: Topical

TRIPLE WARMER (SAN JIAO)
- LOWER BURNER, BLEEDING: Use w/Huai Hua Mi
- LOWER BURNER, BLEEDING W/ DAMP HEAT

Clinical/Pharmaceutical Studies:

- ASTRINGENT: Wounds, Reduces Exudate

ABDOMEN/ GASTROINTESTINAL TOPICS
- GASTROINTESTINAL, UPPER BLEEDING: Equal Amounts Of Di Yu, Tu Jing Jie, 4 Tabs, 0.25 g Each, 3-4x/Day/Radix Fibrosae Coptidis, Di Yu, Ce Bai Ye, Hai Piao Xiao As Cooled, Concentrated Decoction (Not With Stomach Cancer With Prolonged Blood In Stool) / Xiao Xue San, Too

BLOOD RELATED

ENDOCRINE RELATED DISORDERS
- HORMONES: Lengthens Estrus Of Mice

HEMORRHAGIC DISORDERS
- HEMOSTATIC: When Charred/Extract/Powdered

INFECTIOUS DISEASES
- ANTIBIOTIC: Many, Some Flu, Strongly-- Pneumoniae, Pseudomonas, B.Typhi, Shigella Dysenteriae, But Heat Destroys This Effect
- VIRAL, ANTI-: Some Asian Flus

LUNGS

Days, 4 Applications/ Course, Stop For 5 Days Between Courses, Omit Treatment 5 Days Before, After Menstrual Period, Usually 1-3 Courses Needed, About 50% Cured
- UTERINE BLEEDING: With Bai Tou Weng/ Another--Decoct Herb In Vinegar, Water, 1:1

SKIN
- BURNS: Powder For 2nd/ 3rd/May Use In Petroleum Jelly, 3%
- BURNS/SCALDS: Topical--Hong Yu Ointment (Zi Cao, Dang

Petroleum Jelly
- ECZEMA, INFANTILE ACUTE/SUBACUTE, SEBORRHEIC: Roast Herb Over Low Heat, Powder, Make 30% Ointment With Vaseline, May Need To Clean Skin With 1:8000 Potassium Permanganate, Then Apply, May Use Cooled 10% Decoction Of Uncured Herb As Wet Compress
- FUNGAL, ANTI-
- PURPURA, CHILDHOOD
- ULCERS, BLEEDING

STOMACH/DIGESTIVE

Clinical/Pharmaceutical Studies:

DISORDERS/TOPICS
- **BLOOD PRESSURE, LOWERS:** Slightly, Temporarily

BOWEL RELATED DISORDERS
- **DYSENTERY, BACILLARY:** 0.17 g Tabs, 6, 3x/Day, 7 Days

CHILDHOOD DISORDERS
- **PURPURA, CHILDHOOD**

- **TUBERCULOSIS, PULMONARY W/ HEMOPTYSIS**

SEXUALITY, FEMALE: GYNECOLOGICAL
- **CERVIX, EROSION OF:** 2 Pills (Di Yu, Huai Hua, Alum, Long Gu) Inserted Deep Into Vagina In Evening, After 0.1% Potassium Permanganate Solution Cleanse, 1x/2

Gui, Di Yu, Bing Pian, Gan Cao) Plus Antibiotics To Control Infection, Dressing Changed/6-7 Days, If Infection/2-3 Days, Took 6-8 Dressings, Relieved Pain, Too/May Make Ointment With Stir-Fried Herb Powder With 50% Sesame Oil, Good Analgesic Effect
- **ECZEMA:** Soaks/30% Roasted Di Yu And

DISORDERS
- **ANTIEMETIC:** For Digitalis Induced But Not Apomorphine Induced Vomiting
- **DIGESTION, ENHANCES:** 4x Protein Digestion
- **VOMITING:** Antiemetic, For Digitalis Induced But Not Apomorphine Induced Vomiting

Dose
9 - 15 gm

Common Name
Burnet-Bloodwort Root

Contraindications
Not: Cold Def
Not: Large Burns, Ointment Can Cause Toxic Infection If Absorbed
Not: With Qi Descending Bleeding
Not: Cold/Weak Persons

FU LONG GAN
(ZAO XIN TU)

伏龍肝
（伏龙肝）

TERRA FLAVA USTA

Traditional Functions:

1. Warms the Blood and stops bleeding
2. Arrests deficient Spleen diarrhea
3. Warms the Middle, harmonizes the Stomach and controls vomiting

Traditional Properties:

Enters: SP, ST,

Properties: SP, W

Indications:

ABDOMEN/ GASTROINTESTINAL TOPICS
- **SMALL INTESTINE, BLEEDING:** Cold Deficient

BOWEL RELATED DISORDERS
- **DIARRHEA, CHRONIC:** Spleen Deficient

HEMORRHAGIC DISORDERS
- **EPISTAXIS**
- **GASTROINTESTINAL BLEEDING, CHRONIC**

- **HEMAFECIA**
- **HEMATURIA**
- **HEMOPTYSIS**
- **HEMORRHAGE:** Cold Deficient, Warming Channels To Stop

SEXUALITY, FEMALE: GYNECOLOGICAL
- **LEUKORRHEA, BLOOD TINGED**
- **MENSTRUATION, DISORDERS OF:** Calm Chong, Lower Reflux
- **MORNING SICKNESS:**

Gestational Foul Obstruction--Cold
- **UTERINE BLEEDING**

STOMACH/DIGESTIVE DISORDERS
- **HICCUPS:** Qi Deficiency-Cold
- **REGURGITATION**
- **STOMACH, BLEEDING:** Cold Deficient
- **VOMITING:** Qi Deficiency-Cold/ Stomach Cold

Clinical/Pharmaceutical Studies:

HEMORRHAGIC DISORDERS
- **HEMOSTATIC**

KIDNEYS
- **DIURETIC**

LIVER

- **TOXINS, LIVER:** Helps To Detoxify

STOMACH/DIGESTIVE DISORDERS

- **ANTIEMETIC:** Counteracts Digitalis, Not Apomorphine

TRAUMA, BITES, POISONINGS
- **DETOXIFIES:** Acidosis, Liver

Dose
15 - 60 gm

Common Name
Old Clay From Stove

Contraindications
Not: Bleeding With Def Yin w/Heat
Not: Nausea/Vomiting w/Heat

HUA RUI SHI   花蕊石   OPHICALCITUM

Traditional Functions:

1. Stops bleeding and vitalizes congealed blood

Traditional Properties:

Enters: LV,

Properties: SO, A, N

Indications:

**CANCER/TUMORS/SWELLINGS/
LUMPS**
• TUMORS: Blood Stasis, Herbs
  Used Other Than Vitalize Blood
HEMORRHAGIC DISORDERS
• EPISTAXIS
• HEMAFECIA
• HEMATEMESIS

• HEMOPTYSIS
• HEMORRHAGE: Blood Stasis
  Caused, Charred/Fried Herbs
**SEXUALITY, FEMALE:
GYNECOLOGICAL**
• AMENORRHEA: Blood Stasis, In
  Addition To Vitalize Blood Herbs
• POSTPARTUM, ABDOMINAL

PAIN: Blood Stasis
• POSTPARTUM, SYNCOPE:
  Excess Blood Loss
• UTERINE BLEEDING
TRAUMA, BITES, POISONINGS
• TRAUMA, INJURIES: Die Da
• WOUNDS: Topical

Dose

3 - 15 gm

Common Name

Ophicalcite

Contraindications

Not: Pregnancy

Notes

San Qi-Like
Powder: 1-3 gm, Max: 6-9 gm

HUAI HUA MI
(HUAI HUA)   槐花米   FLOS SOPHORAE JAPONICAE IMMATURUS

Traditional Functions:

1. Cools the Blood and stops bleeding, clearing Damp Heat in the Large
Intestine, primarily
2. Cools Liver Heat

Traditional Properties:

Enters: LI, IV,

Properties: BIT, CL

Indications:

**ABDOMEN/
GASTROINTESTINAL TOPICS**
• LARGE INTESTINE, DAMP HEAT
  W/BLEEDNG
BOWEL RELATED DISORDERS
• DYSENTERY-LIKE DISORDERS
  W/BLEEDING: Damp Heat
• HEMORRHOIDS, BLOODY
  STOOL: Damp Heat
• HEMORRHOIDS, PAIN,
  SWELLING

CIRCULATION DISORDERS
• HYPERTENSION
EARS/HEARING DISORDERS
• VERTIGO: Liver Yang/Fire Rising
EYES
• EYES, RED, CONGESTED: Liver
  Heat
HEMORRHAGIC DISORDERS
• EPISTAXIS
• HEMAFECIA
• HEMATEMESIS

• HEMATURIA
• HEMOPTYSIS
• HEMORRHAGE: Cool Blood To
  Stop
LIVER
• LIVER WIND HEAT: Red Eyes/
  Dizziness
**SEXUALITY, FEMALE:
GYNECOLOGICAL**
• MENORRHAGIA
• UTERINE BLEEDING

Clinical/Pharmaceutical Studies:

**ABDOMEN/
GASTROINTESTINAL TOPICS**
• ULCERS, INTESTINAL:
  Stimulates Increase Of Effusion
**BLOOD RELATED DISORDERS/
TOPICS**
• BLOOD PRESSURE, LOWERS
• CHOLESTEROL, LOWERS
CIRCULATION DISORDERS
• CAPILLARIES, DECREASE
  LEAKAGE FROM

HEART
• CARDIOTONIC
• CORONARY ARTERIES,
  DILATES
HEMORRHAGIC DISORDERS
• HEMORRHAGE: Rutin
• HEMOSTATIC: Shortens Bleeding
  Time
**IMMUNE SYSTEM RELATED
DISORDERS/TOPICS**
• ALLERGIC RESPONSE, ARTHUS

ACCIDENTS: Help Prevent With
Vit C
**MUSCULOSKELETAL/
CONNECTIVE TISSUE**
• ANTISPASMODIC: Intestines,
  Bronchi, Stomach
• MUSCLES, SMOOTH RELAXES
  LU/LI: Decrease Tension
**NUTRITIONAL/METABOLIC
DISORDERS/TOPICS**
• RUTIN MAIN INGREDIENT

Clinical/Pharmaceutical Studies:

- HYPERTENSION: (Rutin Content) Use With Vit C
- STROKE: Rutin

FLUID DISORDERS
- EDEMA, REDUCES: Inhibits ATPase In Cell Membrane

PHENOMENON, DECREASES

INFECTIOUS DISEASES
- BACTERIAL, ANTI-

MENTAL STATE/ NEUROLOGICAL DISORDERS
- CEREBROVASCULAR

SKIN
- FUNGAL, ANTI-: Aqueous Extract

TRAUMA, BITES, POISONINGS
- INFLAMMATORY, ANTI-: Inhibits Edema And Reddening

Dose

6 - 15 gm

Common Name

Pagoda Tree Flower Bud

Contraindications

Not: Def SP/ST

Notes

One Known Case Of Anaphylactic Reaction After Oral Dose

JIANG XIANG
(JIANG ZHEN XIAN)

降香

LIGNUM DALBERGIAE ODORIFERAE
(ACRONYCHIAE)

Traditional Functions:

1. Moves stagnation and controls bleeding
2. Vitalizes the Blood, promotes Qi circulation and relieves pain

Traditional Properties:

Enters: SP, ST, LV, PC

Properties: SP, W

Indications:

ABDOMEN/ GASTROINTESTINAL TOPICS
- ABDOMEN, PAIN OF: Stagnant Qi

CHEST
- CHEST, PAIN: Congealed Blood

HEART
- ANGINA PECTORIS: Chest Bi

Strangulating Pain

STOMACH/DIGESTIVE DISORDERS
- EPIGASTRIC PAIN: Stagnant Qi
- GASTROSIS

TRAUMA, BITES, POISONINGS
- CONTUSIONS

- FRACTURES
- LACERATIONS, BLEEDING: Topical
- SPRAINS
- TRAUMA, INTERNAL
- WOUNDS, BLEEDING

Clinical/Pharmaceutical Studies:

HEART
- CARDIOTONIC: Increased Heart

Output

HEMORRHAGIC DISORDERS

- BLEEDING: Clotting Time, Mildly Lengthens From Oral Dose

Dose

3 - 6 gm

Common Name

Acronychia

LIAN FANG

連房
(连房)

RECEPTACULUM NELUMBINIS NUCIFERAE

Traditional Functions:

1. Disperses stagnation and stops bleeding
2. Stops bleeding and calms the restless fetus
3. Controls childhood diarrhea with Summer Heat and Dampness

Traditional Properties:

Enters: SP, KI, LV,

Properties: BIT, A, W

Indications:

ABDOMEN/ GASTROINTESTINAL TOPICS
- ABDOMEN, PAIN OF: Blood Stasis

CANCER/TUMORS/SWELLINGS/

HEMORRHAGIC DISORDERS
- HEMAFECIA
- HEMATURIA
- HEMORRHAGE: Blood Stasis Caused, Charred/Fried Herbs

- MENORRHAGIA
- MISCARRIAGE, THREATENED
- PLACENTA, RETENTION
- UTERINE BLEEDING

SKIN

Indications:

LUMPS
• CERVICAL CANCER
HEAT
• SUMMER HEAT DAMPNESS:
Diarrhea In Children

SEXUALITY, FEMALE:
GYNECOLOGICAL
• FETUS, RESTLESS: Threatened
Abortion, Blood Deficiency

• PEMPHIGUS: Autoimmune
Disease
URINARY BLADDER
• URODYNIA

Clinical/Pharmaceutical Studies:

**HEMORRHAGIC
DISORDERS**

• HEMOSTATIC: Reduces
Bleeding Time, Charred

Herb Even More So
INFECTIOUS DISEASES

• BACTERIAL, ANTI-:
Staph Aureus

Dose
3 - 9 gm

Common Name
Mature Lotus Receptacle

Notes
Fresh For Summer Heat

OU JIE

藕節
（藕节）

RHIZOMA
NELUMBINIS NUCIFERAE
RHIZOMATIS

Traditional Functions:

1. Astringes and arrests bleeding

Traditional Properties:

Enters: LU, ST, LV,

Properties: SW, A, N

Indications:

BOWEL RELATED DISORDERS
• DYSENTERY, BLOODY STOOL
HEMORRHAGIC DISORDERS
• BLEEDING, CHRONIC
• EPISTAXIS
• HEMAFECIA
• HEMATEMESIS

• HEMATURIA
• HEMOPTYSIS
• HEMORRHAGE: Astringe To Stop
LUNGS
• LUNGS, BLEEDING
SEXUALITY, FEMALE:

GYNECOLOGICAL
• MENORRHAGIA
• UTERINE BLEEDING
**STOMACH/DIGESTIVE
DISORDERS**
• STOMACH, BLEEDING

Clinical/Pharmaceutical Studies:

HEMORRHAGIC DISORDERS

• HEMOSTATIC

Dose
9 - 30 gm

Common Name
Lotus Rhizome Node

Notes
Safe: Won't Cause Blood Stasis

Charred Even Stronger For Hemostat Applications

PU HUANG

蒲黄
（蒲黄）

POLLEN
TYPHAE

Traditional Functions:

1. Stops bleeding by cooling and vitalizing Blood
2. Relieves pain, vitalizes and disperses stagnant Blood
3. Promotes urination

Traditional Properties:

Enters: PC, LV,

Properties: SW, N

Indications:

ABDOMEN/ GASTROINTESTINAL TOPICS
- ABDOMEN, PAIN OF: Use Raw
- ABDOMEN, PAIN OF, SHARP

BLOOD RELATED DISORDERS/TOPICS
- BLOOD, QI, SLUGGISH FLOW OF: Raw

BOWEL RELATED DISORDERS
- DYSENTERY, BLOODY STOOL: Fried, Black

CANCER/TUMORS/ SWELLINGS/LUMPS
- SWELLINGS, TOXIC: Raw
- TUMORS: Blood Stasis, Herbs Used Other Than Vitalize Blood

CHEST
- CHEST, PAIN: Blood Stasis

EARS/HEARING DISORDERS
- EARS, BLEEDING: Topical
- EARS, OTITIS MEDIA: Topical

HEART
- ANGINA PECTORIS: Chest Bi Strangulating Pain
- HEART PAIN, SHARP

HEMORRHAGIC DISORDERS
- BLEEDING, SUBCUTANEOUS
- EPISTAXIS: Fried, Black
- HEMAFECIA: Fried, Black
- HEMATEMESIS: Fried, Black
- HEMATURIA
- HEMOPTYSIS
- HEMORRHAGE: Blood Stasis Caused, Charred/ Fried Herbs/Cool Blood To

Stop

INFECTIOUS DISEASES
- SCROFULA

ORAL CAVITY
- ULCERS, ORAL: Topical

SEXUALITY, EITHER SEX
- GENITALS, PRURITUS, DAMP: Topical

SEXUALITY, FEMALE: GYNECOLOGICAL
- AMENORRHEA: Blood Stasis, In Addition To Vitalize Blood Herbs, Use Raw
- DYSMENORRHEA: Blood Stasis
- LEUKORRHEA: Fried, Black
- MENORRHAGIA: Fried, Black
- MENSTRUATION, DISORDERS OF: Constrict Uterus, Stimulate Chong

- POSTPARTUM, ABDOMINAL PAIN: Blood Stasis
- UTERINE BLEEDING

SKIN
- ABSCESS
- CARBUNCLES: Fried Black, Only
- FURUNCLES: Raw

STOMACH/DIGESTIVE DISORDERS
- STOMACH, PAIN: Sharp, Use Raw

TRAUMA, BITES, POISONINGS
- TRAUMA, BLEEDING: Raw
- TRAUMA, INJURIES: Die Da

URINARY BLADDER
- URINATION, PAINFUL, DRIBBLING, CONCENTRATED, RED/ YELLOW/TURBID

Clinical/Pharmaceutical Studies:

ABDOMEN/ GASTROINTESTINAL TOPICS
- ABDOMEN, PAIN OF, CHRONIC COLITIS: With Wu Ling Zhi, Baked Ge Gen, Baked Rou Dou Dou
- PERISTALSIS, INCREASES

BLOOD RELATED DISORDERS/ TOPICS
- BLOOD CLOTTING TIME, SHORTENS: Oral Of Aqueous Extract/50% ETOH Extract, Carbonized Herb Even Stronger
- BLOOD PRESSURE, LOWERS: Large Doses
- CHOLESTEROL, LOWERS: Inhibits Intestinal Absorption, Reduces Platelet Adhesion Rate, Granules Reduces, Too

CIRCULATION DISORDERS
- HYPERTENSION: Pu Huang, Dang Shen, Hong Hua, Jiang Huang, E Zhu, Lignum Dalbergiae Odoriferae/Pu Huang Tab, Excellent For 1ST-2nd Stage, 90% Effective

HEART
- ANGINA PECTORIS: Modified Shi Xiao San
- HEART, HYPERLIPIDEMIC: As Tablet

HEMORRHAGIC DISORDERS

- EPISTAXIS: By Itself/With Xiao Ji, Hua Shi, Charred With, Shu Di, Charred Ce Bai Ye
- HEMAFECIA: By Itself/With Xiao Ji, Hua Shi, Charred With, Shu Di, Charred Ce Bai Ye, *With Wu Ling Zhi, Baked Ge Gen, Baked Rou Dou Dou
- HEMATURIA
- HEMOPTYSIS: By Itself/With Xiao Ji, Hua Shi, Charred With, Shu Di, Charred Ce Bai Ye
- HEMOSTATIC: Water/Alcohol Extracts, Orally, Increase Platelet Count, Speed Coagulation, Charred Even Stronger

INFECTIOUS DISEASES
- BACTERIAL, ANTI-: TB

KIDNEYS
- DIURETIC

LUNGS
- ASTHMA
- TUBERCULOSIS: May Be Used To Cure TB

ORAL CAVITY
- MOUTH, FUNGAL INFECTIONS: From Antibiotic Useage, Topical

SEXUALITY, FEMALE: GYNECOLOGICAL
- ABORTION, INDUCES: Mid-Term

Pregnancy, Give Extra Amniotically, Usually Within 33 Hrs, One Dose, Some May Need 2-3 Doses, Plus Oxytocin
- LEUKORRHEA: By Itself/With Xiao Ji, Hua Shi, Charred With, Shu Di, Charred Ce Bai Ye
- POSTPARTUM, ABDOMINAL CRAMPS: With Wu Ling Zhi
- POSTPARTUM, BLOOD RETENTION: With Wu Ling Zhi
- UTERINE BLEEDING: By Itself/ With Xiao Ji, Hua Shi, Charred With, Shu Di, Charred Ce Bai Ye
- UTERUS, STIMULATES: Especially Non-Pregnant/Postpartum, Large Dose Can Cause Spasmodic Contraction

SKIN
- ECZEMA: Topical Powder, 6-15 Days To Cure

TRAUMA, BITES, POISONINGS
- INFLAMMATORY, ANTI-: Topical Decoction, Striking Effect

URINARY BLADDER
- URETHRITIS: Pu Huang San (Pu Huang, Semen Malval Verticillatae, Sheng Di, Equal Amounts)
- URINATION, PAINFUL

Dose
4.5 - 12.0 gm
Common Name
Cattail Pollen

Precautions
Watch: Pregnancy
Notes
Raw: Stops Pain, Blood Stagnation
Charred: Hemostatic
Some May Have Dizziness, Diarrhea

QIAN CAO GEN
茜草根
RADIX RUBIAE CORDIFOLIAE

Traditional Functions:
1. Cools the Blood and controls bleeding
2. Vitalizes the Blood and expels congealed Blood

Traditional Properties:
Enters: HT, LV,

Properties: BIT, C

Indications:

ABDOMEN/ GASTROINTESTINAL TOPICS
• ABDOMEN, PAIN OF: From Amenorrhea
• FLANK PAIN: Blood Stasis
CANCER/TUMORS/ SWELLINGS/LUMPS
• SWELLINGS, PAIN: Blood Stasis
CHEST
• CHEST, PAIN: Blood Stasis
GALL BLADDER
• GALL BLADDER, STONES

HEMORRHAGIC DISORDERS
• BLEEDING: Blood Heat
• EPISTAXIS
• HEMAFECIA: Blood Heat
• HEMATEMESIS: Blood Heat
• HEMATURIA
• HEMOPTYSIS
• HEMORRHAGE: Blood Stasis Caused, Charred/ Fried Herbs
LIVER
• HEPATOMEGALY
LUNGS

• BRONCHITIS, CHRONIC
MUSCULOSKELETAL/ CONNECTIVE TISSUE
• JOINTS, PAIN
ORAL CAVITY
• ABSCESS, THROAT
SEXUALITY, FEMALE/ GYNECOLOGICAL
• AMENORRHEA
• LOCHIA, DESCENDS
• MENORRHAGIA
• MENSTRUATION, DISORDERS OF: Constrict Uterus, Stimulate Chong

• UTERINE BLEEDING: Blood Heat
SKIN
• ABSCESS, EARLY STAGE
• RASHES, W/PRURITUS: Blood Heat, Wind
SPLEEN
• SPLENOMEGALY
TRAUMA, BITES, POISONINGS
• INJURIES, EXTERNAL
• TRAUMA, PAIN
URINARY BLADDER
• URINARY TRACT STONES

Clinical/Pharmaceutical Studies:

ABDOMEN/ GASTROINTESTINAL TOPICS
• INTESTINES, INHIBITS CONTRACTION
BLOOD RELATED DISORDERS/TOPICS
• BLOOD PRESSURE, LOWERS
HEMORRHAGIC DISORDERS
• EPISTAXIS: From Injury, Local Application
• HEMOSTATIC, MILD: Local Application With Gauze For 35 Seconds, Charred Herb Better
INFECTIOUS DISEASES
• ANTIBIOTIC: Flu, Staph,

Strep, Pneumococci
• VIRAL, ANTI-: Some Flu
KIDNEYS
• DIURETIC
• KIDNEY STONES: Helps Prevent Formation Of
LIVER
• HEPATITIS, CHRONIC: Hepatomegaly/ Splenomegaly
LUNGS
• ANTITUSSIVE: Marked From Oral Decoction, Not Tinctures
• BRONCHITIS, CHRONIC: Decoction With Qing Pi, More Effective With Asthmatic

Than Simple Type, Controlled Rales, Wheezing
• EXPECTORANT: Marked From Oral Decoction, Not Tinctures
ORAL CAVITY
• TOOTH EXTRACTION, BLEEDING OF: Local Application Of Powder, Stopped 1-2 Minutes
SEXUALITY, FEMALE: GYNECOLOGICAL
• MENORRHAGIA: 90 g Decoction Added To Yellow Wine, Brown Sugar, 2 Days Of Daily Treatment

• UTERUS, STIMULATES: Causes Contractions During Labor
SKIN
• FUNGAL, ANTI-: Some Skin
TRAUMA, BITES, POISONINGS
• INFLAMMATORY, ANTI-
URINARY BLADDER
• URINARY BLADDER STONES: Helps Passage Of, Helps To Prevent Formation Of, Especially Calcium Carbonate Stones, But Removes By Stimulation Of Muscles In Bladder

Dose
6 - 15 gm

Common Name
Madder Root

Contraindications
Not: Cold Def SP/ST

Notes
May Cause Urine, Milk To Have Pink Color
Prolonged Nausea, Mild Blood Pressure Increase With
Oral Use

SAN QI HUA   三七花   FLOS PSEUDOGINSENG

Traditional Functions:
1. Pacifies the Liver and reduces hypertension

Traditional Properties:
Enters: LV

Properties: SW, CL

Indications:

CIRCULATION DISORDERS
• HYPERTENSION
EARS/HEARING DISORDERS

• DIZZINESS: Hypertension
• TINNITUS: Hypertension
• VERTIGO: Hypertension

ORAL CAVITY
• THROAT, SORE: Acute

Common Name
Pseudoginseng Flower

SAN QI   三七   RADIX PSEUDOGINSENG
(TIAN QI)

Traditional Functions:
1. Controls bleeding and releases stagnation
2. Vitalizes Blood, reduces swelling and relieves pain

Traditional Properties:
Enters: LI, ST, LV,

Properties: SW, <BIT, <W

Indications:

ABDOMEN/
GASTROINTESTINAL TOPICS
• ABDOMEN, PAIN OF, COLD:
Throbbing, Blood Stasis
BOWEL RELATED DISORDERS
• RECTAL BLEEDING
CANCER/TUMORS/SWELLINGS/
LUMPS
• TUMORS: Blood Stasis, Herbs
Used Other Than Vitalize Blood
CHEST
• CHEST, PAIN: Throbbing
HEART
• ANGINA PECTORIS: Chest Bi
Strangulating Pain
HEMORRHAGIC DISORDERS
• BLEEDING, GENERAL
INTERNAL/EXTERNAL

• EPISTAXIS
• HEMAFECIA
• HEMATEMESIS
• HEMATURIA
• HEMOPTYSIS
• HEMORRHAGE: Blood Stasis
Caused, Charred/Fried Herbs/
Deficiency Caused
LUNGS
• COUGH, LUNG EXHAUSTION W/
HEMORRHAGE
MUSCULOSKELETAL/
CONNECTIVE TISSUE
• JOINTS, PAIN: Blood Stasis/
Ecchymosis
SEXUALITY, FEMALE:
GYNECOLOGICAL
• AMENORRHEA: Blood Stasis, In

Addition To Vitalize Blood Herbs
• MENORRHAGIA: Avalanche &
Leakage (w/Other Herbs)
• POSTPARTUM, ABDOMINAL
PAIN: Blood Stasis
• POSTPARTUM, PROMOTES
BLOOD CIRCULATION
• UTERINE BLEEDING
SKIN
• ABSCESS, PAIN
TRAUMA, BITES, POISONINGS
• CONTUSIONS
• FRACTURES
• SPRAINS
• SWELLING, PAIN, FALLS
• TRAUMA, BLEEDING
• WOUNDS, PAIN, SWELLING

Clinical/Pharmaceutical Studies:

ABDOMEN/
GASTROINTESTINAL
TOPICS
• GASTROINTESTINAL,

HEMORRHAGE: 1%
Solution Into Eyes, 1-6
Days, 2-10% Worked
Better At Stopping

• MYOCARDIAL
INFARCTION: Mycardial
Infarction
HEMORRHAGIC

ml 50% Dextrose,
Injection 1x/Day, 2-4
Weeks
LIVER

Clinical/Pharmaceutical Studies:

CROHN'S DISEASE:
Crohn's Disease--
Powdered, 10 Days For
Acute Condition To Pass
**BLOOD RELATED
DISORDERS/TOPICS**
• BLOOD GLUCOSE,
REDUCES
• BLOOD PRESSURE,
LOWERS: Significantly
• CHOLESTEROL,
LOWERS: Varies, Take
Daily
• HYPERLIPIDEMIA:
Worked Equal To
Clofibrate, No Side Effects
• THROMBOCYTOPENIC
PURPURA
**CANCER/TUMORS/
SWELLINGS/LUMPS**
• TUMOR, ANTI-
EYES
• CORNEAL BURNS
• INTRAOCULAR

Bleeding
HEAD/NECK
• HEAD, TRAUMA: Good
For Mild To Moderate
Cases
HEART
• ANGINA PECTORIS:
San Qi Guan Xin Pian (San
Qi, Yan Hu Suo, Hong Hua,
He Shou Wu, Ji Xue Teng,
Mo Ya) , 73% Stopped/
Reduced Nitroglycerin, 4
Weeks Or Fu Fang San Qi
(San Qi, Chi Shao) w/
Angina
• CORONARY HEART
DISEASE: 1-12 Courses
Of 4 Weeks/Course, 1 gm,
3x/Day Or Fu Fang San Qi
(San Qi, Chi Shao) w/
Angina
• HEART, INCREASES
CORONARY BLOOD
FLOW

DISORDERS
• HEMATURIA: 3 Days,
0.9-1.5 g, 1x/4-8 Hrs, Oral
• HEMOPTYSIS:
Bronchiectasis, TB, Lung
Abscess, 6-9 g, 2-3x/Day, 5
Days
• HEMOSTATIC: Liver
Mediates, Oral Ingestion
**IMMUNE SYSTEM
RELATED DISORDERS/
TOPICS**
• IMMUNE SYSTEM
ENHANCEMENT
INFECTIOUS DISEASES
• ANTIBIOTIC: Norwalk
Virus
• VIRAL, ANTI-
KIDNEYS
• DIURETIC: Increase
Urine Output 5x
• NEPHRITIS, ACUTE
INFANTILE: MEOH
Extract, 20mg/2ml In 50

• HEPATITIS, CHRONIC:
Lowers SGPT, 1 g, 3x/Day,
1 Month
**MUSCULOSKELETAL/
CONNECTIVE TISSUE**
• ARTHRITIS:
Antiinflammatory,
Significant
SKIN
• FUNGAL, ANTI-: Some
**TRAUMA, BITES,
POISONINGS**
• HEAD, TRAUMA: Good
For Mild To Moderate
Cases
• INFLAMMATORY, ANTI-
• TRAUMA, HEAD
INJURIES: Good For
Mild To Moderate Cases, 3
g Orally, 2-3x/Day, 3-10
Days, Max 21 Days,
Accelerated Recovery, 75%
Effective

Dose
0.9 - 9.0 gm

Common Name
Pseudoginseng Root

Contraindications
Not: Pregnancy

Precautions
Watch: Def Blood

Notes
Will Not Congeal Blood

Powder: 1-3 gm, 2-3x/Day

Large (>5g) May Affect Heart Rate

SHAN ZI CAO
(JI CAI)

扇子草

**HERBA
CAPSELLAE**

Traditional Functions:

1. Clears Heat from the Blood and controls bleeding
2. Harmonizes the Spleen
3. Clears Heat and promotes urination
4. Clears the vision and brings the Liver Yang down

Traditional Properties:

Enters: LV, ST, UB

Properties: SW, CL

Indications:

BOWEL RELATED DISORDERS
• DYSENTERY, RED
CIRCULATION DISORDERS
• HYPERTENSION
FLUID DISORDERS
• EDEMA, NEPHRITIC
HEMORRHAGIC DISORDERS

• HEMAFECIA
• HEMATURIA
• HEMOPTYSIS
SEXUALITY, EITHER SEX
• GENITAL BLEEDING,
ABNORMAL
SEXUALITY, FEMALE:

GYNECOLOGICAL
• MENORRHAGIA,
INFLAMMATION DURING
• POSTPARTUM, BLEEDING
• UTERINE BLEEDING
URINARY BLADDER
• URINARY INFECTIONS

Clinical/Pharmaceutical Studies:

**ABDOMEN/
GASTROINTESTINAL TOPICS**
• SMALL INTESTINE,
CONTRACTS SMOOTH
MUSCLES OF
BLOOD RELATED DISORDERS/

TRUNK
HEART
• CORONARY ARTERIES,
DILATES
HEMORRHAGIC DISORDERS
• HEMOSTATIC

**MENTAL STATE/
NEUROLOGICAL DISORDERS**
• SEDATIVE: Synergistic With
Barbituates
SEXUALITY, FEMALE:
GYNECOLOGICAL

Clinical/Pharmaceutical Studies:

TOPICS
- BLOOD PRESSURE, LOWERS

FEVERS
- ANTIPYRETIC

FLUID DISORDERS
- EDEMA, INHIBITS IN LOWER

KIDNEYS
- DIURETIC

LUNGS
- BRONCHI, CONTRACTS SMOOTH MUSCLES OF
- RESPIRATION, EXCITES

- UTERUS, STIMULATES: Similar To Ergot, Oxytocin

STOMACH/DIGESTIVE DISORDERS
- ULCERS, STRESS: Increases Healing Of

Dose
3 - 15 gm

Common Name
Shepherd's Purse

Notes
May Be Used Singly

XIAN HE CAO

仙鶴草
（仙鹤草）

HERBA AGRIMONIAE PILOSAE

Traditional Functions:

1. Cools Blood, arrests bleeding
2. Relieves dysentery
3. Kills parasites
4. Clears Heat from the Liver and dissipates nodules

Traditional Properties:

Enters: LU, SP, LV,

Properties: BIT, SP, N, A

Indications:

BOWEL RELATED DISORDERS
- DIARRHEA: Suppository
- DYSENTERY: Blood Heat

HEMORRHAGIC DISORDERS
- BLEEDING, ANY TYPE: Hot, Cold, Deficient
- EPISTAXIS: Any Etiology
- HEMATEMESIS: Any Etiology
- HEMATURIA: Any Etiology
- HEMOPTYSIS: Any Etiology
- HEMORRHAGE, ALL TYPES/ LOCATIONS: Astringe To Stop/

Deficiency Caused
- MELENA

INFECTIOUS DISEASES
- MALARIA

LUNGS
- COUGH, LUNG EXHAUSTION W/ HEMORRHAGE

ORAL CAVITY
- GUMS, BLEEDING: Any Etiology

PARASITES
- TAPEWORMS: Suppository

SEXUALITY, FEMALE:

GYNECOLOGICAL
- MENORRHAGIA: Avalanche & Leakage (w/Other Herbs)
- TRICHOMONAS, VAGINAL
- UTERINE BLEEDING: Any Etiology

SKIN
- BOILS
- FURUNCLES, TOXIC
- SKIN, ULCERS

TRAUMA, BITES, POISONINGS
- TRAUMA, BLEEDING

Clinical/Pharmaceutical Studies:

- ASTRINGENT

ABDOMEN/ GASTROINTESTINAL TOPICS
- ENTERITIS

BLOOD RELATED DISORDERS/TOPICS
- BLOOD GLUCOSE, REDUCES
- BLOOD PRESSURE: Effect Dose Dependent, Cardiotonic, Peripheral Blood Vessel Constriction

CANCER/TUMORS/ SWELLINGS/LUMPS
- CANCER, ANTI-: Decoction Inhibits Growth Of Some Forms

EYES
- CONJUNCTIVITIS: Alcohol/Aqueous Extract, Antiinflammatory, Decoction Reduces Inflammation Of Chemical Or Bacterial Induced

HEART
- CARDIOTONIC: Regulates Heart Rate

HEMORRHAGIC DISORDERS
- HEMOSTATIC: Used In Surgery/Trauma As Powder, Equivocal Research

INFECTIOUS DISEASES
- ANTIBIOTIC: Gram

Positive, Staph A., Bac. Subtl., TB
- MALARIA: Inhibits Growth
- VIRAL, ANTI-: Alcohol Extract--Columbia Sk Virus

MUSCULOSKELETAL/ CONNECTIVE TISSUE
- MUSCLES, SMOOTH, INHIBITS, RELAXES

PAIN/NUMBNESS/ GENERAL DISCOMFORT
- ANALGESIC: Injected Large Doses, Aqueous/ Acid Extract

SEXUALITY, FEMALE:

GYNECOLOGICAL
- TRICHOMONAS, VAGINAL W/PRURITUS: 120 gm Herb In Decoction (200% Concentration) , Soak Cotton Ball Then In Vagina For 3-4 Hrs, 1x/ Day For 7 Days

STOMACH/DIGESTIVE DISORDERS
- FOOD POISONING: Vibrio Parahemolyticus, 30 g In Decoction

TRAUMA, BITES, POISONINGS
- INFLAMMATORY, ANTI-
- TRAUMA, BLEEDING

Dose

9 - 30 gm

Common Name

Agrimony

Notes

Can Cause Nausea/Vomiting

Use With Di Yu/Huai Hua

May Cause Palpitation, Facial Flushing

XIAO JI

小薊
(小薊)

HERBA CIRSII SEGETI

Traditional Functions:

1. Cools the Blood and controls bleeding in the urine
2. Promotes urination

Traditional Properties:

Enters: HT, LV,

Properties: SW, CL

Indications:

CIRCULATION DISORDERS
• HYPERTENSION
HEMORRHAGIC DISORDERS
• EPISTAXIS
• HEMAFECIA
• HEMATURIA
• HEMOPTYSIS
• HEMORRHAGE: Cool Blood To Stop
KIDNEYS

• NEPHRITIS
LIVER
• HEPATITIS, ACUTE, INFECTIOUS
ORAL CAVITY
• ABSCESS, THROAT
SEXUALITY, FEMALE:
GYNECOLOGICAL
• UTERINE BLEEDING
SKIN

• CARBUNCLES
• SKIN, INFECTIONS
TRAUMA, BITES, POISONINGS
• WOUNDS, BLEEDING
• WOUNDS, TOXIC
URINARY BLADDER
• URINATION, PAINFUL, DRIBBLING, CONCENTRATED, RED/YELLOW/TURBID

Clinical/Pharmaceutical Studies:

BLOOD RELATED DISORDERS/ TOPICS
• CHOLESTEROL, LOWERS
CIRCULATION DISORDERS
• HYPERTENSION: Action Is Long Acting, Strong
GALL BLADDER
• GALL BLADDER,

CHOLAGOGUE
HEMORRHAGIC DISORDERS
• HEMOSTATIC
INFECTIOUS DISEASES
• ANTIBIOTIC: Strep, Diplococcus, Diphtheriae, et al.
MENTAL STATE/

NEUROLOGICAL DISORDERS
• SEDATIVE
SEXUALITY, FEMALE:
GYNECOLOGICAL
• UTERUS, CONTRACTS
TRAUMA, BITES, POISONINGS
• INFLAMMATORY, ANTI-

Dose

9 - 18 gm

Common Name

Field Thistle

XUE YU TAN
(LUAN FA SHUANG)

血余炭

CRINIS CARBONISATUS

Traditional Functions:

1. Arrests bleeding
2. Promotes urination

Traditional Properties:

Enters: ST, KI, LV,

Properties: BIT, N

Indications:

BOWEL RELATED DISORDERS
• DYSENTERY, BLOODY STOOL
HEMORRHAGIC DISORDERS
• BLEEDING, MANY KINDS
• BLEEDING, SKIN

• HEMORRHAGE: Blood Stasis Caused, Charred/Fried Herbs
ORAL CAVITY
• GUMS, BLEEDING
• HOARSENESS

GYNECOLOGICAL
• MENORRHAGIA
• UTERINE BLEEDING
SKIN
• CARBUNCLES

Indications:

- EPISTAXIS
- HEMATEMESIS
- HEMATURIA

SEXUALITY, EITHER SEX
- GENITAL BLEEDING
SEXUALITY, FEMALE:

- FURUNCLES
URINARY BLADDER
- DYSURIA W/HEMATURIA

Clinical/Pharmaceutical Studies:

**HEMORRHAGIC
DISORDERS**
- HEMORRHAGE, ALL

TYPES/LOCATIONS:
Add Ou Jie Juice, 3x/Day
KIDNEYS

- DIURETIC
URINARY BLADDER

- DYSURIA W/
  HEMATURIA: w/Hua Shi

Dose

1.5 - 15.0 gm

Common Name

Charred Human Hair

Notes

When Used As Powder: 1-3 gm

ZI ZHU CAO
(ZI ZHU)

紫珠草

**FOLIUM
CALLICARPAE**

Traditional Functions:

1. Arrests bleeding
2. Treats burns

Traditional Properties:

Enters: SP, LV,

Properties: BIT, N

Indications:

HEMORRHAGIC DISORDERS
- BLEEDING, INTERNAL/
  EXTERNAL

- HEMATURIA: Especially Good
- HEMORRHAGE: Astringe To Stop/
  Cool Blood To Stop

SKIN
- BURNS

Clinical/Pharmaceutical Studies:

BOWEL RELATED DISORDERS
- HEMORRHOIDS: Direct Injection
HEMORRHAGIC DISORDERS
- HEMORRHAGE: Best Digestive,
  Respiratory, Mild Bleeding

- HEMOSTATIC: Increased Platelets,
  Shortens Bleeding Time
INFECTIOUS DISEASES
- ANTIBIOTIC: Shigella, Staph

Aureus
ORAL CAVITY
- TOOTH EXTRACTION: Stops
  Bleeding

Dose

15 - 30 gm

Vitalize The Blood

CHI SHAO YAO
(CHI SHAO)

赤芍藥
(赤芍药)

RADIX
PAEONIAE RUBRA

Traditional Functions:

1. Vitalizes the Blood, expels congealed Blood and reduces swelling
2. Clears Heat and cools the Blood
3. Clears Liver Fire

Traditional Properties:

Enters: SP, LV,

Properties: SO, BIT, <C

Indications:

**ABDOMEN/
GASTROINTESTINAL TOPICS**
• ABDOMEN, MASS, IMMOBILE
• ABDOMEN, PAIN OF
• ACCUMULATION
• APPENDICITIS W/PAIN
• HERNIA
• HERNIA, MASS
• SUBCOSTAL PAIN
BOWEL RELATED DISORDERS
• HEMORRHOIDS
**CANCER/TUMORS/SWELLINGS/
LUMPS**
• MASSES
• TUMORS: Blood Stasis, Herbs
Used Other Than Vitalize Blood
CIRCULATION DISORDERS
• BLOOD CIRCULATION,
OBSTRUCTION
EARS/HEARING DISORDERS
• VERTIGO: Liver Yang/Fire Rising
EYES
• EYES, PAIN, RED, SWOLLEN:
Liver Fire
FEVERS
• FEVER: Blood Heat
HEAD/NECK
• ALOPECIA: Blood Heat Complex

• HAIR, PREMATURE WHITENING:
Blood Heat
HEART
• ANGINA PECTORIS: Chest Bi
Strangulating Pain
HEAT
• BLOOD HEAT-YING STAGE
HEMORRHAGIC DISORDERS
• BLEEDING: Blood Heat
• EPISTAXIS
• HEMATEMESIS
INFECTIOUS DISEASES
• INFECTIONS, LOCALIZED
LIVER
• HEPATOMEGALY
• LIVER QI CONGESTION W/
SUBCOSTAL PAIN
**MUSCULOSKELETAL/
CONNECTIVE TISSUE**
• JOINTS, PAIN, SWELLING, RED:
Hot Bi, Toxic Heat With Stasis
ORAL CAVITY
• THROAT, PAIN, SWOLLEN
**PAIN/NUMBNESS/GENERAL
DISCOMFORT**
• NUMBNESS, PAIN: Blood Stasis
SEXUALITY, FEMALE:

GYNECOLOGICAL
• AMENORRHEA: Blood Stasis, In
Addition To Vitalize Blood Herbs
• BREASTS, SWOLLEN, PAINFUL,
ABSCESS
• DYSMENORRHEA
• GYNECOLOGICAL PROBLEMS
FROM BLOOD HEAT
• POSTPARTUM, ABDOMINAL
PAIN: Blood Stasis
SKIN
• ABSCESS, EARLY STAGE
• ECZEMA: Damp Heat
• HYPEREMIA W/SWELLING
• RASHES: Heat
• RASHES, W/PRURITUS: Blood
Heat, Wind
• SKIN, BLOTCHES: Blood Heat
• SKIN, SORES: Damp Heat
• SKIN, SORES, SWOLLEN, TOXIC:
Blood Stasis, Swelling
SPLEEN
• SPLENOMEGALY
TRAUMA, BITES, POISONINGS
• TRAUMA, INJURIES: Die Da
• TRAUMA, PAIN/SWELLING:
Internal/External

Clinical/Pharmaceutical Studies:

**BLOOD RELATED
DISORDERS/TOPICS**
• BLOOD PRESSURE,
LOWERS
**CIRCULATION
DISORDERS**
• VASODILATES: Mild
FEVERS
• ANTIPYRETIC
HEART

FLOW: Much Less Than
Nitroglycerin, Aqueous
Extract
INFECTIOUS DISEASES
• BACTERIAL, ANTI-: B.
Dysenteriae, Streptococci,
Pneumococci, E.Coli, Et.
Al.
• VIRAL, ANTI-: Common
Cold

• CONVULSIVE, ANTI-:
Strychnine
• SEDATIVE
• TRANQUILIZING: CNS
**MUSCULOSKELETAL/
CONNECTIVE TISSUE**
• ANTISPASMODIC IN
SMOOTH MUSCLE:
Synergistic With Gan Cao
PAIN/NUMBNESS/

Smooth Muscle Spasms
**SEXUALITY, FEMALE:
GYNECOLOGICAL**
• UTERUS, INHIBITS:
Smooth Muscle Inhibitor
**STOMACH/DIGESTIVE
DISORDERS**
• STOMACH: Smooth
Muscle Inhibitor
• ULCERS, GASTRIC:

Clinical/Pharmaceutical Studies:

- CORONARY ARTERIES, DILATES: Aqueous Extract
- HEART, INCREASES CORONARY BLOOD

KIDNEYS
- DIURETIC
MENTAL STATE/ NEUROLOGICAL DISORDERS

GENERAL DISCOMFORT
- ANALGESIC: Abdominal Pain From Small Intestine

Reduces Gastric Secretion
TRAUMA, BITES, POISONINGS
- INFLAMMATORY, ANTI-

Dose
3 - 15 gm

Common Name
Peony Root (Red)

Contraindications
Not: w/LI LU

Precautions
Watch: Def Blood

CHONG WEI ZI
(HUANG WEI ZI/XIAO HU MA)

沖慰子
（沖慰子）

Cyr. IV i XIV
FRUCTUS LEONURI

Traditional Functions:

1. Vitalizes the Blood and regulates the menses
2. Clears the vision
3. Astringes and tonifies Blood

Traditional Properties:

Enters: LV,

Properties: SW, CL

Indications:

EYES
- CONJUNCTIVITIS
- NEBULA

HEMORRHAGIC DISORDERS
- HEMORRHAGE, CONTINUOUS
SEXUALITY, FEMALE:

GYNECOLOGICAL
- MENORRHAGIA
- MENSTRUATION, ABNORMAL

Clinical/Pharmaceutical Studies:

BLOOD RELATED DISORDERS/TOPICS
- BLOOD PRESSURE, LOWERS
CIRCULATION DISORDERS
- HYPERTENSION, REDUCES PRIMARY: Lotion/Syrup With Sang

Zhi
EYES
- CONJUNCTIVITIS
- EYESIGHT, IMPROVES: Probably Because Of Vit A
- NEBULA
INFECTIOUS DISEASES
- BACTERIAL, ANTI-

KIDNEYS
- DIURETIC: Significant
LUNGS
- RESPIRATION, EXCITES CENTER
MENTAL STATE/ NEUROLOGICAL DISORDERS

- SEDATIVE: CNS
SEXUALITY, FEMALE:
GYNECOLOGICAL
- UTERUS, CONTRACTS: With Greater Frequency And Tension
SKIN
- FUNGAL, ANTI-

Dose
3 - 9 gm

Common Name
Leonurus Fruit

Contraindications
Not: Pregnancy
Not: Pupil Dilatation From Liver Blood Def

Notes
Toxic At 30 gm In 4-6 Hrs, General Soreness, Weakness, Legs Weak, Tight Chest

---

CHUAN NIU XI

川牛膝

RADIX CYATHULAE

Traditional Functions:

1. Vitalizes Blood, activates the channels and regulates menses
2. Drains Dampness from the Lower Burner
3. Dispels Wind and Dampness, especially from the Lower Burner

Traditional Properties:

Enters: KI, LV,

Properties: SW, BIT, N

Indications:

ABDOMEN/
GASTROINTESTINAL TOPICS
• ABDOMEN, MASS
HEMORRHAGIC DISORDERS
• HEMATURIA
• HEMORRHAGE: Leading Blood
Down To Stop
MUSCULOSKELETAL/

CONNECTIVE TISSUE
• ARTHRITIS, PAIN, SPASMS
• BACK, LOWER PAIN: Wind
Damp Bi
• JOINTS, PAIN, SWELLING, RED:
Hot Bi
SEXUALITY, FEMALE:

GYNECOLOGICAL
• AMENORRHEA: Blood Stasis
• MENSTRUATION, DISORDERS
OF: Dredge, Regulate Chong, Ren
URINARY BLADDER
• URINATION, PAINFUL, W/
BLOOD

Dose

4.5 - 9.0 gm

Common Name

Cyathula Root

Contraindications

Not: Pregnancy, Excessive Menstruation, Spermatorrhea,
Nocturnal Emission

CHUAN SHAN JIA

穿山甲

SQUAMA
MANITIS PENTADACTYLAE

Traditional Functions:

1. Moves menstruation and promotes lactation
2. Reduces swelling, vitalizes Blood stagnation and dispels pus
3. Expels Wind Damp from the channels
4. Stops bleeding

Traditional Properties:

Enters: ST, LV,

Properties: SA, C

Indications:

CANCER/TUMORS/SWELLINGS/
LUMPS
• TUMORS
IMMUNE SYSTEM RELATED
DISORDERS/TOPICS
• LYMPH GLANDS,
ENLARGEMENT, CHRONIC:
Phlegm Nodules
INFECTIOUS DISEASES
• SCROFULA
• TETANUS
PAIN/NUMBNESS/GENERAL
DISCOMFORT

• BI, WIND: Joint Pain
• BI, WIND DAMP, CHRONIC:
With Blood Stasis, Open The Luo
PARASITES
• BRAIN, CYSTICERCOSIS
SEXUALITY, FEMALE:
GYNECOLOGICAL
• AMENORRHEA
• BREASTS, SWOLLEN, PAINFUL,
ABSCESS
• DYSMENORRHEA
• LACTATION, INSUFFICIENT

SKIN
• ABSCESS: Helps To Drain
• BOILS: Topical, Too
• INFLAMMATION, ACUTE
PURULENT
• SKIN, SORES, SWOLLEN, TOXIC:
Blood Stasis, Swelling
TRAUMA, BITES, POISONINGS
• INFLAMMATION, ACUTE
PURULENT
• TRAUMA, EXTERNAL
• WOUNDS, TOXIC

Clinical/Pharmaceutical Studies:

BLOOD RELATED DISORDERS/
TOPICS
• BLOOD, INCREASES WBC
HEMORRHAGIC DISORDERS

• HEMATURIA: Of Unknown Origin,
3 Doses
• HEMOSTATIC: Excellent, Surgery
IMMUNE SYSTEM RELATED

DISORDERS/TOPICS
• IMMUNE SYSTEM: Raises WBC
Count

Dose

3 - 9 gm

Common Name

Pangolin Scales

Contraindications

Not: Pregnancy

Precautions

Watch: Deficiency Conditions

Watch: Sores Already Ulcerated

Notes

Do Not Use If Abscess Is Draining

CHUAN XIONG

川芎

RADIX LIGUSTICI WALLICHII

Traditional Functions:

1. Vitalizes the Blood and promotes the circulation of Qi
2. Dispels Wind and controls pain
3. Used for headaches: moves the Qi upwards and alleviates pain

Traditional Properties:

Enters: PC, LV, GB,

Properties: SP, W

Indications:

ABDOMEN/ GASTROINTESTINAL TOPICS
• ABDOMEN, PAIN OF
• FLANK, PAIN, SORENESS
• HYPOCHONDRIAC REGION, PAIN, SORENESS
• SUBCOSTAL PAIN
BLOOD RELATED DISORDERS/TOPICS
• BLOOD, CONGEALED W/STAGNANT QI
CHEST
• CHEST, PAIN, SORENESS
EARS/HEARING DISORDERS

• DIZZINESS: Wind
HEAD/NECK
• HEADACHE: Wind, Heat, Cold, Deficient Blood/ Brain Concussion
HEART
• ANGINA PECTORIS: Chest Bi Strangulating Pain
• CORONARY HEART DISEASE
LIVER
• LIVER QI CONGESTION W/SUBCOSTAL PAIN
MENTAL STATE/ NEUROLOGICAL DISORDERS
• CEREBRAL EMBOLISM

MUSCULOSKELETAL/ CONNECTIVE TISSUE
• ARTHRITIS, PAIN: Cold
• JOINTS, PAIN W/ CONTRACTURE: Cold Bi
• SPASMS, TENDONS
PAIN/NUMBNESS/ GENERAL DISCOMFORT
• BI, WIND
• BI, WIND DAMP, CHRONIC: With Blood Stasis, Open The Luo
• BODY ACHES: Wind Cold
SEXUALITY, FEMALE: GYNECOLOGICAL

• AMENORRHEA
• DYSMENORRHEA
• LABOR, DIFFICULT
• LOCHIOSCHESIS
• MENSTRUATION, DISORDERS OF: Constrict Uterus, Stimulate Chong
• MENSTRUATION, IRREGULAR
SKIN
• ABSCESS
• SKIN, FOCAL PROBLEMS
• SKIN, SORES, SWOLLEN, TOXIC: Blood Stasis, Swelling
• ULCERS

Clinical/Pharmaceutical Studies:

ABDOMEN/ GASTROINTESTINAL TOPICS
• INTESTINES, INHIBITS CONTRACTION
CIRCULATION DISORDERS
• HYPERTENSION: Oral, Weak, Injection, Significant, Water Extracts Strongest, Synergises Reserpine
• STROKE, ACUTE: IV Infusion Helped
EARS/HEARING DISORDERS
• VERTIGO: 3-9 g Daily Of Oral Decoction, Extract, Tincture
HEAD/NECK
• HEADACHE: 3-9 g Daily Of Oral Decoction, Extract, Tincture
HEART
• ANGINA PECTORIS: Improved 1/ 3 Cases

INFECTIOUS DISEASES
• ANTIBIOTIC: Shigella, Pseudomonas, Salmonella, Vibrio, B. Dysenteriae, B.Typhi, E.Coli
MENTAL STATE/ NEUROLOGICAL DISORDERS
• CEREBROVASCULAR DISEASE: Acute/Chronic
• CONVULSIVE, ANTI-
• SEDATIVE: Orally, Large Doses (25 gm/kg)
• TRANQUILIZING: Essential Oil Inhibits CNS
MUSCULOSKELETAL/ CONNECTIVE TISSUE
• MUSCLES, SMOOTH, INHIBITS: Large Doses
NUTRITIONAL/METABOLIC DISORDERS/TOPICS

• VITAMIN E DEFICIENCY
SEXUALITY, FEMALE: GYNECOLOGICAL
• ABORTIFACIENT: Repeated Injection Of Solution
• POSTPARTUM, LOCHIA
• UTERUS, STIMULATES: Small Doses Of 10% Solution, Large Doses Inhibits
SKIN
• FUNGAL, ANTI-: Many Skin Fungi
TRAUMA, BITES, POISONINGS
• MOSQUITO REPELLENT: Dried Material Made Into Incense
• RADIATION, DAMAGE: Definite Protection Against Radiation, IP Injections Best Mode, Oral Still Worked

Dose

3 - 9 gm

Common Name

Szechuan Lovage Root

Contraindications

Not: Pregnancy
Not: Def Yin w/Heat
Not: Liver Yang/Yin Def Headache
Not: Def Qi
Not: Profuse Menstrual Flow
Not: During Hemorrhagic Diseases

Notes

Possible Vomiting/Dizziness

DAN SHEN

丹參

RADIX SALVIAE MILTIORRHIZAE

Traditional Functions:

1. Vitalizes the Blood and moves stagnation
2. Clears Heat in the Heart and soothes irritability
3. Cools Blood and eliminates carbuncles
4. Regulates menstruation
5. Generates new tissue

Traditional Properties:

Enters: HT, PC, LV,

Properties: BIT, <C

Indications:

ABDOMEN/ GASTROINTESTINAL TOPICS
- ABDOMEN, PAIN OF: Postpartum Blood Stasis
- ABDOMEN, PAIN OF, POSTMENSTRUAL
- HYPOCHONDRIAC REGION, SORENESS: Liver Qi Stagnation With Blood Stasis

BLOOD RELATED DISORDERS/TOPICS
- BLOOD STASIS/ ECCHYMOSIS

CANCER/TUMORS/ SWELLINGS/LUMPS
- MASSES, PALPABLE
- TUMORS, GYNECOLOGICAL

CHEST
- CHEST, PAIN: Blood Stasis
- RIB SORENESS: Liver Qi Stagnation With Blood Stasis

HEART
- ANGINA PECTORIS:

Chest Bi Strangulating Pain
- CORONARY HEART DISEASE
- HEART KIDNEY YIN DEFICIENCY PATTERNS
- HEART QI DEF-KIDNEY YIN DEFICIENCY
- HEART, RESTLESS: Internal Heat
- PALPITATIONS: Ying Level Heat

HEAT
- YING STAGE HEAT: Insomnia, Palpitations, Restlessness, Irritability

HEMORRHAGIC DISORDERS
- HEMORRHAGE: Cool Blood To Stop

LIVER
- HEPATOMEGALY
- LIVER QI STAGNATION LUMPS

MENTAL STATE/ NEUROLOGICAL DISORDERS

- INSOMNIA: Ying Level Heat
- INSOMNIA, DREAMS, FREQUENT
- IRRITABILITY: Ying Level Heat
- RESTLESSNESS: Ying Level Heat
- SPIRIT, CALMS

MUSCULOSKELETAL/ CONNECTIVE TISSUE
- JOINTS, BONE PAIN
- JOINTS, PAIN: Wind Damp
- JOINTS, PAIN, SWELLING, RED: Hot Bi

PAIN/NUMBNESS/ GENERAL DISCOMFORT
- PAIN: Blood Stasis

SEXUALITY, FEMALE: GYNECOLOGICAL
- AMENORRHEA
- BREASTS, SWOLLEN, PAINFUL, ABSCESS
- DYSMENORRHEA

- LOCHIOSCHESIS
- MENSTRUATION, DISORDERS OF: Constrict Uterus, Stimulate Chong
- MENSTRUATION, IRREGULAR
- METRORRHAGIA

SKIN
- BOILS
- ECZEMA: Damp Heat
- ERYSIPELAS
- RASHES
- RASHES, W/PRURITUS: Blood Heat, Wind
- SKIN, SORES: Damp Heat
- SKIN, SORES, SWOLLEN, TOXIC: Blood Stasis, Swelling
- ULCERS

SPLEEN
- SPLENOMEGALY

STOMACH/DIGESTIVE DISORDERS
- EPIGASTRIC PAIN: Blood Stasis

Clinical/Pharmaceutical Studies:

BLOOD RELATED DISORDERS/TOPICS
- BLOOD GLUCOSE, REDUCES
- BLOOD PRESSURE, LOWERS: Short Term
- BLOOD, COAGULATION: Inhibits
- CHOLESTEROL, LOWERS: Injections, For Some Patients

CANCER/TUMORS/ SWELLINGS/LUMPS
- TUMOR, ANTI-: Inhibits Fibroblast, Tumor Cells

CIRCULATION DISORDERS
- BLOOD CIRCULATION, INCREASES MICROCIRCULATION

EXTREMITIES
- FEET, INFECTIONS OF
- HANDS, INFECTIONS OF

EYES
- CENTRAL RETINITIS
- OPTIC ATROPHY

FEVERS
- FEVER, EPIDEMIC HEMORRHAGIC

HEART
- ANGINA PECTORIS: Treat 1-9 Months, Best If No History Of Heart Attack, With Jiang Huang Injection Even Better, *1-9 Months, Extract Tablet
- CORONARY HEART DISEASE: By Itself/Dan Shen Pills

- INFECTIONS, POSTOPERATIVE
- JOINTS, INFECTIONS OF

KIDNEYS
- KIDNEYS, CHRONIC RENAL INSUFFICIENCY

LIVER
- HEPATITIS, ACUTE, ICTERIC/ PREVENTATIVE FOR INFECTIOUS: Add Tian Ji Huang (Hypericum Japonicum)
- HEPATITIS, CHRONIC PERSISTENT/ACTIVE: Injection

LUNGS
- BRONCHITIS,

PERIARTHRITIS OF JOINT: Injection As Local Block, Followed By Vigorous Massaged With Electropuncture Anesthesia

NUTRITIONAL/ METABOLIC DISORDERS/TOPICS
- METABOLISM, INCREASES: Increase Hypoxia Tolerance, Too
- TISSUES, PROMOTES REGENERATION OF: Promotes Repair, Regeneration

ORAL CAVITY
- TONSILLITIS, ACUTE

PARASITES
- SCHISTOSOMIASIS, ADVANCED W/LIVER

Clinical/Pharmaceutical Studies:

- HYPERTENSION: Significant Lowering, Eliminated Stroke-Like Symptoms
- PHLEBITIS: 30-60 gm
- STROKE, ISCHEMIC: Cerebral Atherosclerosis, IV/IM Injection
- THROMBOANGIITIS OBLITERANS: Tinctures
- VASODILATOR

EARS/HEARING DISORDERS
- EARS, OTITIS EXTERNA

ENDOCRINE RELATED DISORDERS
- HORMONE EFFECTS: No Estrogenic Action

- HEART DISEASE: 1-9 Months, Extract Tablet
- HEART, VASODILATOR
- KESHAN DISEASE

IMMUNE SYSTEM RELATED DISORDERS/ TOPICS
- IMMUNE RESPONSE: Increases
- IMMUNE SYSTEM ENHANCEMENT: Increases Macrophage Activity

INFECTIOUS DISEASES
- ANTIBIOTIC: TB, Flu, Polio, Vibrio Proteus, B. Typhi, Shigella, Staph. Aureus, etc
- CELLULITIS

CHRONIC/ASTHMATIC: Associated With Pulomonary Emphysema, Increases T-Lymphocytes

MENTAL STATE/ NEUROLOGICAL DISORDERS
- INSOMNIA
- NEURASTHENIA
- SEDATIVE

MUSCULOSKELETAL/ CONNECTIVE TISSUE
- BACK, LOWER PAIN
- BONES, INFECTIONS OF
- JOINTS, INFECTIONS OF
- OSTEOMYELITIS
- SHOULDERS,

CIRRHOSIS

SEXUALITY, FEMALE: GYNECOLOGICAL
- MASTITIS

SKIN
- ABSCESS, GLUTEAL
- ACNE
- CARBUNCLES
- ERYSIPELAS
- FUNGAL, ANTI-: Some
- SKIN, DISORDERS: Injection Alone Or With Spatholobus Suberectus Stem

TRAUMA, BITES, POISONINGS
- TRAUMA: Promotes Repair, Regeneration

Dose

6 - 15 gm

Contraindications

Not: w/LI LU

Precautions

Watch: w/o Blood Stasis

Notes

Enhance Invigorate Blood Effect By Wine Frying

Tinctures Can Lead To Pruritus, Anorexia, Stomach Ache

Large Dose: 15-30 gm

Possible: Dry Mouth, Dizziness, Numbness, Chest Tight, Mild Irritability, Nausea, Vomiting, These Disappear Spontaneously Without Stopping Treatment

---

E ZHU

(PENG E ZHU)

莪術
（莪术）

RHIZOMA CURCUMAE ZEDOARIAE

Traditional Functions:

1. Vitalizes stagnant Blood
2. Pomotes Qi circulation and reduces pain
2. Removes food accumulations and controls pain

Traditional Properties:

Enters: SP, LV,

Properties: BIT, SP, W

Indications:

ABDOMEN/ GASTROINTESTINAL TOPICS
- ABDOMEN, MASS
- ABDOMEN, PAIN OF, DISTENTION: Food Stagnation
- ACCUMULATION
- APPENDICITIS W/PAIN

CANCER/TUMORS/SWELLINGS/ LUMPS
- CERVICAL CANCER
- TUMORS, BENIGN

CHEST
- CHEST, DISTENTION, PAIN: Food Stagnation

CHILDHOOD DISORDERS
- NUTRITIONAL IMPAIRMENT, CHILDHOOD

LIVER
- HEPATOMEGALY
- LIVER QI CONGESTION W/ SUBCOSTAL PAIN

QI RELATED DISORDERS/ TOPICS
- QI/BLOOD STAGNATION

SEXUALITY, FEMALE: GYNECOLOGICAL
- AMENORRHEA: Blood Stasis
- CERVIX, CANCINOMA

- DYSMENORRHEA

SPLEEN
- SPLENOMEGALY

STOMACH/DIGESTIVE DISORDERS
- EPIGASTRIC MASSES: Blood Stasis
- EPIGASTRIC PAIN, DISTENTION
- FOOD STAGNATION, PAIN: Overnight
- STOMACH, PAIN, DISTENTION

TRAUMA, BITES, POISONINGS
- INJURIES, TRAUMATIC, PAINFUL

Clinical/Pharmaceutical Studies:

**ABDOMEN/
GASTROINTESTINAL TOPICS**
• GASTROINTESTINAL
STIMULATION: For Distension
• INTESTINES, COLIC: From
Flatulence, Similar To Fresh Ginger
**BLOOD RELATED DISORDERS/
TOPICS**
• BLOOD, COAGULATED:
Decoction Helps To Reabsorb
• BLOOD, WBC: Increases Count
BOWEL RELATED DISORDERS
• FLATULENCE W/SPASMS:
Directly Stimulates GI Tract
CANCER/TUMORS/SWELLINGS/

LUMPS
• CANCER, ANTI-: Injections,
Effective In Treating Some Cancers
• TUMOR, ANTI-: Granuloma,
Cervical, Injection
**IMMUNE SYSTEM RELATED
DISORDERS/TOPICS**
• IMMUNE SYSTEM
ENHANCEMENT: Contributes To
Antineoplastic Effects
INFECTIOUS DISEASES
• ANTIBIOTIC: Essential Oils--
Staph, Strep, Salmonella, E.Coli,
Strep, Cholera

**SEXUALITY, FEMALE:
GYNECOLOGICAL**
• ABORTIFACIENT: ETOH Extract
Shows Marked Effects, 4x/Day
Orally, Equal To 15g/kg, Induces
Abortion Early In Pregnancy
**STOMACH/DIGESTIVE
DISORDERS**
• CARMINATIVE: Stimulate GI
Tract
• STOMACHIC
TRAUMA, BITES, POISONINGS
• ANTIHISTAMINE: Aqueous
Extract

Dose
3 - 9 gm

Common Name
Zedoary Rhizome

Contraindications
Not: Pregnancy

Precautions
Watch: Def Blood/Qi

Watch: Excess Menstruation

Notes
San Leng-Like But E Zhu Is Warm Whereas Other Is
Cold

FAN HONG HUA
(ZANG HONG HUA)

番紅花
（番紅花）

STIGMA
CROCUS
(STIGMA CROCI)

Traditional Functions:

1. Vitalizes Blood and clears channels
2. Cools the Blood and clears toxins

Traditional Properties:

Enters: HT, LV

Properties: SW, C

Indications:

**BLOOD RELATED DISORDERS/
TOPICS**
• BLOOD HEAT
• BLOOD STASIS PAIN
CHEST
• CHEST, FULLNESS
FEVERS
• FEVER, HIGH

**SEXUALITY, FEMALE:
GYNECOLOGICAL**
• AMENORRHEA
• DYSTOCIA
• MENORRHAGIA
• POSTPARTUM, ABDOMINAL
PAIN

• POSTPARTUM, RETENTION OF
LOCHIA
SKIN
• MACULOPAPULES
TRAUMA, BITES, POISONINGS
• TRAUMA, INTERNAL/
EXTERNAL

Clinical/Pharmaceutical Studies:

**ABDOMEN/
GASTROINTESTINAL TOPICS**
• INTESTINES, STIMULATES
**BLOOD RELATED DISORDERS/
TOPICS**
• BLOOD PRESSURE, LOWERS
CIRCULATION DISORDERS
• VASOCONSTRICTOR

**ENDOCRINE RELATED
DISORDERS**
• ESTRUS, PROLONGED, IN MICE
HEART
• HEART, STIMULATES
CONTRACTION, RELAXATION
OF
LUNGS

• BRONCHIAL CONTRACTION
**SEXUALITY, FEMALE:
GYNECOLOGICAL**
• ESTRUS, PROLONGED IN MICE
• UTERUS, STIMULATES: Alcohol
Extract Stimulates, Large Doses Can
Cause Spasms, More So In
Pregnancy

Dose
1.5 - 3.0 gm

Common Name
Saffron

Contraindications
Not: Pregnancy

Notes
Similar To Hong Hua, But Stronger

GUEI YU JIAN
(GUI JIAN YU)

鬼羽箭
（鬼羽箭）

RAMULUS/HERBA
SUBERALATUM EUONYMI
(BUCHNERAE)

Traditional Functions:

1. Moves the Blood and opens the menstruation
2. Disperses and vitalizes stagnant Blood and controls pain
3. Kills intestinal parasites

Traditional Properties:

Enters: LU, SP,

Properties: BIT, C

Indications:

ABDOMEN/
GASTROINTESTINAL TOPICS
• ABDOMEN, PAIN OF: Postpartum
 Stagnant Blood
CANCER/TUMORS/SWELLINGS/

LUMPS
• ABDOMEN, TUMORS
MUSCULOSKELETAL/
 CONNECTIVE TISSUE

• ARTHRITIS
SEXUALITY, FEMALE:
 GYNECOLOGICAL
• AMENORRHEA

Clinical/Pharmaceutical Studies:

BLOOD RELATED DISORDERS/
TOPICS

• BLOOD GLUCOSE, REDUCES:

Decoction

Dose
4.5 - 9.0 gm

Common Name
Winded Spindle Tree

HONG HUA

紅花
（红花）

FLOS
CARTHAMI TINCTORII

Traditional Functions:

1. Vitalizes the Blood and promotes menstruation
2. Dispels congealed Blood and relieves pain

Traditional Properties:

Enters: HT, LV,

Properties: SP, W

Indications:

ABDOMEN/
GASTROINTESTINAL
TOPICS
• ABDOMEN, MASS
• ABDOMEN, PAIN OF
BLOOD RELATED
DISORDERS/TOPICS
• BLOOD STASIS PAIN
CANCER/TUMORS/
SWELLINGS/LUMPS
• TUMORS,
 GYNECOLOGICAL
CHEST
• CHEST BI: Blood Stasis
HEART

• ANGINA PECTORIS:
 Chest Bi Strangulating
 Pain
• HEART DISEASE
INFECTIOUS DISEASES
• MEASLES,
 INCOMPLETE
 EXPRESSION OF RASH
LIVER
• HEPATOMEGALY
MUSCULOSKELETAL/
CONNECTIVE TISSUE
• ARTHRITIS
SEXUALITY, FEMALE:
GYNECOLOGICAL

• AMENORRHEA
• DYSMENORRHEA
• FETUS, DEAD
• LABOR, DIFFICULT
• LOCHIOSCHESIS
• MENSTRUATION,
 DISORDERS OF:
 Constrict Uterus, Stimulate
 Chong
• POSTPARTUM,
 DIZZINESS
SKIN
• CARBUNCLES
• ERYTHEMA, PURPLE
• RASHES, INCOMPLETE

EXPRESSION OF: Blood
 Heat, Wind, Dull Red
• SKIN, SORES,
 SWOLLEN, TOXIC:
 Blood Stasis, Swelling
• SORES, W/O
 SUPPURATION
SPLEEN
• SPLENOMEGALY
TRAUMA, BITES,
POISONINGS
• INJURIES, TRAUMATIC
• TRAUMA, BLEEDING:
 External/Interal

Clinical/Pharmaceutical Studies:

ABDOMEN/
GASTROINTESTINAL
TOPICS
• INTESTINES,
 ADHESIONS,
 POSTOPERATIVE: IM

• VASOCONSTRICTOR,
 PERIPHERAL
HEAD/NECK
• BRAIN: Protects From
 Anoxia, Ischemia, Injury
HEART

• HEPATITIS: IM Injection,
 Lowered SGPT
LUNGS
• BRONCHI, SMOOTH
 MUSCLES STIMULANT
MUSCULOSKELETAL/

Effective, May Cause
 Temporary Irritation
TRAUMA, BITES,
POISONINGS
• FRACTURES, W/
 SWELLING: Hong Hua,

Clinical/Pharmaceutical Studies:

Injection Of Alcohol Extract Hong Hua, Ze Lan, *Use During Operation To Prevent Adhesions
• INTESTINES, SMOOTH MUSCLES STIMULANT
BLOOD RELATED DISORDERS/TOPICS
• BLOOD PRESSURE, LOWERS: Long Term
• CHOLESTEROL, LOWERS: w/Safflower Oil, 1 gm/kg/Day
CIRCULATION DISORDERS
• PHLEBITIS: Injection, Marked Symptom Improvement
• STROKE, CEREBRAL THROMBOSIS: Injection
• THROMBOANGIITIS: Injection, Marked Symptom Improvement

• CORONARY HEART DISEASE: 1-4 Months With Vitalize Blood Herbs, 90% Stopped Nitroglycerin, *ETOH Extract Tab, Good Effects, *Coronary Tablet No.2 (Chi Shao, Chuan Xiong, Hong Hua, Dan Shen, Lignum Dalbergia Odoriferae) , *Hong Hua Jiang Huang Tablet (Hong Hua, Jiang Huang, Dan Shen, Gua Luo) , *Hong Hua-Bai Guo Ye Tablet (Bai Guo Ye, Chuan Xiong, Hong Hua)
• HEART, INCREASES CORONARY BLOOD FLOW
• HEART, STIMULATES: Small Doses Stimulate Heart
LIVER

CONNECTIVE TISSUE
• TENOSYNOVITIS, SUBACUTE: External, 0.5% Tincture, Reduced Swelling Rapidly
SEXUALITY, FEMALE: GYNECOLOGICAL
• MENSTRUATION, DISORDERS OF: Tincture Of Hong Hua, 6.3% , Dang Gui, 12.7%, 2-3 ml 3x/Day, After Food, Best For Post Puberty Women
• UTERUS, STIMULATES: Fast Acting, Long Lasting-- Especially When Pregnant
SKIN
• NEURODERMATITIS: Injection As Local Block
• WARTS: Verruca Plana, Use Tea Of 9 g, 1x/Day For 10 Days, 92%

Flos Impatiens Balsamina, 50 g Ea, Small Amount Of Alum, Macerate In 60 Proof White Wine For 24 Hrs, Apply Externally With Gauze
• SPRAINS: External, 0.5% Tincture, Reduced Swelling Rapidly, *Joints, Paste Of Hong Hua, Bai Shao, Shan Zhi Zi, 9 g Each, Grind Add Egg White
• TRAUMA, MUSCULOSKELETAL: 1% Tinctures For 3-5 Days
• WOUNDS: External, 0.5% Tincture, Reduced Swelling Rapidly, *Topical Application Of Aqueous Extract, 30% Prevented Decubitus Ulcer

Dose

3 - 9 gm

Common Name

Safflower Flower

Contraindications

Not: Pregnancy

Precautions

Watch: Peptic Ulcers, Hemorrhagic Disease

Notes

Small Doses: Vitalizes Blood

Large Dose: Breaks Blood (12-15 g)

Raw: Vitalizes Blood

w/Wine: Breaks Blood

w/Water: Tonifies Blood (1.2-1.5 gm)

No Toxic Effects

Women May Have Slight Increase In Menstrual Flow

HUAI JIAO

槐角

FRUCTUS SOPHORAE JAPONICAE

Traditional Functions:

1. Clears Heat and assists in controlling bleeding
2. Directs the Qi downward, moistens the intestines
3. Benefits the Liver and clears Liver Fire

Traditional Properties:

Enters: LI, LV,

Properties: BIT, CL

Indications:

BOWEL RELATED DISORDERS
• CONSTIPATION
• HEMORRHOIDS, BLOODY STOOL
• HEMORRHOIDS, INFLAMMED
• HEMORRHOIDS, PAIN, SWELLING
CHEST
• CHEST, STUFFINESS

CIRCULATION DISORDERS
• HYPERTENSION: Liver Fire
EARS/HEARING DISORDERS
• DIZZINESS: Liver Fire
• VERTIGO: Liver Yang/Fire Rising
EYES
• EYES, RED: Liver Fire
HEAD/NECK
• HEADACHE: Liver Fire

HEMORRHAGIC DISORDERS
• HEMATURIA
• HEMORRHAGE: Cool Blood To Stop
• HEMOSTATIC
SEXUALITY, FEMALE: GYNECOLOGICAL
• UTERINE BLEEDING

Clinical/Pharmaceutical Studies:

BLOOD RELATED DISORDERS/ TOPICS
• BLOOD GLUCOSE, INCREASES
• BLOOD PRESSURE, LOWERS:

Small Doses
INFECTIOUS DISEASES
• BACTERIAL, ANTI-: E.Coli, Staph

MENTAL STATE/ NEUROLOGICAL DISORDERS
• CNS, EXCITATORY: Respiration, Small Doses

Dose
9 - 15 gm

Common Name
Pagoda Tree Fruit

Contraindications
Not: Pregnancy

JI XING ZI   急性子   SEMEN IMPATIENTIS

Traditional Functions:

1. Softens hard masses and moves stagnant Blood
2. Stops bleeding
3. Promotes digestion
4. Disperses masses and removes toxin

Traditional Properties:

Enters: HT, LV

Properties: BIT, W, SP, <TX

Indications:

**ABDOMEN/
GASTROINTESTINAL TOPICS**
• ABDOMEN, MASS
**CANCER/TUMORS/SWELLINGS/
LUMPS**

• CANCER
ORAL CAVITY
• THROAT, SENSATION OF
OBSTRUCTION
SEXUALITY, FEMALE:

GYNECOLOGICAL
• AMENORRHEA
TRAUMA, BITES, POISONINGS
• CHOKING: From Accidental
Swallowing Of Bones

Clinical/Pharmaceutical Studies:

**ABDOMEN/
GASTROINTESTINAL
TOPICS**
• INTESTINES, INHIBITS:
Aqueous Extract
**CANCER/TUMORS/
SWELLINGS/LUMPS**
• CANCER: Used With
Other Herbs In Various
• ESOPHAGEAL CANCER:
Symptomatic
Improvement, Dysphagia,
Some Lessening Vomiting,
Pain

• STOMACH CANCER:
Symptomatic Improvement,
Dysphagia, Some
Lessening Vomiting, Pain
**SEXUALITY, EITHER
SEX**
• ANTIFERTILITY: Taken
For 10 Days, Probably
Suppresses Ovulation, Pills
From Ji Xing Zi, Bing
Lang, Ling Xiao Hua
(Plant Of) , Ze Lan, Grind
To Fine pwdr, Mix With
Honey, Take 20 g 2x/Day

On Empty Stomach For 10
Days, 68% Contraception
Rate, Increased To 80% If
Started On 3rd Day Of
Menstruation
• CONTRACEPTIVE: Oral
Route Of Extract
**SEXUALITY, FEMALE:
GYNECOLOGICAL**
• ABORTIFACIENT: Ji
Xing Zi, Tao Ren, Gui Zhi,
Da Huang, Ling Xiao Hua,
Ban Mao, San Leng, E Zhu,

Shui Zhi, Zhe Chong,
Anoplophora Chinesnis,
About 50% Had
Termination Of Pregnancy
• UTERUS, STIMULATES:
Strongly Stimulates,
Increase Tonicity
**STOMACH/DIGESTIVE
DISORDERS**
• STOMACH, CANCER:
Symptomatic Improvement,
Dysphagia, Some
Lessening Vomiting, Pain

Dose
0.9 - 3.0 gm

Common Name
Touch-Me-Not

Notes
Cancers: 15-60 g

Possible Dry Mouth, Nausea, Anorexia With Prolonged
Use, But Disappeared When Reduced Or Discontinued
For 2-3 Days

JI XUE TENG
(JI XUE DENG)

雞血藤
(鸡血藤)

CAULIS MUCUNAE
(SPATHOLOBI)

Traditional Functions:

1. Vitalizes the Blood
2. Nourishes and harmonizes the Blood
3. Relaxes and activates the tendons

Traditional Properties:

Enters: SP, HT, KI, LV,

Properties: BIT, SW, W

Indications:

BLOOD RELATED DISORDERS/ TOPICS
- ANEMIA, APLASTIC
- BLOOD DEFICIENCY W/ WITHERING YELLOW COMPLEXION
- DIZZINESS FROM ANEMIA

EARS/HEARING DISORDERS
- VERTIGO W/PARALYSIS, WINDSTROKE: Blood Stasis

EXTREMITIES
- EXTREMITIES, NUMB
- EXTREMITIES, WEAKNESS OF IN ELDERLY

MENTAL STATE/

NEUROLOGICAL DISORDERS
- PARALYSIS W/VERTIGO, WINDSTROKE: Blood Stasis

MUSCULOSKELETAL/ CONNECTIVE TISSUE
- ARTHRITIS: For Opening The Luo Channels
- BACK, LOWER PAIN/NUMB
- JOINTS, SORE: Wind Damp Bi, With Blood Stasis/Deficient
- KNEES, PAIN/NUMB

PAIN/NUMBNESS/GENERAL DISCOMFORT
- BODY, NUMBNESS
- NUMBNESS W/SPASMS,

CONTRACTURES: Blood Deficiency Bi

SEXUALITY, FEMALE: GYNECOLOGICAL
- AMENORRHEA, W/ABDOMINAL PAIN: Blood Deficient
- DYSMENORRHEA: Blood Deficient
- LEUKOPENIA: From Radiotherapy
- MENSTRUATION, IRREGULAR: Blood Deficient
- METRORRHAGIA

WIND DISORDERS
- WINDSTROKE: Paralysis, Vertigo

Clinical/Pharmaceutical Studies:

BLOOD RELATED DISORDERS/ TOPICS
- BLOOD PRESSURE, LOWERS

CIRCULATION DISORDERS
- VASOCONSTRICTOR

MENTAL STATE/

NEUROLOGICAL DISORDERS
- HYPNOTIC: Tincture

- SEDATIVE: Tincture

MUSCULOSKELETAL/ CONNECTIVE TISSUE
- ARTHRITIS: Tincture Has Marked Effect

NUTRITIONAL/METABOLIC DISORDERS/TOPICS
- METABOLISM OF PHOSPHATE,

INCREASES IN KIDNEYS, UTERUS

SEXUALITY, FEMALE: GYNECOLOGICAL
- UTERUS, STIMULATES: Pregnant More Sensitive, Decoction Stronger Than Tincture (Millettia)

Dose
9 - 60 gm

Common Name
Millettia Root And Vine

JIANG HUANG

姜黄
（姜黄）

RHIZOMA CURCUMAE

Traditional Functions:

1. Vitalizes the Blood and promotes Qi circulation
2. Clears Wind from the channels and collaterals and moves Blood, relieving pain
3. Promotes menstruation and stops pain

Traditional Properties:

Enters: SP, LV,

Properties: SP, BIT, W

Indications:

ABDOMEN/ GASTROINTESTINAL TOPICS
- ABDOMEN, PAIN OF: Cold/Deficient Cold Leading To Blood Stasis/ Stagnant Qi
- ABDOMEN, PAIN OF, HERNIA-LIKE: Cold

BLOOD RELATED DISORDERS/TOPICS
- BLOOD STASIS

CANCER/TUMORS/ SWELLINGS/LUMPS
- TUMORS, GYNECOLOGICAL

CHEST
- CHEST, PAIN: Deficient Cold Leading To Blood Stasis

LIVER
- JAUNDICE, YIN

MUSCULOSKELETAL/ CONNECTIVE TISSUE
- ARTHRITIS, SHOULDERS: Cold Type

PAIN/NUMBNESS/ GENERAL DISCOMFORT
- BI, WIND DAMP W/ BLOOD STASIS:

Shoulder, Especially

QI RELATED DISORDERS/TOPICS
- QI STAGNATION

SEXUALITY, FEMALE: GYNECOLOGICAL
- AMENORRHEA: Deficient Cold Leading To Blood Stasis
- DYSMENORRHEA: Deficient Cold Leading To Blood Stasis
- MENSTRUATION, DISORDERS OF: Constrict Uterus, Stimulate

Chong
- POSTPARTUM, HEART INVADED BY FOUL BLOOD

SKIN
- CARBUNCLES

STOMACH/DIGESTIVE DISORDERS
- EPIGASTRIC PAIN: Stagnant Qi

TRAUMA, BITES, POISONINGS
- INJURIES
- TRAUMA, BLEEDING: Blood Stasis

Clinical/Pharmaceutical Studies:

**ABDOMEN/
GASTROINTESTINAL
TOPICS**
• ABDOMEN, PAIN OF,
POSTPARTUM
**BLOOD RELATED
DISORDERS/TOPICS**
• BLOOD PRESSURE,
LOWERS: Alcohol
Extract
• BLOOD,
TRIGLYCERIDES,
LOWERS: Tablets
(Extracts Equivalent To 3.5
g Crude Herb/Tab) 5 Tabs,
3x/Day For 12 Weeks, 62
mg% Lowering, Equal To
Clofibrate
• CHOLESTEROL,
LOWERS: ETOH/Ether
Extract
CIRCULATION

DISORDERS
• ATHEROSCLEROSIS:
Curcumin Inhibits Platelet
Aggregation
• HYPERTENSION
FEVERS
• ANTIPYRETIC
GALL BLADDER
• CHOLAGOGUE:
Decoction/Infusion, ETOH
Extract Better
• CHOLECYSTITIS
• GALL BLADDER,
STONES: Helps To
Resolve Sandy Type
HEART
• ANGINA PECTORIS:
Curcumin Inhibits Platelet
Aggregation, Use As
Powder With Dang Gui,
Mu Xiang, Wu Yao
• MYOCARDIAL

INFARCTION: Curcumin
Inhibits Platelet
Aggregation
• MYOCARDIAL
ISCHEMIA: Oral Doses
Increases Blood Flow
INFECTIOUS DISEASES
• ANTIBIOTIC: Strong:
Staph
• VIRAL, ANTI-: Many
LIVER
• JAUNDICE
• LIVER,
DETOXIFICATION:
Ether/ETOH Extract
**PAIN/NUMBNESS/
GENERAL
DISCOMFORT**
• ANALGESIC
**SEXUALITY, FEMALE:
GYNECOLOGICAL**
• ABORTIFACIENT: Early

Pregnancy, Oral Dose Of
Aqueous Extract Effective,
By Antagonization Of
Progesterone, Uterine
Contraction
• UTERUS, STIMULATES:
Decoction Causes
Contractions, Paroxysmal,
5-7 Hrs
SKIN
• FUNGAL, ANTI-: Oil Of,
Strong Skin Fungi
**STOMACH/DIGESTIVE
DISORDERS**
• APPETITE, INCREASES:
50% Decoction
• STOMACH, ACHE
**TRAUMA, BITES,
POISONINGS**
• FLIES, LETHAL TO
• INFLAMMATORY, ANTI-

Dose
3 - 9 gm

Common Name
Turmeric Rhizome

Contraindications
Not: Pregnancy

Not: Def Blood w/o Stagnant Qi Or Blood Stasis

Notes
Possible Frequent Bowel Movements, Mild Stomach
Upset

JUAN BO
(JUAN BAI YE)

卷柏

HERBA
SELAGINELLAE

Traditional Functions:

1. Benefits the Essence
2. Vitalizes the Blood and disperses stagnation
3. Calms the Heart
4. Promotes urination

Traditional Properties:

Enters: LV, KI

Properties: SP, N

Indications:

**ABDOMEN/
GASTROINTESTINAL TOPICS**
• ABDOMEN, PAIN OF
BOWEL RELATED DISORDERS
• HEMORRHOIDS, INTERNAL

• RECTAL PROLAPSE
HEMORRHAGIC DISORDERS
• HEMAFECIA
LUNGS
• COUGH, GASPING

**MUSCULOSKELETAL/
CONNECTIVE TISSUE**
• ATROPHIC DEBILITIES
TRAUMA, BITES, POISONINGS
• TRAUMA, PAIN, SWELLING

Dose
1.5 - 9.0 gm

Common Name
Selaginella

LA MEI HUA

臘梅花
（腊梅花）

FLOS CHIMONANTHI

Traditional Functions:

1. Circulates the Qi and resolves constrained Liver Qi
2. Promotes tissue regeneration
3. Cools Blood, clears Heat, removes toxin, vitalizes Blood

Traditional Properties:

Enters: LU, LV,

Properties: SP, BIT, N

Indications:

EYES
• EYES, WIND HEAT IRRITATION
HEAD/NECK
• PLUM SEED QI

INFECTIOUS DISEASES
• MEASLES, RECOVERY STAGE
ORAL CAVITY
• PHARYNGITIS

• TONSILLITIS
QI RELATED DISORDERS/
  TOPICS
• PLUM SEED QI

Clinical/Pharmaceutical Studies:

ABDOMEN/
  GASTROINTESTINAL TOPICS
• INTESTINES, STIMULATES
BLOOD RELATED DISORDERS/
  TOPICS

• BLOOD GLUCOSE, REDUCES
MENTAL STATE/
  NEUROLOGICAL DISORDERS
• CONVULSIONS: Can Cause
  Violent

SEXUALITY, FEMALE:
  GYNECOLOGICAL
• UTERUS, STIMULATES: Causes
  Contractions

Dose

3 - 9 gm

Common Name

Lamei

LING XIAO HUA

凌霄花

FLOS CAMPSIS

Traditional Functions:

1. Cools the Blood and disperses Wind
2. Invigorates the Blood and promotes menstruation

Traditional Properties:

Enters: PC, LV,

Properties: SO, C, SW,

Indications:

ABDOMEN/
  GASTROINTESTINAL TOPICS
• ABDOMEN, MASS
MENTAL STATE/
  NEUROLOGICAL DISORDERS
• EPILEPSY: Blood Heat Creating
  Wind

SEXUALITY, FEMALE:
  GYNECOLOGICAL
• AMENORRHEA
• MENORRHAGIA
• POSTPARTUM, BLOOD
  OBSTRUCTION
• UTERINE BLEEDING,

FUNCTIONAL
SKIN
• PRURITUS: Take Internal/
  Externally
• RASHES, W/PRURITUS: Blood
  Heat, Wind

Dose

3 - 9 gm

Common Name

Trumpet Flower

Contraindications

Not: Pregnancy

LIU JI NU

劉寄奴
(刘寄奴)

HERBA ARTEMISIAE ANOMALAE
(SIPHONOSTEGIA)

Traditional Functions:

1. Dispels stagnant Blood, promotes menstruation and controls pain

Traditional Properties:

Enters: SP, HT,

Properties: BIT, W

Indications:

ABDOMEN/
  GASTROINTESTINAL TOPICS
• ABDOMEN, MASS
CHEST
• CHEST, PAIN, FULLNESS
SEXUALITY, FEMALE:

GYNECOLOGICAL
• AMENORRHEA: Blood Stagnation
• POSTPARTUM, ABDOMINAL
  PAIN: Blood Stagnation
SKIN
• BURNS: Topical

TRAUMA, BITES, POISONINGS
• BRUISES: Topical
• CONTUSIONS
• FRACTURES
• SPRAINS
• WOUNDS, BLEEDING: Topical

Clinical/Pharmaceutical Studies:

LIVER
• HEPATITIS, ACUTE, VIRAL:
  Icteric, Non-Icteric–Good, 16 Days

• HEPATITIS, IMPROVES
  APPETITE
SKIN

• BURNS: Ointment Made For 2/3rd
  Degree From Powder

Dose

3 - 9 gm

Common Name

Mugwort

Contraindications

Not: SP Def Diarrhea

Not: Pregnancy

Precautions

Watch: Qi/Blood Weak

LU LU TONG

路路通

FRUCTUS LIQUIDAMBARIS TAIWANIANAE

Traditional Functions:

1. Circulates Qi and Blood and opens the Luo
2. Dispels Wind Damp Bi
3. Promotes urination
4. Promotes lactation

Traditional Properties:

Enters: ST, LV,

Properties: BIT, N

Indications:

ABDOMEN/
  GASTROINTESTINAL TOPICS
• ABDOMEN, DISTENTION OF
BOWEL RELATED DISORDERS
• BOWEL MOVEMENT,
  IRREGULAR
EXTREMITIES
• ARMS, NUMB
• FEET, NUMB
• HANDS, NUMB
• LEGS, NUMB
• LIMBS, CONTRACTURES
FLUID DISORDERS
• EDEMA, ABDOMINAL
  FULLNESS

• EDEMA, PAIN OF
• EDEMA, URINATION
  DIFFICULTY
INFECTIOUS DISEASES
• MEASLES
MUSCULOSKELETAL/
  CONNECTIVE TISSUE
• ARTHRITIS, PAIN
• ARTHRITIS, WHOLE BODY PAIN
PAIN/NUMBNESS/GENERAL
  DISCOMFORT
• ARTHRITIS, WHOLE BODY PAIN
• BI, WIND: Knees, Low Back
• NUMBNESS, BODY

SEXUALITY, FEMALE:
  GYNECOLOGICAL
• BREASTS, DISTENTION
• LACTATION, INSUFFICIENT
• MENSTRUATION, DISORDERS
  OF: Dredge, Regulate Chong, Ren
• MENSTRUATION, IRREGULAR,
  SCANTY
STOMACH/DIGESTIVE
  DISORDERS
• EPIGASTRIC PAIN
URINARY BLADDER
• DYSURIA
• URINATION, SCANTY

Clinical/Pharmaceutical Studies:

IMMUNE SYSTEM RELATED
DISORDERS/TOPICS
• ALLERGIC DISORDERS
NOSE

• RHINITIS, ALLERGIC: Cures
PARASITES
• HOOKWORMS: Tincuture

Prevents From Penetration Of Skin
SKIN
• URTICARIA, ALLERGIC

Dose
3 - 9 gm

Contraindications
Not: Pregnancy

Notes
Hsu Says: Liquidambaris Formosana, This Herb Is Bai
Jiao Xiang

MA BIAN CAO

馬鞭草
(马鞭草)

HERBA
VERBENAE

Traditional Functions:

1. Clears Heat and disperses Blood
2. Kills intestinal parasites
3. Disperses swelling

Traditional Properties:

Enters: SP, LV,

Properties: BIT, C

Indications:

ABDOMEN/
GASTROINTESTINAL TOPICS
• ABDOMEN, DISTENTION OF
• ABDOMEN, TUMORS
BOWEL RELATED DISORDERS
• DYSENTERY
CANCER/TUMORS/SWELLINGS/
LUMPS
• ABDOMEN, TUMORS
FLUID DISORDERS

• EDEMA
INFECTIOUS DISEASES
• INFLUENZA
• MALARIA, CHRONIC
ORAL CAVITY
• GINGIVITIS
SEXUALITY, FEMALE:
GYNECOLOGICAL
• AMENORRHEA
• DYSMENORRHEA

• LEUKORRHEA, MORBID
SKIN
• CARBUNCLES
SPLEEN
• SPLENOMEGALY: From Malaria
TRAUMA, BITES, POISONINGS
• WOUNDS, PURULENT
URINARY BLADDER
• URINATION, SCANTY

Clinical/Pharmaceutical Studies:

HEMORRHAGIC DISORDERS
• HEMOSTATIC: Promotes
Coagulation
INFECTIOUS DISEASES
• BACTERIAL, ANTI-

PAIN/NUMBNESS/GENERAL
DISCOMFORT
• ANALGESIC
PARASITES

• SCHISTOSOMIASIS: Helps To
Eliminate Ascites In
TRAUMA, BITES, POISONINGS
• INFLAMMATORY, ANTI-

Dose
15 - 30 gm

Common Name
Vervain

Contraindications
Not: Pregnancy

MAO DONG QING

毛冬青

RADIX
ILICIS PUBESCENTIS

Traditional Functions:

1. Clears toxic Heat
2. Vitalizes the Blood and removes stasis in the channels
3. Stops cough and circulates Lung Qi

Traditional Properties:

Enters: LU, HT,

Properties: BIT, A, N, (SP, C)

Indications:

BOWEL RELATED DISORDERS
• DYSENTERY
CIRCULATION DISORDERS
• ATHEROSCLEROSIS
• BUERGER'S DISEASE
• HYPERTENSION
• PHLEBITIS: 500 gm Dose Needed
• STROKE
• THROMBOTIC INFARCT
• VASCULITIS: (Inflammation Of
  The Blood/Lymph Vessels)
EYES
• IRIS INFLAMMATION
• RETINITIS, CENTRAL

HEART
• ANGINA PECTORIS: Chest Bi
  Strangulating Pain
• CORONARY HEART DISEASE,
  ATHEROSCLEROSIS
• INFARCTION, ACUTE
  MYOCARDIAC
INFECTIOUS DISEASES
• COMMON COLD: Wind Heat
LUNGS
• BRONCHITIS, ACUTE W/COUGH,
  SPUTUM
• COUGH: Lung Heat

**MENTAL STATE/
NEUROLOGICAL DISORDERS**
• HEMIPLEGIA, NOT STROKES
ORAL CAVITY
• LARYNX, WATER DISTENTION
• TONSILLITIS
SKIN
• ERYSIPELAS
• SCALDS
• SKIN, SUPPURATIVE DISEASES
TRAUMA, BITES, POISONINGS
• GANGRENE, SPONTANEOUS
  PRESENILE

Clinical/Pharmaceutical Studies:

**CIRCULATION
DISORDERS**
• THROMBOANGIITIS
OBLITERANS: With Pig
Trotters Or Bones, Oral
Decoction, Tablet, Syrup
Or Injection, Highly
Effective, Some Cases
Needed Surgery, Too
• VASODILATES
EYES
• CENTRAL RETINITIS:
IM Injections, Favorable
Results
HEART
• ANGINA PECTORIS:
Very Effective
• CARDIOTONIC:
Reduces Oxygen

Consumption, Increases
Blood Flow
• HEART DISEASE:
Decoction, Tablet, Granule
Infusion, 60-150 g/Day, 6-
8 Weeks Or 1-3 Months
• MYOCARDIAL
INFARCTION: Injection +
Oral
**IMMUNE SYSTEM
RELATED DISORDERS/
TOPICS**
• ALLERGIC RHINITIS:
Decoction
INFECTIOUS DISEASES
• BACTERIAL, ANTI-:
Gram Positive/Negative
Bacilli
• LEPROSY, SOLE

ULCERS OF: Decoction
LUNGS
• ANTITUSSIVE
• ASTHMA, BRONCHIAL:
Decoction
• BRONCHITIS, SPASTIC,
IN CHILDREN:
Decoction
• EXPECTORANT
• PNEUMONIA,
CHILDHOOD: Injection,
75% Cure
**MENTAL STATE/
NEUROLOGICAL
DISORDERS**
• CEREBRAL
THROMBOSIS:
Decoction + Injection With
Vasodilators, New

Acupuncture Therapy,
High Cure Rate, 13-52
Days
NOSE
• ALLERGIC RHINITIS:
Decoction
SKIN
• BURNS: 50%
Concentrated Decoction
With Vaseline Gauze,
Change Daily, With Oral
Decoction If Fever
**TRAUMA, BITES,
POISONINGS**
• LIMB, SEVERED
(FINGER) : Injection
Relieved Post Op
Vasospasm, Increased
Rejoining Rate

Dose

30 - 120 gm

Common Name

Hairy Holly

Contraindications

Not: Bleeding Tendency

Notes

For Some: Dry Mouth, Stomach Discomfort, Headache,
Dizziness, Nausea, Abdominal Distention, All Mild,
Stopped With Herbs

MO YAO   没藥   MYRRHA
                        (没药)

Traditional Functions:

1. Vitalizes the Blood and dispels stagnant Blood, reduces swellings and
relieves pain
2. Promotes healing of chronic non-healing sores and wounds--topical

Traditional Properties:

Enters: LV,

Properties: BIT, N

Indications:

**ABDOMEN/
GASTROINTESTINAL TOPICS**
• ABDOMEN, MASS: Blood Stasis
• ABDOMEN, PAIN OF: Blood
Stasis

**PAIN/NUMBNESS/GENERAL
DISCOMFORT**
• BI DISORDERS: Blood Stasis
• BI, WIND DAMP: Pain
• BI, WIND DAMP, CHRONIC:

SKIN
• CARBUNCLES: Pain, Swelling Of
• FURUNCLES: Topical Treatment
• SKIN, SORES, SWOLLEN, TOXIC:
Blood Stasis, Swelling

Indications:

CANCER/TUMORS/SWELLINGS/
LUMPS
• SWELLINGS
CHEST
• CHEST, PAIN: Blood Stasis
ORAL CAVITY
• MOUTH, WASH

With Blood Stasis, Open The Luo
SEXUALITY, FEMALE:
GYNECOLOGICAL
• AMENORRHEA: Blood Stasis
• BREASTS, SWOLLEN, PAINFUL,
ABSCESS
• DYSMENORRHEA

• SORES
• SORES, CHRONIC, NON-
HEALING: Topical
TRAUMA, BITES, POISONINGS
• TRAUMA, PAIN, SWELLING:
Blood Stasis
• WOUNDS

Clinical/Pharmaceutical Studies:

ABDOMEN/
GASTROINTESTINAL TOPICS
• GASTROINTESTINAL,
STIMULATES MOTILITY
BLOOD RELATED DISORDERS/
TOPICS
• CHOLESTEROL, LOWERS
CIRCULATION DISORDERS
• ATHEROSCLEROSIS: Prevent
Plaque Formation

INFECTIOUS DISEASES
• BACTERIAL, ANTI-
LUNGS
• ANTITUSSIVE: Tincture Of,
Suppresses Secretions
• BRONCHI, INHIBITS
SECRETION
• BRONCHITIS, CHRONIC
• EXPECTORANT: Tincture Of

NUTRITIONAL/METABOLIC
DISORDERS/TOPICS
• BODY WEIGHT, DECREASES
SEXUALITY, FEMALE:
GYNECOLOGICAL
• UTERUS, INHIBITS SECRETION
SKIN
• FUNGAL, ANTI-: Aqueous Extract,
Many Skin

Dose

3 - 12 gm

Common Name

Myrrh

Contraindications

Not: Pregnancy

Not: Excess Uterine Bleeding

Notes

Ru Xiang Similar But Warm Property
w/Vinegar To Enhance Analgesic Effect
Large Dose: Up To 15 gm

NIU XI

(HUAI NIU XI)

牛膝

RADIX
ACHYRANTHIS
BIDENTATAE

Traditional Functions:

1. Vitalizes the Blood and releases stagnant Blood
2. Tonifies the Liver and Kidney, strengthens the tendons and bones and
benefits the joints
3. Promotes urination and clears Damp Heat in the Lower Burner
4. Conducts the downward movement of Blood

Traditional Properties:

Enters: KI, LV,

Properties: BIT, SO, N

Indications:

ABDOMEN/
GASTROINTESTINAL TOPICS
• ABDOMEN, MASS
BLOOD RELATED DISORDERS/
TOPICS
• BLOOD PRESSURE, LOWERS
CANCER/TUMORS/SWELLINGS/
LUMPS
• TUMORS, GYNECOLOGICAL:
Raw
CIRCULATION DISORDERS
• HYPERTENSION
EARS/HEARING DISORDERS
• DIZZINESS: Liver Yang Rising
• VERTIGO: Liver Yang/Fire Rising
EXTREMITIES
• LEGS, UPPER THIGHS,

Fire Rising
• HEMATEMESIS: Yin Deficient
With Fire Rising
• HEMATURIA
• HEMORRHAGE: Leading Blood
Down To Stop
LIVER
• LIVER YANG RISING: Headache,
Dizziness, Blurred Vision
MUSCULOSKELETAL/
CONNECTIVE TISSUE
• ARTHRITIS
• BACK, LOWER PAIN: Deficiency/
Damp Heat, Descending/Wind Damp
Bi, Wine Treated
• JOINTS, PAIN: Damp Bi With
Liver Kidney Weakness

GYNECOLOGICAL
• AMENORRHEA: Blood Stasis,
Raw
• DYSMENORRHEA: Blood Stasis
• LABOR, DIFFICULT: Raw
• LEUKORRHEA: Auxillary Herb
• LOCHIOSCHESIS: Blood Stasis
• MENSTRUATION, DISORDERS
OF: Dredge, Regulate Chong, Ren
• POSTPARTUM, ABDOMINAL
PAIN: Blood Stasis, Raw
• WOMEN'S DISEASES,
BLEEDING
SKIN
• CARBUNCLES: Raw
TRAUMA, BITES, POISONINGS
• TRAUMA: Raw

Indications:

WEAKNESS OF
- **LEGS, WEAK, LACK OF SENSATION:** Liver Kidney Deficiency

EYES
- **EYES, BLURRED VISION:** Liver Yang Rising

HEAD/NECK
- **HEADACHE:** Liver Yang Rising

HEMORRHAGIC DISORDERS
- **BLEEDING GUMS:** Yin Deficient With Fire Rising
- **EPISTAXIS:** Yin Deficient With

- **JOINTS, PAIN, ATROPHIC:** Wine Treated
- **KNEES, PAIN:** Deficiency/Damp Heat Descending/Wind Damp, Wine Treated
- **MUSCLES, NUMB**

ORAL CAVITY
- **GUMS, BLEEDING:** Yin Deficient With Fire Rising
- **THROAT, BI PAIN:** Raw
- **TOOTHACHE:** Yin Deficient With Fire Rising

SEXUALITY, FEMALE:

URINARY BLADDER
- **DYSURIA:** Auxillary Herb
- **URINARY STONES, W/ HEAMTURIA, LOWER BACK PAIN:** Raw
- **URINARY TRACT INFECTIONS:** Auxillary Herb
- **URINATION, DRIBBLING:** Raw

YIN RELATED DISORDERS/ TOPICS
- **YIN DEFICIENCY FIRE:** Epistaxis, Hematemesis, Toothaches, Bleeding Gums

Clinical/Pharmaceutical Studies:

ABDOMEN/ GASTROINTESTINAL TOPICS
- **GASTROINTESTINAL TRACT:** More Contractions, Less Motility

BLOOD RELATED DISORDERS/ TOPICS
- **BLOOD PRESSURE, LOWERS:** Both Decoctions, Alcohol Extracts-- Vasodilation, Heart Inhibition, Short Term

IMMUNE SYSTEM RELATED DISORDERS/TOPICS
- **ALLERGIC, ANTI-:** Aqueous Extract

INFECTIOUS DISEASES
- **DIPHTHERIA:** Oral Decoction Or

Spray

KIDNEYS
- **DIURETIC**

LUNGS
- **PNEUMONIA, CHILDHOOD:** Use Fresh Juice

MUSCULOSKELETAL/ CONNECTIVE TISSUE
- **SPRAINS, ANALGESIC FOR:** Much Less Than Morphine

NUTRITIONAL/METABOLIC DISORDERS/TOPICS
- **METABOLISM, STRONG PROTEIN ANABOLISM ACTION**

PAIN/NUMBNESS/GENERAL

DISCOMFORT
- **ANALGESIC, SPRAINS:** Much Less Than Morphine

SEXUALITY, FEMALE: GYNECOLOGICAL
- **ABORTION, INDUCES LABOR:** Directly Insert Piece Into Cervix
- **UTERUS, STIMULATES:** Causes Contractions

TRAUMA, BITES, POISONINGS
- **INFLAMMATORY, ANTI-:** ETOH Extracts

URINARY BLADDER
- **URINARY STONES:** Niu Xi-Ru Xiang Powder

Dose

9 - 15 gm

Contraindications

Not: Pregnancy

Not: Diarrhea w/Def SP

Not: Excess Menstruation Or Spermatorrhea

Notes

Dose: Up To 30 gm

RU XIANG

乳香

GUMMI OLIBANUM

Traditional Functions:

1. Vitalizes the Blood, promotes the circulation of Qi and controls bleeding
2. Relaxes the tendons and muscles, activates the channels, and controls pain
3. Reduces swelling and promotes healing--topical application

Traditional Properties:

Enters: SP, HT, LV,

Properties: SP, BIT, W

Indications:

ABDOMEN/ GASTROINTESTINAL TOPICS
- **ABDOMEN, PAIN OF:** Blood Stasis

CANCER/TUMORS/SWELLINGS/ LUMPS
- **SWELLINGS:** Topical, Early Stage

CHEST
- **CHEST, PAIN:** Blood Stasis

CIRCULATION DISORDERS
- **VASCULAR CONTRACTIONS**

MENTAL STATE/

ORAL CAVITY
- **GUMS, SWOLLEN**
- **MOUTH, PAIN IN**
- **THROAT PAIN**

PAIN/NUMBNESS/GENERAL DISCOMFORT
- **BI, WIND DAMP DISEASES**
- **BI, WIND DAMP, CHRONIC:** With Blood Stasis, Open The Luo
- **PAIN, EARLY STAGE**

SEXUALITY, FEMALE: GYNECOLOGICAL

BLEEDING

SKIN
- **ABSCESS:** Early Stage
- **SKIN, SORES, SWOLLEN, TOXIC:** Blood Stasis, Swelling
- **SORES:** Early Stage, Promotes Healing, Reduces Pain
- **ULCERS, CHRONIC**

STOMACH/DIGESTIVE DISORDERS
- **EPIGASTRIC PAIN:** Blood Stasis

TRAUMA, BITES, POISONINGS

Indications:

NEUROLOGICAL DISORDERS
• RIGIDITY
MUSCULOSKELETAL/
CONNECTIVE TISSUE
• MUSCLES, CONTRACTIONS OF
• SPASMS

• AMENORRHEA
• BREASTS, SWOLLEN, PAINFUL,
  ABSCESS
• DYSMENORRHEA
• WOMEN'S DISEASES,

• TRAUMA, INJURIES: Promotes
  Healing, Reduces Pain
• TRAUMA, PAIN, SWELLING:
  Internal/External
• WOUNDS

Clinical/Pharmaceutical Studies:

CHEST
• CHEST, PAIN: (Sharp/Colicky) w/
  Mo Yao, et al

INFECTIOUS DISEASES
• BACTERIAL, ANTI-: Very Strong

LUNGS
• TUBERCULOSIS, ANTI

Dose
3 - 9 gm
Common Name
Frankincense

Contraindications
Not: Pregnancy
Notes
w/Vinegar To Increase Vitalizing Blood/Stop Pain
Action
May Be Up To 15 gm

SAN LENG   三 稜   *RHIZOMA SPARGANII*

Traditional Functions:

1. Strongly vitalizes stagnant Blood
2. Promotes Qi circulation and reduces pain
3. Helps dissolve food accumulations and moves stagnant Qi

Traditional Properties:

Enters: SP, LV,

Properties: BIT, SP, N

Indications:

ABDOMEN/
GASTROINTESTINAL TOPICS
• ABDOMEN, MASS/TUMOR
• ABDOMEN, PAIN OF,
  DISTENTION, SEVERE: Food
  Stagnation, Qi Stagnation
• ABDOMEN, PAIN OF,
  POSTPARTUM: Blood Stasis
• APPENDICITIS W/PAIN
CANCER/TUMORS/SWELLINGS/
LUMPS
• ABDOMEN, MASS/TUMORS
• MASSES, ABDOMINAL

• TUMORS, GYNECOLOGICAL
CHEST
• CHEST, DISTENTION, PAIN
• CHEST, PAIN
• COSTAL REGION, PAIN
LIVER
• HEPATOMEGALY
• LIVER QI CONGESTION W/
  SUBCOSTAL PAIN
QI RELATED DISORDERS/
TOPICS
• QI, BLOOD STAGNATION
SEXUALITY, FEMALE:

GYNECOLOGICAL
• AMENORRHEA
• DYSMENORRHEA
• LACTATION, INSUFFICIENT
• UTERUS, FIBROSIS
SPLEEN
• SPLENOMEGALY
STOMACH/DIGESTIVE
DISORDERS
• FOOD STAGNATION: Severe
  Abdominal Pain, Distension
• INDIGESTION

Clinical/Pharmaceutical Studies:

CANCER/TUMORS/SWELLINGS/
LUMPS

• CANCER: w/E Zhu-Hepatic Cancer,
  Granuloma, Injections With

Decoctions

Dose
3 - 9 gm
Common Name
Bur-Reed Rhizome
Contraindications
Not: Pregnancy

Not: Profuse Menstrual Flow
Precautions
Watch: Def Conditions
Notes
Vinegar Prepared Helps Stop Pain
Do Not Use Long Term

SHU FU

鼠婦
（鼠妇）

ARMADILLIDIUM

Traditional Functions:

1. Vitalizes the Blood and disperses stagnation
2. Promotes urination
3. Clears toxin and controls pain

Traditional Properties:

Enters: LV, PC

Properties: SO, C

Indications:

ABDOMEN/
GASTROINTESTINAL TOPICS
• ABDOMEN, MASS
INFECTIOUS DISEASES
• MALARIA, CHRONIC

ORAL CAVITY
• STOMATITIS, MYCOTIC: (Mouth,
Throat Fungus Infection, Of
Children)
• TOOTHACHE

SEXUALITY, FEMALE:
GYNECOLOGICAL
• AMENORRHEA
URINARY BLADDER
• DYSURIA

Clinical/Pharmaceutical Studies:

INFECTIOUS DISEASES
• LEPROSY: Topical As Ointment/
Ingested Extract

SEXUALITY, FEMALE:
GYNECOLOGICAL

• UTERUS, STIMULATES: Similar
To Ergot

Dose

3 - 6 gm

Common Name

Wood Louse

SHUI ZHI

水蛭

HIRUDO SEU WHITMANIAE

Traditional Functions:

1. Cracks stagnant Blood, opens menstruation and reduces immobile masses

Traditional Properties:

Enters: UB, LV,

Properties: SA, BIT, N, TX

Indications:

ABDOMEN/
GASTROINTESTINAL TOPICS
• ABDOMEN, LOWER BLOOD
RETENTION
• ABDOMEN, MASS, IMMOBILE:
Stagnant Blood

BLOOD RELATED DISORDERS/
TOPICS
• BLOOD STASIS PAIN
CANCER/TUMORS/SWELLINGS/
LUMPS
• TUMORS, GYNECOLOGICAL

SEXUALITY, FEMALE:
GYNECOLOGICAL
• AMENORRHEA
TRAUMA, BITES, POISONINGS
• FRACTURES
• TRAUMA, INJURIES

Clinical/Pharmaceutical Studies:

BLOOD RELATED DISORDERS/
TOPICS
• ANTICOAGULANT: (Unless
Heated) , Stronger Than Tao Ren,

Alcohol Stronger Than Decoctions,
Contains Heparin, Hirudin
CIRCULATION DISORDERS
• VASODILATOR

EYES
• CONJUNCTIVITIS, ACUTE: Eye
Drops, 1-5 Days

Dose

1.5 - 4.5 gm

Common Name

Leech

Contraindications

Not: Pregnancy

Not: Def Blood/Weakness w/o Stasis

Notes

Very Strong-Not For Long Term Use
Cancers: Max 6-9 gm
Powder: 0.3-0.6 gm

SI GUA LUO

絲瓜蔞
(丝瓜蒌)

FASCICULUS VASCULARIS LUFFAE

Traditional Functions:

1. Expels Wind and promotes circulation through the channels
2. Disperses Phlegm and clears Lung Heat cough
3. Removes Summer Heat and promotes urination
4. Promotes lactation, disperses swelling and benefits the breasts

Traditional Properties:

Enters: LU, ST, LV,

Properties: SW, N

Indications:

ABDOMEN/
GASTROINTESTINAL TOPICS
• ABDOMEN, PAIN OF
• FLANK SORENESS: Wind Damp
Heat In Muscles, Channels
CANCER/TUMORS/SWELLINGS/
LUMPS
• SWELLINGS, PAIN
CHEST
• CHEST, SORENESS: Wind Damp
Heat In Muscles, Channels
FLUID DISORDERS
• EDEMA
HEART
• HEART, PAIN OF: Qi Stasis
HEAT
• SUMMER HEAT W/FEVER,
SCANTY URINE

HEMORRHAGIC DISORDERS
• HEMAFECIA
LIVER
• LIVER QI CONGESTION W/
SUBCOSTAL PAIN
LUNGS
• COUGH, FEVER, CHEST PAIN:
Lung Heat
MUSCULOSKELETAL/
CONNECTIVE TISSUE
• BACK, LOWER PAIN
• JOINTS, PAIN, SWELLING, RED:
Hot Bi
• JOINTS, STIFF: Wind Damp Heat
In Muscles, Channels
• MUSCLES, SORE: Wind Damp
Heat In Muscles, Channels
PAIN/NUMBNESS/GENERAL

DISCOMFORT
• PAIN, CHANNELS
QI RELATED DISORDERS/
TOPICS
• QI, BLOOD STAGNATION
SEXUALITY, FEMALE:
GYNECOLOGICAL
• AMENORRHEA
• BREASTS, ABSCESS OF
• BREASTS, SWOLLEN, PAINFUL
• LACTATION, INSUFFICIENT
• UTERINE BLEEDING
SEXUALITY, MALE:
UROLOGICAL TOPICS
• TESTICLES, SWELLING
TRAUMA, BITES, POISONINGS
• TRAUMA

Clinical/Pharmaceutical Studies:

FEVERS
• ANTIPYRETIC
KIDNEYS

• DIURETIC
LUNGS
• ANTITUSSIVE

• EXPECTORANT
TRAUMA, BITES, POISONINGS
• ANTIDOTE, TOXICS

Dose

6 - 12 gm

Common Name

Luffa Sponge

SU MU

蘇木
(苏木)

LIGNUM SAPPAN

Traditional Functions:

1. Vitalizes the blood, reduces swellings and relieves pain
2. Stops postpartum bleeding

Traditional Properties:

Enters: HT, LV, SP

Properties: SW, SA, N

Indications:

ABDOMEN/
GASTROINTESTINAL TOPICS
• ABDOMEN, PAIN OF: Women's,
In Xue/Qi Portion
BLOOD RELATED DISORDERS/
TOPICS
• ANEMIA
CANCER/TUMORS/SWELLINGS/
LUMPS

Joints
• PAIN: Blood Stasis
QI RELATED DISORDERS/
TOPICS
• QI OBSTRUCTION
SEXUALITY, FEMALE:
GYNECOLOGICAL
• AMENORRHEA: With Surging Of
Qi

SKIN
• CARBUNCLES
• ECZEMA: Damp Heat
• SKIN, SORES: Damp Heat
STOMACH/DIGESTIVE
DISORDERS
• STOMACH, PAIN: Women's, In
Xue/Qi Portion
TRAUMA, BITES, POISONINGS

Indications:

- SWELLINGS, INFLAMMED
HEART
- ANGINA PECTORIS: Chest Bi
Strangulating Pain
- CARDIAC PAIN IN WOMEN
**PAIN/NUMBNESS/GENERAL
DISCOMFORT**
- ANALGESIC: Stomach, Muscles,

- DYSMENORRHEA
- POSTPARTUM, ABDOMINAL
PAIN: Blood Stasis
- POSTPARTUM, BLEEDING,
EXCESS W/DIZZINESS,
SHORTNESS OF BREATH
- WOMEN'S DISEASES,
BLEEDING

- CONTUSIONS
- FRACTURES
- SPRAINS
- TRAUMA, BLEEDING
- TRAUMA, INTERNAL/
EXTERNAL
- TRAUMA, PAIN, SWELLING
- WOUNDS

Clinical/Pharmaceutical Studies:

**BLOOD RELATED DISORDERS/
TOPICS**
- BLOOD CLOTTING TIME,
SHORTENS
CIRCULATION DISORDERS
- VASOCONSTRICTOR
INFECTIOUS DISEASES

- ANTIBIOTIC: Very Strong Inhibits,
Many Bacteria
**MENTAL STATE/
NEUROLOGICAL DISORDERS**
- HYPNOTIC: Coma In Large Doses
(Anti-Strychnine, Cocaine)
- TRANQUILIZING

**PAIN/NUMBNESS/GENERAL
DISCOMFORT**
- ANALGESIC
**SEXUALITY, FEMALE:
GYNECOLOGICAL**
- UTERUS, INHIBITS
CONTRACTION

Dose

3 - 9 gm

Common Name

Sappan Wood

Contraindications

Not: Pregnancy

Notes

May Induce Vomiting, Diarrhea

TAO REN   桃仁   SEMEN PERSICAE

Traditional Functions:

1. Vitalizes the Blood and disperses stagnant Blood.
2. Moistens the intestines and facilitates passage of stool
3. Relieves cough and wheezing

Traditional Properties:

Enters: LU, LI, HT, LV,

Properties: BIT, SW, N

Indications:

**ABDOMEN/
GASTROINTESTINAL
TOPICS**
- ABDOMEN, PAIN OF
- ABDOMEN, TUMORS
- ABSCESS, LARGE
INTESTINE/LUNG
- APPENDICITIS W/PAIN
- FLANK PAIN
**BLOOD RELATED
DISORDERS/TOPICS**
- BLOOD STASIS IN LUO
**BOWEL RELATED
DISORDERS**
- CONSTIPATION:
Intestinal Dryness

**CANCER/TUMORS/
SWELLINGS/LUMPS**
- ABDOMEN, TUMORS
- LUMPS, MASSES
- MASSES, ABDOMINAL
CHEST
- INTERCOSTAL PAIN
HEART
- ANGINA PECTORIS:
Chest Bi Strangulating
Pain
LUNGS
- ABSCESS, LUNG/
LARGE INTESTINE
- ASTHMA
- COUGH: Cold Phlegm

- LUNGS, ABSCESS W/
PURULENT VOMIT
- LUNGS, DYSPNEA:
Cold Phlegm
**MENTAL STATE/
NEUROLOGICAL
DISORDERS**
- MENTAL
DERANGEMENT: Blood
Retention
**PAIN/NUMBNESS/
GENERAL
DISCOMFORT**
- PAIN: Vertex To Teeth
**SEXUALITY, FEMALE:
GYNECOLOGICAL**

- AMENORRHEA
- MENSTRUATION,
CRAMPS OF
- MENSTRUATION,
DISORDERS OF:
Constrict Uterus, Stimulate
Chong
- WOMEN'S DISEASES,
BLEEDING
SKIN
- CARBUNCLES
**TRAUMA, BITES,
POISONINGS**
- TRAUMA, PAIN,
INJURIES, INTERNAL/
EXTERNAL

Clinical/Pharmaceutical Studies:

**BLOOD RELATED DISORDERS/
TOPICS**
- ANTICOAGULANT: Alcohol
Extractions, Weak
- BLOOD PRESSURE, LOWERS
BOWEL RELATED DISORDERS
- LAXATIVE: Emollient

LUNGS
- ANTITUSSIVE: From Hydrolyzed
Amygdalin, Sedates Respiratory
Center
- ASTHMA: From Hydrolyzed
Amygdalin, Sedates Respiratory
Center

- TUBERCULOSIS: Anti
**PAIN/NUMBNESS/GENERAL
DISCOMFORT**
- ANALGESIC
TRAUMA, BITES, POISONINGS
- DETOXIFIES
- INFLAMMATORY, ANTI-

Dose
3 - 9 gm
Common Name
Peach Kernel

Contraindications
Not: Pregnancy
Notes
(Hong Hua & Tao Ren Used Together)
Pound Into Pieces Before Decoction

TU BIE CHONG
(ZHE CHONG)

土鱉蟲
（土鳖虫）

EUPOLYPHAGAE SEU OPISTHOPLATIAE

Traditional Functions:

1. Moves stagnant Blood, promotes healing and relieves pain
2. Dissolves lumps and masses
3. Moves the Qi in the channels

Traditional Properties:

Enters: SP, HT, LV,

Properties: SA, C, TX

Indications:

ABDOMEN/
 GASTROINTESTINAL TOPICS
• ABDOMEN, MASS: Congealed
 Blood
• ABDOMEN, MASS, CANCER: 9-
 15 gm
• ABDOMEN, PAIN OF
• HYPOCHONDRIAC REGION,
 PAIN: Hepatomegaly/Splenomegaly
CANCER/TUMORS/SWELLINGS/
 LUMPS
• ABDOMEN MASS, CANCER:

Cancers, 9-15 gm
• SWELLINGS: Stagnant Blood
• TUMORS, ABDOMINAL: Cancers,
 9-15 gm
MUSCULOSKELETAL/
 CONNECTIVE TISSUE
• BACK, LOWER PAIN
• LIGAMENTS, INJURIES
ORAL CAVITY
• TONGUE, NUMB, SWOLLEN:
 Congealed Blood
SEXUALITY, FEMALE:

GYNECOLOGICAL
• AMENORRHEA: Congealed Blood
STOMACH/DIGESTIVE
 DISORDERS
• FOOD STAGNATION
TRAUMA, BITES, POISONINGS
• CONTUSIONS
• FRACTURES
• LACERATIONS
• SPRAINS
• TRAUMA, INTERNAL,
 EXTERNAL

Dose
3 - 12 gm
Common Name
Wingless Cockroach
Contraindications
Not: Pregnancy

Notes
For Numb, Swollen Tongue: 6 gm + 3 gm Salt. Grind.
Apply
Cancers: 9-15 gm
Powder: 1.2-1.8 gm

WA LENG ZI

瓦楞子

CONCHA ARCAE

Traditional Functions:

1. Vitalizes the Blood, resolves Phlegm and dissipates nodules
2. Neutralizes acids and relieves pain

Traditional Properties:

Enters: SP, ST, LV,

Properties: SW, SA, N

Indications:

ABDOMEN/
 GASTROINTESTINAL TOPICS
• ABDOMEN, MASS, IMMOBILE/
 MOBILE: Blood/Qi Stagnation/
 Phlegm
• GASTROINTESTINAL
 NODULAR SWELLINGS
• ULCERS, DUODENAL
CANCER/TUMORS/SWELLINGS/
 LUMPS

• TUMORS, GYNECOLOGICAL
ENDOCRINE RELATED
 DISORDERS
• GOITER
IMMUNE SYSTEM RELATED
 DISORDERS/TOPICS
• LYMPH GLANDS,
 ENLARGEMENT, CHRONIC:
 Phlegm Nodules
LIVER

• HEPATOMEGALY
SPLEEN
• SPLENOMEGALY
STOMACH/DIGESTIVE
 DISORDERS
• REGURGITATION, ACIDIC W/
 VOMITING, STABBING PAIN:
 Congealed Blood
• STOMACH, HYPERACIDITY
• ULCERS, GASTRIC, PAINFUL

Clinical/Pharmaceutical Studies:

STOMACH/DIGESTIVE DISORDERS

• ULCERS, GASTRIC/DUODENAL: With Gan Cao (5:1) , A Few Had

Edema, Hematuria, Frequent Urinary Tract Infections

Dose
9 - 30 gm

Common Name
Cockle Shell

Notes
Raw: Nodules

Baked: Acid Regurgitation And Pain

3-9 gm Pill/Powder

WANG BU LIU XING

王不留行

SEMEN VACCARIAE SEGETALIS

Traditional Functions:

1. Moves Blood and promotes circulation through the channels, thus encouraging menstruation and lactation
2. Reduces swelling, relieves pain and promotes healing
3. Promotes urination and clears urinary stones

Traditional Properties:

Enters: ST, LV,

Properties: BIT, N

Indications:

CANCER/TUMORS/SWELLINGS/ LUMPS
• BREASTS, TUMORS
• SWELLINGS, PAIN
SEXUALITY, FEMALE: GYNECOLOGICAL
• AMENORRHEA
• BREASTS, TUMORS OF
• DYSMENORRHEA
• LABOR, DIFFICULT

• LACTATION, INSUFFICIENT
• MENSTRUATION, DISORDERS OF: Dredge, Regulate Chong, Ren
• SWELLING, BREASTS/ TESTICLES
SEXUALITY, MALE: UROLOGICAL TOPICS
• SWELLING, BREASTS/ TESTICLES

SKIN
• ABSCESS: Topical
• FURUNCLES, TOXIC
• ULCERS, TOXIC: Topical
TRAUMA, BITES, POISONINGS
• WOUNDS: Topical
URINARY BLADDER
• URINARY TRACT/BLADDER, STONES

Clinical/Pharmaceutical Studies:

INFECTIOUS DISEASES
• HERPES ZOSTER: Pain/Cleared-- Toasted, Powdered, With Sesame Oil, Local, Not Open Sores, 1-2x/Day

For 30 Minutes, Pain Gone In 10-20 Minutes
SEXUALITY, FEMALE:

GYNECOLOGICAL
• UTERUS, STIMULATES: Decoction Strong, Alcohol Stronger

Dose
3 - 30 gm

Contraindications
Not: Pregnancy

WU LING ZHI

五靈脂
(五灵脂)

EXCREMENTUM TROGOPTERORI SEU PTEROMI

Traditional Functions:

1. Circulates stagnant Blood and relieves pain
2. Treats chronic childhood nutritional impairment with abdominal distension

Traditional Properties:

Enters: SP, LV,

Properties: BIT, SW, W

Indications:

ABDOMEN/ GASTROINTESTINAL TOPICS
• ABDOMEN, PAIN OF: Raw, Derangement Of Qi, Blood
CHILDHOOD DISORDERS
• MALNUTRITION BLOATING,

MENTAL STATE/ NEUROLOGICAL DISORDERS
• EPILEPSY
MUSCULOSKELETAL/ CONNECTIVE TISSUE
• SPASMS: Wind

CHRONIC: Fried
• LOCHIOSCHESIS
• MENORRHAGIA: Fried
• MENORRHALGIA
• POSTPARTUM, ABDOMINAL PAIN: Raw, Blood Stasis

Indications:

CHILDHOOD
HEART
• ANGINA PECTORIS: Chest Bi
Strangulating Pain
• CORONARY ARTERY DISEASE
• CORONARY HEART DISEASE
HEMORRHAGIC DISORDERS
• HEMORRHAGE: Blood Stasis
Caused, Charred/Fried Herbs

PAIN/NUMBNESS/GENERAL
DISCOMFORT
• ANALGESIC: Stomach, Muscles,
Joints
SEXUALITY, FEMALE:
GYNECOLOGICAL
• AMENORRHEA
• DYSMENORRHEA
• LEUKORRHEA, BLOOD TINGED,

• UTERINE BLEEDING: Stagnant
Blood
**STOMACH/DIGESTIVE
DISORDERS**
• EPIGASTRIC PAIN
TRAUMA, BITES, POISONINGS
• CENTIPEDE BITE: Topical
• SCORPION BITE: Topical
• SNAKE BITES: Topical

Clinical/Pharmaceutical Studies:

INFECTIOUS DISEASES
• BACTERIAL, ANTI-
• MYCOBACTERIAL, ANTI-
LUNGS
• TUBERCULOSIS: With Lian Qiao
MUSCULOSKELETAL/

CONNECTIVE TISSUE
• MUSCLES, SMOOTH: Releases
Spasms
PAIN/NUMBNESS/GENERAL
DISCOMFORT
• ANALGESIC

SKIN
• FUNGAL, ANTI-
TRAUMA, BITES, POISONINGS
• SNAKE BITES: Powdered With
Xiong Huang, Internally With Wine
And Topical

Dose
3 - 9 gm
Common Name
Flying Squirrel Feces

Notes
Raw: Vitalizes Blood, Stops Pain
w/Vinegar: To Break Blood, Stop Pain
Stir Fry: Stops Bleeding
Wrap For Decoction

XUE JIE   血竭   SANGUIS DRACONIS

Traditional Functions:
1. Vitalizes and disperses stagnant Blood and reduces pain
2. Stops bleeding and promotes tissue regeneration

Traditional Properties:
Enters: HT, LV,

Properties: SW, SA, N

Indications:

BLOOD RELATED DISORDERS/
TOPICS
• BLOOD STASIS PAIN
HEART
• ANGINA PECTORIS: Chest Bi
Strangulating Pain
HEMORRHAGIC DISORDERS
• HEMORRHAGE: Topical

PAIN/NUMBNESS/GENERAL
DISCOMFORT
• ANALGESIC
SKIN
• FURUNCLES
• SKIN, SORES, SWOLLEN, TOXIC:
Blood Stasis, Swelling
• ULCERS, CHRONIC,

NONHEALING
TRAUMA, BITES, POISONINGS
• CONTUSIONS
• FRACTURES
• SPRAINS
• TRAUMA, INJURIES: Die Da
• WOUNDS, PROMOTES
HEALING

Clinical/Pharmaceutical Studies:

BLOOD RELATED DISORDERS/
TOPICS
• BLOOD: Helps To Restore Calcium

Levels In
HEMORRHAGIC DISORDERS
• HEMOSTATIC

SKIN
• FUNGAL, ANTI-: Large Doses,
Aqueous Extract

Dose
0.3 - 1.5 gm
Common Name
Dragon's Blood

Contraindications
Not: Pregnancy
Not: Def Yin Hot Blood
Not: In Absence Of Blood Stagnation

YAN HU SUO   延胡索   *RHIZOMA CORYDALIS YANHUSUO*

Traditional Functions:

1. Vitalizes the Blood and dispels Blood stasis/ecchymosis
2. Promotes the flow of Qi and relieves pain

Traditional Properties:

Enters: SP, LV,

Properties: SP, BIT, W

Indications:

ABDOMEN/ GASTROINTESTINAL TOPICS
• ABDOMEN, PAIN OF: Stagnant Qi
• ABDOMEN, PAIN OF, HERNIA-LIKE: Cold
BLOOD RELATED DISORDERS/ TOPICS
• BLOOD STASIS PAIN
CANCER/TUMORS/SWELLINGS/ LUMPS
• TUMORS, GYNECOLOGICAL
CHEST
• CHEST, PAIN: Stagnant Qi
HEART
• ANGINA PECTORIS: Chest Bi

Strangulating Pain
• HEART, PAIN OF
LIVER
• LIVER QI CONGESTION W/ SUBCOSTAL PAIN
MENTAL STATE/ NEUROLOGICAL DISORDERS
• INSOMNIA
MUSCULOSKELETAL/ CONNECTIVE TISSUE
• BACK, LOWER PAIN
• KNEES, PAIN
PAIN/NUMBNESS/GENERAL DISCOMFORT
• ANALGESIC: Stomach, Muscles,

Joints
• PAIN, GENERAL
SEXUALITY, FEMALE: GYNECOLOGICAL
• DYSMENORRHEA: Stagnant Qi
• MENORRHAGIA
• MENSTRUATION, IRREGULAR
STOMACH/DIGESTIVE DISORDERS
• EPIGASTRIC PAIN: Stagnant Qi
TRAUMA, BITES, POISONINGS
• TRAUMA, INJURIES
URINARY BLADDER
• URINATION, DRIBBLING

Clinical/Pharmaceutical Studies:

ABDOMEN/ GASTROINTESTINAL TOPICS
• ABDOMEN, PAIN OF: 60-120 mg 1-4x/Day Of L-Tetrahydropalmatine, Active Ingredient
CIRCULATION DISORDERS
• HYPERTENSION, EARLY: 50-100 mg Dl-Tetrahydropalmatine, 3-4x/ Day, For 1-2 Months, Relieves Dizziness, Headache With Later Blood Pressure Lowering
ENDOCRINE RELATED DISORDERS
• ACTH, STIMULATES
• THYROID, CAN ENLARGE, WHEN INJECTED
HEAD/NECK
• HEADACHE: 60-120 mg 1-4x/Day Of L-Tetrahydropalmatine, Active Ingredient
• HEADACHE, FROM BRAIN CONCUSSION: 60-120 mg 1-4x/ Day Of L-Tetrahydropalmatine, Active Ingredient
HEART
• ANGINA PECTORIS: 80% Extract

Of Herb, 83% Effective
• CORONARY ARTERIES, DILATES: ETOH Extract
• MYOCARDIAL INFARCTION: Reduced Mortality, Improved Ekg
MENTAL STATE/ NEUROLOGICAL DISORDERS
• HYPNOTIC: Large Doses, 100-200 mg Dl-Tetrahydropalmatine, No Side Effects Such As Dizziness/Vertigo
• NEUROLOGICAL PAIN: 60-120 mg 1-4x/Day Of L-Tetrahydropalmatine, Active Ingredient
• SEDATIVE, LARGE DOSES: 100-200 mg Of Active Ingredient, Tetrahydropalmatine
• TRANQUILIZING: High Doses
MUSCULOSKELETAL/ CONNECTIVE TISSUE
• ANTISPASMODIC: Relaxes Muscles
• BACK, LOWER PAIN
• JOINTS, PAIN
NUTRITIONAL/METABOLIC DISORDERS/TOPICS

• HYPOTHERMIA: Helps
PAIN/NUMBNESS/GENERAL DISCOMFORT
• ANALGESIC: 1% Opium Strength, ETOH/Acetic Acid Extract Strongest, 40% Of Morphine Strength
• ANESTHETIC, LOCAL: 0.2% By Injection
SEXUALITY, FEMALE: GYNECOLOGICAL
• DYSMENORRHEA: 3x/Day Of Extract, Great Relief, Side Effects-- Reduced Flow, Headaches, Fatigue, 60-120 mg 1-4x/Day Of L-Tetrahydropalmatine, Active Ingredient
STOMACH/DIGESTIVE DISORDERS
• GASTRITIS, CHRONIC: Reduces Secretion, 5-10 g Herb, Every Day, 76% Effective
• ULCERS, GASTRIC/DUODENAL: Pain Good For, Especially Aspirin Induced
• VOMITING: Suppresses Emesis

Dose
4.5 - 12.0 gm

Common Name
Corydalis Rhizome

Contraindications
Not: Pregnancy

Notes
First Cook w/Vinegar For Pain

(1.5-3 gm As Powder)

Overdose: Severe Depression, Extreme Sedation, Deep Sleep

No Addiction/Tolerance

Possible Nausea, Fatigue, Skin Rash

Consider Jin Bu Huan (Rx Stephaniae Sinica) As A Substitute For Same Active Ingredient

---

YI MU CAO

益母草
（益母草）

HERBA LEONURI HETEROPHYLLI

Traditional Functions:

1. Vitalizes the Blood and smoothes the menses
2. Vitalizes the Blood, disperses Phlegm and reduces masses
3. Promotes urination and reduces edema
4. Clears toxic Heat from the skin

Traditional Properties:

Enters: HT, KI, LV,

Properties: SP, BIT, <C

Indications:

ABDOMEN/ GASTROINTESTINAL TOPICS
- ABDOMEN, MASS
- ABDOMEN, PAIN OF: Blood Stasis

BOWEL RELATED DISORDERS
- DIARRHEA, BLOODY

CANCER/TUMORS/ SWELLINGS/LUMPS
- SWELLINGS, TOXIC
- TUMORS

FLUID DISORDERS

- EDEMA: Dampness, Evil Fluid
- EDEMA, HEMATURIA
- EDEMA, SYSTEMIC

HEMORRHAGIC DISORDERS
- HEMATURIA

KIDNEYS
- NEPHRITIC EDEMA

SEXUALITY, EITHER SEX
- INFERTILITY

SEXUALITY, FEMALE: GYNECOLOGICAL

- DYSMENORRHEA
- LABOR, DIFFICULT
- MENSTRUATION, DISORDERS OF: Constrict Uterus, Stimulate Chong
- MENSTRUATION, IRREGULAR
- PLACENTA, LEAKAGE
- PMS: Abdominal Pain
- POSTPARTUM, ABDOMINAL PAIN W/ LOCHIOSCHESIS
- UTERINE BLEEDING

SKIN
- ABSCESS, SUPPURATIVE
- ECZEMA: Damp Heat
- SKIN, SORES: Damp Heat
- ULCERS

URINARY BLADDER
- DYSURIA
- URINATION, PAINFUL, DRIBBLING, CONCENTRATED, RED/ YELLOW/TURBID
- URINATION, REDUCED

Clinical/Pharmaceutical Studies:

BLOOD RELATED DISORDERS/TOPICS
- BLOOD PRESSURE, LOWERS: Aqueous Extraction, Short Term
- CHOLESTEROL, HIGH: Hyperlipidemia, Yi Mu Cao, Shan Zha, etc
- HEMOLYTIC: Injection

CIRCULATION DISORDERS
- HYPERTENSION, ESSENTIAL: Compound Chou Wu Tong Tablet (Yi Mu Cao, Chou Wu Tong, Xia Ku Cao, Xi Xian Cao), Lowered BP In 1 Day, Maximal Effects In 10 Days

HEART
- HEART DISEASE: Injection IM Or IV In

LUNGS
- RESPIRATORY CENTER, STIMULATES

MENTAL STATE/ NEUROLOGICAL DISORDERS
- CNS, INHIBITOR

SEXUALITY, FEMALE: GYNECOLOGICAL
- ABORTIFACIENT: Causes Miscarriages
- CERVICITIS, CHRONIC: Xiao Yan Zhi Dai Wan (Yi Mu Cao, Xi Xian Cao, Fried, etc), 10 Days Treatment, Leucorrhea Became Clear, Scanty, Abdominal Pain Less
- ENDOMETRITIS: Xiao Yan Zhi Dai Wan (Yi Mu Cao, Xi Xian Cao, Fried, etc), 10 Days Treatment,

Less
- MENORRHAGIA: Decoction, Resembled Ergot Extract, Slow Onset Of Contraction, 1-2 Hrs, 15-20 g/Day, Fluidextract 2-3 ml 3x/Day
- MENSTRUATION, IRREGULAR: Decoction, Resembled Ergot Extract, Slow Onset Of Contraction, 1-2 Hrs, 15-20 g/Day, Fluidextract 2-3 ml 3x/Day
- POSTPARTUM, CONTRACTS UTERUS: Ergotamine-Like, Safer, Slower
- SALPINGITIS: (Inflammation Of Fallopian Tube) Xiao Yan Zhi Dai Wan (Yi Mu Cao, Xi Xian Cao, Fried, etc), 10 Days

2-3 ml 3x/Day
- UTERUS, INCOMPLETE INVOLUTION: Decoction, Resembled Ergot Extract, Slow Onset Of Contraction, 1-2 Hrs, 15-20 g/Day, Fluidextract 2-3 ml 3x/Day
- UTERUS, STIMULATES: Oxytocin/Ergotamine- Like, Safer, Less Than Pituatary Hormones, Decoction Stronger Than ETOH Extract, Leaf Strongest Part Of Plant
- VAGINITIS: Various Forms, Xiao Yan Zhi Dai Wan (Yi Mu Cao, Xi Xian Cao, Fried, etc), 10 Days Treatment, Leucorrhea Became Clear, Scanty, Abdominal Pain Less

Clinical/Pharmaceutical Studies:

Glucose, Marked Symptom Improvement
• HEART, IMPROVES MICROCIRCULATION
INFECTIOUS DISEASES
• BACTERIAL, ANTI-
KIDNEYS
• DIURETIC: Significant
• GLOMERULO-NEPHRITIS, ACUTE

Leucorrhea Became Clear, Scanty, Abdominal Pain Less
• LEUKORRHEA: Xiao Yan Zhi Dai Wan (Yi Mu Cao, Xi Xian Cao, Fried, etc) , 10 Days Treatment, Leucorrhea Became Clear, Scanty, Abdominal Pain

Treatment, Leucorrhea Became Clear, Scanty, Abdominal Pain Less
• UTERINE BLEEDING, POSTPARTUM: Decoction, Resembled Ergot Extract, Slow Onset Of Contraction, 1-2 Hrs, 15-20 g/Day, Fluidextract

SKIN
• FUNGAL, ANTI-
• URTICARIA: Extract, 30 g 2x/Day, Satisfactory Results
URINARY BLADDER
• URINARY RETENTION, POSTPARTUM: With Acupuncture

Dose

9 - 60 gm

Common Name

Chinese Motherwort

Contraindications

Not: Pregnancy, May Cause Miscarriage

Precautions

Watch: Def Yin/Blood

Notes

For Nephritis: 90-120 gm

No Observed Side Effects In Clinical Use

YU JIN

鬱 金
（郁金）

TUBER CURCUMAE

Traditional Functions:

1. Vitalizes the Blood, disperses stagnant Blood and stops pain
2. Circulates Liver Qi, releasing stagnation
3. Clears the Heart of Hot phlegm and cools the Blood
4. Relieves jaundice and facilitates Gall Bladder function

Traditional Properties:

Enters: LU, HT, LV,

Properties: SP, BIT, C

Indications:

ABDOMEN/GASTROINTESTINAL TOPICS
• ABDOMEN, PAIN OF: Liver Qi Stagnation
• FLANK PAIN: Liver Qi Stagnation
BLOOD RELATED DISORDERS/TOPICS
• BLOOD/QI CONGESTION, STAGNATION
CANCER/TUMORS/SWELLINGS/LUMPS
• TUMORS
CHEST
• CHEST, PAIN: Liver Qi Stagnation
• RIB PAIN
CIRCULATION DISORDERS
• SYNCOPE
GALL BLADDER
• GALL BLADDER, STONES
HEART
• ANGINA PECTORIS: Chest Bi Strangulating Pain
• CORONARY HEART DISEASE
HEAT
• HEAT STROKE
HEMORRHAGIC DISORDERS
• EPISTAXIS
• HEMATEMESIS

• HEMATURIA
• HEMORRHAGE: Blood Stasis Caused, Charred/Fried Herbs/Cool Blood To Stop
LIVER
• HEPATOMEGALY
• JAUNDICE: Heat/Damp Heat
• LIVER QI CONGESTION W/ SUBCOSTAL PAIN
• LIVER QI STAGNATION LUMPS
• LIVER QI STAGNATION W/HEAT
• LIVER, PAIN
MENTAL STATE/NEUROLOGICAL DISORDERS
• AGITATION: Hot Phlegm Obstructing Heart
• ANXIETY: Hot Phlegm Obstructing Heart
• CONVULSIONS, FEVER, ACUTE
• EPILEPSY
• EPILEPSY, FROM FRIGHT
• MADNESS: Hot Phlegm Obstructing Heart
• MANIA W/DELIRIUM, CONVULSIONS
• SEIZURES: Hot Phlegm Obstructing Heart
• UNCONSCIOUSNESS: (Mental

Cloudiness) , Excess Heat (Shut-In)
MUSCULOSKELETAL/CONNECTIVE TISSUE
• SPASMS, W/FEVER, ACUTE
PHLEGM
• PHLEGM, HOT: Blocks Heart
SEXUALITY, FEMALE: GYNECOLOGICAL
• AMENORRHEA
• DYSMENORRHEA: Liver Qi Stagnation
• ENDOMETRIOSIS
• MENORRHAGIA
• MENSTRUATION, VICARIOUS
SKIN
• SORES, CHRONIC: Heals
SPLEEN
• SPLENOMEGALY
STOMACH/DIGESTIVE DISORDERS
• ANOREXIA
• STOMACH, PAIN
TRAUMA, BITES, POISONINGS
• TRAUMA, INJURIES: Topical, Too
URINARY BLADDER
• URINARY TRACT STONES

Clinical/Pharmaceutical Studies:

CIRCULATION DISORDERS
• ARTERIOSCLEROSIS: Decreased Plaque Formation In Arteries
GALL BLADDER
• CHOLAGOGUE
INFECTIOUS DISEASES
• BACTERIAL, ANTI-

KIDNEYS
• DIURETIC
LIVER
• HEPATITIS: Jaundice, Pain, Organomegaly, Powder For 1 Month
PAIN/NUMBNESS/GENERAL DISCOMFORT

• ANALGESIC: Mild
SKIN
• FUNGAL, ANTI-
STOMACH/DIGESTIVE DISORDERS
• STOMACHIC: Essential Oil Increases Appetite

Dose
4.5 - 9.0 gm

Common Name
Turmeric Tuber

Contraindications
Not: Def Yin From Blood Loss

Not: w/o Stagnant Qi/Blood

Not: Combined With Ding Xiang (Cloves)

Precautions
Watch: Pregnancy

Notes
Bake: Reduces Coldness, Toxicity

YUE JI HUA
(YUE YUE HONG)

月季花

FRUCTUS ROSAE CHINENSIS

Traditional Functions:

1. Vitalizes the Blood and regulates menstruation
2. Vitalizes the Blood and reduces swelling

Traditional Properties:

Enters: LV,

Properties: SW, W

Indications:

ABDOMEN/ GASTROINTESTINAL TOPICS
• ABDOMEN, PAIN OF, DISTENTION
CHEST
• CHEST, PAIN, DISTENTION
HEAD/NECK
• NECK, SWELLINGS: Auxillary Herb

INFECTIOUS DISEASES
• SCROFULA: Auxillary Herb
LIVER
• LIVER QI STAGNATION LUMPS
SEXUALITY, FEMALE: GYNECOLOGICAL
• AMENORRHEA
• DYSMENORRHEA
• MENSTRUATION, IRREGULAR

• MENSTRUATION, SCANTY
• METRORRHAGIA
SKIN
• CARBUNCLES: Topical
• FURUNCLES, SWELLING: Topical
TRAUMA, BITES, POISONINGS
• INFLAMMATION

Dose
3 - 9 gm

Common Name
Chinese Tea Rose Flower

Contraindications
Not: Pregnancy

Precautions
Watch: Can Cause Diarrhea w/Excessive Use
Watch: SP/ST Weakness

ZE LAN

澤蘭
(泽兰)

HERBA LYCOPI LUCIDI

Traditional Functions:

1. Vitalizes the Blood and promotes menstruation
2. Dissipates Blood stasis and congealed Blood by vitalizing the Blood
3. Promotes urination and reduces swelling

Traditional Properties:

Enters: SP, LV,

Properties: BIT, SP, <W,

Indications:

ABDOMEN/ GASTROINTESTINAL TOPICS
• ABDOMEN, MASS, IN WOMEN

• EDEMA, POSTPARTUM
• EDEMA, SYSTEMIC
HEART

SKIN
• ABSCESS: Topical, Too
• CARBUNCLES, TOXIC

Indications:

- ABDOMEN, PAIN OF,
  POSTPARTUM: Blood Stasis
- **BLOOD RELATED DISORDERS/
  TOPICS**
- ANEMIA
- **CANCER/TUMORS/SWELLINGS/
  LUMPS**
- TUMORS, GYNECOLOGICAL
- **FLUID DISORDERS**
- EDEMA, FACE

- ANGINA PECTORIS: Chest Bi
  Strangulating Pain
- **SEXUALITY, FEMALE:
  GYNECOLOGICAL**
- AMENORRHEA
- DYSMENORRHEA
- MENSTRUATION, ABNORMAL
- MENSTRUATION, LATE W/PAIN
- POSTPARTUM, ABDOMINAL
  PAIN: Blood Stasis

- SKIN, SORES, SWOLLEN, TOXIC:
  Blood Stasis, Swelling
- **TRAUMA, BITES, POISONINGS**
- TRAUMA, PAIN/SWELLING:
  Topical, Too
- **URINARY BLADDER**
- URINATION, CONTINUOUS
  DRIPPING
- URINATION, PAINFUL:
  Postpartum

Clinical/Pharmaceutical Studies:

HEART
- CARDIOTONIC

KIDNEYS

- DIURETIC

Dose

3 - 9 gm

Precautions

Watch: Pregnancy

Watch: w/o Congealed Blood

Notes

Safe For Long Term Use

ZHI XUE CAO
(JI XUE CAO)

積雪草
（积雪草）

HERBA
CENTELLAE

Traditional Functions:

1. Clears Heat and promotes water metabolism

Traditional Properties:

Enters: LV, SP, KI

Properties: BIT, SP, C

Indications:

- **ABDOMEN/
  GASTROINTESTINAL TOPICS**
- ABDOMEN, PAIN OF
- **BOWEL RELATED DISORDERS**
- DIARRHEA: Summer Heat
- DYSENTERY
- **CANCER/TUMORS/SWELLINGS/
  LUMPS**
- SWELLINGS, TOXIC
- **EYES**
- EYES, IRRITATION
- **HEMORRHAGIC DISORDERS**

- EPISTAXIS
- HEMATURIA
- HEMOPTYSIS
- **LIVER**
- JAUNDICE: Damp Heat
- **ORAL CAVITY**
- PHARYNGITIS
- **SKIN**
- FURUNCLES, DEEP ROOTED,
  NAIL-LIKE
- SCABIES

- SKIN, ERUPTIONS
- **STOMACH/DIGESTIVE
  DISORDERS**
- VOMITING
- **TRAUMA, BITES, POISONINGS**
- TRAUMA, INTERNAL/
  EXTERNAL
- **URINARY BLADDER**
- URINARY BLADDER STONES
- **WIND DISORDERS**
- WIND RASH

Clinical/Pharmaceutical Studies:

- **INFECTIOUS DISEASES**
- BACTERIAL, ANTI-: Water
  Extract
- LEPROSY

- **MENTAL STATE/
  NEUROLOGICAL DISORDERS**
- SEDATIVE

- **SKIN**
- SKIN, TUBERCULOSIS
- SKIN, ULCERS: Wounds

Dose

9 - 15 gm

Common Name

Centella

ZI RAN TONG   自然銅   PYRITUM

Traditional Functions:

1. Disperses stagnant Blood and promotes the healing of bones and tendons

Traditional Properties:

Enters: KI, LV,

Properties: SP, BIT, N

Indications:

ABDOMEN/
  GASTROINTESTINAL TOPICS
• ACCUMULATION
BLOOD RELATED DISORDERS/
  TOPICS
• BLOOD STASIS PAIN
CANCER/TUMORS/SWELLINGS/

LUMPS
• SWELLINGS, PAIN
MUSCULOSKELETAL/
  CONNECTIVE TISSUE
• LIGAMENTS, INJURIES
• TENDONS, INJURY OF

SKIN
• SCALDS
TRAUMA, BITES, POISONINGS
• FRACTURES, HEALING OF
• TRAUMA, INTERNAL/
  EXTERNAL

Clinical/Pharmaceutical Studies:

ENDOCRINE RELATED
  DISORDERS

• GOITER, ENDEMIC
TRAUMA, BITES, POISONINGS

• FRACTURES: With Hu Gu,
  Promotes Healing Of

Dose

3 - 9 gm

Common Name

Pyrite

Relieve Coughing And Wheezing

BAI BU   百部   **RADIX STEMONAE**

Traditional Functions:

1. Moistens the Lungs and stops cough
2. Kills parasites and lice

Traditional Properties:

Enters: LU,

Properties: SW, BIT, <W

Indications:

LUNGS
- BRONCHITIS, ACUTE/CHRONIC
- COUGH: Cold Phlegm/Cold/Lung Heat/Steaming Bone, Consumption/ Wind Cold/Yin Deficient
- COUGH, ACUTE
- COUGH, CHRONIC: Deficient
- COUGH, DIFFICULT EXPECTORATION
- COUGH, LUNG EXHAUSTION:

Tuberculosis
- LUNGS, DYSPNEA: Cold Phlegm/ Lung Heat
- TUBERCULOSIS

PARASITES
- ASCARIASIS
- ENTEROBIASIS: (Pinworm Infestation)
- FLEAS: Topical (Tincture/Decotion)

- HOOKWORMS
- LICE, HEAD/BODY: Topical (Tincture/Decotion)
- PINWORMS: Internal As Enema, * 1-2 Liang Daily, 3 Days For
- TAPEWORMS

SKIN
- FUNGAL INFECTIONS: Topical
- SCABIES: Topical

Clinical/Pharmaceutical Studies:

INFECTIOUS DISEASES
- ANTIBIOTIC: Inhibits Many
- BACTERIAL, ANTI-: B. Dysenteriae, Staph.Aureus, Pseudomanas, Pneumonococci, TB, et al
- PERTUSSIS: Can Also Act As A Preventative
- VIRAL, ANTI-: Decoction Prevents Infection By Asian Flu

LUNGS
- BRONCHITIS, ACTIVATED BY COMMON COLD: Pill From 2:1.5 Of Bai Bu/Honey, 8.75 g/Pill, Take In AM, PM For 14 Days, Then 7 Days Every Month
- BRONCHITIS, CHRONIC: 50% Syrup, 15-100 ml And Extract Tab, 0.5 g 3-4 Tabs, 3x/Day, For 10 Day Course, Each, 1/2 Improved
- COUGH: Can Inhibit Excitatory Action On Respiratory Center, 100% Alkaloid Extract, 0.2 ml Similar In Potency To Aminophylline, Though

Slower Onset And Lasted Longer *
- EXPECTORANT
- TUBERCULOSIS, PULMONARY: Tab From Bai Bu, 30 g, Huang Qin, Dan Shen, 15 g Each, 3-6 Tabs, 3x/ Day, Average 2.5 Years Of Treatment, Can Inject Single Herb, Similar To Streptomycin Plus Isoniazid

PARASITES
- ANTIPARASITIC: Stronger Than DDT For Lice
- HOOKWORMS
- LICE: 20% Herb Extract/50% Decoction, Spray Made With 5 g Herb In 2 oz Of White Wine, With Small Amount Of Soap
- LICE, HEAD/BODY: 20-50% ETOH Tincture, Wash
- PINWORMS: Suppository For Children, 12.5 g Each, One In Rectum At 8PM, Another 10 PM Every Night For 1 Week, *1.5 g Powder, 3x/Day For 3 Days, *50% Decoction With Ku Lian Gen Pi, Wu

Mei As Retention Enema, 5-6 Tblspoons, Each Evening, 2-4 Days, Enema Synergistic With Oral Dose, May Add 20 g Di Gu Pi With Same Amount Zi Cao In 100 g Vaseline For Perianal Application Every Night, *30ml 100% Decoction As Enema Before Sleep, 5 Days

SEXUALITY, FEMALE: GYNECOLOGICAL
- TRICHOMONAS, VAGINAL: 100% Cure After 1-3 Courses, 1 g Di Bai Chong Added To 100 ml Of 50% Decoction, Soak Cotton Ball, Insert Deep In Vagina At Bed Time, Remove In Morning, 4 Days=1 Course

SKIN
- FUNGAL, ANTI-
- SCABIES: 50% Decoction/Extract

TRAUMA, BITES, POISONINGS
- BED BUGS
- INSECTICIDE: Lice, Flies

Dose

3 - 18 gm

Common Name

Stemona Root

Contraindications

Not: Loose BM

Not: Def SP

Notes

Oral May Cause Heartburn, Dry Mouth, Dizziness, Chest Discomfort

Overdose: May Paralyze Respiratory Center

BAO MA ZI

暴馬子
（暴马子）

CORTEX SYRINGAE

Traditional Functions:

1. Relieves coughing and wheezing, reduces fever
2. Promotes urination, circulates fluids

Traditional Properties:

Enters: LU, HT

Properties: BIT, <C

Indications:

FLUID DISORDERS
• EDEMA, CARDIAC

LUNGS
• ASTHMA W/RALES

• BRONCHITIS, CHRONIC

Clinical/Pharmaceutical Studies:

INFECTIOUS DISEASES
• BACTERIAL, ANTI-
LUNGS

• ANTITUSSIVE: Less Than Codeine
• ASTHMA

• BRONCHITIS, CHRONIC
• EXPECTORANT: Similar To Jie Geng

Dose

90 - 180 gm

Common Name

Manchurian Lilac Bark

Precautions

Watch: Acute Febrile Conditions

Notes

Used Singly

KUAN DONG HUA

款冬花

FLOS TUSSILAGI FARFARAE

Traditional Functions:

1. Descends Lung Qi and moistens the Lung
2. Stops cough and disperses sputum

Traditional Properties:

Enters: LU,

Properties: SP, W

Indications:

HEMORRHAGIC DISORDERS
• HEMATEMESIS
• HEMOPTYSIS: Pus, Blood
LUNGS
• ASTHMA
• COUGH: Cold Phlegm/Lung Dryness/Lung Heat/Wind Cold

• COUGH, ALL KINDS
• COUGH, CHRONIC W/PROFUSE SPUTUM
• COUGH, LUNG EXHAUSTION: Tuberculosis
• LUNG ATROPHY
• LUNG FISTULA

• LUNGS, ABSCESS
• LUNGS, DYSPNEA: Cold Phlegm/ Lung Heat
• WHEEZING, MANY ETIOLOGIES
ORAL CAVITY
• THROAT, SORE: Bi Pain

Clinical/Pharmaceutical Studies:

FEVERS
• ANTIPYRETIC: Aqueous Extract
HEART
• HEART, INHIBITS

• ASTHMA W/ EMPHYSEMA
• ASTHMA, BRONCHIAL: Weak, Transient, Less Than Aminophylline.

Used With Other Herbs
• BRONCHITIS, CHRONIC: Cough Of, With Zi Wan As Decoction, 5-10 g Each, *Kuan Dong

Opposite Effect
• EXPECTORANT: Thru Irritation Of Lung Mucosa, Less Than Jie Geng Or Less Than Che Qian Cao

---

Clinical/Pharmaceutical Studies:

LUNGS
• ANTITUSSIVE:
Significant, 40%
Decoction, Volatile Oil

ETOH Extract, 5ml (−6g
Herb), 3x/Day, Marked
Improvement In 1-3 Days,
Antiasthmatic Effect If

Hua, Di Long Injection
Helped After 3-4 Days
• BRONCHODILATORY:
Small Doses, Large

• RESPIRATION,
STIMULATES: Like
Nikethamide

Dose
3 - 9 gm

Common Name
Coltsfoot/Tussilago Flowr

Precautions
Watch: Cough w/Heat

Notes
Nausea Common (30%), Some Irritability, Insomnia
Alkaloid, Sendirkine, In Herb Is Hepatotoxic

MA DOU LING

馬兜鈴
(马兜铃)

FRUCTUS ARISTOLOCHIAE

Traditional Functions:

1. Clears Lungs, descends Qi and clears Heat
2. Stops coughing and soothes asthma

Traditional Properties:

Enters: LU,

Properties: BIT, C

Indications:

BOWEL RELATED DISORDERS
• FISTULA W/PAINFUL
SWELLINGS
• HEMORRHOIDS, BLOODY
STOOL
• HEMORRHOIDS, PAIN,
SWELLING
CIRCULATION DISORDERS
• HYPERTENSION
FLUID DISORDERS
• FLUID, SUPPORTS
HEMORRHAGIC DISORDERS

• HEMOPTYSIS
LUNGS
• ASTHMA, ACUTE: Lung Heat
• COUGH: Lung Heat/Deficient
Lung With Heat
• COUGH, DRY, DIFFICULT
SPUTUM
• LUNG HEAT, CHRONIC W/
BLOODY SPUTM
• LUNGS, DYSPNEA: Lung Heat
• LUNGS, INFLAMMATION OF
MUCOSA

• WHEEZING: Lung Heat/Deficient
Lung With Heat
NOSE
• NOSE, INFLAMMATION OF
ORAL CAVITY
• THROAT, INFLAMMATION
SEXUALITY, FEMALE:
GYNECOLOGICAL
• MORNING SICKNESS
• PREGNANCY, QI STAGNATION
DURING

Clinical/Pharmaceutical Studies:

**BLOOD RELATED DISORDERS/
TOPICS**
• BLOOD PRESSURE, LOWERS:
Sustained Effect, Average Lowering,
15mm Hg Diastolic
**CANCER/TUMORS/SWELLINGS/
LUMPS**
• CANCER, ANTI-: Unique Nitro
Compound
• TUMOR, ANTI-: Used With
Chemo/Radiotherapy
**IMMUNE SYSTEM RELATED
DISORDERS/TOPICS**
• IMMUNE SYSTEM

ENHANCEMENT: Increases
Phagocytosis
INFECTIOUS DISEASES
• ANTIBIOTIC: Staph A.,
Pneumococci, B.Dysenteriae, etc.
• INFECTIOUS DISEASES: Use
With Antibiotics
LUNGS
• BRONCHITIS, CHRONIC: With
Gan Cao Pi, Effective
• BRONCHODILATORY:
Counteracts Pilocarpine,
Acetylcholine, Histamine
• EXPECTORANT: Bronchidilatory,

Weak, Less Than Zi Wan, Tian Nan
Xing, But Greater Than Ammonium
Chloride
**MUSCULOSKELETAL/
CONNECTIVE TISSUE**
• OSTEOMYELITIS, CHRONIC
ORAL CAVITY
• TONSILLITIS
SKIN
• ABSCESS, CHRONIC
• DERMATITIS, BACTERIAL:
(Pyodermia)
• FUNGAL, ANTI-: Various

Dose
3 - 9 gm

Common Name
Birthwort Fruit

Contraindications
Not: Def Cold Cough

Notes
ETOH Extract Can Cause Nausea/Vomiting/Diarrhea
Not w/Diarrhea Def SP
w/Honey To Enhance Antitussive Action

MING DANG SHEN

明黨參
（明党参）

RADIX CHANGII

Traditional Functions:

1. Moistens Lungs and dissolves Phlegm
2. Harmonizes the Stomach and controls vomiting
3. Helps reverse rebellious Qi and stops cough
4. Relieves toxins

Traditional Properties:

Enters: LU, LV,

Properties: SW, BIT, C

Indications:

ENERGETIC STATE
• POST ILLNESS WEAKNESS
LUNGS
• COUGH: Dry, Heat

SKIN
• FURUNCLES, TOXIC
STOMACH/DIGESTIVE
  DISORDERS

• ANOREXIA
• HICCUPS
• STOMACH, UPSET
• VOMITING

Dose

6 - 15 gm

Common Name

Changii

Contraindications

Not: Pregnancy
Not: Qi Def And Ptosis (Organ Drooping From Weak Abdominal Muscles)

MU HU DIE
(QIAN CHENG ZI)

木蝴蝶

SEMEN OROXYLI INDICI

Traditional Functions:

1. Moistens Lungs, controls cough
2. Clears Lung Heat and restores the voice
3. Opens the Liver and regulates the Qi
3. Promotes tissue regeneration
4. Harmonizes the Stomach

Traditional Properties:

Enters: LU, LV, SP

Properties: SW, BL, CL

Indications:

ABDOMEN/
  GASTROINTESTINAL TOPICS
• ABDOMEN, PAIN OF
• FLANK PAIN: Liver Qi Stagnation
LUNGS
• BRONCHITIS
• COUGH, W/LOSS OF VOICE
• WHOOPING COUGH

ORAL CAVITY
• HOARSENESS
• THROAT, PAIN, SWOLLEN
• THROAT, SWOLLEN/
  INFLAMMATION
• VOICE, HOARSENESS/SORE
  THROAT

SKIN
• SORES, ULCERATED,
  SUPPURATIVE
STOMACH/DIGESTIVE
  DISORDERS
• STOMACH, PAIN: Liver Qi
  Stagnation

Clinical/Pharmaceutical Studies:

TRAUMA, BITES, POISONINGS
• INFLAMMATORY, ANTI-:
Aqueous Extract

Dose

0.9 - 4.5 gm

Common Name

Oroxylum

PI PA YE

枇杷葉
（枇杷叶）

FOLIUM ERIOBOTRYAE JAPONICAE

Traditional Functions:

1. Descends Lung Qi, stops cough, clears Heat and resolves Phlegm
2. Harmonizes Stomach, conducts rebellious Qi downward and clears Stomach Heat

Traditional Properties:

Enters: LU, ST,

Properties: BIT, CL

Indications:

FLUID DISORDERS
• THIRST: Lung Heat/Stomach Fire
LUNGS
• ASTHMA, ACUTE
• BRONCHITIS, ACUTE/CHRONIC
• COUGH: Lung Dryness/Lung Heat/ Wind Heat
• COUGH, DRY, STICKY SPUTUM
• LUNG HEAT

• LUNGS, DYSPNEA: Lung Heat
PHLEGM
• PHLEGM FLUID RETENTION
• SPUTUM: Thins
SEXUALITY, FEMALE:
GYNECOLOGICAL
• MORNING SICKNESS:
Gestational Foul Obstruction--Heat
STOMACH/DIGESTIVE

DISORDERS
• BELCHING: Stomach Heat
• GASTRITIS
• HICCUPS: Qi Deficiency--Heat/ Stomach Heat
• NAUSEA: Stomach Heat
• RETCHING
• VOMITING: Qi Deficiency--Heat/ Stomach Fire

Clinical/Pharmaceutical Studies:

INFECTIOUS DISEASES
• BACTERIAL, ANTI-
• VIRAL, ANTI-: Flu
LUNGS
• ANTITUSSIVE: Good, Amygadalin

• ASTHMA: Did Not Stop
• BRONCHITIS, CHRONIC: Short Term Control
• EXPECTORANT: Weak

PAIN/NUMBNESS/GENERAL DISCOMFORT
• ANALGESIC: Amygdalin Ingredient

Dose

3 - 15 gm

Common Name

Loquat Leaf

Contraindications

Not: Vomiting w/Cold ST/Caused By Irritability

Not: Cough From External Cold In LU

Notes

Scrub Leaves Of "Hair" To Prevent Throat Irritaiton
No Side Effects

SANG BAI PI

桑白皮

CORTEX MORI ALBAE RADICIS

Traditional Functions:

1. Reduces Heat from Lungs and soothes asthma
2. Promotes urination and reduces edema

Traditional Properties:

Enters: LU, SP,

Properties: SW, C

Indications:

ABDOMEN/
GASTROINTESTINAL TOPICS
• ABDOMEN, DISTENTION OF
CIRCULATION DISORDERS
• HYPERTENSION
EXTREMITIES
• ARMS, SWELLING
• LEGS, SWELLING
FEVERS
• FEVER, THIRST: Lung Heat
FLUID DISORDERS

• ASCITES
• EDEMA: Dampness, Evil Fluid
• EDEMA, FACE: Lung Heat
• EDEMA, FLOATING: Lung Heat
HEMORRHAGIC DISORDERS
• HEMATEMESIS
LUNGS
• ASTHMA: Mild
• COUGH: Lung Heat
• DYSPNEA: Lung Heat

• LUNG HEAT: Cough/Wheezing
• LUNG QI DESCENT, DISRUPTION OF
• LUNGS, DYSPNEA: Lung Heat
• LUNGS, MOISTENS
STOMACH/DIGESTIVE DISORDERS
• VOMITING, CLEAR FLUIDS
URINARY BLADDER
• DYSURIA: Lung Heat

Clinical/Pharmaceutical Studies:

BLOOD RELATED DISORDERS/
TOPICS
• BLOOD PRESSURE, LOWERS:
Mild, Slow, With Bradycardia,
Chinese Stronger, More Toxic Than
Japanese
BOWEL RELATED DISORDERS
• PURGATIVE: At 3g/kg Causes
Watery Stool
CANCER/TUMORS/SWELLINGS/
LUMPS
• ESOPHAGEAL CANCER: Sang Pi
Ku Jiu/Cu Tang (Sang Bai Pi Bitter
Wine/Vinegar Preparation)
• GASTRIC CANCER: Sang Pi Ku
Jiu/Cu Tang (Sang Bai Pi Bitter
Wine/Vinegar Preparation)

FLUID DISORDERS
• EDEMA, PREGNANCY: Wu Pi
Yin (Sang Bai Pi, Fu Ling Pi, Da Fu
Pi, Chen Pi, Sheng Jiang Pi) , Plus
Yu Mi Xu, In Severe Cases Add Zhu
Ling, Ze Xie, etc
INFECTIOUS DISEASES
• BACTERIAL, ANTI-: 100%
Decoction Inhibits, Staph.Aureus,
Salmonella Typhi, Shigella Flexneri
KIDNEYS
• DIURETIC: For 6 Hours
LUNGS
• ANTITUSSIVE: Weak
• ASTHMA
• BRONCHITIS, ACUTE: Decoction
Of Herb, Huang Qin, Chuan Bei Mu,

Pi Pa Ye, Jie Geng, Xing Ren, Di Gu
Pi, 9 g Each
• BRONCHITIS, ASTHMATIC:
Ding Chuan Tang
• EXPECTORANT
MENTAL STATE/
NEUROLOGICAL DISORDERS
• CONVULSIVE, ANTI-: Slightly
Inhibited Electroshock
• SEDATIVE
• TRANQUILIZING
PAIN/NUMBNESS/GENERAL
DISCOMFORT
• ANALGESIC: Aqueous Extract, 2g/
kg = 0.5 g/kg Of Aspirin
TRAUMA, BITES, POISONINGS
• INFLAMMATORY, ANTI-

Dose
9 - 18 gm

Common Name
Bark Of Mulberry Root

Contraindications
Not: Def LU

Not: Excessive Urination

Not: Wind-Cold Cough

Notes
Large Amounts May Cause Watery Stool

TIAN XIAN TENG   天仙滕   CAULIS ARISTOLOCHIAE

Traditional Functions:

1. Promotes the circulation of Qi
2. Resolves Dampness and promotes water circulation
3. Vitalizes Blood and controls pain

Traditional Properties:

Enters:

Properties: BIT, W

Indications:

ABDOMEN/
GASTROINTESTINAL TOPICS
• ABDOMEN, PAIN OF
• HERNIA
CHEST

• CHEST, PAIN
EARS/HEARING DISORDERS
• DIZZINESS
FEVERS
• FEVER

SEXUALITY, FEMALE:
GYNECOLOGICAL
• PREGNANCY, EDEMA DURING
TRAUMA, BITES, POISONINGS
• SNAKE BITES

Clinical/Pharmaceutical Studies:

BLOOD RELATED DISORDERS/
TOPICS
• BLOOD PRESSURE, LOWERS

CANCER/TUMORS/SWELLINGS/
LUMPS
• CANCER, ANTI-

TRAUMA, BITES, POISONINGS
• WOUNDS: Promotes Regeneration

Dose
6 - 9 gm

Common Name
Birthwort

TIAN XIAN ZI　　　　天仙子　　　　SEMEN HYOSCYAMI

Traditional Functions:

1. Controls cough and wheezing
2. Helps suppress pain

Traditional Properties:

Enters:

Properties: BIT, W

Indications:

BOWEL RELATED DISORDERS
• DIARRHEA, CHRONIC
• DYSENTERY, CHRONIC
• RECTAL PROLAPSE
CANCER/TUMORS/SWELLINGS/ LUMPS
• SWELLINGS, PAIN: Topical
LUNGS
• ASTHMA
• ASTHMA, COUGH

• COUGH, CHRONIC
MENTAL STATE/ NEUROLOGICAL DISORDERS
• CONVULSIONS
• EPILEPSY: Wind
• INSANITY
• MENTAL DISORDERS
MUSCULOSKELETAL/ CONNECTIVE TISSUE

• ARTHRITIS, PAIN
PAIN/NUMBNESS/GENERAL DISCOMFORT
• PAIN, FLUSHING UP
SKIN
• SWEATING, REDUCES
STOMACH/DIGESTIVE DISORDERS
• STOMACH, ACHE

Clinical/Pharmaceutical Studies:

EYES
• MYDRIATIC
LUNGS
• ANTITUSSIVE

MUSCULOSKELETAL/ CONNECTIVE TISSUE
• ANTISPASMODIC
PAIN/NUMBNESS/GENERAL

DISCOMFORT
• ANALGESIC: From Atropine
SKIN
• PERSPIRATION, INHIBITS

Dose
0.6 - 1.5 gm

Common Name
Henbane

XING REN　　　　杏仁　　　　SEMEN PRUNI ARMENIACAE
(BEI XING REN/KU XING REN)

Traditional Functions:

1. Moistens Lungs, controls cough and wheezing
2. Moistens the intestines and facilitates passage of stool

Traditional Properties:

Enters: LU, LI,

Properties: BIT, W, <TX

Indications:

BOWEL RELATED DISORDERS
• CONSTIPATION: Intestinal Dryness/Secondary Use, From Oils
LUNGS
• ASTHMA

• BRONCHITIS, CHRONIC/ACUTE
• COUGH: Cold Phlegm/External Pathogens/Wind Cold/Wind Heat
• COUGH, GENERAL: Hot/Cold, Best Dry

• COUGH, WHEEZING
• LUNG YIN DEFICIENCY, CHRONIC: Moistens In Chronic Yin Deficient
• LUNGS, DYSPNEA: Cold Phlegm

Clinical/Pharmaceutical Studies:

BLOOD RELATED DISORDERS/TOPICS
• ANEMIA, APLASTIC: Caused By Chloramphenicol, Use As Adjunct To Stimulate RBC
BOWEL RELATED DISORDERS
• LAXATIVE: Fatty Oil Of Seed
CANCER/TUMORS/

• CANCER: Hodgkin's Disease, Bronchial Carcinoma, Spindle Cell Sarcoma, Seminoma, Chronic Myelocytic Leukemia, Pleura Cancer, Malignant Lymphoma, Rectal Cancer, Breast Cancer With Bone Metastasis--Amygdalin Given Orally, 0.5-1.0 g On

INFECTIOUS DISEASES
• BACTERIAL, ANTI-: B. Typhi, B.Paratyphi, etc
LUNGS
• ANTITUSSIVE
• ASTHMA
• BRONCHITIS, CHRONIC: Paste Made With Sugar, 3-4 Days
• EXPECTORANT
• RESPIRATORY ILLNESS:

• PINWORMS
• ROUNDWORMS
SEXUALITY, FEMALE: GYNECOLOGICAL
• TRICHOMONAS, VAGINAL: Topical With Water Or Sesame Oil And Sang Ye--Good To Excellent Results, 1 Week
STOMACH/DIGESTIVE DISORDERS

Clinical/Pharmaceutical Studies:

SWELLINGS/LUMPS
• ANTINEOPLASTIC:
Cervical Cancer

1ST Day, Then 0.1 g For
10 Days, Use Sodium
Thiosulfate IV To Detoxify

With Ma Huang
PARASITES
• HOOKWORMS

• DIGESTION, INHIBITS:
Benzaldehyde Inhibits
Pepsin

Dose
3 - 12 gm
Common Name
Almond Kernel
Contraindications
Not: Diarrhea
Notes
Forms Hydrocyanic Acid In ST: Lethal Dose 50-60

Kernals (Child: 10) -Activated Carbon Anecdote
Possible Transient Headache/Nausea
Poisoning: Vomiting, Respiratory Distress, Possible
Coma, Convulsion, Paralysis, Death By Respiratory
Paralysis
Antidotes: Nitrites, Sodium Thiosulfate, Give Nitrates
First

ZI SU ZI

紫蘇子
(紫苏子)

FRUCTUS PERILLAE FRUTESCENTIS

Traditional Functions:

1. Relieves cough and wheezing, descends Qi and resolves Phlegm
2. Moistens the intestines and facilitates the passage of stool

Traditional Properties:

Enters: LU, LI,

Properties: SP, W

Indications:

BOWEL RELATED DISORDERS
• CONSTIPATION:
Intestinal Dryness
• DIARRHEA: Cold
Dampness (Add Warm
Interior Herbs, Too)
CHEST

• CHEST, STUFFINESS
INFECTIOUS DISEASES
• COMMON COLD: Wind
Cold
LUNGS
• ASTHMA
• BRONCHITIS,
CHRONIC W/THIN,

WHITE PHLEGM
• COUGH: Cold Phlegm/
Flushing Up/Wind Cold
• COUGH/WHEEZING:
Copious Phlegm/
Exhalation Difficult
Compared To Inhalation
• LUNGS, DYSPNEA:

Cold Phlegm
QI RELATED DISORDERS/TOPICS
• QI STAGNATION
SKIN
• RASHES, INCOMPLETE
EXPRESSION OF: With
Wind Cold Complex

Dose
3 - 9 gm
Common Name
Purple Perilla Fruit
Contraindications
Not: Chronic Diarrhea
Notes
Only In Cold Conditions

ZI WAN
(CI WAN)

紫菀

RADIX ASTERIS TATARICI

Traditional Functions:

1. Resolves Phlegm and stops cough

Traditional Properties:

Enters: LU,

Properties: BIT, <W

Indications:

CHEST
• CHEST, COLD, HEAT IN
LUNGS
• ASTHMA
• BRONCHITIS, CHRONIC

Copious Sputum
• COUGH, DYSPNEA
• COUGH, LUNG EXHAUSTION:
Tuberculosis
• COUGH, PROLONGED

PHLEGM
• PHLEGM
• PHLEGM, BLOODY
QI RELATED DISORDERS/TOPICS

Indications:

- COUGH: Cold Phlegm/Lung Dryness/Lung Heat/Wind Cold
- COUGH, CHRONIC: Blood Stained Sputum/Cold With Difficult
- COUGH, THICK SPUTUM
- DYSPNEA: Cold Phlegm/Lung Heat
- TUBERCULOSIS
- QI ACCUMULATION **URINARY BLADDER**
- URINATION, SCANTY

Clinical/Pharmaceutical Studies:

CANCER/TUMORS/ SWELLINGS/LUMPS
- CANCER, ANTI-: Especially Ascitic Cancer

INFECTIOUS DISEASES
- ANTIBIOTIC: Shigella, E.Coli, Proteus, Pseudomonas, B. Dysenteriae, et al
- VIRAL, ANTI-: Markedly

Inhibited Flu

KIDNEYS
- DIURETIC: Marked

LUNGS
- ANTITUSSIVE: Decoction Showed None, Isolated Extract Showed Some, IP Injection
- BRONCHITIS, CHRONIC/ACUTE: 6-9 g

With Kuan Dong Hua As Decoction, *Ether Extract Of Zi Wan, MEOH Extract Herba Ardisiae Japonicae (Jin Niu Cao), ETOH Extract Shan Yao, Hyocholic Acid
- EXPECTORANT: Increases Respiratory Tract Secretions, Significant,

Last Greater Than 4 Hrs
- TUBERCULOSIS: Inhibits Bacteria, With Cough Use Zi Wan, Chuan Bei Mu, Zhi Mu, Wu Wei Zi, E Jiao, Gan Cao, Jie Geng

SKIN
- FUNGAL, ANTI-

Dose

3 - 9 gm

Common Name

Purple Aster Root

Precautions

Watch: Def Yin w/Heat Cough

Watch: Excess Heat Patterns

Warm And Transform Cold Phlegm

BAI FU ZI
(GUAN BAI FU)

白附子

RHIZOMA TYPHONII GIGANTEI
(ACONITI COREANI)

Traditional Functions:

1. Expels Wind and Cold Dampness and relieves pain
2. Expesl Wind Phlegm and suppresses spasms
3. Resolves toxic swellings and reduces distension

Traditional Properties:

Enters: ST, LV,

Properties: SP, SW, W, TX

Indications:

CIRCULATION DISORDERS
• STROKE, FACIAL DEVIATIONS FROM
EARS/HEARING DISORDERS
• DIZZINESS: Wind Damp/Cold Damp
• VERTIGO: Wind Phlegm
HEAD/NECK
• FACE, DEVIATIONS FROM STROKE
• FACE, PAIN: Wind Damp/Cold Damp
• FACE, PARALYSIS: Wind Phlegm
• FACE, WEAKNESS: Wind Damp/ Cold Damp
• HEAD, PAIN, ANY: Wind Damp/

Cold Damp
• HEADACHE: Cold Phlegm
• HEADACHE, SEVERE LATERAL: Wind Damp/Cold Damp
INFECTIOUS DISEASES
• SCROFULA
• TETANUS
LUNGS
• COUGH: With Profuse Sputum
MENTAL STATE/ NEUROLOGICAL DISORDERS
• EPILEPSY
• HEMIPLEGIA: Wind Phlegm
PAIN/NUMBNESS/GENERAL DISCOMFORT

• NUMBNESS, EXTREMITIES
PHLEGM
• PHLEGM ACCUMULATION
SEXUALITY, EITHER SEX
• GENITALS, PRURITUS, EXTERNAL: Damp
SKIN
• FUNGAL INFECTIONS: Topical
• SCABIES: Topical
• SKIN, ULCERS: Wind
TRAUMA, BITES, POISONINGS
• BITES, SNAKE
• SNAKE BITES
WIND DISORDERS
• WINDSTROKE: Wind Phlegm

Clinical/Pharmaceutical Studies:

INFECTIOUS DISEASES
• TUBERCULOSIS, ANTI-: Less Than Streptomycin With Injection
MENTAL STATE/

NEUROLOGICAL DISORDERS
• TRANQUILIZING: Similar To Aconite

PAIN/NUMBNESS/GENERAL DISCOMFORT
• ANALGESIC: Less Than Aconite

Dose

3 - 9 gm

Contraindications

Not: Pregnancy

Not: Def Yin w/Heat

Notes

Raw Herb Not Taken Internally, Toxic

BAI JIE ZI

白芥子

SEMEN SINAPIS ALBAE

Traditional Functions:

1. Warms the Lung and resolves Phlegm
2. Vitalizes Qi circulation to disperse nodules
3. Opens the channels and stops pain

Traditional Properties:

Enters: LU, ST,

Properties: SP, W

Indications:

ABDOMEN/
GASTROINTESTINAL TOPICS
• SUBCOSTAL DISTENDED PAIN
CANCER/TUMORS/SWELLINGS/
LUMPS
• SWELLINGS: External
CHEST
• CHEST, DISTENTION, CHRONIC:
  Cold Phlegm
• CHEST, PAIN, CHRONIC: Cold
  Phlegm
• RIB PAIN, SWELLING
IMMUNE SYSTEM RELATED
DISORDERS/TOPICS
• LYMPH NODES, SWELLING
LUNGS

• COUGH: From Tuberculosis
• COUGH, CHRONIC: Cold Phlegm
• LUNGS, DYSPNEA: Cold Phlegm
• PLEURISY: With Stuffy Sensation
  In Chest, Liquid Accumulation In
  Thoracic Cavity
MUSCULOSKELETAL/
CONNECTIVE TISSUE
• JOINTS, PAIN: Cold Phlegm In
  Channels, External Application
• RHEUMATIC PAIN: External
PAIN/NUMBNESS/GENERAL
DISCOMFORT
• BODY ACHES: Cold Phlegm In
  Channels

• NUMB PAIN: External
SKIN
• BEDSORES: Cold Phlegm In
  Channels
• BOILS, YIN TYPE: Cold Phlegm
  In Channels
• SORES, WATERY, OOZING: Cold
  Phlegm In Channels
• ULCERS, SKIN: External
• ULCERS, YIN TYPE WITH
  PHLEGM NODULES
STOMACH/DIGESTIVE
DISORDERS
• REGURGITATION
• VOMITING: Stomach Reflux

Clinical/Pharmaceutical Studies:

INFECTIOUS DISEASES
• BACTERIAL, ANTI-
LUNGS
• BRONCHITIS, CHRONIC:
  (Injection Into Accu-Pts)
• EXPECTORANT: Oil Slightly

Irritates GI, Thus Increasing
Secretions Of Bronchi
SKIN
• ANTIINFLAMMATORY: Apply
  Topically
• FUNGAL, ANTI-: Aqueous Extract,

Many Skin Fungi, At 1:3
Concentration
TRAUMA, BITES, POISONINGS
• INFLAMMATORY, ANTI-: Apply
  Topically

Dose

3 - 9 gm

Common Name

White Mustard Seed

Contraindications

Not: Yin Def Coughs

Not: w/Skin Allergies

Precautions

Watch: Def Individuals, Disperses Qi

Notes

May Cause Vomiting

BAI QIAN

白前

RHIZOMA
CYNANCHII STAUTONI

Traditional Functions:

1. Lowers Lung Qi, expels Phlegm
2. Relieves cough and removes persistent Phlegm

Traditional Properties:

Enters: LU,

Properties: SP, SW, <W

Indications:

LUNGS
• ASTHMA: With Edema,
  Rales/With Profuse
  Sputum, Cough Difficulty

• COUGH: From Wind
  Cold/Wind Heat/With
  Edema, Rales
• COUGH, SPUTUM,

SORE THROAT
• LUNG QI BLOCKAGE &
  STAGNATION
• WHEEZING: Similar To

Ma Huang But Weaker
PHLEGM
• PHLEGM, PROFUSE

Dose

3 - 9 gm

Contraindications

Not: Cough From Def Qi
Not: Cough From KI Not Grasping Qi

BAN XIA
(FA XIA)

半夏

RHIZOMA
PINELLIAE TERNATAE

Traditional Functions:

1. Dries Dampness, transforms phlegm
2. Conducts rebellious Qi downward and Harmonizes the Stomach, stopping vomiting
3. Dispels nodules and reduces distension

Traditional Properties:

Enters: SP, ST,

Properties: SP, W, TX

Indications:

ABDOMEN/
GASTROINTESTINAL TOPICS
• ABDOMEN, DISTENTION OF:
  Damp Heat
• ABDOMEN, DISTENTION OF,
  PAIN
CHEST
• CHEST, DISTENTION: Phlegm/
  Focal Distension
• CHEST, NODULES: Phlegm
• CHEST, PAIN: Phlegm
• CHEST, PRESSURE: Phlegm
CIRCULATION DISORDERS
• STROKE: Phlegm Collapse
• SYNCOPE: Phlegm
EARS/HEARING DISORDERS
• DIZZINESS
• VERTIGO: Wind Phlegm
ENDOCRINE RELATED
DISORDERS
• GOITER
HEAD/NECK

• HEADACHE
• NECK, NODULES: Phlegm
INFECTIOUS DISEASES
• SCROFULA
LUNGS
• COUGH: Cold Phlegm
• COUGH, COPIOUS SPUTUM:
  Lung Cold Phlegm
• LUNGS, DYSPNEA: Cold Phlegm
MENTAL STATE/
NEUROLOGICAL DISORDERS
• INSOMNIA
ORAL CAVITY
• GLOBUS HYSTERICUS
PAIN/NUMBNESS/GENERAL
DISCOMFORT
• FOCAL DISTENTION
PHLEGM
• PHLEGM: Spleen Dampness
• SPUTUM OBSTRUCTIONS
  ANYWHERE
SEXUALITY, FEMALE:

GYNECOLOGICAL
• MENSTRUATION, DISORDERS
  OF: Calm Chong, Lower Reflux/
  Dredge, Regulate Chong, Ren
• MORNING SICKNESS:
  Gestational Foul Obstruction--Cold
SKIN
• CARBUNCLES: External
• ULCERS, DEEP ROOTED, SKIN
SPLEEN
• SPLEEN STOMACH, DAMPNESS
STOMACH/DIGESTIVE
DISORDERS
• HICCUPS: Qi Deficiency-Cold/
  Dampness
• NAUSEA/VOMITING: Stomach
  Damp Phlegm
• STOMACH COLD: Nausea/Vomit
• STOMACH, FOCAL DISTENTION
• VOMITING: Qi Deficiency--
  Dampness/Cold

Clinical/Pharmaceutical Studies:

CANCER/TUMORS/SWELLINGS/
LUMPS
• ANTINEOPLASTIC: Diluted
  Alcohol/Aqueous Extract
• CERVICAL CANCER: Ban Xia
  Water Extract Tablet, Plus Pessary In
  Cervix And Canal, 2 Months
• SKIN, CANCER: Extract Of Ban
  Xia Had Definite Effects
EARS/HEARING DISORDERS
• OTITIS MEDIA: Tincture
EXTREMITIES
• CORNS: Remove Keratinized
  Tissue With Knife, Powder With
  Untreated Then Cover With
  Adhesive Plaster, Sloughed Off In 5-
  7 Days
EYES
• GLAUCOMA, ACUTE: Oral
  Decoction Slightly Reduces Pressure
LUNGS
• ANTITUSSIVE: Hot Water Soluble,
  Lasts Over 5 Hrs, Slightly Weaker

Than Codeine
• BRONCHIECTASIS, W/COUGH,
  THIN SPUTUM: With Jie Geng, Fu
  Ling, Gan Cao (Ju Fang Er Chen
  Tang)
• BRONCHITIS, CHRONIC: With
  Jie Geng, Fu Ling, Gan Cao (Ju Fang
  Er Chen Tang)
• EXPECTORANT
• PNEUMOSILICOSIS: Prevents/
  Slows Progression, The Earlier The
  Better
MENTAL STATE/
NEUROLOGICAL DISORDERS
• PARANOIA: Wen Dan Tang With
  Suan Zao Ren, Yuan Zhi, Zhu LI
• SEDATIVE: Affects Respiratory
  Center Slightly
ORAL CAVITY
• TOOTHACHE: Untreated, 30 g
  Crushed, Soak In 90 ml 90% Alcohol
  For 1 Day, Soak Cotton Ball, 95%
  Effective

SEXUALITY, FEMALE:
GYNECOLOGICAL
• CERVIX, CANCINOMA: Ban Xia
  Water Extract Tablet, Plus Pessary In
  Cervix And Canal, 2 Months
• MORNING SICKNESS: Ban Xia,
  Sheng Jiang, Fu Ling
STOMACH/DIGESTIVE
DISORDERS
• ANTIEMETIC: Hot Water Soluble,
  Strong
• GASTRITIS, CHRONIC,
  VOMITING: Xian Sha Liu Jun Zi
  Tang (Ban Xia, Chen Pi, Mu Xiang,
  Sha Ren, Fu Ling, Dang Shen, Bai
  Zhu, Gan Cao)
• VOMITING, NEUROGENIC: Oral,
  Ban Xia, Xuan Fu Hua, Ren Shen,
  Dai Zhe Shi, Ginger Juice
TRAUMA, BITES, POISONINGS
• ANTIDOTE, TOXICS: Strychnine &
  Acetylcholine

Dose
9 - 12 gm
Contraindications
Not: Bleeding, Def.Yin Coughs, Fluid Def
Not: Phlegm Heat Cough
Not: w/Wu Tou/Hai Zao/Yi Tang
Not: With Aconites

Notes
Unprepaired Is Toxic In Large Doses, Use Fresh Ginger
As Antidote
Treat With Alum To Detoxify
Untreated May Cause Abortion, When Decocted
Becomes Safe
Untreated Antidote: Dilute Vinegar, Concentrated Tea Or
Egg White By Mouth/Decoction Of Ginger, 30 g, Gan
Cao, 15 g, Fang Feng, 60 g, Half As Gargle, Rest Orally

E BU SHI CAO
(SHI HU SUI)

鵝不食草
（鹅不食草）

HERBA CENTIPEDAE

Traditional Functions:

1. Clears Wind and relieves the surface
2. Disperses Cold and Damp Bi
3. Clears the Eyes

Traditional Properties:

Enters: LU, LV

Properties: SW, <W

Indications:

BOWEL RELATED DISORDERS
• DYSENTERY
• HEMORRHOIDS
EYES
• CONJUNCTIVITIS
• CORNEAL OPACITY
• PTERYGIUM
INFECTIOUS DISEASES
• COMMON COLD: Wind Cold
With Headache, Runny Nose

• MALARIA
LUNGS
• COUGH
• COUGH, WHOOPING
**MUSCULOSKELETAL/
CONNECTIVE TISSUE**
• ARTHRITIS, PAIN
NOSE
• NOSE, STUFFY

• RHINITIS, ACUTE/CHRONIC
• SINUSITIS, PARANASAL
ORAL CAVITY
• THROAT, SORE
SKIN
• RASHES
TRAUMA, BITES, POISONINGS
• SNAKE BITES
• TRAUMA

Clinical/Pharmaceutical Studies:

INFECTIOUS DISEASES
• BACTERIAL, ANTI-: TB,
Pseudomonas, Proteus, B.Typhi, B.

Dysenteriae, Staph Aureus
• VIRAL, ANTI-
LUNGS

• ANTITUSSIVE: Tincture
• ASTHMA: Tincture
• EXPECTORANT: Tincture

Dose
4.5 - 9.0 gm

Common Name
Centipeda
Precautions
Watch: Wind Heat Patient

JIE GENG

桔梗

RADIX PLATYCODI GRANDIFLORI

Traditional Functions:

1. Circulates the Lung Qi and expels Phlegm from Wind Heat or Cold
2. Expels pus
3. Clears and benefits the throat
4. Directs effect of other herbs upwards, causing them to affect upper body

Traditional Properties:

Enters: LU,

Properties: BIT, SP, N

Indications:

FLUID DISORDERS
• EDEMA: Smooth Lung Qi
Circulation To Remove
HERBAL FUNCTIONS

Lung Infection
• LUNGS, ABSCESS W/PURULENT
VOMIT
• LUNGS, ABSCESS, W/PUS,

• THROAT, PAIN, SWOLLEN
• THROAT, SORE: Heat/Hot Phlegm/
Deficient Yin Heat
• TONSILLITIS

Indications:

- HERBS, DIRECTS UPWARDS
LUNGS
- COUGH: Cold Phlegm/Wind Heat/ Cold
- COUGH, PROFUSE SPUTUM:

BLOOD
- LUNGS, DYSPNEA: Cold Phlegm
ORAL CAVITY
- THROAT ABSCESS, EXPELS PUS

- VOICE LOSS: Heat/Hot Phlegm/ Deficient Yin Heat
PHLEGM
- SPUTUM, COPIOUS

Clinical/Pharmaceutical Studies:

ABDOMEN/ GASTROINTESTINAL TOPICS
- ABDOMEN, FULLNESS OF, UPPER: Cold, Jie Geng Zhi Ke Tang (Jie Geng, Zhi Ke)
BLOOD RELATED DISORDERS/TOPICS
- BLOOD GLUCOSE, REDUCES: Aqueous/ ETOH Extract, Aqueous Extract Similar To Tolbutamide (At 1/4th Dose) , ETOH Extract More Potent At Inhibiting Dietary Hyperglycemia
- BLOOD PRESSURE, LOWERS
- CHOLESTEROL, LOWERS
- HEMOLYTIC: Only When Injected
CHEST
- CHEST, FULLNESS: Cold, Jie Geng Zhi Ke Tang (Jie Geng, Zhi Ke)
CIRCULATION DISORDERS
- VASODILATES
FEVERS
- ANTIPYRETIC: Inhibits

CNS
IMMUNE SYSTEM RELATED DISORDERS/ TOPICS
- IMMUNE SYSTEM ENHANCEMENT: Aqueous Extract Enhances Phagocytosis
INFECTIOUS DISEASES
- BACTERIAL, ANTI-
- COMMON COLD: With Other Expectorants, Antitussives In Compound Formulae
LUNGS
- ANTITUSSIVE
- BRONCHITIS: With Other Expectorants, Antitussives In Compound Formulae
- COUGH: With Other Expectorants, Antitussives In Compound Formulae
- EXPECTORANT, STRONG: Oral Intake Stimulates Mild Nausea, Causing Bronchi To Secrete By Reflex, Similar In Strength To Ammonium Chloride, Stronger Than Yuan Zhi
- LUNGS, ABSCESS: Jie

Geng Bai San (Jie Geng, Chuan Bei Mu, Fructis Crotonis) Or Jie Geng Tang (With Gan Cao)
- PNEUMONIA, LOBAR: Jie Geng Tang (With Gan Cao)
- RESPIRATORY TRACT, UPPER INFECTION: With Other Expectorants, Antitussives In Compound Formulae
MENTAL STATE/ NEUROLOGICAL DISORDERS
- TRANQUILIZING: Inhibits CNS
ORAL CAVITY
- MOUTH, GINGIVITIS: Powder Of Jie Geng With Yi Yi Ren
- TEETH, DENTAL CARIES: Powder Of Jie Geng With Yi Yi Ren
- THROAT, SORE: Oral Dose
PAIN/NUMBNESS/ GENERAL DISCOMFORT
- ANALGESIC: Inhibits CNS

SEXUALITY, FEMALE: GYNECOLOGICAL
- POSTPARTUM, GASTRIC DYSFUNCTION: Jie Geng Ban Xia Tang (Jie Geng, Chen Pi, Ban Xia, Sheng Jiang)
SKIN
- CARBUNCLES: Either Jie Geng, Gan Cao, Sheng Jiang As Decoction Or Zhi Ke, Bai Shao, Jie Geng As Powder
- FUNGAL, ANTI-: Many Skin Fungi
- FURUNCLES: Either Jie Geng, Gan Cao, Sheng Jiang As Decoction Or Zhi Ke, Bai Shao, Jie Geng As Powder
STOMACH/DIGESTIVE DISORDERS
- ULCERS, PEPTIC: Needs 5 g/kg To Inhibit Gastric Secretion, Prevent Gastric Ulcer, Stronger Than Gan Cao
TRAUMA, BITES, POISONINGS
- INFLAMMATORY, ANTI-

Dose
3 - 9 gm

Common Name
Balloon Flower Root

Contraindications
Not: In Hemoptysis

Not: w/Dry Sputum

Not: Tuberculosis

Notes
Causes Hemolysis If Injected

TIAN NAN XING

天南星

RHIZOMA ARISAEMATIS

Traditional Functions:

1. Dries Dampness and disperses Phlegm
2. Dispels Wind Phlegm and stops spasms
3. Reduces swelling and relieves pain

Traditional Properties:

Enters: LU, SP, LV,

Properties: BIT, SP, W, TX

Indications:

CANCER/TUMORS/SWELLINGS/
LUMPS
- TUMORS
CHEST
- CHEST, TIGHTNESS/
CONSTRICTION: Phlegm
CIRCULATION DISORDERS
- STROKE: Wind Phlegm
EARS/HEARING DISORDERS
- DIZZINESS: Wind Phlegm
EXTREMITIES
- EXTREMITIES, NUMB: Wind
Phlegm
- EXTREMITIES, SPASMS: Wind
Phlegm
EYES

- EYES, DEVIATION OF
HEAD/NECK
- FACE, PARALYSIS: Wind Phlegm
- LOCKJAW: Wind Phlegm
INFECTIOUS DISEASES
- TETANUS
LUNGS
- COUGH: Cold Phlegm
- COUGH, CHRONIC W/PROFUSE
SPUTUM
- LUNGS, DYSPNEA: Cold Phlegm
MENTAL STATE/
NEUROLOGICAL DISORDERS
- CONVULSIONS, HIGH FEVER
- EPILEPTIC SEIZURES
- HEMIPLEGIA

- OPISTHOTONOS: Wind Phlegm
- PARALYSIS
- TRIGEMINAL NEURALGIA
MUSCULOSKELETAL/
CONNECTIVE TISSUE
- SHOULDERS, PAIN, SORENESS
ORAL CAVITY
- MOUTH, DEVIATION OF
PHLEGM
- PHLEGM NODULES
SKIN
- CARBUNCLES: Topical
- SORES, DEEP ROOTED: Topical
- ULCERS, SKIN: Topical
TRAUMA, BITES, POISONINGS
- TRAUMA, SWELLING: Topical

Clinical/Pharmaceutical Studies:

CANCER/TUMORS/

SWELLINGS/LUMPS
- ANTICARCINOGENIC:
Many Cell Types
- CERVICAL CANCER:
Oral (15 g, Then Increase

To 45 g, Decoction) +
Intracervix Application (50
g Pessary Insert Into
Cervical Canal, 2ml (10 g
Of Herb) 4 ml Injected Into
Cervical Area, 1x/1-2 Days,
3-4 Months Course, 78%
Effective, With 20% Short
Term Cures

- TUMOR, ANTI-: Many

Cell Types
CIRCULATION
DISORDERS
- STROKE: With Tian Ma,
(Saposhnikovia Divaricata) ,

Qiang Huo, Oral
HEAD/NECK
- FACE, PARALYSIS:
Fresh Herb With Vinegar,
Ground, Juice Rubbed On
Affected Side Of Neck,
Nightly, Covered With
Gauze
INFECTIOUS DISEASES

- MUMPS: Fresh Soaked In

Vinegar 5 Days, Local
Application, Cure In 5
Days
- TETANUS: With Tian Ma,
(Saposhnikovia Divaricata) ,
Qiang Huo, Oral, •
Injection Slows Disease
Progress
LUNGS
- LUNGS, INCREASES
SECRETIONS
MENTAL STATE/
NEUROLOGICAL
DISORDERS
- EPILEPSY: With Tian Ma,

(Saposhnikovia Divaricata) ,
Qiang Huo, Oral
- SEDATIVE: Aqueous
Extract
- SEIZURES, REDUCES
- TRANQUILIZING
PAIN/NUMBNESS/

GENERAL
DISCOMFORT
- ANALGESIC
SKIN
- NEURODERMATITIS:
Powdered Herb + Paraffin
To Make Ointment For 1-2
Applications

Not: Dry LU Sputum

Dose

3 - 9 gm

Common Name

Jack-In-The-Pulpit

Contraindications

Not: Def Yin
Not: Pregnancy

Notes

Very Drying

Raw Herb Not Used Internally, Damages Oral Cavity

Prepared w/Alum, Ginger

Cancers: 3-15 gm

Use Bile Treated Or Roasted To Avoid Toxicity

XUAN FU HUA   旋復花   FLOS INULAE

Traditional Functions:

1. Redirects the Qi downwards and expels Phlegm and Dampness from the
Lungs
2. Stops vomiting and calms rebellious Qi
3. Softens hardness and masses

Traditional Properties:

Enters: LU, LI, SP, ST,

Properties: BIT, SP, SA, <W

Indications:

ABDOMEN/
GASTROINTESTINAL TOPICS
- ABDOMEN, WATER RETENTION

- COUGH: Cold Phlegm
- COUGH, ASTHMA W/COPIOUS
SPUTUM

STOMACH/DIGESTIVE
DISORDERS
- BELCHING: Unrelievable

Indications:

- SUBCOSTAL FULLNESS, DISTENTION

CHEST
- CHEST, FULLNESS: Phlegm Accumulation
- COSTAL REGION, DISTENTION

FLUID DISORDERS
- ASCITES

LUNGS
- BRONCHITIS, ASTHMATIC W/ COPIOUS PHLEGM

- DYSPNEA
- LUNGS, DYSPNEA: Cold Phlegm
- WHEEZING, COPIOUS SPUTUM

PHLEGM
- SPUTUM, VISCOUS

SEXUALITY, FEMALE: GYNECOLOGICAL
- MENSTRUATION, DISORDERS OF: Calm Chong, Lower Reflux
- MORNING SICKNESS: Gestational Foul Obstruction–Cold

- HICCUPS: Qi Deficiency-Cold/ Spleen Dampness
- HICCUPS, CHRONIC
- STOMACH, FIRM MASS
- STOMACH, STUFFINESS, RIGIDITY
- VOMITING: Qi Deficiency-Cold/ Stomach Cold Deficient/Spleen Dampness
- VOMITING, CHRONIC

Clinical/Pharmaceutical Studies:

ABDOMEN/ GASTROINTESTINAL TOPICS
- INTESTINES, PERISTALSIS, INCREASES

HEART
- HEART RATE, REDUCES: Slows Heart Rate

INFECTIOUS DISEASES
- BACTERIAL, ANTI-: Strongly Inhibits Staph Aureus, Bacillus Anthracis, Shigella, Salmonella, Pseudomonas, Proteus, C.Diphteriae

LUNGS
- ANTITUSSIVE: IP Injection Of 150% Decoction
- ASTHMA: Protects Against, Slower, Weaker Than Aminophylline

- BRONCHITIS, ACUTE/CHRONIC: Honey Pill Of Herb, Jie Geng, Bai Jiang Cao, 3 g/Pill, 3 Ea In 2 Doses/ Day For 10 Days, 3 Courses With 5 Days Between Courses
- BRONCHITIS, CHRONIC: With Sang Bai Pi, Jie Geng, Pu Yan Pian (Radix Rhois Chinensis)
- EXPECTORANT

MENTAL STATE/ NEUROLOGICAL DISORDERS
- CAFFEINE-LIKE: CNS Stimulant, Stomach Secretion Increase

MUSCULOSKELETAL/ CONNECTIVE TISSUE
- MUSCLES, SMOOTH

STIMULATES
STOMACH/DIGESTIVE DISORDERS
- ANTIEMETIC
- HICCUPS: Liver Stomach Disharmoney, Xuan Fu Huan Dai Zhe Shi Tang (Herbs Plus Chen Pi, Ban Xia)
- VOMITING: Liver Stomach Disharmoney, Xuan Fu Huan Dai Zhe Shi Tang (Herbs Plus Chen Pi, Ban Xia)
- VOMITING, INTRACTABLE: Dai Zhe Shi Tang And Six Major Herbs Decoction, Plus Large Dose Dai Zhe Shi

Dose

3 - 9 gm

Contraindications

Not: Wind Heat Cough

Notes

Wrap In Filter Paper Petals Can Irritate Stomach/May Induce Cough

---

YANG JIN HUA

洋金花

FLOS DATURAE ALBAE

Traditional Functions:

1. Relieves asthma and controls cough
2. Dispels Wind Dampness, controls pain

Traditional Properties:

Enters: HT, LU, SP

Properties:

Indications:

ABDOMEN/ GASTROINTESTINAL TOPICS
- ABDOMEN, PAIN OF

LUNGS
- ASTHMA
- COUGH, NO SPUTUM

PAIN/NUMBNESS/GENERAL DISCOMFORT
- BI, WIND DAMP

SKIN
- SWEATING, INHIBITS

STOMACH/DIGESTIVE DISORDERS
- EPIGASTRIC PAIN

TRAUMA, BITES, POISONINGS
- TRAUMA, PAIN

Clinical/Pharmaceutical Studies:

- SHOCK: From Infection, Toxins, IV, Every 10-30 Minutes Until Face Flushes, Extremities Warm, BP Up,

EYES
- MYDRIATIC

LUNGS
- BRONCHITIS,

CHILDHOOD: Used As Adjuvant, Most Effective During Acute Stage

MENTAL STATE/

GENERAL DISCOMFORT
- ANALGESIC
- ANESTHETIC: Usually

Clinical/Pharmaceutical Studies:

Pupils Dilated
CIRCULATION DISORDERS
• THROMBOANGIITIS OBLITERANS: IM/IV With Chlorpromazine, Tetrandrine (Active Ingredient Of Han Fang Ji, 60 mg) , Best In Mild-Moderate Pain, Pain Relief For 2 Days, Needs Continual Treatments For Remission

CHRONIC: Injection Was Highly Efficacious, Control 70%, High Rate Of Side Effects, Less With Liquor, Tablet, Herb Cigarette, Suppository (Keep Dose At 0.01 mg/kg) , *Clinical Control Acheived 63% For Tablet, 0.01 mg/kg Taken At Bed For 5 Courses Of 10 Days Each
• PNEUMONIA,

NEUROLOGICAL DISORDERS
• HALLUCINATIONS: Causes
• PSYCHOSIS: Best With Manic Patients, Used With Chlorpromazine, Allowed Useage Of Smaller Doses
• SEDATIVE
MUSCULOSKELETAL/ CONNECTIVE TISSUE
• ANTISPASMODIC
PAIN/NUMBNESS/

Combined With Chlorpromazine, Pethidine, IV
• PAIN, INTRACTABLE: Good For Severe Pain As In Malignancy Unable To Respond To Morphine, Fentanyl, etc, Use 2 mg IV With Chlorpromazine Or "Artificial Hibernation Mixture" (Literature Unclear On Components)

Dose

0.3 - 0.6 gm

Common Name

Datura Flower, Jimson Weed

Contraindications

Not: Glaucoma

Precautions

Watch: Hypertension, Weakness, Children, Pregnancy

Notes

Toxic: 9 gm Enough To Make One "Tipsy"

Possible: Nausea, Vomiting, Decreased Mental Activity, Amnesia, Hallucination At 45 mg Scopolamine (Main Active Ingredient)

ZAO JIAO
(ZAO JIA)

皂角

FRUCTUS GLEDITSIAE SINENSIS

Traditional Functions:

1. Disperses and expels Phlegm
2. Opens orifices and awakens spirit
3. Moves the stool and expels roundworms--as a suppository
4. Dispels Wind Damp
5. Kills Parasites

Traditional Properties:

Enters: LU, LI,

Properties: SP, W, <TX

Indications:

BOWEL RELATED DISORDERS
• CONSTIPATION: Suppository
CANCER/TUMORS/SWELLINGS/ LUMPS
• SWELLINGS, FROM TOXINS
CIRCULATION DISORDERS
• APOPLEXY W/LOSS OF CONSCIOUSNESS
INFECTIOUS DISEASES
• LEPROSY
LUNGS

• ASTHMA, BRONCHIAL W/ STICKY SPUTUM
• COUGH, COPIOUS SPUTUM
MENTAL STATE/ NEUROLOGICAL DISORDERS
• EPILEPSY
• HEMIPLEGIA
• MENTAL CLOUDINESS: Excess (Shut-In Complex)
• UNCONSCIOUSNESS: Excess (Shut-In Complex)

ORAL CAVITY
• THROAT, SORE
PARASITES
• ROUNDWORMS: Suppository
PHLEGM
• PHLEGM NODULES
• PHLEGM OBSTRUCTION
SKIN
• SKIN, SORES, INTRACTABLE
• TINEA FUNGUS

Clinical/Pharmaceutical Studies:

BLOOD RELATED DISORDERS/ TOPICS
• HEMOLYTIC: (Binds To Cholesterol Which Reduces This Action In Vivo)
INFECTIOUS DISEASES

• ANTIBIOTIC: Gram Negative Bacteria In Intestines, E.Coli, Typhosa, Pseudomonas, Proteus
LUNGS
• EXPECTORANT: Stomach/Lungs, Increases Secretions, Significant,

Less Than Jie Geng
• LUNGS, INCREASES SECRETION: Less Than Jie Geng
SKIN
• FUNGAL, ANTI-: Various

Dose
1.5 - 6.0 gm

Common Name
Chinese Honeylocust Fruit

Contraindications
Not: If Ulcers Have Burst Or Opened Up

Not: Pregnancy

Not: With Hemoptysis

Notes
Powder Or Pill Only

Topical, Too

Overdose: Hemolysis, Respiratory Paralysis

As Powder, Use: 0.6-1.5 gm

ZAO JIAO CI

皂角刺

SPINA GLEDITSIAE SINENSIS

Traditional Functions:

1. Reduces inflammation, discharges pus
2. Expels Wind of the skin
3. Kills parasites

Traditional Properties:

Enters: ST, LV, LU, LI

Properties: SP, W

Indications:

INFECTIOUS DISEASES
* LEPROSY

MENTAL STATE/ NEUROLOGICAL DISORDERS
* MENTAL CLOUDINESS: Excess (Shut-In Complex)
* UNCONSCIOUSNESS: Excess (Shut-In Complex)

ORAL CAVITY
* TONSILLITIS

PARASITES

* PARASITES

SEXUALITY, FEMALE: GYNECOLOGICAL
* BREASTS, SWOLLEN, PAINFUL, ABSCESS
* PLACENTA, RETENTION

SKIN
* ABSCESS, HELPS TO DRAIN
* BOILS
* CARBUNCLES
* FUNGAL INFECTIONS: Topical

* RINGWORM
* SKIN, INFECTIONS, EARLY STAGE TO CAUSE SUPPURATION
* SKIN, LESIONS: Acute Purulent
* SKIN, SORES, INTRACTABLE
* ULCERS, TOXIC

TRAUMA, BITES, POISONINGS
* INFLAMMATION, PURULENT

WIND DISORDERS
* WIND, EPIDEMIC

Dose
3 - 9 gm

Common Name
Chinese Honeylocust Spine

Contraindications
Not: Pregnancy

Not: When Ulcers/Boils Have Burst/Opened Up

Clear And Dissolve The Heated Phlegm

Herbs Eleocharitis

BI QI
(BI JI/WU CAO)

荸薺
（荸荠））

CORMUS
HELEOCHRIS
PLANTAGINEA

Traditional Functions:

1. Dissolves Phlegm and dissipates accumulation
2. Clears Heat, cools Blood and promotes fluid secretion
3. Clears and brightens the eyes

Traditional Properties:

Enters: LU, LI, ST,

Properties: SW, C

Indications:

BOWEL RELATED DISORDERS
• CONSTIPATION
**CANCER/TUMORS/SWELLINGS/
 LUMPS**
• MASSES, HARD
• NODULES: Phlegm

EYES
• CONJUNCTIVITIS
• CORNEAL OPACITY
FLUID DISORDERS
• THIRST: Fluid Injury/Heat
LUNGS

• COUGH: Hot Phlegm
• LUNGS, DRY: Yin Deficiency
**STOMACH/DIGESTIVE
 DISORDERS**
• INDIGESTION

Clinical/Pharmaceutical Studies:

INFECTIOUS DISEASES
• BACTERIAL, ANTI-: Staph.
Aureus, E.Coli, Pseudomonas

Dose
30 - 90 gm

Common Name
Water Chestnut

CHUAN BEI MU

川貝母
（川贝母）

BULBUS
FRITILLARIAE CIRRHOSAE

Traditional Functions:

1. Clears Heat and disperses Phlegm
2. Clears Heat and dissipates accumulations and nodules
3. Stops cough
4. Moistens and nourishes the Lungs

Traditional Properties:

Enters: LU, HT,

Properties: BIT, SW, CL

Indications:

**CANCER/TUMORS/SWELLINGS/
 LUMPS**
• CYSTS
• SWELLINGS, GLANDULAR:
 Phlegm Fire
CHEST
• CHEST, CONGESTION/
 ENTANGLEMENT
**ENDOCRINE RELATED
 DISORDERS**
• THYROID, ENLARGEMENT:
 Phlegm Fire

DISORDERS/TOPICS
• LYMPH GLANDS,
 ENLARGEMENT, CHRONIC:
 Phlegm Nodules
LUNGS
• BRONCHITIS, CHRONIC
• COUGH: Lung Dryness/Lung Heat/
 Yin Deficient With Fire
• COUGH IN CHILDREN
• COUGH, BLOOD STREAKED
 SPUTUM
• COUGH, CHEST CONSTRICTION

• COUGH, DRY
• COUGH, LUNG EXHAUSTION:
 Tuberculosis
• LUNGS, DYSPNEA: Lung Heat
• TUBERCULOSIS
PHLEGM
• SPUTUM, EXCESSIVE
**SEXUALITY, FEMALE:
 GYNECOLOGICAL**
• BREASTS, ABSCESS OF: Phlegm
 Fire
• MASTITIS

Indications:

HEMORRHAGIC DISORDERS
- HEMOPTYSIS

IMMUNE SYSTEM RELATED

- COUGH, CHRONIC
- COUGH, DIFFICULT
  EXPECTORATION

SKIN
- ABSCESS
- SKIN, ULCERS: External Use

Clinical/Pharmaceutical Studies:

**ABDOMEN/
GASTROINTESTINAL
TOPICS**
- INTESTINES,
  PERISTALSIS, INHIBITS
- ULCERS, DUODENAL

**BLOOD RELATED
DISORDERS/TOPICS**
- BLOOD GLUCOSE,
  INCREASES: Increases
- BLOOD PRESSURE,
  LOWERS: Prolonged,
  Profound

CANCER/TUMORS/

SWELLINGS/LUMPS
- CERVICAL CANCER

**HEMORRHAGIC
DISORDERS**
- HEMOPTYSIS,
  TUBERCULOSIS: With
  Sheng Di, Shu Di, Bai He,
  Add Hou PO For Dyspnea

LUNGS
- ANTITUSSIVE: Atropine-
  Like
- BRONCHITIS, ACUTE/
  CHRONIC: 0.5 g/Tab, 4
  Tabs 3x/Day, 1-5 Days

- COUGH,
  TUBERCULOSIS: With
  Pi Pa Ye, Sang Ye, Mai Ya,
  Yu Zhu (Qing Zao Jiu Fei
  Tang)
- EXPECTORANT:
  Decreases Secretion
- RESPIRATORY TRACT
  INFECTION: 0.5 g/Tab, 4
  Tabs 3x/Day, 1-5 Days
- WHOOPING COUGH:
  Snake Bile-Fritillaria Bulb
  Powder

MENTAL STATE/

**NEUROLOGICAL
DISORDERS**
- CNS, INHIBITOR

ORAL CAVITY
- THROAT, SORE,
  PAINFUL: With Lian
  Qiao, Shan Zhi Zi, Jin Yin
  Hua, etc

**SEXUALITY, FEMALE:
GYNECOLOGICAL**
- CERVIX, CANCINOMA
- UTERUS, STIMULATES:
  Causes Contractions

Dose

3 - 9 gm

Contraindications

Not: In Def SP/ST

Not: w/Wu Tou

Notes

0.3-.5 Qian If Powdered

Not Effective For Cold, Damp Coughs

DAN NAN XING

膽南星
(胆南星)

PULVIS
ARISAEMAI CUM FELLE
BOVIS

Traditional Functions:

1. Clears Heat and transforms Phlegm
2. Dispels Wind and stops spasms
3. Calms fear

Traditional Properties:

Enters: LU, SP, LV,

Properties: BIT, CL

Indications:

CHILDHOOD DISORDERS
- PEDIATRICS, FOR FEAR

CIRCULATION DISORDERS
- STROKE: Hot Phlegm

LUNGS

- COUGH: Lung Heat
- LUNGS, DYSPNEA: Lung Heat

**MENTAL STATE/
NEUROLOGICAL DISORDERS**
- CONVULSIONS, FEVER, ACUTE

- SEIZURES: Hot Phlegm

**MUSCULOSKELETAL/
CONNECTIVE TISSUE**
- SPASMS: Hot Phlegm
- SPASMS, W/FEVER, ACUTE

Dose

3 - 9 gm

Common Name

Bile Treated Jack-Pulpit

GUA LOU

瓜蔞
(瓜蒌)

FRUCTUS
TRICHOSANTHIS

Traditional Functions:

1. Clears and disperses Hot Phlegm
2. Circulates the bound Qi in the chest
3. Dissipates nodules and accumulations

Traditional Properties:

Enters: LU, LI, ST,

Properties: SW, BIT, C

Indications:

ABDOMEN/ GASTROINTESTINAL TOPICS
- APPENDICITIS W/PAIN

BOWEL RELATED DISORDERS
- CONSTIPATION: Intestinal Dryness

HEART

- ANGINA PECTORIS: Chest Bi Strangulating Pain

LUNGS
- ABSCESS, LUNG/BREAST
- COUGH: Lung Dryness/Lung Heat w/Difficult Sputum
- LUNG INFECTION

- LUNGS, DYSPNEA: Lung Heat

PAIN/NUMBNESS/GENERAL DISCOMFORT
- PAIN: Chest, Intercostal

SEXUALITY, FEMALE: GYNECOLOGICAL
- BREASTS, ABSCESS OF

Clinical/Pharmaceutical Studies:

CANCER/TUMORS/ SWELLINGS/LUMPS
- ANTINEOPLASTIC: Granuloma, Hepatic Cancer
- LIVER CANCER

CHEST
- COSTAL REGION, CHONDRITIS: Tricosanthes-Allium Decoction
- INTERCOSTAL NEURALGIA: Tricosanthes-Allium Decoction

HEART
- CORONARY ARTERY DISEASE

INFECTIOUS DISEASES
- ANTIBIOTIC: E Coli, Shigell, Pseudomonas

LIVER
- LIVER, CANCER

LUNGS
- COUGH, DRY, THICK SPUTUM: With Zhi Bei Mu, Jie Geng, Chen Pi
- PLEURISY, CHEST PAIN, EXCESSIVE EXPECTORATION: With

Huang Lian, Ban Xia (e.g. Xiao Xian Xion Tang/Chai Xian Tang)
- PNEUMONIA, CHEST PAIN, EXCESSIVE EXPECTORATION: With Huang Lian, Ban Xia (e.g. Xiao Xian Xion Tang/Chai Xian Tang)

SEXUALITY, FEMALE: GYNECOLOGICAL
- AMENORRHEA: Tricosanthes-Dendrobium Decoction (Gua Lou, Shi

Hu, Xuan Shen, Mai Dong, Shu Di, Qu Mai, Che Qian Zi, Yi Mu Cao, Huang Lian, Niu Xi) , Notes--Not A Steroid Substitute, Possible Hypothalamus Regulation
- MASTITIS: As Adjuvant In Treating, With Pu Gong Ying, Chi Shao, Chuan Shan Jia, Jin Yin Hua, etc

SKIN
- FUNGAL, ANTI-: Many Skin Fungi

Dose
9 - 15 gm

Contraindications
Not: Cold Def SP/ST, Cold Phlegm, Damp Phlegm
Not: w/Wu Tou

GUA LOU PI

瓜蔞皮
（瓜蔞皮）

PERICARPIUM TRICHOSANTHIS

Traditional Functions:

1. Clears and disperses Hot Phlegm
2. Circulates the bound Qi in the chest
3. Dissipates nodules and accumulations

Traditional Properties:

Enters: LU, LI, ST,

Properties: SW, C

Indications:

CHEST
- CHEST, PAIN, STUFFINESS

LUNGS

- COUGH, DRY, DIFFICULT SPUTUM: Wind Heat

- LUNGS, HEAT: Infections With Yellow, Thick Sputum

Clinical/Pharmaceutical Studies:

CANCER/TUMORS/SWELLINGS/ LUMPS
- ANTINEOPLASTIC: Granuloma, Hepatic Cancer, Husk Most Potent, ETOH Extract Strongest
- LIVER CANCER

HEART
- ANGINA PECTORIS: Extract From Peel, Seed, Long Term Use, Or Tricosanthes-Allium-Pinellia Decoction, Tricosanthes-Allium

Decoction, etc

LIVER
- LIVER, CANCER

LUNGS
- EXPECTORANT: Good

Dose
9 - 15 gm

Notes
Very Low Toxicity

GUA LOU REN　　瓜蔞仁　　SEMEN TRICHOSANTHIS
（瓜蔞仁）

Traditional Functions:

1. Clears and disperses Hot Phlegm
2. Circulates the bound Qi in the chest and dissipates accumulations
3. Moistens intestines, promoting passage of stool
4. Promotes healing of sores
5. Moistens the Lungs

Traditional Properties:

Enters: LU, LI, ST,

Properties: SW, C

Indications:

BOWEL RELATED DISORDERS
• CONSTIPATION: Dry Stool, Especially Lung Heat Pattern
CHEST
• CHEST, DISTENTION, PAIN/ PRESSURE: Phlegm Accumulation
ENDOCRINE RELATED DISORDERS
• DIABETES

FLUID DISORDERS
• THIRST: Febrile Diseases
LIVER
• JAUNDICE
LUNGS
• COUGH: Hot Phlegm
• COUGH, CHEST PAIN, DIFFICULT EXPECTORATION

ORAL CAVITY
• THROAT, SORE
SEXUALITY, FEMALE: GYNECOLOGICAL
• BREASTS, ABSCESS OF
SKIN
• SKIN, SORES/SWELLINGS
• SORES, W/O SUPPURATION

Clinical/Pharmaceutical Studies:

BLOOD RELATED DISORDERS/TOPICS
• CHOLESTEROL, LOWERS
BOWEL RELATED

DISORDERS
• LAXATIVE: Strong, Fixed Oil
CANCER/TUMORS/ SWELLINGS/LUMPS

• ANTINEOPLASTIC: Granuloma, Hepatic Cancer
• CANCER, ANTI-: 60% Extract Strong Action

Against Cancer Cells, Skin Is Better Than Fruit
• LIVER CANCER
HEART
• CORONARY ARTERY

DISEASE
INFECTIOUS DISEASES
• ANTIBIOTIC: E Coli, Shigell, Pseudomonas, B. Dysenteriae, B.Typhi, et al

LIVER
• LIVER, CANCER
LUNGS
• BRONCHITIS, ACUTE:

With Thick Sputum, Fritillaria Tricosanthes Antitussive Decoction (Gua Lou Ren, Chuan Bei Mu, Bai He, Xing Ren, etc), Short Term Cure, 3-12 Doses
SKIN
• FUNGAL, ANTI-: Many Skin Fungi

Dose

9 - 18 gm

Not: w/Diarrhea From Cold Def SP/ST

Notes

Contraindications

Not: w/Gan Jiang/Niu Xi/Wu Tou

Overdose: Gastric Discomfort, Nausea, Abdominal Pain, Diarrhea

---

HAI FU SHI　　海浮石　　PUMICE
（海浮石）

Traditional Functions:

1. Clears Heat from the Lungs and dissipates Hot Phlegm.
2. Softens hardness and disperses accumulation of Phlegm
3. Promotes urination

Traditional Properties:

Enters: LU

Properties: SA, <C

Indications:

CANCER/TUMORS/SWELLINGS/ LUMPS
• MASSES, HARD
• TUMORS
ENDOCRINE RELATED DISORDERS

DISORDERS/TOPICS
• LYMPH GLANDS, ENLARGEMENT, CHRONIC: Phlegm Nodules
• LYMPH NODES, SWELLING: Phlegm Fire

• COUGH, STICKY PHLEGM: Hot Phlegm
PHLEGM
• PHLEGM FIRE IN LUNG
• PHLEGM, LINGERING
• PHLEGM, THICK IN LUNG

Indications:

- GOITER: Phlegm Fire
HEMORRHAGIC DISORDERS
- HEMOPTYSIS
IMMUNE SYSTEM RELATED

INFECTIOUS DISEASES
- SCROFULA: Phlegm Fire
LUNGS
- COUGH: Lung Heat

URINARY BLADDER
- PAINFUL URINARY
DYSFUNCTION: Hot
- URINARY STONES

Dose

9 - 15 gm

Common Name

Pumice

Contraindications

Not: Def Cold Cough

HAI GE KE
(GE KE/GE QIAO)

海蛤殼
（海蛤壳）

CONCHA
CYCLINAE SINENSIS

Traditional Functions:

1. Clears Heat, dissolves Phlegm and redirects Lung Qi down
2. Removes Dampness by promoting urination
3. Softens the hardness and dissipates nodules

Traditional Properties:

Enters: LU, KI,

Properties: BIT, SA, N

Indications:

**ENDOCRINE RELATED
DISORDERS**
- GOITER: Phlegm Fire
- THYROID, ENLARGEMENT
- THYROID, LUMPS
FLUID DISORDERS
- EDEMA
HEART
- HEART PAIN
**IMMUNE SYSTEM RELATED
DISORDERS/TOPICS**
- LYMPH GLANDS,
ENLARGEMENT, CHRONIC:
Phlegm Nodules
INFECTIOUS DISEASES
- SCROFULA: Phlegm Fire

LUNGS
- COUGH, CHEST, RIB PAIN: Lung
Heat
PHLEGM
- PHLEGM DAMP
- PHLEGM HEAT
- PHLEGM, LINGERING
- PHLEGM, PERSISTENT
SEXUALITY, EITHER SEX
- GENITALS, DISEASES OF
SEXUALITY, FEMALE:
GYNECOLOGICAL
- LEUKORRHEA
- MENORRHAGIA
SEXUALITY, MALE:
UROLOGICAL TOPICS

- SEMINAL INCONTINENCE
- SPERMATORRHEA
SKIN
- BURNS: Topical
SPLEEN
- SPLEEN PAIN
STOMACH/DIGESTIVE
DISORDERS
- ACID REGURGITATION: Use
Calcined Form
- STOMACH, PAIN: Use Calcined
Form
URINARY BLADDER
- URINARY DRIBBLING, WHITE
- URINARY DYSFUNCTION,
PAINFUL, TURBID

Dose

3 - 9 gm

Common Name

Clam Shell

Notes

Powder Usually, Wrap Or Use Strainer

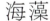

HAI ZAO

海藻

HERBA
SARGASSII

Traditional Functions:

1. Clears Heat and disperses Phlegm accumulations and nodules
2. Decreases goiter size
3. Promotes urination and reduces swelling

Traditional Properties:

Enters: LU, SP, KI, LV,

Properties: BIT, SA, C

Indications:

ABDOMEN/
GASTROINTESTINAL TOPICS
• HERNIA-LIKE CONDITION,
PAIN
CANCER/TUMORS/SWELLINGS/
LUMPS
• THYROID TUMORS
• TUMORS
CIRCULATION DISORDERS
• HYPERTENSION
ENDOCRINE RELATED
DISORDERS
• HYPOTHYROID GOITER:
Phlegm
• THYROID, ENLARGEMENT
• THYROID, TUMORS
EXTREMITIES

• LEG QI: Adjunctive Herb
FLUID DISORDERS
• EDEMA: Adjunctive Herb
HEAT
• HEAT PHLEGM
IMMUNE SYSTEM RELATED
DISORDERS/TOPICS
• GLANDS, SWOLLEN: Phlegm
• LYMPH GLANDS,
ENLARGEMENT, CHRONIC:
Phlegm Nodules
INFECTIOUS DISEASES
• MUMPS: Phlegm
• SCROFULA: Phlegm
LIVER
• HEPATOMEGALY
LUNGS

• BRONCHITIS, CHRONIC
• TUBERCULOSIS OF LYMPH
NODES
MENTAL STATE/
NEUROLOGICAL DISORDERS
• CONVULSIONS, FEVER, ACUTE
MUSCULOSKELETAL/
CONNECTIVE TISSUE
• SPASMS, W/FEVER, ACUTE
PHLEGM
• PHLEGM, HOT
SEXUALITY, MALE:
UROLOGICAL TOPICS
• TESTICLES, INFLAMED
SPLEEN
• SPLENOMEGALY

Clinical/Pharmaceutical Studies:

BLOOD RELATED DISORDERS/
TOPICS
• ANTICOAGULANT: Similar To
Heparin (About 1/2 Of Its Strength,
Occurs After Decoction)
• BLOOD PRESSURE, LOWERS:
Large (0.75g/kg) Doses, Water
Extracts Better
• CHOLESTEROL, LOWERS: Mild
CIRCULATION DISORDERS
• HYPERTENSION

ENDOCRINE RELATED
DISORDERS
• HYPERTHYROID: Temporarily
Inhibits Metabolism And Relieves
Symptoms
• HYPOTHYROID: From Iodine Def,
Form Of Iodine Is Retained By
Body For Long Time
HEMORRHAGIC DISORDERS
• HEMOSTATIC
NUTRITIONAL/METABOLIC

DISORDERS/TOPICS
• WEIGHT CONTROL: Suppresses
Appetite w/o Insomnia
PARASITES
• ANTIPARASITIC: Schistosoma
SKIN
• FUNGAL, ANTI-: Many, Water
Extractions, Inhibits
TRAUMA, BITES, POISONINGS
• DETOXIFIES: Speeds Excretion Of
Radioactive Elements

Dose
9 - 15 gm

Common Name
Seaweed

Contraindications
Not: w/Gan Cao (Traditional) Although Research Shows
No Problem With Gan Cao
Not: w/Cold Def SP/ST

Notes
Single Herb: 15-30 gm

HOU ZAO

猴棗
(猴枣)

CALCULUS
MACACAE MULATTAE

Traditional Functions:

1. Clears the Heat and disperses Phlegm
2. Clears Heat, removes swelling and relieves toxins
3. Calms fright and stops spasms
4. Relieves asthma by clearing Phlegm

Traditional Properties:

Enters: LU, HT, LV, GB,

Properties: BIT, SA, C

Indications:

CHILDHOOD DISORDERS
• CONVULSIONS, CHILDHOOD:
Heat
INFECTIOUS DISEASES
• SCROFULA
LUNGS
• COUGH: Lung Heat

• DYSPNEA
• LUNGS, DYSPNEA: Lung Heat
MENTAL STATE/
NEUROLOGICAL DISORDERS
• EPILEPSY
ORAL CAVITY
• VOICE, HOARSE

PHLEGM
• PHLEGM HEAT
• PHLEGM, HOT OBSTRUCTION
SKIN
• BOILS
• SORES, SUPPURATIVE

Clinical/Pharmaceutical Studies:

MENTAL STATE/
NEUROLOGICAL DISORDERS

• TRANQUILIZING
MUSCULOSKELETAL/

CONNECTIVE TISSUE
• ANTISPASMODIC

Dose
0.6 - 1.5 gm

Common Name
Macaque Gallstone

Notes
Very Expensive

HUANG YAO ZI

黃藥子
(黄药子)

RHIZOMA
DIOSCOREAE BULBIFERAE

Traditional Functions:

1. Softens firm mass and disperses nodules
2. Cools the Blood and stops bleeding
3. Reduces and detoxifies toxic swellings
4. Stops cough
5. Decreases goiter size

Traditional Properties:

Enters: HT, LV,

Properties: BIT, N

Indications:

CANCER/TUMORS/SWELLINGS/
LUMPS
• TUMORS: Esophageal, Stomach,
Uterine
ENDOCRINE RELATED
DISORDERS
• HYPERTHYROID
• HYPOTHYROID GOITER
• THYROID, ENLARGEMENT
HEMORRHAGIC DISORDERS

• HEMATEMESIS
• HEMOPTYSIS
IMMUNE SYSTEM RELATED
DISORDERS/TOPICS
• LYMPH NODES, SWELLING
LUNGS
• ASTHMA: Deficient
• COUGH: Dry Lung
• WHOOPING COUGH
ORAL CAVITY

• THROAT, PAIN, SWOLLEN
SEXUALITY, FEMALE:
GYNECOLOGICAL
• UTERINE BLEEDING
SKIN
• ABSCESS
• SORES: Topical
TRAUMA, BITES, POISONINGS
• BITES, SNAKE, DOGS: Topical
• INSECT BITES: Topical

Clinical/Pharmaceutical Studies:

ABDOMEN/
GASTROINTESTINAL TOPICS
• INTESTINES, STIMULATES:
Tincture/Decoctions
CANCER/TUMORS/SWELLINGS/
LUMPS
• ESOPHAGEAL TUMORS:
Tincture
• GASTRIC TUMORS: Tincture
• THYROID TUMORS: Decoction,
Best For Nonmalignant Of Short

Duration, Nausea/Vomiting Possible
• TUMORS: Dose, 30 g
ENDOCRINE RELATED
DISORDERS
• GOITER, INHIBITS
HEART
• HEART, INHIBITS: Tinctures
Strongest, Fastest
INFECTIOUS DISEASES
• BACTERIAL, ANTI-: Typhoid,
Enteritis, Dysentary, Diplococcus

SEXUALITY, FEMALE:
GYNECOLOGICAL
• UTERUS, STIMULATES: Tincture/
Decoctions
SKIN
• FUNGAL, ANTI-: Aqueous Extract-
-Skin, Tinea
STOMACH/DIGESTIVE
DISORDERS
• GASTRIC TUMORS: Tincture

Dose
3 - 12 gm

Common Name
Yellow Yam Root

Contraindications
Not: Ulcerated Abscess

Notes
Not Long Term Use Of Tinctures: LV Damage/Jaundice
Nausea Possible
Cancers: 30 gm

KUN BU   昆布   *THALLUS ALGAE*

Traditional Functions:

1. Clears Heat and disperses Phlegm accumulations and nodules
2. Promotes urination and reduces swelliing from edema and Leg Qi

Traditional Properties:

Enters: LU, SP, LV,

Properties: SA, C

Indications:

ABDOMEN/
GASTROINTESTINAL TOPICS
• ACCUMULATION
• GROIN AREA PAIN
• HERNIA-LIKE CONDITION,
  PAIN
CANCER/TUMORS/SWELLINGS/
LUMPS
• THYROID TUMORS
ENDOCRINE RELATED
DISORDERS
• HYPOTHYROID GOITER: Hot
  Phlegm
• THYROID, ENLARGEMENT

• THYROID, TUMORS
FLUID DISORDERS
• EDEMA
HEAT
• HEAT PHLEGM
IMMUNE SYSTEM RELATED
DISORDERS/TOPICS
• GLANDS, SWOLLEN: Hot
  Phlegm
• LYMPH GLANDS,
  ENLARGEMENT, CHRONIC:
  Phlegm Nodules
• LYMPH NODES, CHRONIC
  SWOLLEN INFLAMMATION OF

INFECTIOUS DISEASES
• MUMPS: Hot Phlegm
• SCROFULA: Hot Phlegm
LIVER
• HEPATOMEGALY
PHLEGM
• PHLEGM, HOT
SEXUALITY, MALE:
UROLOGICAL TOPICS
• TESTICLES, INFLAMED, PAIN,
  SWELLING
SPLEEN
• SPLENOMEGALY

Clinical/Pharmaceutical Studies:

BLOOD RELATED DISORDERS/
TOPICS
• BLOOD PRESSURE, LOWERS:
  Slightly, Short Term Only
CIRCULATION DISORDERS
• ATHEROSCLEROSIS: Can Reduce
  Lipids In Blood
ENDOCRINE RELATED
DISORDERS
• GOITER: Due To Deficient Iodine

• HYPERTHYROID: Temporarily
  Helps Symptoms, By Reducing
  Metabolism
• HYPOTHYROID: From Low
  Iodine
LUNGS
• ANTITUSSIVE
• ASTHMA
• EXPECTORANT
MUSCULOSKELETAL/

CONNECTIVE TISSUE
• MUSCLES, SMOOTH, INHIBITS
PARASITES
• SCHISTOSOMIASIS: Inhibits
  Growth, Helps Liver To Recover
TRAUMA, BITES, POISONINGS
• DETOXIFIES. Helps Increase
  Excretion Of Radioactive Elements
  From Body
• INFLAMMATORY, ANTI-

Dose

3 - 15 gm

Common Name

Kelp Thallus

Contraindications

Not: In Hyperthyroid Conditions
Not: w/Cold, Damp Def SP/ST

PANG DA HAI   胖大海   *SEMEN STERCULIAE SCAPHIGERAE*

Traditional Functions:

1. Opens Lung Qi and eliminates Heat from the Lungs
2. Moistens intestines, promoting passage of stool
3. Encourages rashes to surface
4. Moistens the Lung and clears the throat
5. Clears Heat and toxins

Traditional Properties:

Enters: LU, LI,

Properties: SW, C

Indications:

BOWEL RELATED DISORDERS
• CONSTIPATION W/HEADACHE &
  RED EYES: Heat

HEAT
• HEAT, INTERNAL
HEMORRHAGIC DISORDERS

• LUNGS, DYSPNEA: Lung Heat
ORAL CAVITY
• HOARSENESS

Indications:

- FISTULA
- HEMORRHOIDS
CANCER/TUMORS/SWELLINGS/
  LUMPS
- TUMORS, FISTULOUS
EYES
- EYES, INFLAMMATION
FEVERS
- BONE STEAMING FEVER

- EPISTAXIS
- HEMAFECIA
- HEMATEMESIS
- HEMOPTYSIS
LUNGS
- COUGH: Hot Phlegm/Lung Heat/
  Wind Heat
- LUNG QI, CONSTRAINED

- LARYNGITIS
- THROAT, PAIN, SWOLLEN
- TONSILLITIS
- TOOTHACHE: Wind Heat, Fire
SKIN
- RASHES, ENCOURAGES
  EXPRESSION OF: Topical
- SORES: San Jiao Fire

Clinical/Pharmaceutical Studies:

BLOOD RELATED DISORDERS/
TOPICS
- BLOOD PRESSURE, LOWERS:
  Decoction, Significant
BOWEL RELATED DISORDERS
- LAXATIVE: Mild, Absorbs Water,
  Thus Increasing Peristalsis

INFECTIOUS DISEASES
- VIRAL, ANTI-: Flu-Strong, Pr3
KIDNEYS
- DIURETIC
ORAL CAVITY
- TONSILLITIS, ACUTE: 4-8 Seeds
  To Make Tea, 30 Minutes Steep,

Every 4 Hrs
PAIN/NUMBNESS/GENERAL
DISCOMFORT
- ANALGESIC
TRAUMA, BITES, POISONINGS
- INFLAMMATORY, ANTI-

Dose

3 - 12 gm

Notes

Take 3-5 Seeds Or Indicated Weight

QIAN HU   前 胡   *RADIX*
PEUCEDANI

Traditional Functions:

1. Redirects Lung Qi downward, disperses Phlegm and stops cough
2. Dispeles Wind Heat or Cold and cough

Traditional Properties:

Enters: LU, SP,

Properties: BIT, SP, CL

Indications:

CHEST
- CHEST, FULLNESS: With Mass
  Sensation, Vomiting
LUNGS
- COUGH: Cold Phlegm/Phlegm
  Heat/Wind Cold
- COUGH, COPIOUS SPUTUM:

Wind Heat/Cold
- COUGH/WHEEZING: Early Lung
  Heat w/Thick Sputum
- LUNGS, DYSPNEA: Cold Phlegm
- LUNGS, UPPER RESPIRATORY
  TRACT INFECTION
PHLEGM

- PHLEGM, HEAT
- SPUTUM, COPIOUS: Wind Heat/
  Cold
STOMACH/DIGESTIVE
DISORDERS
- HICCUPS

Clinical/Pharmaceutical Studies:

CANCER/TUMORS/SWELLINGS/
LUMPS
- SWELLINGS, VIRULENT,
  VARIOUS: Crushed Fresh Root,
  Topical
HEART
- CORONARY ARTERIES,
  DILATES
INFECTIOUS DISEASES

- BACTERIAL, ANTI-
- COMMON COLD W/COUGH:
  With Other Herbs
- VIRAL, ANTI-: 1:1 Herb Decoction
  Inhibited Asian Flu
LUNGS
- ANTITUSSIVE: Weaker Than Jie
  Geng, Some Say None Noted
- BRONCHITIS: With Other Herbs

- COUGH: With Other Herbs
- LUNGS, INCREASES SPUTUM IN
SKIN
- FUNGAL, ANTI-
STOMACH/DIGESTIVE
DISORDERS
- HICCUPS: With Other Herbs
TRAUMA, BITES, POISONINGS
- ANTIHISTAMINE

Dose

3 - 9 gm

Contraindications

Not: Def Cold Sputum
Not: With Zao Jia

TIAN HUA FEN
(GUA LOU GEN)

天花粉

**RADIX
TRICHOSANTHIS**

Traditional Functions:

1. Subdues Heat, generates fluids and quenches thirst
2. Clears Heat and toxins and dissipates pus

Traditional Properties:

Enters: LU, ST,

Properties: BIT, <SW, SO, CL

Indications:

BOWEL RELATED DISORDERS
• FISTULA
• HEMORRHOIDS
**CANCER/TUMORS/SWELLINGS/
  LUMPS**
• SWELLINGS
**ENDOCRINE RELATED
  DISORDERS**
• DIABETES: Internal Heat With
  Exhaustion Thirst
FLUID DISORDERS
• THIRST: Febrile Diseases/Fluid
  Injury/Deficient Yin
• THIRST, CONSUMPTIVE

HEAT
• HEAT: In Yang Ming, Qi Level
HEMORRHAGIC DISORDERS
• HEMOPTYSIS
LIVER
• JAUNDICE
LUNGS
• COUGH: Lung Dryness/Lung Heat
• COUGH, THICK/BLOODY
  SPUTUM
• LUNGS, DYSPNEA: Lung Heat
**MENTAL STATE/
  NEUROLOGICAL DISORDERS**
• IRRITABILITY: Fluid Injury

ORAL CAVITY
• THROAT, SORE
**SEXUALITY, FEMALE:
  GYNECOLOGICAL**
• ABORTION, INDUCES: Injection
• BREASTS, ABSCESS OF
SKIN
• ABSCESS, HELPS TO DRAIN
• BOILS, TOXIC: Heat, Toxins,
  Swellings
• SKIN, INFLAMMATIONS
• SORES, W/O SUPPURATION
TRAUMA, BITES, POISONINGS
• TRAUMA, INJURIES: Die Da

Clinical/Pharmaceutical Studies:

**BLOOD RELATED
DISORDERS/TOPICS**
• BLOOD GLUCOSE,
  INCREASES: Aqueous
  Extracts, Especially When
  Fasting
**CANCER/TUMORS/
SWELLINGS/LUMPS**
• CANCER, ANTI-:
  Inhibits
• CHORIOCARCINOMA:
  (Rare Uterine Cancer)
**ENDOCRINE RELATED
DISORDERS**

• DIABETES MELLITUS:
  Symptom Relief, Reduced
  Urinary Sugar (9gm, 3x/
  Day Oral 3-7 Days, This
  Dose May Cause Mild
  Nausea, Diarrhea) ,
  Marked Short Term
  Reduction
**IMMUNE SYSTEM
RELATED DISORDERS/
TOPICS**
• ANTIGENIC, STRONG
INFECTIOUS DISEASES

• MUMPS: External With
  Thalictrum Ichangense
LUNGS
• BRONCHITIS, ACUTE:
  Symptomatic Relief
• COUGH: Heat Caused
  With Mai Dong, Jie Geng,
  Bei Sha Shen
• PNEUMONIA:
  Symptomatic Relief
**SEXUALITY, FEMALE:
GYNECOLOGICAL**
• ABORTION, INDUCES:

  Injected Intramuscular,
  Takes 3-7 Days
• ECTOPIC PREGNANCY
• HYDATID MOLE,
  MALIGNANT: Injected
  At Site
• MASTITIS: With Jin Yin
  Hua, Chuan Shan Jia, Zao
  Ci (Xian Fan Huo Ming
  Yin)
SKIN
• ECZEMA: External With
  Water

Dose

9 - 15 gm

Contraindications

Not: Diarrhea From Cold Def SP/ST

Not: Pregnacy

Not: Gan Jiang, Niu Xi, Wu Tou

Notes

Protein In Herb Is Strongly Antigenic, Watch Allergic

Reactions, Skin Test Before Injection

TIAN ZHU HUANG

天竹黃
(天竹黃)

**CONCRETIO
SILICEA BAMBUSAE**

Traditional Functions:

1. Clears and disperses Hot Phlegm
2. Cools the Heart, calms fright and stops childhood convulsions

Traditional Properties:

Enters: HT, LV, GB,

Properties: SW, C

Indications:

CHILDHOOD DISORDERS
• CONVULSIONS, CHILDHOOD
CIRCULATION DISORDERS
• STROKE W/HIGH BP
• SYNCOPE
FEVERS
• FEVER, IRRITABILITY
HEMORRHAGIC DISORDERS
• EPISTAXIS
• HEMOPTYSIS
LUNGS

• COUGH, DIFFICULT
  EXPECTORATION: Lung Hot
  Phlegm
MENTAL STATE/
  NEUROLOGICAL DISORDERS
• CONSCIOUSNESS, LOSS OF
• CONVULSIONS, FEVER, ACUTE
• DELIRIUM
MUSCULOSKELETAL/
  CONNECTIVE TISSUE

• SPASMS, W/FEVER, ACUTE
PHLEGM
• PHLEGM HEAT SPASMS/
  CONVULSIONS
SEXUALITY, FEMALE:
  GYNECOLOGICAL
• UTERINE BLEEDING
STOMACH/DIGESTIVE
  DISORDERS
• VOMITING

Clinical/Pharmaceutical Studies:

INFECTIOUS DISEASES

• BACTERIAL, ANTI-: Staph,

Bacillus, E.Coli, B.Typhi

Dose
3 - 9 gm

Common Name
Tabasheer/Bamboo Secretns

Notes
0.5-1 g In Powder

ZE QI

澤溓
(澤溓)

**HERBA
EUPHORBIAE
HELIOSCOPIAE**

Traditional Functions:

1. Disperses Phlegm and dissipates nodules and accumulations
2. Promotes urination and disperses swelling

Traditional Properties:

Enters: LU, LI, SP, SI,

Properties: SP, BIT, CL,

Indications:

BOWEL RELATED DISORDERS
• DYSENTERY
• HEMORRHOIDS
CANCER/TUMORS/SWELLINGS/
  LUMPS
• LYMPHOSARCOMA
FLUID DISORDERS
• EDEMA, EXTREMITIES
• EDEMA, FACE, EYES
• EDEMA, SEVERE: Excess
  Constitution

• EDEMA, UPPER ABDOMEN
INFECTIOUS DISEASES
• MALARIA
• SCROFULA
LUNGS
• ASTHMA, COUGH W/PHLEGM
  RETENTION
• COUGH
• EMPHYSEMA, PULMONARY
  DUE TO HEART
• WHEEZING: Lung Heat w/

Congested Fluids
MUSCULOSKELETAL/
  CONNECTIVE TISSUE
• OSTEOMYELITIS
NUTRITIONAL/METABOLIC
  DISORDERS/TOPICS
• BERIBERI
ORAL CAVITY
• TOOTHACHE
SKIN
• SCABIES

Clinical/Pharmaceutical Studies:

ABDOMEN/
  GASTROINTESTINAL TOPICS
• INTESTINES, STIMULATES
BOWEL RELATED DISORDERS
• DYSENTERY: Bacillary-Good

Orally
CANCER/TUMORS/SWELLINGS/
  LUMPS
• ESOPHAGEAL CANCER: Softens
  Tumor, Injections Of 20% Extract Of

Neutral Saponins
CIRCULATION DISORDERS
• VASODILATES
FEVERS
• ANTIPYRETIC: Very Mild

Dose
3 - 9 gm

Precautions
Watch: Debilitated Patients

Notes
Low Toxicity
Large Doses: Gasrtroenteritis, Palpitations, Dizziness,
Spasms

ZHE BEI MU
(BEI MU)

浙貝母
(浙贝母)

BULBUS
FRITILLARIAE THUNBERGII

Traditional Functions:

1. Clears and disperses Hot Phlegm
2. Clears Heat and dissipates accumulations and nodules

Traditional Properties:

Enters: LU, ST, SJ, LV,

Properties: BIT, C

Indications:

**CANCER/TUMORS/SWELLINGS/
LUMPS**
• SWELLINGS, TOXIC
**ENDOCRINE RELATED
DISORDERS**
• GOITER
HEAD/NECK
• NECK, SWELLINGS: Phlegm Fire
INFECTIOUS DISEASES
• SCROFULA
LUNGS
• BRONCHITIS, ACUTE

• COUGH: Externally Caused
• COUGH, PRODUCTIVE: Phlegm
  Heat/Lung Heat
• LUNG HEAT W/SPUTUM IN
  COUGH
• LUNGS, ABSCESS
• PNEUMONIA
ORAL CAVITY
• LARYNGEAL ULCER
• THROAT, BI
PHLEGM
• PHLEGM, HOT: Obstruct

Pericardium
**SEXUALITY, FEMALE:
GYNECOLOGICAL**
• BREASTS, ABSCESS OF
• BREASTS, SWOLLEN
SKIN
• CARBUNCLES
• SKIN, SORES, SWOLLEN, TOXIC:
  Blood Stasis, Swelling
• ULCERS
TRAUMA, BITES, POISONINGS
• WOUNDS, TOXIC

Clinical/Pharmaceutical Studies:

**ABDOMEN/
GASTROINTESTINAL TOPICS**
• INTESTINES, STIMULATES
  PERISTALSIS
**BLOOD RELATED DISORDERS/
TOPICS**
• BLOOD GLUCOSE, INCREASES:
  Alcohol Extract
• BLOOD PRESSURE, LOWERS
EYES
• MYDRIATIC
**IMMUNE SYSTEM RELATED
DISORDERS/TOPICS**
• LYMPHADENITIS COLLI,
  CHRONIC: Herb Or Chuan Bei Mu,
  Xuan Shen, Mu Li, Xia Ku Cao,

Sheng Di
INFECTIOUS DISEASES
• COMMON COLD: With Cough
  With Dry Mouth, Itchy Throat, Thick
  Yellow Sputum, Herb With Lian
  Qiao, Niu Bang Zi
• SCROFULA: Herb Or Chuan Bei
  Mu, Xuan Shen, Mu Li, Xia Ku Cao,
  Sheng Di, *As Adjuvant With Lian
  Qiao, Ju Hua, Pu Gong Ying, 9-15
  Gr, Max 18-30 g In Scrofula
LUNGS
• ANTITUSSIVE: ETOH Extract,
  Lasts 2 Hrs
• BRONCHITIS, CHRONIC: The
  Flower Extract Tablet, 68% Effective,

0.35 g=1 g Herb, 3 Tabs 3x/Day
• BRONCHODILATORY, LOW
  DOSES
**SEXUALITY, FEMALE:
GYNECOLOGICAL**
• MASTITIS: As Adjuvant With Lian
  Qiao, Ju Hua, Pu Gong Ying, 9-15
  Gr, Max 18-30 g In Scrofula
• UTERUS, STIMULATES: Causes
  Contractions
**STOMACH/DIGESTIVE
DISORDERS**
• ULCERS, GASTRIC/DUODENAL:
  Use Herb/Chuan Bei Mu To Prevent
  Constipation From Hai Piao Xiao
  (Calcium Content May Cause)

Dose

3 - 9 gm

Contraindications

Not: w/Wu Tou (Traditional) , Although Clinical
Research Has Found No Untoward Effects
Not: Def SP/ST Cold, Damp

ZHU LI

竹瀝
(竹沥)

SUCCUS
BAMBUSAE

Traditional Functions:

1. Clears Heat, dissipates Phlegm and alleviates cough and Stomach reflux
2. Clears Phlegm and Heat in the Heart to open the channel

Traditional Properties:

Enters: HT, LU, ST

Properties: SW, >C

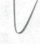

Indications:

CHEST
• CHEST, STUFFINESS
CIRCULATION DISORDERS
• FAINTING: Phlegm Blocking Orifices
• STROKE W/COMA: Phlegm Blocking Orifices
EXTREMITIES
• EXTREMITIES, PARALYSIS OF: Phlegm Blocking Orifices
LUNGS
• COUGH: Lung Heat With Excess Sputum, 9-15 gm/Powerful

Adjunctive For Hot Phlegm, 9-15 gm
• LUNG INFECTION W/HOT SPUTUM
• LUNGS, DYSPNEA: Lung Heat
MENTAL STATE/ NEUROLOGICAL DISORDERS
• CONVULSIONS
• EPILEPSY: Phlegm Blocking Orifices
• HEMIPLEGIA: Phlegm Blocking Orifices
• PARALYSIS, EXTREMITIES:

Phlegm Blocking Orifices
• UNCONSCIOUSNESS: (Mental Cloudiness) Use w/Heat Shut-In Herbs/Phlegm Blocking Orifices
PHLEGM
• PHLEGM BLOCKING HEART ORIFICE
• PHLEGM CONGESTION
STOMACH/DIGESTIVE DISORDERS
• VOMITING: Stomach Heat/Hot Phlegm

Dose

30 - 90 gm

Common Name

Dried Bamboo Sap

Contraindications

Not: Common Cold Cough
Not: Diarrhea From Def SP

Notes

9-15 For Cough
Use Singly Or w/Ginger Juice

ZHU RU   竹茹   CAULIS BAMBUSAE IN TAENIIS

Traditional Functions:

1. Clears and disperses Hot Phlegm in the Lungs
2. Clears Heat and stops vomiting
3. Cools the Blood and arrests bleeding

Traditional Properties:

Enters: LU, ST, GB,

Properties: SW, CL

Indications:

CHEST
• CHEST, CONSTRICTION: Lung Heat
CHILDHOOD DISORDERS
• CONVULSIONS, CHILDHOOD
FEVERS
• FEVER, IRRITABILITY
HEAT
• HEAT, RESTLESS W/VOMITING
HEMORRHAGIC DISORDERS
• HEMATEMESIS: Blood Heat
• HEMOPTYSIS: Lung Heat
LUNGS
• COUGH: Lung Heat
• COUGH, DIFFICULT

EXPECTORATION: Lung Heat Sputm
• LUNG INFECTION: Phlegm Heat
• LUNGS, DYSPNEA: Lung Heat
MENTAL STATE/ NEUROLOGICAL DISORDERS
• EPILEPSY
NOSE
• NOSEBLEED
ORAL CAVITY
• HALITOSIS: Stomach Heat
SEXUALITY, FEMALE: GYNECOLOGICAL
• FETUS, RESTLESS: Damp Heat/ Gestational Heat

• MENORRHAGIA
• MENSTRUATION, DISORDERS OF: Calm Chong, Lower Reflux
• MORNING SICKNESS: Gestational Foul Obstruction--Heat
• UTERINE BLEEDING
STOMACH/DIGESTIVE DISORDERS
• GASTRITIS, CHRONIC
• HICCUPS: Qi Deficiency--Heat
• STOMACH HEAT
• VOMITING: Qi Deficiency--Heat
• VOMITING, BITTER, SOUR: Stomach Heat

Clinical/Pharmaceutical Studies:

INFECTIOUS DISEASES
• ANTIBIOTIC: Powdered Has

Strong Bacteriostatic Action--Staph.

A., E.Coli, Salmonella, B.Typhi

Dose

3 - 9 gm

Common Name

Bamboo Shavings

Contraindications

Not: Cold ST/Cold Food Stagnation (See Ban Xia Instead)

Nourish The Heart And Calms The Spirit

BAI ZI REN   柏子仁   *SEMEN BIOTAE ORIENTALIS*

Traditional Functions:

1. Benefits the Heart Qi and calms the Spirit
2. Moistens the intestines and promotes the passage of stool
3. Eliminates deficient Yin night sweats

Traditional Properties:

Enters: LI, HT, KI, LV,

Properties: SW, SP, N

Indications:

BOWEL RELATED DISORDERS
• CONSTIPATION: Intestinal Dryness
• CONSTIPATION, ELDERLY: Deficient Blood/Yin
• CONSTIPATION, POSTPARTUM: Deficient Blood/Yin

HEART
• HEART BLOOD DEFICIENCY
• PALPITATIONS W/ ANXIETY, RAPID BEATS: Heart Blood Deficient

MENTAL STATE/ NEUROLOGICAL DISORDERS

• FORGETFULNESS: Heart Blood Deficient
• INSOMNIA: Heart Blood Deficient
• INSOMNIA, DREAMS, FREQUENT
• IRRITABILITY: Heart Blood Deficient

SEXUALITY, MALE: UROLOGICAL TOPICS

• SEMINAL EMISSIONS
SKIN
• NIGHT SWEATS: Yin Deficients
• PERSPIRATION, FURTIVE
• PERSPIRATION, RESTING & THIEF
• SWEATING, EXCESSIVE: Deficiency

Clinical/Pharmaceutical Studies:

BOWEL RELATED DISORDERS
• APERIENT

MENTAL STATE/ NEUROLOGICAL DISORDERS

• SEDATIVE

Dose

3 - 9 gm

Common Name

Arbor-Vitae Seeds

Contraindications

Not: Loose BM

Not: Phlegm Disorders

Notes

Smells Bad

HE HUAN HUA   合歡花 (合欢花)   *FLOS ALBIZZIAE*

Traditional Functions:

1. Circulates the Qi and resolves constrained Liver Qi
2. Vitalizes Blood
3. Calms the Spirit

Traditional Properties:

Enters: HT, LV,

Properties: SW, N

Indications:

CHEST
• CHEST, FULLNESS
HEART

• LIVER ATTACKING STOMACH: Pain, Emotions
• LIVER QI STAGNATION LUMPS

• INSOMNIA, DREAMS, FREQUENT
• IRRITABILITY: Constrained

Indications:

- PALPITATIONS: From Anxiety, Anger
  LIVER

MENTAL STATE/
NEUROLOGICAL DISORDERS
- INSOMNIA: From Anxiety, Anger

Emotions (Especially With Epigastric Pain, Chest Pressure)
- MEMORY, POOR

Dose

3 - 9 gm

Common Name

Albizzin Flower

Contraindications

Not: w/o LV Qi Stagnation

HE HUAN PI

合歡皮
（合欢皮）

CORTEX ALBIZZIAE JULIBRISSIN

Traditional Functions:

1. Relieves depression and calms the Spirit
2. Vitalizes Blood and controls pain
3. Unites tendons and bones and reduces swelling
4. Resolves and dissipates abscesses

Traditional Properties:

Enters: LV, HT,

Properties: SW, N

Indications:

CHEST
- CHEST, CONSTRICTION
HEART
- HEART SPIRIT, DISTURBED
- PALPITATIONS: From Anxiety, Anger
LUNGS
- LUNGS, ABSCESS: With Vomiting Of Pus
MENTAL STATE/
NEUROLOGICAL DISORDERS

- EMOTIONS, CONSTRAINED
- INSOMNIA: From Anxiety, Anger
- INSOMNIA, DREAMS, FREQUENT
- IRRITABILITY
- WORRIES, CONGESTED
MUSCULOSKELETAL/
CONNECTIVE TISSUE
- MUSCLES, ACHES: Extremities
SKIN

- ABSCESS, SUPERFICIAL
- BOILS
- ULCERS
STOMACH/DIGESTIVE DISORDERS
- ANOREXIA
- VOMITING, PUS IN
TRAUMA, BITES, POISONINGS
- FRACTURES
- TRAUMA, PAIN/SWELLING

Clinical/Pharmaceutical Studies:

ENERGETIC STATE
- TONIFIES
KIDNEYS
- DIURETIC
MENTAL STATE/
NEUROLOGICAL DISORDERS

- SEDATIVE
PAIN/NUMBNESS/GENERAL DISCOMFORT
- ANALGESIC
PARASITES

- WORMS
SEXUALITY, FEMALE:
GYNECOLOGICAL
- UTERUS, STIMULATES: Oxytocin-Like

Dose

9 - 30 gm

Common Name

Mimosa Tree Bark

LING ZHI CAO
(LING ZHI)

靈芝草
（灵芝草）

GANODERMA

Traditional Functions:

1. Calms and sedates the Spirit
2. Disperses Phlegm and alleviates cough
3. Tonifies and nourishes the Qi and Blood
4. Removes toxins

Traditional Properties:

Enters: LU, SP, HT, KI, LV,

Properties: SW, <W

Indications:

**CANCER/TUMORS/SWELLINGS/
LUMPS**
• CANCER, EARLY STAGE
CIRCULATION DISORDERS
• HYPERTENSION
EARS/HEARING DISORDERS
• DIZZINESS
ENERGETIC STATE
• FATIGUE: Deficiency
HEART
• CORONARY HEART DISEASE

• PALPITATIONS
**IMMUNE SYSTEM RELATED
DISORDERS/TOPICS**
• ALLERGIES
• HIV+
LUNGS
• ASTHMA, ACUTE
• COUGH, BRONCHIAL: Elderly
• COUGH, CHRONIC W/
SHORTNESS OF BREATH/
COPIOUS SPUTUM

**MENTAL STATE/
NEUROLOGICAL DISORDERS**
• FORGETFULNESS: From
Hypertension, Neurasthenia
• INSOMNIA
• INSOMNIA, DREAMS,
FREQUENT
• NEURASTHENIA
**STOMACH/DIGESTIVE
DISORDERS**
• INDIGESTION

Clinical/Pharmaceutical Studies:

**BLOOD RELATED
DISORDERS/TOPICS**
• CHOLESTEROL,
LOWERS
• HYPERLIPIDEMIA:
Satisfactory Results
• LEUKOPENIA
**CIRCULATION
DISORDERS**
• HYPOTENSION
ENERGETIC STATE
• TONIFIES: Enhanced
Protein Synthesis In Liver
EYES
• RETINAL PIGMENTARY
DEGENERATION OF
HEAD/NECK
• BRAIN,
MALDEVELOPMENT
OF
HEART
• ARRHYTHMIAS
• CARDIOTONIC
• CORONARY ARTERIES,
INCREASED FLOW
• HEART DISEASE:
Satisfactory Results
• HEART DISEASE,
KESHAN DISEASE
(ENLARGED HEART) :
Ling Zhi Syrup, 45 g

Crude Herb, 1.5-3 Months
• HEART MUSCLE,
REDUCED OXYGEN
NEEDS
• PULMONARY HEART
DISEASE: Syrup Of Herb
Improved Adrenocortical
Function
**IMMUNE SYSTEM
RELATED DISORDERS/
TOPICS**
• ALLERGIC DISORDERS:
Markedly Inhibits
Reaction
• IMMUNE SYSTEM
ENHANCEMENT:
Enhanced Phagocytic
Function, Herb With Dang
Shen Particularly Effective
INFECTIOUS DISEASES
• ANTIBIOTIC: Bacillus
Pneum, Staph & Strep
LIVER
• HEPATITIS: Best In
Cases With High SGPT
But Liver Still Functioning,
15-106 Days, Ling Zhi
Syrup (Alcohol Extract, 10%
) 20 ml, 2x/Day For 1-3
Months
• HEPATITIS, REDUCES

SYMPTOMS OF
• LIVER, PROTECTANT
LUNGS
• ANTIASTHMATIC:
Tincture, Concentraed
Culture Extract
• ANTITUSSIVE
• ASTHMA, BRONCHIAL:
Inhibits Allergic Reactions
• BRONCHITIS,
CHRONIC: Spleen
Deficiency Type, Treated
With Preparations For 4
Months, Reduced
Excitability Of
Parasympathetic Nerves, *
Concentrated Solution, 2
ml, 4 Weeks Of Herb Plus
Bai Mu Er Spores Helped
Regenerate Bronchial
Epithelium, *After Months
Of Treatment A General
Increase Of Iga, *Best For
Bronchitis Of "Old Age",
Asthmatic Type,
Deficiency-Cold Type, 1-2
Weeks To Marked Effects,
Ling Zhi Syrup Tablet
• EXPECTORANT: Thru
Irritation Of Lung Mucosa
• PULMONARY HEART

DISEASE: Syrup Of Herb
Improved Adrenocortical
Function
**MENTAL STATE/
NEUROLOGICAL
DISORDERS**
• CNS, INHIBITOR/
SEDATIVE: Tincture/
Reflux Percolate, Water
Soluble Portion
• INSOMNIA
• NEURASTHENIA
**MUSCULOSKELETAL/
CONNECTIVE TISSUE**
• MUSCULAR
DYSTROPHY,
PROGRESSIVE/
ATROPHIC
**PAIN/NUMBNESS/
GENERAL
DISCOMFORT**
• ANALGESIC
**TRAUMA, BITES,
POISONINGS**
• ALTITUDE SICKNESS,
ACUTE: Use
Prophylactically
• RADIATION, INJURY:
Protective Action If Taken
Before Exposure

Dose

1.5 - 15.0 gm

Common Name

Lucid Ganoderma

SUAN ZAO REN   酸棗仁
                        （酸枣仁）
                                            **SEMEN
                                    ZIZIPHI SPINOSAE**

Traditional Functions:

1. Nourishes the Blood and Liver and calms the Heart and Spirit
2. Astringes sweat and reinforces the Yin

Traditional Properties:

Enters: SP, HT, LV, GB,

Properties: SW, SO, N

Indications:

BOWEL RELATED DISORDERS
• CONSTIPATION, MILD
FLUID DISORDERS
• THIRST, RESTLESS
HEART
• HEART YIN/BLOOD
DEFICIENCY
• PALPITATIONS W/ANXIETY:

Blood/Yin Deficient
MENTAL STATE/
NEUROLOGICAL DISORDERS
• INSOMNIA: Blood/Yin Deficient
• INSOMNIA, DREAMS,
FREQUENT
• IRRITABILITY: Blood/Yin

Deficient
SKIN
• NIGHT SWEATS
• PERSPIRATION, RESTING &
THIEF
• SWEATING, SPONTANEOUS:
Deficiency

Clinical/Pharmaceutical Studies:

BLOOD RELATED
DISORDERS/TOPICS
• BLOOD PRESSURE,
LOWERS: Persistent
HEART
• HEART, INHIBITS:
Inhibits
MENTAL STATE/
NEUROLOGICAL
DISORDERS
• CONVULSIVE, ANTI-
• HYPNOTIC: Tolerance
Develops, 1 Week Off Will
Allow Effectiveness To

Return
• INSOMNIA: With
Palpitation From Lack Of
Nourishment Of Heart
With Rising Heart Fire,
Suan Zao Ren Tang (With
Fu Shen, Bai Zi Ren, Dan
Shen, Shu Di)
• NEURASTHENIA
• SEDATIVE: Tolerance
Develops In 6 Days, 1
Week Off Will Allow
Effectiveness To Return,
Synergistic w/Barbituates,

Oily Component, Water
Extracts (Active
Components Are
Glycosides) , Raw Seed
Stronger
NUTRITIONAL/
METABOLIC
DISORDERS/TOPICS
• BODY TEMPERATURE,
LOWERS: Oral/Injected
PAIN/NUMBNESS/
GENERAL
DISCOMFORT
• ANALGESIC: Injected

Decoction
SEXUALITY, FEMALE:
GYNECOLOGICAL
• MENOPAUSE
SYNDROME: Bai He
Suan Zao Tang With
Acupuncture
• UTERUS, CONTRACTS
SKIN
• BURNS, EXTENSIVE:
Reduces Deaths/Local
Edema--Use With Wu Wei
Zi

Dose

9 - 18 gm

Common Name

Sour Jujube Seed

Precautions

Watch: Severe Diarrhea

Watch: Excess Heat

Watch: Pregnancy

Notes

Very Low Toxicity When Given Orally

YE JIAO TENG
(SHOU WU TENG)

夜交滕/首
烏藤

CAULIS
POLYGONI MULTIFLORI

Traditional Functions:

1. Nourishes the Heart and calms the Spirit
2. Nourishes the Blood and helps move the Qi through the channels
3. Dissipates Wind and alleviates itching

Traditional Properties:

Enters: HT, LV,

Properties: SW, <BIT, N

Indications:

BLOOD RELATED DISORDERS/
TOPICS
• BLOOD DEFICIENCY W/BODY
ACHE
• BLOOD DEFICIENCY W/
WITHERING YELLOW
COMPLEXION
ENERGETIC STATE
• WEAKNESS, GENERAL:
Deficient Blood
EXTREMITIES
• ARMS, ACHING
• LEGS, ACHING
HEART

• PALPITATIONS: Blood Deficiency
MENTAL STATE/
NEUROLOGICAL DISORDERS
• INSOMNIA, DREAM
DISTURBED: Yin/Blood Deficient
• IRRITABILITY: Yin/Blood
Deficient
• NEURASTHENIA
PAIN/NUMBNESS/GENERAL
DISCOMFORT
• NUMBNESS: Blood Deficient
• NUMBNESS W/SPASMS,
CONTRACTURES: Blood

Deficiency Bi
• PAIN, BODY: Deficient Blood
SKIN
• PERSPIRATION, PROFUSE
• PRURITUS: Topical Wash
• SCABIES: Topical
• SKIN, RASHES: Topical Wash
• SKIN, TINEA: Topical
• SKIN, ULCERS: Wind, Topical
YIN RELATED DISORDERS/
TOPICS
• YIN DEFICIENCY W/EXTERNAL
PATHOGEN

Dose

9 - 30 gm

Common Name

Vine Of Solomon's Seal

Precautions

Watch: Loose Stool

YUAN ZHI   遠志   *RADIX POLYGALAE TENUIFOLIAE*
（远志）

Traditional Functions:

1. Benefits the wisdom and will, calms the Spirit and soothes the mind
2. Resolves Phlegm and clears the orifices of the Heart
3. Dissipates congestion in the Lungs

Traditional Properties:

Enters: LU, HT, KI,

Properties: BIT, SP, W

Indications:

**CANCER/TUMORS/
SWELLINGS/LUMPS**
• SWELLINGS, PAIN:
Damp Phlegm
HEART
• PALPITATIONS W/
ANXIETY
LUNGS
• BRONCHIECTASIS
• BRONCHITIS, ACUTE/
CHRONIC
• COUGH: Cold Phlegm
• COUGH, COPIOUS
SPUTUM: Cold Phlegm
• LUNGS, DYSPNEA:

Cold Phlegm
**MENTAL STATE/
NEUROLOGICAL
DISORDERS**
• BROODING, EXCESS
• DREAMING,
EXCESSIVE
• EMOTIONAL
DISORIENTATION:
Heart Qi Disruption/
Phlegm Enveloping Heart
Orifices
• EMOTIONS, PENT-UP
• FORGETFULNESS

• INSOMNIA
• INSOMNIA, DREAMS,
FREQUENT
• MEMORY, POOR
• MENTAL
DISORIENTATION:
Heart Qi Disruption/
Phlegm Enveloping Heart
Orifices
• NEURASTHENIA
• RESTLESSNESS
• SEIZURES
**SEXUALITY, FEMALE:
GYNECOLOGICAL**

• MENSTRUATION,
DISORDERS OF:
Constrict Uterus, Stimulate
Chong
**SEXUALITY, MALE:
UROLOGICAL TOPICS**
• NOCTURNAL
EMISSIONS
SKIN
• BOILS: External
• SKIN, SORES,
SWOLLEN, TOXIC:
Blood Stasis, Swelling
• SKIN, ULCERS

Clinical/Pharmaceutical Studies:

**BLOOD RELATED
DISORDERS/TOPICS**
• BLOOD PRESSURE,
LOWERS
• HEMOLYTIC: Stronger
Than Jie Geng, Saponin
Content Of Root Bark
INFECTIOUS DISEASES
• BACTERIAL, ANTI-:
ETOH Extract–Staph,
Shigella, B.Tuberculosis,
Diplococcus Pneumoniae
• COMMON COLD W/
COPIUS SPUTUM:
Tincture, 2-5 ml 3x/Day, *
Extract 0.5-2.0 ml, 3x/Day
LUNGS

• BRONCHITIS,
CHRONIC: Pill Of Root,
Gan Cao, Yang Jin Hua,
Honey All Equal Amounts
In 0.3 g Pills, 2x/Day For
10 Days
• EXPECTORANT: Thru
Irritation Of Lung Mucosa,
Need High Concentration
**MENTAL STATE/
NEUROLOGICAL
DISORDERS**
• AMNESIA: Decoction/
Syrup, Yuan Zhi, 9g Plus
Wu Wei Zi, 6 g, *3 g
Powder, 2x/Day
• CONVULSIVE, ANTI-

• DREAMS, FREQUENT:
Decoction/Syrup, Yuan Zhi,
9g Plus Wu Wei Zi, 6 g, *
3 g Powder, 2x/Day
• FEAR: Decoction/Syrup,
Yuan Zhi, 9g Plus Wu Wei
Zi, 6 g, *3 g Powder, 2x/
Day
• HYPNOTIC
• INSOMNIA: Decoction/
Syrup, Yuan Zhi, 9g Plus
Wu Wei Zi, 6 g, *3 g
Powder, 2x/Day
• NEURASTHENIA:
Decoction/Syrup, Yuan Zhi,
9g Plus Wu Wei Zi, 6 g, *
3 g Powder, 2x/Day

• SEDATIVE
**MUSCULOSKELETAL/
CONNECTIVE TISSUE**
• MUSCLE TONE,
INCREASES: Aqueous
Extract
**SEXUALITY, FEMALE:
GYNECOLOGICAL**
• MASTITIS, ACUTE
• UTERUS, STIMULATES:
Decoctions Causes
Significant Contractions
**STOMACH/DIGESTIVE
DISORDERS**
• NAUSEA, INDUCES
MILD

Dose

3 - 9 gm

Common Name

Chinese Senega Root

Contraindications

Not: w/Peptic Ulcer, Gastritis

Not: Def Yin w/Heat

Notes

May Cause Mild Nausea, Add Ban Xia

Strongly Pacify And Stabilize The Spirit

CI SHI   磁石   *MAGNETITUM*

Traditional Functions:

1. Sedates the Heart and pacifies the spirit
2. Pacifies the Liver and subdues the rising Yang
3. Calms asthma and restores Qi by aiding the Kidneys in grasping the Qi

Traditional Properties:

Enters: KI, LV, HT

Properties: SP, C

Indications:

BLOOD RELATED DISORDERS/ TOPICS
• ANEMIA, PERNICIOUS
CHILDHOOD DISORDERS
• FRIGHT CONVULSIONS, CHILDHOOD: Best Liver Yin With Yang Rising
EARS/HEARING DISORDERS
• DIZZINESS: Liver Kidney Yin Deficient With Yang Rising
• HEARING, POOR
• TINNITUS: Liver Kidney Yin Deficient With Yang Rising
• VERTIGO: Liver Kidney Yin Deficient With Yang Rising/Liver Yang/Fire Rising
EYES

• EYES, BLURRED: Liver Kidney Yin Deficient With Yang Rising
HEART
• PALPITATIONS: Best Liver Yin With Yang Rising
LIVER
• LIVER KIDNEY YIN DEFICIENCY W/YANG RISING
• LIVER YIN DEFICIENCY W/ YANG RISING
LUNGS
• ASTHMA, CHRONIC: Kidneys Unable To Grasp Qi
• COUGH, CHRONIC W/DYSPNEA: To Store Qi, Stop Cough
• DYSPNEA: Deficiency

MENTAL STATE/ NEUROLOGICAL DISORDERS
• EPILEPSY
• INSOMNIA: Best Liver Yin With Yang Rising
• INSOMNIA, DREAMS, FREQUENT
• MANIA
• RESTLESSNESS: Best Liver Yin With Yang Rising
• TREMORS: Best Liver Yin With Yang Rising
MUSCULOSKELETAL/ CONNECTIVE TISSUE
• SPASMS, CONVULSIONS: Internal Deficiency Wind

Clinical/Pharmaceutical Studies:

BLOOD RELATED DISORDERS/ TOPICS
• BLOOD FORMATION,

STIMULATES
HEMORRHAGIC DISORDERS
• HEMOSTATIC

MENTAL STATE/ NEUROLOGICAL DISORDERS
• SEDATIVE, CNS

Dose
9 - 30 gm

Common Name
Magnetite

Contraindications
Not: Without Yin Def Symptoms Of HT, KI, LV

Notes
Fire, Dip In Vinegar, Pulverize
Cook 20-30 Minutes Before Other Herbs

DAI ZHE SHI   代赭石   *HAEMATITUM*
(ZHE SHI)

Traditional Functions:

1. Strongly descends Qi and controls vomiting
2. Pacifies the Liver and subdues the rising Yang
3. Cools Blood, controls bleeding and guides Blood downwards

Traditional Properties:

Enters: ST, PC, LV,

Properties: BIT, C

Indications:

EARS/HEARING DISORDERS
- DIZZINESS: Liver Yang Rising
- TINNITUS: Liver Yang Rising
- VERTIGO: Liver Yang/Fire Rising

EYES
- EYES, PRESSURE SENSATION:
Liver Yang Rising

HEAD/NECK
- HEADACHE, HYPERTENSIVE

HEMORRHAGIC DISORDERS
- EPISTAXIS
- HEMAFECIA

- HEMATEMESIS
- HEMOPTYSIS
- HEMORRHAGE W/REFLUX

LIVER
- LIVER YANG RISING: Dizziness,
Vertigo, Eye Pressure, Tinnitus

LUNGS
- ASTHMA, ACUTE: Symptoms Of

SEXUALITY, FEMALE:
GYNECOLOGICAL
- LEUKORRHEA
- MENSTRUATION, DISORDERS

OF: Calm Chong, Lower Reflux
- UTERINE BLEEDING

STOMACH/DIGESTIVE
DISORDERS
- ACID REGURGITATION
- BELCHING
- HICCUPS
- HICCUPS, CHRONIC
- NAUSEA
- VOMITING: Liver Yang Rising
- VOMITING, CHRONIC

Clinical/Pharmaceutical Studies:

ABDOMEN/
GASTROINTESTINAL TOPICS
- GASTROINTESTINAL
PERISTALSIS, INCREASES

BLOOD RELATED DISORDERS/
TOPICS
- BLOOD, HELPS TO GENERATE

MENTAL STATE/
NEUROLOGICAL DISORDERS
- SEDATIVE

Dose
9 - 30 gm

Common Name
Hematite

Precautions
Watch: Pregnancy

Notes
Cook 30 Min Before Rest Of Herbs In Formula
Toxic: Progressive Paralysis, Arsenic 1ppm Probable
Reason

FU SHEN

茯神

SCLEROTIUM
PORIAE COCOS
PARARADICIS

Traditional Functions:

1. Promotes urination and filters out Dampness
2. Reinforces the Spleen and harmonizes the Middle Burner
3. Calms the Heart and pacifies the Spirit

Traditional Properties:

Enters: SP, HT,

Properties: SW, BL, N

Indications:

HEART
- PALPITATIONS

MENTAL STATE/
NEUROLOGICAL DISORDERS

- ANGER
- INSOMNIA
- INSOMNIA, DREAMS,
FREQUENT

- MEMORY, POOR

URINARY BLADDER
- URINATION, DIFFICULT

Clinical/Pharmaceutical Studies:

MENTAL STATE/

NEUROLOGICAL DISORDERS

- SEDATIVE: Not Hypnotic

Dose
6 - 12 gm

Common Name
Tuckahoe Spirit

Contraindications
Not: Polyuria

HU PO

琥珀
（琥珀）

SUCCINUM

Traditional Functions:

1. Sedates the Heart and pacifies the Spirit
2. Circulates water and promotes urination
3. Vitalizes the Blood and promotes menstruation
4. Promotes healing and reduces swelling with topical application

Traditional Properties:

Enters: HT, UB, LV,

Properties: SW, N

Indications:

ABDOMEN/
 GASTROINTESTINAL TOPICS
- ABDOMEN, MASS, PAIN OF
- ABDOMEN, PAIN OF,
 OBSTRUCTION
- ABDOMEN, PAIN OF,
 POSTPARTUM: Blood Stasis

CANCER/TUMORS/SWELLINGS/
 LUMPS
- LUMPS

CHILDHOOD DISORDERS
- CONVULSIONS, CHILDHOOD

GALL BLADDER
- GALL BLADDER, STONES

HEART
- ANGINA PECTORIS: Chest Bi
 Strangulating Pain
- CORONARY HEART DISEASE
- PALPITATIONS W/ANXIETY

HEMORRHAGIC DISORDERS
- HEMATURIA

LIVER
- LIVER QI STAGNATION LUMPS

MENTAL STATE/
 NEUROLOGICAL DISORDERS
- ANXIETY
- CONVULSIONS, CHRONIC
- CONVULSIONS, FEVER, ACUTE
- DREAMING, EXCESSIVE
- EPILEPSY
- FORGETFULNESS
- INSOMNIA
- INSOMNIA, DREAMS,
 FREQUENT
- SEIZURES: Disturbed Spirit

MUSCULOSKELETAL/
 CONNECTIVE TISSUE
- SPASMS, CHRONIC
- SPASMS, W/FEVER, ACUTE

SEXUALITY, FEMALE:
 GYNECOLOGICAL

- AMENORRHEA
- MENORRHALGIA

SEXUALITY, MALE:
 UROLOGICAL TOPICS
- PENIS, PAIN
- SCROTUM, PAIN/SWELLING

SKIN
- BOILS
- SKIN, ULCERS
- SORES

TRAUMA, BITES, POISONINGS
- WOUNDS, INCISED

URINARY BLADDER
- DYSURIA
- URINARY TRACT INFECTIONS,
 ACUTE
- URINARY TRACT STONES
- URINATION, DRIBBLING W/
 BLOOD
- URINATION, RETENTION

Dose

0.9 - 3.0 gm

Common Name

Amber

Contraindications

Not: Def Yin w/Heat

Notes

Topical Or As pwdr
Not Used In Decoctions

LONG CHI

龍齒
（龙齿）

FOSSILIA
DENTIS MASTODI
(DENS DRACONIS)

Traditional Functions:

1. Tranquilizes the Spirit, calms the mind
2. Clears fever and irritability

Traditional Properties:

Enters: LV, HT

Properties: ASTR, CL

Indications:

HEART
- PALPITATIONS W/ANXIETY

MENTAL STATE/
 NEUROLOGICAL DISORDERS
- CONVULSIONS

- EPILEPSY
- EPILEPSY, DREAMFULNESS OF
- FRIGHT
- INSOMNIA
- INSOMNIA, DREAMS,

FREQUENT
- MANIC-DEPRESSIVE STATES
- NEURASTHENIA,
 DREAMFULNESS
- SLEEP, DREAM DISTURBED

Dose
9 - 15 gm

Common Name
Dragon Teeth

Notes
Cook 20-30 Min Before Other Herbs

LONG GU

龍骨
(龙骨)

OS DRACONIS

Traditional Functions:

1. Sedates the Heart and pacifies the Spirit
2. Pacifies the Liver and subdues the rising Yang
3. Astringes leakage of fluids
4. With topical application, it astringes ulcers and generates flesh

Traditional Properties:

Enters: HT, KI, LV

Properties: SW, A, N

Indications:

ABDOMEN/ GASTROINTESTINAL TOPICS
• ABDOMEN, MASS, HARD
• ABDOMINAL QI STAGNATION
BLOOD RELATED DISORDERS/TOPICS
• PYEMIA: (Septicemia, Multiple Abscesses)
BOWEL RELATED DISORDERS
• DYSENTERY
• RECTAL PROLAPSE: Topical
CIRCULATION DISORDERS
• HYPERTENSION W/ HEADACHE, DIZZINESS: Raw
EARS/HEARING DISORDERS
• DIZZINESS: Liver Yin Deficient With Yang Rising
• VERTIGO: Liver Yang/ Fire Rising
EYES
• VISION, BLURRED: Liver Yin Deficient With

Yang Rising
HEAD/NECK
• HEADACHE: Hypertension Caused
HEART
• HEART QI STAGNATION
• PALPITATIONS W/ ANXIETY
HEMORRHAGIC DISORDERS
• EPISTAXIS
• HEMORRHAGE: Astringe To Stop
LIVER
• LIVER YIN DEFICIENCY W/YANG RISING: Irritability, Dizziness, Blurred Vision, Temper
MENTAL STATE/ NEUROLOGICAL DISORDERS
• CONVULSIONS, FRIGHT
• DREAMS, FREQUENT, MANY
• EMOTIONAL DISTRESS
• EPILEPSY, CHILDHOOD: Fright, Fever
• INSOMNIA

• INSOMNIA, DREAMS, FREQUENT
• IRRITABILITY: Liver Yin Deficient With Yang Rising
• MANIC-DEPRESSIVE STATES
• RESTLESSNESS
• SEIZURES
• TEMPER: Liver Yin Deficient With Yang Rising
QI RELATED DISORDERS/TOPICS
• ABDOMINAL QI STAGNATION
SEXUALITY, FEMALE: GYNECOLOGICAL
• LEUKORRHEA: Cold, Damp
• LEUKORRHEA, BLOODY: Calcined
• LEUKORRHEA, WHITE
• MENSTRUATION, DISORDERS OF: Consolidate, Astringe Chong, Ren
• UTERINE BLEEDING: Better Calcined
SEXUALITY, MALE:

UROLOGICAL TOPICS
• NOCTURNAL EMISSIONS
• SCROTUM, PRURITUS, DAMP: Topical
• SEMINAL EMISSIONS: Calcined
• SPERMATORRHEA
SKIN
• NIGHT SWEATS: From Fear, Calcined
• PERSPIRATION, RESTING & THIEF
• PERSPIRATION, SPONTANEOUS
• SORES, CHRONIC, NON-HEALING: Topical
• SWEATING, SPONTANEOUS
• ULCERS, SKIN: Topical
• ULCERS, UMBILICAL: Topical
STOMACH/DIGESTIVE DISORDERS
• HICCUPS
URINARY BLADDER
• URINARY INCONTINENCE
• URINATION, FREQUENT

Clinical/Pharmaceutical Studies:

• ASTRINGENT
HEMORRHAGIC DISORDERS
• HEMOSTATIC

LUNGS
• EXPECTORANT

TRAUMA, BITES, POISONINGS
• INFLAMMATORY, ANTI-

Dose
15 - 30 gm

Common Name
Fossilized Bones

Contraindications
Not: Damp Heat

Not: External Excess Conds

Notes
Cook 20-30 Min. Before Other Herbs

MU LI

牡蠣
(牡蛎)

CONCHA OSTREAE

Traditional Functions:

1. Sedates the Heart and pacifies the Spirit
2. Astringes leakage of fluids
3. Softens firm mass and disperses hard lumps and nodules
4. Reduces acidity and controls pain
5. Subdues the floating Yang and benefits the Yin
6. Clears internal Heat due to Yin deficiency

Traditional Properties:

Enters: KI, LV,

Properties: SA, A, <C

Indications:

BOWEL RELATED DISORDERS
• DIARRHEA

CANCER/TUMORS/ SWELLINGS/LUMPS
• NODULES, SUBCUTANEOUS

CIRCULATION DISORDERS
• HYPERTENSION, HEADACHE

EARS/HEARING DISORDERS
• DIZZINESS: Yin Deficient With Yang Rising
• TINNITUS: Yin Deficient With Yang Rising
• VERTIGO: Liver Yang/ Fire Rising

ENDOCRINE RELATED DISORDERS
• GOITER
• THYROID, ENLARGEMENT

ENERGETIC STATE
• FATIGUE, DEFICIENCY

EYES
• VISION, BLURRED: Yin Deficient With Yang

Rising

FEVERS
• FEVER, CHILLS
• FEVER, IRRITABILITY
• SWEATING, POST FEBRILE

HEAD/NECK
• FACE, FLUSHED: Yin Deficient With Yang Rising
• HEADACHE: Yin Deficient With Yang Rising

HEART
• PALPITATIONS W/ ANXIETY

IMMUNE SYSTEM RELATED DISORDERS/ TOPICS
• LYMPH GLANDS, ENLARGEMENT, CHRONIC: Phlegm Nodules

INFECTIOUS DISEASES
• SCROFULA
• SWEATING, POST FEBRILE

LIVER
• HEPATOMEGALY

MENTAL STATE/

NEUROLOGICAL DISORDERS
• CONVULSIONS
• INSOMNIA: Yin Deficient With Yang Rising
• INSOMNIA, DREAMS, FREQUENT
• IRRITABILITY: Yin Deficient With Yang Rising
• NEURASTHENIA
• RESTLESSNESS: Heat
• TEMPER: Yin Deficient With Yang Rising
• TREMORS

MUSCULOSKELETAL/ CONNECTIVE TISSUE
• SPASMS

SEXUALITY, FEMALE: GYNECOLOGICAL
• LEUKORRHEA
• MENORRHAGIA
• MENSTRUATION, DISORDERS OF: Consolidate, Astringe Chong, Ren
• UTERINE BLEEDING: Deficient

SEXUALITY, MALE:

UROLOGICAL TOPICS
• NOCTURNAL EMISSIONS
• SPERMATORRHEA

SKIN
• PERSPIRATION, RESTING & THIEF
• SWEATING: All Types/ Steaming Bone Syndrome
• SWEATING, POST FEBRILE
• SWEATING, SPONTANEOUS

SPLEEN
• SPLENOMEGALY

STOMACH/DIGESTIVE DISORDERS
• STOMACH, ACHE, SOUR TASTE: Excess
• ULCERS, PEPTIC

URINARY BLADDER
• URINARY INCONTINENCE
• URINATION, FREQUENT

YIN RELATED DISORDERS/TOPICS
• YIN DEFICIENCY W/ YANG RISING

Clinical/Pharmaceutical Studies:

CANCER/TUMORS/SWELLINGS/ LUMPS
• CANCER, ANTI-

LUNGS
• TUBERCULOSIS, NIGHT

SWEATS: Decoction, 3-4 Days, Continue 2 Days After Sweating Stops, May Add Long Gu, Suan Zao Ren

MENTAL STATE/

NEUROLOGICAL DISORDERS
• SEDATIVE

PAIN/NUMBNESS/GENERAL DISCOMFORT
• ANALGESIC

Dose

9 - 30 gm

Common Name

Oyster Shell

Contraindications

Not: w/Ma Huang, Wu Zhu Yu, Xi Xin

Not: High Fever w/o Sweat

Notes

Neck Lymphadenits: 90-120 gm
Powder: 3-6 gm

NAO YANG HUA

鬧羊花
(闹羊花)

FOLIUM RHODODENDRI MOLLES

Traditional Functions:

1. Dispels Wind and Dampness, relieving pain
2. Strongly calms the Heart

Traditional Properties:

Enters:

Properties: SP, BIT, W, TX

Indications:

HEAD/NECK
• HEADACHE
MUSCULOSKELETAL/
  CONNECTIVE TISSUE

• ARTHRITIS
SKIN
• TINEA, PERSISTENT

TRAUMA, BITES, POISONINGS
• FRACTURES, PAIN
• TRAUMA, PAIN

Clinical/Pharmaceutical Studies:

BLOOD RELATED DISORDERS/
  TOPICS
• BLOOD PRESSURE, LOWERS
HEART

• HEART RATE, REDUCES
PAIN/NUMBNESS/GENERAL
  DISCOMFORT
• ANALGESIC: Decoction Has

Pronounced Effects
TRAUMA, BITES, POISONINGS
• INSECTICIDE: Very Toxic To

Dose

0.3 - 0.9 gm

Common Name

Yellow Azalea

Notes

Taken As Powder Or Pellets

ZHEN ZHU

珍珠

MARGARITA USTA

Traditional Functions:

1. Calms the Spirit, stabilizes fright
2. Clears vision
3. Generates tissue and helps heal wounds
4. Clears Heat, removes toxins and benefits Yin

Traditional Properties:

Enters: HT, LV,

Properties: SW, SA, C

Indications:

CHILDHOOD DISORDERS
• CONVULSIONS, CHILDHOOD
EYES
• CORNEAL OPACITY: External
• EYES, CLOUDY
• NEBULA: Topical
• PTERYGIUM: External
• VISION, OBSTRUCTIONS
FEVERS
• FEVER, IRRITABLE W/THIRST
FLUID DISORDERS
• THIRST, EXCESSIVE

HEART
• PALPITATIONS
MENTAL STATE/
  NEUROLOGICAL DISORDERS
• ANGERED EASILY
• CONVULSIONS: Wind
• EPILEPSY
• FRIGHTENED EASILY
• INSOMNIA, DREAMS,
  FREQUENT
• RESTLESSNESS, OF MIND,

SPIRIT
• SEIZURES
MUSCULOSKELETAL/
  CONNECTIVE TISSUE
• SPASMS
ORAL CAVITY
• MOUTH, ULCERS
• THROAT, SORE: Deficient Heat
SKIN
• SKIN, ULCERS, CHRONIC:
  Topical

Clinical/Pharmaceutical Studies:

ABDOMEN/
  GASTROINTESTINAL TOPICS
• INTESTINES, PERISTALSIS,
  INHIBITS
IMMUNE SYSTEM RELATED

DISORDERS/TOPICS
• ALLERGIC, ANTI-
KIDNEYS
• DIURETIC
STOMACH/DIGESTIVE

DISORDERS
• GASTRIC ACID, NEUTRALIZES
TRAUMA, BITES, POISONINGS
• ANTIHISTAMINE: When
  Catalyzed By Sulfuric Acid

Dose
0.3 - 0.9 gm

Common Name
Pearl

Notes
Usually Pills/Powder

Topical In Eye Drops

ZHEN ZHU MU   珍珠母   CONCHA MARARITAFERAE

Traditional Functions:

1. Subdues Liver Yang and calms the Spirit
2. Clears the vision
3. Calms the Heart and Spirit

Traditional Properties:

Enters: HT, LV,

Properties: SW, SA, C

Indications:

EARS/HEARING DISORDERS
• DIZZINESS: Liver Yang Rising
• TINNITUS: Liver Yang Rising
• VERTIGO: Liver Yang/Fire Rising
EYES
• CATARACTS
• EYES, BLOOD SHOT
• NIGHT BLINDNESS
• VISION, SUPERFICIAL

OBSTRUCTIONS: Liver Yang
Rising
HEAD/NECK
• HEADACHE, HYPERTENSIVE:
Liver Yang Rising
HEART
• PALPITATIONS
LIVER
• LIVER YANG RISING

MENTAL STATE/
NEUROLOGICAL DISORDERS
• INSANITY: Liver Yang Rising
• INSOMNIA: Liver Yang Rising
• INSOMNIA, DREAMS,
FREQUENT
• MANIA: Liver Yang Rising
• SEIZURES: Liver Yang Rising

Dose
9 - 60 gm

Common Name
Mother Of Pearl

Precautions
Watch: Cold Abdomen

Notes
Less Strong Than Pearl For Sedation, Stronger For
Other Effects

ZHU SHA   朱砂   CINNABARIS

Traditional Functions:

1. Sedates the Heart and pacifies the Spirit
2. Relieves toxin and prevents putrefaction
3. Expels Phlegm and clears Heat
4. Stabilizes convulsions

Traditional Properties:

Enters: HT,

Properties: SW, C, TX

Indications:

CHILDHOOD DISORDERS
• CONVULSIONS, CHILDHOOD:
From High Fever
HEART
• PALPITATIONS W/ANXIETY: ,
Excess Heat, Hot Phlegm, Blood
Deficient
LUNGS
• LUNG HEAT W/SPUTUM IN
COUGH
MENTAL STATE/
NEUROLOGICAL DISORDERS
• CONVULSIONS: Excess Heat, Hot
Phlegm, Blood Deficient

• CONVULSIONS, CHRONIC
• CONVULSIONS, FEVER, ACUTE
• INSOMNIA: Excess Heat, Hot
Phlegm, Blood Deficient
• INSOMNIA, DREAMS,
FREQUENT
• MENTAL DERANGEMENT
• NIGHTMARES
• RESTLESSNESS: Excess Heat,
Hot Phlegm, Blood Deficient
MUSCULOSKELETAL/
CONNECTIVE TISSUE
• SPASMS, CHRONIC
• SPASMS, W/FEVER, ACUTE

ORAL CAVITY
• MOUTH, SORES: Topical
• THROAT, SORE: Topical
SKIN
• BOILS: Topical, Heat, Toxins,
Swellings
• SKIN, SORES, SWOLLEN: Heat,
Toxins, Swelling
• SKIN, ULCERS, TOXIC: Topical
TRAUMA, BITES, POISONINGS
• SNAKE BITES: Topical
WIND DISORDERS
• WIND PHLEGM DIZZINESS

Clinical/Pharmaceutical Studies:

INFECTIOUS DISEASES
• BACTERIAL, ANTI-: Topical
MENTAL STATE/
 NEUROLOGICAL DISORDERS
• SEDATIVE, INHIBITS CNS

MUSCULOSKELETAL/
 CONNECTIVE TISSUE
• SPASMS
NUTRITIONAL/METABOLIC
 DISORDERS/TOPICS

BODY WEIGHT, INCREASES
PARASITES
• ANTIPARASITIC: Topical
SKIN
• FUNGAL, ANTI-: Topical

Dose
0.3 - 1.8 gm

Common Name
Cinnabar

Notes
Topical For Sores/Bites, etc
Do Not Heat--Releases Mercury
Avoid Long Term Use

ZI SHI YING   紫石英   FLUORITUM

Traditional Functions:

1. Sedates the Heart and calms fright
2. Descends Lung Qi and warms the Lungs
3. Warms the uterus

Traditional Properties:

Enters: HT, LV, KI, LU

Properties: SW, W

Indications:

ENERGETIC STATE
• FATIGUE, DEFICIENCY
HEART
• PALPITATIONS W/
 ANXIETY: Liver Yang
 Rising/Heart Blood
 Deficient
LUNGS
• COUGH/WHEEZING:

Lung Cold, Deficient
• WHEEZING, COPIOUS
 SPUTUM
MENTAL STATE/
 NEUROLOGICAL
 DISORDERS
• CONVULSIONS: Liver
 Yang Rising/Heart Blood
 Deficient

• INSOMNIA: Liver Yang
 Rising/Heart Blood
 Deficient
• MENTAL
 DISORIENTATION:
 Liver Yang Rising/Heart
 Blood Deficient
• RESTLESSNESS
SEXUALITY, EITHER

SEX
• INFERTILITY: Cold
 Womb
SEXUALITY, FEMALE:
 GYNECOLOGICAL
• MENORRHAGIA: Cold
 Deficient Womb
• UTERINE BLEEDING:
 Cold Deficient Womb

Clinical/Pharmaceutical Studies:

MENTAL STATE/

NEUROLOGICAL DISORDERS

• TRANQUILIZING

Dose
6 - 15 gm

Common Name
Fluorite

Notes
Cook 20-30 Minutes Before Other Herbs/Substances

Pacifies Liver, Extinguishes Wind

BAI JI LI
(CI JI LI)

白蒺藜

FRUCTUS TRIBULI TERRESTRIS

Traditional Functions:

1. Calms the Liver and subdues the Yang
2. Extinguishes Wind, alleviates pain and clears the vision
3. Expels exterior Wind and stops itching
4. Promotes the smooth flow of Liver Qi and releases stagnation

Traditional Properties:

Enters: LU, LV,

Properties: SP, BIT, W

Indications:

ABDOMEN/ GASTROINTESTINAL TOPICS
• ABDOMEN, MASS
• FLANK PAIN/DISTENTION: Liver Qi Stagnation
CHEST
• CHEST, FULLNESS
• CHEST, PAIN/DISTENTION: Liver Qi Stagnation
EARS/HEARING DISORDERS
• DIZZINESS: Liver Wind/Heat
• VERTIGO: Liver Yang/Fire Rising
EYES

• EYES, RED, CONGESTED: Liver Heat
• EYES, RED, SWOLLEN, PAINFUL: Liver Wind/Heat
HEAD/NECK
• HEADACHE: Hypertensive/Liver Wind/Heat
LIVER
• LIVER YANG RISING: Headache, Dizziness, Red, Swollen Eyes
SEXUALITY, FEMALE: GYNECOLOGICAL
• LACTATION, INSUFFICIENT:

Liver Qi Stagnation
• MASTITIS
SKIN
• HIVES
• PRURITUS
• RASHES, W/PRURITUS: Clears Wind
• VITILIGO
WIND DISORDERS
• WIND HEAT IN LIVER CHANNEL: Headache, Dizziness, Red, Swollen Eyes

Clinical/Pharmaceutical Studies:

BLOOD RELATED DISORDERS/ TOPICS
• BLOOD PRESSURE, LOWERS: Decoction/Alcohol Extract

INFECTIOUS DISEASES
• BACTERIAL, ANTI-: Staph. Aureus, E.Coli
KIDNEYS

• DIURETIC
MENTAL STATE/ NEUROLOGICAL DISORDERS
• SEDATIVE

Dose
6 - 12 gm
Common Name
Caltrop Fruit

Precautions
Watch: Pregnancy
Watch: Def Qi/Blood

DAI MAO

玳瑁

CARAPAX ERETHMOCHELYAS

Traditional Functions:

1. Causes the Yang to descend, suppressing Liver Wind
2. Clears toxic Heat

Traditional Properties:

Enters: HT, LV,

Properties: SW, SA, C

Indications:

CHILDHOOD DISORDERS
• CONVULSIONS, CHILDHOOD
CIRCULATION DISORDERS
• STROKE
EARS/HEARING DISORDERS
• VERTIGO: Liver Yang/Fire Rising
EYES
• TEARING, EXCESSIVE
FLUID DISORDERS
• EDEMA
HEAT
• HEAT: Extreme With Agitation
IMMUNE SYSTEM RELATED DISORDERS/TOPICS
• LYMPH NODES, SWELLING: Wind Pain
INFECTIOUS DISEASES

• FEBRILE DISEASES, SEQUELAE OF
LIVER
• JAUNDICE
MENTAL STATE/ NEUROLOGICAL DISORDERS
• CONVULSIONS, FEBRILE DISEASES
• DELIRIUM
• EPILEPSY
• HEMIPLEGIA
• MANIC AGITATION
• MENTAL CLOUDINESS: Use w/ Heat Shut-In Herbs
ORAL CAVITY
• THROAT, NUMB
SKIN

• ABSCESS
• ABSCESS, W/MENTAL DULLNESS, HIGH FEVER, SPASMS: Blood Heat
• BOILS
• RASHES, INCOMPLETE EXPRESSION OF: Blood Heat, Wind
• SKIN, SORE W/MENTAL DULLNESS, HIGH FEVER, SPASMS: Blood Heat
• ULCERS, TOXIC
URINARY BLADDER
• URINARY OBSTRUCTION
WIND DISORDERS
• WIND HEAT: Red Eyes

Clinical/Pharmaceutical Studies:

MENTAL STATE/ NEUROLOGICAL DISORDERS

• SEDATIVE, LARGE DOSES
TRAUMA, BITES, POISONINGS

• INFLAMMATORY, ANTI-: Arthritis

Dose

3 - 6 gm

Common Name

Hawksbill Turtle Shell

DI LONG
(QIU YIN)

地龍
（地龙）

LUMBRICUS

Traditional Functions:

1. Subdues Heat and stops spasms and fright
2. Expels Wind and clears the Luo channels of the body
3. Promotes urination
4. Soothes asthma, especially Lung Heat

Traditional Properties:

Enters: LU, SP, UB, LV

Properties: SA, C

Indications:

CHILDHOOD DISORDERS
• FRIGHT CONVULSIONS, CHILDHOOD
• INFANTILE CONVULSIONS
CIRCULATION DISORDERS
• HYPERTENSION
EARS/HEARING DISORDERS
• VERTIGO: Liver Yang/Fire Rising
EYES
• EYES, RED: Wind Heat
FLUID DISORDERS
• EDEMA, SEVERE
HEAD/NECK
• TICS: With High Fever
HEAT
• HEAT: Extreme
IMMUNE SYSTEM RELATED DISORDERS/TOPICS
• LYMPH NODES, PAIN: Wind
INFECTIOUS DISEASES
• FEBRILE DISEASES, WARM: Convulsions/Seizures From

• TETANUS
LIVER
• JAUNDICE
LUNGS
• ASTHMA
• COUGH: Lung Heat
• LUNGS, DYSPNEA: Lung Heat
• WHEEZING: Especially Lung Heat
MENTAL STATE/ NEUROLOGICAL DISORDERS
• CONVULSIONS: From High Fever
• EPILEPSY
• HEMIPLEGIA
• IRRITABILITY
• RESTLESSNESS
• SEIZURES: High Fever
MUSCULOSKELETAL/ CONNECTIVE TISSUE
• ARTHRITIS: Pain Of
• RHEUMATISM
• SPASMS, W/FEVER, ACUTE
ORAL CAVITY

• THROAT, NUMB
• THROAT, SORE
PAIN/NUMBNESS/GENERAL DISCOMFORT
• BI, STIFFNESS OF EXTREMITIES
• BI, WIND DAMP, CHRONIC: Open Luo, Arrest Pain
SKIN
• BURNS: Topical
• ECZEMA: Topical
• ERYSIPELAS: Topical
• HYPEREMIA
• ULCERS, EXTERNAL, LOWER LIMBS: Topical
URINARY BLADDER
• URINARY OBSTRUCTION, PARTIAL
• URINARY TRACT INFECTIONS: Hot
WIND DISORDERS
• WINDSTROKE, STIFFNESS

Clinical/Pharmaceutical Studies:

**ABDOMEN/
GASTROINTESTINAL
TOPICS**
• INTESTINES,
STIMULATES
CONTRACTION
**BLOOD RELATED
DISORDERS/TOPICS**
• BLOOD PRESSURE,
LOWERS: No Tolerance
With Oral, Slow But
Persistent Action
**CIRCULATION
DISORDERS**
• HYPERTENSION,
ESSENTIAL: No Side
Effects, Very Effective,
Hot Aqueous/Alcohol
Extract, Peaks 90 Mins,
Lasts 2-3 Hours/40%
Tincture 10 ml, 3x/Day/2
ml Of Acid Soluble
Fraction (B1) , Containing
8 g Di Long, 3x/Day PO /
Di Long, Chou Wu Tong

Tablet, 0.5 g/Tablet, 5 Tabs,
3x/Day For 4-6 Weeks,
Best For Stage I, II
EYES
• CONJUNCTIVITIS,
CHRONIC: External With
Paste And Sugar/Eye
Drops Of Saline Extract
(Trachoma)
FEVERS
• ANTIPYRETIC: Must Be
Decomposed By Heat Or
Enzyme
• FEVER, HIGH W/
CONVULSIONS: From
Flu, Lung Infection,
Pneumonia, Bronchitis–
Injection, 2 ml Amp Of 1:5,
IM, Fast Onset
INFECTIOUS DISEASES
• HERPES ZOSTER:
External With Paste And
Sugar
• MUMPS: Local
Application Of Sugar And

Di Long Liquid
• VIRAL INFECTIONS: In
Eyes:External With Paste
And Surgar/Eye Drops Of
Saline Extract
LUNGS
• ASTHMA, BRONCHIAL:
w/Huang Qin, 40%
Effective/90% Alcohol
Extract
• BRONCHITIS,
CHRONIC: Chuan Shu
Ning Pian (Di Long,
Ammonium Chloride) , 1-2
Tabs/Day/Di Long Powder,
3-4 g, 3-4x/Day, Orally/
Compound Ephedra-
Pheretima Tablet (Ma
Huang, Fried Di Long,
Dan Nan Xing, Ye Qiao
Mai, Pu Gong Ying, Rough
Extract With Alcohol,
Then Made Into Tabs) , 10
Day Courses

• BRONCHODILATORY:
Marked, Oral
Administration, Inhibits
Histamine
**MENTAL STATE/
NEUROLOGICAL
DISORDERS**
• CONVULSIVE, ANTI-:
ETOH Extract
• MENTAL DISORDERS:
Schizophrenia:Oral/IM
Injection With
Chlorpromazine
• SEDATIVE: Inhibits
Caffeine, Not Strychnine
**SEXUALITY, FEMALE:
GYNECOLOGICAL**
• UTERUS, STIMULATES
SKIN
• ECZEMA: 100% Prep
Injection, Acupoint
**TRAUMA, BITES,
POISONINGS**
• ANTIHISTAMINE

Dose
4.5 - 12.0 gm

Common Name
Earthworm

Contraindications
Not: w/o True Heat

Notes
Low Toxicity
Pellets/Powder: 0.6-1.2 gm
Possible Anaphylactic Shock If Injected

GOU TENG

鉤藤
（钩藤）

RAMULUS UNCARIAE CUM UNCIS

Traditional Functions:

1. Extinguishes Wind, reduces spasms and calms nervous excitement
2. Clears Heat and calms the Liver
3. Releases the surface and disperses Wind Heat

Traditional Properties:

Enters: HT, LV,

Properties: SW, CL

Indications:

CHILDHOOD DISORDERS
• FEVER, CONVULSIONS,
CHILDHOOD
CIRCULATION DISORDERS
• HYPERTENSION
EARS/HEARING DISORDERS
• DIZZINESS: Liver Fire With Liver
Yang Rising
• VERTIGO: Liver Yang/Fire Rising
EYES
• EYES, RED: Liver Fire With Liver
Yang Rising
HEAD/NECK
• HEADACHE: Liver Fire With
Liver Yang Rising/Nervous/

Hypertensive/Wind Heat
LIVER
• LIVER FIRE W/YANG RISING
• LIVER HEAT W/WIND
**MENTAL STATE/
NEUROLOGICAL DISORDERS**
• CONVULSIONS: With High Fever
• CONVULSIONS, INFANTILE
• DELIRIUM: Liver Heat With Wind
• EPILEPSY, CHILDHOOD
• IRRITABILITY: Liver Fire With
Liver Yang Rising
• SEIZURES: Liver Heat With Wind
• TREMORS: Liver Heat With Wind
MUSCULOSKELETAL/

CONNECTIVE TISSUE
• SPASMS, CONVULSIONS:
Internal Deficiency Wind
• SPASMS, W/FEVER, ACUTE
**SEXUALITY, FEMALE:
GYNECOLOGICAL**
• ECLAMPSIA: Liver Heat With
Wind
SKIN
• RASHES, INCOMPLETE
EXPRESSION OF: Early Stage
WIND DISORDERS
• WIND HEAT: Headache, Fever,
Red Eyes

Clinical/Pharmaceutical Studies:

CIRCULATION DISORDERS
• HYPERTENSION: If Cooked Less 20 Min, Include Thorns, ETOH Extract/Decoction Active, Decoction Stronger, Action Lasts 3-4 Hrs, Usually Used With Other Herbs, e. g. Tian Ma Gou Teng Yin,

Ling Yang Gou Teng Tang, Most Effective With Yin Deficient With Yang Rising With Headache, Insomnia, Palpitation, Tinnitus, Constipation

INFECTIOUS DISEASES
• VIRAL, ANTI-: Inhibits Flu, Other Respiratory Viruses

MENTAL STATE/ NEUROLOGICAL DISORDERS
• EPILEPSY: Side Effect Of Sedation At Effective Doses, May Cause Motor Paralysis, Respiratory Inhibition (No Other Source Supports This, Low

Toxicity Even At 5 g/kg For 50 Days) , 2 g/kg Could Prevent Attacks, But Started 3 Days After Stopping Treatment
• SEDATIVE: Not Hypnotic, Significant, Injected, Both ETOH Extract/Decoction

Dose
6 - 15 gm

Common Name
Gambir Vine Stems/Thorns

Notes
Do Not Cook For >10 Minutes

JIANG CAN
(BAI JIANG CAN)

僵蠶
(僵蚕)

BOMBYX BATRYTICATUS

Traditional Functions:

1. Calms Liver Wind and controls spasms
2. Relieves pain from Wind Heat
3. Expels exterior Wind rash
3. Resolves Phlegm and disperse nodules
4. Clears and benefits the throat

Traditional Properties:

Enters: LU, LV,

Properties: SP, SA, N

Indications:

CHILDHOOD DISORDERS
• CONVULSIONS, CHILDHOOD
CIRCULATION DISORDERS
• STROKE
EARS/HEARING DISORDERS
• VERTIGO
EYES
• EYES, CONGESTED, BLOOD SHOT
HEAD/NECK
• FACE, PARALYSIS
• HEADACHE
INFECTIOUS DISEASES
• PAROTITIS
• RUBELLA

• SCROFULA: Phlegm Heat
• TETANUS
LUNGS
• TUBERCULOSIS, LYMPHATIC
MENTAL STATE/ NEUROLOGICAL DISORDERS
• CONVULSIONS
• CONVULSIONS, FEVER, ACUTE
• EPILEPSY
MUSCULOSKELETAL/ CONNECTIVE TISSUE
• SPASMS
• SPASMS, W/FEVER, ACUTE
ORAL CAVITY

• APHONIA
• LARYNGITIS
• THROAT, SORE: Wind Heat
PHLEGM
• PHLEGM NODULES
SKIN
• ERYSIPELAS
• PRURITUS
• RASHES, W/PRURITUS: Clears Wind
• SKIN, LESIONS: Wind Rash
• URTICARIA
WIND DISORDERS
• WIND PHLEGM HEAT SEIZURES

Clinical/Pharmaceutical Studies:

BLOOD RELATED DISORDERS/TOPICS
• CHOLESTEROL, LOWERS: 20-30 Days Of Medication
CANCER/TUMORS/ SWELLINGS/LUMPS
• TUMOR, ANTI-
CIRCULATION DISORDERS
• ARTERIOSCLEROSIS: Heart Disease
• HYPERTENSION

HEMORRHAGIC DISORDERS
• HEMATURIA
INFECTIOUS DISEASES
• BACTERIAL, ANTI-: Weak Against E.Coli, Staph.Aureus, Pseudomonas
• ENCEPHALITIS B, EPIDEMIC
• ENCEPHALITIS, SEQUELAE OF
• MUMPS: 7 Days Tablet,

• BRONCHITIS, CHRONIC: Alleviated Cough, Thinned Sputum, Did Not Cure, Though
• RESPIRATORY TRACT INFECTION, UPPER: Tablet Caused Body Temperature To Drop 1-2 Days
MENTAL STATE/ NEUROLOGICAL DISORDERS
• CONVULSIONS: Inhibits

• EPILEPSY: Defatted Tablet, 0.9-1.5 g/Tab, 3x/ Day, Similar Results With Ammonium Oxalate
• HYPNOTIC: ETOH, Water Extracts Synergizes Chloral Hydrate, Barbituates
ORAL CAVITY
• PHARYNGITIS, SEVERE: As Tablet, Throat Swellin, Pain Disappeared After 2 Days

---

Clinical/Pharmaceutical Studies:

ENDOCRINE RELATED DISORDERS
• DIABETES MELLITUS: Best For Mild, Moderate Severe Patients Who Did Not Respond To Diet Therapy

HEAD/NECK
• NECK, LYMPH GLANDS SWOLLEN

Fever Dropped 1-2 Days, Swelling Down In 2-3 Days

KIDNEYS
• NEPHRITIS

LIVER
• LIVER, DISEASES, CHRONIC

LUNGS

Strychnine, Caffeine
• CONVULSIONS, INFANTILE: Tetanus, Chronic/Acute, With Quan Xie, Wu Gong, etc, Or Gou Teng, Pearl Powder, See Wu Hu Zhui Feng San And Silkworm Pearl Sedative Decoction

SKIN
• CARBUNCLES: Lian Qiao, Ban Lan Gen, Huang Qin
• FURUNCLES: Lian Qiao, Ban Lan Gen, Huang Qin
• URTICARIA

URINARY BLADDER
• ENURESIS

Dose

3 - 9 gm

Common Name

Silkworm Sick, Dead Body

Notes

Raw: Wind Heat Syndrome

Fried: Other Applications w/Honey, Flour To Reduce Smell

Ammonium Oxalate Active Principle

Some May Have Dry Mouth, Nausea, Lassitude, Upset Stomach

LING YANG JIAO

羚羊角
（羚羊角）

CORNU ANTELOPIS

Traditional Functions:

1. Subdues Liver Wind and extinguishes Wind
2. Clears Heat and relieves toxins
3. Clears Damp Heat and Wind Damp Heat Bi
4. Clears Liver Heat and clears eyes

Traditional Properties:

Enters: HT, LV,

Properties: SA, C

Indications:

CHILDHOOD DISORDERS
• FEVER, CONVULSIONS, CHILDHOOD

EARS/HEARING DISORDERS
• DIZZINESS: Heat/Liver Yang Rising Creates Wind
• VERTIGO: Liver Yang/Fire Rising

EYES
• EYES, RED: Heat/Liver Yang Rising Creates Wind
• PHOTOPHOBIA: Heat/Liver Yang Rising Creates Wind
• VISION, BLURRED: Heat/Liver Yang Rising Creates Wind

FEVERS
• FEVER, HIGH

HEAD/NECK
• HEADACHE: Heat/Liver Yang Rising Creates Wind

HEAT

• HEAT IN PERICARDIUM

INFECTIOUS DISEASES
• TETANUS

LIVER
• LIVER FIRE BLAZING
• LIVER WIND HEAT
• LIVER YANG RISING

MENTAL STATE/ NEUROLOGICAL DISORDERS
• AGITATION
• CONVULSIONS: Heat/Liver Yang Rising Creates Wind
• CONVULSIONS, FEVER, ACUTE
• DELIRIUM: From High Fever
• EPILEPSY: Fright Induced
• MANIC BEHAVIOR: From High Fever
• UNCONSCIOUSNESS: From High Fever
• UNCONSCIOUSNESS, (MENTAL

CLOUDINESS) : Use w/Heat Shut-In Herbs

MUSCULOSKELETAL/ CONNECTIVE TISSUE
• SPASMS: Heat/Liver Yang Rising Creates Wind
• SPASMS, W/FEVER, ACUTE

PAIN/NUMBNESS/GENERAL DISCOMFORT
• BI, WIND DAMP HEAT

SKIN
• ABSCESS, W/MENTAL DULLNESS, HIGH FEVER, SPASMS: Blood Heat
• RASHES, INCOMPLETE EXPRESSION OF: Blood Heat, Wind
• SKIN, SORE W/MENTAL DULLNESS, HIGH FEVER, SPASMS: Blood Heat

Clinical/Pharmaceutical Studies:

BLOOD RELATED DISORDERS/TOPICS
• THROMBOCYTOPENIC PURPURA, BLEEDING OF: Ling Yang San Huang Decoction (Ling Yang Jiao,

Liver Fire Rising, With Che Qian Zi, Huang Qin, Xuan Shen, Zhi Mu, Fu Ling, Fang Feng, Xi Xin

FEVERS
• FEVER, HIGH: From Flu,

Teng, Sheng Di, Ju Hua)
• CONVULSIVE, ANTI-: ETOH Extract, To Caffeine, Does Not Cause Muscles To Relax
• SEDATIVE: Reduces

OXYGEN

PAIN/NUMBNESS/ GENERAL DISCOMFORT
• ANALGESIC: No Relaxation, Some Effect

Clinical/Pharmaceutical Studies:

Sheng Di, Jin Yin Hua, Mu Dan Pi, Chen Pi, Huang Bai, Huang Lian, Shan Zhi Zi, Bai Shao, Bai Mao Gen, Gan Cao, E Jiao) , Bleeding Stopped 3-7 Days

CIRCULATION DISORDERS
• HYPERTENSION

EYES
• GLAUCOMA, PAIN OF:

Measles, Pneumonia, et al, Use Injection
• FEVER, REDUCES: Starts In 2 Hours, Lasts 6 Hours

MENTAL STATE/ NEUROLOGICAL DISORDERS
• CONVULSIONS, HIGH FEVER: Ling Yang Gou Teng Tang, (With Gou

Effect Of Strychnine, Caffeine
• TRANQUILIZING: ETOH Extract

NUTRITIONAL/ METABOLIC DISORDERS/TOPICS
• OXYGEN METABOLISM, INCREASED RESISTANCE TO LOW

SEXUALITY, FEMALE: GYNECOLOGICAL
• ECLAMPSIA: In Pregnancy, Liver Yin Deficient, With Suan Zao Ren, Mai Dong, Sang Ji Sheng, E Jiao, Mu LI

SKIN
• ECZEMA, INFANTILE: Powder Of

Dose

1.5 - 4.5 gm

Common Name

Antelope Horn

Notes

0.3-0.5 As pwdr (Expensive) Can Use Goat Horn (Shan Yang Jiao, 3-5 Qian, Cook 30 Min, First)

LUO BU MA
(ZE QI MA)

羅布麻
（罗布麻）

FOLIUM APOCYNI VENETI

Traditional Functions:

1. Calms and balances the Yin and Yang of the Liver and clears Heat
2. Lowers the rising Liver Yang
3. Promotes urination

Traditional Properties:

Enters: LV, KI

Properties: SW, BIT, CL

Indications:

ABDOMEN/ GASTROINTESTINAL TOPICS
• ABDOMEN, DISTENTION OF

CIRCULATION DISORDERS
• HYPERTENSION

EARS/HEARING DISORDERS
• DIZZINESS
• VERTIGO

FLUID DISORDERS

• EDEMA, NEPHRITIC

HEAD/NECK
• HEADACHE, HYPERTENSIVE

HEART
• CARDIAC DISEASE

KIDNEYS
• NEPHRITIS

LIVER
• HEPATITIS

MENTAL STATE/ NEUROLOGICAL DISORDERS
• INSOMNIA
• IRRITABILITY
• NEURASTHENIA

URINARY BLADDER
• DYSURIA
• OLIGURIA

Clinical/Pharmaceutical Studies:

BLOOD RELATED DISORDERS/TOPICS
• BLOOD PRESSURE, LOWERS IN RENAL HYPERTENSION

CIRCULATION DISORDERS
• HYPERTENSION: 3-6 g As Tea, Effective Rate Increased With Duration Of Treatment, 4-8 Weeks

FLUID DISORDERS
• EDEMA, ANY TYPE: 12-

15 Gr Of Root, In 2 Doses Daily As Decoction

HEART
• HEART DISEASE, RHEUMATIC W/HEART FAILURE
• HEART FAILURE, CHRONIC CONGESTIVE: 8% Decoction, 100 ml, 2x/ Day Or 5 ml Of Fluid Extract (8 g Crude Herb) , 2x/Day, When Heart Slowed Reduce To 50 ml/3

ml Respectively
• HEART RATE, REDUCES: Orally, Recovers In 30 Minutes
• HEART, INCREASES CORONARY BLOOD FLOW

INFECTIOUS DISEASES
• COMMON COLD: Decreased Incidence, 52%, When Used Prophylactically, 20% Decoction, 50-100 ml, 2x/

Day, As Cure Can Be 90% Effective

KIDNEYS
• DIURETIC: Renal Or Cardiac Edema Or Ascites Of Cirrhosis

LUNGS
• BRONCHITIS, CHRONIC: Cigarette From Leaves Useful In Prevention/Treatment, Help Cough And Other Symptoms

Dose
3 - 9 gm

Common Name
Dogbane

Notes
Can Use Singly As Tea

Possible Nausea, Vomiting, Diarrhea, Abdominal Discomfort, Heart Beat Changes

From Cigarette: Possible Headache, Dizziness, Cough, Insomina, Nausea

---

QUAN XIE

全蠍
(全蝎)

BUTHUS MARTENSI

Traditional Functions:

1. Suppresses Liver Wind and controls spasms
2. Dispels Wind from the channels and stops pain
3. Relieves toxins and disperses lump and sores by topical application

Traditional Properties:

Enters: LV,

Properties: SP, TX, N

Indications:

CANCER/TUMORS/SWELLINGS/ LUMPS
• SWELLINGS, TOXIC: Topical
CHILDHOOD DISORDERS
• CONVULSIONS, CHILDHOOD: Liver Wind Phlegm
CIRCULATION DISORDERS
• STROKE, MUSCLE SPASMS OF
EYES
• EYES, DEVIATION OF
HEAD/NECK
• FACE, PARALYSIS
• HEADACHE, SEVERE
• TICS: Liver Wind Phlegm
IMMUNE SYSTEM RELATED DISORDERS/TOPICS
• LYMPH NODES, SWELLING

INFECTIOUS DISEASES
• SCROFULA: Topical
• TETANUS: Liver Wind Phlegm
LIVER
• LIVER WIND PHLEGM
MENTAL STATE/ NEUROLOGICAL DISORDERS
• EPILEPSY
• HEMIPLEGIA
• OPISTHOTONOS: Liver Wind Phlegm
• SEIZURES: Liver Wind Phlegm
• TRIGEMINAL NEURALGIA
MUSCULOSKELETAL/ CONNECTIVE TISSUE
• ARTHRITIS, PAIN
• SPASMS: Liver Wind Phlegm

ORAL CAVITY
• MOUTH, DEVIATION OF
PAIN/NUMBNESS/GENERAL DISCOMFORT
• BI, WIND DAMP, CHRONIC: Open Luo, Arrest Pain
• BI, WIND DAMP, SEVERE
SKIN
• ABSCESS
• SKIN, INFLAMMATIONS
• SKIN, SORES, SWOLLEN, TOXIC: Topical
• ULCERS, TOXIC
TRAUMA, BITES, POISONINGS
• WOUNDS, INCISED, PURULENT
WIND DISORDERS
• WINDSTROKE

Clinical/Pharmaceutical Studies:

BLOOD RELATED DISORDERS/ TOPICS
• BLOOD PRESSURE, LOWERS: Oral, Significant For Long Periods Of Time (1-3 Hrs)
MENTAL STATE/ NEUROLOGICAL DISORDERS

• CONVULSIVE, ANTI-: Strychnine, Nicotine, Not Cocaine-Wu Gong Stronger, Use With Wu Gong (Zi Qing San) Equal Amounts, 1 gm/ Day
• SEIZURES: Honey With Wu Gong

• TRANQUILIZING: Not Hypnotic
SEXUALITY, FEMALE: GYNECOLOGICAL
• UTERUS, STIMULATES
SKIN
• FUNGAL, ANTI-: Aqueous Extract

Dose
2.4 - 9.0 gm

Common Name
Scorpion

Contraindications
Not: Pregnancy

Precautions
Watch: Def Blood Wind

Notes
Toxic, Watch Overdose

Use Less In Powder Form (0.6-1 gm)

SHI JUE MING

石决明

CONCHA HALIOTIDIS

Traditional Functions:

1. Calms the Liver and subdues the Yang
2. Relieves Liver Fire and clears the eyes

Traditional Properties:

Enters: LV,

Properties: SA, <C

Indications:

CIRCULATION DISORDERS
• HYPERTENSION
EARS/HEARING DISORDERS
• DIZZINESS: Liver Fire/Yang Rising
• VERTIGO: Liver Wind/Liver Yang/ Fire Rising
EXTREMITIES
• LIMBS, CONVULSIONS
EYES
• CATARACTS
• EYES, RED: Liver Fire/Yang Rising

• GLAUCOMA
• PHOTOPHOBIA: Liver Heat
• PTERYGIUM: Liver Heat
• VISION, BLURRED: Liver Heat
• VISION, SUPERFICIAL OBSTRUCTIONS: Liver Heat
FEVERS
• FEVER: Overwork/Yin Deficient
HEAD/NECK
• HEADACHE: Liver Fire/Yang Rising
HEMORRHAGIC DISORDERS
• HEMOPTYSIS

LIVER
• LIVER FIRE
• LIVER FIRE BLAZING
• LIVER YANG RISING
MENTAL STATE/ NEUROLOGICAL DISORDERS
• CONVULSIONS, FEVER, ACUTE
MUSCULOSKELETAL/ CONNECTIVE TISSUE
• SPASMS, CONVULSIONS: Internal Deficiency Wind
• SPASMS, W/FEVER, ACUTE

Clinical/Pharmaceutical Studies:

MENTAL STATE/

NEUROLOGICAL DISORDERS

• SEDATIVE

Dose
9 - 30 gm
Common Name
Abalone Shell

Notes
Cook 1 Hr Before Decoction
Powder Ok
Fine Powder For Eyes
Bao Yu Is The Abalone Meat

TIAN MA

天麻
(天麻)

RHIZOMA GASTRODIAE ELATAE

Traditional Functions:

1. Calms the Liver, subdues the Yang and stops spasms
2. Dissipates Wind and reduces pain from Wind Phlegm
3. Circulates the channels and Disperses Wind Damp Bi

Traditional Properties:

Enters: LV,

Properties: SW, <W

Indications:

ABDOMEN/ GASTROINTESTINAL TOPICS
• WAIST, PAIN, SORE
CHILDHOOD DISORDERS
• CONVULSIONS, CHILDHOOD: Liver Wind
EARS/HEARING DISORDERS
• DIZZINESS: Liver Wind (Good) / Wind Stroke/Wind Phlegm
• VERTIGO: Liver Yang/Fire Rising
EXTREMITIES
• EXTREMITIES, CRAMPS/ SPASMS: Liver Wind
• EXTREMITIES, PAIN/NUMB: Wind Damp Bi

• HEADACHE: Liver Wind/Wind Phlegm
• MIGRAINE: Wind Phlegm
INFECTIOUS DISEASES
• TETANUS: Liver Wind
LIVER
• LIVER WIND HEAT
MENTAL STATE/ NEUROLOGICAL DISORDERS
• CONVULSIONS, CHRONIC
• EPILEPSY: Liver Wind
• HEMIPLEGIA: Wind Stroke
• OPISTHOTONOS: Liver Wind
MUSCULOSKELETAL/ CONNECTIVE TISSUE

Bi
• KNEES, PAIN, SORE
• SPASMS
• SPASMS, CHRONIC
ORAL CAVITY
• SPEECH, DIFFICULTY IN
• VOICE, LOSS OF
PAIN/NUMBNESS/GENERAL DISCOMFORT
• BI, LOW BACK/LIMBS
• BI, WIND DAMP: Pain, Numb Lower Back/Extremities
• NUMBNESS, EXTREMITIES: Wind Stroke/Wind Damp Bi, Stroke, Hypertension

Indications:

EYES
• VISION, BLURRED
HEAD/NECK
• FACE, PARALYSIS

• ARTHRITIS, RHEUMATIC
• BACK, LOWER PAIN/NUMB:
Wind Damp Bi
• JOINTS, PAIN: Wind Cold Damp

WIND DISORDERS
• WIND PHLEGM DIZZINESS
• WINDSTROKE: Liver Wind/Wind
Phlegm

Clinical/Pharmaceutical Studies:

CIRCULATION DISORDERS
• HYPERTENSION, ESSENTIAL/
RENAL: Helps Symptoms Of
Dizziness, Tinnitus, Extremity
Numbness
EARS/HEARING DISORDERS
• DEAFNESS: Ear/Neurological
Diseases
• TINNITUS: Ear/Neurological
Diseases
• VERTIGO: Ear/Neurological
Diseases

EYES
• EYES, PAIN, SUPRAORBITAL:
20% Solution Injection, IM, 1-3x/
Day, Marked Effects After 1-4
Injections
GALL BLADDER
• BILE SECRETION, INCREASES
**MENTAL STATE/
NEUROLOGICAL DISORDERS**
• CONVULSIVE, ANTI-: Epilepsy,
Not Strychnine, Not As Strong As
Phenobarbital (Vanillyl Alcohol,

Active Ingredient)
• SEDATIVE
• TRANQUILIZING
**MUSCULOSKELETAL/
CONNECTIVE TISSUE**
• SCIATICA: 20% Solution Injection,
IM, 1-3x/Day, Marked Effects After
1-4 Injections
**PAIN/NUMBNESS/GENERAL
DISCOMFORT**
• ANALGESIC: Heat

Dose

3 - 9 gm

Common Name

Gastrodia Rhizome

Precautions

Watch: Yin Deficiency

Notes

May Use Mi Huan Jun, (Armillaria Mellea) As
Substitute

WU GONG
(BAI JU)

蜈蚣

SCOLOPENDRA
SUBSPINIPES

Traditional Functions:

1. Subdues Liver Wind and reduces spasms
2. Dispels toxins and disperses lumps or hardenings by topical application
3. Clears the channels and relieves pain

Traditional Properties:

Enters: LV,

Properties: SP, W, TX

Indications:

• UMBILICAL WIND
**CANCER/TUMORS/SWELLINGS/
LUMPS**
• CANCER: Decoct With Jin Yin Hua
• NECK LUMPS: Topical
• NODULES, TOXIC: Topical
• TUMORS
CHILDHOOD DISORDERS
• CONVULSIONS, CHILDHOOD
HEAD/NECK
• HEAD, SCALDED
• HEAD, SORES: Topical
• HEADACHE, PERSISTENT
• LOCKJAW
• NECK, LUMPS: Topical
• TICS

**IMMUNE SYSTEM RELATED
DISORDERS/TOPICS**
• LYMPH NODES, SWELLING:
Topical
INFECTIOUS DISEASES
• JOINT TUBERCULOSIS
• TETANUS, NEONATAL
• TUBERCULOSIS, BONES
**MENTAL STATE/
NEUROLOGICAL DISORDERS**
• EPILEPSY
• OPISTHOTONOS
• SEIZURES
• TREMORS
**MUSCULOSKELETAL/
CONNECTIVE TISSUE**

• ARTHRITIS, PAIN
• JOINTS, TUBERCULOSIS
• SPASMS
ORAL CAVITY
• TOOTHACHE
**PAIN/NUMBNESS/GENERAL
DISCOMFORT**
• BI DISORDERS
SKIN
• BOILS: Topical
• SKIN, ULCERS
• SORES, INFECTED: Topical
TRAUMA, BITES, POISONINGS
• BUG BITES
• SNAKE BITES, POISONOUS:
Topical

Clinical/Pharmaceutical Studies:

**BLOOD RELATED DISORDERS/
TOPICS**
• BLOOD PRESSURE, LOWERS:
10% ETOH Extract

DISORDERS/TOPICS
• LYMPHADENITIS, ACUTE
SUBMANDIBULAR: Decoctions
INFECTIOUS DISEASES

**MENTAL STATE/
NEUROLOGICAL DISORDERS**
• CONVULSIVE, ANTI-: Cocaine,
Caffeine, Nicotine, Camphor, Not

Clinical/Pharmaceutical Studies:

CANCER/TUMORS/SWELLINGS/
LUMPS
• TUMOR, ANTI-
IMMUNE SYSTEM RELATED

• BACTERIAL, ANTI-: Aqueous
Extract Inhibits TB
• DIPHTHERIA: Powdered w/Gan
Cao, 90%

Strychnine
SKIN
• FUNGAL, ANTI-: Strong

Dose

1.5 - 4.5 gm

Common Name

Centipede

Contraindications

Not: Pregnancy

Notes

Toxic, Watch Overdose
Topical Tincture For Bites
0.6-1 gm In pwdr

Fragrant Herbs For Opening The Orifices

AN XI XIANG   安息香   *BENZOINUM*

Traditional Functions:

1. Opens the orifices and transform Phlegm
2. Regulates and moves the Qi and Blood

Traditional Properties:

Enters: LU, SP, ST, HT,

Properties: BIT, SP, N

Indications:

ABDOMEN/
  GASTROINTESTINAL TOPICS
• ABDOMEN, PAIN OF
CHEST
• CHEST, PAIN
CIRCULATION DISORDERS
• FAINTING

• STROKE
HEART
• ANGINA PECTORIS: Chest Bi
  Strangulating Pain
MENTAL STATE/
  NEUROLOGICAL DISORDERS
• CONSCIOUSNESS, MENTAL

CLOUDINESS: Excess (Shut-In
  Complex)
SEXUALITY, FEMALE:
  GYNECOLOGICAL
• POSTPARTUM, BLOOD LOSS/
  FAINTING

Clinical/Pharmaceutical Studies:

INFECTIOUS DISEASES
• BACTERIAL, ANTI-
LUNGS
• BRONCHITIS: Inhale, Watch Large
  Amounts Which Can Irritate Eyes,

Nose, Throat
• EXPECTORANT: Tincture, In
  Water, Boiled, Direct Inhalation,
  Watch Irritation
MENTAL STATE/

NEUROLOGICAL DISORDERS
• STIMULANT, CNS
SKIN
• FUNGAL, ANTI-: Tinea, Topical

Dose

1.5 - 3.0 gm

Common Name

Benzoin

Contraindications

Not: Yin Def w/Excess Fire

Precautions

Watch: People With Liver Malfunction, Detoxified In
Liver

BING PIAN   冰片   *BORNEOL*
(LONG NAO)

Traditional Functions:

1. Aromatically opens the orifices and clears the mind
2. Dissipates congested Fire, controls pain and removes swelling & nodules
3. Moves the Qi and vitalizes Blood
4. Removes visual opacity and clears the vision

Traditional Properties:

Enters: LU, HT,

Properties: SP, BIT, CL

Indications:

BOWEL RELATED DISORDERS
• HEMORRHOIDS
CIRCULATION DISORDERS
• FAINTING: High Fever
• STROKE
• STROKE, MOUTH TIGHTNESS

MENTAL STATE/
  NEUROLOGICAL DISORDERS
• CONVULSIONS: High Fever
• MENTAL CLOUDINESS: Excess
  Heat, Shut-In
• UNCONSCIOUSNESS: (Mental

• TOOTHACHE: External
PHLEGM
• PHLEGM OBSTRUCTION
SKIN
• BOILS: Topical
• FUNGAL INFECTIONS

Indications:

EYES
- CORNEAL OPACITY: Topical
- EYES, DISEASES OF: Topical
- PHOTOPHOBIA: Topical
- TEARING, EXCESSIVE: Topical

HEART
- ANGINA PECTORIS: Chest Bi Strangulating Pain

Cloudiness) , Excess Heat (Shut-In)
ORAL CAVITY
- CANKERS
- MOUTH, SPASMS: (Trismus)
- THROAT, SWOLLEN/PAIN: Topical
- TONSILLITIS

- PRURITUS
- SCABIES: Topical
- SKIN, DISORDERS: Topical
- SKIN, SORES, SWOLLEN, TOXIC: Topical

TRAUMA, BITES, POISONINGS
- TRAUMA, INJURIES: Die Da

Clinical/Pharmaceutical Studies:

EARS/HEARING DISORDERS
- EARS, OTITIS MEDIA/EXTERNA, ECZEMA W/PUS DISCHARGE: w/Alum & Boric Acid

INFECTIOUS DISEASES
- BACTERIAL, ANTI-: ETOH Extract, Staph, E.Coli, Strep, et al-

Needs 0.5% Solution
MENTAL STATE/ NEUROLOGICAL DISORDERS
- STIMULANT, CNS: Higher Centers, Like Camphor

PAIN/NUMBNESS/GENERAL DISCOMFORT

- ANALGESIC: Topical
- NEURALGIA: Topical

SKIN
- FUNGAL, ANTI-: Tinea Alba

TRAUMA, BITES, POISONINGS
- INFLAMMATORY, ANTI-

Dose
0.3 - 0.9 gm

Common Name
Borneol Camphor Resin

Contraindications
Not: Def Qi/Blood

Precautions
Watch: Pregnancy

Notes
Absorbed Thru Skin, Mucous Membranes

JIU JIE CHANG PU

九節菖蒲
（九节菖蒲）

RHIZOMA ANEMONI ALTAICAE

Traditional Functions:

1. Harmonizes the Stomach
2. Dispels Wind Phlegm and Dampness

Traditional Properties:

Enters: HT, ST

Properties: SP, W

Indications:

MENTAL STATE/ NEUROLOGICAL DISORDERS
- CONSCIOUSNESS, IMPAIRED
- EPILEPSY

- INSANITY
- MELANCHOLIA

STOMACH/DIGESTIVE

DISORDERS
- ANOREXIA
- STOMACH, DISTENTION

Dose
3 - 6 gm

Common Name
Altaica

Contraindications
Not: Excess Perspiration

Not: Spermatorrhea

Notes
May Be Used Singly

NIU HUANG

牛黃
（牛黃）

CALCULUS BOVIS

Traditional Functions:

1. Opens the orifices and transform Phlegm
2. Subdues Liver Wind by calming fright and tremors
3. Subdues Heat and relieves toxic Heat

Traditional Properties:

Enters: HT, LV,

Properties: >BIT, SW, CL

Indications:

**CANCER/TUMORS/SWELLINGS/
LUMPS**
• SWELLINGS, INFLAMMED
FEVERS
• FEVER, LOSS OF
CONSCIOUSNESS FROM
INFECTIOUS DISEASES
• TETANUS
**MENTAL STATE/
NEUROLOGICAL DISORDERS**
• COMA: Hot Phlegm Blocking The
Pericardium/Liver Wind

• CONVULSIONS, FEVER, ACUTE
• CONVULSIONS, INFANTILE
• DELIRIUM: Hot Phlegm Blocking
The Pericardium
• EPILEPSY
• MANIA
• TREMORS: Liver Wind
• UNCONSCIOUSNESS: (Mental
Cloudiness) , Excess Heat (Shut-In)
**MUSCULOSKELETAL/
CONNECTIVE TISSUE**
• SPASMS: Liver Wind

• SPASMS, W/FEVER, ACUTE
ORAL CAVITY
• THROAT, SORE, RED, PAINFUL,
SWELLING/ULCERATED
PHLEGM
• PHLEGM, HOT, OBSTRUCT
PERICARDIUM
SKIN
• BOILS
• SORES, OOZING YIN SORES
WIND DISORDERS
• WINDSTROKE

Clinical/Pharmaceutical Studies:

**ABDOMEN/
GASTROINTESTINAL
TOPICS**
• INTESTINES, INHIBITS:
Alcohol/Water Extracts,
Water More So, Some
Components Stimulate,
Though
**BLOOD RELATED
DISORDERS/TOPICS**
• ANEMIA: Increase RBC,
In Small Doses
• BLOOD PRESSURE,
LOWERS: Marked (Up
To 50mmhg) For 2-3 Days
**BOWEL RELATED
DISORDERS**
• CONSTIPATION
• LAXATIVE, MILD
**CIRCULATION
DISORDERS**
• HYPERTENSION:
Lowers BP Long Term
EYES
• EYES, INFLAMMATION
FEVERS
• ANTIPYRETIC
GALL BLADDER
• GALL BLADDER,
CHOLAGOGUE: Bile
Secretion, Increases
HEAD/NECK

• FACE, MAXILLARY
INFLAMMATION: Niu
Huang Jiedu Wan, 100%
Effective 3-5 Days
HEART
• HEART, STIMULATES:
Stimulates, But
Vasocontrictive
**IMMUNE SYSTEM
RELATED DISORDERS/
TOPICS**
• ALLERGIES, TO
CLAMS: 0.1 g Tab, 3
Tabs 3x/Day
INFECTIOUS DISEASES
• DIPHTHERIA: Bai Hou
San--Niu Huang, Pearl,
Bing Pian, Ho PO, Sal
Ammoniac, Resina
Drasaenae, Corium
Elephantis, Long Gu,
Catechu, Mo Yao, Wu Bai
Zi, Local Spray 2-3x/Day,
Pseudomembrane Gone 1-
3 Days
• ENCEPHALITIS B: Best
When Combined With Shi
Gao, Wu Gong, Quan Xie,
Xi Jiao, Ling Yang Jiao
• INFECTIONS W/HIGH
FEVER, COMA,
DELIRUIUM: Use An

Gong Niu Huang Wan
• INFLUENZA
LUNGS
• BRONCHITIS
• RESPIRATORY TRACT
INFECTION, UPPER
• WHOOPING COUGH:
Mix With Sugar, Less Than
2 Yrs, 0.12-.24 g/Day, 2-5
Years, 0.24-.36 g, 5+Yrs,
0.36-.49 g For 1-2 Weeks
**MENTAL STATE/
NEUROLOGICAL
DISORDERS**
• CONVULSIVE, ANTI-:
Cocaine, Caffeine,
Camphor, Not Strychnine,
Strengthens Barbituates
• HYPNOTIC: Synergizes
Chloral Hydrate,
Barbituates
**MUSCULOSKELETAL/
CONNECTIVE TISSUE**
• MUSCLES, SMOOTH
STIMULATES
ORAL CAVITY
• MOUTH, ULCERS
• THROAT, SORE: Topical
Spray Powder (Chui Hou
San--Niu Huang, Alunite
Powder, She Xiang, Borax,
Hu PO, Zhu Sha, Bing

Pian, Huang Lian, Fructus
Malus Asiaticae) , 1-2 X/
Day
• TONSILLITIS
SKIN
• BOILS: Niu Huang Xing
Xiao Wan--Niu Huang,
Realger, She Xiang, Ru
Xiang, Mo Yao, 1.5-3.0 1-
2x/Day, Effective Even
With Drug Resistant Staph
Strains
• FURUNCLES
• SKIN, ULCERS,
CHRONIC: Niu Huang
San--Niu Huang, She
Xiang, Pearl, Bing Pian,
Mercurous Chloride,
Xiong Dan, Long Gu, Mu
LI, Ru Xiang, Mo Yao, Shi
Jui Ming, Huang Lian
**STOMACH/DIGESTIVE
DISORDERS**
• FAT, IMPROVES
DIGESTION OF:
Activates Pacreatic
Enzymes
**TRAUMA, BITES,
POISONINGS**
• DETOXIFIES: Combines
With Many Organics

Dose

0.15 - 1.50 gm

Common Name

Cattle/Water Buffalo

Contraindications

Not: Pregnancy
Not: Cold Phlegm

Not: Def SP/ST

Notes

Usually Pills/Powders Only

Causes Diarrhea

May Cause Skin Allergy, Relieved With Histamine
Antagonists

Generally Artificial Made Today

SHE XIANG

麝香
（麝香）

SECRETIO MOSCHUS MOSCHIFERI

Traditional Functions:

1. Aromatically opens the orifices and clears the mind
2. Vitalizes the Blood, disperses nodules and inflammation
3. Facilitates child delivery or the downward passage of stillborns
4. Promotes the flow of the Luo channels and stops pain

Traditional Properties:

Enters: SP, HT, LV,

Properties: SP, W,

Indications:

ABDOMEN/ GASTROINTESTINAL TOPICS
• ABDOMEN, PAIN OF, VIOLENT

CANCER/TUMORS/SWELLINGS/ LUMPS
• MASSES, PALPABLE, IMMOBILE: Topical, Too
• TUMORS: Blood Stasis, Herbs Used Other Than Vitalize Blood

CIRCULATION DISORDERS
• APOPLEXY
• BUERGER'S DISEASE
• FAINTING: Febrile Diseases/Heat In Pericardium
• STROKE SYNDROME

FEVERS
• FEVER, HIGH W/LOSS OF CONSCIOUSNESS

HEART
• ANGINA PECTORIS: Chest Bi Strangulating Pain

• HEART PAIN, VIOLENT

HEAT
• HEAT IN PERICARDIUM

IMMUNE SYSTEM RELATED DISORDERS/TOPICS
• LYMPH GLANDS, ENLARGEMENT, CHRONIC: Phlegm Nodules

MENTAL STATE/ NEUROLOGICAL DISORDERS
• CLOSED SYNDROME
• CONVULSIONS: Heat In Pericardium
• DELIRIUM: Heat In Pericardium
• EPILEPSY
• STUPOR: Heat In Pericardium
• UNCONSCIOUSNESS: Excess (Shut-In Complex)

PAIN/NUMBNESS/GENERAL DISCOMFORT
• BI DISORDERS: Topical

• BI, WIND DAMP, CHRONIC: With Blood Stasis, Open The Luo

PHLEGM
• PHLEGM COLLAPSE
• PHLEGM OBSTRUCTION

SEXUALITY, FEMALE: GYNECOLOGICAL
• AMENORRHEA: Blood Stasis, In Addition To Vitalize Blood Herbs
• FETUS, DEAD: Afterbirth Fails To Descend
• LOCHIA, RETENTION
• POSTPARTUM, ABDOMINAL PAIN: Blood Stasis

SKIN
• BOILS: Topical, Too
• SKIN, SORES, SWOLLEN, TOXIC: Blood Stasis, Swelling

TRAUMA, BITES, POISONINGS
• TRAUMA, INJURIES: Die Da, Clears Channels

Clinical/Pharmaceutical Studies:

• SECRETION, INCREASES OF MULTIPLE GLANDS

BLOOD RELATED DISORDERS/TOPICS
• BLOOD PRESSURE, RAISES

BOWEL RELATED DISORDERS
• FLATULENCE

CANCER/TUMORS/ SWELLINGS/LUMPS
• CANCER: Esophagus, Stomach, Liver, Colan, Rectum, Treated With Musk Implants, Good

ENDOCRINE RELATED DISORDERS
• ANDROGEN-LIKE EFFECT: In Natural Musk

HEAD/NECK
• HEADACHE, VASCULAR: Sublingual Tabs, 1.5 mg (Muscone) / Tab, 2-3x/Day, Take At First Indication Of Attack, Then 1+ Tabs During Attack, 80% Improved

HEART
• ANGINA PECTORIS: Sublingual Tabs, 4.5mg Synth Musk Each, 1-2

INFECTIOUS DISEASES
• ANTIBIOTIC: Staph A., E.Coli

KIDNEYS
• DIURETIC

LUNGS
• RESPIRATION, STIMULATES
• WHOOPING COUGH

MENTAL STATE/ NEUROLOGICAL DISORDERS
• CEREBRAL PALSY
• EPILEPSY
• SEDATIVE, LARGE DOSES

ORAL CAVITY
• EPIGLOTTIS SPASMS

PAIN/NUMBNESS/ GENERAL DISCOMFORT
• ANALGESIC

SEXUALITY, FEMALE: GYNECOLOGICAL
• UTERUS, STIMULATES: Especially Late Stage Pregnant

SKIN
• DIAPHORETIC

TRAUMA, BITES, POISONINGS
• INFLAMMATORY, ANTI-

Clinical/Pharmaceutical Studies:

Effect For Mid-Stage Cancer, Not For Advanced Cancer
• TUMOR, ANTI-
CIRCULATION DISORDERS
• STROKE

Tags, Effect In 5-10 Minutes, Effective To Relieve Suffocation, But Weaker Slower Than Nitroglycerin For Pain
• HEART, STIMULATES

• STIMULANT, CNS, SMALL DOSES
MUSCULOSKELETAL/ CONNECTIVE TISSUE
• CATECHOLAMINE-LIKE ON MUSCLES

: Strong, 3x Rutin, 40x Aspirin, Liu Shen Pill (Has Musk) Greater Than Hydrocortisone, Synergistic With Chan Su, Niu Huang

Dose
0.03 - 0.15 gm

Common Name
Musk Deer Navel Secretns

Contraindications
Not: Pregnancy

Not: Def Yin w/Heat

Notes
Do Not Cook

SHI CHANG PU
(CHANG PU)

石菖蒲

RHIZOMA
ACORI GRAMINEI

Traditional Functions:

1. Opens the orifices, expels Phlegm and disperses Wind
2. Transforms turbid Dampness and harmonizes the Stomach
3. Benefits wisdom and helps to tranquilize the mind
4. Kills worms

Traditional Properties:

Enters: SP, HT, LV,

Properties: SP, <W, ARO

Indications:

ABDOMEN/ GASTROINTESTINAL TOPICS
• ABDOMEN, DISTENTION OF: Damp Heat
• ABDOMEN, PAIN OF: Spleen Stomach Damp
• GASTROINTESTINAL DISTENTION
BOWEL RELATED DISORDERS
• DIARRHEA, SEVERE
• DYSENTERY W/ANOREXIA
CHEST
• CHEST, FULLNESS/ DISCOMFORT: Spleen Stomach Damp
EARS/HEARING DISORDERS
• DEAFNESS: Phlegm Blocking Rising Of Clear Yang
• DIZZINESS: Phlegm Blocking Rising Of Clear Yang
HEAD/NECK
• LOCKJAW
HEART

• PERICARDIUM, HEAT PHLEGM
HEAT
• HEAT, SEVERE W/ NEUROLOGICAL SYMPTOMS
MENTAL STATE/ NEUROLOGICAL DISORDERS
• AMNESIA
• COMA: Phlegm Accumulation
• DREAMING EXCESSIVE
• INSOMNIA, DREAMS, FREQUENT
• MELANCHOLIA
• MEMORY, POOR
• MENTAL CLOUDINESS: Excess, Shut-In Complex
• SEIZURES: Phlegm Blocking Rising Of Clear Yang
• SENSES, DULLED: Phlegm Blocking Rising Of Clear Yang
• STUPOR: Phlegm Blocking Rising Of Clear Yang
• UNCONSCIOUSNESS: Excess (Shut-In Complex)

MUSCULOSKELETAL/ CONNECTIVE TISSUE
• JOINTS, PAIN: Wind, Cold, Damp Bi
PAIN/NUMBNESS/GENERAL DISCOMFORT
• BI, WIND DAMP COLD
PHLEGM
• PHLEGM HEAT IN PERICARDIUM
QI RELATED DISORDERS/ TOPICS
• QI OBSTRUCTION
SKIN
• CARBUNCLES: Topical
• ULCERS, SKIN: Damp, Topical
SPLEEN
• SPLEEN DAMPNESS W/PAIN
STOMACH/DIGESTIVE DISORDERS
• ANOREXIA
• EPIGASTRIC DISTENTION: Spleen Stomach Damp

Clinical/Pharmaceutical Studies:

ABDOMEN/ GASTROINTESTINAL TOPICS
• GASTROINTESTINAL SECRETIONS INCREASES
• GASTROINTESTINAL, RELAXES SPASMS

• ASTHMA, BRONCHIAL: Volatile Oil Preparations, 120 mg 1x/Day, For Greater Than 20 Days
MENTAL STATE/ NEUROLOGICAL DISORDERS
• COMA: Pulmonary Brain

Day For Greater Than 3 Months, Synergistic
• SEDATIVE: Volatile Oils, Reduces Effects Of Ephedrine, Prolongs Barbituates
MUSCULOSKELETAL/ CONNECTIVE TISSUE

Muscle Of Intestine
PARASITES
• WORMS, ASCARIASIS: Kills And Paralyzes 70% In Culture
SKIN
• FUNGAL, ANTI-: Aqueous Extract, Inhibits

Clinical/Pharmaceutical Studies:

- INTESTINES, SPASMS, RELIEVES

CANCER/TUMORS/ SWELLINGS/LUMPS
- CANCER: Kills Ascitic Carcinoma Cells In Mice

INFECTIOUS DISEASES
- BACTERIAL, ANTI-

KIDNEYS
- DIURETIC

LUNGS

Diseases/Encephalitis/ Liver Cirrhosis/Cerebral Hemorhage--Injection Of Volatile Oil 10 mg/2 ml, 2-4 ml IM, 2-6x/Day
- EPILEPSY, GRAND MAL: Primary/Cranio Cerebral Trauma, Patients Less Than 20 Yrs With Less Than 5 Yrs History, 33% Decoction, 10 ml, 3x/

- ANTISPASMODIC

NUTRITIONAL/ METABOLIC DISORDERS/TOPICS
- BODY TEMPERATURE, LOWERS
- HYPOTHERMIA

PAIN/NUMBNESS/ GENERAL DISCOMFORT
- ANALGESIC: Smooth

Many, Trichopytons, Skin Fungi, Use High Concentration Of Maceration Extract
- SKIN, IRRITATES: Topical

STOMACH/DIGESTIVE DISORDERS
- STOMACHIC: Stimulates Digestive Secretion

Dose

3 - 9 gm

Common Name

Sweetflag Rhizome

Contraindications

Not: Excess Perspiration

Precautions

Watch: Def Yin w/Heat

Notes

Add Last 5-10 Min Of Decoction

Toxic In Large Doses, No Side Effect At 10 g/Day

Decoction For Long Term

Skin Irritation With Topical Application

For Eyes/Throat: 1.5-3 gm

For Constipation, Dysuria: 9 gm

SU HE XIANG

蘇合香
(苏合香)

STYRAX LIQUIDIS

Traditional Functions:

1. Opens the orifices and expels Phlegm turbidity
2. Clears the mind and relieves depression
3. Clears foul odor
4. Stops pain

Traditional Properties:

Enters: SP, HT,

Properties: SW, SP, W

Indications:

ABDOMEN/ GASTROINTESTINAL TOPICS
- ABDOMEN, PAIN OF, STUFFY

CHEST
- CHEST, PAIN, STUFFY

CHILDHOOD DISORDERS
- INFANTS, REGURGITATION OF MILK

CIRCULATION DISORDERS
- FAINTING: Sudden Qi Congestion
- STROKE: Closed Syndrome

HEART
- ANGINA PECTORIS: Chest Bi Strangulating Pain
- HEART DISEASE

INFECTIOUS DISEASES
- EPIDEMIC TOXIC DISEASES

MENTAL STATE/ NEUROLOGICAL DISORDERS
- CONVULSIONS, SUDDEN
- MENTAL DISORDERS

- UNCONSCIOUSNESS: Closed Syndrome Stroke

PHLEGM
- PHLEGM BLOCKAGE

STOMACH/DIGESTIVE DISORDERS
- GAS, FOUL IN STOMACH/ INTESTINES

WIND DISORDERS
- WIND PHLEGM

Clinical/Pharmaceutical Studies:

CIRCULATION DISORDERS
- STROKE

HEART
- ANGINA PECTORIS

INFECTIOUS DISEASES
- BACTERIAL, ANTI-: Especially

Respiratory

LUNGS
- EXPECTORANT: Thru Irritation Of Lung Mucosa

SKIN
- ECZEMA: In Olive Oil, Some

Effect
- SCABIES: With Olive Oil
- ULCERS, PROMOTES HEALING OF

TRAUMA, BITES, POISONINGS
- INFLAMMATORY, ANTI-: Topical

Dose

0.3 - 0.9 gm

Common Name

Rose Maloes Resin

Contraindications

Not: High Fever/Coma

Not: Spontaneous Sweat/Collapse

Not: Yin Deficiency

Precautions

Watch: Pregnancy

Tonify The Qi

BAI ZHU

白 術
（白术）

RHIZOMA ATRACTYLODIS MACROCEPHALAE

Traditional Functions:

1. Strenthens the Spleen and tonifies the Qi
2. Strengthens the Yang of the Spleen and dries Dampness
3. Consolidates the surface, controls sweating
4. Harmonizes the Spleen and Stomach
5. Prevents miscarriage and calms the fetus

Traditional Properties:

Enters: SP, ST,

Properties: BIT, SW, W

Indications:

- PROLAPSE OF ORGANS: Sinking Of Central Qi

ABDOMEN/ GASTROINTESTINAL TOPICS
- ABDOMEN, DISTENTION OF
- GASTROINTESTINAL PROBLEMS

BOWEL RELATED DISORDERS
- DIARRHEA: Cold Dampness (Add Warm Interior Herbs, Too) /Evil Fluid Dampness/Spleen Stomach Deficiency
- DIARRHEA, CHRONIC

EARS/HEARING DISORDERS
- DIZZINESS

ENERGETIC STATE
- FATIGUE: Spleen Stomach Deficiency
- WEAKNESS: Qi Deficiency

FLUID DISORDERS

- EDEMA: Fluid Retention/Spleen Deficiency
- FLUID RETENTION

KIDNEYS
- DIURETIC: Mild

LIVER
- JAUNDICE, YIN

PAIN/NUMBNESS/GENERAL DISCOMFORT
- BI, DAMP: Auxillary Herb

PHLEGM
- PHLEGM FLUID

SEXUALITY, FEMALE: GYNECOLOGICAL
- FETUS, RESTLESS, CALMS: w/ SP Deficient/Qi Deficiency With Dampness
- LEUKORRHEA: Cold, Damp
- SWELLING DURING PREGNANCY

SKIN
- PERSPIRATION, RESTING & THIEF
- PERSPIRATION, SPONTANEOUS: Deficient Qi

SPLEEN
- SPLEEN DEFICIENCY
- SPLEEN STOMACH, DAMPNESS

STOMACH/DIGESTIVE DISORDERS
- ANOREXIA: Spleen Stomach Deficiency
- DIGESTIVE DISORDERS: Spleen Yang Not Rising
- DYSPEPSIA
- VOMITING: Spleen Stomach Deficiency

URINARY BLADDER
- URINATION, DECREASED: Spleen Deficient

Clinical/Pharmaceutical Studies:

BLOOD RELATED DISORDERS/TOPICS
- BLOOD CLOTTING TIME, LENGHTHENS: Decoction Better Than Alchohol Extract, 1:20 Solution, 1 Tbl Spoon, 3x/ Day
- BLOOD GLUCOSE, REDUCES PLASMA, INCREASE ASSIMILATION OF, ORAL
- LEUKOPENIA

BOWEL RELATED DISORDERS

Most

EARS/HEARING DISORDERS
- VERTIGO: With Fu Zi, Gan Cao (Roasted) (In Jin Xiao Zhu Fu Tang) , Reduced After 1 Dose, 3 Doses To Disappear

ENDOCRINE RELATED DISORDERS
- ENDOCRINE EFFECTS: Increases Glucose Assimilation, Lowers Plasma Glu

ENERGETIC STATE
- ENDURANCE,

IMMUNE SYSTEM RELATED DISORDERS/ TOPICS
- IMMUNE SYSTEM ENHANCEMENT

INFECTIOUS DISEASES
- BACTERIAL, ANTI-

KIDNEYS
- DIURETIC: Significant, Prolonged

LIVER
- LIVER, PROTECTANT

MENTAL STATE/ NEUROLOGICAL DISORDERS
- SEDATIVE: Small Doses,

INDUCES

ORAL CAVITY
- SALIVATION: Huang Qi, Bai Zhu, Wheat Grain, Or Singly As Powder

SEXUALITY, FEMALE: GYNECOLOGICAL
- FETUS, RESTLESS: For Deficiency--Ren Shen, Bai Zhu, For Heat--Huang Qin, Bai Zhu, For Cold--Bai Zhu, Ai Ye

SKIN
- PERSPIRATION: Huang Qi, Bai Zhu, Wheat Grain, Or Singly As Powder

Clinical/Pharmaceutical Studies:

- CONSTIPATION, POST GYNECOLOGICAL OPERATION: Daily Decoction--Bai Zhu 60 g, Shu Di 30 g, Sheng Ma 3 g, 1-2 Doses Needed For

INCREASES FLUID DISORDERS
- EDEMA, FACE/LEGS/ ARMS/PREGNANCY: Wu Pi Yin With Bai Zhu

Essential Oil NUTRITIONAL/ METABOLIC DISORDERS/TOPICS
- WEIGHT GAIN,

STOMACH/DIGESTIVE DISORDERS
- DYSPEPSIA: LI Zhong Tang (Bai Zhu, Ren Shen, Gan Jiang, Gan Cao)

Dose

3 - 12 gm

Contraindications

Not: w/Thirst & Fluid Loss

Precautions

Watch: Mild Anemia/Lymphopenia If Used In Large Qty/ Long Term

Notes

Raw: Used For Dampness, Promotes Water Metabolism
Fried: Used To Strengthen Qi/SP

DA ZAO
(HONG ZAO)

大棗/紅棗
(大枣/红枣)

FRUCTUS ZIZIPHI JUJUBAE

Traditional Functions:

1. Tonifies the Spleen and benefits the Stomach
2. Nourishes the Blood, calms the Spirit
3. Moderates and harmonizes the actions of herbs
4. Moistens the Lungs and Heart

Traditional Properties:

Enters: SP, ST,

Properties: SW, W

Indications:

BLOOD RELATED DISORDERS/ TOPICS
- ANEMIA
- BLOOD INSUFFICIENCY
BOWEL RELATED DISORDERS
- DIARRHEA
ENERGETIC STATE
- WEAKNESS: Spleen Stomach Deficient
HEART
- HEART SPLEEN DEFICIENCY
- PALPITATIONS
HERBAL FUNCTIONS
- HERBS, HARSH: Harmonizes And Moderates
IMMUNE SYSTEM RELATED DISORDERS/TOPICS
- ALLERGIES

- ANAPHYLACTIC PURPURA
LIVER
- LIVER QI CONGESTION: Emotional Symptoms
LUNGS
- BREATH, SHORTNESS OF: Spleen Stomach Deficient
MENTAL STATE/ NEUROLOGICAL DISORDERS
- CONVULSIONS: Restless Organ Syndrome
- EMOTIONAL DEBILITY, SEVERE
- INSOMNIA
- INSOMNIA, DREAMS, FREQUENT
- IRRITABILITY: Spleen Heart

Deficiency/Liver Qi Stagnation
- LASSITUDE: Spleen Stomach Deficient
- MALAISE
- RESTLESSNESS
QI RELATED DISORDERS/ TOPICS
- QI INSUFFICIENCY
SKIN
- PURPURA, ANAPHYLACTIC
SPLEEN
- SPLEEN STOMACH DEFICIENCY: Weakness, Lassitude, Shortness Of Breath
STOMACH/DIGESTIVE DISORDERS
- ANOREXIA

Clinical/Pharmaceutical Studies:

- BODY: Increases Weight, Muscle Strength
ENERGETIC STATE
- ENDURANCE, INCREASES: Daily For 3 Weeks
IMMUNE SYSTEM RELATED DISORDERS/TOPICS
- ALLERGIC, ANTI-: Cyclic-Amp In Aqueous Extract

LIVER
- LIVER, RECOVERY FROM TOXIC EXPOSURE: Take For 1 Week
- LIVER, REDUCES ENZYMES: Reduces Serum Transaminase Levels In Hepatic Diseases:With Peanuts, Brown Sugar At Bedtime For 1 Month

NUTRITIONAL/METABOLIC DISORDERS/TOPICS
- WEIGHT GAIN, INDUCES: Daily For 3 Weeks
STOMACH/DIGESTIVE DISORDERS
- ULCERS, STRESS: ETOH Extract Helps

Dose

9 - 30 gm

Common Name

Jujube Fruit

Contraindications

Not: Excess Dampness, Causes Bloating

Not: With Intestinal Parasites

Precautions

Watch: Damp Sputum

DANG SHEN

黨 參
(党参)

RADIX CODONOPSIS PILOSULAE

Traditional Functions:

1. Strengthens the Spleen and Stomach
2. Tonifies the Lung and Spleen Qi
3. Nourishes fluids and promotes the secretion of fluids
4. Harmonizes the Spleen and Stomach

Traditional Properties:

Enters: LU, SP,

Properties: SW, N

Indications:

- PROLAPSED ORGAN: Uterus, Stomach, Anus:Spleen Qi Collapsed

BLOOD RELATED DISORDERS/ TOPICS
- ANEMIA
- BLOOD DEFICIENCY W/ WITHERING YELLOW COMPLEXION

BOWEL RELATED DISORDERS
- DIARRHEA: Spleen Qi Deficient

ENDOCRINE RELATED DISORDERS
- WASTING & THIRSTING SYNDROME

ENERGETIC STATE
- FATIGUE: Spleen Qi Deficient
- WEAKNESS: Qi Deficiency

EXTREMITIES
- LIMBS, TIRED: Spleen Qi

Deficient

FLUID DISORDERS
- THIRST: Fluid Injury

HEAD/NECK
- ALOPECIA: Deficiency Complex

HEART
- PALPITATIONS

HEMORRHAGIC DISORDERS
- BLEEDING, CHRONIC

LUNGS
- BREATH, SHORTNESS OF: Lung Deficient
- COUGH, CHRONIC: Lung Deficient
- LUNG QI DEFICIENCY

PHLEGM
- SPUTUM, COPIOUS: Spleen Deficient

QI RELATED DISORDERS/ TOPICS
- QI DEFICIENCY: Sinking Of Central Qi

SEXUALITY, FEMALE: GYNECOLOGICAL
- LACTATION, INSUFFICIENT: Qi, Blood Deficiency

SKIN
- SKIN, SORES, SWOLLEN, TOXIC: Helps Healing, Deficiency

SPLEEN
- SPLEEN STOMACH DEFICIENCY: Chronic Illness

STOMACH/DIGESTIVE DISORDERS
- ANOREXIA: Spleen Qi Deficient
- VOMITING: Spleen Qi Deficient

Clinical/Pharmaceutical Studies:

BLOOD RELATED DISORDERS/TOPICS
- ANEMIA: Increases RBC
- BLOOD GLUCOSE, INCREASES: Orally, 6 g/ kg, Increases, Related To Sugar Content, Though
- BLOOD PRESSURE, LOWERS: Dilates Peripheral Blood Vessels, Inhibits Adrenalin, Transient Only
- BLOOD, INCREASES RBC, HEMOGLOBIN, DECREASES WBC: Oral Powder/IV Of ETOH/

Aqueous Extract, Short-Lived--Only 2 Days For Effect
- CHLOROSIS

ENERGETIC STATE
- FATIGUE, REDUCES
- INDURANCE, INCREASES
- STRENGTH, INCREASES

IMMUNE SYSTEM RELATED DISORDERS/ TOPICS
- IMMUNE SYSTEM ENHANCEMENT: Oral, 0.25 g/Day 1-2 Weeks, Increased Phagocytosis, Similar To Huang Qi, Ling Zhi Cao, Synergistic With Ling Zhi

KIDNEYS
- NEPHRITIS, CHRONIC: Decreases Protein In Urine, *Dang Shen With Huang

NEUROLOGICAL DISORDERS
- NEUROSIS: Injection, Contains 1 g Plus 50 mg Vit B/ml, 2ml/Day IM, 2 Weeks, Some Effectiveness
- STIMULANT, CNS: 6-7 Mcg/kg

NUTRITIONAL/ METABOLIC DISORDERS/TOPICS
- METABOLISM, PROMOTES
- TEMPERATURE, INCREASES TOLERANCE TO HIGH

SEXUALITY, FEMALE: GYNECOLOGICAL
- PREGNANCY, MORNING SICKNESS:

50% After Only 2 Doses

SPLEEN
- SPLEEN STOMACH DEFICIENCY: Best As 2: 1 Dang Shen, Gou Qi Zi

STOMACH/DIGESTIVE DISORDERS
- ANOREXIA, LOOSE/ MUSHY STOOL: Best As 2:1 Dang Shen, Gou Qi Zi
- DIGESTION, ENHANCES
- ULCERS, GASTRIC: Liu Wei Tang (Dang Shen, Bai Zhu, Fu Ling, Mu Xiang, Sha Ren, Roasted Gan Cao), Benefited, 10% Had Short Term Cure

TRAUMA, BITES, POISONINGS
- INFLAMMATION,

Clinical/Pharmaceutical Studies:

- THROMBOCYTOPENIA
CANCER/TUMORS/
SWELLINGS/LUMPS
- CHEMOTHERAPY:
Increases WBC
- LEUKEMIA

Qi, *Dang Shen Gui LU
Wan (Dang Shen, Gui Ban
Jiao, LU Jiao Jiao, E Jiao,
Shu Di, Dang Gui)
MENTAL STATE/

Liu Jun Zi Tang (Dang
Shen, Bai Zhu, Fu Ling,
Chen Pi, Ban Xia, Roasted
Gan Cao) , Vomiting
Stopped After 2-14 Doses,

INHIBITS
- OPERATION, POST: SI
Jun Zi Tang, Especially If
On Stomach, 16-24 Hrs
After Surgery

Dose

3 - 30 gm

Common Name

"Relative Root"

Contraindications

Not: LI LU, Counteracts

Notes

About 10x < Ren Shen

Single Herb: 90-120 gm

No Ill Effects, Extremely Large Doses (>60 g/Dose)

May Cause Epigastric Discomfort

GAN CAO

(SHENG GAN CAO)

甘草

RADIX
GLYCYRRHIZAE
URALENSIS

Traditional Functions:

1. Tonifies the Spleen and replenishes the Qi
2. Moistens the Lungs and controls coughs
3. Clears Heat and resolves toxic Heat
4. Moderates and harmonizes the actions of other herbs
5. Relaxes spasms and stops acute pain
6. Antidote to toxic substances, internally or topically

Traditional Properties:

Enters: SP, ST,

Properties: SW, N

Indications:

**BLOOD RELATED DISORDERS/
TOPICS**
- BLOOD DEFICIENCY W/BI
BOWEL RELATED DISORDERS
- DIARRHEA: Loose Stools, Spleen
Deficiency
**CANCER/TUMORS/SWELLINGS/
LUMPS**
- SWELLINGS, TOXIC
CHILDHOOD DISORDERS
- TOXICOSIS, CHILDHOOD
**ENDOCRINE RELATED
DISORDERS**
- ADDISON'S DISEASE
ENERGETIC STATE
- WEAKNESS: Qi Deficient
FEVERS
- FEVER, FROM EXHAUSTION
FLUID DISORDERS
- THIRST: Stomach Deficiency
HEART
- PALPITATIONS: Deficient Qi/

Blood
HERBAL FUNCTIONS
- HERBS, GUIDING TO ALL 12 CH
- HERBS, MODERATING,
HARMONIZES
INFECTIOUS DISEASES
- INFECTIONS: Topical, Too
LUNGS
- ASTHMA
- COUGH: Hot/Cold Dry Lung
**MENTAL STATE/
NEUROLOGICAL DISORDERS**
- MALAISE: Qi Deficient
**MUSCULOSKELETAL/
CONNECTIVE TISSUE**
- SPASMS, PAINFUL IN ABDOMEN
& LEGS
ORAL CAVITY
- THROAT, SORE: Topical, Too
**PAIN/NUMBNESS/GENERAL
DISCOMFORT**
- NUMBNESS W/SPASMS,

CONTRACTURES: Blood
Deficiency Bi
**QI RELATED DISORDERS/
TOPICS**
- QI DEFICIENCY
**SEXUALITY, FEMALE:
GYNECOLOGICAL**
- FETAL TOXICOSIS
SKIN
- CARBUNCLES: Topical, Too
- SORES: Topical, Too
SPLEEN
- SPLEEN STOMACH
DEFICIENCY
**STOMACH/DIGESTIVE
DISORDERS**
- STOMACH, ACHE
- ULCERS, PEPTIC
TRAUMA, BITES, POISONINGS
- TOXINS, ANTIDOTE: Topical,
Too

Clinical/Pharmaceutical Studies:

**ABDOMEN/
GASTROINTESTINAL
TOPICS**
- INTESTINES, REDUCES
SPASMS
BLOOD RELATED

EFFECT
- DIABETES INSIPIDUS:
Herb Powder, 5g, 4x/Day
Helped
- GLUCOCORTICOID
EFFECT: Similar To And

Hepatomegaly, Pain
- JAUNDICE: Hepatitis
- LIVER, REDUCES
TOXIC EFFECTS:
Prevents Fat Deposition In,
Fibrin Proliferation

Effects
SKIN
- ULCERS: Helps To
Control
- ULCERS, INHIBITS
FORMATION, PAIN:

Clinical/Pharmaceutical Studies:

DISORDERS/TOPICS
- CHOLESTEROL LOWERS IN HYPERTENSION
- THROMBOCYTOPENIC PURPURA: Decoction, 30 g, 2x/Day

CANCER/TUMORS/ SWELLINGS/LUMPS
- GRANULOMA: Inhibits
- HEPATIC CANCER, ASCITIC: Inhibits
- OBERLING-GUERIN MYELOMA: Inhibits

CIRCULATION DISORDERS
- ATHEROSCLEROSIS: Stopped Progression Of Lesions, Reduced Cholesterol

EARS/HEARING DISORDERS
- EARS, PROTECTS AGAINST STREPTOMYCIN TOXICITY

ENDOCRINE RELATED DISORDERS
- ADDISON'S DISEASE: 15 ml Extract 1/Day, Improved Symptoms, But Could Not Stop Crisis Development, Patients Developed Sensitivity To Gan Cao, After Several Weeks Reduce Dose To 1/10 As Initial
- ADDISON'S DISEASE, EARLY STAGE: Best Used With Corticosteroids
- ALDOSTERONE

Synergistic With Cortisone
- GOITER: With Kun Bu/ Hai Zao
- PITUITARY, POSTPARTUM ANTERIOR INSUFFICIENCY: Cured By Gan Cao, Ren Shen

EXTREMITIES
- LEGS, SPASMS: Gastrocnemius Muscle:10-15 ml, 2x/Day Of Herb Extract, 3-6 Days

EYES
- EYES, INFLAMMATION: Herpeti Keratitis, Keratoconjunctivitis, Fasicular Keratitis, etc, Eye Drops Of 10-30% Extract, 3-4x/Day, 2-7 Days To Cure

FEVERS
- ANTIPYRETIC

GALL BLADDER
- GALL BLADDER, CHOLAGOGUE

IMMUNE SYSTEM RELATED DISORDERS/ TOPICS
- ALLERGIC DISORDERS: Inhibits Histamine Induced Capillary Permeability

LIVER
- HEPATIC CANCER, ASCITIC: Inhibits
- HEPATITIS, INFECTIOUS: 100% Decoction, 15-20 ml, 3x/ Day For 10-20 Days, Helped Jaundice, Bile,

LUNGS
- ANTITUSSIVE: Reduces Stimuli On Throat Mucosa, Similar In Strength To Codeine
- ASTHMA, BRONCHIAL, CHRONIC: Powdered, 3-11 Days
- EXPECTORANT
- TUBERCULOSIS, PULMONARY: As Adjunct To Anti-TB Drugs, Very Effective, 18 g Decocted To 150 ml, Given 3x/Day With TB Drugs, Good For Patients With Poor Results From Previous Treatment

MENTAL STATE/ NEUROLOGICAL DISORDERS
- CONVULSIVE, ANTI-: Synergistic With Bai Shao

MUSCULOSKELETAL/ CONNECTIVE TISSUE
- MUSCLES, SPASMS, PARAMYOTONIA CONGENITA: 15 Day Course

PAIN/NUMBNESS/ GENERAL DISCOMFORT
- ANALGESIC: Weak

SEXUALITY, MALE: UROLOGICAL TOPICS
- TESTICLES, UNDERDEVELOPMENT, SHEEHAN'S SYNDROME: Herb Powder 10 g, 3x/Day With Methyl-Testosterone, Good

Very Effective, 1-3 Weeks, Powder, Possible Edema, Not Useful With Complications

STOMACH/DIGESTIVE DISORDERS
- STOMACH: Reduces Gastric Acid
- ULCERS, PEPTIC: Herb Extract, 15 ml, 4x/Day For 6 Weeks, Good Effects, Herb Powder Best, 2.5-5.0 g, 3x/Day For 3-4 Weeks, Also Gan Cao, Honey, Wa Leng Zi, Chen Pi And Shell Of Sepiella Maindroni

TRAUMA, BITES, POISONINGS
- ANTIHISTAMINE
- FROSTBITE: Yuan Hua, Gan Cao, 9 g Each, Decocted In 2000 ml Water, Wash Affected Parts 3x/ Day, 75% Cure In 1-3 Treatments
- INFLAMMATORY, ANTI-: Less Than Cortisone, Similar Action, Synergistic With, Inhibits Breakdown Of
- SNAKE BITES: Abolishes Lethal Effect Of Toxins Of
- TOXINS, ANTIDOTE FOR MANY SUBSTANCES: Varies-- Strychnine, Histamine, Diptheria, Tetanus, Streptomycin

Dose

1.5 - 9.0 gm

Common Name

Raw Licorice Root

Contraindications

Not: Excess Dampness w/Distension In Chest/Abdomen/ Vomit

Precautions

Watch: Diabetes, Elderly, Heart, Renal Disease Patients

Notes

Very Low Toxiciy

HUANG JING

黄精
（黃精）

RHIZOMA POLYGONATI

Traditional Functions:

1. Tonifies the Spleen and Stomach
2. Moistens the Lungs and relieves coughing
3. Tonifies the Essence and marrow after prolonged illness

Traditional Properties:

Enters: LU, SP,

Properties: SW, N

Indications:

BLOOD RELATED DISORDERS/ TOPICS
- BLOOD DEFICIENCY W/ WITHERING YELLOW COMPLEXION

ENDOCRINE RELATED DISORDERS
- DIABETES: Internal Heat With Exhaustion Thirst
- WASTING & THIRSTING SYNDROME

ENERGETIC STATE
- BODY WEAKNESS, DEFICIENT

- DEBILITY, GENERAL
- FATIGUE
- RECOVERY, LONG ILLNESS

FLUID DISORDERS
- THIRST

HEAD/NECK
- ALOPECIA: Deficiency Complex

LUNGS
- BRONCHITIS, CHRONIC COUGH OF
- COUGH: Lung Dryness
- COUGH, TUBERCULOSIS
- LUNG QI DEFICIENCY COUGH

- LUNG YIN DEFICIENCY COUGH

SEXUALITY, FEMALE: GYNECOLOGICAL
- MENSTRUATION, DISORDERS OF: Tonify Chong, Ren, Essence, Blood

SPLEEN
- SPLEEN STOMACH DEFICIENCY

STOMACH/DIGESTIVE DISORDERS
- ANOREXIA

Clinical/Pharmaceutical Studies:

BLOOD RELATED DISORDERS/TOPICS
- BLOOD GLUCOSE: Slowly Increases Then Decreases
- BLOOD PRESSURE, LOWERS: Both Alcohol, Decoctions
- BLOOD, TRIGLYCERIDES: Markedly Decreases, 100% Decoction, 2x/Day, 30 Days

CIRCULATION DISORDERS

- ATHEROSCLEROSIS: Helps To Prevent, Mild

HEART
- ANGINA PECTORIS: With Bai Shao, Helps Pain, Improves Blood Flow
- HEART DISEASE: With Bai Shao
- HEART, INCREASES CORONARY BLOOD FLOW: ETOH Preparation, 0.2 g/kg, Equal To Aminophylline, 0.75mg/kg

INFECTIOUS DISEASES
- ANTIBIOTIC: TB, B. Typhi, Staph.Aureus

LIVER
- LIVER, REDUCES TOXIC EFFECTS: Protects Fatty Infiltration Of

LUNGS
- TUBERCULOSIS: Oral, 1 g/kg 1x/Day, 60 Days, Start When Lymph Glands Begin To Swell, Significant Effect Against

TB, Did Not Cure, *Fluid Extract For 2 Months, Excellent Therapeutic Effects, Some Cured
- TUBERCULOSIS, PULMONARY: Inhibits In Vivo, 2 Months, Much Improvement

SKIN
- FUNGAL, ANTI-: Many
- SKIN, TINEA: Topical, Cure In 2-30 Days, Acute Responds Better, Helps Genital, Foot Tinea, Too

Dose

6 - 30 gm

Contraindications

Not: Def SP w/Dampness Or Poor Digestion
Not: Cough With Profuse Sputum
Not: Diarrhea From SP/ST Cold

HUANG QI

黄芪
（黃芪））

RADIX ASTRAGALI

Traditional Functions:

1. Replenishes the Qi of the Spleen and Stomach
2. Causes the Yang Qi of the Spleen and Stomach to ascend
3. Benefits the Qi and consolidates the surface, controls sweating
4. Promotes urination and disperses swelling caused by a deficiency pattern
5. Promotes the discharge of pus and speeds healing
6. Tonifies and nourishes the Qi and Blood
7. Used for Wasting and Thirsting syndrome

Traditional Properties:

Enters: LU, SP,

Properties: SW, <W

Indications:

- PROLAPSE OF ORGANS: Sinking Of Central Qi

BLOOD RELATED DISORDERS/ TOPICS
- BLOOD DEFICIENCY W/ WITHERING YELLOW COMPLEXION
- BLOOD LOSS, SEVERE: Used In

- NEPHRITIS, CHRONIC: With Edema, Proteinuria--30-60 gm

LUNGS
- LUNG DEFICIENCY
- SHORTNESS OF BREATH: Lung Deficient

PAIN/NUMBNESS/GENERAL DISCOMFORT

SINKING OF
- CARBUNCLES, PREMATURE
- DIAPHORESIS, PROMOTES: When Diaphoretics Do Not Work
- PERSPIRATION, RESTING & THIEF
- SKIN, SORES, SWOLLEN, TOXIC: Helps Healing, Deficiency

Indications:

Recovery Phase
BOWEL RELATED DISORDERS
• ANAL PROLAPSE
• DIARRHEA: Spleen Deficiency
ENDOCRINE RELATED DISORDERS
• DIABETES: Internal Heat With Exhaustion Thirst
• WASTING & THIRSTING SYNDROME
ENERGETIC STATE
• FATIGUE: Spleen Deficient
• WEAKNESS: Qi Deficiency
FLUID DISORDERS
• EDEMA: Spleen Deficiency
HEAD/NECK
• ALOPECIA: Deficiency Complex
INFECTIOUS DISEASES
• COMMON COLD, FREQUENT
KIDNEYS

• BI DISORDERS
• NUMBNESS: 30-60 gm
QI RELATED DISORDERS/ TOPICS
• QI DEFICIENCY: Original Qi
• QI DEFICIENCY BLOOD DETACHMENT
SEXUALITY, FEMALE: GYNECOLOGICAL
• LACTATION, INSUFFICIENT: Qi, Blood Deficiency
• MENSTRUATION, DISORDERS OF: Tonify Qi Of Chong, Ren
• POSTPARTUM, FEVER: Qi And Blood Deficient
• UTERINE BLEEDING
• UTERUS, PROLAPSE
SKIN
• ABSCESS, YIN, INTERNAL

• SORES, SUPPURATIVE: But Not Drained Or Healed Well
• SURFACE DEFICIENCY
• SWEATING, EXCESSIVE: Deficient Qi/Yang/Yin
• SWEATING, FURTIVE
• SWEATING, SPONTANEOUS: Deficient
• ULCERS, CHRONIC, NONHEALING: Topical
SPLEEN
• SPLEEN DEFICIENCY: Anorexia, Fatigue, Diarrhea
STOMACH/DIGESTIVE DISORDERS
• ANOREXIA: Spleen Deficient
• STOMACH, PROLAPSE
TRAUMA, BITES, POISONINGS
• WOUNDS, INTRACTABLE

Clinical/Pharmaceutical Studies:

BLOOD RELATED DISORDERS/TOPICS
• BLOOD GLUCOSE: Decreases
• BLOOD PRESSURE, LOWERS: Vasodilator
• LEUKOPENIA, CHRONIC: Injection IM, 100% 2ml/Day, 1-2 Weeks
CIRCULATION DISORDERS
• STROKE, POST
• VASODILATOR: Renal In Hypertension, Skin
ENDOCRINE RELATED DISORDERS
• HORMONE-LIKE: Prolongs Estrus In Mice
ENERGETIC STATE
• ENDURANCE, INCREASES
GERIATRIC TOPICS
• AGING PROCESS: Reduced At Cell Level
HEART
• CARDIOTONIC: Significant In Cardiac Failure From Poisoning Or

Fatigue
IMMUNE SYSTEM RELATED DISORDERS/ TOPICS
• IMMUNE SYSTEM ENHANCEMENT: Increases Phagocytosis, Size Of Spleen, Plasma Cells And Antibodies, 32% Decoction PO For 2 Weeks, Use As Ling Zhi Cao Mixture (Herb, Dang Shen, Ling Zhi Cao), Resembled Interferon Mediator, Tilorone
INFECTIOUS DISEASES
• BACTERIAL, ANTI-: Active Against Staph, Strep, Pneumococci, Coryn, Diphtheriae, B. Dysenteriae
• COMMON COLD: Oral Or Nasal Spray Protects Against, Especially If Susceptible Then Use 2-8 Weeks To Increase SIGA, * For Prophylactic Effect Huang Qi, Shan Yao, Bai

Zhu, Shu Di, Chen Pi, Fu Ling, Shorten Course, Reduces Incidence
• LEPROSY
• VIRAL, ANTI-: In Sense That Could Inhibit Pathogenicity Of Virus
KIDNEYS
• DIURETIC: Moderate, Prolonged
• PYELONEPHRITIS, CHRONIC
LIVER
• HEPATITIS, CHRONIC/ PERSISTENT: Injection, 1-2 Months, SGPT Levels Normalized 80% Of Responsive Patients
• HEPATITIS, TOXIC: Oral 100% Decoction Protects Liver
LUNGS
• BRONCHITIS, CHRONIC
MENTAL STATE/ NEUROLOGICAL DISORDERS
• CNS, STIMULANT

NUTRITIONAL/ METABOLIC DISORDERS/TOPICS
• METABOLISM: Increased Life Of Cells And Induced Vigorous Growth
• WEIGHT GAIN, INDUCES
SEXUALITY, FEMALE: GYNECOLOGICAL
• UTERUS, CONTRACTS
STOMACH/DIGESTIVE DISORDERS
• ULCERS, GASTRIC/ DUODENAL: Injection Of Alcohol Precipitated Decoction, 1g/ml IM 2 ml 2x/Day For 1 Month, * Huang Qi Jian Zhong Tang 25 Days, 50% Cured
URINARY BLADDER
• CHYLURIA
• PROTEINURIA, REDUCES: Needs High Doses
• URINARY RETENTION, POSTPARTUM

Not: Qi Stagnation, Dampness, Food Retention, Early Boils

Dose
9 - 30 gm

Common Name
Milk-Vetch Root

Contraindications
Not: Def Yin w/Heat
Not: Exterior Excess Heat

Notes
Prepare With Honey To Tonify Spleen Stomach Qi
w/Wine To Tonify The Essence
w/Salt To Tonify The Kidney

JING MI   粳米   SEMEN ORYZAE

Traditional Functions:

1. Strengthens the Spleen and tonifies the Stomach
2. Promotes urination and removes edema from deficiency

Traditional Properties:

Enters: SP, ST,

Properties: SW, N

Indications:

BOWEL RELATED DISORDERS
• DIARRHEA FROM SUMMER HEAT
ENERGETIC STATE
• FATIGUE
FLUID DISORDERS

• THIRST, DEFICIENT YIN
SKIN
• SWEATING, SPONTANEOUS
STOMACH/DIGESTIVE DISORDERS
• ANOREXIA

• DYSPEPSIA
URINARY BLADDER
• OLIGURIA
YIN RELATED DISORDERS/ TOPICS
• THIRST, DEFICIENT YIN

Clinical/Pharmaceutical Studies:

CANCER/TUMORS/SWELLINGS/   LUMPS

• TUMORS: Liver w/Ascites

Dose

As Decoctn

Common Name

Rice

Contraindications

Not: w/o ST Weakness/Def

REN SHEN   人參   RADIX CHINESE GINSENG

Traditional Functions:

1. Strongly tonifies the original Qi
2. Tonifies the Spleen and Lungs
3. Benefits the Lung Yin and promotes bodily fluids of all Yin organs
4. Calms the spirit and benefits the Heart

Traditional Properties:

Enters: LU, SP,

Properties: SW, <BIT, <W

Indications:

• PROLAPSE OF ORGANS: Sinking Of Central Qi
• SHOCK: 30 Gms
ABDOMEN/ GASTROINTESTINAL TOPICS
• ABDOMEN, DISTENTION OF
• GASTROINTESTINAL DISORDERS
BOWEL RELATED DISORDERS
• DIARRHEA: Spleen Deficiency
• DIARRHEA, CHRONIC
• RECTAL PROLAPSE
CHEST
• CHEST, DISTENTION
ENDOCRINE RELATED DISORDERS
• DIABETES: Internal Heat With Exhaustion Thirst
ENERGETIC STATE
• FATIGUE
• WEAKNESS: Qi Deficiency
EXTREMITIES
• LIMBS, COLD: Collapsed Qi

HEART
• ANGINA PECTORIS: Chest Bi Strangulating Pain
• PALPITATIONS W/ANXIETY: Blood/Qi Deficient
HEMORRHAGIC DISORDERS
• BLEEDING, SEVERE LOSS
LUNGS
• ASTHMA, ACUTE
• COUGH, DEFICIENT W/ DYSPNEA
• RESPIRATION SHALLOW: Collapsed Qi
• SHORTNESS OF BREATH: Collapsed Qi/Lung Qi Deficient
• WHEEZING: Lung Qi Deficient With Kidneys Unable To Grasp Qi
MENTAL STATE/ NEUROLOGICAL DISORDERS
• CONVULSIONS, CHILDHOOD CHRONIC
• FORGETFULNESS: Blood/Qi Deficient

• RESTLESSNESS: Blood/Qi Deficient
QI RELATED DISORDERS/ TOPICS
• COLLAPSED QI
• QI, BLOOD FLUID INSUFFICIENCY
• QI, ZHONG DEFICIENCY
SEXUALITY, EITHER SEX
• INFERTILITY: Uterine Cold Palace
SEXUALITY, FEMALE: GYNECOLOGICAL
• MENORRHAGIA
• MENSTRUATION, DISORDERS OF: Tonify Qi Of Chong, Ren
• UTERUS, PROLAPSE
SEXUALITY, MALE: UROLOGICAL TOPICS
• IMPOTENCE
SKIN
• PERSPIRATION, RESTING
• SWEATING, PROFUSE: Collapsed Qi

Indications:

FEVERS
- FEVER, HIGH W/FLUIDS DAMAGED

FLUID DISORDERS
- THIRST: Fluid Injury
- THIRST, RELENTLESS

- INSOMNIA: Blood/Qi Deficient
- INSOMNIA, DREAMS, FREQUENT
- LETHARGY
- MEMORY, POOR

STOMACH/DIGESTIVE DISORDERS
- ANOREXIA
- STOMACH REFLUX
- STOMACH, PROLAPSE

Clinical/Pharmaceutical Studies:

- ANTIBIOTICS, REDUCES LOSS OF INTESTINAL FLORA
- SHOCK, ACUTE: Large Doses To Stabilize Blood Pressure

ABDOMEN/ GASTROINTESTINAL TOPICS
- INTESTINES, FLORA, REDUCES LOSS OF, BY ANTIBIOTICS

BLOOD RELATED DISORDERS/TOPICS
- BLOOD PRESSURE: Small Doses, Lowers, Large Doses, Slight Increase
- BLOOD, INCREASES RBC
- CHOLESTEROL, LOWERS: In Those With High Cholesterol Readings
- CHOLESTEROL, W/ HIGH LIPIDS: Aqueous Extract Concentrated 5x, 40 mg Daily

BOWEL RELATED DISORDERS
- DIARRHEA, INFANTILE

CANCER/TUMORS/ SWELLINGS/LUMPS
- INTESTINAL CANCER: Synergistic With Chemotherapy
- STOMACH CANCER: Synergistic With Chemotherapy
- TUMORS: Increases Resistance Of Patient To And Inhibits Growth

CIRCULATION DISORDERS
- HYPOTENSION: Extract/ Tincture

ENDOCRINE RELATED DISORDERS
- DIABETES MELLITUS: Aqueous Extract, Reduced Glucose 40-50 mg%, Lasted 2 Weeks After Drug, May Allow Reduction Of Insulin Dose, w/Shu Di

Helped Symptoms
- ENDOCRINE: Increases Basal Metabolic Rate With Large Doses For Short Term
- INSULIN: Synergistic
- PITUITARY GLAND, ANTERIOR HYPOFUNCTION: Gan Cao + Ginseng
- THYROID, INCREASE FUNCTION OF: Short Term With Large Doses

ENERGETIC STATE
- FATIGUE, REDUCES

FLUID DISORDERS
- ANTIDIURETIC

HEART
- ANGINA PECTORIS
- ARRHYTHMIAS: Catecholamine-Induced
- CORONARY HEART DISEASE, ATHEROSCLEROSIS
- HEART DISEASE: Helps To Utilize Nutrients And Improves Function
- HEART, STRENGTHENS: More From Alcohol Extracts Than Water Extracts
- MITRAL VALVULAR DEFECT
- MYOCARDIAL DYSTROPHY
- SHOCK, CARDIOGENIC/ SEPTIC: Sheng Mai Zhu She Ye, Injection Gave Excellent Results

HEMORRHAGIC DISORDERS
- SHOCK, HEMORRHAGE: Du Shen Tang (Ren Shen + Fu Zi)

IMMUNE SYSTEM RELATED DISORDERS/ TOPICS
- ALLERGIES: Reduces Anaphylactic Shock, Inhibits Alllergic Edema, Antihistamine Action
- IMMUNE RESPONSE:

Increases WBC Production And Reduces Their Decrease, *Long Term, Small Dose Helps Reticuloendothelial System Where Large Doses Hinders Response, * Inflammatory Response Lowered

INFECTIOUS DISEASES
- FEBRILE DISEASES, ACUTE/CHRONIC: Du Shen Tang (Ren Shen + Fu Zi)
- POLIOMYELITIS, SEQUELAE OF: Acupoint Injection--Helped Affect Limbs Improve
- SHOCK, CARDIOGENIC/ SEPTIC: Sheng Mai Zhu She Ye, Injection Gave Excellent Results

KIDNEYS
- NEPHRITIS, ACUTE W/ HEART FAILURE: Du Shen Tang (Ren Shen + Fu Zi)

LIVER
- HEPATITIS, VIRAL: Helps Cure, And Keeps From Becoming Chronic, Reduced Jaundice

LUNGS
- TUBERCULOSIS, PULMONARY: Dates Treated With Ren Shen

MENTAL STATE/ NEUROLOGICAL DISORDERS
- CNS, ENHANCES ADAPTABILITY
- CNS, ENHANCES CONDITIONED REFLEX
- CNS, INCREASES ABILITY OF ANALYSIS
- LEARNING ABILITY: One Fraction (Rg1) Can Increase
- MEMORY LOSS: Geriatric
- NEURASTHENIA
- PSYCHOSIS

- SEDATIVE, LARGE DOSES
- STIMULANT, SMALL DOSES
- STRESS: Long Term Ingestion Helps To Adapt To Extremes In Stimuli
- STRESS, ANTI-

MUSCULOSKELETAL/ CONNECTIVE TISSUE
- RHEUMATISM

NUTRITIONAL/ METABOLIC DISORDERS/TOPICS
- PROTEIN SYNTHESIS, INCREASES
- TEMPERATURE EXTREMES: Helps Body To Withstand

SEXUALITY, EITHER SEX
- SEX HORMONE: Stimulates Pituitary To Secrete More Hormones

SEXUALITY, MALE: UROLOGICAL TOPICS
- IMPOTENCE
- INFERTILITY, MALE
- SPERM, LACK OF: (Male Infertility)

STOMACH/DIGESTIVE DISORDERS
- APPETITE, INCREASES: Promote Digestion, Absorption
- GASTRITIS, CHRONIC
- ULCERS, GASTRIC: Aqueous Extract, Increased Recovery
- ULCERS, PEPTIC: Preventative And Helps
- ULCERS, PEPTIC BLEEDING

TRAUMA, BITES, POISONINGS
- INJURIES: Increases Period Of Healing Response By Body
- SURGERY, POST: Tonic To Restore Body
- TOXICITY, REDUCES OF SOME CHEMICALS

Dose

1.5 - 9.0 gm

(1.5-3 g)

Not: w/Tea, LI LU, Zao Jia, Wu Ling Zhi

Common Name

Ginseng Root

Notes

Too Much: GI Tract Symptoms, Hypertension-Dai Kon

(Large Turnip) Antidote

Contraindications

Not: Heat/Excess Signs w/o Def, Or Use Small Dose

REN SHEN YE

人參葉
(人参叶)

GINSENG FOLIUM CUM CAULE

Traditional Functions:

1. Promotes body fluid secretion
2. Clear Heat: alleviates Summer Heat, reduces deficiency Fire and opens the voice
3. Resolves alcoholic intoxication

Traditional Properties:

Enters: LU, ST

Properties: SW, BL, CL

Indications:

ORAL CAVITY
• APHONIA
• HOARSENESS: Lung Heat

• THROAT, SORE, SWOLLEN
TRAUMA, BITES, POISONINGS

• ALCOHOLIC INTOXICATION
• HANGOVER

Clinical/Pharmaceutical Studies:

**ENDOCRINE RELATED
  DISORDERS**
• ADDISON'S DISEASE: Stems And

Leaves
SKIN

• BOILS: External Treatment With
  Aqueous Extract

Dose

3 - 9 gm

Common Name

Ginseng Leaf

SHAN YAO
(HUAI SAN)

山藥
(山药)

RADIX DIOSCOREAE OPPOSITAE

Traditional Functions:

1. Strengthens the Spleen and tonifies the Stomach
2. Benefits the Lungs and nourishes the Kidneys
3. Astringes the vital Essence

Traditional Properties:

Enters: LU, SP, KI,

Properties: SW, N

Indications:

BOWEL RELATED DISORDERS
• DIARRHEA: Spleen Stomach
  Deficient
• DIARRHEA, CHRONIC
**ENDOCRINE RELATED
  DISORDERS**
• DIABETES: Internal Heat With
  Exhaustion Thirst
• THIRST, DIABETES
• WASTING & THIRSTING
  SYNDROME
ENERGETIC STATE

• THIRST: Fluid Injury
• THIRST, DIABETES
LUNGS
• ASTHMA
• COUGH: Lung Dryness
• COUGH, CHRONIC: General
  Debility
• COUGH, LUNG EXHAUSTION:
  Tuberculosis
• SHORTNESS OF BREATH
**SEXUALITY, FEMALE:
  GYNECOLOGICAL**

• SPERMATORRHEA
SKIN
• ABSCESS: Topical Poultice
• BOILS: Topical Poultice
• SWEATING, SPONTANEOUS:
  Spleen Stomach Deficient
**STOMACH/DIGESTIVE
  DISORDERS**
• ANOREXIA: Spleen Stomach
  Deficiency
• INDIGESTION
URINARY BLADDER

Indications:

- FATIGUE: Spleen Stomach Deficient
- WEAKNESS: Qi Deficiency

FLUID DISORDERS

- LEUKORRHEA: Cold, Damp

SEXUALITY, MALE:
UROLOGICAL TOPICS

- ENURESIS
- URINARY INCONTINENCE
- URINATION, FREQUENT

Clinical/Pharmaceutical Studies:

NUTRITIONAL/METABOLIC

DISORDERS/TOPICS

- NUTRITIVE

Dose

9 - 30 gm

Common Name

Chinese Yam Root

Contraindications

Not: Excess Conditions, Food Stagnation

Notes

Use w/Children
May Be Increased To 60-120 gm

TAI ZI SHEN
(HAI ER SHEN)

太子參

RADIX PSEUDOSTELLARIAE HETEROPHYLLAE

Traditional Functions:

1. Tonifies the Qi
2. Generates fluids
3. Nourishes the Blood

Traditional Properties:

Enters: LU, SP,

Properties: SW, N, <BIT

Indications:

BOWEL RELATED DISORDERS
- DIARRHEA

ENERGETIC STATE
- DISEASE, CHRONIC, QI DEFICIENCY FROM
- FATIGUE: Spleen Stomach Deficient
- WEAKNESS: Qi Deficiency

FEVERS
- FEVER, UNREMITTING

FLUID DISORDERS
- FLUID DAMAGE: Post Febrile Disease
- THIRST: Tuberculosis

HEAT

- SUMMER HEAT IN CHILDREN

INFECTIOUS DISEASES
- FEBRILE DISEASES, THIRST, FLUID DAMAGE AFTER

LUNGS
- COUGH: Lung Deficiency
- COUGH, DRY
- HYPERPNEA

MENTAL STATE/ NEUROLOGICAL DISORDERS
- FATIGUE, MENTAL
- MALAISE

QI RELATED DISORDERS/ TOPICS

- QI DEFICIENCY FROM CHRONIC DISEASE

SKIN
- SWEATING, SPONTANEOUS: Lung Qi Deficient

SPLEEN
- SPLEEN DEFICIENCY: With Lethargy, Fluid Insufficiency
- SPLEEN STOMACH DEFICIENCY

STOMACH/DIGESTIVE DISORDERS
- ANOREXIA: Spleen Stomach Deficient

Clinical/Pharmaceutical Studies:

MENTAL STATE/ NEUROLOGICAL DISORDERS

- INSOMNIA: (Neurasthenia) , w/Wu   Wei Zi, Good

Dose

6 - 30 gm

Common Name

Prince Ginseng

WU JIA SHEN
(CI WU JIA)

五加參

RADIX ACANTHOPANAX SENTICOSUS
(ELEUTHEROCOCCUS)

Traditional Functions:

1. Tonifies the Qi
2. Disperses Wind Dampness
3. Controls Liver Wind

Traditional Properties:

Enters: LV, KI

Properties: SP, W

Indications:

ENERGETIC STATE
• FATIGUE
EXTREMITIES
• LEGS, SWELLING
FLUID DISORDERS
• EDEMA
HEART
• ANGINA PECTORIS: Chest Bi Strangulating Pain

MENTAL STATE/ NEUROLOGICAL DISORDERS
• DREAMS, FREQUENT
• INSOMNIA
MUSCULOSKELETAL/ CONNECTIVE TISSUE
• ARTHRITIS
• BACK, LOWER WEAK

• KNEES, WEAK
SPLEEN
• SPLEEN KIDNEY DEFICIENCY
STOMACH/DIGESTIVE DISORDERS
• ANOREXIA
URINARY BLADDER
• DYSURIA

Clinical/Pharmaceutical Studies:

BLOOD RELATED DISORDERS/TOPICS
• BLOOD GLUCOSE, REDUCES
• BLOOD PRESSURE, REGULATES HIGH/LOW
• LEUKOPENIA: From Radiation, Chemotherapy, Unknown Etiology, Tablet Given, Best For Chemo Induced
CANCER/TUMORS/ SWELLINGS/LUMPS
• TUMOR, ANTI-: Inhibited Growth, Metastasis
EARS/HEARING DISORDERS
• DIZZINESS
• HEARING, POWER: Improves In Stressful Conditions
ENDOCRINE RELATED DISORDERS
• DIABETES MELLITUS
• ENDOCRINE DISORDERS: Helped Thyroid, Adrenal, Diabetic Related Disorders
• HORMONE-LIKE: Male, Female Organs Increased Weight
ENERGETIC STATE
• ADAPTOGEN: Stronger

Than Ginseng
• DISEASES, CHRONIC: Reduced Fatigue, Increased Strength
• FATIGUE: Similar To Ren Shen
EYES
• EYES, BLURRED VISION
• VISION: Improves In Stressful Conditions
FLUID DISORDERS
• ANTIDIURETIC
HEAD/NECK
• HEADACHE
HEART
• HEART DISEASE: Injection, 66% Effective Rate For Symptom Improvement, Tablet, 1.5 g, 3x/Day, In 14 Days Improvement Of Angina, Mental State, Sleep, Appetite, 77% Improvement
• PALPITATIONS
HEAT
• HIGH TEMPERATURE: Protects Against
IMMUNE SYSTEM RELATED DISORDERS/ TOPICS
• IMMUNE SYSTEM

ENHANCEMENT: Enhanced Phagocytosis, Increased Antibody Formation
LIVER
• LIVER, PROTECTANT
LUNGS
• ANTITUSSIVE: Water Soluble, Alcohol Extract
• BRONCHITIS, CHRONIC, GERIATRIC: As Tablet/Tincture, 8-22 g/ Day In 3 Doses, Increased Lung Capacity, Stronger, Improved Appetite
• EXPECTORANT
MENTAL STATE/ NEUROLOGICAL DISORDERS
• CEREBRAL THROMBOSIS, ACUTE: IV Injection, In 10% Glucose, High Cure Rate
• CNS, HELPS TO REGULATE EXCITATORY/ INHIBITORY CONTROL
• DREAMS, FREQUENT
• INSOMNIA
• IRRITABILITY
• LASSITUDE
• MEMORY, IMPAIRED
• MENTAL POWER,

IMPROVES
• NEURASTHENIA: Marked Amelioration In 20 Days With Tablet, Tincture, Some Cured In 6 Months
• SEDATIVE: Does Not Affect Normal Sleep
• STIMULANT: Stronger Than Ginseng
• STRESS, HELPS REDUCE
MUSCULOSKELETAL/ CONNECTIVE TISSUE
• ARTHRITIS, RHEUMATIC: Relieved Pain
NUTRITIONAL/ METABOLIC DISORDERS/TOPICS
• BODY WEIGHT, INCREASES: Anabolic
• HYPOXIA PROTECTION
TRAUMA, BITES, POISONINGS
• ALTITUDE SICKNESS, ACUTE, PREVENTION: Use Herb Tablet Or Dang Shen
• INFLAMMATORY, ANTI- : Oral, Water Soluble Portion
• RADIATION, PROTECTION

Dose

9 - 15 gm

Common Name

Siberian Ginseng

Notes

Very Low Toxicity, Similar To Ginseng

YI TANG   飴糖   *SACCHARUM GRANORUM*
                    （饴糖）

Traditional Functions:

1. Tonifies the Qi of the Spleen and Stomach and relieves pain
2. Moistens the Lungs and controls coughing

Traditional Properties:

Enters: LU, SP, ST,

Properties: SW, <W

Indications:

ABDOMEN/
GASTROINTESTINAL TOPICS
• ABDOMEN, COLD
• ABDOMEN, PAIN OF, ACUTE
• ABDOMEN, PAIN OF, CHRONIC
  W/EXCESS SALIVA: Middle Jiao
  Deficient Cold
• ABDOMEN, PAIN OF, SPASMS
BOWEL RELATED DISORDERS

• CONSTIPATION
FLUID DISORDERS
• THIRST
LUNGS
• COUGH: Lung Deficient Dry
MENTAL STATE/
  NEUROLOGICAL DISORDERS
• MALAISE
ORAL CAVITY

• THROAT, SORE
• VOICE, WEAK: Lung Deficient
QI RELATED DISORDERS/
TOPICS
• QI DEFICIENCY: Zhong Qi
TRIPLE WARMER (SAN JIAO)
• MIDDLE BURNER, COLD,
  DEFICIENT

Dose

30 - 60 gm

Common Name

Barley Malt Sugar

Contraindications

Not: Internal Damp Heat

Not: Vomiting

ZHI GAN CAO   炙甘草   *RADIX GLYCYRRHIZAE URALENSIS PREP.*

Traditional Functions:

1. Tonifies the Spleen and benefits the Qi
2. Moistens the Lungs and relieves coughing
3. Clears Heat and resolves toxic Heat
4. Moderates and harmonizes the characteristics of other herbs
5. Soothes spasms
6. Antidote to toxic substances, internally and topically

Traditional Properties:

Enters: SP, ST,

Properties: SW, W

Indications:

ENERGETIC STATE
• WEAKNESS: Qi Deficiency

SPLEEN
• SPLEEN DEFICIENCY

PATTERNS

Dose

1.5 - 9.0 gm

Common Name

Toasted Licorice Root

Precautions

Watch: Congests Dampness

Notes

Warmer, Stronger Tonifying Than Raw

Tonify The Yang

BA JI TIAN
(BA JI)

巴戟天

RADIX
MORINDAE OFFICINALIS

Traditional Functions:

1. Tonifies the Kidneys and strengthens the Yang
2. Strengthens the bones and tendons
3. Dispels Wind Cold Dampness

Traditional Properties:

Enters: KI, LV,

Properties: SP, SW, W

Indications:

ABDOMEN/
GASTROINTESTINAL TOPICS
• ABDOMEN, PAIN OF, LOWER:
Cold
EXTREMITIES
• LEG QI, PAIN
• THIGHS, INNER, PAIN
KIDNEYS
• KIDNEY DEFICIENCY
MUSCULOSKELETAL/
CONNECTIVE TISSUE
• ARTHRITIS, WITH WALKING
DIFFICULTY
• BACK, WEAK/SORE

• JOINTS, PAIN: Damp Bi With
Liver Kidney Weakness/Wind Damp
Cold Bi
• KNEES, SORE
• MUSCLES, ATROPHY
NUTRITIONAL/METABOLIC
DISORDERS/TOPICS
• BERIBERI
PAIN/NUMBNESS/GENERAL
DISCOMFORT
• BI, WIND DAMP COLD
SEXUALITY, FEMALE:
GYNECOLOGICAL

• INFERTILITY, FEMALE
• LEUKORRHEA: Kidney Spleen
Yang Deficiency
• MENSTRUATION, DISORDERS
OF: Tonify Qi Of Chong, Ren
SEXUALITY, MALE:
UROLOGICAL TOPICS
• IMPOTENCE
• PREMATURE EJACULATION
• SPERMATORRHEA
URINARY BLADDER
• URINARY INCONTINENCE
• URINATION, FREQUENT

Clinical/Pharmaceutical Studies:

BLOOD RELATED DISORDERS/
TOPICS
• BLOOD PRESSURE, LOWERS
ENDOCRINE RELATED

DISORDERS
• ANDROGEN-LIKE EFFECT:
None Noted
• HORMONE-LIKE: Acts Likes

Cortical Hormones
INFECTIOUS DISEASES
• BACTERIAL, ANTI-: ETOH
Extract Inhibits B.Subtilis

Dose

4.5 - 15.0 gm

Not: w/Difficult Urination

Notes

Safe, Mild

Contraindications

Not: Def Yin w/Heat, Damp Heat

BU GU ZHI

補骨脂
(补骨脂)

FRUCTUS
PSORALEAE
CORYLIFOLIAE

Traditional Functions:

1. Tonifies the Kidneys and strengthens the Yang
2. Astringes and nourishes the Essence
3. Warms the Spleen Yang and stops diarrhea
4. Calms asthma by aiding the Kidneys in grasping the Qi

Traditional Properties:

Enters: SP, KI,

Properties: SP, BIT, W

Indications:

ABDOMEN/ GASTROINTESTINAL TOPICS
- ABDOMEN, PAIN OF
- BORBORYGMUS

BOWEL RELATED DISORDERS
- DIARRHEA, CHRONIC: Spleen/Kidney Yang Deficient
- DIARRHEA, EARLY MORNING: Kidney Spleen Yang Deficiency

EXTREMITIES
- LOINS, COLD

HEAD/NECK

- ALOPECIA: Topical Application

KIDNEYS
- KIDNEY YANG DEFICIENCY

LUNGS
- ASTHMA: Kidneys Not Grasping Qi
- COUGH, CHRONIC W/ DYSPNEA: To Store Qi, Stop Cough

MUSCULOSKELETAL/ CONNECTIVE TISSUE
- BACK, LOWER PAIN: Cold
- KNEES, COLD

SEXUALITY, EITHER SEX
- INFERTILITY: Uterine Cold Palace

SEXUALITY, FEMALE: GYNECOLOGICAL
- LEUKORRHEA: Kidney Spleen Yang Deficiency
- MENSTRUATION, DISORDERS OF: Consolidate, Astringe Chong, Ren

SEXUALITY, MALE: UROLOGICAL TOPICS
- IMPOTENCE
- PREMATURE

EJACULATION
- SPERMATORRHEA

SKIN
- PSORIASIS: Topical
- VITILIGO: Topical

SPLEEN
- SPLEEN DEFICIENCY, COLD

URINARY BLADDER
- ENURESIS
- URINARY INCONTINENCE
- URINATION, FREQUENT
- UROGENITAL DISEASES

Clinical/Pharmaceutical Studies:

ABDOMEN/ GASTROINTESTINAL TOPICS
- INTESTINES, STIMULATES

BLOOD RELATED DISORDERS/TOPICS
- LEUKOPENIA: Honeyed Pill Of Herb

CANCER/TUMORS/ SWELLINGS/LUMPS
- ANTINEOPLASTIC: Volatile Oil
- TUMOR, ANTI-

ENDOCRINE RELATED DISORDERS
- HORMONE-LIKE: Estrogen, Feeding Of Dried Powder, Strong

EXTREMITIES
- CORNS: Alcohol Extract, Topical Application Or Inject In Center
- NAILS, FUNGAL INFECTION OF: Tinea Unguium (Onychomycosis), Injection Of Equal Amounts Tu Si Zi, Herb

HEAD/NECK
- ALOPECIA: Inject w/Uv Exposure--Six Months For Significant Re-Growth

HEART
- CARDIOTONIC
- HEART, VASODILATOR: Coronary Arteries

HEMORRHAGIC DISORDERS
- EPISTAXIS: Hemostatic In
- HEMOPHILIA: Hemostatic In
- HEMOSTATIC

INFECTIOUS DISEASES
- ANTIBIOTIC: Staph A. (Penicillin-Resistant Strains), TB

LUNGS
- BRONCHODILATORY: Wine Extract Of Herb

SEXUALITY, FEMALE: GYNECOLOGICAL
- ABORTIFACIENT: Antiimplantation, Intrauterine Injection, Required
- GENITALS, FEMALE, LEUKOPLAKIA VULVAE: Alcohol Extract, Good Effect
- MENORRHAGIA: w/Chi Shi Zhi, 90% Stopped
- MENSTRUATION, DISORDERS OF: Volatile

Oil, Orally As Tonic
- UTERINE BLEEDING: From Steroidal (Oral) Contraceptives, Following Abortion, From Iud's, 90% Effective, Needs Other Hemostatic Herbs In Profuse, Serious Cases Because Of Slow Onset Of Herb, Zhi Xie Ling (Herb, Chi Shi Zhi), 90% Effective
- UTERUS, STIMULATES

SEXUALITY, MALE:

UROLOGICAL TOPICS
- IMPOTENCE: Volatile Oil, Orally As Tonic

SKIN
- CALLOUSES
- PSORIASIS: Injected With Local Pruritis Treatment, *More Effective With Progressive Stage Than Quiescent/ Regressive Stage, Injected Psoralen, High Short Term

Rate, Relapse In 1 Year High Then Needs Retreatment, Uv Light Shortens Treatment
- SKIN,

PHOTOSENSITIVITY: Topical Application Causes Photosensitivity To Uv Light And Makes It More Likely To Pigment
- SKIN, PIGMENTATION: Internal/External Use Then Exposure To Uv/Sunlight Causes New, Local Pigment
- TINEA VERSICOLOR: Therapeutic Against
- VITILIGO: Injection, Local Application,

Exposure To Uv Light--3-6 Months, 33% Significant (66-100% Repigmentation), *Herb Plus Tu Si Zi Orally With Sunlight/Uv Irradiation
- WARTS

STOMACH/DIGESTIVE DISORDERS
- PEPTIC ULCER, BLEEDING: Hemostatic In

URINARY BLADDER
- ENURESIS, CHILDHOOD: Herb Powder

Dose

3 - 9 gm

Common Name

Scuffy Pea Fruit

Contraindications

Not: Def Yin w/Heat

Not: With Constipation

Notes

With Salt To Increase Kidney Tonification

DONG CHONG XIA CAO 冬蟲夏草 (冬虫夏草) CORDYCEPS SINENSIS

Traditional Functions:

1. Noursihes the Lungs and strengthens the Kidneys
2. Protects the Lung, controls cough and asthma and helps resolve Phlegm
3. Stops bleeding

Traditional Properties:

Enters: LU, KI,

Properties: SW, W

Indications:

ENERGETIC STATE
• ILLNESS, RECOVERY FROM
• RECOVERY FROM ILLNESS
EXTREMITIES
• LOINS, PAIN
HEMORRHAGIC DISORDERS
• HEMATEMESIS
• HEMOPTYSIS
INFECTIOUS DISEASES
• CONSUMPTION, CHRONIC
LUNGS

• COUGH
• COUGH, CHRONIC: With
Hemoptysis
• COUGH, CHRONIC W/DYSPNEA:
To Store Qi, Stop Cough
• COUGH, LUNG EXHAUSTION:
Tuberculosis
• WHEEZING
MUSCULOSKELETAL/
CONNECTIVE TISSUE
• KNEES, PAIN

• LUMBAGO
SEXUALITY, MALE:
UROLOGICAL TOPICS
• IMPOTENCE
• NOCTURNAL EMISSIONS
• SPERMATORRHEA
SKIN
• NIGHT SWEATS
• PERSPIRATION, EXCESS
• SWEATING, SPONTANEOUS

Clinical/Pharmaceutical Studies:

ABDOMEN/
GASTROINTESTINAL TOPICS
• INTESTINES, INHIBITS
CONTRACTION
CANCER/TUMORS/SWELLINGS/
LUMPS
• CANCER, ANTI-: Nasopharyngeal
ENERGETIC STATE
• DEBILITY AFTER SICKNESS
HEART
• HEART, AFFECTS
CONTRACTION: Inhibits Muscle
Contraction
HEMORRHAGIC DISORDERS
• HEMOPTYSIS, TUBERCULOSIS:
With Bei Sha Shen, Mai Dong, Shu
Di
INFECTIOUS DISEASES
• ANTIBIOTIC: Tuberculosis, Very

Dilute Solutions, Strep.Pneum., B.
Subtilis
LUNGS
• BRONCHODILATORY: Significant,
Through Adrenal Glands
• COUGH, CONSUMPTIVE W/
BLOODY SPUTUM
• LUNG CANCER: Significant
Anticancer Effect, 3 Months
MENTAL STATE/
NEUROLOGICAL DISORDERS
• HYPNOTIC: Coma In Large Doses
(Anti-Strychnine, Cocaine)
• SEDATIVE
• TRANQUILIZING
MUSCULOSKELETAL/
CONNECTIVE TISSUE
• BACK, LOWER PAIN/SORE
• KNEES, SORE

• MUSCLES, SMOOTH, INHIBITS
SEXUALITY, FEMALE:
GYNECOLOGICAL
• UTERUS, INHIBITS
CONTRACTION
SEXUALITY, MALE:
UROLOGICAL TOPICS
• IMPOTENCE: With Gou Qi Zi,
Shan Yu Ru, Shan Yao, 3-9 g As
Decoction
• NOCTURNAL EMISSIONS: With
Gou Qi Zi, Shan Yu Ru, Shan Yao, 3-
9 g As Decoction
SKIN
• FUNGAL, ANTI-: Inhibits
STOMACH/DIGESTIVE
DISORDERS
• GASTRIC ATONY
• GASTRIC SPASMS

Dose
4.5 - 15.0 gm

Common Name
Cordyceps

Precautions
Watch: External Pathogens

Notes
Safe, Can Be Taken Over Long Periods
Cooked With Duck To Increase Action
Boiled Extract Has No Toxicity

DU ZHONG 杜仲 CORTEX EUCOMMIAE ULMOIDIS

Traditional Functions:

1. Tonifies the Liver and Kidneys, strengthens the bones and tendons
2. Aids in the smooth flow of Qi and Blood
3. Calms the fetus to prevent miscarriages
4. Lowers blood pressure

Traditional Properties:

Enters: KI, LV,

Properties: SW, <SP, W

Indications:

CIRCULATION DISORDERS
- HYPERTENSION: Single Herb, 15-30 gm

ENERGETIC STATE
- FATIGUE: Kidney Liver Deficient

EXTREMITIES
- LEGS, WEAK
- LOINS, PAIN

HEMORRHAGIC DISORDERS
- BLEEDING, DURING PREGNANCY

LIVER
- LIVER KIDNEY DEFICIENCY

MUSCULOSKELETAL/ CONNECTIVE TISSUE
- BACK, PAIN: Kidney Liver Deficient
- BONES, SINEWS, PROMOTES

CIRCULATION
- JOINTS, PAIN: Damp Bi With Liver Kidney Weakness
- KNEES, WEAK: Kidney Liver Deficient

PAIN/NUMBNESS/GENERAL DISCOMFORT
- NUMBNESS W/SPASMS, CONTRACTURES: Blood Deficiency Bi

SEXUALITY, EITHER SEX
- GENITALS, PRURITUS: Dampness

SEXUALITY, FEMALE: GYNECOLOGICAL
- FETUS, RESTLESS: Liver Kidney Deficiency
- MENSTRUATION, DISORDERS

OF: Tonify Qi Of Chong, Ren
- MISCARRIAGE, PREVENTION: Kidney, Cold, Deficient
- PREGNANCY, DEFICIENT CONDITION DURING
- PREGNANCY, LOW BACK PAIN DURING

SEXUALITY, MALE: UROLOGICAL TOPICS
- IMPOTENCE
- SPERMATORRHEA: Kidney Liver Deficient

URINARY BLADDER
- ENURESIS
- URINATION, DRIBBLING
- URINATION, FREQUENT: Kidney Liver Deficient

Clinical/Pharmaceutical Studies:

BLOOD RELATED DISORDERS/TOPICS
- BLOOD PRESSURE, LOWERS: Strong (Decoction Of Fried Better)
- CHOLESTEROL, REDUCES ABSORPTION

CIRCULATION DISORDERS
- ATHEROSCLEROSIS: Lowers Blood Pressure Long Term By Tincture
- HYPERTENSION: Not For Severe Cases, Improves Symptoms Better Than Reserpine, 10%

Tincture Used But Water Extracts Of Fried Better, Use Bark/Leaf Extracts, Best Used With Jin Yin Hua, Huang Qin, Xia Ku Cao, Sang Ji Sheng, Relieves Symptoms (Headache, Dizziness, Palpitation, Intractable Insomnia) Markedly In 1 Week

IMMUNE SYSTEM RELATED DISORDERS/ TOPICS
- IMMUNE SYSTEM ENHANCEMENT:

Increased Phagocytosis, Similar To Huang Qi/Dang Shen, But Different Route

KIDNEYS
- DIURETIC

MENTAL STATE/ NEUROLOGICAL DISORDERS
- CNS, SEDATIVE: Large Doses, Oral

MUSCULOSKELETAL/ CONNECTIVE TISSUE
- ARTHRITIS, RHEUMATIC
- BACK, LOWER PAIN: IM Injection, Leaf 0.3 g/ml,

2-4 ml 1-2x/Day, 3-4 Months, *Qing E Pill (Du Zhong, Bu Gu Zhi, Hu Tao Ren

PAIN/NUMBNESS/ GENERAL DISCOMFORT
- ANALGESIC

SEXUALITY, FEMALE: GYNECOLOGICAL
- UTERUS, INHIBITS: Inhibits Contraction

TRAUMA, BITES, POISONINGS
- INFLAMMATORY, ANTI-: Large Doses

Dose
6 - 15 gm

Common Name
Eucommia Bark

Contraindications
Not: Def Yin w/Heat

Notes
Fried: More Effective Than Raw

DU ZHONG YE

杜仲葉
（杜仲叶）

FOLIUM EUCOMMIAE ULMOIDIS

Traditional Functions:

1. Tonifies the Liver and Kidneys, strengthens the bones and tendons
2. Aids in the smooth flow of Qi and Blood
3. Calms the fetus to prevent miscarriages
4. Lowers blood pressure

Traditional Properties:

Enters: KI, LV,

Properties: SP, SW, W

Common Name
Eucommia

E GUAN SHI
(ZHUNG SHUEI SHI)

鵝管石
（鹅管石）

STALACTITUM

Traditional Functions:

1. Strengthens the Yang, warms the Lungs, transforms the Phlegm and relieves asthma
2. Benefits the Qi and promotes lactation

Traditional Properties:

Enters: LU, KI

Properties: SW, W

Indications:

ENERGETIC STATE
• WEAKNESS, GENERAL
LUNGS
• COUGH, COLD
• COUGH, DYSPNEA

• COUGH, WHEEZING: Yang Deficient With Phlegm
SEXUALITY, FEMALE:
GYNECOLOGICAL

• LACTATION, INSUFFICIENT
SEXUALITY, MALE:
UROLOGICAL TOPICS
• IMPOTENCE

Dose
9 - 30 gm
Common Name
Tublular Stalactite Tips

Notes
Stomach Qi Stagnation Can Result From Too Much/Too Long Useage
Boil 30 Min Before Herbs

GE JIE

蛤蚧

GECKO

Traditional Functions:

1. Tonifies the Lungs and nourishes the Kidneys
2. Stops cough and relieves asthma
3. Nourishes the Blood and Essence

Traditional Properties:

Enters: LU, KI,

Properties: SA, N

Indications:

BOWEL RELATED DISORDERS
• DIARRHEA, EARLY MORNING
ENDOCRINE RELATED
  DISORDERS
• DIABETES
FLUID DISORDERS
• THIRST
HEMORRHAGIC DISORDERS
• HEMOPTYSIS
KIDNEYS

• KIDNEY YANG DEFICIENCY
LUNGS
• ASTHMA, CHRONIC: Kidney Qi Type/Weak LU/KI Qi
• COUGH
• COUGH, CHRONIC W/DYSPNEA: To Store Qi, Stop Cough: Tuberculosis
• LUNG ATROPHY
• LUNG FISTULA

• WHEEZING: Kidney Unable To Grasp Qi
SEXUALITY, MALE:
UROLOGICAL TOPICS
• IMPOTENCE
URINARY BLADDER
• URINATION, FREQUENT: Kidney Yang Deficient
• UROGENITAL PROBLEMS

Clinical/Pharmaceutical Studies:

ENDOCRINE RELATED
  DISORDERS

• ANDROGEN-LIKE EFFECT: Weak

• ESTROGEN-LIKE: Alcohol Extract

Dose
9 - 15 gm
Common Name
Gecko

Contraindications
Not: External Heat
Not: External Wind Cold Wheezing
Not: Cough/Asthma From Excess Heat
Notes
1.5-6 g As Powder

GOU JI

狗脊

RHIZOMA CIBOTII BAROMETZ

Traditional Functions:

1. Tonifies the Liver and Kidneys, strengthens the back and knees
2. Dispels Wind and Dampness
3. Helps Kidneys to restrain the Essence

Traditional Properties:

Enters: KI, LV,

Properties: BIT, SW, W

Indications:

ABDOMEN/ GASTROINTESTINAL TOPICS
• WAIST, PAIN
EXTREMITIES
• FEET, DEBILITY OF
• LEGS, SORE, STIFF: Liver Kidney Deficient
• LEGS, SWELLING: Post Illness
MUSCULOSKELETAL/ CONNECTIVE TISSUE
• ARTHRITIS: For Expelling Cold, Dampness

• BACK, LUMBAR STRAIN
• BACK, RHEUMATIC PAIN
• BACK, SORE, STIFF: Liver Kidney Deficient
• JOINTS, PAIN: Damp Bi With Liver Kidney Weakness
• KNEES, PAIN
• STIFFNESS
PAIN/NUMBNESS/GENERAL DISCOMFORT
• BI, WIND DAMP DISEASES: Pain,

Sore, Numb
SEXUALITY, FEMALE: GYNECOLOGICAL
• LEUKORRHEA
SKIN
• ULCERS, BLEEDING
URINARY BLADDER
• ENURESIS
• URINARY INCONTINENCE
• URINATION, FREQUENT: In Elderly Men

Dose

4.5 - 15.0 gm

Common Name

Lamb Of Tartary Rhizome

Precautions

Watch: Def Yin w/Heat

Watch: w/Difficult Urination, Dry Tongue

GU SUI BU

骨碎補
(骨碎补)

RHIZOMA DRYNARIA

Traditional Functions:

1. Tonifies the Kidneys
2. Promotes healing of bones and tendons
3. Stimulates the growth of hair
4. Vitalizes Blood and stops bleeding and pain

Traditional Properties:

Enters: KI, LV,

Properties: BIT, W

Indications:

BLOOD RELATED DISORDERS/ TOPICS
• BLOOD STASIS PAIN
BOWEL RELATED DISORDERS
• DIARRHEA, CHRONIC: Kidney Deficient
EARS/HEARING DISORDERS
• TINNITUS: Kidney Deficient
EXTREMITIES
• ARMS, PAIN: Arthritic Pain
• CORNS
• LEGS, PAIN: Arthritic Pain
• LOINS, PAIN
HEAD/NECK

• ALOPECIA: Topical Application
• BALDNESS, STIMULATE HAIR GROWTH: Topical, Tincture
KIDNEYS
• KIDNEY YANG DEFICIENCY
MUSCULOSKELETAL/ CONNECTIVE TISSUE
• BACK, LOWER PAIN: Arthritic Pain
• BACK, LOWER WEAK
• JOINTS, PAIN: Damp Bi With Liver Kidney Weakness
• KNEES, WEAK
• LIGAMENTS, INJURIES

ORAL CAVITY
• GUMS, BLEEDING: Kidney Deficient
• TOOTHACHE: Kidney Deficient
TRAUMA, BITES, POISONINGS
• FRACTURES, TRAUMA: Especially Simple
• SPRAINS
• TRAUMA, CONVALESCENT PHASE, TO REGAIN STRENGTH
• TRAUMA, INJURIES: Die Da
• TRAUMA, LIGAMENTOUS INJURIES, ESPECIALLY

Clinical/Pharmaceutical Studies:

EXTREMITIES
- CORNS: Repeated Tincture Application, Every 2 Hrs, 15 Days

INFECTIOUS DISEASES
- BACTERIAL, ANTI-: Inhibits Staph.

SKIN
- WARTS: Repeated Tincture Application, Every 2 Hrs, 3 Days

TRAUMA, BITES, POISONINGS
- STREPTOMYCIN TOXICITY/

SENSITIVIY: 3 Days To Control Tinnitus, Hearing Loss, Stopped Headache, Dizziness, Numb Lips, Tongue–May Need To Continue Herb

Dose
6 - 15 gm

Precautions
Watch: Def Yin w/Heat

Contraindications
Not: Symptoms w/o Blood Stasis

Notes
To Reinforce Kidneys: 30 gm

HAI GOU SHEN

海狗腎
（海狗肾）

TESTES/PENIS OTORIAE

Traditional Functions:

1. Strengthens the Kidney Yang and nourishes the Essence

Traditional Properties:

Enters: KI, LV,

Properties: SA, H

Indications:

ENERGETIC STATE
- DEBILITY, GENERAL

EXTREMITIES
- LIMBS, COLD: Kidney Yang Deficiency

MENTAL STATE/

NEUROLOGICAL DISORDERS
- STRESS, CAUSING INTERNAL IMPAIRMENT

SEXUALITY, EITHER SEX
- HYPOGONADISM
- INFERTILITY: Uterine Cold Palace

- SEXUAL DRIVE, DECREASED: Kidney Yang Deficiency

SEXUALITY, MALE: UROLOGICAL TOPICS
- IMPOTENCE: Kidney Yang Deficiency

Clinical/Pharmaceutical Studies:

SEXUALITY, EITHER SEX

- SEXUAL NERVES, STIMULATES

Dose
3 - 15 gm

Common Name
Male Seal Sexual Organs

Contraindications
Not: Def Yin With Heat

Not: Those With Hyperactive Sex Drive

Notes
Take Directly As Powder (1-1.2gm)

HAI LONG

海龍
（海龙）

HAILONG

Traditional Functions:

1. Tonifies the Kidneys and nourishes the Yin
2. Disperses stagnant Blood, nodules and swellings

Traditional Properties:

Enters: KI, LV

Properties: SW, SA, <W

Indications:

**ENDOCRINE RELATED
DISORDERS**
• THYROID, DISEASES
ENERGETIC STATE
• DEBILITY, IN ELDERLY
GERIATRIC TOPICS

• DEBILITY, IN ELDERLY
• IMPOTENCE, IN ELDERLY
**IMMUNE SYSTEM RELATED
DISORDERS/TOPICS**
• LYMPHADENITIS, CHRONIC

INFECTIOUS DISEASES
• SCROFULA
**SEXUALITY, MALE:
UROLOGICAL TOPICS**
• IMPOTENCE, IN ELDERLY

Dose

3 - 9 gm

Common Name

Pipe-Fish

Contraindications

Not: Pregnancy

Not: Yin Def Heat

Notes

Take 1.5-2.0 gm pwdr

HAI MA

海馬
(海马)

HIPPOCAMPUS

Traditional Functions:

1. Tonifies the Kidneys and strengthens the Yang
2. Promotes Blood circulation and removes stagnant Blood

Traditional Properties:

Enters: KI, LV,

Properties: SW, SA, W

Indications:

**ABDOMEN/
GASTROINTESTINAL TOPICS**
• ABDOMEN, LUMPS/MASSES
• ABDOMEN, PAIN OF
**CANCER/TUMORS/SWELLINGS/
LUMPS**
• TUMORS
GERIATRIC TOPICS
• DEFICIENCY, IN ELDERLY
INFECTIOUS DISEASES
• SCROFULA
KIDNEYS

• KIDNEY QI DEFICIENCY, COLD
LUNGS
• WHEEZING: Deficiency
**MUSCULOSKELETAL/
CONNECTIVE TISSUE**
• BACK, LOWER PAIN
**SEXUALITY, FEMALE:
GYNECOLOGICAL**
• CHILDBIRTH, DIFFICULT
DELIVERY
SEXUALITY, MALE:

UROLOGICAL TOPICS
• IMPOTENCE
SKIN
• FURUNCLES: Topical
• SWELLING SORES/BOILS:
Topical
TRAUMA, BITES, POISONINGS
• TRAUMA, BLEEDING
URINARY BLADDER
• URINARY INCONTINENCE
• URINATION, FREQUENT

Clinical/Pharmaceutical Studies:

**ENDOCRINE RELATED
DISORDERS**
• ANDRONERGIC:
Alcohol Extracts, Increase

Erection Of Male Mice
• ENDOCRINE EFFECTS:
Alcohol Extracts Estrogen-

Like, Androgen-Like, Less
Than Yin Yang Huo/She
Chuang Zi, But Greater

Than Ge Jie, Increases
Weight Of Female/Male
Organs And Glands

Dose

4.5 - 12.0 gm

Common Name

Sea Horse

Contraindications

Not: Pregnancy

Not: Def Yin w/Heat

HAI SHEN

海參

STICHOPUS JAPONICUS, SELENKA

Traditional Functions:

1. Awakens the Kidney, strengthens the Yang
2. Moistens dryness by nourishing the Blood

Traditional Properties:

Enters: HT, KI,

Properties: SA, W

Indications:

BLOOD RELATED DISORDERS/
TOPICS
• BLOOD DEFICIENCY
SYNDROME
BOWEL RELATED DISORDERS
• CONSTIPATION: Dry
ENERGETIC STATE
• WEAKNESS, DEBILITY
HEMORRHAGIC DISORDERS

• HEMOPHILIA
KIDNEYS
• ESSENCE DEFICIENCY
LUNGS
• TUBERCULOSIS, PULMONARY
MENTAL STATE/
NEUROLOGICAL DISORDERS
• NEURASTHENIA
SEXUALITY, FEMALE:

GYNECOLOGICAL
• FETAL DEVELOPMENT
• POSTPARTUM, DEBILITY
SEXUALITY, MALE:
UROLOGICAL TOPICS
• IMPOTENCE
• NOCTURNAL EMISSIONS
URINARY BLADDER
• URINATION, FREQUENT

Dose

Up To 30 g

Common Name

Sea Cucumber

Contraindications

Not: SP Qi Def Diarrhea

Not: Copius Sputum In LU

Notes

Often Used In Soups

HU LU BA

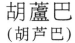
胡蘆巴
(胡芦巴)

SEMEN TRIGONELLAE FOENI-GRAECI

Traditional Functions:

1. Warms Life Gate Fire of the Kidneys
2. Dissipates Cold Dampness and relieves pain

Traditional Properties:

Enters: KI,

Properties: BIT, W

Indications:

ABDOMEN/
GASTROINTESTINAL TOPICS
• ABDOMEN, DISTENTION OF/
PAIN: From GI Spasms:Cold
• ABDOMEN, PAIN OF, HERNIA-
LIKE: Cold
• FLANK DISTENTION/PAIN
• HERNIA, PAIN: Cold Qi
CHEST

• COSTAL REGION, DISTENTION
EXTREMITIES
• LEGS, EDEMA: Cold Damp
KIDNEYS
• KIDNEY YANG DEFICIENCY:
Cold
QI RELATED DISORDERS/
TOPICS
• QI STAGNATION: Cold

SEXUALITY, FEMALE:
GYNECOLOGICAL
• LEUKORRHEA: Kidney Spleen
Yang Deficiency
SEXUALITY, MALE:
UROLOGICAL TOPICS
• IMPOTENCE
• TESTICLES, COLD PAIN IN

Clinical/Pharmaceutical Studies:

BOWEL RELATED DISORDERS
• LAXATIVE
ENDOCRINE RELATED
DISORDERS
• HORMONE-LIKE: None Found

PARASITES
• ROUNDWORMS
SEXUALITY, FEMALE:
GYNECOLOGICAL

• LACTATION, INCREASES
TRAUMA, BITES, POISONINGS
• MOUNTAIN SICKNESS:
Prophylaxis/Treatment

Dose
3 - 9 gm
Common Name
Fenugreek Seed

Contraindications
Not: Def Yin w/Heat
Notes
(May Damage Yin)

HU TAO REN

胡桃仁

SEMEN JUGLANDIS REGIAE

Traditional Functions:

1. Warms and tonifies the Lung and Kidney Yang
2. Relieves asthma by helping the Kidneys to grasp the Qi
3. Astringes the Lungs, dissolves Phlegm
4. Moistens the intestines and facilitates passage of stool

Traditional Properties:

Enters: LU, KI,

Properties: SW, W

Indications:

BOWEL RELATED
DISORDERS
• CONSTIPATION:
Geriatric/Post Febrile/Yin
Deficient/Intestinal
Dryness
EXTREMITIES
• LEGS, WEAK IN BOTH
LUNGS
• ASTHMA: Lung/Kidney

Deficient
• COUGH, CHRONIC:
Lung Deficient/Cold
• DYSPNEA: Deficiency
Cold
MUSCULOSKELETAL/
CONNECTIVE TISSUE
• BACK, LOWER PAIN:
Cold

• KNEES, PAIN: Cold
NUTRITIONAL/
METABOLIC
DISORDERS/TOPICS
• BERIBERI
SEXUALITY, MALE:
UROLOGICAL TOPICS
• IMPOTENCE
• SPERMATORRHEA

SKIN
• DERMATITIS: Paste
Form
• ECZEMA: Paste Form
URINARY BLADDER
• URINARY TRACT
STONES
• URINATION,
FREQUENT

Clinical/Pharmaceutical Studies:

NUTRITIONAL/METABOLIC
DISORDERS/TOPICS
• WEIGHT GAIN: With Oil
SKIN

• DERMATITIS, CONTACT/
SEBORRHEOIC, ATOPIC: Paste
Of With Other Herbs
URINARY BLADDER

• URINARY STONES, EXPULSION:
Use Paste, In Few Days As Milky
Urine

Dose
9 - 30 gm
Common Name
Walnut Nut

Contraindications
Not: Phlegm Fire/Hot Cough
Not: w/Watery BM
Not: Def Yin w/Heat

JIU CAI ZI
(JIU ZI)

菲菜子
(菲菜子)

SEMEN ALLII TUBEROSI

Traditional Functions:

1. Tonifies Liver and Kidneys
2. Strengthens the Yang and astringes the Essence
3. Warms and strengthens the back and knees
4. Warms the Stomach and stops vomiting

Traditional Properties:

Enters: KI, LV,

Properties: SP, SW, W

Indications:

EXTREMITIES
• LOINS, WEAK
MUSCULOSKELETAL/
CONNECTIVE TISSUE
• BACK, WEAK/SORE

• LEUKORRHEA: Kidney Spleen
Yang Deficiency
SEXUALITY, MALE:
UROLOGICAL TOPICS
• IMPOTENCE

• VOMITING: Stomach Cold
URINARY BLADDER
• ENURESIS
• URINARY INCONTINENCE
• URINATION, FREQUENT

Indications:

- KNEES, WEAK/SORE
SEXUALITY, FEMALE:
  GYNECOLOGICAL

- SPERMATORRHEA
STOMACH/DIGESTIVE
  DISORDERS

- URINATION, TURBID, WHITE
- UROGENITAL DISEASES: Cold,
  Damp

Dose

3 - 9 gm

Common Name

Chinese Leek Seed

Contraindications

Not: Yin Def With Excess Fire

LU JIAO   鹿角   *CERVI CORNU*

Traditional Functions:

1. Benefits the Liver and Kidneys
2. Strengthens the sinews and bones
3. Vitalizes Blood, decreases swelling

Traditional Properties:

Enters: KI, LV,

Properties: SA, W

Indications:

BLOOD RELATED DISORDERS/
  TOPICS
- BLOOD STASIS PAIN
CANCER/TUMORS/SWELLINGS/
  LUMPS
- SWELLINGS
COLD
- COLD, INTOLERANCE TO
ENERGETIC STATE
- WEAKNESS, DEBILITY
KIDNEYS
- KIDNEY YANG DEFICIENCY

MUSCULOSKELETAL/
  CONNECTIVE TISSUE
- BACK, LOWER PAIN
- BONES, PAIN
- TENDONS, PAIN
PAIN/NUMBNESS/GENERAL
  DISCOMFORT
- PAIN: Blood Stagnation
SEXUALITY, FEMALE:
  GYNECOLOGICAL
- MASTITIS

SEXUALITY, MALE:
  UROLOGICAL TOPICS
- IMPOTENCE
- SEMINAL EMISSIONS,
  SPONTANEOUS
SKIN
- SKIN, SORES, SWOLLEN, TOXIC:
  Blood Stasis, Swelling
- ULCERS
TRAUMA, BITES, POISONINGS
- TRAUMA: Wounds

Dose

3 - 9 gm

Common Name

Deer Horn, Male Ossified

Contraindications

Not: Yin Def w/Excess Fire

Notes

Similar To LU Rong But Less Active

LU JIAO JIAO   鹿角膠
（鹿角胶）   *CERVI COLLA CORNUS*

Traditional Functions:

1. Tonifies Kidney Yang
2. Nourishes the Essence and Blood
3. Stops bleeding
4. Promotes regeneration of bodily tissues

Traditional Properties:

Enters: KI, LV

Properties: SW, SA, W

Indications:

ABDOMEN/
  GASTROINTESTINAL TOPICS
- ABDOMEN, COLD
BLOOD RELATED DISORDERS/
  TOPICS
- BLOOD DEFICIENCY W/
  WITHERING YELLOW
  COMPLEXION

- HEMATURIA: Cold, Deficient
- HEMORRHAGE: Deficiency
  Caused
MUSCULOSKELETAL/
  CONNECTIVE TISSUE
- BACK, LOWER PAIN
SEXUALITY, FEMALE:
  GYNECOLOGICAL

- IMPOTENCE
- SEMINAL EMISSIONS,
  SPONTANEOUS
SKIN
- ABSCESS, YIN, INTERNAL
  SINKING OF
- SKIN, SORES, SWOLLEN, TOXIC:
  Helps Healing, Deficiency

Indications:

ENERGETIC STATE
• DEBILITY, WEAKNESS
HEAD/NECK
• ALOPECIA: Deficiency Complex
HEMORRHAGIC DISORDERS
• EPISTAXIS
• HEMATEMESIS: Cold, Deficient

• LEUKORRHEA
• MENSTRUATION, DISORDERS
OF: Tonify Chong, Ren, Essence, Blood
• UTERINE BLEEDING
SEXUALITY, MALE:
UROLOGICAL TOPICS

STOMACH/DIGESTIVE DISORDERS
• EPIGASTRIC PAIN: Cold, Deficient
• REGURGITATION: Cold, Deficient
• VOMITING

Dose
6 - 12 gm
Common Name
Deer Horn Gelatin

Notes
Stronger Than LU Jiao For Nourishing Kidney
Weaker Than LU Rong
Use In Melted Form

LU JIAO SHUANG 陸角霜 CORNU CERVI DEGLATINATUM

Traditional Functions:
1. Tonifies Essence and Blood
2. Stops bleeding when applied topically
3. Astringes the Essence

Traditional Properties:
Enters: LV, KI

Properties: SW, <W

Indications:

ABDOMEN/ GASTROINTESTINAL TOPICS
• ABDOMEN, COLD/PAIN
ENERGETIC STATE
• DEBILITY, WEAKNESS
HEMORRHAGIC DISORDERS
• HEMORRHAGE: External Injury, Topical
MUSCULOSKELETAL/

CONNECTIVE TISSUE
• BACK, LOWER PAIN
SEXUALITY, FEMALE: GYNECOLOGICAL
• FRIGIDITY
• LEUKORRHEA: Cold Deficient/Kidney Spleen Yang Deficiency
• MENSTRUATION, DISORDERS OF: Consolidate, Astringe

Chong, Ren
• UTERINE BLEEDING: Cold Deficient
SEXUALITY, MALE: UROLOGICAL TOPICS
• IMPOTENCE
• SEMINAL EMISSIONS, SPONTANEOUS
SKIN
• BOILS
• ULCERS

SPLEEN
• SPLEEN STOMACH DEFICIENCY, COLD
STOMACH/DIGESTIVE DISORDERS
• ANOREXIA
• REGURGITATION: Deficiency Cold
• VOMITING: Spleen Stomach Cold/Kidney Yang Deficient

Dose
15 - 30 gm
Common Name
Deglued Antler Powder

Notes
Less Effective, Less Greasey, But Similar To LU Jiao Jiao

LU RONG 鹿茸 CORNU CERVI PARVUM

Traditional Functions:
1. Tonifies the Essence and nourishes Blood
2. Tonifies Kidney Yang
3. Strengthen bones and muscles
4. Tonifies the Du channel
5. Supports the Chong and Ren channels and strengthens the Dai channel

Traditional Properties:
Enters: KI, LV,

Properties: SW, SA, W

Indications:

CHILDHOOD DISORDERS
• DEVELOPMENT, POOR MENTAL/PHYSICAL,

• HEARING, POOR
• VERTIGO
ENERGETIC STATE
• DEBILITY

WEAK
• JOINTS, PAIN: Damp Bi With Liver Kidney Weakness

Qi Of Chong, Ren
• UTERINE BLEEDING: Cold, Deficient
SEXUALITY, MALE:

Indications:

- CHILDHOOD
- GROWTH, INSUFFICIENT, CHILDHOOD: Essence/Blood Deficiency
- LEARNING DISABILITIES, CHILDHOOD: Essence/Blood Deficiency
- MALNUTRITION, CHILDHOOD
- SKELETAL DEFORMITIES, CHILDHOOD: Essence/Blood Deficiency

COLD
- COLD, INTOLERANCE TO

EARS/HEARING DISORDERS

- DEFICIENCY DAMAGE, ALL TYPES

EXTREMITIES
- EXTREMITIES, COLD

EYES
- VISION, POOR

KIDNEYS
- KIDNEY YANG DEFICIENCY

MENTAL STATE/NEUROLOGICAL DISORDERS
- MENTAL RETARDATION, ESPECIALLY CHILDREN: Essence/Blood Deficiency

MUSCULOSKELETAL/CONNECTIVE TISSUE
- BACK, LOWER SORE,

- KNEES, SORE, WEAK

NUTRITIONAL/METABOLIC DISORDERS/TOPICS
- RICKETS: Essence/Blood Deficiency

SEXUALITY, EITHER SEX
- INFERTILITY: Uterine Cold Palace

SEXUALITY, FEMALE: GYNECOLOGICAL
- LEUKORRHEA: Deficiency Cold/Kidney Spleen Yang Deficiency
- MENORRHAGIA: Deficiency Cold
- MENSTRUATION, DISORDERS OF: Tonify

UROLOGICAL TOPICS
- IMPOTENCE
- SEMINAL EMISSIONS, NOCTURNAL
- SEMINAL EMISSIONS, SPONTANEOUS

SKIN
- SKIN, INFECTIONS W/ PUS
- SKIN, ULCERS, CHRONIC

URINARY BLADDER
- URINARY INCONTINENCE
- URINATION, CLEAR, COPIOUS: Kidney Yang Deficient
- URINATION, FREQUENT

Clinical/Pharmaceutical Studies:

BLOOD RELATED DISORDERS/TOPICS
- BLOOD, INCREASES RBC/WBC

CANCER/TUMORS/SWELLINGS/LUMPS
- CANCER: One Study Showed Accelerated Multiplication Of Cells

CIRCULATION DISORDERS
- CIRCULATORY DISORDER, CHRONIC
- HYPOTENSION

EARS/HEARING DISORDERS
- VERTIGO

ENDOCRINE RELATED DISORDERS
- ENDOCRINE SYSTEM: ETOH Extract Stimulates
- HORMONE-LIKE: None Found

ENERGETIC STATE
- FATIGUE: Reduces
- ILLNESS, POST: To Increase Strength
- STRENGTHENING, GENERAL

GERIATRIC TOPICS
- GERIATRIC TONIC

HEAD/NECK
- BRAIN: Increase Oxygen Uptake, Also Other Organs

HEART
- CARDIOTONIC: Strengthens Pulse, Blood Pressure
- HEART, REGULATES: Regulates Arrhythmias

IMMUNE SYSTEM RELATED DISORDERS/TOPICS
- IMMUNE RESPONSE: Desensitizing On Reexposure Of Presensitized Animals
- IMMUNE SYSTEM ENHANCEMENT: Promotes Lymphocyte Transformation

KIDNEYS
- DIURETIC
- KIDNEY DEFICIENCY
- KIDNEYS, PROMOTES FUNCTION OF

MENTAL STATE/NEUROLOGICAL DISORDERS
- CONVULSIVE, ANTI-: In Audiogenic
- SLEEP: Improves

MUSCULOSKELETAL/CONNECTIVE TISSUE
- BACK, LOWER WEAK
- BONES, PROMOTES HEALING OF FRACTURES

- KNEES, WEAK

NUTRITIONAL/METABOLIC DISORDERS/TOPICS
- GROWTH, INCREASES
- HEALING, HELPS
- METABOLISM, INCREASES
- WEIGHT GAIN AID

SEXUALITY, FEMALE: GYNECOLOGICAL
- METRORRHAGIA
- UTERUS, INCREASES MUSCLE TENSION, RHYTHMIC CONTRACTIONS

SEXUALITY, MALE: UROLOGICAL TOPICS
- IMPOTENCE
- SPERMATORRHEA

SKIN
- ULCERS, INTRACTABLE: Promotes Regeneration

STOMACH/DIGESTIVE DISORDERS
- APPETITE, INCREASES

TRAUMA, BITES, POISONINGS
- FRACTURES, HEALING OF: Promotes Regeneration
- WOUNDS: Promotes Regeneration

Dose

0.5 - 9.0 gm

Common Name

Young Deer Horn Velvet

Contraindications

Not: Def Yin w/Heat, Blood Heat, Excess ST Fire, LU Phlegm Heat, Febrile Disease

Notes

1-3 g As Powder

Overdose May Cause: Dizziness, Red Eyes, Consume Yin

"Pantocrin"=ETOH Extract

ROU CONG RONG

肉蓯蓉
（肉苁蓉）

HERBA CISTANCHES

Traditional Functions:

1. Tonifies the Kidneys and strengthens the Yang of the Life Gate
2. Nourishes the Essence and Blood
3. Warms the womb
4. Moistens the intestines and facilitates passage of stool

Traditional Properties:

Enters: LI, KI,

Properties: SW, SA, W

Indications:

BOWEL RELATED DISORDERS
• CONSTIPATION: Geriatric/Ill/ Postpartum/Blood/Qi Deficient/ Intestinal Dryness
EXTREMITIES
• LOINS, COLD OBSTRUCTION OF
MUSCULOSKELETAL/ CONNECTIVE TISSUE
• BACK, PAIN, COLD

• KNEES, PAIN, COLD
SEXUALITY, FEMALE: GYNECOLOGICAL
• INFERTILITY, FEMALE: Uterine Cold Palace
• LEUKORRHEA: Cold Deficient Womb
• MENSTRUATION, DISORDERS OF: Tonify Qi Of Chong, Ren
• UTERINE BLEEDING

SEXUALITY, MALE: UROLOGICAL TOPICS
• IMPOTENCE
• PREMATURE EJACULATION
• SPERMATORRHEA
URINARY BLADDER
• URINARY INCONTINENCE
• URINATION, FREQUENT
• URINATION, POST-URINE DRIPS

Clinical/Pharmaceutical Studies:

BLOOD RELATED DISORDERS/ TOPICS
• BLOOD PRESSURE, LOWERS: ETOH/Aqueous Extracts
BOWEL RELATED DISORDERS
• LAXATIVE

ENERGETIC STATE
• TONIFIES
LUNGS
• BREATHING RATE: Slows Respiration By Paralysis
NUTRITIONAL/METABOLIC

DISORDERS/TOPICS
• GROWTH, INCREASES OF IMMATURE: Alcohol Extract
ORAL CAVITY
• SALIVATION, INCREASES: Aqueous Extract

Dose

6 - 18 gm

Common Name

Broomrape Fleshy Stem

Contraindications

Not: w/Diarrhea From Def SP/ST

Not: Constipation From ST/Intestine Heat

Not: Def Yin w/Heat

Notes

Mild

For Constipation: 12-18 gm

SHA YUAN ZI
(TONG JI LI)

沙苑子

SEMEN ASTRAGALI COMPLANATI

Traditional Functions:

1. Tonifies the Liver and Kidneys and clears the eyes
2. Tonifies the Kidneys and astringes the Essence

Traditional Properties:

Enters: KI, LV,

Properties: SW, W

Indications:

EARS/HEARING DISORDERS
• TINNITUS: Kidney Yang Deficient
• VERTIGO
EXTREMITIES
• LOINS, PAIN
EYES
• VISION, BLURRED: Liver Kidney Deficient
• VISION, REDUCED ACUITY

CONNECTIVE TISSUE
• BACK, LOWER PAIN: Kidney Yang Deficient
• BACK, PAIN
• KNEES, PAIN
SEXUALITY, EITHER SEX
• INFERTILITY: Uterine Cold Palace
SEXUALITY, FEMALE: GYNECOLOGICAL

UROLOGICAL TOPICS
• IMPOTENCE
• PREMATURE EJACULATION: Kidney Yang Deficient
• SPERMATORRHEA: Kidney Yang Deficient
URINARY BLADDER
• ENURESIS
• URINARY INCONTINENCE:

Indications:

LIVER
- **LIVER KIDNEY INSUFFICIENCY**

MUSCULOSKELETAL/

- **LEUKORRHEA:** Kidney Spleen Yang Deficiency/Cold, Damp

SEXUALITY, MALE:

Kidney Yang Deficient
- **URINATION, FREQUENT:** Kidney Yang Deficient

Clinical/Pharmaceutical Studies:

FLUID DISORDERS
- **ANTIDIURETIC**

SEXUALITY, FEMALE:

GYNECOLOGICAL

- **UTERUS, STIMULATES**

Dose

6 - 15 gm

Contraindications

Not: Def Yin w/Heat
Not: w/Hyperactive Sex Drive
Not: Dysuria

SUO YANG

鎖陽
(锁阳)

HERBA/CAULIS CYNOMORRI SONGARICI

Traditional Functions:

1. Tonifies the Kidneys and Liver and strengthens the Yang
2. Nourishes the Blood and Essence
3. Strengthens the waist and knees
4. Moistens the intestines and facilitates passage of stool

Traditional Properties:

Enters: KI, LV,

Properties: SW, W

Indications:

BLOOD RELATED DISORDERS/ TOPICS
- **BLOOD EXHAUSTION**

BOWEL RELATED DISORDERS
- **CONSTIPATION:** Intestinal Dryness/Qi/Blood Deficient

EXTREMITIES
- **LIMBS, ATROPHY OF TENDONS:** Kidney Yang Deficient
- **LOINS, WEAK**

MENTAL STATE/

NEUROLOGICAL DISORDERS
- **PARALYSIS:** Essence, Blood Deficient

MUSCULOSKELETAL/ CONNECTIVE TISSUE
- **BACK, WEAK:** Kidney Deficient
- **KNEES, WEAK:** Kidney Deficient
- **MOTOR IMPAIRMENT**
- **MUSCLES, WEAK**
- **WALKING DIFFICULTY**

SEXUALITY, FEMALE:

GYNECOLOGICAL
- **INFERTILITY, FEMALE:** Uterine Cold Palace

SEXUALITY, MALE:

UROLOGICAL TOPICS
- **IMPOTENCE**
- **PREMATURE EJACULATION**
- **SEMINAL EMISSIONS**
- **SPERMATORRHEA**

URINARY BLADDER
- **URINATION, FREQUENT**

Dose

4.5 - 15.0 gm

Contraindications

Not: Def Yin w/Heat
Not: w/Diarrhea

TU SI ZI

菟絲子
(菟丝子)

SEMEN CUSCUTAE

Traditional Functions:

1. Tonifies the Kidneys and astringes the Essence
2. Calms the fetus and prevents miscarriage
3. Warms the Spleen and Kidneys and stops diarrhea
4. Nourishes the Liver and clears the eyes

Traditional Properties:

Enters: KI, LV,

Properties: SP, SW, N

Indications:

BOWEL RELATED DISORDERS
- **DIARRHEA:** Spleen Deficiency
- **DIARRHEA, CHRONIC W/**

- **EYES, SPOTS IN FRONT OF:** Essence Deficient/Liver Kidney Yin, Yang Deficient

- **LEUKORRHEA:** Kidney Yang Deficient
- **MENSTRUATION, DISORDERS**

Indications:

ANOREXIA: Spleen Kidney
Deficient
EARS/HEARING DISORDERS
• DIZZINESS: Essence Deficient/
Liver Kidney Yin, Yang Deficient
• HEARING LOSS
• TINNITUS: Kidney Yang Deficient/
Essence Deficient/Liver Kidney Yin,
Yang Deficient
• VERTIGO
ENDOCRINE RELATED
DISORDERS
• DIABETES: Internal Heat With
Exhaustion Thirst
EXTREMITIES
• LOINS, PAIN
EYES

• VISION, BLURRED: Essence
Deficient/Liver Kidney Yin, Yang
Deficient
HEAD/NECK
• ALOPECIA: Topical Application
KIDNEYS
• KIDNEY YANG DEFICIENCY
MUSCULOSKELETAL/
CONNECTIVE TISSUE
• BACK, LOWER SORE, PAIN
• KNEES, PAIN
SEXUALITY, EITHER SEX
• INFERTILITY: Uterine Cold Palace
SEXUALITY, FEMALE:
GYNECOLOGICAL
• FETUS, RESTLESS: Liver Kidney
Deficiency

OF: Tonify Qi Of Chong, Ren
• MISCARRIAGE, THREATENED/
HABITUAL: Important For
SEXUALITY, MALE:
UROLOGICAL TOPICS
• IMPOTENCE
• INFERTILITY, MALE: Kidney
Deficient Cold Sperm
• NOCTURNAL EMISSIONS
• PREMATURE EJACULATION
• SPERMATORRHEA
URINARY BLADDER
• ENURESIS
• URINARY INCONTINENCE
• URINATION, DRIBBLING
• URINATION, FREQUENT: Kidney
Yang Deficient

Clinical/Pharmaceutical Studies:

ABDOMEN/
GASTROINTESTINAL TOPICS
• INTESTINES, INHIBITS
BLOOD RELATED DISORDERS/
TOPICS

• BLOOD PRESSURE, LOWERS
HEART
• CARDIOTONIC: Tincture Of
SEXUALITY, FEMALE:

GYNECOLOGICAL
• UTERUS, STIMULATES
SPLEEN
• SPLEEN, DECREASES SIZE OF

Dose

9 - 18 gm

Common Name

Dodder Seeds

Contraindications

Not: Yin Def With Excess Fire, Constipation, Red,
Scanty Urine

Notes

Wrap For Herb Formula

XIAN MAO   仙茅   *RHIZOMA CURCULIGINIS ORCHIOIDIS*

Traditional Functions:

1. Warms the Kidneys and strengthens the Yang
2. Dispels Cold and Dampness
3. Strengthens bones and tendons

Traditional Properties:

Enters: KI, LV,

Properties: SP, H, TX

Indications:

ABDOMEN/
GASTROINTESTINAL TOPICS
• ABDOMEN, COLD
BOWEL RELATED DISORDERS
• DIARRHEA
CIRCULATION DISORDERS
• HYPERTENSION DURING
MENOPAUSE
COLD
• COLD ESSENCE
EXTREMITIES
• ARMS, PAIN, SPASMS
• LEGS, COLD, NUMB BI
• LEGS, PAIN, SPASMS
• LOINS, PAIN: Cold

Dampness
• BACK, LOWER PAIN: Obstinate
Cold Damp Bi
• BONES, SINEWS, WEAKNESS:
Obstinate Cold Damp Bi
• JOINTS, PAIN: Damp Bi With
Liver Kidney Weakness
• KNEES, PAIN: Obstinate Cold
Damp Bi
NUTRITIONAL/METABOLIC
DISORDERS/TOPICS
• BODY, COLD
PAIN/NUMBNESS/GENERAL
DISCOMFORT
• BI, COLD, DAMP

SEXUALITY, EITHER SEX
• INFERTILITY: Uterine Cold Palace
• INFERTILITY, MEN/WOMEN:
Cold Essence/Womb
SEXUALITY, FEMALE:
GYNECOLOGICAL
• LEUKORRHEA: Kidney Spleen
Yang Deficiency
• MENSTRUATION, DISORDERS
OF: Tonify Qi Of Chong, Ren
SEXUALITY, MALE:
UROLOGICAL TOPICS
• IMPOTENCE
• NOCTURNAL EMISSIONS
• SPERMATORRHEA

Indications:

MUSCULOSKELETAL/
CONNECTIVE TISSUE
• ARTHRITIS: For Expelling Cold,

• NUMBNESS
• PAIN, GENERAL: Obstinate Cold
  Damp Bi

URINARY BLADDER
• URINARY INCONTINENCE
• URINATION, FREQUENT

Dose
3 - 9 gm

Common Name
Golden Eye-Grass Rhizome

Contraindications
Not: Def Yin w/Heat

Notes
Warmest Yang Agent

XU DUAN

續斷
(续断)

RADIX
DIPSACI

Traditional Functions:

1. Tonifies the Liver and Kidneys, fuses the tendons and bones
2. Promotes the circulation of Blood, opens the channels and stops pain
3. Calms the fetus and prevents miscarriage

Traditional Properties:

Enters: KI, LV,

Properties: BIT, SP, <W

Indications:

BOWEL RELATED DISORDERS
• HEMORRHOIDS
EXTREMITIES
• FEET, DEBILITY OF
• LEGS, WEAK
MUSCULOSKELETAL/
CONNECTIVE TISSUE
• BACK, LOWER SORE, PAIN
• JOINTS, PAIN: Damp Bi With
  Liver Kidney Weakness
• KNEES, PAIN, SORE
• LIGAMENTS, INJURIES
• STIFFNESS

PAIN/NUMBNESS/GENERAL
DISCOMFORT
• ANALGESIC: Stomach, Muscles,
  Joints
• BI DISORDERS
SEXUALITY, FEMALE:
GYNECOLOGICAL
• FETUS, RESTLESS: Liver Kidney
  Deficiency
• LEUKORRHEA: Deficient
• MENORRHAGIA
• MENSTRUATION, DISORDERS
  OF: Tonify Qi Of Chong, Ren

• MISCARRIAGE, THREATENED
• RESTLESS FETUS
• UTERINE BLEEDING: Deficient
SEXUALITY, MALE:
UROLOGICAL TOPICS
• SEMINAL FLUID
  INCONTINENCE
SKIN
• CARBUNCLES
TRAUMA, BITES, POISONINGS
• FRACTURES
• TRAUMA, BACK/LIMBS
• WOUNDS

Clinical/Pharmaceutical Studies:

NUTRITIONAL/METABOLIC
DISORDERS/TOPICS
• TISSUES, PROMOTES
  REGENERATION OF

SKIN
• BOILS: Induces Eruption,
  Analgesic

TRAUMA, BITES, POISONINGS
• INFLAMMATORY, ANTI-:
  Infectious Processes

Dose
6 - 15 gm

Common Name
Japanese Teasel Root

Notes
Fried: Uterine Bleeding
Powdered: External Use
w/Wine To Tonify Liver, Kidney
w/Salt To Descend

YANG QI SHI

陽起石
(阳起石)

ACTINOLITUM

Traditional Functions:

1. Warms and tonifies the Life Gate Fire of the Kidneys
2. Tonifies the Kidney Yang

Traditional Properties:

Enters: KI,

Properties: SA, W

Indications:

ABDOMEN/
GASTROINTESTINAL TOPICS
• ABDOMEN, PAIN OF
CANCER/TUMORS/SWELLINGS/
LUMPS
• TUMORS, GYNECOLOGICAL
EXTREMITIES
• LEGS, COLD
• LOINS, DEBILITY OF
HEMORRHAGIC DISORDERS
• HEMORRHAGE, INTERNAL
MUSCULOSKELETAL/
CONNECTIVE TISSUE
• BACK, LOWER PAIN, NUMB:
Kidney Yang Deficient, Cold

• KNEES, DEBILITY, COLD,
NUMB
SEXUALITY, EITHER SEX
• INFERTILITY: Cold Womb
SEXUALITY, FEMALE:
GYNECOLOGICAL
• AMENORRHEA
• LEUKORRHEA: Kidney Spleen
Yang Deficiency
• MENORRHAGIA
• UTERINE BLEEDING: Cold
Womb
• UTERUS, COLD, DEFICIENT
• UTERUS, SPASMS

SEXUALITY, MALE:
UROLOGICAL TOPICS
• IMPOTENCE W/SORE/WEAK
LOWER BACK/KNEES
• NOCTURNAL EMISSIONS
• PREMATURE EJACULATION W/
SORE/WEAK LOWER BACK/
KNEES
• PROSTATITIS
• SPERMATORRHEA W/SORE/
WEAK LOWER BACK/KNEES
TRIPLE WARMER (SAN JIAO)
• LOWER BURNER, DEFICIENCY
COLD

Dose

3.00 - 6.00 gm

Common Name

Actinolite

Contraindications

Not: Def Yin w/Heat

YI ZHI REN

益智仁
（益智仁）

FRUCTUS
ALPINIAE OXYPHYLLAE

Traditional Functions:

1. Warms the Spleen amd Kidney Yang and stops diarrhea
2. Fortifies the Qi and astringes the Essence by holding in urine and stopping diarrhea

Traditional Properties:

Enters: SP, KI,

Properties: SP, W

Indications:

ABDOMEN/
GASTROINTESTINAL TOPICS
• ABDOMEN, PAIN OF: Spleen
Deficient, Cold
BOWEL RELATED DISORDERS
• DIARRHEA: Spleen Deficient,
Cold/Spleen Kidney Yang Deficient
ORAL CAVITY
• SALIVATION, EXCESS W/THICK,
UNPLEASANT TASTE: Spleen
Deficient, Cold
SEXUALITY, FEMALE:

GYNECOLOGICAL
• LEUKORRHEA: Kidney Spleen
Yang Deficiency
• MENORRHAGIA
• PREGNANCY, BLEEDING
DURING
SEXUALITY, MALE:
UROLOGICAL TOPICS
• SEMINAL EMISSIONS
STOMACH/DIGESTIVE
DISORDERS
• GASTRALGIA

• VOMITING: Cold
URINARY BLADDER
• ENURESIS
• NOCTURIA
• URINARY INCONTINENCE
• URINATION, DRIBBLING:
Kidney Yang Deficient
• URINATION, FREQUENT/
COPIOUS: Kidney Yang Deficient
• URINATION, PAINFUL,
DRIBBLING: With Deficiency Cold

Clinical/Pharmaceutical Studies:

FLUID DISORDERS
• ANTIDIURETIC
ORAL CAVITY

• SALIVATION, INHIBITS
STOMACH/DIGESTIVE

DISORDERS
• STOMACHIC

Dose

3 - 9 gm

Contraindications

Not: Yin Def With Heat, Seminal Emissions, Leukorrhea,

Frequent Urination, Uterine Bleeding From Heat

Notes

Add Shan Yao To Reduce Def.Heat Development
Baked Reduces Spicy, Warm Property

YIN YANG HUO
(XIAN LING PI)

淫羊霍

HERBA EPIMEDII

Traditional Functions:

1. Tonifies the Kidney Yang and strengthens the bones and tendons
2. Dispels Wind Cold Damp with Qi weakness
3. Controls ascending Liver Yang
4. Helps control cough and asthma

Traditional Properties:

Enters: KI, LV,

Properties: SP, W

Indications:

CIRCULATION DISORDERS
• HYPERTENSION
COLD
• COLD WIND W/QI EXERTION
EARS/HEARING DISORDERS
• DIZZINESS: Liver Kidney Deficient With Liver Yang Rising
EXTREMITIES
• ARMS, NUMB, WEAK
• FEET, SPASMS/CRAMPS: Wind Cold Damp
• HANDS, SPASMS/CRAMPS: Wind Cold Damp
• LEGS, NUMB, WEAK
• LOINS, WEAK

KIDNEYS
• KIDNEY YANG DEFICIENCY
LUNGS
• BRONCHITIS, CHRONIC
MENTAL STATE/ NEUROLOGICAL DISORDERS
• CONVULSIONS
• FORGETFULNESS
• HEMIPLEGIA
• MALAISE
• PARALYSIS, GENERAL
• WITHDRAWAL, EMOTIONAL
MUSCULOSKELETAL/ CONNECTIVE TISSUE
• ARTHRITIS: For Expelling Cold, Dampness

• BACK, LOWER PAIN: Liver Kidney Deficient With Liver Yang Rising
• BACK, LOWER PAIN, COLD
• JOINTS, PAIN: Damp Bi With Liver Kidney Weakness/Wind Cold Damp
• KNEES, PAIN, COLD
• SPASMS, SUDDEN
• SPASMS/NUMBNESS IN EXTREMTY
PAIN/NUMBNESS/ GENERAL DISCOMFORT
• BI DISORDERS
SEXUALITY, EITHER SEX
• INFERTILITY: Uterine

Cold Palace
SEXUALITY, FEMALE: GYNECOLOGICAL
• LEUKORRHEA: Kidney Spleen Yang Deficiency
• MENSTRUATION, DISORDERS OF: Tonify Qi Of Chong, Ren
• MENSTRUATION, IRREGULAR: Liver Kidney Deficient With Liver Yang Rising
SEXUALITY, MALE: UROLOGICAL TOPICS
• IMPOTENCE
• SEMINAL EMISSIONS
• SPERMATORRHEA
URINARY BLADDER
• URINATION, FREQUENT

Clinical/Pharmaceutical Studies:

BLOOD RELATED DISORDERS/TOPICS
• BLOOD GLUCOSE, REDUCES: Extract 10 mg/kg
• BLOOD PRESSURE, LOWERS: Decoction/ Ethanol Fractionated Decoction Injected IV, *Er Xian Mixture (Yin Yang Huo, Huang Bai, Zhi Mu, Xian Mao, Ba Ji Tian, Dang Gui)
• CHOLESTEROL, LOWERS: 100% Decoction
CIRCULATION DISORDERS
• HYPERTENSION: Extract Tab, 30 g Crude Herb/Day In 3 Doses For 1 Month, Better In Stage I, * Er Xian Decoction (1:15), 15-30 ml, 2x/Day, Good For Stage III, Yin Deficiency With Yang Rising/Yin-Yang Deficiency
• HYPERTENSION,

• ESTROGEN-LIKE: None Noted
HEART
• ANGINA PECTORIS: 4-6 Tabs (0.3 g/Tab), 2x/. Day, 1 Month/Course, 7-10 Days Between Courses
• HEART, INCREASES CORONARY BLOOD FLOW: Marked By 75%
IMMUNE SYSTEM RELATED DISORDERS/ TOPICS
• IMMUNE SYSTEM ENHANCEMENT: Increased Phagocytosis
INFECTIOUS DISEASES
• ANTIBIOTIC: Marked Polio, Staph, TB, B. Influenzae, Pneumococci, Neisseria
• POLIOMYELITIS, ACUTE: 10% Injection 2 ml IM Injection, 1x/Day For 10 Days, * Antiparalytic Injection (Herb, Sang Ji Sheng) For Sequelae, Acute Stase, 2 ml IM 2x/Day For 20 Days

• ASTHMA, BRONCHIAL: Yang Huo Gan Chuan Ping Tablet (Yin Yang Huo, Mu Li, Hai Piao Xiao, Yuan Zhi, Qian Cao Gen, Xiao Hui Xiang, Lycorine, Clorprenaline Glycyrrhizinate)
• BRONCHITIS, ASTHMATIC: Yang Huo Gan Chuan Ping Tablet (Yin Yang Huo, Mu LI, Hai Piao Xiao, Yuan Zhi, Qian Cao Gen, Xiao Hui Xiang, Lycorine, Clorprenaline Glycyrrhizinate)
• BRONCHITIS, CHRONIC: Increases Lung Capacity, *75% From Herb Pill Alone
• BRONCHITIS, CHRONIC W/ EMPHYSEMA: Yang Huo Gan Chuan Ping Tablet (Yin Yang Huo, Mu LI, Hai Piao Xiao, Yuan Zhi, Qian Cao Gen, Xiao Hui Xiang, Lycorine, Clorprenaline

NUTRITIONAL/ METABOLIC DISORDERS/TOPICS
• HYPOXIA: Reduces Effects Of, 100% Decoction
SEXUALITY, EITHER SEX
• SEXUAL NEURASTHENIA: Decoction 3-9 g/Day, Or Small Oral Doses Of 60 g Herb In 1 L Wine
SEXUALITY, FEMALE: GYNECOLOGICAL
• HYPERTENSION, CLIMACTERIC: Er Xian Tang
• MENOPAUSE SYNDROME: Er Xian Tang
SEXUALITY, MALE: UROLOGICAL TOPICS
• SEMEN, INCREASES SECRETION OF
• SEXUAL ACTIVITY, INCREASED: Increased Semen Secretion, Leaf/ Root Strongest

Clinical/Pharmaceutical Studies:

CLIMACTERIC: Er Xian
Tang
ENDOCRINE RELATED
DISORDERS
• ANDROGEN-LIKE
EFFECT: Moderate On
Testes, Prostate, Levator
Ani

• VIRAL, ANTI-: Inhibits
Polio, Echo, Coxsackie
KIDNEYS
• DIURETIC: Low Doses
LUNGS
• ANTITUSSIVE
• ASTHMA: MEOH
Extract

Glycyrrhizinate)
• EXPECTORANT
MENTAL STATE/
NEUROLOGICAL
DISORDERS
• NEURASTHENIA
• SEDATIVE: Injection IP

• SPERM PRODUCTION
INCREASED
TRAUMA, BITES,
POISONINGS
• INFLAMMATORY, ANTI-
: Injection/Oral MEOH
Extract

Dose
3 - 15 gm

Contraindications
Not: Yin Def Fire, Hyperactive Sex, Wet Dreams

Notes
Can Damage Yin Fluid With Time
Large Doses May Cause Mild Spasm
Very Large: Respiratory Arrest

ZI HE CHE
(TAI YI)

紫河車
(紫河车)

PLACENTA HOMINIS

Traditional Functions:

1. Powerfully tonifies the Qi, nourishes the Blood and benefits the Essence

Traditional Properties:

Enters: LU, HT, KI, LV,

Properties: SW, SA, W

Indications:

BLOOD RELATED DISORDERS/
TOPICS
• BLOOD DEFICIENCY W/
WITHERING YELLOW
COMPLEXION
ENERGETIC STATE
• DEBILITY: Tuberculosis
• WEAKNESS: Qi Deficiency
HEAD/NECK
• ALOPECIA: Deficiency Complex
INFECTIOUS DISEASES
• CONSUMPTION, DEFICIENCY
WITH EMACIATION
LUNGS

• ASTHMA, ALLERGIC
• COUGH, WHEEZING, CHRONIC/
RECURRENT
• DYSPNEA
NUTRITIONAL/METABOLIC
DISORDERS/TOPICS
• EMACIATION: Tuberculosis
QI RELATED DISORDERS/
TOPICS
• QI/BLOOD INSUFFICIENCY
SEXUALITY, EITHER SEX
• INFERTILITY: Blood Deficiency/
Uterine Cold Palace

SEXUALITY, FEMALE:
GYNECOLOGICAL
• LACTATION, INSUFFICIENT
• MENSTRUATION, DISORDERS
OF: Tonify Qi Of Chong, Ren
• MISCARRIAGE, HABITUAL
SEXUALITY, MALE:
UROLOGICAL TOPICS
• IMPOTENCE
• NOCTURNAL EMISSIONS
SKIN
• NIGHT SWEATS: Tuberculosis
• SWEATING, FURTIVE

Clinical/Pharmaceutical Studies:

BLOOD RELATED DISORDERS/
TOPICS
• ANEMIA
• BLOOD CLOTTING, ENHANCES:
Factor XIII Def
ENDOCRINE RELATED
DISORDERS
• HORMONE-LIKE: Stimulates
Chorionic Hormones, Testes,
Estrogen
ENERGETIC STATE
• ENDURANCE, INCREASES
IMMUNE SYSTEM RELATED
DISORDERS/TOPICS
• ALLERGIES
• IMMUNE SYSTEM
ENHANCEMENT: Oral
Administration, Injected Contains

Substance
• INFLUENZA: Enhances Immune
Response Against
• MEASLES: Injected Contains
Gamma-Globulin, Enhances Immune
Response Against
LIVER
• LIVER, TOXICITY, REDUCES:
Reduces Fatty Cells
LUNGS
• ASTHMA: UB13, ST16 Injection
• LUNGS, CHRONIC
OBSTRUCTIVE PULMONARY
DISEASE, SEVERE,
RECALCITRANT: Injections,
Helped
• TUBERCULOSIS: Can Slow
Disease By Enhancing Immune

• LACTATION, INCREASES:
Powder, 4-7 Days
• UTERINE ATROPHY
• UTERINE BLEEDING
• UTERUS, MYOMETRITIS:
(Inflammed Uterine Muscle Wall)
• UTERUS, STIMULATES
• UTERUS, UNDEVELOPED
SEXUALITY, MALE:
UROLOGICAL TOPICS
• TESTICLES: Stimulates
SKIN
• SKIN, ULCERS: Powder Of
Sterilized, Inhibits, Cures In Few
Weeks
STOMACH/DIGESTIVE
DISORDERS
• ULCERS, GASTRIC: Can Treat/

Clinical/Pharmaceutical Studies:

Gamma-Globulin, Interferon

INFECTIOUS DISEASES
- ANTIBIOTIC: Flu, Measles (Injected)
- INFECTIONS: A-Globulin-Like

System

SEXUALITY, FEMALE: GYNECOLOGICAL
- AMENORRHEA, FUNCTIONAL

Prevent

TRAUMA, BITES, POISONINGS
- WOUNDS, PROMOTES HEALING

Dose

2.4 - 9.0 gm

Common Name

Human Placenta

Precautions

Watch: May Cause Yin Def/Drying

Notes

Don't Boil
Add Qi/Blood Herbs
Use Cautiously

Tonify The Blood

BAI SHAO
(BAI SHAO YAO)

白芍

RADIX PAEONIAE LACTIFLORAE
(ALBA)

Traditional Functions:

1. Nourishes the Blood and consolidates the Yin
2. Soothes the Liver Yang
3. Calms the Liver and relieves pain
3. Adjusts the Ying and Wei levels

Traditional Properties:

Enters: SP, LV,

Properties: BIT, SO, CL

Indications:

ABDOMEN/ GASTROINTESTINAL TOPICS
- ABDOMEN, PAIN OF, DULL: Liver Qi Stagnation/Liver Spleen Disharmony
- ABDOMEN, PAIN OF, SPASMS
- FLANK PAIN: Liver Qi Stagnation/Liver Spleen Disharmony
- SUBCOSTAL PAIN

BLOOD RELATED DISORDERS/TOPICS
- BLOOD DEFICIENCY SYNDROME: Weakly Tonifies
- BLOOD DEFICIENCY W/ WITHERING YELLOW COMPLEXION

BOWEL RELATED DISORDERS
- DIARRHEA
- DYSENTERY: Blood Heat
- DYSENTERY, ABDOMINAL PAIN

FROM CHEST
- CHEST, PAIN: Liver Qi Stagnation/Liver Spleen Disharmony
- INTERCOSTAL PAIN: Liver Qi Stagnation/Liver Spleen Disharmony

EARS/HEARING DISORDERS
- DIZZINESS: Liver Yang Rising
- TINNITUS
- VERTIGO: Liver Yang/ Fire Rising

EXTREMITIES
- CALF MUSCLE SPASMS
- FEET, SPASMS, CRAMPS
- HANDS, SPASMS, CRAMPS

HEAD/NECK
- ALOPECIA: Deficiency Complex
- FACE, COMPLEXION, WITHERING YELLOW
- HEADACHE: Hypertension/Liver Yang

Rising
LIVER
- HEPATOMEGALY
- LIVER QI CONGESTION W/SUBCOSTAL PAIN
- LIVER QI STAGNATION/ LIVER SPLEEN DISHARMONY: Abdominal Pain, Flank Pain, Chest Pain

MENTAL STATE/ NEUROLOGICAL DISORDERS
- IRRITABILITY

MUSCULOSKELETAL/ CONNECTIVE TISSUE
- SPASMS, CONVULSIONS: Internal Deficiency Wind

PAIN/NUMBNESS/ GENERAL DISCOMFORT
- NUMBNESS W/SPASMS, CONTRACTURES: Blood Deficiency Bi

SEXUALITY, FEMALE: GYNECOLOGICAL
- DYSMENORRHEA:

Blood Deficient
- GYNECOLOGICAL CONDITIONS, GENERAL: Blood Deficient
- LEUKORRHEA
- MENORRHAGIA
- UTERINE BLEEDING

SEXUALITY, MALE: UROLOGICAL TOPICS
- SPERMATORRHEA

SKIN
- PERSPIRATION, RESTING & THIEF
- SWEATING, CONTINUED W/ EXTERIOR CONDITIONS
- SWEATING, FURTIVE
- SWEATING, INHIBITS
- SWEATING, NIGHT: Floating Yang
- SWEATING, RESTING
- SWEATING, SPONTANEOUS: Floating Yang

SPLEEN
- SPLENOMEGALY

Clinical/Pharmaceutical Studies:

BLOOD RELATED DISORDERS/TOPICS
- BLOOD PRESSURE, LOWERS

CIRCULATION DISORDERS
- VASODILATES: Mild

FEVERS
- ANTIPYRETIC: Lowers

FLOW: Much Less Than Nitroglycerin
INFECTIOUS DISEASES
- BACTERIAL, ANTI-: B. Dysenteriae, Strep, Pneum, Pseudomonas, Staph, et al

KIDNEYS
- DIURESIS, INHIBITS

MENTAL STATE/

Camphor, Not Strychnine
- SEDATIVE, CNS
- TRANQUILIZING

MUSCULOSKELETAL/ CONNECTIVE TISSUE
- ANTISPASMODIC IN SMOOTH MUSCLE: Synergistic With Gan Cao

PAIN/NUMBNESS/

GYNECOLOGICAL
- UTERUS, INHIBITS: Inhibits Spasms Of

STOMACH/DIGESTIVE DISORDERS
- STOMACH, INHIBITS SECRETIONS, PREVENTS STRESS ULCERS

Clinical/Pharmaceutical Studies:

Body Temperature, With/
With Out Fever
HEART
• HEART, INCREASES
CORONARY BLOOD

**NEUROLOGICAL
DISORDERS**
• CNS, INHIBITOR
• CONVULSIVE, ANTI-:
Cocaine, Caffeine,

**GENERAL
DISCOMFORT**
• ANALGESIC
SEXUALITY, FEMALE:

**TRAUMA, BITES,
POISONINGS**
• INFLAMMATORY, ANTI-
, REDUCES EDEMA

Dose

3 - 12 gm

Common Name

Peony Root

Contraindications

Not: Cold, Yang Def Syndromes

Precautions

Watch: Cold, Def Diarrhea

Notes

Not With: LI LU

Pain: Use 15 gm

DANG GUI

當歸
(当归)

RADIX ANGELICAE SINENSIS

Traditional Functions:

1. Nourishes the Blood and regulates menstruation
2. Vitalizes and harmonizes the Blood and helps to relieve pain
3. Moistens the intestines and facilitates passage of stool
4. The head of the root is more tonifying, root tips more Blood vitalizing, body used to tonify and vitalize the Blood

Traditional Properties:

Enters: SP, HT, LV,

Properties: SW, SP, BIT, W

Indications:

**BLOOD RELATED DISORDERS/
TOPICS**
• ANEMIA
• BLOOD DEFICIENCY
SYNDROME
• BLOOD DEFICIENCY W/BI
• BLOOD DEFICIENCY W/
WITHERING YELLOW
COMPLEXION
BOWEL RELATED DISORDERS
• CONSTIPATION: Moist (Like:Zhi
Ke) , For Aged, Debilitated
**CANCER/TUMORS/SWELLINGS/
LUMPS**
• TUMORS, GYNECOLOGICAL
CHEST
• CHEST, PAIN
EARS/HEARING DISORDERS
• TINNITUS: Blood Deficient
EYES
• VISION, BLURRED: Blood
Deficient
HEAD/NECK
• ALOPECIA: Deficiency Complex
• FACE, PALE: Blood Deficient
• HAIR, PREMATURE WHITENING

• HEADACHE: Blood Deficient
HEART
• HEART DISEASE: Coronary
• PALPITATIONS: Blood Deficient
HEMORRHAGIC DISORDERS
• HEMORRHAGE: Deficiency
Caused
LUNGS
• ASTHMA: Deficient
• COUGH, CHRONIC
**MUSCULOSKELETAL/
CONNECTIVE TISSUE**
• BACKACHE
**PAIN/NUMBNESS/GENERAL
DISCOMFORT**
• ANALGESIC: Stomach, Muscles,
Joints
• BI, WIND DAMP, CHRONIC:
With Blood Stasis, Open The Luo
• NUMBNESS W/SPASMS,
CONTRACTURES: Blood
Deficiency Bi
**SEXUALITY, FEMALE:
GYNECOLOGICAL**
• AMENORRHEA: Blood Deficient

• DYSMENORRHEA: Blood
Deficient
• GYNECOLOGICAL PROBLEMS
W/BLOOD DEFICIENCY
• LACTATION, INSUFFICIENT: Qi,
Blood Deficiency
• MENORRHAGIA
• MENSTRUATION, DISORDERS
OF: Dredge, Regulate Chong, Ren
• MENSTRUATION, IRREGULAR:
Blood Deficient
• POSTPARTUM, PAIN
• UTERINE BLEEDING
SKIN
• ABSCESS, YIN, INTERNAL
SINKING OF
• CARBUNCLES: Blood Stagnation
• SKIN, INFECTIONS
• SKIN, SORES, SWOLLEN, TOXIC:
Blood Stasis, Swelling
**STOMACH/DIGESTIVE
DISORDERS**
• EPIGASTRIC PAIN
TRAUMA, BITES, POISONINGS
• TRAUMA, INJURIES: Die Da

Clinical/Pharmaceutical Studies:

**ABDOMEN/
GASTROINTESTINAL
TOPICS**
• HERNIA, INGUINAL: SI

TOPICS
• IMMUNE SYSTEM
ENHANCEMENT,
PHAGOCYTOSIS

• JOINTS, PAIN,
SWELLING FROM
ALLERGIC RESPONSE:
Yi Shen Tang (Dang Gui,

• MASTITIS: Xiao Yao San
• MENOPAUSE
SYNDROME W/
AUTONOMIC NERVOUS

Clinical/Pharmaceutical Studies:

Ni Tang With Dang Gui

BLOOD RELATED DISORDERS/TOPICS
- ANEMIA: Dang Gui Bai Shao San
- ANEMIA, PERNICIOUS: Has Folic Acid, Vit B12
- BLOOD PRESSURE, LOWERS
- THROMBOCYTOPENIC PURPURA: Dangui Bu Xue Tang

BOWEL RELATED DISORDERS
- DYSENTERY, BACILLARY: Dang Gui Bai Shao San, Satisfactory Results
- IRRITABLE BOWEL SYNDROME: SI Ni Tang With Dang Gui

CIRCULATION DISORDERS
- ATHEROSCLEROSIS: Reduces Plaque Formation
- CEREBRAL ARTERIOSCLEROSIS: Injection
- ISCHEMIC PAIN
- THROMBOANGIITIS OBLITERANS: Injection, *Dang Gui Huo Xue Tang (Dang Gui, Hong Hua, Tao Ren, Ru Xiang, Gan Cao) For Early Stage

ENDOCRINE RELATED DISORDERS
- HYPERTHYROIDISM: Injection 25% Solution Into Thyroid Gland

EXTREMITIES
- FINGERS, DIGITAL ARTERIAL SPASM: SI Ni Tang With Dang Gui
- LEGS, PAIN

HEAD/NECK
- BRAIN, CONCUSSION: Injection
- OCCIPITAL NEURALGIA
- TEMPOROMANDIBULAR JOINT DISORDER: Injection

HEART
- AORTITIS, CONSTRICTIVE: IV Infusion
- CORONARY ARTERIES, INCREASED FLOW
- CORONARY HEART

- IMMUNE SYSTEM, INHIBITS: Similar To Azathioprine
- JOINTS, PAINFUL, SWOLLEN FROM ALLERGIC RESPONSE: Yi Shen Tang (Dang Gui, Chi Shao, Chuan Xiong, Hong Hua, Dan Shen, Tao Ren)

INFECTIOUS DISEASES
- ANTIBIOTIC: Many, Strep, Shegella, E.Coli, B. Dysenteriae
- HERPES ZOSTER: Tablet Of Extract
- POLIOMYELITIS: Volatile Oil, 0.5 g/ml Injection In Acupoints, Shen Shu, Xia Qu, Zu San Li, Da Zui, Jian Jin , Nei Guan, 1 ml/Point, Every 5 Days, Good Results

KIDNEYS
- DIURETIC
- NEPHRITIS, CHRONIC: Yi Shen Tang, Shen Yan Hua Yu Tang, 1 Dose/Day For 2-12 Months, Some Needed Prednisone, Too

LIVER
- HEPATITIS, ACUTE, ICTERIC: Xiao Yao San
- LIVER, HELPS METABOLISM OF
- LIVER, PROTECTANT

LUNGS
- ASTHMATICUS, STATUS: Ether Extract, No Other Medication, 2-10 Hrs To Get Benefit
- BRONCHITIS, CHRONIC W/ EMPHYSEMA/HEART DISEASE, EARLY/ REMISSION STAGE: Extract

MENTAL STATE/ NEUROLOGICAL DISORDERS
- CEREBRAL ISCHEMIC STROKE
- SEDATIVE: Volatile Oil, Inhibits Brain, Mild, Synergistic With Datura Metel (Yang Jin Hua) , Chinese Herbal Anesthetic

MUSCULOSKELETAL/ CONNECTIVE TISSUE
- ARTHRITIS, PAIN: 25%

Chi Shao, Chuan Xiong, Hong Hua, Dan Shen, Tao Ren)
- MUSCLES, SMOOTH, INHIBITS: Small Intestines
- MYALGIA: 25% Injection
- RHEUMATOID ARTHRITIS
- SCIATICA IN PREGNANCY: Dang Gui Bai Shao San

NUTRITIONAL/ METABOLIC DISORDERS/TOPICS
- METABOLISM, INCREASES
- VITAMIN E DEFICIENCY

ORAL CAVITY
- PERIODONTITIS: Injection
- VOCAL CORDS, WEAK: Solution Of Alum, Dang Gui

PAIN/NUMBNESS/ GENERAL DISCOMFORT
- ANALGESIC: Not For Acute, Sprains, Infections, Tumors, But All Others, About 1.7 X Aspirin
- ANESTHETIC, HERBAL: With Yang Jin Hua
- NEURALGIA: 25% Injection, Into Acu-Points
- NEURALGIA, OCCIPITAL

SEXUALITY, EITHER SEX
- SEX HORMONE: No Female Action
- STERILITY: Dang Gui Bai Shao San

SEXUALITY, FEMALE: GYNECOLOGICAL
- ADNEXITIS: Dang Gui Bai Shao San
- BREASTS, PAIN, PREMENSTRUAL: Xiao Yao San
- CERVICITIS: Dang Gui Bai Shao San
- DYSMENORRHEA: 3-15 g, *SI Wu Tang, *Better With Xiang Fu, Ai Ye, Tao Ren, Hong Hua
- FETUS, ABNORMAL MOVEMENTS: Dang Gui

DISTURBANCES: Dang Gui Bai Shao San (Dang Gui, Bai Shao, Chuan Xiong, Bai Zhu, Ze Xie, Fu Ling) , 70% Effective
- MENSTRUATION, DISORDERS OF
- OVARIAN SURGICAL REMOVAL, POST SYNDROME: Dang Gui Bai Shao San (Dang Gui, Bai Shao, Chuan Xiong, Bai Zhu, Ze Xie, Fu Ling) , 70% Effective
- PELVIC INFLAMMATORY INFECTION: Dang Gui Bai Shao San
- PREMENSTRUAL TENSION: Xiao Yao San
- SCIATICA IN PREGNANCY: Dang Gui Bai Shao San
- UTERUS: Water Soluble/ Non-Volatile--Stimulates, Volatile Component-- Relaxes
- UTERUS, CONTRACTIONS, REGULATES
- UTERUS, PROLAPSE: Injection

SEXUALITY, MALE: UROLOGICAL TOPICS
- PENIS, FIBROTIC CAVERNITIS: Injection Of 10% Solution
- SPERMATIC VARICOSITY: SI Ni Tang With Dang Gui

SKIN
- NEURODERMATITIS, DISCOID: Injection
- SCLERODERMA: Injection Of Dang Gui, Mao Dong Qing
- SKIN, DISORDERS: Many e.g. Urticaria, Eczema, Neurodermatitis, Pruritus, Vitiligo, Pigment Diseases, Rosacea, Alopecia--Ear Point Injection In Shen Shang Xian, Nei Fen Mi, Shen Men, Pi Zhi Xia

TRAUMA, BITES, POISONINGS
- BRAIN CONCUSSION: Injection
- INFLAMMATORY, ANTI-

Clinical/Pharmaceutical Studies:

DISEASE: Can Regulate
Auricular Fibrillation
**IMMUNE SYSTEM
RELATED DISORDERS/**

Injection
• BACK, LOWER PAIN
• JOINTS, PAIN: 25%
Injection

Bai Shao San
• LOCHIA, PROLONGED:
SI Wu Tang

: 1.1 X Aspirin
URINARY BLADDER
• ENURESIS

Dose

3 - 15 gm

Common Name

Tangkuei Root

Contraindications

Not: Def Yin w/Heat

Precautions

Watch: w/Diarrhea

Watch: Abdominal Distension From Dampness

Notes

Mix w/Wine To Enhance Vitalize Blood

For Exterior Symptoms/Signs: 3-9 gm
Blood Circulation/Move Stool: 12-30gm
May Cause Mild Lassitude

E JIAO
(A JIAO)

阿膠
（阿胶）

GELATINUM
ASINI

Traditional Functions:

1. Nourishes the Blood and controls bleeding
3. Nourishes the Yin and moistens the Lungs

Traditional Properties:

Enters: LU, KI, LV,

Properties: SW, N

Indications:

**BLOOD RELATED DISORDERS/
TOPICS**
• BLOOD DEFICIENCY
SYNDROME: All Types/
Postpartum
• BLOOD DEFICIENCY W/
WITHERING YELLOW
COMPLEXION
BOWEL RELATED DISORDERS
• CONSTIPATION: Intestinal
Dryness
EARS/HEARING DISORDERS
• DIZZINESS: Blood Deficient
ENERGETIC STATE
• DEFICIENCY EXHAUSTION
FEVERS
• STEAMING BONE FEVER: Yin
Deficient Heat
HEAD/NECK
• FACE, SALLOW COMPLEXION:
Blood Deficient
HEART
• PALPITATIONS: Blood Deficient
HEMORRHAGIC DISORDERS

• BLEEDING, ANY TYPE: (Best
Consumptive Types)
• HEMATEMESIS
• HEMOPTYSIS
• HEMORRHAGE: Deficiency
Caused
INFECTIOUS DISEASES
• FEBRILE DISEASES, SEQUELAE
OF
LUNGS
• COUGH: Lung Dryness
• COUGH, DEFICIENT
• COUGH, DRY W/BLOODY
SPUTUM
• COUGH, LUNG EXHAUSTION:
Tuberculosis
**MENTAL STATE/
NEUROLOGICAL DISORDERS**
• INSOMNIA: Yin Deficient Post
Febrile Disease
• INSOMNIA, RESTLESS
• IRRITABILITY: Yin Deficient Post
Febrile Disease
• PARALYSIS

• RESTLESSNESS
**MUSCULOSKELETAL/
CONNECTIVE TISSUE**
• SPASMS, CONVULSIONS:
Deficiency Wind–Liver Kidney
**SEXUALITY, FEMALE:
GYNECOLOGICAL**
• FETUS, RESTLESS: Liver Kidney
Deficiency/Threatened Abortion,
Blood Deficiency
• MENORRHAGIA: Avalanche &
Leakage (w/Other Herbs)
• MENSTRUATION, DISORDERS
OF: Tonify Chong, Ren, Essence,
Blood
• POSTPARTUM, BLOOD
DEFICIENCY
TRAUMA, BITES, POISONINGS
• WOUNDS
**YIN RELATED DISORDERS/
TOPICS**
• YIN DAMAGE FROM HEAT
• YIN DEFICIENCY W/DEFICIENT
FIRE

Clinical/Pharmaceutical Studies:

**ABDOMEN/
GASTROINTESTINAL
TOPICS**
• GASTROINTESTINAL,
UPPER BLEEDING:
Various Herb Formulas
BLOOD RELATED

SUBSTITUTE: As
Injection, Superior To
Normal Saline Because Of
Colloids, May Be
Antigenic
• LEUKOPENIA: With
Gou Qi Zi, Dang Shen,

Huang Liang E Jiao Tang
**HEMORRHAGIC
DISORDERS**
• HEMOSTATIC
**MUSCULOSKELETAL/
CONNECTIVE TISSUE**
• MUSCLES, ATROPHY

Promotes Calcium
Absorption
**SEXUALITY, FEMALE:
GYNECOLOGICAL**
• ABORTION, HABITUAL:
SI Wu Tang Plus E Jiao,
Ai Ye

Clinical/Pharmaceutical Studies:

DISORDERS/TOPICS
• ANEMIA, APLASTIC: Sheng Xue Pian (Zi He Che, Zao Fan (Melanteritum) , Rou Gui, E Jiao, Hai Piao Xiao) 2 Tabs, 3x/Day
• ANEMIA, POST HEMORRHAGE
• BLOOD PRESSURE, RAISES: Injection
• BLOOD, INCREASES RBC
• BLOOD, PLASMA

Dan Shen, Vine Spatholobus Suberectus)
• THROMBOCYTOPENIC PURPURA HEMORRHAGICA: Xin Jia Fu Mai Tang (E Jiao, Mai Dong, Sheng Di, Bai Shao, Dang Gui, Huang Qi, Zhi Gan Cao, *Jiao Ai SI Wu Tang (Ai Ye, E Jiao, SI Wu Tang, Zhi Gan Cao)

EYES
• EYES, BLEEDING IN:

• MUSCULAR DYSTROPHY, NUTRITIONAL OR PROGRESSIVE: Prevents Vit E Oxidation, Amino Acids, 6-10 Weeks Treatment
NUTRITIONAL/ METABOLIC DISORDERS/TOPICS
• CALCIUM UPTAKE, INCREASES: From Glycine Content Which

• ABORTION, THREATENED: SI Wu Tang Plus E Jiao, Ai Ye
• MENORRHAGIA: Gui LU Er Xian Jiao (Gui Ban, E Jiao Gelatin)
• UTERINE BLEEDING: SI Wu Tang Plus E Jiao, Ai Ye
TRAUMA, BITES, POISONINGS
• WOUNDS, PREVENTS SHOCK FROM

Dose
9 - 15 gm

Common Name
Ass Skin Glue

Contraindications
Not: w/Exterior Conditions

Precautions
Watch: Weak Stomachs, Diarrhea

GOU QI ZI   枸杞子   *FRUCTUS LYCII CHINENSIS*

Traditional Functions:

1. Nourishes and tonifies the Liver and Kidney Yin
2. Benefits the Essence and clears the eyes
3. Nourishes Blood and replinishes the Yin
4. Moistens the Lungs

Traditional Properties:

Enters: KI, LV,

Properties: SW, N

Indications:

ABDOMEN/. GASTROINTESTINAL TOPICS
• ABDOMEN, PAIN OF, MILD: Yin/Blood Deficient
BLOOD RELATED DISORDERS/TOPICS
• BLOOD DEFICIENCY W/ WITHERING YELLOW COMPLEXION
EARS/HEARING DISORDERS
• DIZZINESS: Liver Kidney Essence/Blood Deficient
ENDOCRINE RELATED DISORDERS
• DIABETES: Internal Heat With Exhaustion Thirst/ Yin/Blood Deficient

EXTREMITIES
• LEGS, SORE: Yin/Blood Deficient
• LEGS, UPPER, WEAK: Loins
EYES
• TEARING, EXCESSIVE
• VISION, BLURRED: Liver Kidney Essence/ Blood Deficient
FEVERS
• STEAMING BONE FEVER: Yin Deficient Heat
FLUID DISORDERS
• THIRST, EXHAUSTION
HEAD/NECK
• HAIR, PREMATURE WHITENING
INFECTIOUS DISEASES
• CONSUMPTION: Yin/

Blood Deficient
KIDNEYS
• ESSENCE/KI QI DEFICIENCY
LIVER
• LIVER/KIDNEY YIN DEFICIENCY
LUNGS
• COUGH: Lung Dryness
• COUGH, DEFICIENT CONSUMPTIVE
MUSCULOSKELETAL/ CONNECTIVE TISSUE
• BACK, PAIN: Yin/Blood Deficient
• KNEES, WEAK
• SPASMS, CONVULSIONS: Deficiency Wind--Liver Kidney

SEXUALITY, FEMALE: GYNECOLOGICAL
• MENSTRUATION, DISORDERS OF: Tonify Chong, Ren, Essence, Blood
SEXUALITY, MALE: UROLOGICAL TOPICS
• IMPOTENCE: Yin/Blood Deficient
• NOCTURNAL EMISSIONS: Yin/Blood Deficient
SKIN
• SWEATING, SPONTANEOUS
TRIPLE WARMER (SAN JIAO)
• LOWER BURNER, DEFICIENCY

Clinical/Pharmaceutical Studies:

ABDOMEN/ GASTROINTESTINAL TOPICS
• INTESTINES, STIMULATES

Slightly Inhibits
EARS/HEARING DISORDERS
• DIZZINESS
• TINNITUS

100% ETOH Extract IM Injection Markedly Increased Phagocytosis, * Use With Dang Shen, 1:2, Also

Wan (Herb, Shu Di, Shan Yao, Rou Gui Pi, Fu Zi, Du Zhong, Dang Gui, Tuber Of Colocasia Esculenta)
MUSCULOSKELETAL/

Clinical/Pharmaceutical Studies:

BLOOD RELATED DISORDERS/TOPICS
- BLOOD GLUCOSE, REDUCES: Marked, Sustained
- BLOOD PRESSURE, LOWERS
- BLOOD, HELPS TO GENERATE: 10% Decoction, 10 Days Enhanced Blood Cell Generation, Especially WBC
- CHOLESTEROL, LOWERS

CIRCULATION DISORDERS
- ATHEROSCLEROSIS:

EXTREMITIES
- LEGS, WEAK

EYES
- EYES, DECREASED VISION

FEVERS
- FEVER, YIN DEFICIENCY

HEART
- HEART RATE, REDUCES: Reduces Output Volume, Too

IMMUNE SYSTEM RELATED DISORDERS/TOPICS
- IMMUNE SYSTEM ENHANCEMENT: Aqueous Extract Orally/

LIVER
- HEPATITIS, CHRONIC
- LIVER, CHRONIC DISEASES
- LIVER, CIRRHOSIS
- LIVER, PROMOTES REGENERATION
- LIVER, PROTECTANT: Water Extract

MENTAL STATE/ NEUROLOGICAL DISORDERS
- CHOLINERGIC, CNS
- NEURASTHENIA: Kidney And Jing/Blood Deficiency–Herb, Ju Hua, Shu Di, Shan Zhu Yu, Shan Yao, Ze Xie Or You Gui

CONNECTIVE TISSUE
- BACK, LOWER PAIN

NUTRITIONAL/ METABOLIC DISORDERS/TOPICS
- GROWTH STIMULANT: 1:10 Dang Shen/Herb Oral Decoction For 4 Days Markedly Increased Body Weight In Animals, Betaine Active Ingredient
- METABOLISM, LIPIDS INCREASES

SEXUALITY, MALE: UROLOGICAL TOPICS
- NOCTURNAL EMISSIONS

Not: External Excess Heat

Dose

6 - 18 gm

Common Name

Matrimony Vine Fruit

Contraindications

Not: SP Def w/Loose BM

Precautions

Watch: Internal Heat

Notes

Very Low Toxicity

HE SHOU WU
(SHOU WU)

何首烏
（何首乌）

RADIX POLYGONI MULTIFLORI

Traditional Functions:

1. Nourishes the Blood, tonifies the Liver and Kidneys
2. Astringes and nourishes the Essence and stops leakage
3. Detoxifies toxic Heat swellings
4. Moistens the intestines and facilitates passage of stool
5. Expels Wind from the skin by nourishing the Blood

Traditional Properties:

Enters: KI, LV,

Properties: BIT, SW, A, <W

Indications:

ABDOMEN/ GASTROINTESTINAL TOPICS
- INTESTINAL WIND

BLOOD RELATED DISORDERS/ TOPICS
- ANEMIA
- BLOOD DEFICIENCY W/BI
- BLOOD DEFICIENCY W/ WITHERING YELLOW COMPLEXION
- CHOLESTEROL, LOWERS

BOWEL RELATED DISORDERS
- CONSTIPATION: Heat Entanglement/Intestinal Dryness
- CONSTIPATION W/DEFICIENT BLOOD

CANCER/TUMORS/SWELLINGS/ LUMPS
- NECK LUMPS

Deficient
- LOINS, SORE

EYES
- VISION, BLURRED: Yin/Blood Deficient

HEAD/NECK
- ALOPECIA: Deficiency Complex
- HAIR, PREMATURE GREYING: Yin/Blood Deficient
- NECK, LUMPS

HEART
- PALPITATIONS: Yin/Blood Deficient

IMMUNE SYSTEM RELATED DISORDERS/TOPICS
- LYMPH GLANDS, ENLARGEMENT, CHRONIC: Phlegm Nodules

INFECTIOUS DISEASES

- NEURASTHENIA

MUSCULOSKELETAL/ CONNECTIVE TISSUE
- BACK, LOWER WEAK: Yin/ Blood Deficient
- BACKACHE
- KNEES, SORE
- KNEES, WEAK: Yin/Blood Deficient

SEXUALITY, FEMALE: GYNECOLOGICAL
- LEUKORRHEA
- MENORRHAGIA

SEXUALITY, MALE: UROLOGICAL TOPICS
- NOCTURNAL EMISSIONS
- SPERMATORRHEA

SKIN
- BOILS, TOXIC: Heat, Toxins,

Indications:

CIRCULATION DISORDERS
• HYPERTENSION
EARS/HEARING DISORDERS
• DIZZINESS: Yin/Blood Deficient
ENDOCRINE RELATED
 DISORDERS
• GOITER
EXTREMITIES
• EXTREMITIES, SORE: Yin/Blood

• LEPROSY
• MALARIA, CHILLS, FEVER OF
• MALARIA, CHRONIC
LIVER
• LIVER KIDNEY YIN
 DEFICIENCY
MENTAL STATE/
 NEUROLOGICAL DISORDERS
• INSOMNIA: Yin/Blood Deficient

Swellings
• RASHES
• RASHES, W/PRURITUS: Blood
 Heat, Wind (Raw)
• SKIN, INFECTIONS
• SKIN, SORES, INTRACTABLE
• SKIN, SORES, SWOLLEN: Heat,
 Toxins, Swelling
• SKIN/SCALP FUNGUS: Topical

Clinical/Pharmaceutical Studies:

ABDOMEN/
 GASTROINTESTINAL
 TOPICS
• INTESTINES,
 PERISTALSIS,
 INCREASES
BLOOD RELATED
 DISORDERS/TOPICS
• BLOOD GLUCOSE,
 INCREASES: Decoctions
 Of Prepared Herb
• CHOLESTEROL,
 LOWERS: May Have
 Increased Bowel
 Movements Or Facial
 Flushing, Reduces
 Absorption, High Lecithin
 Content, *Shou Wu Yan
 Shou Dan (He Shou Wu,
 Jin Yin Hua, Du Zhong,
 Sang Shen, Jin Ying Zi) ,
 Seems That Du Zhong,

Sang Shen Are Main
Active Ingredients To
Reduce Cholesterol, *5-6
Tabs, 1 g Crude Herb Per
Tab, 3x/Day
BOWEL RELATED
 DISORDERS
• LAXATIVE
CIRCULATION
 DISORDERS
• ARTERIOSCLEROSIS:
 Reduces Lipid Deposition
ENDOCRINE RELATED
 DISORDERS
• DIABETES MELLITUS,
 PERIPHERAL NEURITIS
 OF
• HORMONE-LIKE:
 Similar To
 Adrenalcorticoids
HEAD/NECK
• ALOPECIA

• HEAD, INJURY,
 SEQUELAE OF
HEART
• CARDIOTONIC
INFECTIOUS DISEASES
• ANTIBIOTIC: TB,
 Shigella, B.Dysenteriae
• MALARIA: With Gan
 Cao, Possible Diarrhea
 And Mild Abdominal Pain
 As Side Effects
• VIRAL, ANTI-
LUNGS
• BRONCHITIS,
 CHRONIC
MENTAL STATE/
 NEUROLOGICAL
 DISORDERS
• EPILEPSY
• INSOMNIA,
 NEURASTHENIA: 5-7

Tabs, 2-3x/Day Of 1 g
Tabs, For 15-20 Days
• PARAPLEGIA
• SCHIZOPHRENIA:
 Decoction, 90 g, With Ye
 Jiao Teng, 90 g, Da Zao, 2-
 6 Pieces, Divided In 2
 Doses, Morning, Afternoon,
 15 Days
• SLEEP WALKING
• STIMULANT, CNS
MUSCULOSKELETAL/
 CONNECTIVE TISSUE
• ANTISPASMODIC
• MUSCLES, ATROPHY
NUTRITIONAL/
 METABOLIC
 DISORDERS/TOPICS
• HYPOTHERMIA:
 Enhances Ability To
 Withstand

Dose
9 - 30 gm

Contraindications
Not: Def SP
Not: w/Severe Phlegm-Damp, Diarrhea

Notes
Use Raw For Constipation
Most Will Have Mushy Stool
Rare Skin Rash
Numbness After Large Dose For Some

LONG YAN ROU
(GUI YUAN ROU)

龍眼肉
(龙眼肉)

ARILLUS
EUPHORIAE LONGANAE

Traditional Functions:

1. Tonifies and calms the Heart
2. Tonifies the Spleen and benefits the Qi
3. Nourishes the Blood

Traditional Properties:

Enters: SP, HT,

Properties: SW, W

Indications:

EARS/HEARING DISORDERS
• DIZZINESS: Heart Spleen
 Deficient
HEART
• PALPITATIONS: Heart Spleen
 Deficient/Fright
MENTAL STATE/

NEUROLOGICAL DISORDERS
• FORGETFULNESS: Heart Spleen
 Deficient
• INSOMNIA: Heart Spleen
 Deficient
• INSOMNIA, DREAMS,
 FREQUENT

QI RELATED DISORDERS/
 TOPICS
• QI/BLOOD DEFICIENCY
SEXUALITY, FEMALE:
 GYNECOLOGICAL
• POSTPARTUM, WEAKNESS

Clinical/Pharmaceutical Studies:

INFECTIOUS DISEASES
• BACTERIAL, ANTI-: Aqueous

Extract-Microsporon Audouini
SKIN

• FUNGAL, ANTI-: Many, In
Concentrated Extracts

Not: Dampness In Middle Jiao

Dose

6 - 15 gm

Common Name

Longan Fruit Flesh

Contraindications

Not: Phlegm-Fire

Precautions

Watch: Def Heat-Add Cool Herbs

Notes

Large Dose: 30-60 gm

SANG SHEN ZI
(SANG REN)

桑椹子

FRUCTUS
MORI ALBAE

Traditional Functions:

1. Nourishes Blood and replenishes the Yin
2. Moistens the intestines and facilitates passage of stool
3. Nourishes and tonifies the Liver and Kidney Yin

Traditional Properties:

Enters: HT, KI, LV,

Properties: SW, <C

Indications:

**BLOOD RELATED DISORDERS/
TOPICS**
• BLOOD BI: Qi, Blood Blockage
• BLOOD DEFICIENCY
SYNDROME
• BLOOD DEFICIENCY W/
WITHERING YELLOW
COMPLEXION
BOWEL RELATED DISORDERS
• CONSTIPATION: Blood Deficient
CIRCULATION DISORDERS
• BLOOD CIRCULATION,
OBSTRUCTION
• HYPERTENSION,

NEURASTHENIA
EARS/HEARING DISORDERS
• DIZZINESS: Blood Deficient
• TINNITUS
**ENDOCRINE RELATED
DISORDERS**
• DIABETES, YIN DEFICIENCY
EYES
• VISION, OBSTRUCTIONS
FLUID DISORDERS
• THIRST
HEAD/NECK
• ALOPECIA: Deficiency Complex

• HAIR, PREMATURE GREYING:
Blood Deficient
LIVER
• LIVER KIDNEY BLOOD
DEFICIENCY
**MENTAL STATE/
NEUROLOGICAL DISORDERS**
• HYPERTENSION,
NEURASTHENIA
• INSOMNIA: Blood Deficient
**YIN RELATED DISORDERS/
TOPICS**
• YIN/BLOOD DEFICIENCY

Clinical/Pharmaceutical Studies:

**BLOOD RELATED DISORDERS/
TOPICS**
• ANEMIA: Sang Shen With Honey
BOWEL RELATED DISORDERS
• CONSTIPATION, ELDERLY: Sang
Shen With Honey
EXTREMITIES
• LEGS, WEAK, SORE: Sang Shen
With Honey
HEAD/NECK

• HAIR, PREMATURE GREYING:
Sang Shen With Honey
**IMMUNE SYSTEM RELATED
DISORDERS/TOPICS**
• IMMUNE SYSTEM
ENHANCEMENT: Modest
**MENTAL STATE/
NEUROLOGICAL DISORDERS**
• INSOMNIA: Sang Shen With

Honey
• RESTLESSNESS: Sang Shen With
Honey
**MUSCULOSKELETAL/
CONNECTIVE TISSUE**
• ARTHRITIS, PAIN: Blood Stasis,
Sang Shen With Honey
• BACK, LOWER SORE, WEAK:
Sang Shen With Honey

Dose

9 - 30 gm

Common Name

Mulberry Fruit Bud

Contraindications

Not: w/Diarrhea Def, Cold SP
Not: Def KI w/Heat

SHU DI HUANG
(SHU DI)

熟地黃
（熟地黃）

RADIX REHMANNIAE GLUTINOSAE CONQUITAE

Traditional Functions:

1. Nourishes the Blood
2. Benefits the Liver and Kidney Yin

Traditional Properties:

Enters: HT, KI, LV,

Properties: SW, <W

Indications:

BLOOD RELATED DISORDERS/ TOPICS
• ANEMIA
• BLOOD DEFICIENCY SYNDROME: Pregnancy, Postpartum
• BLOOD DEFICIENCY W/ WITHERING YELLOW COMPLEXION
EARS/HEARING DISORDERS
• DIZZINESS: Blood Deficient
ENDOCRINE RELATED DISORDERS
• DIABETES: Internal Heat With Exhaustion Thirst
ENERGETIC STATE
• FATIGUE
FEVERS
• FEVER, TIDAL, CHRONIC
FLUID DISORDERS
• SPUTUM DEFICIENCY
HEAD/NECK
• ALOPECIA: Deficiency Complex
• FACE, PALE: Blood Deficient
• HAIR, PREMATURE WHITENING

HEART
• PALPITATIONS: Blood Deficient
HEAT
• HEAT, DEFICIENT
HEMORRHAGIC DISORDERS
• EPISTAXIS
• HEMATEMESIS
• HEMORRHAGE: Deficiency Caused
LIVER
• LIVER KIDNEY YIN DEFICIENCY
LUNGS
• ASTHMA, DYSPNEA
• COUGH, DRY
• COUGH, LUNG EXHAUSTION: Tuberculosis
• HYPERPNEA
MENTAL STATE/ NEUROLOGICAL DISORDERS
• INSOMNIA: Blood Deficient
MUSCULOSKELETAL/ CONNECTIVE TISSUE
• BACKACHE: Yin Deficient

• KNEES, WEAK
SEXUALITY, FEMALE: GYNECOLOGICAL
• LACTATION, INSUFFICIENT: Qi, Blood Deficiency
• MENORRHAGIA
• MENSTRUATION, DISORDERS OF: Tonify Chong, Ren, Essence, Blood
• MENSTRUATION, IRREGULAR
• POSTPARTUM, BLEEDING
• UTERINE BLEEDING
SEXUALITY, MALE: UROLOGICAL TOPICS
• NOCTURNAL EMISSIONS: Yin Deficient
• SPERM, LOSS/INSUFFICIENCY
SKIN
• ABSCESS, YIN, INTERNAL SINKING OF
• SWEATING, NIGHT
YIN RELATED DISORDERS/ TOPICS
• YIN DEFICIENCY

Clinical/Pharmaceutical Studies:

BLOOD RELATED DISORDERS/ TOPICS
• CHOLESTEROL, LOWERS: 2 Weeks For Improvement
• HYPOGLYCEMIA, REDUCES
CANCER/TUMORS/SWELLINGS/ LUMPS

• TUMOR, ANTI-: Granuloma, Marked
CIRCULATION DISORDERS
• BRAIN, BLOOD FLOW TO: 2 Weeks For Improvement
• HYPERTENSION: 2 Weeks For Improvement

ENERGETIC STATE
• TONIFIES, NUTRITIVE
HEART
• CARDIOTONIC
KIDNEYS
• DIURETIC

Dose
9 - 30 gm

Common Name
Chinese Foxglove-Wine Cooked

Precautions
Watch: Def SP/ST

Watch: Stagnation Of Qi/Phlegm, Epigastric/Abdominal Distension/Pain, Anorexia, Diarrhea

Notes
Greasy-Add Sha Ren

Overuse: Loose BM

Up To 45-60 gm

Tonify The Yin

BAI HE   百合   BULBUS LILII

Traditional Functions:

1. Moistens the Lungs, clears Heat and controls cough
2. Clears Heat in the Heart and calms the Spirit
3. Promotes urination

Traditional Properties:

Enters: LU, HT,

Properties: SW, <C

Indications:

FEVERS
- FEVER, AFTERMATH TO SPIRIT DISTURBANCES
- FEVER, LOW GRADE: Post Febrile Diseases
FLUID DISORDERS
- THIRST, DEFICIENT YIN
HEART
- PALPITATIONS: Qi/Yin Weak
HEMORRHAGIC DISORDERS
- HEMATEMESIS

- HEMOPTYSIS
LUNGS
- COUGH: Deficiency Consumption/ Dry/Lung Heat/Lung Dryness
- COUGH, LUNG EXHAUSTION: Tuberculosis
MENTAL STATE/ NEUROLOGICAL DISORDERS
- FRIGHT, PALPITATIONS
- INSOMNIA: Post Febrile Diseases
- INSOMNIA, DREAMS,

FREQUENT
- IRRITABILITY: Post Febrile Diseases
- RESTLESSNESS: Post Febrile Diseases
ORAL CAVITY
- THROAT, SORE: Lung Heat/Dry
YIN RELATED DISORDERS/ TOPICS
- THIRST, DEFICIENT YIN

Clinical/Pharmaceutical Studies:

LUNGS
- ANTITUSSIVE

- ASTHMA: Reduces Histamine

Induced

Dose

9 - 30 gm

Contraindications

Not: Cough From Wind Cold/Phlegm

Not: Def, Cold SP/ST Diarrhea

Common Name

Lily Bulb

BAI MU ER   白木耳   FRUCTIFICATIO TREMELLAE FUCIFORMIS

Traditional Functions:

1. Nourishes Stomach Yin and generates fluids
2. Moistens and nourishes Lung Yin in Lung Heat patterns

Traditional Properties:

Enters: LU, ST, KI,

Properties: SW, BL, N

Indications:

ENERGETIC STATE
- CHRONIC DISEASES, NOURISHMENT
HEAT
- EMACIATION W/HEAT IN FIVE

TUBERCULOSIS
- LUNG DRYNESS
- LUNG HEAT WITH DRY COUGH AND BLOODY SPUTUM
NUTRITIONAL/METABOLIC

STOMACH/DIGESTIVE DISORDERS
- STOMACH YIN DEFICIENCY, YANG RISING
YIN RELATED DISORDERS/

Indications:

CENTERS
LUNGS
• COUGH, PULMONARY

DISORDERS/TOPICS
• EMACIATION W/HEAT IN FIVE
  CENTERS

TOPICS
• YIN DEFICIENCY W/RISING
  YANG

Dose

3 - 9 gm

BAO YU

鮑魚
(鲍鱼)

HALIOTIS

Traditional Functions:

1. Benefits the Liver and Kidney Yin

Traditional Properties:

Enters:

Properties: SP, SA, W, N

Indications:

**BLOOD RELATED DISORDERS/
TOPICS**
• BLOOD STASIS
CIRCULATION DISORDERS
• BLOOD CIRCULATION
  DISORDERS

EXTREMITIES
• LEGS, FRACTURE
EYES
• OPTIC NERVE DISORDERS
LUNGS
• TUBERCULOSIS

**SEXUALITY, FEMALE:
GYNECOLOGICAL**
• UTERINE BLEEDING
URINARY BLADDER
• URINARY DISORDERS

Clinical/Pharmaceutical Studies:

INFECTIOUS DISEASES
• BACTERIAL, ANTI-: Staph.

Aureus

• VIRAL, ANTI-: Inhibits Polio

Dose

3 - 9 gm

Common Name

Abalone Body

Notes

As Powder: 1.2-1.5 gm

Shi Jue Ming Is The Abalone Shell

BEI SHA SHEN

北沙参

RADIX
GLEHNIAE LITTORALIS

Traditional Functions:

1. Clears and dispels Lung Heat, tonifies Yin and stops cough
2. Strengthens the Stomach and increases fluids
3. Moistens the skin

Traditional Properties:

Enters: LU, ST,

Properties: SW, BIT, BL, <C

Indications:

BOWEL RELATED DISORDERS
• CONSTIPATION: Yin Deficiency/
  Febrile Diseases
**ENDOCRINE RELATED
DISORDERS**
• DIABETES: Internal Heat With
  Exhaustion Thirst
FEVERS
• STEAMING BONE FEVER: Yin
  Deficient Heat

FLUID DISORDERS
• THIRST: Deficient Yin
INFECTIOUS DISEASES
• COMMON COLD: Substitute For
  Feng Fang
LUNGS
• COUGH: Lung Dryness
• COUGH, DRY, NON-
  PRODUCTIVE: Lung Yin Deficient
• COUGH, LUNG EXHAUSTION:

Tuberculosis
ORAL CAVITY
• HOARSENESS: Chronic Cough
• MOUTH, DRY: Yin Deficiency/
  Febrile Diseases
• THROAT, DRY: Yin Deficiency/
  Febrile Diseases
SKIN
• SKIN, DRY, ITCHY: Especially If
  Worsened By Dry, Cold Weather

Clinical/Pharmaceutical Studies:

HEART
• CARDIOTONIC: Dilute Decoctions
LUNGS
• EXPECTORANT, SLIGHT

NUTRITIONAL/METABOLIC DISORDERS/TOPICS
• BODY TEMPERATURE, LOWERS: Alcohol Extracts

PAIN/NUMBNESS/GENERAL DISCOMFORT
• ANALGESIC: ETOH Extract, Tooth Extraction

Dose
9 - 15 gm

Common Name
Beech Silver-Top Root

Contraindications
Not: Cough From Wind-Cold

Not: Cold Def SP

Notes
Not With: LI LU

BIE JIA

鱉 甲
(鳖甲)

CARAPAX AMYDAE SINENSIS

Traditional Functions:

1. Nourishes the Yin and subdues the Yang
2. Softens hardness and disperses nodules
3. Clears Heat, pacifies the Liver and disperses Blood
3. Vitalizes the Blood, promotes menstruation, and dissipates nodules

Traditional Properties:

Enters: SP, KI, LV,

Properties: SA, <C

Indications:

ABDOMEN/ GASTROINTESTINAL TOPICS
• FLANK ACCUMULATIONS, PAIN
CANCER/TUMORS/SWELLINGS/ LUMPS
• ABDOMEN, MASS/TUMORS
• LUMPS, SUBCOSTAL
CHEST
• CHEST, ACCUMULATIONS, PAIN
CHILDHOOD DISORDERS
• CONVULSIONS, CHILDHOOD
EARS/HEARING DISORDERS
• VERTIGO: Liver Yang/Fire Rising
FEVERS
• FEVER, LOW GRADE: Deficient

Fire
• POST FEBRILE DISEASE
• STEAMING BONE SYNDROME: Yin Deficient With Heat
INFECTIOUS DISEASES
• CONSUMPTION: Yin Deficient With Heat
• MALARIA W/MASSES
• MALARIA, CHRONIC
LIVER
• HEPATOMEGALY
MENTAL STATE/ NEUROLOGICAL DISORDERS
• AGITATION: Yin Deficient
MUSCULOSKELETAL/

CONNECTIVE TISSUE
• BACK, LOWER PAIN
• SPASMS, CONVULSIONS: Internal Deficiency Wind
SEXUALITY, FEMALE: GYNECOLOGICAL
• AMENORRHEA
• MENORRHAGIA: Blood Heat
• MENSTRUATION, IRREGULAR
SKIN
• NIGHT SWEATS: Yin Deficient With Heat
SPLEEN
• SPLENOMEGALY

Clinical/Pharmaceutical Studies:

BLOOD RELATED DISORDERS/ TOPICS
• BLOOD: Increases Plasma Protein

MUSCULOSKELETAL/ CONNECTIVE TISSUE

• CONNECTIVE TISSUE: Inhibits Proliferation

Dose
9 - 30 gm

Common Name
Chinese Soft-Shell Turtle

Contraindications

Not: External Conditions

Not: Def, Cold SP/ST

Not: With Diarrhea

Precautions
Watch: Pregnancy

Watch: w/Def SP Yang/ST Qi

Watch: w/Impotence

Notes
Bake w/Vinegar For Masses

GUI BAN

龜板
（龟板）

PLASTRUM TESTUDINIS

Traditional Functions:

1. Nourishes the Yin and subdues the Yang
2. Nourishes the Kidneys and strengthens the tendons and bones
3. Cools Blood and stops uterine bleeding
4. Aids in the healing of sores and ulcerations

Traditional Properties:

Enters: KI, LV,

Properties: SA, SW, N

Indications:

BOWEL RELATED DISORDERS
• DYSENTERY, CHRONIC
• FISTULA
• HEMORRHOIDS
CHILDHOOD DISORDERS
• FONTANEL, LATE CLOSURE
EARS/HEARING DISORDERS
• DIZZINESS: Yin Deficient With Yang Rising
• TINNITUS: Yin Deficient With Yang Rising
• VERTIGO: Liver Yang/ Fire Rising
EXTREMITIES
• FEET, TREMORS: Liver Kidney Yin Deficient With Wind
• HANDS, TREMORS: Liver Kidney Yin Deficient With Wind

• LEGS, SORE/WEAK: Kidney Yin Deficient
• LOINS, WEAK
FEVERS
• FEVER, LOW GRADE: Deficient Fire
• FEVER, TIDAL, CHRONIC
• STEAMING BONE FEVER: Yin Deficient Heat
HEAD/NECK
• FACE, SPASMS OF: Liver Kidney Yin Deficient With Wind
INFECTIOUS DISEASES
• MALARIA, CHRONIC
KIDNEYS
• KIDNEY YIN DEFICIENCY
• KIDNEY YIN, INSUFFICIENT
LUNGS
• COUGH, CHRONIC
• COUGH, LUNG

EXHAUSTION:
Tuberculosis
MENTAL STATE/ NEUROLOGICAL DISORDERS
• AGITATION: Yin Deficiency Wind
• CONVULSIONS: Internal Deficiency Wind
MUSCULOSKELETAL/ CONNECTIVE TISSUE
• BACK, LOWER SORE: Kidney Yin Deficient
• KNEES, SORE W/ WEAKNESS
• OSTEOMALACIA: (Adult Rickets)
• SPASMS, CONVULSIONS: Internal Deficiency Wind
NUTRITIONAL/ METABOLIC DISORDERS/TOPICS
• GROWTH, DELAYED: Kidney Yin Deficient

• RICKETS
ORAL CAVITY
• MOUTH, DRY
• THROAT, DRY
SEXUALITY, FEMALE: GYNECOLOGICAL
• LABOR, DIFFICULT
• LEUKORRHEA
• MENSTRUATION, DISORDERS OF: Consolidate, Astringe Chong, Ren
• UTERINE BLEEDING: Blood Heat, w/Vinegar
SEXUALITY, MALE: UROLOGICAL TOPICS
• INCONTINENCE, SEMINAL
• SPERMATORRHEA
SKIN
• NIGHT SWEATS: Yin Deficient With Yang Rising
• SORES, CHRONIC NON-HEALING

Clinical/Pharmaceutical Studies:

FEVERS
• ANTIPYRETIC

PAIN/NUMBNESS/GENERAL DISCOMFORT

• ANALGESIC

Dose

9 - 30 gm

Common Name

Land Tortise Shell

Contraindications

Not: Pregnancy

Not: Cold Damp ST
Not: w/External Condtions
Not: Def Yang Diarrhea

Notes

Cook First, 30 Min Before

HAN LIAN CAO
(MO HAN LIAN)

旱蓮草
（旱莲草）

HERBA ECLIPTAE PROSTRATAE

Traditional Functions:

1. Nourishes the Yin of the Liver and Kidneys
2. Cools the Blood and controls bleeding

Traditional Properties:

Enters: KI, LV,

Properties: SW, SO, C

Indications:

**BLOOD RELATED
DISORDERS/TOPICS**
• BLOOD IN SPUTUM:
Yin Deficient With Blood
Heat
**BOWEL RELATED
DISORDERS**
• BOWEL MOVEMENT,
BLOODY: Yin Deficient
With Blood Heat
• DYSENTERY W/ OR W/
O BLOOD
**EARS/HEARING
DISORDERS**
• DIZZINESS: Liver
Kidney Yin Deficient
• TINNITUS
• VERTIGO: Liver Kidney

Yin Deficient
**ENDOCRINE RELATED
DISORDERS**
• DIABETES: Internal Heat
With Exhaustion Thirst
EYES
• VISION, BLURRED:
Liver Kidney Yin Deficient
HEAD/NECK
• ALOPECIA: Blood Heat
Complex/Deficiency
Complex
• HAIR, PREMATURE
GREYING: Liver Kidney
Yin Deficient/Blood Heat
**HEMORRHAGIC
DISORDERS**

• BLEEDING, SKIN
LESIONS
• EPISTAXIS: Yin
Deficient With Blood Heat
• HEMATEMESIS: Yin
Deficient With Blood Heat
• HEMATURIA: Yin
Deficient With Blood Heat
• HEMORRHAGE: Cool
Blood To Stop/Deficiency
Caused
• HEMOSTATIC
KIDNEYS
• KIDNEY YIN
DEFICIENCY: Dizziness,
Vertigo, Blurred Vision
MENTAL STATE/

**NEUROLOGICAL
DISORDERS**
• NEUROSIS
ORAL CAVITY
• TEETH, LOSS/LOOSE
**SEXUALITY, FEMALE:
GYNECOLOGICAL**
• MENSTRUATION,
DISORDERS OF:
Consolidate, Astringe
Chong, Ren
• UTERINE BLEEDING:
Yin Deficient With Blood
Heat
SKIN
• DERMATITIS: Extrernal
As Protection

Clinical/Pharmaceutical Studies:

• ASTRINGENT
HEMORRHAGIC DISORDERS
• HEMOSTATIC
INFECTIOUS DISEASES

• BACTERIAL, ANTI-: Strong
Against Staph And B-Group
Dysentery
• DIPHTHERIA: Fresh Herb With

Supportive Treatment
TRAUMA, BITES, POISONINGS
• INFLAMMATORY, ANTI-

Dose

9 - 15 gm

Common Name

Eclipta

Contraindications

Not: Def Cold Of SP/KI

Not: Diarrhea From Cold, Def SP/ST

HEI DOU

黑豆

**SEMEN
GLYCINE SOJAE**

Traditional Functions:

1. Tonifies the Yin and nourishes the Blood
2. Benefits the Essence and clears the vision

Traditional Properties:

Enters:

Properties: SW, N

Indications:

EARS/HEARING DISORDERS
• DIZZINESS
**MUSCULOSKELETAL/
CONNECTIVE TISSUE**

• ARTHRITIS, PAIN: Wind
SKIN
• NIGHT SWEATS
• SWEATING, EXCESSIVE

**YIN RELATED DISORDERS/
TOPICS**
• YIN DEFICIENCY HEAT

Dose

9 - 30 gm

Common Name

Soybean

HEI ZHI MA
(HU MA REN/ZHI MA)

黑芝麻
（黑芝麻）

SEMEN
SESAMI INDICI

Traditional Functions:

1. Nourishes Liver and Kidney Yin and Essence
2. Nourishes the Blood and extinguishes Wind
3. Moistens and lubricates the intestines facilitating the passage of the stool

Traditional Properties:

Enters: KI, LV,

Properties: SW, N

Indications:

BLOOD RELATED
DISORDERS/TOPICS
• BLOOD DEFICIENCY W/
WITHERING YELLOW
COMPLEXION
BOWEL RELATED
DISORDERS
• CONSTIPATION: Dry
Intestines/Blood Deficient
EARS/HEARING
DISORDERS
• DIZZINESS: Liver
Kidney Yin Deficiency/

Blood Def
• TINNITUS: Liver Kidney
Yin Deficiency
ENERGETIC STATE
• DEBILITY, GENERAL
• ILLNESS, RECOVERY
FROM, SEVERE
EYES
• VISION, BLURRED:
Liver Kidney Yin
Deficiency
HEAD/NECK

• ALOPECIA: Deficiency
Complex
• HEADACHE: Blood Def/
Yin Deficient
LIVER
• LIVER KIDNEY YIN
DEFICIENCY: Blurred
Vision, Tinnitus, Dizziness
• LIVER STOMACH
DEFICIENCY
MENTAL STATE/
NEUROLOGICAL

DISORDERS
• PARALYSIS: Wind Damp
PAIN/NUMBNESS/
GENERAL
DISCOMFORT
• NUMBNESS: Blood Def/
Yin Deficient
SEXUALITY, FEMALE:
GYNECOLOGICAL
• LACTATION,
INSUFFICIENT: Qi,
Blood Deficiency

Clinical/Pharmaceutical Studies:

BLOOD RELATED DISORDERS/
TOPICS
• BLOOD: Raises Hematocrit With
Injection Of Oil
• BLOOD GLUCOSE, REDUCES:

Oral--Lowers Serum Levels,
Increases Glycogen
BOWEL RELATED DISORDERS
• LAXATIVE
ENDOCRINE RELATED

DISORDERS
• ADRENAL CORTEX: Decreases
Function Of With Oil In Large Doses
For 10 Days

Dose

9 - 30 gm

Common Name

Black Sesame Seeds

Contraindications

Not: Def SP Diarrhea

HUA QI SHEN
(XI YANG SHEN)

花旗參

RADIX
PANACIS QUINQUEFOLII

Traditional Functions:

1. Tonifies the Qi and increases body fluids
2. Nourishes Yin and clears Heat
3. Tonifies Lung Yin and nutures the Stomach

Traditional Properties:

Enters: LU, ST, KI,

Properties: SW, <BIT, CL

Indications:

ENDOCRINE RELATED
DISORDERS
• DIABETES: Internal Heat With
Exhaustion Thirst
ENERGETIC STATE
• FATIGUE FROM CHONIC
DISEASE
• WEAKNESS: Qi Deficiency

HEART
• HEART DEFICIENCY
HEMORRHAGIC DISORDERS
• HEMOPTYSIS: Lung Yin Deficient
INFECTIOUS DISEASES
• FEBRILE DISEASES,
AFTERMATH: Weakness,
Irritability, Thirst

• DYSPNEA
• LUNG YIN DEFICIENCY
• TUBERCULOSIS
ORAL CAVITY
• VOICE LOSS: Lung Yin Deficient
SKIN
• NIGHT SWEATS
• SWEATING, SPONTANEOUS

Indications:

FEVERS
- FEVER, CHRONIC, UNABATING

FLUID DISORDERS
- THIRST: Fluid Injury

LUNGS
- COUGH, CHRONIC: Lung Yin Deficient

YIN RELATED DISORDERS/ TOPICS
- YIN DEFICIENCY W/HEAT

Clinical/Pharmaceutical Studies:

ENERGETIC STATE
- FATIGUE

HEART
- CARDIOTONIC

MENTAL STATE/ NEUROLOGICAL DISORDERS
- CNS, INHIBITS CEREBRAL

CORTEX
- CNS, STIMULANT, SUBCORTICAL AREAS

Dose

2.4 - 9.0 gm

Common Name

American Ginseng Root

Contraindications

Not: Cold Damp ST

Not: LI LU

Not: Cooked In Iron Pot/Pan

Notes

Cook Separately, Then Add

JI ZI HUANG

雞子黃
（鸡子黄）

GALLUS

Traditional Functions:

1. Nourishes the Yin and moistens dryness
2. Benefits the Blood
3. Subdues internal Wind

Traditional Properties:

Enters: HT, KI

Properties: SW, N

Indications:

BOWEL RELATED DISORDERS
- DYSENTERY

CHILDHOOD DISORDERS
- INDIGESTION, CHILDHOOD

HEMORRHAGIC DISORDERS
- HEMAFECIA
- HEMOPTYSIS: General Debility

INFECTIOUS DISEASES
- FEBRILE DISEASES, SYNCOPE

DURING

LIVER
- HEPATITIS

MENTAL STATE/ NEUROLOGICAL DISORDERS
- CONVULSIONS
- INSOMNIA, FROM FIDGETS

SEXUALITY, FEMALE: GYNECOLOGICAL

- PREGNANCY, BLEEDING DURING

SKIN
- BURNS
- FURUNCLES
- SCALDS

STOMACH/DIGESTIVE DISORDERS
- VOMITING

Common Name

Chicken Egg Yolk

KU DING CHA

苦丁茶

FOLIUM ILICIS LATIFOLIAE

Traditional Functions:

1. Disperses Wind Heat and clears the head and eyes
2. Controls fidgets and thirst

Traditional Properties:

Enters: SP, LU, ST

Properties: SW, BIT, C

Indications:

BOWEL RELATED DISORDERS
• DYSENTERY
EARS/HEARING DISORDERS
• EARS, WAX IN
EYES

• EYES, IRRITATION, REDNESS
FLUID DISORDERS
• THIRST: Febrile Diseases
HEAD/NECK
• HEADACHE

MENTAL STATE/
 NEUROLOGICAL DISORDERS
• IRRITABILITY
ORAL CAVITY
• TOOTHACHE

Dose
3 - 9 gm

Common Name
Chinese Holly

LUO HAN GUO

羅漢果
（罗汉果）

*FRUCTUS
MOMORDICAE
GROSVENORI*

Traditional Functions:

1. Moistens the Lungs, clears Heat and alleviates cough
2. Dissipates Phlegm swellings and nodules

Traditional Properties:

Enters: LU, SP,

Properties: SW, N

Indications:

HEAD/NECK
• NECK, NODULES: Phlegm
INFECTIOUS DISEASES

• SCROFULA
LUNGS
• COUGH: Lung Heat/Lung Yin

Deficient
• COUGH, WHOOPING

Dose
9.0 - 15.0 gm

Notes
Leaf (Luo Han He) Is Good For Throat

MAI MEN DONG
(MAI DONG)

麥門冬
（麦门冬）

*TUBER
OPHIOPOGONIS JAPONICI*

Traditional Functions:

1. Nourishes the Yin and clears Heat
2. Moistens the Lungs and controls coughing
3. Nourishes Stomach Yin and increases body fluids
4. Nourish the Heart, clears Heat and calms the Spirit

Traditional Properties:

Enters: LU, ST, HT,

Properties: SW, <BIT, <C

Indications:

BOWEL RELATED DISORDERS
• CONSTIPATION: Intestinal
Dryness/Yin Deficient/Febrile
Disease
ENDOCRINE RELATED
DISORDERS
• DIABETES: Internal Heat With
Exhaustion Thirst
FEVERS
• STEAMING BONE FEVER: Yin
Deficient Heat
FLUID DISORDERS
• THIRST: Fluid Injury/Yin Deficient
With Heat/Febrile Illness
HEART
• ANGINA PECTORIS: Chest Bi

• HEAT: Deficiency Consumption
HEMORRHAGIC DISORDERS
• HEMATEMESIS
• HEMOPTYSIS
INFECTIOUS DISEASES
• FEBRILE DISEASES W/FLUID
INJURY
LUNGS
• COUGH: Lung Dryness
• COUGH, DRY W/THIN/BLOODY
SPUTUM
• COUGH, LUNG EXHAUSTION:
Tuberculosis
• LUNG HEART IMBALANCE:
Spirit Affected
• LUNG YIN DAMAGE

• INSOMNIA
• INSOMNIA, DREAMS,
FREQUENT
• IRRITABILITY: Yin Deficient With
Heat/Febrile Illness
• RESTLESSNESS
MUSCULOSKELETAL/
CONNECTIVE TISSUE
• SPASMS, CONVULSIONS:
Deficiency Wind–Liver Kidney
ORAL CAVITY
• MOUTH, DRY
• THROAT, DRY
PHLEGM
• SPUTUM, THICK, DIFFICULT TO
EXPECTORATE

Indications:

Strangulating Pain
• PALPITATIONS
HEAT

MENTAL STATE/
NEUROLOGICAL DISORDERS
• FEARFULNESS

YIN RELATED DISORDERS/
TOPICS
• YIN DEFICIENCY W/HEAT

Clinical/Pharmaceutical Studies:

BLOOD RELATED
DISORDERS/TOPICS
• BLOOD GLUCOSE,
REDUCES: Alcohol/
Water Extracts For A Long
Period
ENDOCRINE RELATED
DISORDERS
• DIABETES: Speeded
Recovery Of Islets Of
Langerhans, Lowered
Blood Glucose:Alcohol/

Water Extracts
FEVERS
• ANTIPYRETIC
HEART
• ANGINA PECTORIS: 25
g, 3x/Day For 3-18 Months
• CORONARY HEART
DISEASE: 25 g, 3x/Day
For 3-18 Months
INFECTIOUS DISEASES
• ANTIBIOTIC: (Topical)
Staph Albus, E.Coli, B.

Typhi
KIDNEYS
• DIURETIC
LUNGS
• ANTITUSSIVE
• COUGH: Dry Heat, Lung
Deficiency, Pulmonary
Tuberculosis, Chronic
Bronchitis, Chronic
Pharyngitis:Use Ban Xia
As Expectorant,
Antitussive, Add Ren Shen

To Increase Qi
• EXPECTORANT
NUTRITIONAL/
METABOLIC
DISORDERS/TOPICS
• HYPOXIA TOLERANCE,
INCREASES
TRAUMA, BITES,
POISONINGS
• INFLAMMATORY, ANTI-
: ETOH Extract

Dose

3 - 18 gm

Common Name

Lily Turf Root

Contraindications

Not: Def Cold SP/ST

Not: Congested Fluids, Turbid Damp, Phlegm Fluid

Not: Cough From Wind Cold Common Cold

Not: Def Diarrhea

Notes

Stir-Fry To Reduce Coldness

w/Zhu Sha For Sedative Effect

NAN SHA SHEN

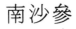
南沙參

RADIX
ADENOPHORAE
TETRAPHYLLA

Traditional Functions:

1. Expels Phlegm and clears Lung Heat
2. Controls cough and nourishes Lung Yin

Traditional Properties:

Enters: LU, LV,

Properties: SW, <C

Indications:

BOWEL RELATED DISORDERS
• CONSTIPATION: Yin Deficiency/
Febrile Diseases
FLUID DISORDERS
• THIRST, DEFICIENT YIN
LUNGS
• COUGH: Lung Heat
• COUGH, DRY, NON-

PRODUCTIVE: Lung Yin Deficient
• LUNGS, DYSPNEA: Lung Heat
ORAL CAVITY
• HOARSENESS: Chronic Cough
• MOUTH, DRY: Yin Deficiency/
Febrile Diseases
• THROAT, DRY: Yin Deficiency/

Febrile Diseases
SKIN
• SKIN, DRY, ITCHY: Especially If
Worsened By Dry, Cold Weather
YIN RELATED DISORDERS/
TOPICS
• THIRST, DEFICIENT YIN

Clinical/Pharmaceutical Studies:

HEART
• CARDIOTONIC
LUNGS

• ANTITUSSIVE
• EXPECTORANT
SKIN

• FUNGAL, ANTI-: Various
Dermatophytes, Microsporons

Dose

9 - 15 gm

Common Name

Ladybell Root

Notes

Similar To Bei Sha Shen, But Weaker

NU ZHEN ZI

女貞子
（女贞子）

FRUCTUS LIGUSTRI LUCIDI

Traditional Functions:

1. Nourishes Liver and Kidney Yin
2. Strengthens back and knees
3. Clears Heat and clears the eyes
4. Darkens hair

Traditional Properties:

Enters: KI, LV,

Properties: BIT, SW, N

Indications:

ABDOMEN/ GASTROINTESTINAL TOPICS
• WAIST, WEAK
EARS/HEARING DISORDERS
• DEAFNESS
• DIZZINESS: Liver Kidney Yin Deficient
• TINNITUS: Liver Kidney Yin Deficient
• VERTIGO
ENDOCRINE RELATED DISORDERS
• DIABETES: Internal Heat With Exhaustion Thirst
EYES
• EYES, BENEFITS
• EYES, SPOTS BEFORE: Liver

Kidney Yin Deficient
• EYESIGHT, DECREASED
FEVERS
• STEAMING BONE FEVER: Yin Deficient Heat
HEAD/NECK
• ALOPECIA: Deficiency Complex
• HAIR, PREMATURE GREYING: Liver Kidney Yin Deficient
HEART
• PALPITATIONS
HEAT
• HEAT, INTERNAL
INFECTIOUS DISEASES
• CONSUMPTION W/HEAT: Liver Kidney Yin Deficient

LIVER
• LIVER KIDNEY YIN DEFICIENCY
MENTAL STATE/ NEUROLOGICAL DISORDERS
• INSOMNIA
• NEURASTHENIA
MUSCULOSKELETAL/ CONNECTIVE TISSUE
• BACK, LOWER PAIN: Liver Kidney Yin Deficient
• KNEES, WEAK
YIN RELATED DISORDERS/ TOPICS
• YIN DEFICIENCY
• YIN DEFICIENCY W/HEAT

Clinical/Pharmaceutical Studies:

BLOOD RELATED DISORDERS/ TOPICS
• BLOOD, INCREASES WBC
• HYPERLIPIDEMIA
• LEUKOPENIA: 2-4 ml 100% Injection, 1-2x/Day Treats WBC Loss From Radiation/Chemotherapy, Can Use Sheng Bai Tablet
BOWEL RELATED DISORDERS
• PURGATIVE
CANCER/TUMORS/SWELLINGS/ LUMPS
• CHEMOTHERAPY: Increases WBC
• RADIOTHERAPY: Incrases WBC
• TUMOR, ANTI-: Aqueous Extract Inhibits Growth Of
CIRCULATION DISORDERS
• HYPERTENSION, II STAGE: 10 Doses Of Er Zhi Pill (Nu Zhen Zi +

Han Lian Cao)
EYES
• CATARACTS, EARLY
• CENTRAL RETINITIS/EARLY CATARACT: Wang Mo Yan Fang (Retinitis Prescription) /Ming Mu Zi Shen Pian (Vision Improving And Kidney Tonic Tablet)
• RETINITIS, CENTRAL: See Central Retinitis/Early Cataract For More Information For Herb
HEART
• CARDIOTONIC
INFECTIOUS DISEASES
• BACTERIAL, ANTI-: Staph. Aureus, E.Coli, B.Dysenteriae
KIDNEYS
• DIURETIC
LIVER
• HEPATITIS, ACUTE, ICTERIC

• LIVER, REDUCES ENYZMES: Oleanolic Acid, Lowers SGPT
LUNGS
• BRONCHITIS, CHRONIC: Equivalent 50 g Of Raw Herb Or Nu Zhen Zi, Dong Gua Ren, Promethazine
MENTAL STATE/ NEUROLOGICAL DISORDERS
• PARKINSON'S DISEASE: Yang Gan Xi Feng Tang (Hepatotonic And Sedative Decoction) Effective Treats
ORAL CAVITY
• PHARYNGITIS, CHRONIC: Nu Zhen Zi, Pu Gong Ying, Yan Hu Suo, Chen Pi, Han Lian Cao, He Huan Pi (Compound Nu Zhen Zi Decoction)
TRAUMA, BITES, POISONINGS
• TOXINS, BENZENE POISONING CHRONIC

Dose

4.5 - 15.0 gm

Common Name

Privet Fruit

Contraindications

Not: Def Yang

Not: Cold Def SP Diarrhea

Notes

Lightly Tonifies

SANG JI SHENG
(HU JI SHENG)

桑寄生

RAMULUS LORANTHI SEU VISCI

Traditional Functions:

1. Tonifies the Liver and Kidneys and strengthens the tendons and muscles
2. Nourishes the Blood, calms the fetus and prevents miscarriages
3. Dispels Wind Damp
4. Nourishes the Blood and makes the skin glow
5. Lowers ascendent Liver Yang

Traditional Properties:

Enters: KI, LV,

Properties: BIT, N

Indications:

BLOOD RELATED DISORDERS/ TOPICS
- BLOOD DEFICIENCY W/ WITHERING YELLOW COMPLEXION

CIRCULATION DISORDERS
- HYPERTENSION

EXTREMITIES
- LEGS, ACHING: Arthritis

HEART
- CORONARY HEART DISEASE

MUSCULOSKELETAL/ CONNECTIVE TISSUE
- BACK, LOWER SORE, PAIN: Liver Kidney Yin Weak
- BACK, STIFF
- JOINTS, PAIN: Damp Bi With

Liver Kidney Weakness
- JOINTS, PROBLEMS: Liver Kidney Yin Weak
- KNEES, PAIN, SORE: Liver Kidney Yin Weak
- MUSCLES, PAIN
- MUSCLES, WEAK, ATROPHY: Liver Kidney Yin Weak
- TENDONS, PAIN

PAIN/NUMBNESS/GENERAL DISCOMFORT
- BI, WIND DAMP DISEASES W/ LIVER KIDNEY YIN WEAK
- NUMBNESS: Liver Kidney Yin Weak
- NUMBNESS W/SPASMS,

CONTRACTURES: Blood Deficiency Bi

SEXUALITY, FEMALE: GYNECOLOGICAL
- DYSMENORRHEA
- FETUS, RESTLESS: Liver Kidney Deficiency/Threatened Abortion, Blood Deficiency
- LACTATION, INSUFFICIENT
- MENSTRUATION, DISORDERS OF: Tonify Qi Of Chong, Ren
- MISCARRIAGE, THREATENED
- UTERINE BLEEDING DURING PREGNACY

SKIN
- DRY, SCALY: Blood Deficient

Clinical/Pharmaceutical Studies:

BLOOD RELATED DISORDERS/TOPICS
- BLOOD PRESSURE, LOWERS: Temporarily, Alcohol Extracts
- CHOLESTEROL: Lowers

CIRCULATION DISORDERS
- HYPERTENSION

HEART
- ANGINA PECTORIS: Granule Infusion, 4-5 Months With Effects And Symptom Improvement In

1-2 Weeks
- ARRHYTHMIAS: Injection, IM 2-4 ml, 2x/ Day, For 14 Days, Ineffective Against Chronic Atrial Fibrillation, Similar To Verapamil/ Lidocaine In Effects
- CARDIOTONIC: Similar To Digitalis
- CORONARY ARTERIES, DILATES: Coronary Artery Dilation

INFECTIOUS DISEASES

- BACTERIAL, ANTI-: B. Typhi, Staph.
- VIRAL, ANTI-: Echo, Coxsackie, Polio (More Pronounced With Yin Yang Huo) , Flu

KIDNEYS
- DIURETIC: Marked

MENTAL STATE/ NEUROLOGICAL DISORDERS
- SEDATIVE: Inhibits Caffeine Stimulation

- TRANQUILIZING

TRAUMA, BITES, POISONINGS
- FROSTBITE: Local Ointment First Degree-- From Decoction Dried Over Low Heat Then Reconstituted With Distilled Water, Alcohol, White Clay, 2nd Degree-- Extract, Glycerin, Ointment Base, Zinc Oxide Powder

Dose

9 - 30 gm

Notes

Large Overdoses Can Cause Diarrhea/Vomiting/Death

Normal Doses May Cause: Dizziness, Blurred Vision, Malaise, Anorexia, Abdominal Distention, Mild Diarrhea, Dry Mouth

---

SHI HU

石斛

HERBA DENDROBII

Traditional Functions:

1. Nourishes the Yin and clears Heat
2. Moistens Lung and Stomach Yin
3. Generates fluids and quenches thirst

Traditional Properties:

Enters: LU, ST, KI,

Properties: SW, <SA, BL, <C

Indications:

ENDOCRINE RELATED DISORDERS
- DIABETES: Internal Heat With Exhaustion Thirst

FEVERS
- FEVER W/FLUID DAMAGE
- FEVER, RECURRENT: Yin Deficient
- POST FEBRILE

DISEASE: Dry Mouth, Severe Thirst, Recurrent Fever
- STEAMING BONE FEVER: Yin Deficient Heat
- TIDAL FEVER, CHRONIC

FLUID DISORDERS
- THIRST: Fluid Injury

- THIRST, SEVERE/ RESTLESS: Yin Deficient

HEAT
- HEAT, FLUID DAMAGE

LUNGS
- COUGH: Lung Dryness
- COUGH, LUNG EXHAUSTION: Tuberculosis

MENTAL STATE/

NEUROLOGICAL DISORDERS
- RESTLESSNESS

ORAL CAVITY
- MOUTH, DRY: Yin Deficient

STOMACH/DIGESTIVE DISORDERS
- DRY HEAVES
- STOMACH, ACHE

Clinical/Pharmaceutical Studies:

ABDOMEN/ GASTROINTESTINAL TOPICS
- INTESTINES: Stimulates From Dilute Solutions, Inhibits In Concentrated Solutions
- INTESTINES, SMALL STIMULATES PERISTALSIS

BLOOD RELATED DISORDERS/

TOPICS
- BLOOD GLUCOSE, INCREASES: Induces High Levels In Animals
- BLOOD PRESSURE, LOWERS: Large Doses

FEVERS
- ANTIPYRETIC: Mild

HEART

- HEART MUSCLE, INHIBITS

PAIN/NUMBNESS/GENERAL DISCOMFORT
- ANALGESIC: Mild

STOMACH/DIGESTIVE DISORDERS
- DIGESTION, ENHANCES

Dose

6 - 21 gm

Common Name

Dendrobium Stem

Contraindications

Not: Def w/o Heat

Not: Excess Heat

Not: w/Abdominal Distension/Thick, Greasy Tongue

Not: Early Febrile Disease

Notes

Cook First

Overdose: May Induce Convulsions

TIAN MEN DONG

天門冬
(天门冬)

TUBER ASPARAGI COCHINCHINENSIS

Traditional Functions:

1. Nourishes the Yin, clears Lung Heat and controls cough
2. Moistens the Lung and nourishes the Kidney Essence

Traditional Properties:

Enters: LU, KI,

Properties: SW, BIT, C

Indications:

BOWEL RELATED DISORDERS
- CONSTIPATION: Drying Of Fluid/ Intestinal Dryness

ENDOCRINE RELATED DISORDERS
- DIABETES: Internal Heat With Exhaustion Thirst

ENERGETIC STATE
- THIRST, EXHAUSTION

FEVERS
- FEVER, LOW GRADE, AFTERNOON
- FEVER, TIDAL

FLUID DISORDERS
- THIRST: Fluid Injury
- THIRST, DEFICIENT YIN
- THIRST, EXHAUSTION

HEMORRHAGIC DISORDERS

- HEMATEMESIS
- HEMOPTYSIS

INFECTIOUS DISEASES
- CONSUMPTION: Lung Kidney Yin Deficient

LUNGS
- COUGH: Lung Dryness
- COUGH, DRY/BLOODY SPUTUM
- COUGH, LUNG EXHAUSTION: Tuberculosis
- EXPECTORANT
- LUNG KIDNEY YIN DEFICIENCY
- LUNGS, ABSCESS
- LUNGS, WEAK

MUSCULOSKELETAL/ CONNECTIVE TISSUE
- MUSCLES, ATROPHY

ORAL CAVITY
- MOUTH, DRY: Yin Deficient With Heat/Dry Lung
- THROAT, DRY

PHLEGM
- SPUTUM, THICK, BLOOD STAINED: Dry Lung

SEXUALITY, MALE: UROLOGICAL TOPICS
- NOCTURNAL EMISSIONS
- SEMINAL EMISSIONS

SKIN
- NIGHT SWEATS

YIN RELATED DISORDERS/ TOPICS
- YIN DEFICIENCY W/FIRE RISING
- YIN DEFICIENCY W/HEAT

Clinical/Pharmaceutical Studies:

BOWEL RELATED DISORDERS
- LAXATIVE

CANCER/TUMORS/SWELLINGS/ LUMPS
- ANTINEOPLASTIC: Leukemia
- TUMOR, ANTI-

INFECTIOUS DISEASES

- ANTIBIOTIC: Gram Positive And Many Bacteria

KIDNEYS
- DIURETIC

LUNGS
- ANTITUSSIVE
- BRONCHITIS: L-Asparagine

Component
- EXPECTORANT

SEXUALITY, FEMALE: GYNECOLOGICAL
- ABORTION, INDUCES: Helps By Dilating, Softening Cervix

Dose
6 - 24 gm

Common Name
Chinese Asparagus Tuber

Contraindications
Not: Cold Def Diarrhea, Def SP/ST

Not: Wind-Cold Cough

YU ZHU

玉竹

RHIZOMA POLYGONATI ODORATI

Traditional Functions:

1. Nourishes the Lung and Stomach Yin
2. Increases body fluids
3. Extinguishes Wind and softens and moistens the tendons

Traditional Properties:

Enters: LU, ST,

Properties: SW, <C

Indications:

EARS/HEARING DISORDERS
- DIZZINESS: Yin Deficient With Wind

ENDOCRINE RELATED DISORDERS
- DIABETES: Internal Heat With Exhaustion Thirst
- DIABETES, HUNGER/ CONSTIPATION, THIRST, COUGH

FEVERS
- FEVER, INJURED YIN
- STEAMING BONE FEVER: Yin Deficient Heat
- STEAMING BONE FEVER W/ SWEAT

FLUID DISORDERS
- THIRST: Fluid Injury

- THIRST, RESTLESS: Yin Deficient

HEART
- CORONARY HEART DISEASE: Need 30-60 gm To Stimulate

HEAT
- HEAT SENSATION

LUNGS
- COUGH, DRY: Lung Heat
- COUGH, LUNG EXHAUSTION: Tuberculosis
- LUNG STOMACH DRY HEAT

MENTAL STATE/ NEUROLOGICAL DISORDERS
- IRRITABILITY: Yin Deficient
- RESTLESSNESS

MUSCULOSKELETAL/ CONNECTIVE TISSUE

- SPASMS: Wind From Insufficient Fluids

ORAL CAVITY
- MOUTH, DRY
- THROAT, DRY: Yin Deficient

STOMACH/DIGESTIVE DISORDERS
- HUNGER, INSATIABLE

WIND DISORDERS
- WIND HEAT, YIN DEFICIENCY

YIN RELATED DISORDERS/ TOPICS
- YIN DEFICIENCY FROM FEVERS
- YIN DEFICIENCY W/EXTERNAL PATHOGEN
- YIN DEFICIENCY WIND

Clinical/Pharmaceutical Studies:

BLOOD RELATED DISORDERS/ TOPICS
- BLOOD GLUCOSE, REDUCES
- BLOOD PRESSURE, LOWERS: Temporarily
- HYPERLIPIDEMIA: 100% Decoction, 3x/Day For 1 Month/Yu Zhu, Dang Shen Pill, 7.5 g Each
- HYPOGLYCEMIA, REDUCES: Oral Administration

BOWEL RELATED DISORDERS
- LAXATIVE

CIRCULATION DISORDERS
- ATHEROSCLEROSIS: 100%

Decoction, 3x/Day For 1 Month
ENDOCRINE RELATED DISORDERS
- HORMONE-LIKE: Adrenocortical- Like, Effects Liver Glycogen

HEART
- ANGINA PECTORIS
- CARDIOTONIC: Small Doses Decoctions/Tinctures-Lasts 20 Hrs, 5x Digitoxin
- CORONARY HEART DISEASE, HYPERTENSIVE: 10 Doses Of Decoction, No Relapse In 9 Months
- HEART FAILURE: From

Rheumatic, Coronary, Pulmonary Heart Disease--5-10 Days Control, 25 g, 1x/Day As Decoction, Able To Discontinue Digitalis
- MYOCARDIAL ISCHEMIA

KIDNEYS
- DIURETIC

LUNGS
- TUBERCULOSIS: Lengthens Life Of Rats

SEXUALITY, FEMALE: GYNECOLOGICAL
- UTERUS, STIMULATES: Mild

Dose

9 - 30 gm

Common Name

Solomon's Seal Rhizome

Contraindications

Not: Phlegm-Damp In ST

Not: Cold In Middle

Not: Qi Stagnation

Precautions

Watch: w/Hypertension/Tachycardia

Notes

To Stimulate Heart: 30-60 gm

Astringent Herbs

BAI GUO YE
(YIN XING YE)

白果葉
(白果叶)

FOLIUM
GINKO

Traditional Functions:

1. Benefits the Heart
2. Astringes the Lungs
3. Transforms Dampness and stops diarrhea

Traditional Properties:

Enters: LU

Properties: SW, BIT, A, N

Indications:

BOWEL RELATED DISORDERS
• DIARRHEA
CHEST
• CHEST, STIFLING SENSATION
HEART

• ANGINA PECTORIS
• PALPITATIONS
LUNGS
• ASTHMA, COUGH OF, W/

PHLEGM
SEXUALITY, FEMALE:
GYNECOLOGICAL
• LEUKORRHEA

Clinical/Pharmaceutical Studies:

• GRAFTS, ORGANS: Inhibits PAF
BLOOD RELATED DISORDERS/ TOPICS
• BLOOD CLOTS, REDUCES
• BLOOD PRESSURE, LOWERS IN HIGH BP
• CHOLESTEROL, LOWERS: "Guan Xin Tong Tablet" (Aqueous Extract) , 4 Tabs, 3x/Day, 1-5 Months, 39 mg% Avg Reduction
CIRCULATION DISORDERS
• BRAIN, INCREASES BLOOD FLOW
• CIRCULATION DISEASES, PERIPHERAL
• STROKE, MAY BE ABLE TO REDUCE, HELPS RECOVERY
EARS/HEARING DISORDERS
• DEAFNESS, COCHLEAR: From Lowered Blood Circulation
• TINNITUS
• VERTIGO, CHRONIC: Three Month Treatment
EXTREMITIES
• CALF, PAIN: Helps Reduce Pain

From Intermittent Claudication
EYES
• MACULAR DEGENERATION, HELPS RECOVER
GERIATRIC TOPICS
• EMOLLIENT FOR ELDERLY: Ginkgetin Extract Increases Sebaceous Secretion, Helping Senile Skin
HEART
• CORONARY HEART DISEASE, ATHEROSCLEROSIS: "Shu Xue Ning Tablet", 2 Tabs, 3x/Day, 3 Months
• HEART, IMPROVES CIRCULATION IN
IMMUNE SYSTEM RELATED DISORDERS/TOPICS
• ALLERGIES: Respiratory Effects Of
INFECTIOUS DISEASES
• BACTERIAL, ANTI-: Decoction Inhibits Staph Aureus, Shigella, Pseudomonas
LUNGS

• ASTHMA, ATTACKS OF: Inhibits PAF
• BRONCHITIS, CHRONIC, GERIATRIC: As Decoction, Or Tablet (Yin Guo Ye, Swine Bile) Or Liang Ye Tang (Herb, Ai Ye, Sheng Jiang)
MENTAL STATE/ NEUROLOGICAL DISORDERS
• ALZHEIMER'S DISEASE: Possible Help In
• CEREBRAL THROMBOSIS
• CEREBROVASCULAR SPASM
• MEMORY, IMPROVES
• PARKINSON'S DISEASE: Oral Use Of Extact Helped Symptoms
SEXUALITY, MALE: UROLOGICAL TOPICS
• IMPOTENCE: Helps When Caused By Arterial Insufficiency
SKIN
• EMOLLIENT FOR ELDERLY: Ginkgetin Extract Increases Sebaceous Secretion, Helping Senile Skin

Dose
4.5 - 9.0 gm
Common Name
Maidenhair Tree Leaf

Notes
Large Doses May Cause Irritability, Diarrhea, Nausea, Dizziness, Headache, Dry Mouth, Lassitude

BAI GUO
(YIN GUO/YIN XING)

白果
（白果）

SEMEN
GINKGO BILOBAE

Traditional Functions:

1. Expels Phlegm, stops cough and soothes asthma
2. Stops discharge, especially from Damp Heat
3. Astringes and stabilizes the Lower Burner
4. Astringes Lungs and benefits the Lung Qi

Traditional Properties:

Enters: LU, KI,

Properties: SW, BIT, A, N, <TX

Indications:

LUNGS
• ASTHMA: Phlegm
• COUGH: Persistent
• COUGH, CHRONIC W/
  DYSPNEA: Astringe
  Lung Qi
• WHEEZING, COUGH,

COPIOUS SPUTUM
SEXUALITY, FEMALE:
GYNECOLOGICAL
• LEUKORRHEA: Damp
  Heat
• MENSTRUATION,
  DISORDERS OF:

Consolidate, Astringe
Chong, Ren
SEXUALITY, MALE:
UROLOGICAL TOPICS
• SPERMATORRHEA
URINARY BLADDER

• URINARY
  INCONTINENCE
• URINATION,
  FREQUENT
• URINATION, TURBID,
  WHITISH: Damp Heat

Clinical/Pharmaceutical Studies:

• ASTRINGENT
ABDOMEN/
  GASTROINTESTINAL
  TOPICS
• INTESTINES,
  CONTRACTIONS,
  INHIBITS
• PERISTALSIS, INHIBITS
INFECTIOUS DISEASES
• ANTIBIOTIC: Many
  Pathogenic, TB

LUNGS
• BRONCHITIS,
  CHRONIC: With Di Long,
  Huang Qin Or Di Long,
  Pu Gong Ying, 90-100%
  Effective, 1ST Group
  Better As Tablet, •
  Antiasthmatic Decoction
  (Yin Guo, Ma Huang, Ban
  Xia, Kuan Dong Hua, Sang
  Bai Pi, Zi Su Zi, Xing Ren,

Huang Qin)
• COUGH: Improved
  Secretion Of Bronchial
  Mucous Membrane,
  Reduces Goblet Cells
• EXPECTORANT:
  Possible
• TUBERCULOSIS: Strong
  In Vitro
MENTAL STATE/
NEUROLOGICAL

DISORDERS
• CEREBRAL ISCHEMIA:
  Extract Helped
SEXUALITY, FEMALE:
GYNECOLOGICAL
• UTERUS, STIMULATES:
  Causes Contractions
SKIN
• SKIN, DISORDERS:
  Overdose Causes

Dose

3 - 15 gm

Common Name

Ginkgo Nut

Contraindications

Not: Excess Condtions

Notes

Slight Toxic: Antidote-60 g Gan Cao/Or 30 g Shells Of
Yin Guo

Overdoses: Skin Disorders

Toxic Dose: 40-300 Pcs, Adults

Juice/ETOH Extract Irritates Skin

May Cause GI Irritation

Toxic Reaction: (More Common In Young Children)

Foamy Saliva, Vomiting, Diarrhea, High Fever,

Twitching, Pupil Size Changes, Pallor/Flushing

Treatment: Induce Vomiting, Sedatives, Diuretics, Keep
Warm

CHI SHI ZHI
(BAI SHI ZHI)

赤石脂

HALLOYSITUM RUBRUM
(ALBUM)

Traditional Functions:

1. Astringes the intestines and controls diarrhea
2. Arrests bleeding and holds Blood in
3. Promotes tissue regeneration and contracts lesions
4. Absorbs Dampness

Traditional Properties:

Enters: LI, SP, ST,

Properties: SW, A, W

Indications:

BOWEL RELATED
DISORDERS
• DIARRHEA, CHRONIC:
  Cold Deficient

• DYSENTERY, CHRONIC:
  w/Mucus/Blood In BM
• RECTAL PROLAPSE
• RECTAL PROLAPSE W/

Astringe To Stop
SEXUALITY, FEMALE:
GYNECOLOGICAL
• LEUKORRHEA: Cold,

• UTERINE BLEEDING
SEXUALITY, MALE:
UROLOGICAL TOPICS
• SEMINAL

Indications:

- DIARRHEA, CHRONIC W/INCONTINENCE
- DIARRHEA, LINGERING
- DIARRHEA, UNCONTROLLABLE

BLOODY STOOL: Cold Deficient Lower Jiao

HEMORRHAGIC DISORDERS
- HEMAFECIA
- HEMORRHAGE:

Damp
- MENORRHAGIA
- MENSTRUATION, DISORDERS OF: Consolidate, Astringe Chong, Ren

INCONTINENCE
SKIN
- SKIN, ULCERS: Topical
- ULCERS, CHRONIC, NONHEALING: Topical

Clinical/Pharmaceutical Studies:

BOWEL RELATED DISORDERS
- DIARRHEA: Protects GI Membranes

HEMORRHAGIC DISORDERS
- GASTROINTESTINAL BLEEDING: Stops Bleeding,

Protects Membranes
- HEMOSTATIC: Stops GI Bleeding

STOMACH/DIGESTIVE DISORDERS
- FOOD STAGNATION: Adheres To Toxic Substances, Unusual

Fermentative Products From Food

TRAUMA, BITES, POISONINGS
- TOXIC, ANTI-: Adsorbs Toxins & Fermented Food Products
- TOXINS: Adheres To Toxic Substances

Dose

9 - 30 gm

Common Name

Halloysite (Red Or White)

Contraindications

Not: Damp Heat Dysentery

Not: Excess Heat

Not: With Rou Gui Pi, Gui Zhi

Precautions

Watch: Pregnancy

CI WEI PI

刺謂皮
(刺谓皮)

CORIUM ERINACEI

Traditional Functions:

1. Moves the Qi and alleviates pain
2. Vitalizes Blood and stops bleeding
3. Fortifies sperm and controls urination
4. Removes Wind, disperses Cold and removes Phlegm
5. Lowers the Qi and cools the Blood

Traditional Properties:

Enters: LI, ST,

Properties: BIT, N

Indications:

ABDOMEN/ GASTROINTESTINAL TOPICS
- ABDOMEN, PAIN OF, COLD
- HERNIATED ACCUMULATION
- INTESTINAL WIND
- INTESTINES, BLEEDING

BOWEL RELATED DISORDERS
- ANAL PROLAPSE
- DYSENTERY, RED
- FISTULA
- HEMORRHOIDS

- HEMORRHOIDS, BLOODY STOOL

HEMORRHAGIC DISORDERS
- HEMAFECIA
- HEMORRHAGE: Astringe To Stop
- HEMORRHAGE, INTERNAL
- INTESTINAL BLEEDING

SEXUALITY, FEMALE: GYNECOLOGICAL
- MASTITIS

- UTERINE BLEEDING

SEXUALITY, MALE: UROLOGICAL TOPICS
- SPERMATORRHEA

STOMACH/DIGESTIVE DISORDERS
- REGURGITATION
- STOMACH REFLUX
- STOMACH, ACHE
- VOMITING

Clinical/Pharmaceutical Studies:

- ASTRINGENT

Dose

3 - 6 gm

Common Name

Hedge Hog Skin

Contraindications

Not: Pregnancy

FU PEN ZI

復盆子
(复盆子)

FRUCTUS RUBI

Traditional Functions:

1. Benefits the Kidneys by reducing urination and astringing semen
2. Tonifies the Liver and Kidneys
3. Benefits the Liver by improving vision

Traditional Properties:

Enters: KI, LV,

Properties: SW, A, <W

Indications:

EARS/HEARING DISORDERS
• DIZZINESS
EYES
• VISION, BLURRED
HEAD/NECK
• HAIR, PREMATURE GREYING
KIDNEYS
• KIDNEY YANG DEFICIENCY: Urination, Urogenital Symptoms
LIVER
• LIVER KIDNEY DEFICIENCY
SEXUALITY, EITHER SEX

• STERILITY
SEXUALITY, FEMALE:
GYNECOLOGICAL
• MENSTRUATION, DISORDERS OF: Tonify Qi Of Chong, Ren
SEXUALITY, MALE:
UROLOGICAL TOPICS
• IMPOTENCE: Kidney Yang Deficient
• PREMATURE EJACULATION: Kidney Yang Deficient
• SEMINAL EMISSIONS

• SPERMATORRHEA: Kidney Yang Deficient
• WET DREAMS: Kidney Yang Deficient
URINARY BLADDER
• ENURESIS: Kidney Yang Deficient
• URINATION, FREQUENT
• URINATION, INCONTINENT
• URINATION, NIGHT FREQUENCY: Kidney Yang Deficient

Clinical/Pharmaceutical Studies:

• ASTRINGENT
ENDOCRINE RELATED DISORDERS

• ESTROGEN-LIKE: Effects Vagina Mucosa
INFECTIOUS DISEASES

• BACTERIAL, ANTI-: Inhibits Vibrio Cholerae

Dose

4.5 - 15.0 gm

Common Name

Chinese Raspberry Fruit

Contraindications

Not: w/Difficult Urinination

Precautions

Watch: Def Yin w/Heat

Notes

Won't Cause Yin Damage Or Dampness

FU XIAO MAI

浮小麥
(浮小麦)

SEMEN TRITICI AESTIVI LEVIS

Traditional Functions:

1. Tonifies Qi and removes deficiency Heat
2. Arrests excessive sweating from deficient Qi or Yin conditions
3. Benefits the Heart Qi and calms the Spirit
4. Helps control bedwetting in children

Traditional Properties:

Enters: LU, HT,

Properties: SW, CL

Indications:

CHILDHOOD DISORDERS
• ENURESIS, CHILDHOOD
HEART
• HEART, RESTLESS
• PALPITATIONS: Restless Organ Syndrome
HEAT
• HEAT, DEFICIENT
MENTAL STATE/

NEUROLOGICAL DISORDERS
• EMOTIONAL INSTABILITY: Restless Organ Syndrome
• INSOMNIA: Restless Organ Syndrome
• INSOMNIA, DREAMS, FREQUENT
• IRRITABILITY: Restless Organ Syndrome

• MENTAL DISORIENTATION: Restless Organ Syndrome
SKIN
• PERSPIRATION, RESTING & THIEF
• SWEATING, DEFICIENT
• SWEATING, NIGHT: Yin Deficient
• SWEATING, SPONTANEOUS: Qi Deficient

Dose

9 - 30 gm

Common Name

Wheat Grain

Contraindications

Not: Cold, Dampness

HAI PIAO XIAO
(WU ZEI GU)

海螵蛸
（海螵蛸）

OS
SEPIAE SEU SEPIELLAE

Traditional Functions:

1. Astringes Essence and relieves leukorrhea
2. Controls hyperacidity and stops pain
3. Helps absorb lumps and abscesses and promotes healing
4. Astringes the intestines and controls diarrhea
5. Astringes and controls bleeding

Traditional Properties:

Enters: ST, KI, LV,

Properties: SA, <W

Indications:

ABDOMEN/
GASTROINTESTINAL
TOPICS
• ABDOMEN, PAIN OF
BLOOD RELATED
DISORDERS/TOPICS
• BLOOD
ACCUMULATION
• BLOOD, WITHERING
OF
BOWEL RELATED
DISORDERS
• DIARRHEA, CHRONIC
W/NAVEL PAIN
EARS/HEARING
DISORDERS
• OTITIS MEDIA W/PUS:
Topical
ENDOCRINE RELATED
DISORDERS
• GOITER
EXTREMITIES

• LEGS, SWOLLEN,
PAINFUL (BERIBERI,
LEG QI) : Cold Dampness
EYES
• CORNEAL OPACITY:
Topical
HEMORRHAGIC
DISORDERS
• EPISTAXIS
• HEMAFECIA
• HEMATEMESIS
• HEMOPTYSIS
• HEMORRHAGE:
Astringe To Stop
NUTRITIONAL/
METABOLIC
DISORDERS/TOPICS
• BERIBERI: Cold
Dampness
SEXUALITY, EITHER
SEX
• GENITALS, PAIN,

SWELLING
SEXUALITY, FEMALE:
GYNECOLOGICAL
• AMENORRHEA
• LEUKORRHEA: All
Types
• MENORRHAGIA:
Avalanche & Leakage (w/
Other Herbs)
• MENSTRUATION,
DISORDERS OF:
Consolidate, Astringe
Chong, Ren
• UTERINE BLEEDING:
All Types
SEXUALITY, MALE:
UROLOGICAL TOPICS
• NOCTURNAL
EMISSIONS: Kidney
Deficient
• PREMATURE
EJACULATION: Kidney

Deficient
• SEMINAL EMISSIONS
• SPERMATORRHEA
SKIN
• BOILS
• ECZEMA: Cold
Dampness
• SKIN, SORES: Cold
Damp
• SKIN, ULCERS,
CHRONIC, LEGS
• ULCERS, SKIN: Topical
STOMACH/DIGESTIVE
DISORDERS
• ACID REGURGITATION
• BELCHING,
DISTASTEFUL
• STOMACH, ANTIACID
TRAUMA, BITES,
POISONINGS
• TRAUMA, BLEEDING:
Topical Powder

Clinical/Pharmaceutical Studies:

• ASTRINGENT
HEMORRHAGIC
DISORDERS
• HEMOSTATIC:
Powdered w/Starch For
Tooth Extraction, Epistaxis,

Surgery
INFECTIOUS DISEASES
• MALARIA: Powdered
With Rice Wine,
Symptoms Gone, Few

Relapses
STOMACH/DIGESTIVE
DISORDERS
• ANTIACID: Contains
Calcium Carbonate

• ULCERS, GASTRIC/
DUODENAL: With Ba Ji,
Powdered, Symptoms,
Hemoccult Test Gone/
Negative 3-7 Days

Dose

4.5 - 12.0 gm

Common Name

Cuttle-Fish Bone

Contraindications

Not: Yin Def With Excess Heat

Notes

Can Lead To Constipation If Used Too Long

HE ZI

荷子

FRUCTUS TERMINALIAE CHEBULAE

Traditional Functions:

1. Astringes the intestines and controls diarrhea
2. Astringes Lung Qi and stops coughing by lowering the Qi
3. Benefits the throat

Traditional Properties:

Enters: LU, LI,

Properties: BIT, SO, A, N

Indications:

ABDOMEN/ GASTROINTESTINAL TOPICS
• INTESTINES, BLEEDING
BOWEL RELATED DISORDERS
• ANAL PROLAPSE
• DIARRHEA, CHRONIC W/ INCONTINENCE
• DYSENTERY-LIKE DISORDERS, CHRONIC
HEMORRHAGIC DISORDERS
• HEMAFECIA

LUNGS
• COUGH: Phlegm Fire Blocking Lungs (Use With Other Herbs)
• COUGH, CHRONIC W/DYSPNEA: Astringe Lung Qi
• COUGH, CHRONIC, PERSISTENT
• WHEEZING, CHRONIC
ORAL CAVITY
• HOARSENESS
• VOICE LOSS: From Long Standing

Cough
SEXUALITY, FEMALE: GYNECOLOGICAL
• LEUKORRHEA
• MENORRHAGIA
SEXUALITY, MALE: UROLOGICAL TOPICS
• SPERMATORRHEA
SKIN
• SWEATING, NIGHT

Clinical/Pharmaceutical Studies:

• ASTRINGENT: Tannin
ABDOMEN/ GASTROINTESTINAL TOPICS
• ENTERITIS: Protects Ulceration From
• INTESTINES, ULCERS, PROTECTS MUCOSA
BOWEL RELATED DISORDERS

• DIARRHEA: Astringes, Tannin Content
• DYSENTERY: Retention Enemas With Oral Administration Of Capsules, 3 Days/Protects Ulceration From
• LAXATIVE
INFECTIOUS DISEASES

• ANTIBIOTIC: Shigella, Pseudo Aerug, Salmonella, Coryn Diphth, Staph, Typhoid
• VIRAL, ANTI-: Flu
MUSCULOSKELETAL/ CONNECTIVE TISSUE
• ANTISPASMODIC: Papaverine-Like, Alcohol Extracts

Dose

3 - 9 gm

Common Name

Myrobalan Fruit

Contraindications

Not: Acute Diarrhea

Not: Cough From External Pathogen

Not: Internal Damp Heat

Notes

Large Dose: 6-9 gm

JI GUAN HUA

雞冠花
（鸡冠花）

FLOS CELOSIAE CRISTATAE

Traditional Functions:

1. Cools the Blood and controls bleeding

Traditional Properties:

Enters: KI, LI, LV

Properties: SW, CL

Indications:

BOWEL RELATED DISORDERS
• DIARRHEA
• HEMORRHOIDS, BLOODY STOOL
HEMORRHAGIC DISORDERS

• HEMAFECIA
• HEMATURIA
• HEMOPTYSIS
• HEMORRHAGE: Astringe To Stop
SEXUALITY, FEMALE:

GYNECOLOGICAL
• LEUKORRHEA: Cold, Damp
• LEUKORRHEA, PINK
• UTERINE BLEEDING

Clinical/Pharmaceutical Studies:

HEMORRHAGIC DISORDERS
• HEMOSTATIC
INFECTIOUS DISEASES

• BACTERIAL, ANTI-
PARASITES
• ANTIPARASITIC: Trichomonas-

Very Effective, Extract Completely
Eliminates 10-15 Mins

Dose

6 - 15 gm

Common Name

Cockscomb

JIN YING ZI

金櫻子
(金樱子)

FRUCTUS ROSAE LAEVIGATAE

Traditional Functions:

1. Stabilizes the Kidneys by astringing semen
2. Astringes the intestines and controls diarrhea
3. Consolidates the Kidney Qi by concentrating urine

Traditional Properties:

Enters: LI, KI, UB,

Properties: SO, A, N

Indications:

BOWEL RELATED DISORDERS
• DIARRHEA, CHRONIC: Spleen
Deficiency
• DIARRHEA, CHRONIC W/
INCONTINENCE
• DYSENTERY-LIKE DISORDERS
SEXUALITY, FEMALE:
GYNECOLOGICAL

• LEUKORRHEA: Kidney Deficient/
Cold, Damp
• MENSTRUATION, DISORDERS
OF: Consolidate, Astringe Chong,
Ren/Constrict Uterus, Stimulate
Chong
• PROLAPSE OF UTERUS: Weak,
But Effective

SEXUALITY, MALE:
UROLOGICAL TOPICS
• SPERMATORRHEA: Kidney
Deficient
URINARY BLADDER
• URINARY INCONTINENCE:
Kidney Deficient
• URINATION, FREQUENT

Clinical/Pharmaceutical Studies:

BLOOD RELATED DISORDERS/
TOPICS
• CHOLESTEROL, LOWERS: 2-3
Weeks
BOWEL RELATED DISORDERS
• DIARRHEA: Reduces Intestinal
Secretions
CIRCULATION DISORDERS

• ATHEROSCLEROSIS: 2-3 Weeks,
Reduces Cholesterol, Lesions
INFECTIOUS DISEASES
• ANTIBIOTIC: Staph A., E.Coli--
Strong, Proteus Vulgaris, Shigella
• VIRAL, ANTI-: Some Flu
SEXUALITY, FEMALE:
GYNECOLOGICAL

• UTERUS, PROLAPSE: Decoction
Good, Best When Mild, w/o
Leukorrhea
STOMACH/DIGESTIVE
DISORDERS
• STOMACHIC: Increases Gastric
Secretions

Dose

4.5 - 30.0 gm

Common Name

Cherokee Rose Fruit

Contraindications

Not: Excess Heat

Not: Excess Pathogens

LIAN XU

蓮須
(莲须)

NELUMBINIS STAMEN

Traditional Functions:

1. Benefits the Kidneys and retains Essence
2. Controls bleeding
3. Dispels Heat in the Heart

Traditional Properties:

Enters: HT, KI,

Properties: SW, A, N

Indications:

BOWEL RELATED DISORDERS
• DYSENTERY
HEMORRHAGIC DISORDERS

• KIDNEYS, STABILIZES
SEXUALITY, FEMALE:
GYNECOLOGICAL

• SPERMATORRHEA: Kidney
Deficient
URINARY BLADDER

Indications:

- EPISTAXIS
- HEMOPTYSIS
- HEMORRHAGE: Astringe To Stop
KIDNEYS
- ESSENCE, RETENTION: Helps

- LEUKORRHEA: Kidney Deficient
- UTERINE BLEEDING
SEXUALITY, MALE:
UROLOGICAL TOPICS

- INCONTINENCE: Kidney Deficient
- URINATION, FREQUENT: Kidney Deficient

Clinical/Pharmaceutical Studies:

INFECTIOUS DISEASES

- VIRAL, ANTI-: Flu, Strong

Dose

6 - 9 gm

Common Name

Lotus Stamen

Contraindications

Not: Patients w/Difficult Urination

LIAN ZI

蓮子
(莲子)

SEMEN NELUMBINIS NUCIFERAE

Traditional Functions:

1. Benefits the Kidneys and controls the Essence
2. Nourishes the Blood and calms the Spirit
3. Tonifies the Spleen and controls diarrhea

Traditional Properties:

Enters: SP, HT, KI,

Properties: SW, A, N

Indications:

BOWEL RELATED
DISORDERS
- DIARRHEA, CHRONIC: Spleen Deficient
- DIARRHEA, CHRONIC W/INCONTINENCE
ENERGETIC STATE
- WEAKNESS: Qi Deficiency
HEART
- PALPITATIONS: Kidney Heart Discommunication
KIDNEYS
- KIDNEY HEART DISCOMMUNICATION:

Irritability, Restlessness, Insomnia, Palpitations, etc
MENTAL STATE/
NEUROLOGICAL
DISORDERS
- DREAMING, EXCESSIVE: Kidney Heart Discommunication
- DREAMS, FREQUENT
- INSOMNIA: Kidney Heart Discommunication
- IRRITABILITY: Kidney Heart Discommunication
- RESTLESSNESS: Kidney Heart

Discommunication
ORAL CAVITY
- MOUTH, DRY: Kidney Heart Discommunication
SEXUALITY, FEMALE:
GYNECOLOGICAL
- LEUKORRHEA: Cold, Damp
- MENSTRUATION, DISORDERS OF: Consolidate, Astringe Chong, Ren
- UTERINE BLEEDING
SEXUALITY, MALE:
UROLOGICAL TOPICS

- SPERMATORRHEA
- WET DREAMS: Kidney Heart Discommunication
STOMACH/DIGESTIVE
DISORDERS
- ANOREXIA
URINARY BLADDER
- URINARY INCONTINENCE
- URINATION, DARK: Kidney Heart Discommunication
- URINATION, FREQUENT

Clinical/Pharmaceutical Studies:

MUSCULOSKELETAL/
CONNECTIVE TISSUE
- SMOOTH MUSCLE, RELAXES: Uterus, Coronary Arteries

NOSE
- NOSE INFECTION, SWELLING: Reduces
ORAL CAVITY

- THROAT, INFECTION, SWOLLEN: Reduces
TRAUMA, BITES, POISONINGS
- TOXINS, NEUTRALIZES

Dose

6 - 18 gm

Common Name

Lotus Seed

Contraindications

Not: Constipation

Not: Abdominal Distension

MA HUANG GEN

麻黄根
（麻黃根）

RADIX EPHEDRAE

Traditional Functions:

1. Arrests excessive sweating from deficient Qi or Yin conditions

Traditional Properties:

Enters: LU,

Properties: SW, N

Indications:

SEXUALITY, FEMALE:
  GYNECOLOGICAL
• SWEATING, POSTPARTUM
SKIN

• PERSPIRATION, RESTING &
  THIEF
• SWEATING, DEFICIENT: All
  Types

• SWEATING, NIGHT: Yin Deficient
• SWEATING, POSTPARTUM
• SWEATING, SPONTANEOUS: Qi
  Deficient

Clinical/Pharmaceutical Studies:

ABDOMEN/
  GASTROINTESTINAL TOPICS
• INTESTINES, CONSTRICTS:
  Constricts Smooth Muscle
BLOOD RELATED DISORDERS/

TOPICS
• BLOOD PRESSURE, LOWERS:
  Injection
CIRCULATION DISORDERS
• BLOOD VESSELS, DILATES,

PERIPHERAL
SEXUALITY, FEMALE:
  GYNECOLOGICAL
• UTERUS, STIMULATES:
  Constricts Smooth Muscle

Dose

3 - 9 gm

Contraindications

Not: w/External Pathogens

NUO DAO GEN
(NUO DAO GEN XU/NUO MI GEN)

糯稻根

RADIX/RHIZOMA ORYZAE GLUTINOSAE

Traditional Functions:

1. Arrests excessive sweating from deficient Qi or Yin conditions
2. Reduces deficient fevers

Traditional Properties:

Enters: LU, KI, LV, SP, ST

Properties: SW, N

Indications:

ENDOCRINE RELATED
  DISORDERS
• DIABETES
FEVERS
• FEVER: Yin Deficient
• TOXINS, FEBRILE
LIVER
• HEPATITIS, INFECTIOUS
LUNGS

• PNEUMONIA, CHRONIC
• TUBERCULOSIS
ORAL CAVITY
• THROAT, OBSTRUCTION
PARASITES
• FILARIASIS
SKIN
• ABSCESS, PERINEAL
• PERSPIRATION, RESTING &

THIEF
• SWEATING, DEFICIENT
• SWEATING, NIGHT
• SWEATING, SPONTANEOUS
STOMACH/DIGESTIVE
  DISORDERS
• INDIGESTION
URINARY BLADDER
• URINATION, TURBID, WHITISH

Clinical/Pharmaceutical Studies:

• ASTRINGENT
ENERGETIC STATE
• TONIFIES

MENTAL STATE/
  NEUROLOGICAL DISORDERS
• SEDATIVE

SKIN
• ANTISUDORIFIC

Dose

15 - 60 gm

Common Name

Glutinous Rice Root

Contraindications

Not: Sweating From External Pathogens

Notes

Use Singly With Sugar/Other Herbs

QIAN SHI
(QIAN REN)

芡實
(芡实)

SEMEN
EURYALES FEROX

Traditional Functions:

1. Tonifies the Spleen and controls diarrhea
2. Strengthens the Kidneys and controls Essence
3. Dispels Dampness and leukorrhea

Traditional Properties:

Enters: SP, KI,

Properties: SW, A, N

Indications:

BOWEL RELATED DISORDERS
• DIARRHEA: Spleen Deficiency
• DIARRHEA, CHRONIC: Spleen Deficient-Especially Children
KIDNEYS
• KIDNEY QI DEFICIENCY
MUSCULOSKELETAL/

CONNECTIVE TISSUE
• BACK, NUMB PAIN OF
• KNEES, PAIN, NUMB
SEXUALITY, FEMALE: GYNECOLOGICAL
• LEUKORRHEA: Cold, Damp/Deficiency/Damp Heat
• MENSTRUATION, DISORDERS OF:

Consolidate, Astringe Chong, Ren
SEXUALITY, MALE: UROLOGICAL TOPICS
• NOCTURNAL EMISSIONS: Kidney Qi Deficient
• PREMATURE EJACULATION: Kidney Qi Deficient

• SPERMATORRHEA: Kidney Qi Deficient
URINARY BLADDER
• URINARY INCONTINENCE
• URINATION, FREQUENT: Kidney Qi Deficient
• URINATION, TURBID, WHITISH

Dose

9 - 18 gm

Notes

Good For Cold Or Hot Cases
Helps SP/KI w/o Antagonism To Either

ROU DOU KOU

肉豆蔻

SEMEN
MYRISTICAE
FRAGRANTICIS

Traditional Functions:

1. Astringes the intestines and controls diarrhea
2. Warms the Spleen and Stomach, circulates the Qi and reduces pain

Traditional Properties:

Enters: LI, SP, ST,

Properties: SP, W

Indications:

ABDOMEN/ GASTROINTESTINAL TOPICS
• ABDOMEN, PAIN OF, DISTENTION: Cold
BOWEL RELATED DISORDERS
• DIARRHEA: Spleen Kidney Yang Deficient

• DIARRHEA, CHRONIC W/ INCONTINENCE
• DIARRHEA, CHRONIC, INTRACTABLE
• DIARRHEA, EARLY MORNING: Deficient Spleen Kidney

STOMACH/DIGESTIVE DISORDERS
• ANOREXIA: Spleen Stomach Cold Deficient
• EPIGASTRIC PAIN, DISTENTION
• FOOD STAGNATION

Clinical/Pharmaceutical Studies:

• ASTRINGENT
ABDOMEN/ GASTROINTESTINAL TOPICS
• GASTROINTESTINAL TRACT STIMULANT: Small Doses
• PERISTALSIS, INCREASES: Small Doses

BOWEL RELATED DISORDERS
• DIARRHEA
LIVER
• LIVER, TOXIC TO
MENTAL STATE/ NEUROLOGICAL DISORDERS
• HALLUCINOGENIC

• MONOAMINE OXIDASE INHIBITOR
PAIN/NUMBNESS/GENERAL DISCOMFORT
• ANESTHETIC: Oil Of, But Toxic At Proper Dose

Dose

1.5 - 9.0 gm

Common Name

Nutmeg Seeds

Contraindications

Not: Damp Heat Diarrhea-Like Disorders

Notes

Toxic: >7.5 gm Stupor, Can Cause Death

SANG PIAO XIAO

桑螵蛸

OOTHECA MANTIDIS

Traditional Functions:

1. Benefits the Kidney Yang, fortifies and retains the semen and urine

Traditional Properties:

Enters: KI, LV,

Properties: SW, SA, N

Indications:

EARS/HEARING DISORDERS
• DIZZINESS
KIDNEYS
• KIDNEY YANG DEFICIENCY
SEXUALITY, FEMALE: GYNECOLOGICAL
• AMENORRHEA
• LEUKORRHEA, BLOOD TINGED

• LEUKORRHEA, CLEAR: Kidney Yang Deficient
• MENSTRUATION, DISORDERS OF: Consolidate, Astringe Chong, Ren
SEXUALITY, MALE: UROLOGICAL TOPICS
• IMPOTENCE
• NOCTURNAL EMISSIONS, W/O

DREAMS: Kidney Yang Deficient
• SPERMATORRHEA
URINARY BLADDER
• ENURESIS, CHILDHOOD: Kidney Yang Deficient
• URINARY INCONTINENCE
• URINATION,

DRIBBLING: Kidney Yang Deficient
• URINATION, FREQUENT.
• URINATION, FREQUENT, IN ELDERLY: Kidney Yang Deficient
• URINATION, TURBID, WHITISH, DRIBBLING

Clinical/Pharmaceutical Studies:

FLUID DISORDERS
• ANTIDIURETIC

SKIN

• ANTISUDORIFIC

Dose

3 - 9 gm

Common Name

Praying Mantis Egg Case

Contraindications

Not: Def Yin w/Heat

Not: Frequent Urination With Damp Heat

Notes

Toasted As pwdr, Raw Induces Diarrhea

SHAN ZHU YU
(SHAN YU ROU)

山茱萸

FRUCTUS CORNI OFFICINALIS

Traditional Functions:

1. Astringes the Essence of the Kidneys
2. Stabilizes the menses and controls bleeding
3. Astringes excessive perspiration and supports collapsed Yang or Qi
4. Tonifies Liver and Kidneys--Yin and Yang

Traditional Properties:

Enters: KI, LV,

Properties: SO, <W

Indications:

• SHOCK
ABDOMEN/ GASTROINTESTINAL TOPICS
• GROIN AREA PAIN
BLOOD RELATED DISORDERS/TOPICS
• BLOOD DEFICIENCY W/ WITHERING YELLOW COMPLEXION
EARS/HEARING DISORDERS
• DIZZINESS: Liver Kidney Deficient
• HEARING, IMPAIRED/

• VERTIGO
ENDOCRINE RELATED DISORDERS
• DIABETES: Internal Heat With Exhaustion Thirst
ENERGETIC STATE
• WEAKNESS: Qi Deficiency
EXTREMITIES
• LOINS, PAIN
HEMORRHAGIC DISORDERS
• HEMORRHAGE: Astringe To Stop/ Deficiency Caused

CONNECTIVE TISSUE
• BACK, LOWER PAIN: Liver Kidney Deficient
• KNEES, PAIN: Liver Kidney Deficient
SEXUALITY, EITHER SEX
• INFERTILITY: Uterine Cold Palace
SEXUALITY, FEMALE: GYNECOLOGICAL
• MENORRHAGIA
• MENSTRUATION, DISORDERS OF: Consolidate, Astringe

UROLOGICAL TOPICS
• IMPOTENCE: Liver Kidney Deficient
• SPERMATORRHEA: Liver Kidney Deficient
SKIN
• PERSPIRATION, RESTING & THIEF
• SWEATING, EXCESSIVE
• SWEATING, SPONTANEOUS
URINARY BLADDER
• URINARY INCONTINENCE

Indications:

REDUCED ACUITY:
Liver Kidney Deficient
• TINNITUS: Liver Kidney
Deficient

KIDNEYS
• KIDNEY LIVER
DEFICIENCY
MUSCULOSKELETAL/

Chong, Ren
• MENSTRUATION,
PROLONGED
SEXUALITY, MALE:

• URINATION, EXCESS
• URINATION,
FREQUENT

Clinical/Pharmaceutical Studies:

**BLOOD RELATED DISORDERS/
TOPICS**
• BLOOD CELLS, WHITE,
INCREASES
**CANCER/TUMORS/SWELLINGS/
LUMPS**
• TUMOR, ANTI-
CIRCULATION DISORDERS

• HYPERTENSION
INFECTIOUS DISEASES
• ANTIBIOTIC: Staph A., B.
Dysenteriae
KIDNEYS
• DIURETIC: Marked
MENTAL STATE/

NEUROLOGICAL DISORDERS
• PARASYMPATHOMIMETIC,
MILD
SKIN
• FUNGAL, ANTI-
TRAUMA, BITES, POISONINGS
• ANTIHISTAMINE

Dose

4.5 - 12.0 gm

Common Name

Asiatic Cornelian Cherry

Contraindications

Not: Dysuria, Damp Heat

Precautions

Watch: Def KI Yang

Notes

30-60 g For Shock

For Collapse: 60-120 gm

SHI LIU PI

石榴皮
（石榴皮）

PERICARPIUM GRANATI

Traditional Functions:

1. Astringes the intestines and controls diarrhea
2. Kills parasites

Traditional Properties:

Enters: LI, KI

Properties: SO, A, W, TX

Indications:

**ABDOMEN/
GASTROINTESTINAL TOPICS**
• ABDOMEN, PAIN OF: Ascarias
Infestation
BOWEL RELATED DISORDERS
• DIARRHEA, CHRONIC: Deficient
Cold
• DIARRHEA, CHRONIC W/
INCONTINENCE
• DYSENTERY-LIKE DISORDERS

• HEMORRHOIDS, BLOODY
STOOL
• RECTAL PROLAPSE
HEMORRHAGIC DISORDERS
• HEMAFECIA
• HEMORRHAGE: Astringe To Stop
PARASITES
• HOOKWORMS
• PINWORMS

• ROUNDWORMS
• TAPEWORMS
**SEXUALITY, FEMALE:
GYNECOLOGICAL**
• LEUKORRHEA: Cold, Damp
• UTERINE BLEEDING
**SEXUALITY, MALE:
UROLOGICAL TOPICS**
• SPERMATORRHEA

Clinical/Pharmaceutical Studies:

• ASTRINGENT: Contracts
Intestines
**BLOOD RELATED DISORDERS/
TOPICS**
• BLOOD: Increases Coagulation
BOWEL RELATED DISORDERS
• DYSENTERY, AMOEBIC: 6 Days
To Clear

INFECTIOUS DISEASES
• ANTIBIOTIC: Staph Aureus, Strep,
Shigella, Salmonella Typhi,
Pseudomonas
• VIRAL, ANTI-: Flu, Some Other
Common
PARASITES

• ANTIPARASITIC: Strong,
Hookworm
SEXUALITY, EITHER SEX
• CONTRACEPTIVE: In Female
Rats, Guinea Pigs
SKIN
• FUNGAL, ANTI-

Dose
3 - 15 gm
Common Name
Pomegranate Husk
Contraindications
Not: w/Excess Fire

Notes
Very Toxic, Especially Root Cortex

Do Not Mix With Oil/Fats When Taken

Common Side Effects: Dizziness, Weakness, Tremors,

Calf Spasms, Visual Disturbances

As Fine Powder: 6 gm/Dose

WU BEI ZI   五蓓子   GALLA CHINENSIS

Traditional Functions:
1. Astringes Lung Qi and stops coughing
2. Astringes the intestines and controls diarrhea
3. Reabsorbs sweat or moisture, reduces swellings and relieves Heat and toxins
4. Controls bleeding

Traditional Properties:
Enters: LU, LI, KI,

Properties: SO, SA, C

Indications:

BOWEL RELATED DISORDERS
• DIARRHEA, CHRONIC
• DIARRHEA, CHRONIC W/INCONTINENCE
• DYSENTERY-LIKE DISORDERS
• HEMORRHOIDS, BLOODY STOOL
• RECTAL PROLAPSE W/ BLOODY STOOL: Chronic Diarrhea
HEMORRHAGIC DISORDERS
• EPISTAXIS
• HEMAFECIA
• HEMATEMESIS
• HEMATURIA, CHRONIC

• HEMOPTYSIS
• HEMORRHAGE: Astringe To Stop
INFECTIOUS DISEASES
• INFECTIONS W/PUS
LUNGS
• COUGH, BLOODY SPUTUM
• COUGH, CHRONIC: Lung Deficient
• COUGH, CHRONIC W/ DYSPNEA: Astringe Lung Qi
ORAL CAVITY
• MOUTH, ULCERS
SEXUALITY, FEMALE: GYNECOLOGICAL
• LEUKORRHEA: Cold,

Damp
• MENSTRUATION, DISORDERS OF: Consolidate, Astringe Chong, Ren
• UTERINE BLEEDING
SEXUALITY, MALE: UROLOGICAL TOPICS
• SPERMATORRHEA
SKIN
• BOILS
• BURNS
• RINGWORM: Topical As Wash/Powder
• SCARS: Topical
• SKIN, ULCERS, DAMP: Topical As Wash/Powder

• SORES, OOZING YIN SORES
• SWEATING, FURTIVE
• SWEATING, NIGHT: From TB Or TB With Silicosis, Powdered Into Paste On Navel Before Bedtime
• SWEATING, RESTING
• SWEATING, SPONTANEOUS
STOMACH/DIGESTIVE DISORDERS
• VOMITING
TRAUMA, BITES, POISONINGS
• WOUNDS, BLEEDING

Clinical/Pharmaceutical Studies:

• ASTRINGENT: From Tannic Acid
BLOOD RELATED DISORDERS/ TOPICS
• BLOOD PRESSURE, LOWERS
BOWEL RELATED DISORDERS
• DIARRHEA: Reduces Inflammation
HEART
• HEART, REGULATES: Improves Blood Circulation

HEMORRHAGIC DISORDERS
• HEMOSTATIC: Forms Thin Membrane Over Skin
INFECTIOUS DISEASES
• BACTERIAL, ANTI-: Strong-- Staph A., Strep Pneum, Salmonella, Shigella, et al
• VIRAL, ANTI-: Flu, et al
MENTAL STATE/

NEUROLOGICAL DISORDERS
• CNS, STIMULANT: Increases Efficiency
SEXUALITY, FEMALE: GYNECOLOGICAL
• UTERUS, STIMULATES: Regulates
SKIN
• FUNGAL, ANTI-

Dose
1.5 - 9.0 gm
Common Name
Chinese Sumac Gallnut

Contraindications
Not: Cough From Excess Heat/Wind Cold
Notes
Decoction Safe

May Cause Abdominal Pain, Diarrhea/Constipation, If Taken On Empty Stomach

WU MEI

烏梅
（乌梅）

FRUCTUS PRUNI MUME

Traditional Functions:

1. Astringes Lung Qi and stops coughing
2. Astringes the intestines and controls diarrhea
3. Expels roundworms and reduces pain
4. Arrests bleeding
5. Generates bodily fluids and alleviates thirst in diabetics
6. Treats corns and warts with topical application

Traditional Properties:

Enters: LU, LI, SP, LV,

Properties: SO, W

Indications:

ABDOMEN/
GASTROINTESTINAL TOPICS
• ABDOMEN, PAIN OF: Ascariasis
BOWEL RELATED DISORDERS
• DIARRHEA, CHRONIC
• DIARRHEA, CHRONIC W/
INCONTINENCE
• DYSENTERY-LIKE DISORDERS
ENDOCRINE RELATED
DISORDERS
• DIABETES: Internal Heat With
Exhaustion Thirst
ENERGETIC STATE
• DEFICIENT HEAT/DEFICIENT

YIN/QI/FLUID INJURY
EXTREMITIES
• CORNS: Soften In Hot Water, Then
Topical
FLUID DISORDERS
• THIRST: Heat
HEMORRHAGIC DISORDERS
• HEMAFECIA
• HEMORRHAGE: Astringe To Stop
LUNGS
• COUGH, CHRONIC: Lung
Deficient
• COUGH, CHRONIC W/DYSPNEA:
Astringe Lung Qi

SEXUALITY, FEMALE:
GYNECOLOGICAL
• MENORRHAGIA W/DEFICIENT
BLOOD THIRST, DRYNESS
SKIN
• TINEA FUNGUS
• WARTS: Soften In Hot Water, Then
Topical
STOMACH/DIGESTIVE
DISORDERS
• VOMITING/PAIN FROM
ROUNDWORMS
URINARY BLADDER
• URINATION, BLOODY

Clinical/Pharmaceutical Studies:

ABDOMEN/
GASTROINTESTINAL TOPICS
• ENTERITIS, CHRONIC: Seeded
Fruit
• INTESTINES, FUNGI AFTER
ANTIBIOTIC TREATMENT: 18 g
In Decoction Plus Acacia Catechu
Tablet, 1 g 3x/Day, Marked Results,
Negative Stools After Treatment
• INTESTINES, OBSTRUCTION:
Ascariasis, Decoction
BLOOD RELATED DISORDERS/
TOPICS
• LEUKOPENIA
BOWEL RELATED DISORDERS
• DIARRHEA, CHILDHOOD: Wu
Mei, Shan Zha Equal Amounts As
Decoction, 90% Effective
• DYSENTERY, BACILLARY: Wu
Mei, 18 g Crushed, Water Extracts
With 12 g, Xiang Fu Decoct Over
Low Heat, Concentrate To 50 ml, 2
Doses, Or Decoction 3 Days
CANCER/TUMORS/SWELLINGS/
LUMPS
• CERVICAL CANCER: Inhibits
Growth
• NASOPHARYNGEAL CANCER
• POLYPS, VARIOUS: Rectal,
Vaginal, Nasal, Laryngeal, Laryngeal
Nodules, Esophageal, Uterine,
Myoma Of Uterus–Stir Fry Wu Mei,

Bai Jiang Can, Stir Fry To Yellow,
248 g Each, Grind, Mix With Honey,
Make Pills, 6 g 3x/Day
• RECTAL CANCER
• UTERINE CANCER
EXTREMITIES
• CORNS: External, With Vinegar,
Salt To Make Paste, First Soak In
Warm Water, Remove Thick Skin
GALL BLADDER
• BILE DUCT: Roundworm In, With
Other Herbs
• BILE STIMULANT: Production/
Contraction Of Bile Duct, Relaxes
Oddi's Sphincter
IMMUNE SYSTEM RELATED
DISORDERS/TOPICS
• ALLERGIC DISORDERS:
Counteracts Histamine Shock,
Protein Sensitization
• IMMUNE SYSTEM
ENHANCEMENT
INFECTIOUS DISEASES
• ANTIBIOTIC: Many, Probably
From Acid–TB, B.Typhi,
Pseudomonas, B.Dysenteriae, E.Coli,
V.Choloerae
NOSE
• NASAL POLYPS: See Polyps,
Various For Rx
ORAL CAVITY

• GUMS, SWOLLEN: Kidney Qi
Weak
• TEETH, LOOSE: Kidney Qi Weak
PARASITES
• ASCARIASIS, BILIARY:
Decoction, Pill, etc
• HOOKWORMS: Decoctions Best,
5-23 Days
SEXUALITY, FEMALE:
GYNECOLOGICAL
• LEUKORRHEA: Oral
Concentrated Decoction, 3-5 ml, 3x/
Day, Not With Blood Stasis
• LOCHIA: Oral Concentrated
Decoction, 3-5 ml, 3x/Day, Not With
Blood Stasis
SEXUALITY, MALE:
UROLOGICAL TOPICS
• PROSTATIC HYPERTROPHY
SKIN
• CALLOUSES: External, With
Vinegar, Salt To Make Paste, First
Soak In Warm Water, Remove Thick
Skin
• FUNGAL, ANTI-
• PSORIASIS: External Or Linctus 1
To 5, 9 g, 3x/Day
STOMACH/DIGESTIVE
DISORDERS
• DYSPEPSIA, CHILDHOOD: Wu
Mei, Da Qing Ye Equal Amounts

Dose
3 - 15 gm

Contraindications
Not: Exterior Conditions
Not: Excess Heat In Interior

WU WEI ZI
五味子
FRUCTUS SCHISANDRAE CHINENSIS

Traditional Functions:
1. Astringes Lung Qi and nourishes the Kidneys
2. Restrains the Essence and stops diarrhea--astringes Kidneys
3. Arrests excessive sweating from Yin or Yang deficiency
4. Calms the Spirit by tonification of Heart and Kidney
5. Generates bodily fluids and alleviates thirst

Traditional Properties:
Enters: LU, HT, KI,

Properties: SO, W

Indications:

BLOOD RELATED DISORDERS/
TOPICS
• BLOOD DEFICIENCY W/
WITHERING YELLOW
COMPLEXION
BOWEL RELATED DISORDERS
• DIARRHEA: Spleen Kidney Yang
Deficient
• DIARRHEA, CHRONIC W/
INCONTINENCE
• DIARRHEA, EARLY MORNING:
Spleen Kidney Deficient
ENDOCRINE RELATED
DISORDERS
• DIABETES: Internal Heat With
Exhaustion Thirst
ENERGETIC STATE
• WEAKNESS: Qi Deficiency
FLUID DISORDERS
• THIRST: Fluid Injury
HEART
• ANGINA PECTORIS: Chest Bi
Strangulating Pain

• PALPITATIONS
LUNGS
• ASTHMA: Lung Kidney Deficient
• COUGH: Cold Phlegm
• COUGH, CHRONIC: Lung
Deficiency
• COUGH, CHRONIC W/DYSPNEA:
Astringe Lung Qi/To Store Qi, Stop
Cough
• COUGH, DRY
• COUGH/WHEEZING: Lung
Kidney Deficient
• LUNGS, DYSPNEA: Cold Phlegm
MENTAL STATE/
NEUROLOGICAL DISORDERS
• FORGETFULNESS
• INSOMNIA
• INSOMNIA, DREAMS,
FREQUENT
• NEURASTHENIA
ORAL CAVITY
• MOUTH, DRY

SEXUALITY, FEMALE:
GYNECOLOGICAL
• LEUKORRHEA: Kidney Deficient
• MENSTRUATION, DISORDERS
OF: Consolidate, Astringe Chong,
Ren/Tonify Qi Of Chong, Ren
SEXUALITY, MALE:
UROLOGICAL TOPICS
• NOCTURNAL EMISSIONS:
Kidney Deficient
• SPERMATORRHEA: Kidney
Deficient
SKIN
• NIGHT SWEATS: Yin Deficient
• PERSPIRATION, RESTING
• PERSPIRATION, THIEF
• SWEATING, SPONTANEOUS:
Yang Deficient
URINARY BLADDER
• URINARY INCONTINENCE
• URINATION, FREQUENT: Kidney
Deficient

Clinical/Pharmaceutical Studies:

BLOOD RELATED DISORDERS/
TOPICS
• BLOOD PRESSURE, LOWERS:
Large Doses, IV
BOWEL RELATED DISORDERS
• DIARRHEA, EARLY MORNING:
Wu Wei Zi San (Wu Zhu Yu + Wu
Wei Zi)
• DYSENTERY, INFANTILE: 0.25-2
gm Herb/90% Tincture, 30-40 Drops/
Extract 0.5 gm
CIRCULATION DISORDERS
• BLOOD CIRCULATION,
INCREASES
• STROKE: Help Mild Spastic
Paralysis, 2-4 Days Post Stroke, May
Add Da Zao, Tai Zi Shen
• VASODILATES: Alcohol Extract
EARS/HEARING DISORDERS
• MENIERES SYNDROME: 4-5
Doses With Da Zao, Dang Gui, Long

HEART
• HEART, AFFECTS CIRCULATION:
Regulates, Improves Blood
Circulation--Tincture Strongest
• PALPITATIONS,
NEURASTHENIA: Alcohol
Extractions
INFECTIOUS DISEASES
• BACTERIAL, ANTI-: Strongly
Inhibits--Mycobacteria, B.Subtilis,
Shigella, B.Typhi, Staph.Aureus, Et,
Al.
LIVER
• HEPATITIS, ANICTERIC: Powder,
25 Days
• TOXINS, LIVER: Lowers SGPT,
Powder, 25 Days
LUNGS
• EXPECTORANT: Ether Extract
• RESPIRATION, STIMULATES:
Can Help Morphine Respiratory

Relieved Insomnia, Headache,
Dizziness, Blurred Vision,
Palpitation, Nocturnal Emission
• PARKINSON'S DISEASE: May
Add Da Zao, Tai Zi Shen, Too
• PSYCHOSIS: Helps Symptoms Of
Hallucination, Paranoia, Neurosis
• SENSORY ACUITY, INCREASES:
Visual, Tactile
• STIMULANT, CNS: Quickens
Reflexes, Increases Work Efficiency--
Less Than Caffeine, Tincture
Strongest
• TRANQUILIZING: Ether Extract
NUTRITIONAL/METABOLIC
DISORDERS/TOPICS
• METABOLISM, INCREASES
PAIN/NUMBNESS/GENERAL
DISCOMFORT
• ANALGESIC
SEXUALITY, FEMALE:

Clinical/Pharmaceutical Studies:

Yan Rou

ENERGETIC STATE
• ADAPTOGEN: Less Than Ginseng, But Safer
• ENDURANCE, INCREASES

EYES
• VISION IMPROVEMENT: For Night Vision, Too

GALL BLADDER
• BILE SECRETION, STIMULATES

HEAD/NECK
• HEADACHE, NEURASTHENIA: Alcohol Extractions

Depression

MENTAL STATE/ NEUROLOGICAL DISORDERS
• CEREBELLAR ATAXIA: May Add Da Zao, Tai Zi Shen, Too
• DIZZINESS, NEURASTHENIA: Alcohol Extractions
• INSOMNIA, NEURASTHENIA: Alcohol Extractions
• NEURASTHENIA: Alcohol Extractions
• NEUROSIS: 40-100% Tincture, 2.5 ml/2-3x/Day For 2-4 Weeks,

GYNECOLOGICAL
• LABOR, INDUCES, IN PROLONGED LABOR: 70% Tincture, 20-25 Drops 1 Every Hr, 3x, Good Effect When Uterus Has Proper Muscle Tone
• UTERUS, MUSCLE, STIMULATES

STOMACH/DIGESTIVE DISORDERS
• STOMACH, REGULATES GASTRIC SECRETION

Dose

1.5 - 9.0 gm

Common Name

Schisandra Fruit

Contraindications

Not: Internal Excess Heat w/External Syndrome

Not: In Early Stage Cough, Rash, Rubella

Not: Peptic Ulcer, Epileptic Seizure, Hypertension, Intercranial Pressure

Notes

To Support LU/Relieve Cough: 1.5-3 gm

Yin Def: 6-9 gm

YING SU KE
(YING SU QIAO)

罌 粟 殼
（罂 粟 壳）

PERICARPIUM PAPAVERIS SOMNIFERI

Traditional Functions:

1. Astringes Lung Qi and stops coughing
2. Astringes the intestines and controls diarrhea
3. Astringes and stabilizes the Lower Burner
4. Stops pain: especially in tendons, bones or epigastrium

Traditional Properties:

Enters: LU, LI, KI,

Properties: SO, N

Indications:

ABDOMEN/ GASTROINTESTINAL TOPICS
• ABDOMEN, PAIN OF

BOWEL RELATED DISORDERS
• DIARRHEA, CHRONIC
• DIARRHEA, CHRONIC W/ INCONTINENCE
• DYSENTERY W/ABDOMINAL PAIN
• DYSENTERY-LIKE DISORDERS
• RECTAL PROLAPSE

HEART

• HEART PAIN

LUNGS
• ASTHMA
• COUGH, CHRONIC

MUSCULOSKELETAL/ CONNECTIVE TISSUE
• BONES, PAIN
• LIGAMENTS, PAIN

PAIN/NUMBNESS/GENERAL DISCOMFORT
• ANALGESIC: Stomach, Muscles, Joints

• PAIN, GENERAL

SEXUALITY, FEMALE: GYNECOLOGICAL
• LEUKORRHEA

SEXUALITY, MALE: UROLOGICAL TOPICS
• SPERMATORRHEA

STOMACH/DIGESTIVE DISORDERS
• STOMACH, PAIN

URINARY BLADDER
• POLYURIA

Clinical/Pharmaceutical Studies:

BOWEL RELATED DISORDERS
• CONSTIPATION, CAUSES
• DIARRHEA: Inhibits Peristalsis

CIRCULATION DISORDERS
• ORTHOSTATIC HYPOTENSION, CAUSES

GALL BLADDER
• BILE DUCT, CAUSES PRESSURE IN

LUNGS
• RESPIRATION, DEPRESSES

MENTAL STATE/

NEUROLOGICAL DISORDERS
• HYPNOTIC: Induces Light, Restless Sleep

PAIN/NUMBNESS/GENERAL DISCOMFORT
• ANALGESIC

Dose

1.5 - 9.0 gm

Common Name

Opium Poppy Husk

Contraindications

Not: Acute Coughs/Diarrhea

Notes

Morphine Extremely Toxic, Highly Addictive

YU YU LIANG
(YU LIANG SHI/TAI YI YU LIANG)

禹余糧
（禹余粮）

LIMONITUM

Traditional Functions:

1. Astringes the intestines and controls diarrhea
2. Controls bleeding

Traditional Properties:

Enters: LI, ST,

Properties: SW, N, A

Indications:

BOWEL RELATED DISORDERS
• DIARRHEA, CHRONIC
• RECTAL PROLAPSE W/BLOODY
  STOOL

HEMORRHAGIC DISORDERS
• HEMAFECIA
• HEMORRHAGE: Astringe To Stop
SEXUALITY, FEMALE:

GYNECOLOGICAL
• LEUKORRHEA: Cold, Damp
• UTERINE BLEEDING,
  FUNCTIONAL

Dose

9 - 15 gm

Common Name

Clay Ironstone

Emetics

GUA DI

瓜蒂
(瓜蒂)

MELO PEDICELUS
(MELONIS CALYX)

Traditional Functions:

1. Induces expectoration and vomiting of accumulated undigested food

Traditional Properties:

Enters: ST,

Properties: BIT, C, <TX

Indications:

CIRCULATION DISORDERS
• APOPLEXY
MENTAL STATE/

NEUROLOGICAL DISORDERS
• EPILEPSY
PHLEGM

• PHLEGM ACCUMULATION:
  Stroke

Clinical/Pharmaceutical Studies:

STOMACH/DIGESTIVE

DISORDERS

• EMETIC: Excites Vomiting Center

Dose

1.5 - 4.5 gm

Common Name

Young Melon Stalk

LI LU

黎蘆
(黎芦)

RHIZOMA ET RADIX VERATRI NIGRI

Traditional Functions:

1. Induces vomiting
2. Expels Wind Phlegm
3. Kills intestinal parasites

Traditional Properties:

Enters: LU, ST, LV,

Properties: BIT, SP, C, TX

Indications:

CHEST
• CHEST, OBSTRUCTION
CIRCULATION DISORDERS
• APOPLEXY
LUNGS
• DYSPNEA
MENTAL STATE/

NEUROLOGICAL DISORDERS
• EPILEPSY
ORAL CAVITY
• THROAT OBSTRUCTION
• THROAT, SORE
PARASITES

• PARASITES, INTESTINAL
PHLEGM
• PHLEGM ACCUMULATION
• SPUTUM, PROFUSE
SKIN
• SCABIES: Topical

Clinical/Pharmaceutical Studies:

BLOOD RELATED DISORDERS/
  TOPICS
• BLOOD PRESSURE, LOWERS
HEART
• HEART RATE, REDUCES

LUNGS
• TUBERCULOSIS: Strongly
  Inhibits
SKIN
• FUNGAL, ANTI-: Varies

STOMACH/DIGESTIVE
  DISORDERS
• EMETIC: Sneezing, Vomiting Thru
  Irritation

Dose
1.5 - 3.0 gm

Common Name
False Hellebore

REN SHEN LU

人參蘆
(人参芦)

CERVIX
GINSENG

Traditional Functions:
1. Mildly induces vomiting and expectoration of phlegm and fluid in cases of deficiency

Traditional Properties:
Enters: LU,

Properties: BIT, BL, W

Indications:

CHEST
• CHEST, OBSTRUCTION W/ PHLEGM
FLUID DISORDERS
• THIRST, DEFICIENT YIN
HEMORRHAGIC DISORDERS

• HEMOPTYSIS
STOMACH/DIGESTIVE DISORDERS
• FOOD STAGNATION, PHLEGM: Deficiency
• STOMACH DEFICIENCY

• VOMITING, OBSTRUCTION OCCURING
YIN RELATED DISORDERS/ TOPICS
• THIRST, DEFICIENT YIN

Dose
3 - 6 gm

Common Name
Ginseng Root Neck

Notes
Do Not Use As A Tonic

Substances For External Application

BAI FAN
(MING FAN)

白礬
（白矾）

ALUM

Traditional Functions:

1. Dries Dampness and Heat and relieves itching
2. Expels Wind Phlegm
3. Controls bleeding and diarrhea
4. Reduces swelling of eyes or throat

Traditional Properties:

Enters: LU, LI, SP, ST,

Properties: SO, A, C, TX

Indications:

BOWEL RELATED DISORDERS
- DIARRHEA, CHRONIC
- DYSENTERY
- HEMORRHOIDS, BLOODY
  STOOL: Topical

EYES
- EYES, SWOLLEN, PAINFUL: As
  A Wash

GALL BLADDER
- CHOLELITHIASIS

HEMORRHAGIC DISORDERS
- EPISTAXIS: Topical
- HEMAFECIA
- HEMOPTYSIS
- HEMORRHAGE: Astringe To Stop

LIVER
- HEPATITIS
- JAUNDICE

LUNGS

- COUGH, DIFFICULT
  EXPECTORATION

**MENTAL STATE/
NEUROLOGICAL DISORDERS**
- CONVULSIONS: Wind Phlegm
- DELIRIUM: Wind Phlegm
- EPILEPSY
- IRRITABILITY: Wind Phlegm
- NEURASTHENIA

ORAL CAVITY
- GUMS, BLEEDING: Topical
- MOUTH, ULCERS
- THROAT, SWOLLEN, PAINFUL

PHLEGM
- PHLEGM, EXCESS
  ACCUMULATION

**SEXUALITY, FEMALE:
GYNECOLOGICAL**

- LEUKORRHEA
- UTERINE BLEEDING

SKIN
- BURNS: As A Wash
- ECZEMA: As A Wash
- PRURITUS: Damp Rashes
- RASHES: Damp
- RASHES, W/PRURITUS: External
  Application
- RINGWORM: Damp Rashes
- SCABIES: Damp Rashes
- SKIN, DISORDERS

TRAUMA, BITES, POISONINGS
- TRAUMA, BLEEDING: Topical

WIND DISORDERS
- WIND PHLEGM W/
  PERICARDIUM ENVOLVEMNT:
  Irritability, Delirium, Convulsions

Clinical/Pharmaceutical Studies:

- ASTRINGENT

BOWEL RELATED DISORDERS
- DIARRHEA: Inhibits Mucosal
  Secretion
- HEMORRHOIDS: Astringent

EARS/HEARING DISORDERS
- OTITIS MEDIA, CHRONIC: 10%
  Solution, Topical As Drops

HEMORRHAGIC DISORDERS

- HEMOSTATIC: Topical

INFECTIOUS DISEASES
- ANTIBIOTIC: Trich Vaginalis,
  Strep, Diphteriae, Pseudomonas,
  Pneumococci, Meningococcci
- CANDIDA ALBICANS

**SEXUALITY, FEMALE:
GYNECOLOGICAL**
- LEUKORRHEA: Astringent

SKIN
- PERSPIRATION, EXCESS:
  Astringent
- ULCERS, SKIN: Astringent

**STOMACH/DIGESTIVE
DISORDERS**
- EMETIC

TRAUMA, BITES, POISONINGS
- INFLAMMATORY, ANTI-

Dose
0.6 - 9.0 gm

Common Name
Alum/Potassium Alum

Precautions
Watch: Internal Use-Over Dose May Cause Ulceration,
Vomit, Diarrhea, Shock, Burning Of Mouth And Throat

Notes
External Use

BAN MAO

班蝥

MYLABRIS

Traditional Functions:

1. Detoxifies poison
2. Breaks up congealed blood

Traditional Properties:

Enters: LI, SI, KI, LV,

Properties: SP, C, TX

Indications:

CANCER/TUMORS/SWELLINGS/
LUMPS
• MASSES, PALPABLE, IMMOBILE
HEAD/NECK
• ALOPECIA: Topical Application
IMMUNE SYSTEM RELATED
DISORDERS/TOPICS
• SWELLINGS, LYMPH: Topical
INFECTIOUS DISEASES
• RABIES: Topical On Swollen

Glands
• SCROFULA: Topical
PAIN/NUMBNESS/GENERAL
DISCOMFORT
• FOCAL DISTENTION: Blood
Stasis
SEXUALITY, FEMALE:
GYNECOLOGICAL
• FETUS, DEAD RETENTION
SKIN

• BOILS: Topical
• FURUNCLES, DEEP ROOTED
• FURUNCLES, MALIGNANT
• NEURODERMATITIS: Topical
• PSORIASIS: Topical
• SCABIES
• SORES: Topical
• ULCERS, SKIN: Topical
TRAUMA, BITES, POISONINGS
• INSECT BITES

Clinical/Pharmaceutical Studies:

BLOOD RELATED
DISORDERS/TOPICS
• BLOOD, INCREASES
WBC: Stimulates Bone
Marrow
CANCER/TUMORS/
SWELLINGS/LUMPS
• ANTINEOPLASTIC:
Liver Cancer
• CANCER: Esophageal,
Cardiac, Gastric, Hepatic,
Tablet Of Substance (As

Cantharidin, 0.25 mg) , Ba
Ji Powder, Aluminum
Hydroxide, Magnesium
Trisilicate, 2-6 Tabs/Day In
3 Doses, 45-60% Effective
• TUMORS
ENDOCRINE RELATED
DISORDERS
• HORMONE EFFECTS:
Increases Estrogen Levels,
Oral Administration

HEAD/NECK
• FACE, NEURALGIA
INFECTIOUS DISEASES
• VIRAL, ANTI-:
Newcastle Disease, 90%
Effective
LIVER
• HEPATITIS, VIRAL
NOSE
• RHINITIS, ALLERGIC:
Symptomatic Relief,

Topical To Yin Tang
Acupoint
SEXUALITY, EITHER
SEX
• APHRODISIAC: Irritates
Urethral Mucosa, Which
Induces Erection
SKIN
• BLISTERS FORMATION:
Strong, Slow, Shallow
• FUNGAL, ANTI-: Many

Dose

0.03 - 0.06 gm

Common Name

Cantharides

Contraindications

Not: Pregnancy

Precautions

Watch: Irritates Skin, May Blister, Can Cause Permanent
Damage To Broken Skin

Notes

Very Toxic: Oral Ingestion May Cause Gastroenteritis,

Glomerulonephrits

Lethal Dose: 0.03gm Of Pure Cantharidin

As Little As 0.6 g Of Ban Mao May Cause Serious

Toxic Reaction, 1.3-3 g Is Lethal

Toxic Symptoms: Burning Sensation In Mouth, Thirst,

Tongue Blisters, Difficult Breathing, Nausea, Vomiting,

Stomach Bleeding, Intestinal Colic, Diarrhea,

Abdominal Pain, Many Urination Problems

Does Not Induce Abortion!

CHAN SU

蟾酥
(蟾酥)

SECRETIO BUFONIS

Traditional Functions:

1. Disperses swelling and clears toxins
2. Controls pain with topical application
3. Expels Summer Heat and Dampness and opens the orifices

Traditional Properties:

Enters: ST, HT, KI,

Properties: SW, SP, W, TX

Indications:

ABDOMEN/ GASTROINTESTINAL TOPICS
- ABDOMEN, PAIN OF: Summer Heat, Turbid

BOWEL RELATED DISORDERS
- DIARRHEA: Summer Heat, Turbid

CANCER/TUMORS/ SWELLINGS/LUMPS
- SWELLINGS, SORE: Topical, Too
- TUMORS

CHILDHOOD DISORDERS
- MALNUTRITION,

CHILDHOOD CIRCULATION DISORDERS
- SYNCOPE: Summer Heat, Turbid

HEART
- ANGINA PECTORIS: Chest Bi Strangulating Pain

HEAT
- SUMMER HEAT, EXTREMELY TURBID: Abdominal Pain, Nausea/ Vomiting

MENTAL STATE/ NEUROLOGICAL

DISORDERS
- MENTAL CLOUDINESS: Excess, Shut-In Complex
- SHUT-IN COMPLEX: Unconsciousness, Mental Cloudiness, Excess
- UNCONSCIOUSNESS: Excess, Mental Cloudiness, (Shut-In Complex)

MUSCULOSKELETAL/ CONNECTIVE TISSUE
- JOINTS, PAIN, SWELLING
- OSTEOMYELITIS, CHRONIC

ORAL CAVITY

- CANKERS: Topical, Too
- LARYNGITIS
- THROAT, SORE: w/ Swelling/Pain
- TONSILLITIS, ACUTE
- TOOTHACHE

SKIN
- BACK, BOILS ON
- BOILS: Topical, Too
- SWEATING, INHIBITS
- ULCERS, SKIN: Topical, Too

STOMACH/DIGESTIVE DISORDERS
- VOMITING: Summer Heat, Turbid

Clinical/Pharmaceutical Studies:

ABDOMEN/ GASTROINTESTINAL TOPICS
- INTESTINES, CONTRACTS

BLOOD RELATED DISORDERS/TOPICS
- BLOOD GLUCOSE, REDUCES: Enhances Glycogenesis

CANCER/TUMORS/ SWELLINGS/LUMPS
- ANTINEOPLASTIC: Synergistic With Cyclophosphamide, etc
- CANCER: Lungs, Liver, Breast, Lymphosarcoma, etc, 2% In Sesame Oil, Injection IM, 2 ml, 1-2x/ Day, 8-26 Days, May Use With Other Chemotherapies
- CANCER, ANTI-: Leukemia
- SKIN, CANCER: Effective, Even More So With Radio, Chemotherapy, Side Effects Reduced, 23% Short Term Cured With Topical 20% Ointment Application
- TUMOR, ANTI-: Increases Reticuloendothelium Cell Function, ETOH Extract, Effect Varies

HEAD/NECK

- HAIR LOSS FROM RADIATION: Protected

HEART
- CARDIOTONIC: Digitalis-Like, Quicker But Shorter, Toxic, Not Accumulative
- HEART FAILURE: 4-8 mg, 2-3x/Day, Improvement In 2-48 Hrs, * Cardiotonic Powder (Chan Su, Fu Ling, 1:9), 87% Effective

HEMORRHAGIC DISORDERS
- HEMOSTATIC: Topical

IMMUNE SYSTEM RELATED DISORDERS/ TOPICS
- ALLERGIES: Antihypersensitivity Effect
- IMMUNE SYSTEM ENHANCEMENT

INFECTIOUS DISEASES
- INFECTIONS, ACUTE SUPPURATIVE

KIDNEYS
- DIURETIC

LUNGS
- ANTITUSSIVE: Weak, Too Toxic, Aqueous Extract, Less Than Morphine, Stronger Than Expectorant Effect
- ASTHMA
- RESPIRATION,

STIMULATES: Stronger Than Lobeline
- RESPIRATORY CENTER: Excitatory Via CNS
- RESPIRATORY FAILURE: From Hypnotic Poisoning
- TUBERCULOSIS, PULMONARY: Injection Of Aqueous Extract, Improved Symptoms, Did Not Close Cavities, Better If Used With Isoniazid

MENTAL STATE/ NEUROLOGICAL DISORDERS
- CNS, EFFECTS: Analgesic, Hallucinogenic-- Short Duration, Convulsions, Stimulant

MUSCULOSKELETAL/ CONNECTIVE TISSUE
- MUSCLES, STRIATED, STIMULANT: Bufotenidine, Active Ingredient, Greater Than Nicotine, Less Than Acetylcholine

ORAL CAVITY
- GINGIVITIS: Topical Application Of Tincture
- GUMS, BLEEDING: Topical Application Of Tincture
- PERIODONTITIS, ACUTE: Topical

Application Of Tincture
- STOMATITIS, NECROTIC: Topical Application Of Tincture
- THROAT, SORE: Topical Application Of Tincture
- TOOTH EXTRACTION: Anesthesia In 3 Minutes When Tincture Applied To Gingiva, Periodontal Sac Of Tooth, Good Alternative To Procaine

PAIN/NUMBNESS/ GENERAL DISCOMFORT
- ANESTHETIC, LOCAL: 80% Alcohol Solution Injected Or Local, May Cause Vomiting, Slower But Longer Than Cocaine, Several Hundred Times Procaine

SEXUALITY, FEMALE: GYNECOLOGICAL
- UTERUS, STIMULATES: Induces Contractions, Caused Abortion In Lab Animals

TRAUMA, BITES, POISONINGS
- INFLAMMATORY, ANTI- : Through Adrenals, Steroid-Like Substance
- RADIATION, SICKNESS: Oil Solution Reduces Or Treats

Dose

0.03 - 0.06 gm

Common Name

Toad Dried Skin Secretion

Contraindications

Not: Pregnancy

Not: In Eyes-Zi Cao Antidote

Precautions

Watch: Internal Use, May Cause Exfoliative Dermatitis

Notes

Easily Absorbed Orally

DA FENG ZI

大楓子
（大枫子）

SEMEN HYDNOCARPI ANTHELMINTHICAE

Traditional Functions:

1. Dispels Wind and dries Dampness
2. Kills parasites and clears toxins

Traditional Properties:

Enters: SP, KI, LV,

Properties: SP, H, TX

Indications:

INFECTIOUS DISEASES
• LEPROSY
• SYPHILIS

SKIN
• BOILS, TOXIC
• SCABIES

• SKIN, DAMP SORES
• SKIN, SORES, INTRACTABLE
• TINEA FUNGUS

Clinical/Pharmaceutical Studies:

INFECTIOUS DISEASES
• ANTIBIOTIC: Acid Fast Bact, TB

• LEPROSY: Oil Of
• TUBERCULOSIS, ANTI-: Oil Of

SKIN
• FUNGAL, ANTI-

Dose

0.3 - 0.9 gm

Common Name

Chaulmoogra Seeds

Notes

Toxic: Headache

Induces Vomiting-Increase In Small Doses

Do Not Inject

Topical Use

ER CHA

(HAI ER CHA/A XIAN YAO)

兒茶
（儿茶）

ACACIA SEU UNCARIA

(GAMBIR)

Traditional Functions:

1. Drains and absorbs dampness and seepage
2. Contols bleeding
3. Stops diarrhea
4. Stimulates growth of body tissue
5. Clears Heat and generates fluids
6. Clears Hot Phlegm

Traditional Properties:

Enters: LU, HT,

Properties: BIT, A, CL

Indications:

BOWEL RELATED DISORDERS
• DIARRHEA
• DIARRHEA, BLOODY
• DYSENTERY
• HEMORRHOIDS
CHILDHOOD DISORDERS
• INDIGESTION, CHILDHOOD
FLUID DISORDERS
• THIRST

• HEMOPTYSIS
• HEMORRHAGE: Astringe To Stop/
  Topical
LUNGS
• COUGH, SPUTUM: Heat
ORAL CAVITY
• COLD SORES
• LARYNGITIS
• SORES, ORAL CAVITY

• UTERINE BLEEDING
SKIN
• BOILS, TOXIC: Heat, Toxins,
  Swellings
• ECZEMA: Topical
• SKIN, SORES, SWOLLEN: Heat,
  Toxins, Swelling
• SORES, NON-HEALING
• SORES, W/PUS

Indications:

HEMORRHAGIC DISORDERS
- EPISTAXIS
- HEMAFECIA

- STOMATITIS
SEXUALITY, FEMALE:
GYNECOLOGICAL

- ULCERS, SKIN: Topical
TRAUMA, BITES, POISONINGS
- TRAUMA, INJURIES: Die Da

Clinical/Pharmaceutical Studies:

- ASTRINGENT
- FIBRINOLYSIS, INHIBITS FROM
  STREPTOKINASE
ABDOMEN/
  GASTROINTESTINAL TOPICS
- PERISTALSIS, INHIBITS: Small
  Intestines, Duodenum
BOWEL RELATED DISORDERS
- DIARRHEA: Astringes

CHILDHOOD DISORDERS
- INDIGESTION, CHILDHOOD: 90%
CIRCULATION DISORDERS
- CAPILLARIES, INCREASES
  RESISTANCE
INFECTIOUS DISEASES
- BACTERIAL, ANTI-: Staph,
  Pseudo, Diphtheria, Salmonella
NUTRITIONAL/METABOLIC

DISORDERS/TOPICS
- VITAMIN C, INCREASES
  ABSORPTION
TRAUMA, BITES, POISONINGS
- ANTIHISTAMINE
URINARY BLADDER
- BLADDER STONES, PREVENTS
  FORMATION OF

Dose
0.9 - 3.0 gm

Common Name
Black/White Cutch Bark, Extract

Contraindications
Not: Cold, Damp

FENG LA

蜂蠟
（蜂蜡）

CERA FLAVA

Traditional Functions:

1. Promotes tissue growth and relieves pain
2. Removes toxin

Traditional Properties:

Enters: SP, ST, LI

Properties: SW, N

Indications:

BOWEL RELATED DISORDERS
- DIARRHEA, CHRONIC
- DYSENTERY
HEART
- HEART, ACUTE PAIN

INFECTIOUS DISEASES
- BOILS, INTERNAL
SEXUALITY, FEMALE:
GYNECOLOGICAL
- FETUS, RESTLESS, W/VAGINAL

BLEEDING
SKIN
- BURNS
- SCALDS
- ULCERS, PERSISTENT

Dose
4.5 - 9.0 gm

Common Name
Bees Wax

Notes
Dose Is For Oral Intake

LIU HUANG

硫黄
（硫黄）

SULPHUR

Traditional Functions:

1. Clears toxins and kills parasites when applied topically
2. Tonifies the Yang and the Life Gate fire
3. Dispels Cold and benefits the Large Intestine

Traditional Properties:

Enters: SP, KI,

Properties: SO, H, TX

Indications:

- INTERIOR COLD YIN
BOWEL RELATED DISORDERS
- CONSTIPATION, ELDERLY: Cold,

- COUGH, CHRONIC W/DYSPNEA:
  To Store Qi, Stop Cough
- COUGH/WHEEZING: Lung

- BOILS, YIN TYPE: Topical
- CARBUNCLES, DAMP,
  FESTERING: Topical

Indications:

Weakness
- DIARRHEA, CHRONIC, GERIATIRIC
HEAD/NECK
- HEAD, SCALDED
KIDNEYS
- KIDNEY YANG DEFICIENCY
LUNGS
- ASTHMA, CHRONIC: Spleen Kidney Deficient, Cold

Deficiency
MUSCULOSKELETAL/ CONNECTIVE TISSUE
- BACK, LOWER PAIN, COLD
- KNEES, PAIN, COLD
SEXUALITY, MALE: UROLOGICAL TOPICS
- IMPOTENCE: Kidney Yang Deficient
SKIN

- PRURITUS, DAMP SORES: Topical
- RINGWORM: Topical
- SCABIES: Topical
- SCALP, SCABBY
- SKIN, DISORDERS: Tinea, et al
- SORES, DAMP, FESTERING: Topical
URINARY BLADDER
- URINATION, FREQUENT

Clinical/Pharmaceutical Studies:

ABDOMEN/ GASTROINTESTINAL TOPICS
- GASTROINTESTINAL, PERISTALSIS INCREASES: Increases Peristalsis, Diarrhea
BOWEL RELATED DISORDERS

- PURGATIVE, MILD: In Intestines Forms Hydrogen Sulfide Which Stimulate Peristalsis
HEAD/NECK
- HAIR: Can Cause To Fall Out

When Applied Topically
SKIN
- FUNGAL, ANTI-
- SKIN, PARASITES OF
- SKIN, SOFTENS

Dose

1.5 - 6.0 gm

Common Name

Sulfur

Contraindications

Not: Pregnancy

Not: Def w/Heat

Precautions

Watch: Internal Use

Notes

Powder/Paste-External Use
Pill/Powders Used Usually

LU FENG FANG
(FENG FANG)

露蜂房

NIDUS VESPAE

Traditional Functions:

1. Dispels Wind, removes toxins and reduces pain when applied topically
2. Controls pain and helps dispel Wind Damp Bi

Traditional Properties:

Enters: LU, ST, LV,

Properties: SW, N, TX

Indications:

CANCER/TUMORS/SWELLINGS/ LUMPS
- CERVICAL CANCER
- GASTRIC CANCER
- TUMORS
LUNGS
- COUGH, CHRONIC
MENTAL STATE/ NEUROLOGICAL DISORDERS
- CONVULSIONS
- EPILEPSY

MUSCULOSKELETAL/ CONNECTIVE TISSUE
- JOINTS, PAIN, SWELLING
ORAL CAVITY
- GUMS, PAIN, SWELLING: Gargle
- TOOTHACHE, ACUTE: Warm Gargle
PAIN/NUMBNESS/GENERAL DISCOMFORT
- BI, WIND DAMP DISEASES
SKIN

- BOILS: Topical
- FURUNCLES, MALIGNANT
- ITCHING, GENERAL: Topical
- RINGWORM: Topical
- SCABIES: Topical
- SKIN, RASHES: Topical
- SKIN, SUPPURATIVE DISEASES: Topical
- SORES: Topical
- ULCERS, PERSISTENT

Clinical/Pharmaceutical Studies:

BLOOD RELATED DISORDERS/ TOPICS
- BLOOD PRESSURE, LOWERS: Temporarily
HEART
- CARDIOTONIC: Low Concentrations
HEMORRHAGIC DISORDERS

- BLEEDING, SHORTENS COAGULATION TIME: Alcohol/ Ether/Acetone Extracts--Strongest Of 3
KIDNEYS
- DIURETIC
PARASITES

- TAPEWORMS: Not Used, Toxic, May Cause Acute Nephritis
SEXUALITY, FEMALE: GYNECOLOGICAL
- MASTITIS: Not Suppurative, 30 gm Toasted In Wine Every 4 Hrs, 2-3 Days, No Side Effects

Dose

2.4 - 6.0 gm

Common Name

Hornet Nest

Contraindications

Not: For Burst Sores

Precautions

Watch: Def Qi/Blood

Notes

Very Toxic If Taken Internally

LU GAN SHI

爐甘石

(炉甘石)

SMITHSONITUM
(CALAMINA)

Traditional Functions:

1. Clears the eyes and removes film
2. Dries Dampness, promotes tissue regeneration and helps control bleeding

Traditional Properties:

Enters: LU, SP, ST, LV,

Properties: SW, N

Indications:

EYES
- BLEPHARITIS: (Eyelids Inflammation) Wind
- EYES, RED, SWOLLEN: External
- KERATITIS: External
- NEBULA

- PTERYGIUM: External
- VISION, SUPERFICIAL OBSTRUCTIONS: External

SKIN
- ECZEMA: External
- PUS, DRAINAGE FROM OPEN

SORES
- SKIN, SORES, SWOLLEN, TOXIC: Topical
- ULCERS, CHRONIC, SKIN

TRAUMA, BITES, POISONINGS
- WOUNDS, POOR HEALING

Clinical/Pharmaceutical Studies:

- ASTRINGENT: Absorbs Wound Secretions
- PRESERVATIVE

INFECTIOUS DISEASES
- BACTERIAL, ANTI-

SKIN
- ANTISEPTIC

Dose

6 - 30 gm

Common Name

Smithsonite/Calamine

Notes

External Use Only, As Fine Pwder, After Calcined

MA QIAN ZI
(FAN MU BIE)

馬錢子

(马钱子)

SEMEN
STRYCHNOTIS

Traditional Functions:

1. Awakens Spirit
2. Moves and circulates the Qi in the channels
3. Eliminates accumulations and swellings and controls pain by moving the Blood

Traditional Properties:

Enters: SP, LV,

Properties: >BIT, C, TX

Indications:

ABDOMEN/
  GASTROINTESTINAL TOPICS
- ABDOMEN, MASS
INFECTIOUS DISEASES
- FEBRILE DISEASES
MUSCULOSKELETAL/
  CONNECTIVE TISSUE
- SPASMS

ORAL CAVITY
- THROAT, SORE, SWOLLEN
PAIN/NUMBNESS/GENERAL
  DISCOMFORT
- BI, WIND DAMP: Arthritis
- BI, WIND DAMP, CHRONIC: Open Luo, Arrest Pain
SKIN

- CARBUNCLES
- FURUNCLES, MALIGNANT
- ULCERS, SKIN: Yin
TRAUMA, BITES, POISONINGS
- CONTUSIONS, SWELLING OF
- FRACTURES, SWELLING OF
- SPRAINS, SWELLING OF
- TRAUMA, INJURIES

Clinical/Pharmaceutical Studies:

ABDOMEN/ GASTROINTESTINAL TOPICS
• PERISTALSIS, INCREASES

BLOOD RELATED DISORDERS/TOPICS
• ANEMIA, APLASTIC, CHRONIC

CHILDHOOD DISORDERS
• INFANTILE PARALYSIS: Injection

ENDOCRINE RELATED DISORDERS
• MYASTHENIA GRAVIS: Powdered Seed

HEAD/NECK
• FACE, PARALYSIS: Topical Paste, Cut Seeds Into Thin Slices, 18-24 Slices/3.5 g Of Seeds, Set On Zinc Oxide Plaster, Apply To Paralyzed Parts Of Face, Change Every 7-

10 Days Until Better, Usually 2 Applications Enough

INFECTIOUS DISEASES
• MENINGITIS SEQUELAE: Injection

LUNGS
• BRONCHITIS, CHRONIC: Brucine Tablet, 10-50 mg, 3x/Day For 10 Days With 3 Day Rest Mid-Course, 3 Courses Needed To Cure, Better After 3 Days
• TUBERCULOSIS, LYMPH NODE, PERITONITIS, PULMONARY: Hen Egg With Ma Qian Zi, Found Effective

MENTAL STATE/ NEUROLOGICAL DISORDERS
• HEMIPLEGIA, FROM CEREBRAL

THROMBOSIS: Injection
• PARAPLEGIA: Injection
• SCHIZOPHRENIA, DEPRESSED, PARANOID TYPES: Ma Qian Zi + Chlorpormazine, Did Not Help Mania
• STIMULANT: Cerebral, Rapidly Absorbed Orally, Affects Cortex, Respiratory, Sensory Centers

MUSCULOSKELETAL/ CONNECTIVE TISSUE
• BACK, PAIN, HYPERTOPHIC ARTHIRITIS OF LUMBAR SPINES: 300 g Of Ma Qian Zi, 35 g Each, Niu Xi, Gan Cao, Cang Zhu, Ma Huang, Bai Jian Can, Ru Xiang, Mo Yao, Quan Xie Powder, 1 g Each Night With White Wine, 20 Days/Course, 90% Marked Effect

• MUSCLES, TETANY
• SCIATICA: Injection

SEXUALITY, FEMALE: GYNECOLOGICAL
• CERVIX, EROSION OF: Make Ointment, Local Application, Daily/ Alternate Days, 5 Applications

SKIN
• CARBUNCLES: 1 Seed Makes 4 Caps, 3-4 Caps/ Day, Marked Effects
• DERMATITIS: Extract Ma Qian Zi, She Chuang Zi, Wu Gong, Ban Mao Macerated In Vinegar, Topical
• FUNGAL, ANTI-

STOMACH/DIGESTIVE DISORDERS
• ANOREXIA: Tincture, 0.6-2.0 ml Oral Before Meal

Dose

0.06 - 0.09 gm

Common Name

Nux-Vomica Seeds

Contraindications

Not: Pregnancy, Weak

Notes

Very Toxic!

If Poisoned: Mild Ether Anesthesia, IV Pentobarbital, Chloral Hydrate, Follow With Gastric Lavage By Potassium Permanganate Solution

---

MI TUO SENG

密陀僧
(密陀僧)

LITHARGYRUM

Traditional Functions:

1. Kills intestinal parasites
2. Contols sweating, removes Phlegm
3. Absorbs fluids, reduces swelling and stops bleeding

Traditional Properties:

Enters: SP, LV,

Properties: SA, SP, N, TX

Indications:

BOWEL RELATED DISORDERS
• DYSENTERY-LIKE DISORDERS, CHRONIC
• HEMORRHOIDS, SWELLING

MENTAL STATE/ NEUROLOGICAL DISORDERS
• CONVULSIONS: Take Internally

PHLEGM
• PHLEGM ACCUMULATION: Take Internally

SKIN
• ECZEMA
• SCABIES
• SKIN, SORES, DAMP

• TINEA FUNGUS
• ULCERS/SORES
• UNDERARM ODOR
• VITILIGO

TRAUMA, BITES, POISONINGS
• WOUNDS, INCISED: Take Internally

Clinical/Pharmaceutical Studies:

SKIN

• FUNGAL, ANTI-: Many

Dose

0.9 - 3.0 gm

Common Name

Litharge/Galena

Contraindications

Not: Weak Patients

Precautions

Watch: Internal Use

MU BIE ZI

木鱉子

（木鱉子）

SEMEN MOMORDICAE COCHINCHINENSIS

Traditional Functions:

1. Relieves toxic swellings when applied topically
2. Decreases swelling of masses and vitalizes the Blood

Traditional Properties:

Enters: LI, LV,

Properties: <SW, W, TX

Indications:

BOWEL RELATED DISORDERS
• ANAL PAIN
• HEMORRHOIDS, BLOODY
  STOOL
**CANCER/TUMORS/SWELLINGS/
LUMPS**
• SWELLINGS, TOXIC
INFECTIOUS DISEASES
• SCROFULA
• SYPHILIS

**MUSCULOSKELETAL/
  CONNECTIVE TISSUE**
• BACK, LOWER PAIN
**PAIN/NUMBNESS/GENERAL
DISCOMFORT**
• BI, WIND DAMP, CHRONIC:
  Open Luo, Arrest Pain
**SEXUALITY, FEMALE:
  GYNECOLOGICAL**

• BREASTS, ABSCESS OF
SKIN
• SORES, NON-HEALING
TRAUMA, BITES, POISONINGS
• CONTUSIONS
• FRACTURES
• SNAKE BITES
• SPRAINS
• TRAUMA, PAIN, SWELLING

Clinical/Pharmaceutical Studies:

**ABDOMEN/
  GASTROINTESTINAL TOPICS**
• INTESTINES, POTENTIATES
  ACETYLCHOLINE
**BLOOD RELATED DISORDERS/
TOPICS**
• BLOOD PRESSURE, LOWERS:

But Toxic
EXTREMITIES
• LEGS, EDEMA
HEART
• HEART, POTENTIATES
  ACETYLCHOLINE
MENTAL STATE/

NEUROLOGICAL DISORDERS
• PARASYMPATHETIC
  STIMULANT
SKIN
• PSORIASIS: Paste Of-Good
• RINGWORM: Paste Of-Good

Dose

0.6 - 1.2 gm

Common Name

Vegetable Turtle

Contraindications

Not: Pregnancy, Weak Patients

Notes

Topical For Swellings

PENG SHA

硼砂

BORAX

Traditional Functions:

1. Clears Heat and toxins when used as a gargle
2. Removes Phlegm and clears Heat in the Lung when taken internally
3. Dries Dampness when applied topically
4. Transforms stones

Traditional Properties:

Enters: LU, ST,

Properties: SW, SA, CL

Indications:

EXTREMITIES
• TOES, BLISTERS BETWEEN:
  Damp Toxin
EYES
• EYES, DISEASES OF
LUNGS
• COUGH, THICK SPUTUM

• THROAT, BONE OBSTRUCTION
• THROAT, PAIN, SWOLLEN: Take
  Internal/External
• TONSILLITIS, ACUTE
PHLEGM
• PHLEGM ACCUMULATION
• PHLEGM, HOT: With Difficult To

• VAGINAL LESIONS: White,
  Draining
SKIN
• SKIN, SORES, SWOLLEN, TOXIC:
  Topical
• ULCERS
STOMACH/DIGESTIVE

Indications:

ORAL CAVITY
- GINGIVITIS
- HOARSENESS, WITH THICK PHLEGM
- MOUTH, SORES, OPEN

Expectorate Sputum
SEXUALITY, FEMALE:
GYNECOLOGICAL
- CANDIDIASIS, VAGINAL: Severe

DISORDERS
- DYSPHAGIA: Orally
URINARY BLADDER
- DYSURIA W/STONES

Clinical/Pharmaceutical Studies:

INFECTIOUS DISEASES
- BACTERIAL, ANTI-: E.Coli, B. Antracis, P.Aeruginosa, Candida Albicans, etc
LUNGS

- EXPECTORANT
SKIN
- FUNGAL, ANTI-
- ULCER, ANTI-

TRAUMA, BITES, POISONINGS
- INFLAMMATORY, ANTI-
URINARY BLADDER
- URINATION, MAKES ALKALINE

Dose

0.9 - 6.0 gm

Common Name

Borax

Contraindications

Not: Pregnancy

Precautions

Watch: Internal Use

Notes

Best Blown Directly On Oral Sores

QIAN DAN   鉛丹   *MINIUM*

Traditional Functions:

1. Removes toxins, vitalizes muscles and aids in tissue regeneration
2. Disperses stagnancy, expels accumulation and kills intestinal parasites
3. Directs Phlegm downward and suppresses spasms

Traditional Properties:

Enters: SP, HT, LV,

Properties: SP, SA, CL, TX

Indications:

BOWEL RELATED DISORDERS
- DYSENTERY
CHILDHOOD DISORDERS
- MALNUTRITION, CHILDHOOD
INFECTIOUS DISEASES
- MALARIA
MENTAL STATE/

NEUROLOGICAL DISORDERS
- EPILEPSY, INDUCED BY FRIGHT
- INSANITY
- SEIZURES: Phlegm Induced
SKIN
- FURUNCLES, MALIGNANT
- PUS, HELPS TO EXPEL

- SKIN, SORES, SWOLLEN, TOXIC: Topical
- ULCERS, SWOLLEN, TOXIC
STOMACH/DIGESTIVE DISORDERS
- REGURGITATION
- VOMITING

Clinical/Pharmaceutical Studies:

- ASTRINGENT

TRAUMA, BITES, POISONINGS

- TOXIC, ANTI-

Dose

0.3 - 0.9 gm

Common Name

Lead Oxide, Red

Contraindications

Not: Cold, Deficient

Notes

Topical Use!
Internal Use For Short Time Only

QING FEN   輕粉 (轻粉)   *CALOMELAS*

Traditional Functions:

1. Kills parasites when applied topically
2. Strongly promotes urination and helps move the stool
3. Disperses accumulations and resolves Phlegm

Traditional Properties:

Enters: LI, SI,

Properties: SP, C, TX

Indications:

BOWEL RELATED DISORDERS
- BOWEL MOVEMENT, DECREASED
- CONSTIPATION: Excess

FLUID DISORDERS
- EDEMA: Excess Type

INFECTIOUS DISEASES
- SYPHILIS

- SYPHILITIC CHANCRES: Topical Wash

PHLEGM
- PHLEGM ACCUMULATION

SKIN
- NEURODERMATITIS
- SCABIES: Topical Wash

- SKIN, DAMP SORES
- TINEA FUNGUS: Topical Wash

STOMACH/DIGESTIVE DISORDERS
- DISTENTION

URINARY BLADDER
- URINATION, DECREASED

Clinical/Pharmaceutical Studies:

BOWEL RELATED DISORDERS
- DIARRHEA: Induces By Inhibiting Absorption

INFECTIOUS DISEASES
- BACTERIAL, ANTI-

- SYPHILIS: Inhibits, Increases Patients Resistance, Too Toxic

KIDNEYS
- DIURETIC

PARASITES

- ANTIPARASITIC

SKIN
- FUNGAL, ANTI-: Many

TRAUMA, BITES, POISONINGS
- TOXIC TO GI TRACT, KIDNEYS

Dose

0.06 - 1.50 gm

Common Name

Calomel (Mercurous Chloride)

Contraindications

Not: Internal Use In Pregnancy

Not: Internal Use In Weak Patients

Notes

Contains Mercury

Generally External

May Cause Abdominal Pain, Tenesmus

Overdose: Acute Nephritis

SHAN CI GU
(YI BI JIAN/CAO BEI MU)

山慈菇

BULBUS SANTSIGU

Traditional Functions:

1. Clears toxic Heat
2. Disperses accumulation and dissipates swellings

Traditional Properties:

Enters: SP, LV,

Properties: SW, C, TX

Indications:

CANCER/TUMORS/SWELLINGS/ LUMPS
- ESOPHAGEAL CANCER
- LYMPHATIC CANCER
- SWELLINGS, TOXIC: Excess Heat
- TUMORS, SALIVARY GLAND

INFECTIOUS DISEASES

- SCROFULA: Excess Heat

LUNGS
- ASTHMA
- BRONCHITIS

MUSCULOSKELETAL/ CONNECTIVE TISSUE
- GOUT

SKIN
- CARBUNCLES: Excess Heat
- SORES: Excess Heat
- ULCERS, SKIN: Excess Heat

TRAUMA, BITES, POISONINGS
- INSECT BITES
- SNAKE BITES

Clinical/Pharmaceutical Studies:

CANCER/TUMORS/ SWELLINGS/LUMPS
- ANTINEOPLASTIC: Leukemia, Lymphocytic, Granulocytic, Breast, Cerivix, Esophagus, Lung, Stomach--Colchincine/

Cholchicinamide, See Source Text For More Details (Chang, But)

HEART
- CARDIOTONIC

INFECTIOUS DISEASES
- VIRAL, ANTI-: Flu Virus

LIVER
- HEPATITIS, CHRONIC PERSISTENT/ACTIVE: Colchicine Tablet, 0.5 mg/ Tab, 1 Tab 3x/Day Until Symptoms Gone

MUSCULOSKELETAL/

CONNECTIVE TISSUE
- GOUT, ACUTE: Responds In Few Hours, 0.5 mg/Tab, 2 Tabs Initially, 1tab/2 Hrs Thereafter, Do Not Exceed 6 mg/24 Hrs

Dose

3 - 15 gm

Common Name

Chinese Tulip Bulb

Precautions

Watch: Weak Patients

Notes

Has Colchicine

Slow Onset, 3-6 Hrs Post Ingestion, Nausea, Vomiting, Diarrhea

Large Overdose Is Fatal, No Antidote

SHE CHUANG ZI

蛇床子

SEMEN CNIDII MONNIERI

Traditional Functions:

1. Warms the Kidneys and strengthens the Yang
2. Dries Dampness and stops itch
3. Kills intestinal parasites

Traditional Properties:

Enters: SP, KI,

Properties: SP, BIT, W

Indications:

EXTREMITIES
• LEGS, PAIN, SWELLING:
(Beriberi, Leg Qi) , Cold Dampness
MUSCULOSKELETAL/
CONNECTIVE TISSUE
• ARTHRITIS: For Expelling Cold,
Dampness
• BACK, LOWER PAIN
SEXUALITY, EITHER SEX
• GENITALS, PRURITUS
• INFERTILITY: Kidney Yang

Deficient
SEXUALITY, FEMALE:
GYNECOLOGICAL
• LEUKORRHEA: Kidney Spleen
Yang Deficiency
• MENSTRUATION, DISORDERS
OF: Tonify Qi Of Chong, Ren
SEXUALITY, MALE:
UROLOGICAL TOPICS
• IMPOTENCE: Kidney Yang
Deficient

SKIN
• ECZEMA: Cold Dampness
• RASHES, W/PRURITUS: External
Application
• RINGWORM
• SCABIES
• SKIN, LESIONS, ITCHY,
WEEPING
• SKIN, SORES: Cold Damp
URINARY BLADDER
• URINATION, FREQUENT

Clinical/Pharmaceutical Studies:

INFECTIOUS DISEASES
• VIRAL, ANTI-: Flu, etc
PARASITES
• ROUNDWORMS
SEXUALITY, EITHER SEX
• SEX GLANDS, INCREASES
WEIGHT OF
• SEX HORMONE-LIKE: Male/
Female
SEXUALITY, FEMALE:
GYNECOLOGICAL

• LEUKORRHEA, PROFUSE:
Nontrichomonal, Reduces
Leukorrhea Discharge, Alleviates
Pruritus
• TRICHOMONAS, VAGINAL:
Decoctions (Must Be 50% Or
Stronger) , Powders
• VAGINITIS: Nontrichomonal,
Reduces Leukorrhea, Alleviates
Pruritus, Use Vaginal Application Of
Decoction, Powder, Extract

SKIN
• ECZEMA: Topically
• ECZEMA, INFANTILE: Topical,
Had Astringent Effect
• FUNGAL, ANTI-: Many
• PRURITUS: Topically
• SKIN, CANDIDIASIS: 20%
Ointment To Effectively Treat
TRAUMA, BITES, POISONINGS
• FLIES: Powder Will Kill

Dose

3 - 15 gm

Contraindications

Not: Damp Heat Of Lower Jiao
Not: Def Yin w/Heat

SONG XIANG

松香

RESINA PINI
(COLORHONIUM)

Traditional Functions:

1. Dries Dampness and dispels Wind
2. Removes toxin, discharges pus
3. Controls pain and promotes regeneration of tissue

Traditional Properties:

Enters: LV, SP

Properties: SW, W

Indications:

MUSCULOSKELETAL/
CONNECTIVE TISSUE
• ARTHRITIS: Wind Damp
PAIN/NUMBNESS/GENERAL
DISCOMFORT

• BI, WIND DAMP
SKIN
• BOILS
• FURUNCLES: Damp

• PRURITUS
• SCABIES
• SKIN, SORES, SWOLLEN, TOXIC:
Topical

Common Name

Pine Resin

Notes

Grind Into Powder For Topical Application

XIONG HUANG

雄黃
(雄黃)

REALGAR

Traditional Functions:

1. Clears toxins and controls pain
2. Kills parasites when applied topically

Traditional Properties:

Enters: ST, LI, LV,

Properties: SP, W, TX

Indications:

BOWEL RELATED DISORDERS
• DIARRHEA
INFECTIOUS DISEASES
• MALARIA, CHRONIC
MENTAL STATE/
  NEUROLOGICAL DISORDERS
• EPILEPSY
PARASITES

• BRAIN, CYSTICERCOSIS
• PARASITES, INTESTINAL
• ROUNDWORMS
SKIN
• ABSCESS
• RASHES, DAMP: Topical
• RINGWORM: Topical
• SCABIES: Topical

• SKIN, ITCHING: Soak
• SKIN, SORES, SWOLLEN, TOXIC:
  Topical
• ULCERS, SKIN
TRAUMA, BITES, POISONINGS
• INFLAMMATION, SUPPURATIVE
• INSECT BITES
• SNAKE BITES

Clinical/Pharmaceutical Studies:

INFECTIOUS DISEASES
• BACTERIAL, ANTI-
PARASITES

• ANTIPARASITIC: Ascaris, Blood
  Fluke, Schistosome
SKIN

• FUNGAL, ANTI-: Many
• NEURODERMATITIS: Topical
  Paste

Dose

0.15 - 0.60 gm

Common Name

Realgar (Arsenic Sulfide)

Contraindications

Not: Pregnancy

Not: Blood/Yin Deficiency

Notes

When Burned Becomes Extremely Toxic

ZAO FAN
(LU FAN)

皂礬
(皂矾)

MELANTERITUM

Traditional Functions:

1. Dries Dampness and transforms Phlegm
2. Dispels accumulations by killing intestinal parasites
3. Nourishes the Blood and arrests bleeding
4. Detoxifies poison and reduces swelling

Traditional Properties:

Enters: SP, LV,

Properties: SO, A, CL

Indications:

BOWEL RELATED DISORDERS
• DYSENTERY, CHRONIC: Mucus/
  Blood In BM
EYES
• BLEPHARITIS ULCEROSA
FLUID DISORDERS
• EDEMA, GENERALIZED W/

  YELLOWISH SKIN
HEMORRHAGIC DISORDERS
• HEMAFECIA
LIVER
• JAUNDICE: Blood Deficient
NUTRITIONAL/METABOLIC
  DISORDERS/TOPICS

• MALNUTRITION
ORAL CAVITY
• ORAL LESIONS
• PHARYNGITIS
SKIN
• ECZEMA
• SCABIES

Dose

1.5 - 4.5 gm

Common Name

Green Vitriol (Ferrous Sulfate)

ZHANG NAO 樟腦 （樟腦） CAMPHORA

Traditional Functions:

1. Removes Wind Dampness and kills parasites
2. Opens the orifices and removes turbidity
3. Vitalizes the Blood, reduces pain and disperses swellings

Traditional Properties:

Enters: SP, HT,

Properties: SP, H, TX

Indications:

ABDOMEN/
GASTROINTESTINAL TOPICS
• ABDOMEN, PAIN OF, SWELLING
CANCER/TUMORS/SWELLINGS/
LUMPS
• SWELLINGS: Blood Stasis
CHEST
• CHEST, PAIN, SWELLING
INFECTIOUS DISEASES
• FEBRILE DISEASES, FAINTING
MENTAL STATE/
NEUROLOGICAL DISORDERS

• COMA
• DELIRIUM
• MENTAL CLOUDINESS: Excess
  (Shut-In Complex)
• UNCONSCIOUSNESS: Excess
  (Shut-In Complex)
NUTRITIONAL/METABOLIC
DISORDERS/TOPICS
• BERIBERI
ORAL CAVITY
• TOOTHACHE
SKIN

• PRURITUS: Topical
• RINGWORM: Topical
• SCABIES: Topical
• SKIN, DISORDERS
• SORES, ITCHY: Topical
TRAUMA, BITES, POISONINGS
• CONTUSIONS: Topical
• FRACTURES: Topical
• SPRAINS: Topical
• TRAUMA, INJURIES, PAIN:
  Topical

Clinical/Pharmaceutical Studies:

ABDOMEN/
GASTROINTESTINAL TOPICS
• GASTROINTESTINAL,
  IRRITATES: Ingestion, Causing
  Warm Sensation In Small Doses
HEART
• CARDIOTONIC: In Weak Hearts,
  Slight
• HEART FAILURE

MENTAL STATE/
NEUROLOGICAL DISORDERS
• STIMULANT, CNS: Small Doses
ORAL CAVITY
• COLD SORES
PAIN/NUMBNESS/GENERAL
DISCOMFORT
• ANALGESIC: Topical
• ANESTHETIC: Topical, Local

SKIN
• ABSORBED THROUGH ANY
  BODY SURFACE
• ANTISEPTIC, WARMING TO
  SKIN
• FUNGAL, ANTI-: Strongly Inhibits
  Some
• SKIN, ITCHING

Dose

0.3 - 1.5 gm

Common Name

Camphor

Contraindications

Not: Pregnancy

Not: Def Qi

Notes

0.5-1 gm: Dizziness, Headache, Warmth, Restlessness, 2
gm Spasms, Possible Respiratory Arrest, 7-15 gm Fatal

Anomalous Herbs

CAO MIAN HUA ZI 草棉花子 SEMEN GOSSYPII

Traditional Functions:

1. Warms and benefits the Kidneys
2. Controls bleeding

Traditional Properties:

Enters: KI,

Properties: SP, H, <TX

Indications:

BOWEL RELATED DISORDERS
• HEMORRHOIDS
• RECTAL PROLAPSE: From
  Uterine Bleeding
SEXUALITY, FEMALE:

GYNECOLOGICAL
• LACTATION, INSUFFICIENT
• LEUKORRHEA, MORBID
SEXUALITY, MALE:
UROLOGICAL TOPICS

• IMPOTENCE
• TESTICLES, PROLAPSE
URINARY BLADDER
• ENURESIS

Clinical/Pharmaceutical Studies:

SEXUALITY, FEMALE:

GYNECOLOGICAL

• LACTATION, PROMOTES

Dose

6 - 9 gm

Common Name

Gossypium/Cotton Seed

Notes

See Mian Hua Gen For More Uses, Clinical
Applications

LING LING XIANG 零陵香 (零陵香) HERBA LYSIMACHIAE

Traditional Functions:

1. Clears evil Qi pain and fullness in Heart and abdomen
2. Relieves focal distension in chest and stomach

Traditional Properties:

Enters:

Properties: SW, SP, N

Indications:

ABDOMEN/
  GASTROINTESTINAL TOPICS
• ABDOMEN, PAIN OF, FULLNESS
CHEST
• CHEST, OPRESSION IN

HEART
• HEART PAIN, FULLNESS
NOSE
• NOSE, STUFFY

STOMACH/DIGESTIVE
  DISORDERS
• ANOREXIA
• STOMACH, WEAK

Dose

4.5 - 9.0 gm

Common Name

Sweet Basil

MAN SHAN HONG

滿山紅
(满山红)

FOLIUM RHODODENDORI DAURICI

Traditional Functions:

1. Controls cough and disperses Phlegm

Traditional Properties:

Enters:

Properties: BIT, C

Indications:

LUNGS   • BRONCHITIS, CHRONIC   • COUGH

Clinical/Pharmaceutical Studies:

HEART	• ANTITUSSIVE: Decoction/Volatile	Suppresses Bronchial Spasm
• CARDIOTONIC: Digitalis-Like	Oil Suppresses Cough	• EXPECTORANT: Alcohol Infusion
LUNGS	• ASTHMA: Ethanol Extract Injected	Dramatic

Dose

15 - 30 gm

Common Name

Daurian Rhododendron

Notes

Fresh Leaf Used

MIAN HUA GEN

棉花根

RADIX GOSSYPII

Traditional Functions:

1. Benefits deficiency, calms coughing and wheezing
2. Regulates menstruation

Traditional Properties:

Enters:

Properties:

Indications:

ABDOMEN/	• ASTHMA: Deficiency	GYNECOLOGICAL
GASTROINTESTINAL TOPICS	• COUGH: Deficiency	• UTERINE BLEEDING
• HERNIA	SEXUALITY, FEMALE:	• UTERUS, PROLAPSE
LUNGS		

Clinical/Pharmaceutical Studies:

CANCER/TUMORS/ SWELLINGS/LUMPS	Greater Than Amantadine LUNGS	SEXUALITY, EITHER SEX	Tab, 2 Tabs/Day For 1 Month, 1-4 Courses
• TUMOR, ANTI-: Strongly Suppresses Yoshida Tumor, Solid Tumors, Melanoma When Applied Topically	• ANTITUSSIVE: Dramatic	• ANTIFERTILITY: Oral, 2-4 Weeks, Persisted 3-5 Weeks After Discontinuation	• UTERUS, MYOMA: Gossypol Tablet, 4.5 mg/ Tab, 2 Tabs/Day For 1 Month, 1-4 Courses
	• ASTHMA: Suppresses Wheezing	SEXUALITY, FEMALE: GYNECOLOGICAL	• UTERUS, STIMULATES: Weaker Than Ergot
INFECTIOUS DISEASES	• BRONCHITIS, CHRONIC: Symptomatic	• ABORTIFACIENT: Weak Oxytocic Action, Less	SEXUALITY, MALE: UROLOGICAL TOPICS
• ANTIBIOTIC: Bacteriostatic To Many, Long Term Treatment Can Change GI Tract Bacterial Flora	Treatment, Good For Cough, Expectoration	Than Ergot	• CONTRACEPTION, MALE: Reversible, Fertility Not Affected
	• EXPECTORANT: Dramatic, Especially ETOH Extract, Resin Fraction	• ENDOMETRIOSIS: Gossypol Tablet, 4.5 mg/ Tab, 2 Tabs/Day For 1 Month, 1-4 Courses	• TESTICLES, EPIDIDYMIS, SWOLLEN: Shrinks In 2 Months Or So
• COMMON COLD/FLU: Nose Drops Of Active Ingredient Helped	• PNEUMONIA, VIRAL: Nose Drops Of Active Ingredient Helped With Cure	• UTERINE BLEEDING: Gossypol Tablet, 4.5 mg/	
• VIRAL, ANTI-: Inhibits Several, Inhibits Flu			

Dose

30 - 60 gm

Common Name

Cotton Root Bark

Notes

Large Doses May Cause Vomiting, Clinical Doses May Cause Short Term, Mild Lassitude, A Few Reports Of Nausea

Gossypol Main Active Agent, Root Bark Has 0.56-2.05%

SUAN JIANG

酸漿

RHIZOMA ET RADIX PHYSALITIS

Traditional Functions:

1. Dispels fever and calms the mind
2. Supplements the Qi
3. Promotes diuresis
4. Clears the vision

Traditional Properties:

Enters:

Properties: BIT, C

Indications:

**ABDOMEN/
 GASTROINTESTINAL TOPICS**
• HERNIA
FEVERS
• FEVER: Wind Heat

LUNGS
• COUGH
• WHOOPING COUGH
**SEXUALITY, FEMALE:
 GYNECOLOGICAL**

• MISCARRIAGE: Lack Of Uterine
 Contraction After
URINARY BLADDER
• UROPENIA: (Lack Of Urination)

Clinical/Pharmaceutical Studies:

FEVERS
• ANTIPYRETIC
HEART

• CARDIOTONIC
**SEXUALITY, FEMALE:
 GYNECOLOGICAL**

• UTERUS, STIMULATES:
 Increases Contractions, Used As
 Abortificient In Ancient China

Common Name

Physalis

Notes

Steep In Hot Water, Decoct Or Cook In Gruel For Oral Intake

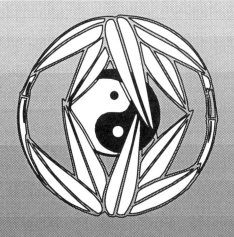

PART III
Appendices

Pin Yin (Chinese) Herb Name	Pharmaceutical Herb Name	Page No.	Pin Yin (Chinese) Herb Name	Pharmaceutical Herb Name	Page No.
A Jiao	*Gelatinum Asini*	797	Bai Ji Li 白蒺藜	*Fructus Tribuli Terrestris*	743
A Wei 阿魏	*Asafoetida*	637	Bai Jiang Can	*Bombyx Batryticatus*	746
A Xian Yao	*Acacia Seu Uncaria/Gambir*	839	Bai Jiang Cao 敗醬草	*Herba Patrinia/Thlaspi*	512
Ai Ye 艾葉	*Folium Artemisiae Vulgaris/Argyi*	651	Bai Jie Zi 白芥子	*Semen Sinapis Albae*	708
An Xi Xiang 安息香	*Benzoinum*	753	Bai Ju	*Scolopendra Subspinipes*	751
Ba Dou 巴豆	*Semen Crotonis*	550	Bai Lian 白蔹	*Radix Ampelopsis*	513
Ba Ji	*Radix Morindae Officinalis*	773	Bai Mao Gen 白茅根	*Rhizoma Imperatae Cylindricae*	653
Ba Ji Tian 巴戟天	*Radix Morindae Officinalis*	773	Bai Mao Gen Hua 白茅根花	*Flos Imperatae Cylindriae*	653
Ba Jiao Gen 芭蕉根	*Musae Caudex*	510	Bai Mao Teng	*Herba Solani Lyrati*	535
Ba Jiao Hui Xiang 八角茴香	*Fructus Illicius*	608	Bai Mu Er 白木耳	*Fructificatio Tremellae Fuciformis*	803
Ba Jiao Lian 八角連	*Rhizoma Podophylli*	510	Bai Qian 白前	*Rhizoma Cynanchii Stautoni*	709
Ba Jiao Wu Tong	*Folium Clerondendri, Ramulus Et*	560	Bai Shao 白芍	*Radix Paeoniae Lactiflorae/Alba*	794
Bai Bian Dou 白扁豆	*Semen Dolichoris Lablab*	506	Bai Shao Yao	*Radix Paeoniae Lactiflorae/Alba*	794
Bai Bu 百部	*Radix Stemonae*	699	Bai Shi Zhi	*Halloysitum Rubrum/Album*	818
Bai Dou Kou 白豆蔻	*Fructus Amomi Cardamomi*	577	Bai Tou Weng 白頭翁	*Radix Pulsatillae Chinensis*	514
Bai Fan 白礬	*Alum*	836	Bai Wei 白薇	*Radix Cynanchi Atrati*	495
Bai Fu Ling	*Sclerotium Poriae Cocos*	594	Bai Xian Pi 白鮮皮	*Cortex Dictamni Dasycarpi Radicis*	515
Bai Fu Zi 白附子	*Rhizoma Typhonii Gigantei/Aconiti Coreani*	708	Bai Zhi 白芷	*Radix Angelicae*	441
Bai Guo 白果	*Semen Ginkgo Bilobae*	818	Bai Zhu 白術	*Rhizoma Atractylodis Macrocephalae*	760
Bai Guo Ye 白果葉	*Folium Ginko*	817	Bai Zi Ren 柏子仁	*Semen Biotae Orientalis*	730
Bai He 百合	*Bulbus Lilii*	803	Ban Bian Lian 半邊蓮	*Herba Lobeliae Chinensis Cum Radice*	586
Bai Hua Lian 白花連	*Radix Rauwolfiae Verticillatae*	511	Ban Lan Gen 板籃根	*Radix Isatidis Seu Baphicacanthi*	515
Bai Hua She 白花蛇	*Agkistrodon Seu Bungarus*	558	Ban Mao 班螯	*Mylabris*	837
Bai Hua She She Cao 白花蛇舌草	*Herba Oldenlandiae Diffusae/Hedyotis Diffusae*	511	Ban Xia 半夏	*Rhizoma Pinelliae Ternatae*	710
Bai Ji 白芨	*Rhizoma Bletillae Striatae*	652	Ban Zhi Lian 半枝蓮	*Herba Scutellariae Barbatae*	516

Pin Yin (Chinese) Herb Name	Pharmaceutical Herb Name	Page No.	Pin Yin (Chinese) Herb Name	Pharmaceutical Herb Name	Page No.
Bao Ma Zi 暴馬子	*Cortex Syringae*	700	Cao Dou Kou 草豆蔻	*Semen Alpiniae Katsumadai*	579
Bao Yu 鮑魚	*Haliotis*	804	Cao Guo 草果	*Fructus Amomi Tsao-ko*	580
Bei Mu	*Bulbus Fritillariae Thunbergii*	728	Cao He Che 草河車	*Rhizoma Polygoni Bistortae*	517
Bei Sha Shen 北沙參	*Radix Glehniae Littoralis*	804	Cao Jue Ming	*Semen Cassiae Torae*	471
Bei Xie 萆解	*Rhizoma Dioscoreae Sativae*	587	Cao Mian Hua Zi 草棉花子	*Semen Gossypii*	850
Bei Xing Ren	*Semen Pruni Armeniacae*	705	Cao Wu 草烏	*Radix Aconiti Kusnezoffii*	609
Bei Yin Chen	*Herba Origani/Artemisia*	602	Ce Bai Ye 側柏葉	*Cacumen Biotae Orientalis*	654
Bi Ba 蓽茇	*Fructus Piperis Longi*	608	Ce Bo Ye	*Cacumen Biotae Orientalis*	654
Bi Bo	*Fructus Piperis Longi*	608	Cha Chi Huang 茶匙潢	*Herba Malachii*	517
Bi Cheng Qie 蓽澄茄	*Fructus Litseae*	609	Cha Ye 茶葉	*Folium Camelliae*	589
Bi Ji	*Cormus Heleochris Plantaginea*	717	Chai Hu 柴胡	*Radix Bupleuri*	457
Bi Ma Zi 蓖麻子	*Semen Ricini*	547	Chan Su 蟾酥	*Secretio Bufonis*	837
Bi Qi 荸薺:荸荠 . . .	*Cormus Heleochris Plantaginea*	717	Chan Tui 蟬蛻	*Periostracum Cicadae*	458
Bi Xie	*Rhizoma Dioscoreae Sativae*	587	Chang Pu	*Rhizoma Acori Graminei*	757
Bi Zi Cao 筆仔草	*Herba Pogonatheri*	587	Chang Shan 常山	*Radix Dichorae Febrifugae*	518
Bian Dou	*Semen Dolichoris Lablab*	506	Che Qian Cao 車前草	*Herba Plantaginis*	589
Bian Xu 萹蓄	*Herba Polygoni Avicularis*	588	Che Qian Zi 車前子	*Semen Plantaginis*	590
Bie Jia 鱉甲	*Carapax Amydae Sinensis*	805	Chen Pi 陳皮	*Pericarpium Citri Reticulatae*	621
Bing Lang 檳榔	*Semen Arecae Catechu*	643	Chen Xiang 沉香	*Lignum Aquilariae*	622
Bing Lang Zi	*Semen Arecae Catechu*	643	Chen Zong Tan 陳棕炭	*Vagina Trachycarpi Carbonista*	655
Bing Pian 冰片	*Borneol*	753	Cheng Liu	*Cacumen Tamaricis*	451
Bo He 薄荷	*Herba Menthae*	456	Chi Fu Ling 赤茯苓	*Sclerotium Poriae Cocos Rubrae*	483
Bu Gu Zhi 補骨脂	*Fructus Psoraleae Corylifoliae*	773	Chi Shao	*Radix Paeoniae Rubra*	668
Can Sha 蠶砂	*Excrementum Bombycis Mori*	558	Chi Shao Yao 赤芍藥	*Radix Paeoniae Rubra*	668
Cang Er Zi 蒼耳子	*Fructus Xanthii*	559	Chi Shi Zhi 赤石脂	*Halloysitum Rubrum/Album*	818
Cang Zhu 蒼術	*Rhizoma Atractylodis*	578	Chi Xiao Dou 赤小豆	*Semen Phaseoli Calcarati*	591
Cao Bei Mu	*Bulbus Santsigu*	846	Chong Lou	*Rhizoma Paris*	540
			Chong Wei Zi 沖蔚子	*Fructus Leonuri*	669

Pin Yin (Chinese) Herb Name	Pharmaceutical Herb Name	Page No.	Pin Yin (Chinese) Herb Name	Pharmaceutical Herb Name	Page No.
Chou Wu Tong 臭梧桐......	Folium Clerondendri, Ramulus Et	560	Da Ji 大薊........	Herba Cirsii Japonici	655
Chuan Bei Mu 川貝母......	Bulbus Fritillariae Cirrhosae	717	Da Ji	Radix Knoxiae/Euphorbia Pekinesis	551
Chuan Jiao 川椒........	Fructus Zanthoxyli Bungeani	610	Da Ji	Radix Euphorbiae Pekinensis	552
Chuan Lian Zi 川楝子.....	Fructus Meliae Toosendan	623	Da Qing Ye 大青葉......	Folium Daqingye	519
Chuan Niu Xi 川牛膝......	Radix Cyathulae	669	Da Suan 大蒜........	Sublus Alli Sativi	644
Chuan Po	Cortex Magnoliae Officinalis	581	Da Xue Teng....	Caulis Sargentodoxae	497
Chuan Po Hua ..	Flos Magnolia Officianlis	580	Da Zao 大棗/紅棗...	Fructus Ziziphi Jujubae	761
Chuan Shan Jia 穿山甲......	Squama Manitis Pentadactylae	670	Dai Mao 玳瑁........	Carapax Erethmochelyas	743
Chuan Shan Long 川山龍......	Rhizoma Dioscoreae Nipponicae	442	Dai Zhe Shi 代赭石.....	Haematitum	735
Chuan Wu 川烏........	Radix Aconitii	611	Dan Dou Chi 淡豆豉......	Semen Sojae Praeparatum	459
Chuan Xin Lian 穿心蓮......	Herba Andrographis Paniculatae	518	Dan Nan Xing 膽南星......	Pulvis Arisaemai Cum Felle Bovis	718
Chuan Xiong 川芎........	Radix Ligustici Wallichii	671	Dan Shen 丹參........	Radix Salviae Miltiorrhizae	672
Chui Si Liu	Cacumen Tamaricis	451	Dan Zhu Ye 淡竹葉......	Herba Lophatheri Gracilis	470
Chun Bai Pi.....	Cortex Ailanthi	483	Dang Gui 當歸........	Radix Angelicae Sinensis	795
Chun Pi 椿皮........	Cortex Ailanthi	483	Dang Shen 黨參........	Radix Codonopsis Pilosulae	762
Ci Ji Li	Fructus Tribuli Terrestris	743	Dao Ya	Fructus Oryzae Sativae Germinantus	637
Ci Shi 磁石........	Magnetitum	735	Deng Xin Cao 燈心草......	Medulla Junci Effusi	592
Ci Wan	Radix Asteris Tatarici	706	Di Dan Tou 地膽頭......	Herba Elephantopi	520
Ci Wei Pi 刺謂皮......	Corium Erinacei	819	Di Fu Zi 地膚子......	Fructus Kochiae Scopariae	592
Ci Wu Jia	Radix Acanthopanax Senticosus/Eleutheroc occus	771	Di Gu Pi 地骨皮......	Cortex Lycii Chinensis Radicis	495
Cong Bai 蔥白........	Herba Allii Fistulosi	442	Di Jiao 地椒........	Herba Thymi Serpylli	443
Da Dou Huang Juan 大豆黃卷 ...	Semen Glycines Germinatum	506	Di Long 地龍........	Lumbricus	744
Da Feng Zi 大楓子......	Semen Hydnocarpi Anthelminthicae	839	Di Yu 地榆........	Radix Sanguisorbae Officinalis	656
Da Fu Pi 大腹皮......	Pericarpium Arecae Catechu	624	Ding Xiang 丁香........	Flos Caryophylli	612
Da Huang 大黃........	Rhizoma Rhei	542	Dong Bei Guan Zhong 東北貫衆....	Rhizoma Dryopteridis Crassirhizomae	645

Pin Yin (Chinese) Herb Name	Pharmaceutical Herb Name	Page No.	Pin Yin (Chinese) Herb Name	Pharmaceutical Herb Name	Page No.
Dong Chong Xia Cao 冬蟲夏草	Cordyceps Sinensis	775	Feng Mi 蜂蜜.........	Mel	548
Dong Gua Pi 冬瓜皮	Exocarpium Benincasae	593	Feng Wei Cao 鳳尾草.......	Herba Pteris	496
Dong Gua Ren 冬瓜仁	Semen Benincasae Hispidae	593	Fo Shou 佛手	Fructus Citri Sarcodactylis	624
Dong Gua Zi .... 冬瓜子	Semen Benincasae Hispidae	593	Fo Shou Gan.....	Fructus Citri Sarcodactylis	624
Dong Kui Zi 冬葵子	Semen Abutiloni Seu Malvae	594	Fu Ling 茯苓.........	Sclerotium Poriae Cocos	594
Dou Chi Jiang 豆豉姜	Ramus/Radix Litseae Cubebae	612	Fu Ling Pi 茯苓皮......	Cortex Poriae Cocos	595
Dou Juan	Semen Glycines Germinatum	506	Fu Long Gan 伏龍肝.......	Terra Flava Usta	657
Dou Kou........	Semen Alpiniae Katsumadai	579	Fu Pen Zi 復盆子.......	Fructus Rubi	820
Dou Kou........	Fructus Amomi Cardamomi	577	Fu Ping 浮萍.........	Herba Lemnae Seu Spirodelae	460
Du Huo 獨活........	Radix Duhuo	561	Fu Shen 茯神.........	Sclerotium Poriae Cocos Pararadicis	736
Du Zhong 杜仲........	Cortex Eucommiae Ulmoidis	775	Fu Xiao Mai 浮小麥......	Semen Tritici Aestivi Levis	820
Du Zhong Ye 杜仲葉	Folium Eucommiae Ulmoidis	776	Fu Zi 附子.........	Radix Aconiti Carmichaeli Praeparata	613
E Bu Shi Cao 鵝不食草	Herba Centipedae	711	Gan Cao 甘草........	Radix Glycyrrhizae Uralensis	763
E Guan Shi 鵝管石	Stalactitum	777	Gan Jiang 干姜.........	Rhizoma Zingiberis Officinalis	614
E Jiao 阿膠........	Gelatinum Asini	797	Gan Lan 橄欖	Fructus Canarii	484
E Wei	Asafoetida	637	Gan Song Xiang 甘松香.......	Rhizoma Nardostachytis	580
E Zhu 莪術........	Rhizoma Curcumae Zedoariae	673	Gan Sui 甘遂.........	Radix Euphorbiae Kansui	551
Er Cha 兒茶........	Acacia Seu Uncaria/Gambir	839	Gan Sung	Rhizoma Nardostachytis	580
Fa Xia	Rhizoma Pinelliae Ternatae	710	Gao Ben 藁本	Radix Ligustici Sinensis	444
Fan Hong Hua 番紅花	Stigma Crocus/Stigma Croci	674	Gao Liang Jiang 高良姜.......	Rhizoma Alpiniae Officinari	615
Fan Mu Bie......	Semen Strychnotis	842	Ge Gen 葛根........	Radix Puerariae	460
Fan Xie Ye 番瀉葉	Folium Sennae	544	Ge Hua 葛花........	Flos Puerariae	521
Fang Feng 防風........	Radix Sileris/Ledebouriellae Sesloidis	444	Ge Jie 蛤蚧........	Gecko	777
Fang Ji	Radix Stephaniae Tetrandrae	596	Ge Ke	Concha Cyclinae Sinensis	721
Fei Zi 榧子........	Semen Torreyae Grandis	645	Ge Qiao	Concha Cyclinae Sinensis	721
Feng Fang	Nidus Vespae	841	Gou Ji 狗脊........	Rhizoma Cibotii Barometz	778
Feng La 蜂蠟	Cera Flava	840			

Pin Yin (Chinese) Herb Name	Pharmaceutical Herb Name	Page No.	Pin Yin (Chinese) Herb Name	Pharmaceutical Herb Name	Page No.
Gou Qi Zi 枸杞子......	*Fructus Lycii Chinensis*	798	Hai Fu Shi 海浮石......	*Pumice*	720
Gou Teng 鉤藤........	*Ramulus Uncariae Cum Uncis*	745	Hai Ge Ke 海蛤殼......	*Concha Cyclinae Sinensis*	721
Gu Jing Cao 谷精草......	*Scapus Eriocaulonis Buergeriani*	461	Hai Gou Shen 海狗腎......	*Testes/Penis Otoriae*	779
Gu Sui Bu 骨碎補......	*Rhizoma Drynaria*	778	Hai Jin Sha 海金沙......	*Spora Lygodii*	522
Gu Ya 谷芽........	*Fructus Oryzae Sativae Germinantus*	637	Hai Jin Sha Cao 海金砂草....	*Herba Lygodii Japonici*	522
Gua Di 瓜蒂........	*Melo Pedicelus/Melonis Calyx*	834	Hai Long 海龍........	*Hailong*	779
Gua Lou 瓜蔞........	*Fructus Trichosanthis*	718	Hai Ma 海馬........	*Hippocampus*	780
Gua Lou Gen....	*Radix Trichosanthis*	726	Hai Piao Xiao 海螵蛸......	*Os Sepiae Seu Sepiellae*	821
Gua Lou Pi 瓜蔞皮......	*Pericarpium Trichosanthis*	719	Hai Shen 海參......	*Stichopus Japonicus, Selenka*	781
Gua Lou Ren 瓜蔞仁......	*Semen Trichosanthis*	720	Hai Tong Pi 海桐皮......	*Cortex Erythrinae Variegatae*	562
Guan Bai Fu	*Rhizoma Typhonii Gigantei/Aconiti Coreani*	708	Hai Zao 海藻........	*Herba Sargassii*	721
Guan Chong	*Rhizoma Guanzhong/Blechni/Et. Al.*	521	Han Fang Ji 漢防己......	*Radix Stephaniae Tetrandrae*	596
Guan Zhong 貫衆........	*Rhizoma Guanzhong/Blechni/Et. Al.*	521	Han Lian Cao 旱蓮草......	*Herba Ecliptae Prostratae*	806
Guang Fang Ji 廣防己......	*Radix Aristolochiae Seu Cocculi*	595	Han Lian Ye	*Folium Nelumbinis Nuciferae*	507
Guei Yu Jian 鬼羽箭......	*Ramulus/Herba Suberalatum Euonymi/Buchnerae*	675	Han Shui Shi 寒水石......	*Calcitum*	471
Gui Ban 龜板........	*Plastrum Testudinis*	806	He Huan Hua 合歡花......	*Flos Albizziae*	730
Gui Jian Yu	*Ramulus/Herba Suberalatum Euonymi/Buchnerae*	675	He Huan Pi 合歡皮......	*Cortex Albizziae Julibrissin*	731
Gui Yuan Rou ...	*Arillus Euphoriae Longanae*	800	He Shi 鶴虱........	*Fructus Carpesii Abrotanoidis/Dauci*	646
Gui Zhen Cao 鬼針草......	*Herba Bidentis Bipinnatae*	462	He Shou Wu 何首烏......	*Radix Polygoni Multiflori*	799
Gui Zhi 桂枝........	*Ramulus Cinnamomi Cassiae*	445	He Ye 荷葉........	*Folium Nelumbinis Nuciferae*	507
Hai Bai	*Bulbus Allii*	634	He Zi 荷子........	*Fructus Terminaliae Chebulae*	822
Hai Er Cha	*Acacia Seu Uncaria/Gambir*	839	Hei Dou 黑豆........	*Semen Glycine Sojae*	807
Hai Er Shen	*Radix Pseudostellariae Heterophyllae*	770	Hei Zhi Ma 黑芝麻......	*Semen Sesami Indici*	808
Hai Feng Teng 海風藤......	*Caulis Piperis*	562	Hong Da Ji 紅大薊......	*Radix Knoxiae/Euphorbia Pekinesis*	551
			Hong Hua 紅花........	*Flos Carthami Tinctorii*	675

Pin Yin (Chinese) Herb Name	Pharmaceutical Herb Name	Page No.	Pin Yin (Chinese) Herb Name	Pharmaceutical Herb Name	Page No.
Hong Teng 紅藤	Caulis Sargentodoxae	497	Huang Jing 黃精	Rhizoma Polygonati	764
Hong Zao	Fructus Ziziphi Jujubae	761	Huang Lian 黃連	Rhizoma Coptidis	486
Hou Po 厚樸	Cortex Magnoliae Officinalis	581	Huang Qi 黃芪:黃芪	Radix Astragali	765
Hou Po Hua 厚樸花	Flos Magnolia Officianlis	580	Huang Qin 黃芩	Radix Scutellariae Baicalensis	489
Hou Zao 猴棗	Calculus Macacae Mulattae	722	Huang Wei Zi	Fructus Leonuri	669
Hu Chang	Rhizoma Polygoni Cuspidati	497	Huang Yao Zi 黃藥子	Rhizoma Dioscoreae Bulbiferae	723
Hu Gu 虎骨	Os Tigris	563	Hui Xiang	Fructus Foeniculi Vulgaris	619
Hu Huang Lian 胡黃連	Rhizoma Picrorrhizae	484	Huo Ma Ren 火麻仁	Semen Cannabis Sativae	548
Hu Ji Sheng	Ramulus Loranthi Seu Visci	813	Huo Tan Mu Cao 火炭母草	Herba Polygoni Chinese	498
Hu Jiao 胡椒	Fructus Piperis Nigri	615	Huo Xiang 藿香	Herba Agastaches Seu Pogostemi	582
Hu Lu Ba 胡蘆巴	Semen Trigonellae Foeni-graeci	781	Ja Lang	Herba Eupatorii Fortunei	583
Hu Ma Ren	Semen Sesami Indici	808	Ji Cai	Herba Capsellae	664
Hu Po 琥珀	Succinum	737	Ji Gu Cao 雞骨草	Herba Abri	564
Hu Sui 胡荽	Herba /Fructus Coriandri	446	Ji Guan Hua 雞冠花	Flos Celosiae Cristatae	822
Hu Tao Ren 胡桃仁	Semen Juglandis Regiae	782	Ji Nei Jin 雞內金	Endothelium Corneum Gigeraiae Galli	638
Hu Zhang 虎杖	Rhizoma Polygoni Cuspidati	497	Ji Xing Zi 急性子	Semen Impatientis	677
Hua Qi Shen 花旗參	Radix Panacis Quinquefolii	808	Ji Xue Cao	Herba Centellae	697
Hua Rui Shi 花蕊石	Ophicalcitum	658	Ji Xue Deng	Caulis Mucunae/Spatholobi	677
Hua Shan Jiao	Fructus Zanthoxyli Bungeani	610	Ji Xue Teng 雞血藤	Caulis Mucunae/Spatholobi	677
Hua Shi 滑石	Talcum	597	Ji Zi Huang 雞子黃	Gallus	809
Huai Hua	Flos Sophorae Japonicae Immaturus	658	Jiang Can 僵蠶	Bombyx Batryticatus	746
Huai Hua Mi 槐花米	Flos Sophorae Japonicae Immaturus	658	Jiang Huang 姜黃	Rhizoma Curcumae	678
Huai Jiao 槐角	Fructus Sophorae Japonicae	676	Jiang Xiang 降香	Lignum Dalbergiae Odoriferae/Acronychia e	659
Huai Niu Xi	Radix Achyranthis Bidentatae	684	Jiang Zhen Xian	Lignum Dalbergiae Odoriferae/Acronychia e	659
Huai San	Radix Dioscoreae Oppositae	769	Jie Geng 桔梗	Radix Platycodi Grandiflori	711
Huang Bai 黃柏	Cortex Phellodendri	485	Jin Di Luo 錦地羅	Herba Droserae	523
Huang Bo	Cortex Phellodendri	485			

Pin Yin (Chinese) Herb Name	Pharmaceutical Herb Name	Page No.	Pin Yin (Chinese) Herb Name	Pharmaceutical Herb Name	Page No.
Jin Guo Lan 金果攬	*Radix Tinosporae*	523	Kun Bu 昆布	*Thallus Algae*	724
Jin Qian Cao 金錢草	*Herba Desmodii Styracifolii*	598	La Mei Hua 臘梅花	*Flos Chimonanthi*	680
Jin Sha Teng	*Herba Lygodii Japonici*	522	Lai Fu Zi 萊菔子	*Semen Raphani Sativi*	639
Jin Yin Hua 金銀花	*Flos Lonicerae Japonicae*	524	Lao Gong Xu	*Radix Fici Aerius*	570
Jin Yin Hua Teng	*Caulis/Folium Lonicerae*	531	Lao Guan Cao 老鸛草	*Herba Erodii Seu Geranii*	565
Jin Ying Zi 金櫻子	*Fructus Rosae Laevigatae*	823	Lei Wan 雷丸	*Fructificato Omphalia/Polypori Mylittae*	647
Jing Da Ji 京大戟	*Radix Euphorbiae Pekinensis*	552	Li Lu 黎蘆	*Rhizoma Et Radix Veratri Nigri*	834
Jing Jie 荊芥	*Flos Schizonepetae Tenuifoliae*	447	Li Zhi He 荔枝核	*Semen Litchi Chinensis*	626
Jing Mi 粳米	*Semen Oryzae*	767	Lian Fang 連房	*Receptaculum Nelumbinis Nuciferae*	659
Jiu Bai	*Bulbus Allii*	634			
Jiu Bi Ying 救必應	*Cortex Olocus Rotundae*	625	Lian Jiao	*Fructus Forsythiae Suspensae*	525
Jiu Cai Zi 菲菜子	*Semen Allii Tuberosi*	782	Lian Qiao 連翹	*Fructus Forsythiae Suspensae*	525
Jiu Jie Chang Pu 九節菖蒲	*Rhizoma Anemoni Altaicae*	754	Lian Xin	*Plumula Nelumbinis Nuciferae*	472
Jiu Li Ming	*Herba Senecionis*	474	Lian Xu 蓮須	*Nelumbinis Stamen*	823
Jiu Zi	*Semen Allii Tuberosi*	782			
Ju He 橘核	*Semen Citri Reticulatae*	626	Lian Zi 蓮子	*Semen Nelumbinis Nuciferae*	824
Ju Hong 橘紅	*Exocarpium Citri Grandis*	626	Lian Zi Xin 蓮子心	*Plumula Nelumbinis Nuciferae*	472
Ju Hua 菊花	*Flos Chrysanthemi Morifolii*	463	Liao Diao Zhu 了刁竹	*Herba Pycnostelmae*	565
Ju Pi	*Pericarpium Citri Reticulatae*	621	Ling Ling Xiang 零陵香	*Herba Lysimachiae*	850
Juan Bai Ye	*Herba Selaginellae*	679	Ling Xiao Hua 凌霄花	*Flos Campsis*	680
Juan Bo 卷柏	*Herba Selaginellae*	679	Ling Yang Jiao 羚羊角	*Cornu Antelopis*	747
Jue Ming Zi 決明子	*Semen Cassiae Torae*	471	Ling Zhi	*Ganoderma*	731
Ku Ding Cha 苦丁茶	*Folium Ilicis Latifoliae*	809	Ling Zhi Cao 靈芝草	*Ganoderma*	731
Ku Lian Gen Pi 苦楝根皮	*Cortex Meliae Radicis*	646	Liu Huang 硫黃	*Sulphur*	840
Ku Shen 苦參	*Radix Sophorae Flavescentis*	491	Liu Ji Nu 劉寄奴	*Herba Artemisiae Anomalae/Siphonostegia*	681
Ku Xing Ren	*Semen Pruni Armeniacae*	705	Liu Qu	*Massa Fermentata*	642
Kuan Dong Hua 款冬花	*Flos Tussilagi Farfarae*	700	Long Chi 龍齒	*Fossilia Dentis Mastodi/Dens Draconis*	737
Kuan Jin Teng 寬筋藤	*Ramus Tinosporae Sinensis*	564			

Pin Yin (Chinese) Herb Name	Pharmaceutical Herb Name	Page No.	Pin Yin (Chinese) Herb Name	Pharmaceutical Herb Name	Page No.
Long Dan Cao 龍膽草	Radix Gentianae Scabrae	492	Ma Chi Xian 馬齒莧	Herba Portulacae Oleraceae	528
Long Gu 龍骨	Os Draconis	738	Ma Dou Ling 馬兜鈴	Fructus Aristolochiae	701
Long Kui 龍葵	Herba Solani	526	Ma Huang 麻黃	Herba Ephedrae	448
Long Nao	Borneol	753	Ma Huang Gen 麻黃根	Radix Ephedrae	825
Long Yan Rou 龍眼肉	Arillus Euphoriae Longanae	800	Ma Qian Zi 馬錢子	Semen Strychnotis	842
Lou Lu 漏蘆	Radix Rhapontici Seu Echinops	527	Ma Zi Ren	Semen Cannabis Sativae	548
Lu Dou 綠豆	Semen Phaseoli Radiati	508	Mai Dong	Tuber Ophiopogonis Japonici	810
Lu Fan	Melanteritum	848	Mai Men Dong 麥門冬	Tuber Ophiopogonis Japonici	810
Lu Feng Fang 露蜂房	Nidus Vespae	841	Mai Ya 麥芽	Fructus Hordei Vulgaris Geminantus	640
Lu Gan Shi 爐甘石	Smithsonitum/Calamina	842	Man Jing Zi 蔓荊子	Fructus Viticis	464
Lu Gen 蘆根	Rhizoma Phragmitis Communis	472	Man Shan Hong 滿山紅	Folium Rhododendori Daurici	851
Lu Han Cao	Herba Pyrolae	566	Mang Xiao 芒硝	Mirabilitum	545
Lu Hui 蘆薈	Herba Aloes	544	Mao Dong Qing 毛冬青	Radix Ilicis Pubescentis	682
Lu Jiao 鹿角	Cervi Cornu	783	Mao Hua	Flos Imperatae Cylindriae	653
Lu Jiao Jiao 鹿角膠	Cervi Colla Cornus	783	Mei Gui Hua 玫瑰花	Flos Rosae Rugosae	627
Lu Jiao Shuang 陸角霜	Cornu Cervi Deglatinatum	784	Mi Meng Hua 密蒙花	Flos Buddleiae Officinalis	474
Lu Jing 蘆莖/葦莖	Ramulus Phragmitis	473	Mi Tuo Seng 密陀僧	Lithargyrum	843
Lu Lu Tong 路路通	Fructus Liquidambaris Taiwanianae	681	Mian Hua Gen 棉花根	Radix Gossypii	851
Lu Rong 鹿茸	Cornu Cervi Parvum	784	Mian Yin Chen	Herba Artemesiae Capillaris	603
Lu Ti Cao	Herba Pyrolae	566	Ming Dang Shen 明黨參	Radix Changii	702
Lu Xian Cao 鹿銜草	Herba Pyrolae	566	Ming Fan	Alum	836
Luan Fa Shuang	Crinis Carbonisatus	666	Mo Han Lian	Herba Ecliptae Prostratae	806
Luo Bu Ma 羅布麻	Folium Apocyni Veneti	748	Mo Li Hua	Flos Jasmini Officinalis	631
Luo Han Guo 羅漢果	Fructus Momordicae Grosvenori	810	Mo Yao 沒藥	Myrrha	683
Luo Le 羅勒	Herba Ocimi	583	Moxa	Folium Artemisiae Vulgaris/Argyi	651
Luo Shi Teng 絡石藤	Caulis Trachelospermi Jasminoidis	566	Mu Bie Zi 木鱉子	Semen Momordicae Cochinchinensis	844
Ma Bian Cao 馬鞭草	Herba Verbenae	682			
Ma Bo 馬勃	Frucificatio Lasiosphaerae	528			

Pin Yin (Chinese) Herb Name	Pharmaceutical Herb Name	Page No.	Pin Yin (Chinese) Herb Name	Pharmaceutical Herb Name	Page No.
Mu Dan Pi 牡丹皮	Cortex Moutan Radicis	499	Pi Pa Ye 枇杷葉	Folium Eriobotryae Japonicae	703
Mu Gua 木瓜	Fructus Chaenomelis Lagenariae	567	Pu Gong Ying 蒲公英	Herba Taraxaci Mongolici Cum Radice	529
Mu Hu Die 木蝴蝶	Semen Oroxyli Indici	702	Pu Huang 蒲黄	Pollen Typhae	660
Mu Li 牡蠣	Concha Ostreae	739	Qi Ye Lian 七葉蓮	Radix/Caulis/Folium Schefflera	568
Mu Mian Hua 木棉花	Flos Gossampini	529	Qi Ye Yi Zhi Hua	Rhizoma Paris	540
Mu Tong 木通	Caulis Akebiae/Mutong	599	Qian Cao Gen 茜草根	Radix Rubiae Cordifoliae	662
Mu Xiang 木香	Radix Saussureae Seu Vladimiriae	628	Qian Cheng Zi	Semen Oroxyli Indici	702
Mu Zei 木賊	Herba Equiseti Hiemalis	464	Qian Dan 鉛丹	Minium	845
Nan Gua Zi 南瓜子	Semen Cucurbitae Moschatae	648	Qian Hu 前胡	Radix Peucedani	725
Nan Sha Shen 南沙參	Radix Adenophorae Tetraphylla	811	Qian Li Guang 千里光	Herba Senecionis	474
Nao Yang Hua 鬧羊花	Folium Rhododendri Molles	740	Qian Nian Jian 千年健	Rhizoma Homalomenae Occultae	568
Nian Shen Cao	Herba Bidentis Bipinnatae	462	Qian Niu Zi 牽牛子	Semen Pharbitidis	553
Ning Ma Gen	Radix Boehmeriae	607	Qian Ren	Semen Euryales Ferox	826
Niu Bang Zi 牛蒡子	Fructus Arctii Lappae	465	Qian Shi 芡實	Semen Euryales Ferox	826
Niu Huang 牛黄	Calculus Bovis	755	Qiang Huo 羌活	Radix Notopterygii	449
Niu Xi 牛膝	Radix Achyranthis Bidentatae	684	Qin Jiao 秦艽	Radix Gentianae Macrophyllae	569
Nu Zhen Zi 女貞子	Fructus Ligustri Lucidi	812	Qin Pi 秦皮	Cortex Fraxini	493
Nuo Dao Gen 糯稻根	Radix/Rhizoma Oryzae Glutinosae	825	Qing Dai 青黛	Indigo Pulverata Levis	531
Nuo Dao Gen Xu	Radix/Rhizoma Oryzae Glutinosae	825	Qing Fen 輕粉	Calomelas	845
Nuo Mi Gen	Radix/Rhizoma Oryzae Glutinosae	825	Qing Hao 青蒿	Herba Artemisiae Apiaceae	508
Ou Jie 藕節	Rhizoma Nelumbinis Nuciferae Rhizomatis	660	Qing Mu Xiang 青木香	Radix Aristolochiae	628
			Qing Pi 青皮	Pericarpium Citri Reticulatae Viride	629
Pang Da Hai 胖大海	Semen Sterculiae Scaphigerae	724	Qing Xiang Zi 青葙子	Semen Celosiae Argenteae	475
Pei Lan 佩蘭	Herba Eupatorii Fortunei	583	Qiu Yin	Lumbricus	744
Peng E Zhu	Rhizoma Curcumae Zedoariae	673	Qu Mai 瞿麥	Herba Dianthi	600
Peng Sha 硼砂	Borax	844	Quan Shen	Rhizoma Polygoni Bistortae	517
			Quan Xie 全蠍	Buthus Martensi	749

Pin Yin (Chinese) Herb Name	Pharmaceutical Herb Name	Page No.	Pin Yin (Chinese) Herb Name	Pharmaceutical Herb Name	Page No.
Ren Dong Teng 忍冬藤	Caulis/Folium Lonicerae	531	Shan Zhi Zi 山梔子	Fructus Gardeniae Jasminoidis	476
Ren Shen 人參	Radix Chinese Ginseng	767	Shan Zhu Yu 山茱萸	Fructus Corni Officinalis	827
Ren Shen Lu 人參蘆	Cervix Ginseng	835	Shan Zi Cao 扇子草:扇子草	Herba Capsellae	664
Ren Shen Ye 人參葉	Ginseng Folium Cum Caule	769	Shang Lu 商陸	Radix Phytolaccae	554
Rong Shu Xu 榕樹鬚	Radix Fici Aerius	570	She Chuang Zi 蛇床子	Semen Cnidii Monnieri	847
Rou Cong Rong 肉蓯蓉	Herba Cistanches	786	She Gan 射干	Rhizoma Belamcandae Chinensis	533
Rou Dou Kou 肉豆蔻	Semen Myristicae Fragranticis	826	She Shen	Radix Aristolochiae	628
Rou Gui 肉桂	Cortex Cinnamomi Cassiae	616	She Tui 蛇蛻	Periostracum Serpentis	571
Rou Gui Pi 肉桂皮	Cortex Cinnamoni	617	She Xiang 麝香	Secretio Moschus Moschiferi	756
Ru Xiang 乳香	Gummi Olibanum	685	Shen Jin Cao 伸筋草	Herba Lycopodii	571
San Leng 三稜	Rhizoma Sparganii	686	Shen Qu 神曲	Massa Fermentata	642
San Qi 三七	Radix Pseudoginseng	663	Sheng Di	Radix Rehmanniae Glutinosae	500
San Qi Hua 三七花	Flos Pseudoginseng	663	Sheng Di Huang 生地黃	Radix Rehmanniae Glutinosae	500
Sang Bai Pi 桑白皮	Cortex Mori Albae Radicis	703	Sheng Gan Cao	Radix Glycyrrhizae Uralensis	763
Sang Ji Sheng 桑寄生	Ramulus Loranthi Seu Visci	813	Sheng Jiang 生姜	Rhizoma Zingiberis Officinalis Recens	450
Sang Piao Xiao 桑螵蛸	Ootheca Mantidis	827	Sheng Jiang Pi 生姜皮	Cortex Zingiberis Officinalis Recens	600
Sang Ren	Fructus Mori Albae	801	Sheng Ma 升麻	Rhizoma Cimicifugae	467
Sang Shen Zi 桑椹子	Fructus Mori Albae	801	Shi Bing 柿餅	Fructus Diospyros	630
Sang Ye 桑葉	Folium Mori Albae	466	Shi Chang Pu 石菖蒲	Rhizoma Acori Graminei	757
Sang Zhi 桑枝	Ramulus Mori Albae	570	Shi Di 柿蒂	Calyx Diospyros Kaki	630
Sha Ren 砂仁	Fructus/Semen Amomi	584	Shi Gao 石膏	Gypsum	477
Sha Yuan Zi 沙苑子	Semen Astragali Complanati	786	Shi Hu 石斛	Herba Dendrobii	813
Shan Ci Gu 山慈菇	Bulbus Santsigu	846	Shi Hu Sui	Herba Centipedae	711
Shan Dou Gen 山豆根	Radix Sophorae Subprostratae	532	Shi Jue Ming 石決明	Concha Haliotidis	750
Shan Yao 山藥	Radix Dioscoreae Oppositae	769	Shi Jun Zi 使君子	Fructus Quisqualis Indicae	648
Shan Yu Rou	Fructus Corni Officinalis	827	Shi Liu Gen Pi 石榴根皮	Radix Granati	649
Shan Zha 山楂	Fructus Crataegi	641			

Pin Yin (Chinese) Herb Name	Pharmaceutical Herb Name	Page No.	Pin Yin (Chinese) Herb Name	Pharmaceutical Herb Name	Page No.
Shi Liu Pi 石榴皮......	Pericarpium Granati	828	Suo Sha........	Fructus/Semen Amomi	584
Shi Shang Bai 石上柏......	Herba Selaginellae Doederleinii	534	Suo Yang 鎖陽........	Herba/Caulis Cynomorri Songarici	787
Shi Wei 石葦........	Folium Pyrrosiae	601	Tai Wau	Radix Linderae Strychnifoliae	632
Shou Wu	Radix Polygoni Multiflori	799	Tai Yi	Placenta Hominis	792
Shou Wu Teng ..	Caulis Polygoni Multiflori	733	Tai Yi Yu Liang ..	Limonitum	833
Shu Di	Radix Rehmanniae Glutinosae Conquitae	802	Tai Zi Shen 太子參......	Radix Pseudostellariae Heterophyllae	770
Shu Di Huang 熟地黃......	Radix Rehmanniae Glutinosae Conquitae	802	Tan Xiang 檀香........	Lignum Santali Albi	632
Shu Fu 鼠婦........	Armadillidium	687	Tao Ren 桃仁........	Semen Persicae	689
Shu Qi 蜀漆........	Folium /Plantula Dichorae Febrifugae	534	Tian Hua Fen 天花粉......	Radix Trichosanthis	726
Shu Yang Quan 蜀羊泉/白毛藤............	Herba Solani Lyrati	535	Tian Ji Huang 田基黃......	Herba Hyperici	536
Shui Niu Jiao 水牛角......	Cornu Bubali	501	Tian Ma 天麻........	Rhizoma Gastrodiae Elatae	750
Shui Xian Gen 水仙根......	Bulbus Narcissi	535	Tian Men Dong 天門冬......	Tuber Asparagi Cochinchinensis	814
Shui Zhi 水蛭........	Hirudo Seu Whitmaniae	687	Tian Nan Xing 天南星......	Rhizoma Arisaematis	712
Si Gua Luo 絲瓜蔞......	Fasciculus Vascularis Luffae	688	Tian Qi	Radix Pseudoginseng	663
Song Jie 松節........	Lignum Pini Nodi	572	Tian Xian Teng 天仙滕......	Caulis Aristolochiae	704
Song Xiang 松香........	Resina Pini/Colorhonium	847	Tian Xian Zi 天仙子......	Semen Hyoscyami	705
Song Zi 松子仁......	Fructus Pini Tabulaeformis	546	Tian Zhu Huang 天竹黃......	Concretio Silicea Bambusae	726
Su Geng 蘇梗........	Caulis Perillae Acutae	451	Ting Li Zi 葶藶子......	Semen Lepidii	555
Su He Xiang 蘇合香......	Styrax Liquidis	758	Tong Cao 通草........	Medulla Tetrapanacis Papyriferi	601
Su Mu 蘇木........	Lignum Sappan	688	Tong Ji Li	Semen Astragali Complanati	786
Su Xin Hua 素馨花......	Flos Jasmini Officinalis	631	Tsao Wu	Radix Aconiti Kusnezoffii	609
Su Ye	Folium Perillae Frutescentis	454	Tu Bie Chong 土鱉蟲......	Eupolyphagae Seu Opisthoplatiae	690
Suan Jiang 酸漿........	Rhizoma Et Radix Physalitis	852	Tu Fu Ling 土茯苓......	Rhizoma Smilacis Glabrae	536
Suan Zao Ren 酸棗仁......	Semen Ziziphi Spinosae	732	Tu Niu Xi 土牛膝......	Radix Achyranthis	537
Suo Luo Zi 娑羅子......	Fructus Aesculi	631	Tu Si Zi 菟絲子......	Semen Cuscutae	787
			Tu Xiang Ju.....	Herba Origani/Artemisia	602

Pin Yin (Chinese) Herb Name	Pharmaceutical Herb Name	Page No.	Pin Yin (Chinese) Herb Name	Pharmaceutical Herb Name	Page No.
Tu Yin Chen 土茵陳	Herba Origani/Artemisia	602	Xi Jiao 犀角	Cornu Rhinoceri	502
Wa Leng Zi 瓦楞子	Concha Arcae	690	Xi Xian Cao 稀薟草	Herba Siegesbeckiae Orientalis	575
Wang Bu Liu Xing 王不留行	Semen Vaccariae Segetalis	691	Xi Xin 細辛	Herba Asari Cum Radice	452
Wei Jing	Ramulus Phragmitis	473	Xi Yang Shen	Radix Panacis Quinquefolii	808
Wei Ling Xian 威靈仙	Radix Clemetidis Chinensis	572	Xia Ku Cao 夏枯草	Spica Prunellae Vulgaris	478
Wo Niu 蝸牛	Eulotae	537	Xian Feng Cao . . .	Herba Bidentis Bipinnatae	462
Wu Bei Zi 五蓓子	Galla Chinensis	829	Xian He Cao 仙鶴草	Herba Agrimoniae Pilosae	665
Wu Cao	Cormus Heleochris Plantaginea	717	Xian Ling Pi	Herba Epimedii	791
Wu Gong 蜈蚣	Scolopendra Subspinipes	751	Xian Mao 仙茅	Rhizoma Curculiginis Orchioidis	788
Wu Huan Zi 無患子	Semen Sapindi	538	Xiang Fu 香附	Rhizoma Cyperi Rotundi	633
Wu Jia Pi 五加皮	Cortex Acanthopanacis Radicis	574	Xiang Fu Zi	Rhizoma Cyperi Rotundi	633
Wu Jia Shen 五加參	Radix Acanthopanax Senticosus/Eleutheroc occus	771	Xiang Ru 香薷	Herba Elsholtziae Splendentis	453
Wu Jiu Gen Pi 烏桕根皮:乌桕根皮	Cortex Radicis Sapii	555	Xiao Hu Ma	Fructus Leonuri	669
			Xiao Hui Xiang 小茴香	Fructus Foeniculi Vulgaris	619
Wu Ling Zhi 五靈脂	Excrementum Trogopterori Seu Pteromi	691	Xiao Ji 小薊	Herba Cirsii Segeti	666
Wu Mei 烏梅	Fructus Pruni Mume	830	Xie Bai 薤白	Bulbus Allii	634
Wu Shao She 烏梢蛇	Zaocys Dhumnades	574	Xin Yi Hua 辛夷花	Flos Magnoliae Liliflorae	453
Wu Tou	Radix Aconitii	611	Xing Ren 杏仁	Semen Pruni Armeniacae	705
Wu Wei Zi 五味子	Fructus Schisandrae Chinensis	831	Xiong Dan 熊膽	Fel Ursi	479
Wu Yao 烏藥	Radix Linderae Strychnifoliae	632	Xiong Huang 雄黃	Realgar	848
Wu Yi 蕪夷	Pasta Ulmi Macrocarpi	649	Xu Chang Qing . . .	Herba Pycnostelmae	565
			Xu Duan 續斷	Radix Dipsaci	789
Wu Zei Gu	Os Sepiae Seu Sepiellae	821	Xu Sui Zi 續隨子	Semen Euphorbia Lathyridis	556
Wu Zhu Yu 吳茱萸	Fructus Evodiae Rutaecarpae	618	Xuan Fu Hua 旋復花	Flos Inulae	713
Xi Gua 西瓜	Fructus Citrullus Vulgaris	509	Xuan Shen 玄參	Radix Scrophulariae Ningpoensis	503
Xi He Liu 西河柳	Cacumen Tamaricis	451	Xue Jie 血竭	Sanguis Draconis	692
Xi Jian Cao	Herba Siegesbeckiae Orientalis	575	Xue Yu Tan 血余炭	Crinis Carbonisatus	666

Pin Yin (Chinese) Herb Name	Pharmaceutical Herb Name	Page No.	Pin Yin (Chinese) Herb Name	Pharmaceutical Herb Name	Page No.
Xun Gu Feng 尋骨風......	Herba Aristolochiae	576	Yu Yu Liang 禹余糧......	Limonitum	833
Ya Dan Zi 鴉膽子......	Fructus Brucae Javanicae	538	Yu Zhu 玉竹........	Rhizoma Polygonati Odorati	815
Yan Hu Suo 延胡索......	Rhizoma Corydalis Yanhusuo	693	Yuan Hua 芫花........	Flos Daphnes Genkwa	556
Yang Jin Hua 洋金花......	Flos Daturae Albae	714	Yuan Sui Zi.....	Herba /Fructus Coriandri	446
Yang Qi Shi 陽起石......	Actinolitum	789	Yuan Zhi 遠志........	Radix Polygalae Tenuifoliae	734
Ye Jiao Teng 夜交滕/首烏 藤...........	Caulis Polygoni Multiflori	733	Yue Ji Hua 月季花......	Fructus Rosae Chinensis	696
Ye Ju Hua 野菊花......	Flos Chrysanthemi Indici	468	Yue Yue Hong...	Fructus Rosae Chinensis	696
Ye Ming Sha 夜明砂......	Excrementum Vespertilii Murini	480	Zang Hong Hua .	Stigma Crocus/Stigma Croci	674
Yi Bi Jian.......	Bulbus Santsigu	846	Zao Fan 皂礬........	Melanteritum	848
Yi Mu Cao 益母草......	Herba Leonuri Heterophylli	694	Zao Jia	Fructus Gleditsiae Sinensis	715
Yi Tang 飴糖........	Saccharum Granorum	772	Zao Jiao 皂角........	Fructus Gleditsiae Sinensis	715
Yi Yi Ren 薏苡仁......	Semen Coicis Lachryma-jobi	602	Zao Jiao Ci 皂角刺......	Spina Gleditsiae Sinensis	716
Yi Zhi Ren 益智仁......	Fructus Alpiniae Oxyphyllae	790	Zao Xin Tu.....	Terra Flava Usta	657
Yin Chai Hu 銀柴胡......	Radix Stellariae Dichotomae	504	Zao Xiu 蚤休........	Rhizoma Paris	540
Yin Chen 茵陳........	Herba Artemesiae Capillaris	603	Ze Lan 澤蘭........	Herba Lycopi Lucidi	696
Yin Chen Hao ...	Herba Artemesiae Capillaris	603	Ze Qi 澤漆........	Herba Euphorbiae Helioscopiae	727
Yin Guo	Semen Ginkgo Bilobae	818	Ze Qi Ma.......	Folium Apocyni Veneti	748
Yin Xing	Semen Ginkgo Bilobae	818	Ze Xie 澤瀉........	Rhizoma Alismatis	605
Yin Xing Ye.....	Folium Ginko	817	Zhang Nao 樟腦........	Camphora	849
Yin Yang Huo 淫羊霍......	Herba Epimedii	791	Zhe Bei Mu 浙貝母......	Bulbus Fritillariae Thunbergii	728
Ying Su Ke 罌粟殼......	Pericarpium Papaveris Somniferi	832	Zhe Chong	Eupolyphagae Seu Opisthoplatiae	690
Ying Su Qiao ...	Pericarpium Papaveris Somniferi	832	Zhe Shi	Haematitum	735
You Song Jie....	Lignum Pini Nodi	572	Zhen Zhu 珍珠........	Margarita Usta	740
Yu Jin 鬱金........	Tuber Curcumae	695	Zhen Zhu Mu 珍珠母......	Concha Mararitaferae	741
Yu Li Ren 鬱李仁......	Semen Pruni	549	Zhi Gan Cao 炙甘草......	Radix Glycyrrhizae Uralensis Prep.	772
Yu Liang Shi....	Limonitum	833	Zhi Ke 枳殼........	Fructus Aurantii	635
Yu Mi Xu 玉米須......	Stylus Zeae Mays	605	Zhi Ma	Semen Sesami Indici	808
Yu Xing Cao 魚腥草......	Herba Houttuyniae Cordatae	539			

Pin Yin (Chinese) Herb Name	Pharmaceutical Herb Name	Page No.
Zhi Mu 知母	*Radix Anemarrhenae Asphodeloidis*	480
Zhi Qiao	*Fructus Aurantii*	635
Zhi Shi 枳實	*Fructus Aurantii Immaturus*	635
Zhi Xue Cao 積雪草	*Herba Centellae*	697
Zhi Zi	*Fructus Gardeniae Jasminoidis*	476
Zhong Lou	*Rhizoma Polygoni Bistortae*	517
Zhong Lu Tan	*Vagina Trachycarpi Carbonista*	655
Zhu Li 竹瀝	*Succus Bambusae*	728
Zhu Ling 豬苓	*Sclerotium Polypori Umbellati/Grifola*	606
Zhu Ma Gen 苧麻根	*Radix Boehmeriae*	607
Zhu Pi	*Pericarpium Citri Reticulatae*	621
Zhu Ru 竹茹	*Caulis Bambusae In Taeniis*	729
Zhu Sha 朱砂	*Cinnabaris*	741
Zhu Ye 竹葉	*Folium Bambusae*	482
Zhuan Lian Zi	*Fructus Meliae Toosendan*	623
Zhung Shuei Shi	*Stalactitum*	777
Zi Cao 紫草	*Radix Lithospermi Seu Arnebiae*	504
Zi He Che 紫河車	*Placenta Hominis*	792
Zi Hua Di Ding 紫花地丁	*Herba Violae Cum Radice*	541
Zi Ran Tong 自然銅	*Pyritum*	698
Zi Shi Ying 紫石英	*Fluoritum*	742
Zi Su Geng	*Caulis Perillae Acutae*	451
Zi Su Ye 紫蘇葉	*Folium Perillae Frutescentis*	454
Zi Su Zi 紫蘇子	*Fructus Perillae Frutescentis*	706
Zi Wan 紫菀	*Radix Asteris Tatarici*	706
Zi Zhu	*Folium Callicarpae*	667
Zi Zhu Cao 紫珠草	*Folium Callicarpae*	667

Pharmaceutical Herb Name	Pin Yin (Chinese) Herb Name	Page No.	Pharmaceutical Herb Name	Pin Yin (Chinese) Herb Name	Page No.
Abri, Herba	Ji Gu Cao 雞骨草	564	Albizziae, Flos	He Huan Hua 合歡花	730
Abutiloni, Semen	Dong Kui Zi 赤石脂	594	Albizziae Julibrissin, Cortex	He Huan Pi 合歡皮	731
Acacia	Er Cha/Hai Er Cha/A Xian Yao 兒茶	839	Album	Chi Shi Zhi/Bai Shi Zhi 赤石脂	818
Acanthopanacis Radicis, Cortex	Wu Jia Pi 五加皮	574	Algae, Thallus	Kun Bu 昆布	724
Acanthopanax Senticosus, Radix	Wu Jia Shen/Ci Wu Jia 五加參	771	Alismatis, Rhizoma	Ze Xie 澤瀉	605
Achyranthis, Radix	Tu Niu Xi 土牛膝	537	Alli Sativi, Sublus	Da Suan 大蒜	644
Achyranthis Bidentatae, Radix	Niu Xi/Huai Niu Xi 牛膝	684	Allii, Bulbus	Xie Bai/Jiu Bai/Hai Bai 薤白	634
Aconiti Carmichaeli Praeparata, Radix	Fu Zi 附子	613	Allii Fistulosi, Herba	Cong Bai 蔥白	442
Aconiti Coreani, Rhizoma	Bai Fu Zi/Guan Bai Fu 白附子	708	Allii Tuberosi, Semen	Jiu Cai Zi/Jiu Zi 菲菜子	782
Aconiti Kusnezoffii, Radix	Cao Wu/Tsao Wu 草烏	609	Aloes, Herba	Lu Hui 蘆薈	544
Aconitii, Radix	Chuan Wu/Wu Tou 川烏	611	Alpiniae Katsumadai, Semen	Cao Dou Kou/Dou Kou 草豆蔻	579
Acori Graminei, Rhizoma	Shi Chang Pu/Chang Pu 石菖蒲	757	Alpiniae Officinari, Rhizoma	Gao Liang Jiang 高良姜	615
Acronychiae, Lignum	Jiang Xiang/Jiang Zhen Xian 降香	659	Alpiniae Oxyphyllae, Fructus	Yi Zhi Ren 益智仁	790
Actinolitum	Yang Qi Shi 陽起石	789	Alum	Bai Fan/Ming Fan 白礬	836
Adenophorae Tetraphylla, Radix	Nan Sha Shen 南沙參	811	Amomi, Fructus/Semen	Sha Ren/Suo Sha 砂仁	584
Aesculi, Fructus	Suo Luo Zi 娑羅子	631	Amomi Cardamomi, Fructus	Bai Dou Kou/Dou Kou 白豆蔻	577
Agastaches, Herba	Huo Xiang 紅大薊	582	Amomi Tsao-ko, Fructus	Cao Guo 草果	580
Agkistrodon	Bai Hua She 白附子	558	Ampelopsis, Radix	Bai Lian 白蘞	513
Agrimoniae Pilosae, Herba	Xian He Cao 仙鶴草	665	Amydae Sinensis, Carapax	Bie Jia 鱉甲	805
Ailanthi, Cortex	Chun Pi/Chun Bai Pi 椿皮	483	Andrographis Paniculatae, Herba	Chuan Xin Lian 穿心蓮	518
Akebiae, Caulis	Mu Tong 木通	599	Anemarrhenae Asphodeloidis, Radix	Zhi Mu 知母	480
Alba, Radix	Bai Shao/Bai Shao Yao 白芍	794	Anemoni Altaicae, Rhizoma	Jiu Jie Chang Pu 九節菖蒲	754

Pharmaceutical Herb Name	Pin Yin (Chinese) Herb Name	Page No.	Pharmaceutical Herb Name	Pin Yin (Chinese) Herb Name	Page No.
Angelicae, Radix	*Bai Zhi* 白芷	441	Artemisiae Apiaceae, Herba	*Qing Hao* 青蒿	508
Angelicae Sinensis, Radix	*Dang Gui* 當歸	795	Artemisiae Vulgaris, Folium	*Ai Ye/Moxa* 艾葉	651
Antelopis, Cornu	*Ling Yang Jiao* 羚羊角	747	Asafoetida	*A Wei/E Wei* 阿魏	637
Apocyni Veneti, Folium	*Luo Bu Ma/Ze Qi Ma* 羅布麻	748	Asari Cum Radice, Herba	*Xi Xin* 細辛	452
Aquilariae, Lignum	*Chen Xiang* 沉香	622	Asini, Gelatinum	*E Jiao/A Jiao* 阿膠	797
Arcae, Concha	*Wa Leng Zi* 瓦楞子	690	Asparagi Cochinchinensis, Tuber	*Tian Men Dong* 天門冬	814
Arctii Lappae, Fructus	*Niu Bang Zi* 牛蒡子	465	Asteris Tatarici, Radix	*Zi Wan/Ci Wan* 紫菀	706
Arecae Catechu, Pericarpium	*Da Fu Pi* 大腹皮	624	Astragali, Radix	*Huang Qi* 黃芪:黃芪	765
Arecae Catechu, Semen	*Bing Lang/Bing Lang Zi* 檳榔	643	Astragali Complanati, Semen	*Sha Yuan Zi/Tong Ji Li* 沙苑子	786
Argyi, Folium	*Ai Ye/Moxa* 艾葉	651	Atractylodis, Rhizoma	*Cang Zhu* 蒼術	578
Arisaemai Cum Felle Bovis, Pulvis	*Dan Nan Xing* 膽南星	718	Atractylodis Macrocephalae, Rhizoma	*Bai Zhu* 白術	760
Arisaematis, Rhizoma	*Tian Nan Xing* 天南星	712	Aurantii, Fructus	*Zhi Ke/Zhi Qiao* 枳殼	635
Aristolochiae, Herba	*Xun Gu Feng* 尋骨風	576	Aurantii Immaturus, Fructus	*Zhi Shi* 枳實	635
Aristolochiae, Radix	*Qing Mu Xiang/She Shen* 青木香	628	Bambusae, Succus	*Zhu Li* 竹瀝	728
Aristolochiae, Radix	*Guang Fang Ji* 貫眾	595	Bambusae, Folium	*Zhu Ye* 竹葉	482
Aristolochiae, Caulis	*Tian Xian Teng* 天仙滕	704	Bambusae In Taeniis, Caulis	*Zhu Ru* 竹茹	729
Aristolochiae, Fructus	*Ma Dou Ling* 馬兜鈴	701	Baphicacanthi, Radix	*Ban Lan Gen* 白芍	515
Armadillidium	*Shu Fu* 鼠婦	687	Belamcandae Chinensis, Rhizoma	*She Gan* 射干	533
Arnebiae, Radix	*Zi Cao* 豬苓	504	Benincasae, Exocarpium	*Dong Gua Pi* 冬瓜皮	593
Artemesiae Capillaris, Herba	*Yin Chen/Mian Yin Chen/Yin Chen Hao* 茵陳	603	Benincasae Hispidae, Semen	*Dong Gua Ren/Dong Gua Zi* 冬瓜仁	593
Artemisia, Herba	*Tu Yin Chen/Bei Yin Chen/Tu Xiang Ju* 土茵陳	602	Benzoinum	*An Xi Xiang* 安息香	753
Artemisiae Anomalae, Herba	*Liu Ji Nu* 劉寄奴	681	Bidentis Bipinnatae, Herba	*Gui Zhen Cao/Xian Feng Cao/Nian Shen Cao* 鬼針草	462

Pharmaceutical Herb Name	Pin Yin (Chinese) Herb Name	Page No.	Pharmaceutical Herb Name	Pin Yin (Chinese) Herb Name	Page No.
Biotae Orientalis, Semen	Bai Zi Ren 柏子仁	730	Camphora	Zhang Nao 樟腦	849
Biotae Orientalis, Cacumen	Ce Bai Ye/Ce Bo Ye 側柏葉	654	Campsis, Flos	Ling Xiao Hua 凌霄花	680
Blechni, Rhizoma	Guan Zhong/Guan Chong 貫衆	521	Canarii, Fructus	Gan Lan 橄欖	484
Bletillae Striatae, Rhizoma	Bai Ji 白芨	652	Cannabis Sativae, Semen	Huo Ma Ren/Ma Zi Ren 火麻仁	548
Boehmeriae, Radix	Zhu Ma Gen/Ning Ma Gen 苧麻根	607	Capsellae, Herba	Shan Zi Cao/Ji Cai 扇子草:扇子草	664
Bombycis Mori, Excrementum	Can Sha 蠶砂	558	Carpesii Abrotanoidis, Fructus	He Shi 鶴虱	646
Bombyx Batryticatus	Jiang Can/Bai Jiang Can 僵蠶	746	Carthami Tinctorii, Flos	Hong Hua 紅花	675
Borax	Peng Sha 硼砂	844	Caryophylli, Flos	Ding Xiang 丁香	612
Borneol	Bing Pian/Long Nao 冰片	753	Cassiae Torae, Semen	Jue Ming Zi/Cao Jue Ming 決明子	471
Bovis, Calculus	Niu Huang 牛黃	755	Celosiae Argenteae, Semen	Qing Xiang Zi 青葙子	475
Brucae Javanicae, Fructus	Ya Dan Zi 鴉膽子	538	Celosiae Cristatae, Flos	Ji Guan Hua 雞冠花	822
Bubali, Cornu	Shui Niu Jiao 水牛角	501	Centellae, Herba	Zhi Xue Cao/Ji Xue Cao 積雪草	697
Buchnerae, Ramulus/Herba	Guei Yu Jian /Gui Jian Yu 鬼羽箭	675	Centipedae, Herba	E Bu Shi Cao/Shi Hu Sui 鵝不食草	711
Buddleiae Officinalis, Flos	Mi Meng Hua 密蒙花	474	Cervi Cornu	Lu Jiao 鹿角	783
Bufonis, Secretio	Chan Su 蟾酥	837	Cervi Parvum, Cornu	Lu Rong 鹿茸	784
Bungarus	Bai Hua She 白附子	558	Chaenomelis Lagenariae, Fructus	Mu Gua 木瓜	567
Bupleuri, Radix	Chai Hu 柴胡	457	Changii, Radix	Ming Dang Shen 明黨參	702
Buthus Martensi	Quan Xie 全蠍	749	Chimonanthi, Flos	La Mei Hua 臘梅花	680
Calamina	Lu Gan Shi 爐甘石	842	Chinensis, Galla	Wu Bei Zi 五蓓子	829
Calcitum	Han Shui Shi 寒水石	471	Chinese Ginseng, Radix	Ren Shen 人參	767
Callicarpae, Folium	Zi Zhu Cao/Zi Zhu 紫珠草	667	Chrysanthemi Indici, Flos	Ye Ju Hua 野菊花	468
Calomelas	Qing Fen 輕粉	845	Chrysanthemi Morifolii, Flos	Ju Hua 菊花	463
Camelliae, Folium	Cha Ye 茶葉	589			

Pharmaceutical Herb Name	Pin Yin (Chinese) Herb Name	Page No.	Pharmaceutical Herb Name	Pin Yin (Chinese) Herb Name	Page No.
Cibotii Barometz, Rhizoma	*Gou Ji* 狗脊	778	Colorhonium, Resina	*Song Xiang* 松香	847
Cicadae, Periostracum	*Chan Tui* 蟬蛻	458	Coptidis, Rhizoma	*Huang Lian* 黃連	486
Cimicifugae, Rhizoma	*Sheng Ma* 升麻	467	Cordyceps Sinensis	*Dong Chong Xia Cao* 冬蟲夏草	775
Cinnabaris	*Zhu Sha* 朱砂	741	Coriandri, Herba /Fructus	*Hu Sui /Yuan Sui Zi* 胡荽	446
Cinnamomi Cassiae, Cortex	*Rou Gui* 肉桂	616	Corneum Gigeraiae Galli, Endothelium	*Ji Nei Jin* 雞內金	638
Cinnamomi Cassiae, Ramulus	*Gui Zhi* 桂枝	445	Corni Officinalis, Fructus	*Shan Zhu Yu/Shan Yu Rou* 山茱萸	827
Cinnamoni, Cortex	*Rou Gui Pi* 肉桂皮	617	Cornu Cervi Deglatinatum	*Lu Jiao Shuang* 陸角霜	784
Cirsii Japonici, Herba	*Da Ji* 大薊	655	Corydalis Yanhusuo, Rhizoma	*Yan Hu Suo* 延胡索	693
Cirsii Segeti, Herba	*Xiao Ji* 小薊	666	Crataegi, Fructus	*Shan Zha* 山楂	641
Cistanches, Herba	*Rou Cong Rong* 肉蓯蓉	786	Crinis Carbonisatus	*Xue Yu Tan/Luan Fa Shuang* 血余炭	666
Citri Grandis, Exocarpium	*Ju Hong* 橘紅	626	Crocus, Stigma	*Fan Hong Hua/Zang Hong Hua* 番紅花	674
Citri Reticulatae, Pericarpium	*Chen Pi/Ju Pi/Zhu Pi* 陳皮	621			
Citri Reticulatae, Semen	*Ju He* 橘核	626	Crotonis, Semen	*Ba Dou* 巴豆	550
Citri Reticulatae Viride, Pericarpium	*Qing Pi* 青皮	629	Cucurbitae Moschatae, Semen	*Nan Gua Zi* 南瓜子	648
Citri Sarcodactylis, Fructus	*Fo Shou/Fo Shou Gan* 佛手	624	Curculiginis Orchioidis, Rhizoma	*Xian Mao* 仙茅	788
Citrullus Vulgaris, Fructus	*Xi Gua* 西瓜	509	Curcumae, Tuber	*Yu Jin* 鬱金	695
Clemetidis Chinensis, Radix	*Wei Ling Xian* 威靈仙	572	Curcumae, Rhizoma	*Jiang Huang* 姜黃	678
Clerondendri, Ramulus Et, Folium	*Chou Wu Tong/Ba Jiao Wu Tong* 臭梧桐	560	Curcumae Zedoariae, Rhizoma	*E Zhu/Peng E Zhu* 莪術	673
Cnidii Monnieri, Semen	*She Chuang Zi* 蛇床子	847	Cuscutae, Semen	*Tu Si Zi* 菟絲子	787
Cocculi, Radix	*Guang Fang Ji* 貫眾	595	Cyathulae, Radix	*Chuan Niu Xi* 川牛膝	669
Codonopsis Pilosulae, Radix	*Dang Shen* 黨參	762	Cyclinae Sinensis, Concha	*Hai Ge Ke/Ge Ke/Ge Qiao* 海蛤殼	721
Coicis Lachrymajobi, Semen	*Yi Yi Ren* 薏苡仁	602	Cynanchi Atrati, Radix	*Bai Wei* 白薇	495
Colla Cornus, Cervi	*Lu Jiao Jiao* 鹿角膠	783	Cynanchii Stautoni, Rhizoma	*Bai Qian* 白前	709

Pharmaceutical Herb Name	Pin Yin (Chinese) Herb Name	Page No.	Pharmaceutical Herb Name	Pin Yin (Chinese) Herb Name	Page No.
Cynomorri Songarici, Herba/Caulis	*Suo Yang* 鎖陽	787	Dolichoris Lablab, Semen	*Bai Bian Dou/Bian Dou* 白扁豆	506
Cyperi Rotundi, Rhizoma	*Xiang Fu/Xiang Fu Zi* 香附	633	Draconis, Os	*Long Gu* 龍骨	738
Dalbergiae Odoriferae, Lignum	*Jiang Xiang/Jiang Zhen Xian* 降香	659	Droserae, Herba	*Jin Di Luo* 錦地羅	523
			Drynaria, Rhizoma	*Gu Sui Bu* 骨碎補	778
Daphnes Genkwa, Flos	*Yuan Hua* 芫花	556	Dryopteridis Crassirhizomae, Rhizoma	*Dong Bei Guan Zhong* 東北貫衆	645
Daqingye, Folium	*Da Qing Ye* 大青葉	519	Duhuo, Radix	*Du Huo* 獨活	561
Daturae Albae, Flos	*Yang Jin Hua* 洋金花	714	Echinops, Radix	*Lou Lu* 龍齒	527
Dauci, Fructus	*He Shi* 鶴虱	646	Ecliptae Prostratae, Herba	*Han Lian Cao/Mo Han Lian* 旱蓮草	806
Dendrobii, Herba	*Shi Hu* 石斛	813	Elephantopi, Herba	*Di Dan Tou* 地膽頭	520
Dens Draconis, Fossilia	*Long Chi* 龍齒	737	Eleutherococcus, Radix	*Wu Jia Shen/Ci Wu Jia* 五加參	771
Dentis Mastodi, Fossilia	*Long Chi* 龍齒	737	Elsholtziae Splendentis, Herba	*Xiang Ru* 香薷	453
Desmodii Styracifolii, Herba	*Jin Qian Cao* 金錢草	598	Ephedrae, Radix	*Ma Huang Gen* 麻黃根	825
Dianthi, Herba	*Qu Mai* 瞿麥	600	Ephedrae, Herba	*Ma Huang* 麻黃	448
Dichorae Febrifugae, Folium /Plantula	*Shu Qi* 蜀漆	534	Epimedii, Herba	*Yin Yang Huo/Xian Ling Pi* 淫羊霍	791
Dichorae Febrifugae, Radix	*Chang Shan* 常山	518	Equiseti Hiemalis, Herba	*Mu Zei* 木賊	464
Dictamni Dasycarpi Radicis, Cortex	*Bai Xian Pi* 白鮮皮	515	Erethmochelyas, Carapax	*Dai Mao* 玳瑁	743
Dioscoreae Bulbiferae, Rhizoma	*Huang Yao Zi* 黃藥子	723	Erinacei, Corium	*Ci Wei Pi* 刺謂皮	819
Dioscoreae Nipponicae, Rhizoma	*Chuan Shan Long* 川山龍	442	Eriobotryae Japonicae, Folium	*Pi Pa Ye* 枇杷葉	703
Dioscoreae Oppositae, Radix	*Shan Yao/Huai San* 山藥	769	Eriocaulonis Buergeriani, Scapus	*Gu Jing Cao* 谷精草	461
Dioscoreae Sativae, Rhizoma	*Bei Xie/Bi Xie* 萆解	587	Erodii, Herba	*Lao Guan Cao* 降香	565
Diospyros, Fructus	*Shi Bing* 柿餅	630	Erythrinae Variegatae, Cortex	*Hai Tong Pi* 海桐皮	562
Diospyros Kaki, Calyx	*Shi Di* 柿蒂	630	Eucommiae Ulmoidis, Cortex	*Du Zhong* 杜仲	775
Dipsaci, Radix	*Xu Duan* 續斷	789			

Pharmaceutical Herb Name	Pin Yin (Chinese) Herb Name	Page No.	Pharmaceutical Herb Name	Pin Yin (Chinese) Herb Name	Page No.
Eucommiae Ulmoidis, Folium	Du Zhong Ye 杜仲葉	776	Gambir	Er Cha/Hai Er Cha/A Xian Yao 兒茶	839
Eulotae	Wo Niu 蝸牛	537	Ganoderma	Ling Zhi Cao/Ling Zhi 靈芝草	731
Eupatorii Fortunei, Herba	Pei Lan/Ja Lang 佩蘭	583	Gardeniae Jasminoidis, Fructus	Shan Zhi Zi/Zhi Zi 山梔子	476
Euphorbia Lathyridis, Semen	Xu Sui Zi 續隨子	556	Gastrodiae Elatae, Rhizoma	Tian Ma 天麻	750
Euphorbia Pekinesis, Radix	Hong Da Ji/Da Ji 紅大薊	551	Gecko	Ge Jie 蛤蚧	777
Euphorbiae Helioscopiae, Herba	Ze Qi 澤漆	727	Gentianae Macrophyllae, Radix	Qin Jiao 秦艽	569
Euphorbiae Kansui, Radix	Gan Sui 甘遂	551	Gentianae Scabrae, Radix	Long Dan Cao 龍膽草	492
Euphorbiae Pekinensis, Radix	Jing Da Ji/Da Ji 京大戟	552	Geranii, Herba	Lao Guan Cao 降香	565
Euphoriae Longanae, Arillus	Long Yan Rou/Gui Yuan Rou 龍眼肉	800	Ginkgo Bilobae, Semen	Bai Guo/Yin Guo/Yin Xing 白果	818
Eupolyphagae	Tu Bie Chong/Zhe Chong 木通	690	Ginko, Folium	Bai Guo Ye/Yin Xing Ye 白果葉	817
Euryales Ferox, Semen	Qian Shi/Qian Ren 芡實	826	Ginseng, Cervix	Ren Shen Lu 人參蘆	835
Evodiae Rutaecarpae, Fructus	Wu Zhu Yu 吳茱萸	618	Ginseng Folium Cum Caule	Ren Shen Ye 人參葉	769
Fasciculus Vascularis Luffae	Si Gua Luo 絲瓜蔓	688	Gleditsiae Sinensis, Spina	Zao Jiao Ci 皂角刺	716
Fici Aerius, Radix	Rong Shu Xu/Lao Gong Xu 榕樹鬚	570	Gleditsiae Sinensis, Fructus	Zao Jiao /Zao Jia 皂角	715
Flava, Cera	Feng La 蜂蠟	840	Glehniae Littoralis, Radix	Bei Sha Shen 北沙參	804
Fluoritum	Zi Shi Ying 紫石英	742	Glycine Sojae, Semen	Hei Dou 黑豆	807
Foeniculi Vulgaris, Fructus	Xiao Hui Xiang/Hui Xiang 小茴香	619	Glycines Germinatum, Semen	Da Dou Huang Juan/Dou Juan 大豆黃卷	506
Forsythiae Suspensae, Fructus	Lian Qiao/Lian Jiao 連翹	525	Glycyrrhizae Uralensis, Radix	Gan Cao/Sheng Gan Cao 甘草	763
Fraxini, Cortex	Qin Pi 秦皮	493	Glycyrrhizae Uralensis Prep., Radix	Zhi Gan Cao 炙甘草	772
Fritillariae Cirrhosae, Bulbus	Chuan Bei Mu 川貝母	717	Gossampini, Flos	Mu Mian Hua 木棉花	529
Fritillariae Thunbergii, Bulbus	Zhe Bei Mu/Bei Mu 浙貝母	728	Gossypii, Radix	Mian Hua Gen 棉花根	851
Fructificatio Tremellae Fuciformis	Bai Mu Er 白木耳	803	Gossypii, Semen	Cao Mian Hua Zi 草棉花子	850
Gallus	Ji Zi Huang 雞子黃	809			

Pharmaceutical Herb Name	Pin Yin (Chinese) Herb Name	Page No.	Pharmaceutical Herb Name	Pin Yin (Chinese) Herb Name	Page No.
Granati, Pericarpium	Shi Liu Pi 石榴皮	828	Illicius, Fructus	Ba Jiao Hui Xiang 八角茴香	608
Granati, Radix	Shi Liu Gen Pi 石榴根皮	649	Impatientis, Semen	Ji Xing Zi 急性子	677
Grifola, Sclerotium	Zhu Ling 豬苓	606	Imperatae Cylindriae, Flos	Bai Mao Gen Hua/Mao Hua 白茅根花	653
Guanzhong, Rhizoma	Guan Zhong/Guan Chong 貫眾	521	Imperatae Cylindricae, Rhizoma	Bai Mao Gen 白茅根	653
Gypsum	Shi Gao 石膏	477	Indigo Pulverata Levis	Qing Dai 青黛	531
Haematitum	Dai Zhe Shi/Zhe Shi 代赭石	735	Inulae, Flos	Xuan Fu Hua 旋復花	713
Hailong	Hai Long 海龍	779	Isatidis, Radix	Ban Lan Gen 白芍	515
Haliotidis, Concha	Shi Jue Ming 石決明	750	Jasmini Officinalis, Flos	Su Xin Hua/Mo Li Hua 素馨花	631
Haliotis	Bao Yu 鮑魚	804			
Halloysitum Rubrum	Chi Shi Zhi/Bai Shi Zhi 赤石脂	818	Juglandis Regiae, Semen	Hu Tao Ren 胡桃仁	782
			Junci Effusi, Medulla	Deng Xin Cao 燈心草	592
Hedyotis Diffusae, Herba	Bai Hua She She Cao 白花蛇舌草	511	Knoxiae, Radix	Hong Da Ji/Da Ji 紅大薊	551
Heleochris Plantaginea, Cormus	Bi Qi/Bi Ji Ji/Wu Cao 荸薺·荸荠	717	Kochiae Scopariae, Fructus	Di Fu Zi 地膚子	592
Hippocampus	Hai Ma 海馬	780	Lasiosphaerae, Frucificatio	Ma Bo 馬勃	528
Hirudo	Shui Zhi 木通	687	Ledebouriellae Sesloidis, Radix	Fang Feng 防風	444
Homalomenae Occultae, Rhizoma	Qian Nian Jian 千年健	568	Lemnae, Herba	Fu Ping 防風	460
Hordei Vulgaris Geminantus, Fructus	Mai Ya 麥芽	640	Leonuri, Fructus	Chong Wei Zi/Huang Wei Zi/Xiao Hu Ma 沖慰子	669
Houttuyniae Cordatae, Herba	Yu Xing Cao 魚腥草	539	Leonuri Heterophylli, Herba	Yi Mu Cao 益母草	694
Hydnocarpi Anthelminthicae, Semen	Da Feng Zi 大楓子	839	Lepidii, Semen	Ting Li Zi 葶藶子	555
Hyoscyami, Semen	Tian Xian Zi 天仙子	705	Ligustici Sinensis, Radix	Gao Ben 藁本	444
Hyperici, Herba	Tian Ji Huang 田基黃	536	Ligustici Wallichii, Radix	Chuan Xiong 川芎	671
Ilicis Latifoliae, Folium	Ku Ding Cha 苦丁茶	809	Ligustri Lucidi, Fructus	Nu Zhen Zi 女貞子	812
Ilicis Pubescentis, Radix	Mao Dong Qing 毛冬青	682	Lilii, Bulbus	Bai He 百合	803

Pharmaceutical Herb Name	Pin Yin (Chinese) Herb Name	Page No.	Pharmaceutical Herb Name	Pin Yin (Chinese) Herb Name	Page No.
Limonitum	Yu Yu Liang/Yu Liang Shi/Tai Yi Yu Liang 禹余糧	833	Magnetitum	Ci Shi 磁石	735
Linderae Strychnifoliae, Radix	Wu Yao/Tai Wau 烏藥	632	Magnolia Officianlis, Flos	Hou Po Hua/Chuan Po Hua 厚樸花	580
Liquidambaris Taiwanianae, Fructus	Lu Lu Tong 路路通	681	Magnoliae Liliflorae, Flos	Xin Yi Hua 辛夷花	453
Litchi Chinensis, Semen	Li Zhi He 荔枝核	626	Magnoliae Officinalis, Cortex	Hou Po/Chuan Po 厚樸	581
Lithargyrum	Mi Tuo Seng 密陀僧	843	Malachii, Herba	Cha Chi Huang 茶匙黃	517
Lithospermi, Radix	Zi Cao 豬苓	504	Malvae, Semen	Dong Kui Zi 赤石脂	594
Litseae, Fructus	Bi Cheng Qie 蓽澄茄	609	Manitis Pentadactylae, Squama	Chuan Shan Jia 穿山甲	670
Litseae Cubebae, Ramus/Radix	Dou Chi Jiang 豆豉姜	612	Mantidis, Ootheca	Sang Piao Xiao 桑螵蛸	827
Lobeliae Chinensis Cum Radice, Herba	Ban Bian Lian 半邊蓮	586	Mararitaferae, Concha	Zhen Zhu Mu 珍珠母	741
Lonicerae, Caulis/Folium	Ren Dong Teng/Jin Yin Hua Teng 忍冬藤	531	Margarita Usta	Zhen Zhu 珍珠	740
Lonicerae Japonicae, Flos	Jin Yin Hua 金銀花	524	Massa Fermentata	Shen Qu/Liu Qu 神曲	642
Lophatheri Gracilis, Herba	Dan Zhu Ye 淡竹葉	470	Mel	Feng Mi 蜂蜜	548
Loranthi, Ramulus	Sang Ji Sheng/Hu Ji Sheng 木通	813	Melanteritum	Zao Fan/Lu Fan 皂礬	848
Lumbricus	Di Long/Qiu Yin 地龍	744	Meliae Radicis, Cortex	Ku Lian Gen Pi 苦楝根皮	646
Lycii Chinensis, Fructus	Gou Qi Zi 枸杞子	798	Meliae Toosendan, Fructus	Chuan Lian Zi/Zhuan Lian Zi 川楝子	623
Lycii Chinensis Radicis, Cortex	Di Gu Pi 地骨皮	495	Melo Pedicelus	Gua Di 瓜蒂	834
Lycopi Lucidi, Herba	Ze Lan 澤蘭	696	Melonis Calyx	Gua Di 瓜蒂	834
Lycopodii, Herba	Shen Jin Cao 伸筋草	571	Menthae, Herba	Bo He 薄荷	456
Lygodii, Spora	Hai Jin Sha 海金沙	522	Minium	Qian Dan 鉛丹	845
Lygodii Japonici, Herba	Hai Jin Sha Cao/Jin Sha Teng 海金砂草	522	Mirabilitum	Mang Xiao 芒硝	545
Lysimachiae, Herba	Ling Ling Xiang 零陵香	850	Momordicae Cochinchinensis, Semen	Mu Bie Zi 木鱉子	844
Macacae Mulattae, Calculus	Hou Zao 猴棗	722	Momordicae Grosvenori, Fructus	Luo Han Guo 羅漢果	810
			Mori Albae, Folium	Sang Ye 桑葉	466

Pharmaceutical Herb Name	Pin Yin (Chinese) Herb Name	Page No.	Pharmaceutical Herb Name	Pin Yin (Chinese) Herb Name	Page No.
Mori Albae, Fructus	*Sang Shen Zi/Sang Ren* 桑椹子	801	Ocimi, Herba	*Luo Le* 羅勒	583
Mori Albae, Ramulus	*Sang Zhi* 桑枝	570	Oldenlandiae Diffusae, Herba	*Bai Hua She She Cao* 白花蛇舌草	511
Mori Albae Radicis, Cortex	*Sang Bai Pi* 桑白皮	703	Olibanum, Gummi	*Ru Xiang* 乳香	685
Morindae Officinalis, Radix	*Ba Ji Tian/Ba Ji* 巴戟天	773	Olocus Rotundae, Cortex	*Jiu Bi Ying* 救必應	625
Moschus Moschiferi, Secretio	*She Xiang* 麝香	756	Omphalia, Fructificato	*Lei Wan* 雷丸	647
Moutan Radicis, Cortex	*Mu Dan Pi* 牡丹皮	499	Ophicalcitum	*Hua Rui Shi* 花蕊石	658
Mucunae, Caulis	*Ji Xue Teng/Ji Xue Deng* 雞血藤	677	Ophiopogonis Japonici, Tuber	*Mai Men Dong/Mai Dong* 麥門冬	810
Musae Caudex	*Ba Jiao Gen* 芭蕉根	510	Opisthoplatiae	*Tu Bie Chong/Zhe Chong* 木通	690
Mutong, Caulis	*Mu Tong* 木通	599	Origani, Herba	*Tu Yin Chen/Bei Yin Chen/Tu Xiang Ju* 土茵陳	602
Mylabris	*Ban Mao* 班蝥	837	Oroxyli Indici, Semen	*Mu Hu Die/Qian Cheng Zi* 木蝴蝶	702
Myristicae Fragranticis, Semen	*Rou Dou Kou* 肉豆蔻	826	Oryzae, Semen	*Jing Mi* 粳米	767
Myrrha	*Mo Yao* 沒藥	683	Oryzae Glutinosae, Radix/Rhizoma	*Nuo Dao Gen /Nuo Dao Gen Xu/Nuo Mi Gen* 糯稻根	825
Narcissi, Bulbus	*Shui Xian Gen* 水仙根	535	Oryzae Sativae Germinantus, Fructus	*Gu Ya/Dao Ya* 谷芽	637
Nardostachytis, Rhizoma	*Gan Song Xiang/Gan Sung* 甘松香	580	Ostreae, Concha	*Mu Li* 牡蠣	739
Nelumbinis Nuciferae, Receptaculum	*Lian Fang* 連房	659	Otoriae, Testes/Penis	*Hai Gou Shen* 海狗腎	779
Nelumbinis Nuciferae, Plumula	*Lian Zi Xin/Lian Xin* 蓮子心	472	Paeoniae Lactiflorae, Radix	*Bai Shao/Bai Shao Yao* 白芍	794
Nelumbinis Nuciferae, Folium	*He Ye/Han Lian Ye* 荷葉	507	Paeoniae Rubra, Radix	*Chi Shao Yao/Chi Shao* 赤芍藥	668
Nelumbinis Nuciferae, Semen	*Lian Zi* 蓮子	824	Panacis Quinquefolii, Radix	*Hua Qi Shen/Xi Yang Shen* 花旗參	808
Nelumbinis Nuciferae Rhizomatis, Rhizoma	*Ou Jie* 藕節	660	Papaveris Somniferi, Pericarpium	*Ying Su Ke/Ying Su Qiao* 罌粟殼	832
Nelumbinis Stamen	*Lian Xu* 蓮須	823			
Nidus Vespae	*Lu Feng Fang/Feng Fang* 露蜂房	841			
Notopterygii, Radix	*Qiang Huo* 羌活	449			

Pharmaceutical Herb Name	Pin Yin (Chinese) Herb Name	Page No.	Pharmaceutical Herb Name	Pin Yin (Chinese) Herb Name	Page No.
Paris, Rhizoma	Zao Xiu/Chong Lou/Qi Ye Yi Zhi Hua 蚤休	540	Placenta Hominis	Zi He Che/Tai Yi 紫河車	792
Patrinia, Herba	Bai Jiang Cao 敗醬草	512	Plantaginis, Herba	Che Qian Cao 車前草	589
Perillae Acutae, Caulis	Su Geng/Zi Su Geng 蘇梗	451	Plantaginis, Semen	Che Qian Zi 車前子	590
Perillae Frutescentis, Folium	Zi Su Ye/Su Ye 紫蘇葉	454	Platycodi Grandiflori, Radix	Jie Geng 桔梗	711
Perillae Frutescentis, Fructus	Zi Su Zi 紫蘇子	706	Podophylli, Rhizoma	Ba Jiao Lian 八角連	510
Persicae, Semen	Tao Ren 桃仁	689	Pogonatheri, Herba	Bi Zi Cao 筆仔草	587
Peucedani, Radix	Qian Hu 前胡	725	Pogostemi, Herba	Huo Xiang 紅大薊	582
Pharbitidis, Semen	Qian Niu Zi 牽牛子	553	Polygalae Tenuifoliae, Radix	Yuan Zhi 遠志	734
Phaseoli Calcarati, Semen	Chi Xiao Dou 赤小豆	591	Polygonati, Rhizoma	Huang Jing 黃精	764
Phaseoli Radiati, Semen	Lu Dou 綠豆	508	Polygonati Odorati, Rhizoma	Yu Zhu 玉竹	815
Phellodendri, Cortex	Huang Bai/Huang Bo 黃柏	485	Polygoni Avicularis, Herba	Bian Xu 褊蓄	588
Phragmitis, Ramulus	Lu Jing/Wei Jing 蘆莖/葦莖	473	Polygoni Bistortae, Rhizoma	Cao He Che/Zhong Lou /Quan Shen 草河車	517
Phragmitis Communis, Rhizoma	Lu Gen 蘆根	472	Polygoni Chinese, Herba	Huo Tan Mu Cao 火炭母草	498
Physalitis, Rhizoma Et Radix	Suan Jiang 酸漿	852	Polygoni Cuspidati, Rhizoma	Hu Zhang/Hu Chang 虎杖	497
Phytolaccae, Radix	Shang Lu 商陸	554	Polygoni Multiflori, Radix	He Shou Wu/ Shou Wu 何首烏	799
Picrorrhizae, Rhizoma	Hu Huang Lian 胡黃連	484	Polygoni Multiflori, Caulis	Ye Jiao Teng/Shou Wu Teng 夜交籐/首烏藤	733
Pinelliae Ternatae, Rhizoma	Ban Xia/Fa Xia 半夏	710			
Pini, Resina	Song Xiang 松香	847	Polypori Mylittae, Fructificato	Lei Wan 雷丸	647
Pini Nodi, Lignum	Song Jie/You Song Jie 松節	572	Polypori Umbellati, Sclerotium	Zhu Ling 豬苓	606
Pini Tabulaeformis, Fructus	Song Zi 松子仁	546	Poriae Cocos, Cortex	Fu Ling Pi 茯苓皮	595
Piperis, Caulis	Hai Feng Teng 海風藤	562	Poriae Cocos, Sclerotium	Fu Ling /Bai Fu Ling 茯苓	594
Piperis Longi, Fructus	Bi Ba/Bi Bo 華芨	608	Poriae Cocos Pararadicis, Sclerotium	Fu Shen 茯神	736
Piperis Nigri, Fructus	Hu Jiao 胡椒	615	Poriae Cocos Rubrae, Sclerotium	Chi Fu Ling 赤茯苓	483

Pharmaceutical Herb Name	Pin Yin (Chinese) Herb Name	Page No.	Pharmaceutical Herb Name	Pin Yin (Chinese) Herb Name	Page No.
Portulacae Oleraceae, Herba	Ma Chi Xian 馬齒莧	528	Rauwolfiae Verticillatae, Radix	Bai Hua Lian 白花連	511
Prunellae Vulgaris, Spica	Xia Ku Cao 夏枯草	478	Realgar	Xiong Huang 雄黃	848
Pruni, Semen	Yu Li Ren 鬱李仁	549	Rehmanniae Glutinosae, Radix	Sheng Di Huang/Sheng Di 生地黃	500
Pruni Armeniacae, Semen	Xing Ren/Bei Xing Ren/Ku Xing Ren 杏仁	705	Rehmanniae Glutinosae Conquitae, Radix	Shu Di Huang/Shu Di 熟地黃	802
Pruni Mume, Fructus	Wu Mei 烏梅	830	Rhapontici, Radix	Lou Lu 龍齒	527
Pseudoginseng, Radix	San Qi/Tian Qi 三七	663	Rhei, Rhizoma	Da Huang 大黃	542
Pseudoginseng, Flos	San Qi Hua 三七花	663	Rhinoceri, Cornu	Xi Jiao 犀角	502
Pseudostellariae Heterophyllae, Radix	Tai Zi Shen/Hai Er Shen 太子參	770	Rhododendori Daurici, Folium	Man Shan Hong 滿山紅	851
Psoraleae Corylifoliae, Fructus	Bu Gu Zhi 補骨脂	773	Rhododendri Molles, Folium	Nao Yang Hua 鬧羊花	740
Pteris, Herba	Feng Wei Cao 鳳尾草	496	Ricini, Semen	Bi Ma Zi 蓖麻子	547
Pteromi, Excrementum	Wu Ling Zhi 五加參	691	Rosae Chinensis, Fructus	Yue Ji Hua/Yue Yue Hong 月季花	696
Puerariae, Radix	Ge Gen 葛根	460	Rosae Laevigatae, Fructus	Jin Ying Zi 金櫻子	823
Puerariae, Flos	Ge Hua 葛花	521	Rosae Rugosae, Flos	Mei Gui Hua 玫瑰花	627
Pulsatillae Chinensis, Radix	Bai Tou Weng 白頭翁	514	Rubi, Fructus	Fu Pen Zi 復盆子	820
Pumice	Hai Fu Shi 海浮石	720	Rubiae Cordifoliae, Radix	Qian Cao Gen 茜草根	662
Pycnostelmae, Herba	Liao Diao Zhu/Xu Chang Qing 了刁竹	565	Saccharum Granorum	Yi Tang 飴糖	772
Pyritum	Zi Ran Tong 自然銅	698	Salviae Miltiorrhizae, Radix	Dan Shen 丹參	672
Pyrolae, Herba	Lu Xian Cao/Lu Han Cao/Lu Ti Cao 鹿銜草	566	Sanguis Draconis	Xue Jie 血竭	692
Pyrrosiae, Folium	Shi Wei 石葦	601	Sanguisorbae Officinalis, Radix	Di Yu 地榆	656
Quisqualis Indicae, Fructus	Shi Jun Zi 使君子	648	Santali Albi, Lignum	Tan Xiang 檀香	632
Radicis Sapii, Cortex	Wu Jiu Gen Pi 烏桕根皮:烏桕根皮	555	Santsigu, Bulbus	Shan Ci Gu/Yi Bi Jian/Cao Bei Mu 山慈菇	846
Raphani Sativi, Semen	Lai Fu Zi 萊菔子	639	Sapindi, Semen	Wu Huan Zi 無患子	538
			Sappan, Lignum	Su Mu 蘇木	688

Pharmaceutical Herb Name	Pin Yin (Chinese) Herb Name	Page No.	Pharmaceutical Herb Name	Pin Yin (Chinese) Herb Name	Page No.
Sargassii, Herba	Hai Zao 海藻	721	Siphonostegia, Herba	Liu Ji Nu 劉寄奴	681
Sargentodoxae, Caulis	Hong Teng/Da Xue Teng 紅藤	497	Smilacis Glabrae, Rhizoma	Tu Fu Ling 土茯苓	536
Saussureae, Radix	Mu Xiang 木通	628	Smithsonitum	Lu Gan Shi 爐甘石	842
Schefflera, Radix/Caulis/Folium	Qi Ye Lian 七葉蓮	568	Sojae Praeparatum, Semen	Dan Dou Chi 淡豆豉	459
Schisandrae Chinensis, Fructus	Wu Wei Zi 五味子	831	Solani, Herba	Long Kui 龍葵	526
Schizonepetae Tenuifoliae, Flos	Jing Jie 荊芥	447	Solani Lyrati, Herba	Shu Yang Quan/Bai Mao Teng 蜀羊泉/白毛藤	535
Scolopendra Subspinipes	Wu Gong/Bai Ju 蜈蚣	751	Sophorae Flavescentis, Radix	Ku Shen 苦參	491
Scrophulariae Ningpoensis, Radix	Xuan Shen 玄參	503	Sophorae Japonicae, Fructus	Huai Jiao 槐角	676
Scutellariae Baicalensis, Radix	Huang Qin 黃芩	489	Sophorae Japonicae Immaturus, Flos	Huai Hua Mi/Huai Hua 槐花米	658
Scutellariae Barbatae, Herba	Ban Zhi Lian 半枝蓮	516	Sophorae Subprostratae, Radix	Shan Dou Gen 山豆根	532
Selaginellae, Herba	Juan Bo/Juan Bai Ye 卷柏	679	Sparganii, Rhizoma	San Leng 三稜	686
Selaginellae Doederleinii, Herba	Shi Shang Bai 石上柏	534	Spatholobi, Caulis	Ji Xue Teng/Ji Xue Deng 雞血藤	677
Senecionis, Herba	Qian Li Guang/Jiu Li Ming 千里光	474	Spirodelae, Herba	Fu Ping 防風	460
Sennae, Folium	Fan Xie Ye 番瀉葉	544	Stalactitum	E Guan Shi/Zhung Shuei Shi 鵝管石	777
Sepiae, Os	Hai Piao Xiao/Wu Zei Gu 鬼羽箭	821	Stellariae Dichotomae, Radix	Yin Chai Hu 銀柴胡	504
Sepiellae, Os	Hai Piao Xiao/Wu Zei Gu 鬼羽箭	821	Stemonae, Radix	Bai Bu 百部	699
Serpentis, Periostracum	She Tui 蛇蛻	571	Stephaniae Tetrandrae, Radix	Han Fang Ji/Fang Ji 漢防己	596
Sesami Indici, Semen	Hei Zhi Ma/Hu Ma Ren/Zhi Ma 黑芝麻	808	Sterculiae Scaphigerae, Semen	Pang Da Hai 胖大海	724
Siegesbeckiae Orientalis, Herba	Xi Xian Cao/Xi Jian Cao 稀薟草	575	Stichopus Japonicus, Selenka	Hai Shen 海參	781
Sileris, Radix	Fang Feng 防風	444	Stigma Croci, Stigma	Fan Hong Hua/Zang Hong Hua 番紅花	674
Silicea Bambusae, Concretio	Tian Zhu Huang 天竹黃	726	Strychnotis, Semen	Ma Qian Zi/Fan Mu Bie 馬錢子	842
Sinapis Albae, Semen	Bai Jie Zi 白芥子	708			

Pharmaceutical Herb Name	Pin Yin (Chinese) Herb Name	Page No.	Pharmaceutical Herb Name	Pin Yin (Chinese) Herb Name	Page No.
Styrax Liquidis	Su He Xiang 蘇合香	758	Trichosanthis, Semen	Gua Lou Ren 瓜蔞仁	720
Suberalatum Euonymi, Ramulus/Herba	Guei Yu Jian /Gui Jian Yu 鬼羽箭	675	Trichosanthis, Pericarpium	Gua Lou Pi 瓜蔞皮	719
Succinum	Hu Po 琥珀	737	Trichosanthis, Radix	Tian Hua Fen/Gua Lou Gen 天花粉	726
Sulphur	Liu Huang 硫黃	840	Trigonellae Foenigraeci, Semen	Hu Lu Ba 胡蘆巴	781
Syringae, Cortex	Bao Ma Zi 暴馬子	700	Tritici Aestivi Levis, Semen	Fu Xiao Mai 浮小麥	820
Talcum	Hua Shi 滑石	597	Trogopterori, Excrementum	Wu Ling Zhi 五加參	691
Tamaricis, Cacumen	Xi He Liu/Chui Si Liu/Cheng Liu 西河柳	451	Tussilagi Farfarae, Flos	Kuan Dong Hua 款冬花	700
Taraxaci Mongolici Cum Radice, Herba	Pu Gong Ying 蒲公英	529	Typhae, Pollen	Pu Huang 蒲黃	660
Terminaliae Chebulae, Fructus	He Zi 荷子	822	Typhonii Gigantei, Rhizoma	Bai Fu Zi/Guan Bai Fu 白附子	708
Terra Flava Usta	Fu Long Gan/Zao Xin Tu 伏龍肝	657	Ulmi Macrocarpi, Pasta	Wu Yi 蕪夷	649
Testudinis, Plastrum	Gui Ban 龜板	806	Uncaria	Er Cha/Hai Er Cha/A Xian Yao 兒茶	839
Tetrapanacis Papyriferi, Medulla	Tong Cao 通草	601	Uncariae Cum Uncis, Ramulus	Gou Teng 鉤藤	745
Thlaspi, Herba	Bai Jiang Cao 敗醬草	512	Ursi, Fel	Xiong Dan 熊膽	479
Thymi Serpylli, Herba	Di Jiao 地椒	443	Vaccariae Segetalis, Semen	Wang Bu Liu Xing 王不留行	691
Tigris, Os	Hu Gu 虎骨	563	Veratri Nigri, Rhizoma Et Radix	Li Lu 黎蘆	834
Tinosporae, Radix	Jin Guo Lan 金果攬	523	Verbenae, Herba	Ma Bian Cao 馬鞭草	682
Tinosporae Sinensis, Ramus	Kuan Jin Teng 寬筋藤	564	Vespertilii Murini, Excrementum	Ye Ming Sha 夜明砂	480
Torreyae Grandis, Semen	Fei Zi 榧子	645	Violae Cum Radice, Herba	Zi Hua Di Ding 紫花地丁	541
Trachelospermi Jasminoidis, Caulis	Luo Shi Teng 絡石藤	566	Visci, Ramulus	Sang Ji Sheng/Hu Ji Sheng 木通	813
Trachycarpi Carbonista, Vagina	Chen Zong Tan/Zhong Lu Tan 陳棕炭	655	Viticis, Fructus	Man Jing Zi 蔓荊子	464
Tribuli Terrestris, Fructus	Bai Ji Li/Ci Ji Li 白蒺藜	743	Vladimiriae, Radix	Mu Xiang 木通	628
Trichosanthis, Fructus	Gua Lou 瓜蔞	718	Whitmaniae	Shui Zhi 木通	687
			Xanthii, Fructus	Cang Er Zi 蒼耳子	559

Pharmaceutical Herb Name	Pin Yin (Chinese) Herb Name	Page No.
Zanthoxyli Bungeani, Fructus	*Chuan Jiao/Hua Shan Jiao* 川椒	610
Zaocys Dhumnades	*Wu Shao She* 烏梢蛇	574
Zeae Mays, Stylus	*Yu Mi Xu* 玉米須	605
Zingiberis Officinalis, Rhizoma	*Gan Jiang* 干姜	614
Zingiberis Officinalis Recens, Rhizoma	*Sheng Jiang* 生姜	450
Zingiberis Officinalis Recens, Cortex	*Sheng Jiang Pi* 生姜皮	600
Ziziphi Jujubae, Fructus	*Da Zao/Hong Zao* 大棗/紅棗	761
Ziziphi Spinosae, Semen	*Suan Zao Ren* 酸棗仁	732

Turn the Page to Order Your Copy of *The Chinese Herb Selection Guide*

Start making more effective Chinese herb preparations for your clients. Order today!

Order Form

The Chinese Herb Selection Guide

A Traditional and Modern Clinical Repertory
with
A Summary Materia Medica
for the Health Care Practitioner

Charles A. Belanger, L.Ac., M. S.

Name _____

Street/P.O. Box _____

City, State, Zip _____

I understand that I may return any books for a full refund (less shipping costs), for any reason. (Assumes books are in like-new condition.)

Books are \$59.95 each.   Total Books   _____
California residents, please add 8.25% sales tax   Total Tax   _____
Book rate & handling is \$5.00 for the first book;   Total Shipping   _____
\$3.00 for each book up to five; UPS for more than five books (\$3.00/book)
                                                          Total Enclosed   _____
Student Buying Clubs are welcome. Please write or call for more information concerning quantity discounts.
(*The Chinese Herb Selection Guide* (ISBN 0-9657310-3-0) is also available through Redwing Book Co. and fine book stores.)

Ask for a **Phytotech Herb Extract** information packet for making your custom herb formula into an extract to offer your clients.
High quality, high potency, whole herb liquid extracts for professionals

Send check or money
order to: **Phytotech**
1620 Olive Ave.
Richmond, California 94805
(510) 215-9525 email: 72050.2415@compuserve.com

Start making more effective Chinese herb preparations for your clients—Order today!